W0082692

Manual of
Clinical
Medicine

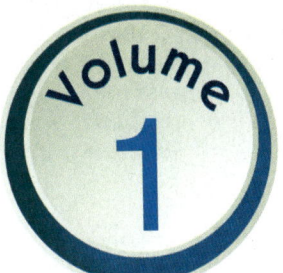

Volume
1

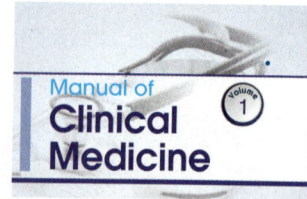

Manual of
**Clinical
Medicine**
Volume 1

Two-volume set

Manual of Clinical Medicine

Volume 1

Chapters 1–5

Ashis Kumar Saha

MD (Cal), DTM & H (Cal), FICP, FACP (USA), FRCP (EDINBURGH), FRCP (GLASGOW), MNAMS (INDIA)

Professor and Head
Department of General Medicine
KPC Medical College and Hospital
Jadavpur, Kolkata
West Bengal

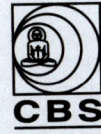

CBS

CBS Publishers & Distributors Pvt Ltd

New Delhi • Bengaluru • Chennai • Kochi • Kolkata • Mumbai
Bhubaneswar • Hyderabad • Jharkhand • Nagpur • Patna • Pune • Uttarakhand

Disclaimer
Science and technology are constantly changing fields. New research and experience broaden the scope of information and knowledge. The author has tried his best in giving information available to him while preparing the material for this book. Although all efforts have been made to ensure optimum accuracy of the material, yet it is quite possible some errors might have been left uncorrected. The publisher, the printer and the author will not be held responsible for any inadvertent errors or inaccuracies.

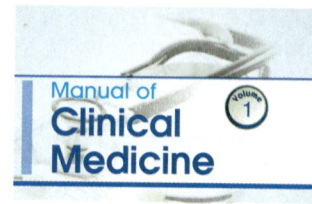

Two-volume set

ISBN: 978-93-86478-31-3

Copyright © Author and Publisher

First Edition: 2018

All rights reserved. No part of this book may be reproduced or transmitted in any form or by any means, electronic or mechanical, including photocopying, recording, or any information storage and retrieval system without permission, in writing, from the author and the publisher.

Published by Satish Kumar Jain and Produced by Varun Jain for

CBS Publishers & Distributors Pvt Ltd

4819/XI Prahlad Street, 24 Ansari Road, Daryaganj, New Delhi 110 002, India.
Ph: 23289259, 23266861, 23266867   Fax: 011-23243014   Website: www.cbspd.com
                                              e-mail: delhi@cbspd.com; cbspubs@airtelmail.in.

Corporate Office: 204 FIE, Industrial Area, Patparganj, Delhi 110 092
Ph: 4934 4934   Fax: 4934 4935   e-mail: publishing@cbspd.com; publicity@cbspd.com

Branches

- **Bengaluru:** Seema House 2975, 17th Cross, K.R. Road,
  Banasankari 2nd Stage, Bengaluru 560 070, Karnataka
  Ph: +91-80-26771678/79   Fax: +91-80-26771680   e-mail: bangalore@cbspd.com
- **Chennai:** 7, Subbaraya Street, Shenoy Nagar, Chennai 600 030, Tamil Nadu
  Ph: +91-44-26680620, 26681266   Fax: +91-44-42032115   e-mail: chennai@cbspd.com
- **Kochi:** Ashana House, No. 39/1904, AM Thomas Road, Valanjambalam,
  Ernakulam 682 016, Kochi, Kerala
  Ph: +91-484-4059061-65   Fax: +91-484-4059065   e-mail: kochi@cbspd.com
- **Kolkata:** 6/B, Ground Floor, Rameswar Shaw Road, Kolkata-700 014, West Bengal
  Ph: +91-33-22891126, 22891127, 22891128   e-mail: kolkata@cbspd.com
- **Mumbai:** 83-C, Dr E Moses Road, Worli, Mumbai-400018, Maharashtra
  Ph: +91-22-24902340/41   Fax: +91-22-24902342   e-mail: mumbai@cbspd.com

Representatives

- **Bhubaneswar** 0-9911037372   • **Hyderabad** 0-9885175004   • **Jharkhand** 0-9811541605   • **Nagpur** 0-9021734563
- **Patna** 0-9334159340   • **Pune** 0-9623451994   • **Uttarakhand** 0-9716462459

Printed at Rashtriya Printers, Dilshad Garden, Delhi, India

to

---

my parents, my wife, my teachers,
my beloved students and sons, lastly
my philosopher and guide
Dr KP Chowdhury

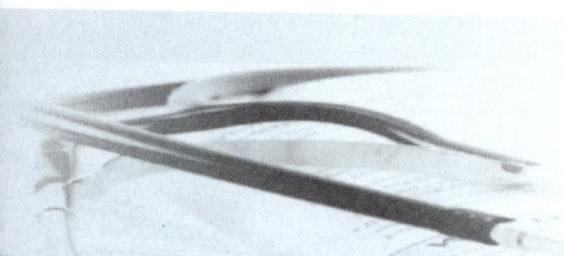

Foreword

It is with great pleasure I introduce the great endeavour by Prof (Dr) Ashis Kumar Saha in writing this *Manual of Clinical Medicine*. The book which covers altogether 14 chapters will be full of fun to read and foster the understanding of difficult diagnoses and common pitfalls in diagnoses of difficult clinical scenarios related to medicine. Each chapter is lucidly depicted with innumerable pictorials—needless to say students and practitioners will be benefitted immensely.

Sir William Osler said " To study the phenomenon of disease without books is to sail an uncharted sea, while to study books without patients is to not go to sea at all". The chapters in this book represent "real-life" experiences in the life of a physician. The most poignant questions in the mind of a physician "how does this information help us to devise a treatment plan?" and "what is the precise relationship about the anticipated course and prognosis?" The questions are raised in each section and follows in a beautiful way to incorporate answers in relation to pathogenesis, diagnosis, treatment and prognosis where a knowledge-base exists. Wherever possible, the discussions are based on latest medical evidence available in world literature. The chapter of gene therapy is an added inclusion for students. However, a further elaboration and bibliographic database will add flavour to this daunting effort by the author.

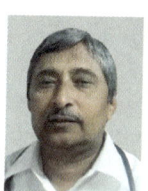

I understand that time is precious and, therefore, the author wanted to create a resource that is precise and trustworthy. This can never be a substitute of textbook and that was not the intention of the author either. This treatise is easy to follow, unpretentious and above all helpful.

I hope the readers will enjoy reading this book. Both undergraduates and postgraduates will be benefitted and this book will find a place in the library of medical practitioners at large.

Prof Anup Kr Bhattacharya MD, DM, FRCP (Edinburgh)
Past Hony Editor, *JIMA* 2014–15
President, Indian Science Congress–Medical Section
105th Indian Science Congress–2018

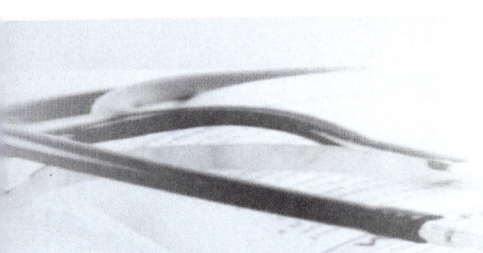

Foreword

It gives me a great pleasure to present this work of art by a prolific author of present day—Prof (Dr) Ashis Kumar Saha. I have known Dr. Saha for the last 10 years. His contribution to internal medicine is simply astounding. Despite being practicing gastro-enterologist, his footsteps remain equally in nephrology to hematology. He is just the prototype internist who takes responsibility of whole human organism. I sincerely hope that this book will certainly create ripples all over the world of academic medicine.

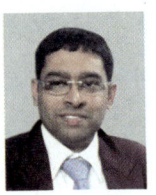

(Prof) Dr Nirmalya Roy

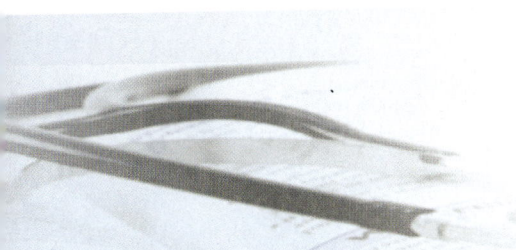

Preface

Writing a book on internal medicine is currently the most daunting task, more so when a single author makes such an attempt. Nevertheless I have made this Herculean attempt. It has to be understood that patients would certainly appreciate when a single physician takes the charge of their whole body. Even though it is not quite practical, an astute internist should be capable to deal with most common problems that a patient encounters. This book is a challenge to factory-line medicine that has become vogue currently where each subspecialist takes care of individual organ while neglecting the human face of the sick patient. Every attempt has been made to make the information as up-to-date as possible when the book was sent to press. I sincerely believe that internists are lifelong students and would be highly grateful if this *Manual* becomes one of the most thumbed books in a physician's library. I believe this *Manual* will upgrade the knowledge of undergraduate as well as postgraduate students.

Ashis Kumar Saha

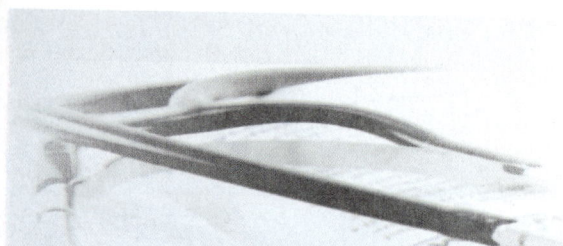

Acknowledgements

At last I finished my herculean work of writing this book *Manual of Clinical Medicine* and I kept the word given to my mother Late Radharani Saha of being within the mindframe of teacher and student community all over the world. My father, my lifelong inspiration Prof (Dr) Tushar Kanti Saha, has always been with me during my work.

Our Chairman Dr KP Chowdhury always inspired and guided me in my work throughout the teaching profession at our renowned KPC Medical College and Hospital. He loved me very much and inspired me to do more and more academic work for the students as well as for the hospital—the result is this book. He always tells me what is right and what is wrong and I should try to follow his word.

Our Medical Director, Dr Sourav Ghosh, and our Principal, Prof Siddhartha Chakraborty, have also inspired me to do new innovative work for the students. So I thought this was the way by which I could help my students, and I started writing this book and finished it.

I also acknowledged teacher and guide Prof Maloy Maitra, cheerful endocrinologist Prof Anirban Majumdar, my respected guide Prof Debasish Basu, Prof PK Ganguly, Prof Sagar Basu, retired Prof Subhas Chandra Hazra, my colleague Prof Santanu Bhakta, and Dr Rishad Ahmed. Prof Nirmalya Roy helped me to edit and add new part in my book and gave constant inspiration for writing this book.

Dr SK Saha, my father-in-law, constantly inspired me to do more and more new academic work.

A human being has two lungs and one heart. He can breathe fresh air and continue his life by the composite functions of the above three organs. Here two lungs are my two sons, Subhra Kanti beloved and Abhra Kanti beloved, and heart is my wife Mrs Kalyani most Saha. So, without their constant inspiration, support and a lot of sacrifice, I could not take breath and it was not possible for me to write the book of more than one thousand pages.

I do not like praise but constant inspiration will help me in making progress further and achieve the summit.

Ashis Kumar Saha

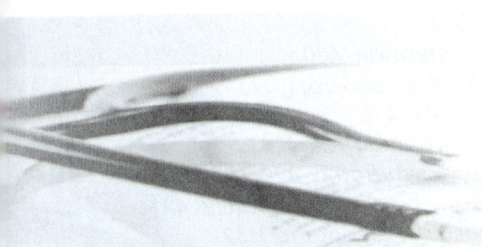

Contents

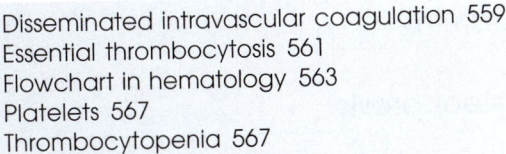

VOLUME 2

Volume 1

Cardiology

VALVULAR DISEASE

MITRAL STENOSIS

Key points to Diagnosis

1. **Symptoms included:** Exertional dyspnea, paroxysmal nocturnal dyspnea, orthopnea, or fatigue.
2. **Signs included:** Opening snap, mid-diastolic rumbling murmur with presystolic accentuation, with breath held in expiration, with or without pulmonary hypertension, loud pulmonary component of 2nd heart sound and right parasternal lift due to right ventricular hypertrophy.
3. **ECG evidence of** (i) left atrial enlargement, (ii) atrial fibrillation, (iii) right ventricular hypertrophy.
4. **Chest radiographic** evidence of left atrial enlargement fullness of pulmonary bay, no left ventricular enlargement.
5. **Echocardiographic evidence** of thickened mitral valve leaflet with restricted valve motion and reduced orifice size.
6. **Doppler echocardiographic evidence** of transvalvular pressure gradient across the mitral valve.
7. **Interventions indicated** for symptoms of pulmonary hypertension with valve area <1.5 cm².

Etiopathology

Causes

1. Rheumatic heart disease
2. Congenital—parachute mitral valve
3. Systemic diseases—producing valvular fibrosis:
   i. SLE
   ii. Rheumatoid arthritis
   iii. Mucopolysaccharidosis
   iv. Healed endocarditis
   v. Mitral annular calcification

Pathology (Fig. 1.1)

In rheumatic heart disease
Valve leaflets are thickened by fibrous tissue and calcific deposits
↓
Mitral commissure fuse
Chordae tendineae fuse and shorten
Valve cusps are rigid
↓
Leads to narrowing at the apex of the funnel-shaped valve called fish mouth valve.

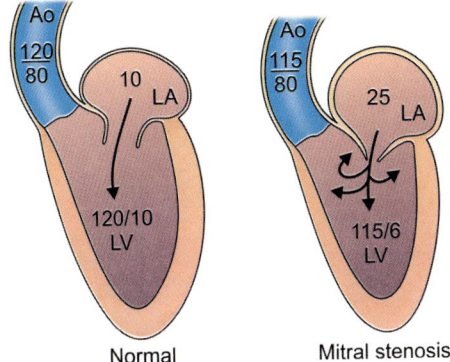

Fig. 1.1: Shape of mitral valve

The shape of mitral valve orifice in mitral stenosis is due to:
i. Initially rheumatic process
ii. Latter change is due to trauma to the valve due to altered flow pattern.

Thrombus formation—occurs in case of atrial fibrillation. It occurs mainly in left atrium, particularly in left atrial appendage.

Hemodynamics

Flowchart 1.1 depicts hemodynamics in mitral stenosis.

Pathophysiology

Normal valve orifice is 4–6 cm²
↓

1. **When the orifice size <2 cm²**—blood flow from left atrium to left ventricle depends on left atrioventricular pressur gradient—this is hemodynamic hallmark of mit stenosis.
2. **When the orifice size is <1 cm²**—blood will flow from atrium to left ventricle only when left atrial pressure will be ≥25 mmHg.
3. Elevated pulmonary venous pressure and pulmonary capillary wedge pressure lead to reduced pulmonary compliance—responsible for exertional dyspnea.

Flowchart 1.1: *Hemodynamics in mitral stenosis*

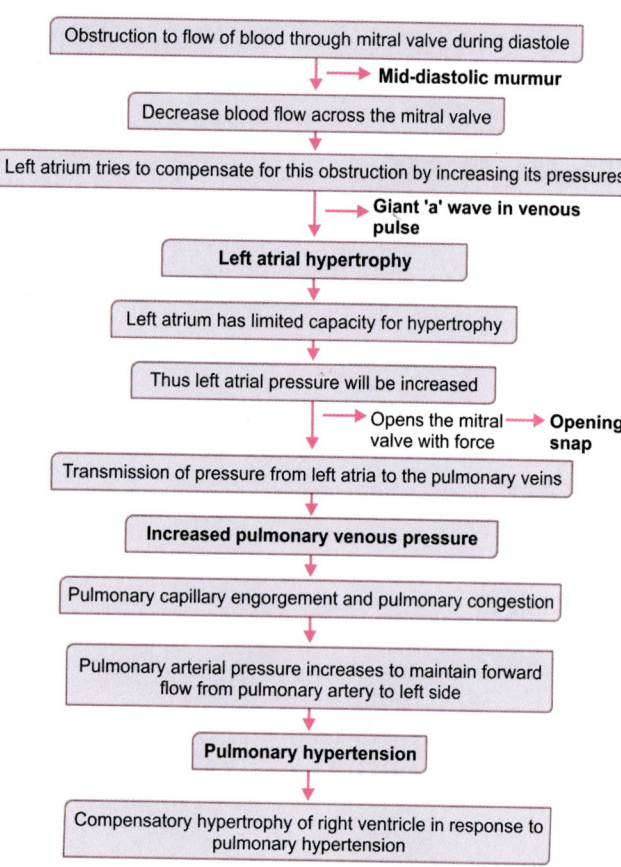

4. Severity of mitral valvular obstruction can be assessed by:
   i. Transvalvular pressure gradient
   ii. Flow rate across the valve—depends upon:
      - Cardiac output
      - Heart rate

   If heart rate is increased: Diastolic interval will be shortened than systolic interval—which in turn reduces the time available for flow across the mitral valve—hence elevation of left atrial pressure.
5. Elevation of left atrial pressure and pulmonary artery wedge pressure—leads to effective left atrial contraction (in absence of atrial fibrillation)—exhibits prominent 'a' wave.
6. **In case of mitral stenosis**—increased left atrial pressure is transmitted to pulmonary vasculature:
   - *In case acute elevation of LV pressure,* there is elevation pulmonary capillary pressure—leads to pulmonary congestion—producing pulmonary edema.
   - *In case chronic elevation of pulmonary venous pressure*—leads to pulmonary vascular resistance (reactive pulmonary hypertension)
   - It can be reversible, **if it is not long-standing MS.** But **in long-standing severe mitral stenosis**—obliterative changes occur in pulmonary vasculature—leading to non-**reversible pulmonary hypertension.**
   - This leads to right ventricular hypertrophy and right-sided heart failure.

Pulmonary hypertension in mitral stenosis results from:
i. *Passive backward transmission* of left atrial pressure
ii. *Pulmonary arteriolar constriction (so-called second stenosis)* which probably triggered by left atrial and

pulmonary venous hypertension (reactive pulmonary hypertension)
iii. *Interstitial edema* around walls of small pulmonary vessels
iv. *In last stage*—organic obliterative changes in the wall of pulmonary vasculature.

Severe PH—leads to pulmonary regurgitation, tricuspid regurgitation.

Clinical Features

Symptoms in Mitral Stenosis

1. In temperate climate, latent period between the initial attack of rheumatic fever and development of mitral stenosis is 2 decades.

   Patient develops symptoms since 4th decade.
2. **Dyspnea**
   i. In case of **mild mitral stenosis** with mild elevation of left atrial pressure—usually produces no symptom. But, sudden change in heart rate, volume status and cardiac output (by severe exertion, fever, severe anemia, thyrotoxicosis, pregnancy)—produces marked elevation of left atrial pressure leading to dyspnea and cough.
   ii. **As mitral stenosis progresses**—patient develops gradually:
      a. Marked exertional dyspnea
      b. Paroxysmal exertional dyspnea
      c. Orthopnea
      d. Ultimately dyspnea at rest.
3. **Hemoptysis:** It occurs in patients with elevated left atrial pressure without marked by increased pulmonary vascular resistance, it results front rupture of pulmonary–bronchial venous connections secondary to pulmonary venous hypertension.
4. **Recurrent pulmonary emboli**—sometimes with infarction—occur late in the course of mitral stenosis.
5. **Pulmonary infections**—commonly occur in winter months. The infective diseases are:
   i. Bronchitis
   ii. Bronchopneumonia
   iii. Lobar pneumonia
6. **Symptoms due to embolization** originating from left atrium in patient with atrial fibrillation—originating in:
   i. Brain—producing different levels of unconsciousness with or without paralysis or aphasia.
   ii. Kidney
   iii. Coronary artery in heart
   iv. Lower limb

   It usually occurs in persons having:
      a. >65 years age
      b. Reduced cardiac output.
7. **Hoarseness of voice** due to compression of recurrent laryngeal nerve (Ortner's syndrome)
8. **Fatigue** due to low cardiac output.
9. **Anginal pain** due to low cardiac output.

Physical Findings in Mitral Stenosis

Inspection and palpation:
1. *Facies*—malar flush—with pinched and blue facies.
2. *Jugular venous wave* shows prominent 'a' wave—provided patient is in sinus rhythm.

3. *Peripheral cyanosis* due to low cardiac output
4. In case right ventricular hypertrophy—**left parasternal heaves.**
5. *Carotid artery*—amplitude is low due to low cardiac output
6. *Palpable P2* in case of pulmonary hypertension.
7. *Apex beats* tapping in character—site little inside left mid-clavicular line.
8. *Rarely diastolic thrill* may be palpable in left recumbent position.

Auscultation (Fig. 1.2)

1. **1st heart sound** is loud and accentuated.
2. In case of pulmonary hypertension—**P2 component** is loud—gap between A2 and P2 will be close.
3. **Opening snap** of mitral valve—heard during expiration and patient will be in left lateral position. This sound occurs 0.05–0.12 seconds after aortic component of 2nd heart sound.
4. **Murmur:** Low-pitched rumbling mid-diastolic murmur heard at the apex with the bell of stethoscope, in left latest position and in deep expiration.

    It may be associated with pre-systolic accentuation—due to forceful left atrial contraction—if patient is in sinus rhythm.

    But in case of atrial fibrillation, this pre-systolic component will not be present.

    Severity of murmur can be assessed by:

    i. **Duration of murmur**—longer the duration of murmur, more severe the stenosis.
    ii. **Distance between A2 and opening snap**—time interval varies inversely with the severity of stenosis. More closer OS to A2 component, more severe is the stenosis.

       Loud 1st heart sound signifies—valve is pliable and not calcified.

       Conditions that reduce the blood flow across the mitral valve—also reduce the diastolic murmur:
       i. Congestive heart failure
       ii. Pulmonary hypertension
       iii. Aortic stenosis

Associated Lesions

1. In case of severe pulmonary hypertension—a pansystolic murmur audible along left sternal border of heart—

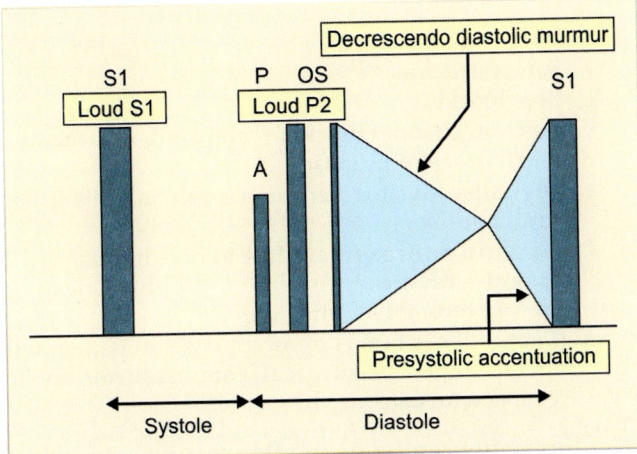

Fig. 1.2: Heart sounds (mitral stenosis)

suggests **tricuspid regurgitation**—this murmur is louder during inspiration, diminished during forced expiration (Carvallo's sign).

2. In case of severely depressed cardiac output, diastolic rumble may not be detected—this **is silent mitral stenosis**—murmur reappears when cardiac output will be restored.
3. High-pitched diastolic, decrescendo, blowing murmur heard along the left sterna border—due to dilatation of pulmonary valve ring—in patient with mitral valve disease associated with pulmonary hypertension.
4. **Graham Steell murmur**, this murmur will be increased during inspiration, accompanied by loud P2.

Laboratory Investigations

ECG (Fig. 1.3)

i. Tall, peaked P wave in LII, wide notched or biphasic wave with more downward stroke in V_1—P mitrale seen in normal sinus rhythm—suggest enlarged left atrium.
ii. In case of atrial fibrillation—fibrillation wave.
iii. In case of pulmonary hypertension—evidence of right ventricular hypertrophy with right axis deviation.

Echocardiography (Fig. 1.4)

Transthoracic echocardiography with color Doppler studies provides the following informations:

a. Mitral inflow velocity during early and late diastolic ventricular filling
b. Transvalvular peak and mean pressure gradient.
c. Mitral orifice area
d. Presence and severity of associated mitral regurgitation
e. Extent of leaflet calcification
f. Restriction of valve leaflet movements
g. Degree of distortion of subvalvular apparatus
h. Anatomic suitability for percutaneous mitral balloon valvoplasty or valvotomy

Transthoracic echocardiography gives following information:

i. Left ventricular or right ventricular function
ii. Chamber size
iii. Estimation of pulmonary hypertension
iv. Presence and severity of associated valvular lesion.

Chest X-ray (Fig. 1.5)

Earliest changes are:

a. Straightening of the upper left border of the cardiac silhouette
b. Prominence of main pulmonary arteries
c. Dilatation of upper lobe pulmonary veins.
d. Posterior displacement of the esophagus by enlarged left atrium
e. Kerley's B lines are fine, dense, opaque, horizontal lines—most prominent in lower and mid-lung fields. Kerley's B lines result from—distension of interlobular septa and lymphatics with edema when left atrial mean pressure ≈ 20 mmHg.

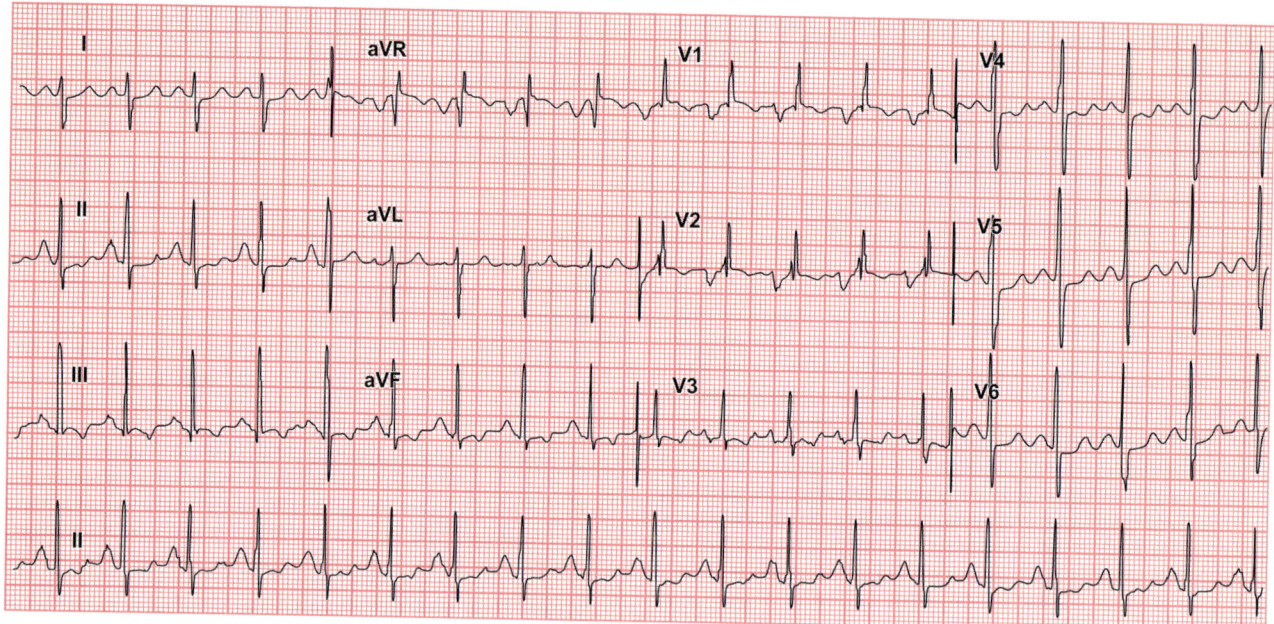

Fig. 1.3: ECG in mitral stenosis

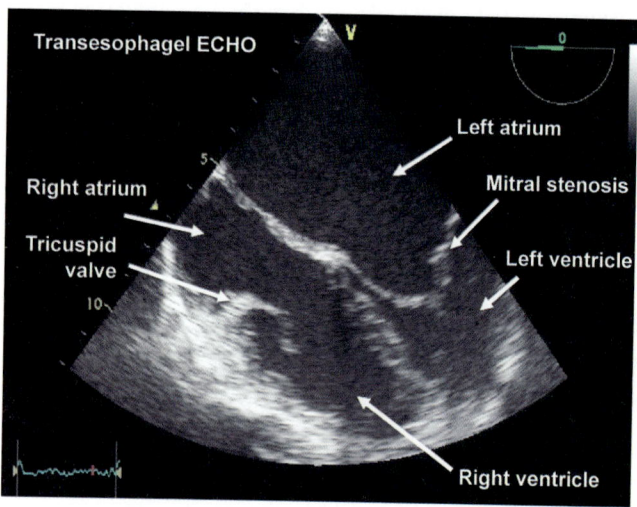

Fig. 1.4: Echocardiography in MS

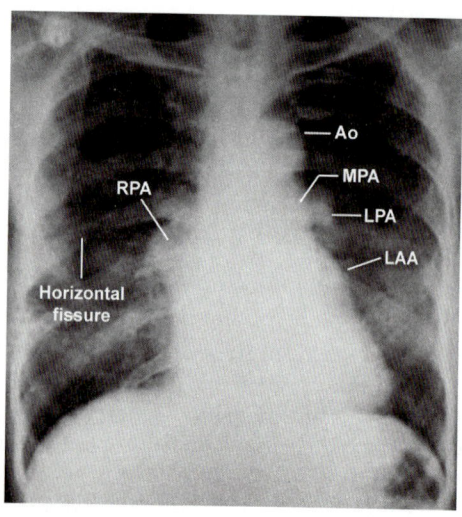

Fig. 1.5: Chest X-ray in mitral stenosis

Gradation of mitral stenosis—given by American Society of Echocardiography:

A. *Severe stenosis:*
   i. Mean transvalvular gradient >10 mmHg
   ii. PA pressure >50 mmHg
   iii. Valve area <1 cm^2

B. *Moderate stenosis:*
   i. Mean transvalvular gradient 5–10 mmHg
   ii. PA pressure—30–50 mmHg
   iii. Valve area—1–1.5 cm^2

C. *Mild stenosis:*
   i. Mean transvalvular gradient <5 mmHg
   ii. PA pressure <30 mmHg
   iii. Valve area >1.5 cm^2

Treatment

I. Medical Therapy

   i. Penicillin prophylaxis against group A β hemolytic *Streptococcus* for secondary prevention of rheumatic fever
   ii. In symptomatic patient:
      a. **Salt restriction**
      b. **Beta blocker**
      c. **Calcium channel blocker (verapamil, diltiazem)**
      d. **Small doses of diuretics**
      e. **Digitalis**—to slow ventricular rate in patient with atrial fibrillation
      f. **Warfarin anticoagulant** has to be administered in patient with atrial fibrillation prophylactically to prevent thrombus formation.
      g. If atrial fibrillation is of recent onset in patient with mitral stenosis—**surgical commissurotomy** for reversion to sinus rhythm.

Cardioversion can be done after complete 3 weeks of anticoagulation treatment.

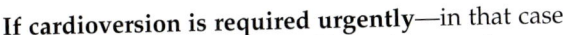

If cardioversion is required urgently—in that case:
a. Intravenous heparin should be given, and
b. Transesophageal echocardiography to exclude the presence of left atrial thrombus.

Converted sinus rhythm is not sustained in case of severe mitral stenosis.

II. Surgical Treatment

A. Mitral valvotomy—indication: Symptomatic NYHA functional class II–IV patients with isolated mitral stenosis, whose effective orifices are <1 cm/m² —valvotomy can be done in two techniques:

1. *Percutaneous mitral balloon valvotomy:*

Contraindication:
i. Commissural calcification
ii. Subvalvular structures should not be scarred or thickness
iii. Left atrial thrombus

Short- and long-term result of PMBV is similar to surgical valvotomy.

Prognostic factors:
a. <45 years of age
b. Pliable mitral valve

2. *Surgical valvotomy:*

Indication:
i. In patient in whom PMBV is not possible
ii. Restenosis post-PMBV

What are the indications of percutaneous mitral balloon valvotomy?
Successful valvotomy is defined by:
i. 50% reduction in mean mitral valve gradient
ii. Doubling of mitral valve area
iii. Striking symptomatic and hemodynamic improvement and prolonged survival

B. Valve replacement
Risk:
i. Thromboembolism
ii. Endocarditis
iii. Primary valve failure

Differential diagnosis (Fig. 1.6):
1. *Functional mitral diastolic murmur* in patient with isolated mitral regurgitation:
   i. S1 is soft
   ii. No opening snap
   iii. Diastolic murmur commences slightly later than in patient with MS
   iv. P2 is normal
   v. Evidence of left ventricular hypertrophy.

Recommendations for percutaneous mitral balloon valvotomy[†]	
Indication	**Class**
1. Symptomatic patients (NYHA functional Class II, III or IV), moderate or severe mitral stenosis (MS) (mitral valve area ≤1.5 cm²)[*] and valve morphology favorable for percutaneous balloon valvotomy in the absence of left atrial thrombus or moderate to severe mitral regurgitation (MR)	I
2. Asymptomatic patients with moderate or severe MS (mitral valve area ≤1.5 cm²)[*] and valve morphology favorable for percutaneous balloon valvotomy who have pulmonary hypertension (pulmonary artery systolic pressure >50 mmHg at rest or 60 mmHg with exercise) in the absence of left atrial thrombus or moderate to severe MR	IIa
3. Patients with NYHA functional Class III–IV symptoms, moderate or severe MS (mitral valve area ≤1.5 cm²)[*] and a nonpliable calcified valve who are at high risk for surgery in the absence of left atrial thrombus or moderate to severe MR	IIa
4. Aysmptomatic patients, moderate or severe MS (mitral valve area ≤1.5 cm²), and valve morphology favorable for percutaneous balloon valvotomy who have new onset of atrial fibrillation in the absence of left atrial thrombus or moderate to severe MR	IIb
5. Patients in NYHA functional Class III–IV, moderate or severe MS (mitral valve area ≤1.5 cm²), and a nonpliable calcified valve who are low-risk cadidates for surgery	IIb
6. Patients with mild MS	

[*]The committee recognizes that there may be variability in the measurement of mitral valve area and that the mean transmitral gradient, pulmonary artery wedge pressure, and pulmonary artery pressure at rest or during exercise should also be taken into consideration.

ACC/AHA Classification

Class I: Conditions for which there is evidence and/or general agreement that a given procedure or treatment is useful and effective.

Class II: Conditions for which there is conflicting evidence and/or a divergence of opinion about the usefulness/efficacy of a procedure or treatment.

Class IIa: Weight of evidence/opinion is a favor of usefulness/efficacy.

Class IIb: Usefulness/efficacy less well established by evidence/opinion.

Class III: Conditions for which there is evidence and/or general agreement that the procedure/ treatment is not useful and in some cases may be harmful.

[†] Data from Bonow, RV, Carabello, B, De Leon, AC, et al, Circulation 1998;98:1949.

Write the algorithm of management of mitral stenosis

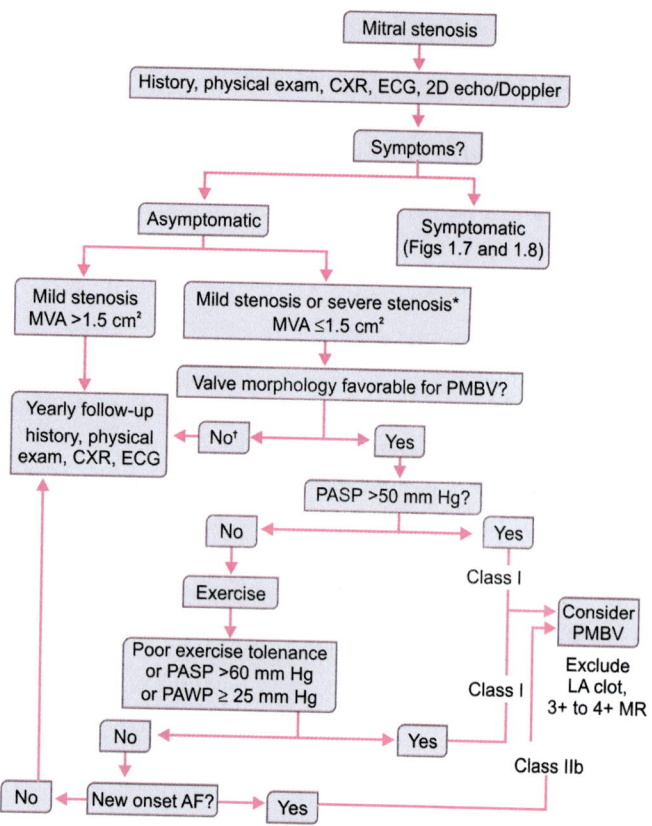

Fig. 1.6: Diagnostic algorithm in MS

* The writing committee recognizes that there may be variability in the measurement of mitral valve area (MVA) and that the mean transmitral gradients, pulmonary artery wedge pressure (PAWP), and pulmonary artery systolic pressure (PASP) should also be taken into consideration.

† There is controversy as to whether patients with severe mitral stenosis (MVA <1.0 cm²) and severe pulmonary hypertension (pulmonary artery pressure >60 mmHg) should undergo percutaneous mitral balloon valvotomy (PMBV) or mitral valve replacement to prevent right ventricular failure.

‡ Assuming no other cause for pulmonary hypertension is present.

AF=atrial fibrillation; **CXR**=chest X-ray;
ECG=electrocardiogram; **echo**=echocardiography;
LA=left atrial; **MR**=mitral regurgitation; **2D**=2-dimensional.

2. *Austin Flint murmur:*
   i.   No presystolic accentuation
   ii. Softer with administration of amyl nitrate
   iii. Associated aortic regurgitation
   iv. No opening snap.
3. *Tricuspid stenosis:*
   i.   Site—lower left border of sternum
   ii. Associated with MS
   iii. Increase in intensity during inspiration
4. *Atrial septal defect:*
   i.   Fixed split of 2nd heart sound
   ii. Grade II to III mid-systolic murmur heard in upper left border of sternum, increases during inspiration
   iii. Absence of left atrial hypertrophy
   iv. Absence of Kerley's B lines.
5. *Left atrial myxoma:*
   i.   Feature of systemic manifestation—fever, weight loss, anemia, systemic emboli, elevated serum IgG and interleukin-6 concentration

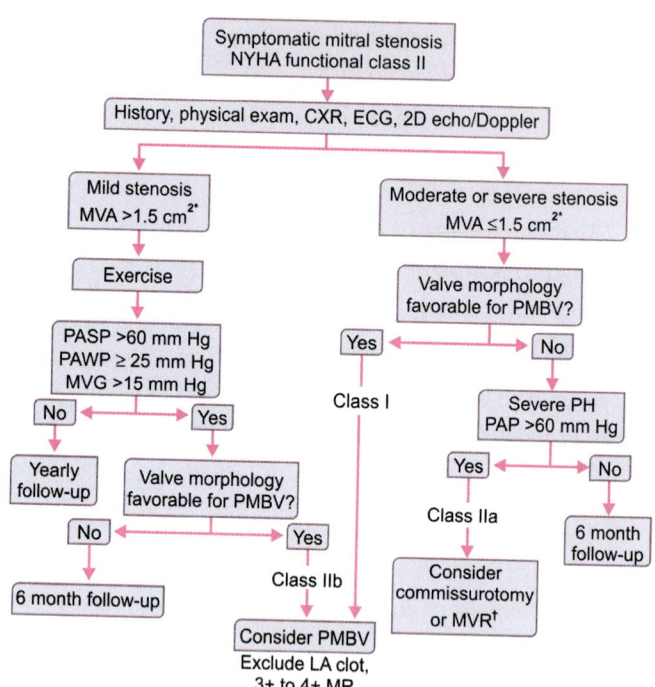

Fig. 1.7: Management strategy for patients with mitral stenosis and mild symptoms.

* The writing committee recognizes that there may be variability in the measurement of mitral valve area (MVA) and that the mean transmitral gradients, pulmonary artery wedge pressure (PAWP), and pulmonary artery systolic pressure (PASP) should also be taken into consideration.

† There is controversy as to whether patients with severe mitral stenosis (MVA <1.0 cm²) and severe pulmonary hypertension (pH; PASP >60 mmHg) should undergo percutaneous mitral balloon valvotomy (PMBV) or mitral valve replacement (MVR) to prevent right ventricular failure.

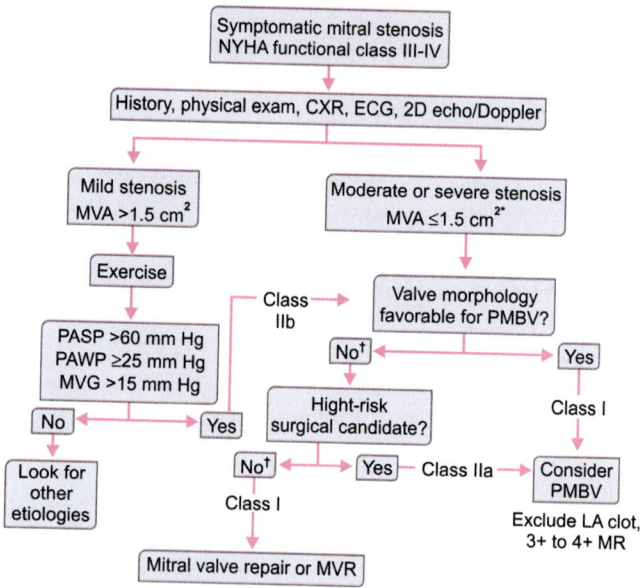

Fig. 1.8: Management strategy for patients with mitral stenosis and moderate to severe symptoms.

* The writing committee recognizes that there may be variability in the measurement of mitral valve area (MVA) and that the mean transmitral gradients, pulmonary artery wedge pressure (PAWP), and pulmonary artery systolic pressure (PASP) should also be taken into consideration.

† It is controversial as to which patients with less favorable value morphology should undergo percutaneous mitral balloon valvotomy (PMBV) rather than mitral valve surgery (*see text*).

ii. Murmur intensity changes with body position

iii. Echo producing mass in left atrium.

iv. Tumor plop may be audible

MITRAL REGURGITATION

Key Points to Diagnosis

1. **Symptoms:** Dyspnea, orthopnea, may be asymptomatic for year.
2. **Signs:** Characteristic pansystolic murmur on apical area with radiation to axilla, accentuated in expiration, loud pulmonary 2nd heart sound, left parasternal lift.
3. **Color Doppler echocardiography** shows evidence of systolic regurgitation into left atrium.
4. **For chronic mitral regurgitation,** surgery is indicated for symptoms or when LVEF <60% or echocardiographic LV endsystolic diameter >4 cm.

Mitral Valve Disease (Figs 1.9 and 1.10)

Mitral Valve Apparatus

It consists of:

i. Anterior and posterior leaflets   ii. Mitral annulus

iii. Chordae tendineae   iv. Papillary muscles

Mitral Regurgitations

It occurs as a result of malfunction of any of above components.

Causes of Mitral Regurgitation

I. Leaflet abnormalities:
1. *Rheumatic fever*—scarring and contraction leaflets to loss of renal tissue.
2. *Endocarditis*—can cause perforations and retraction of valve tissue
3. *Myxomatous degeneration* of leaflets with excursive motion
4. *Aneurysm*—usually from aortic valve endocarditis.
5. *Congenital:*
   i. Cleft mitral valve   ii. Double orifice mitral valve
6. *Hypertrophic cardiomyopathy*—systolic anterior motion of mitral valve.

II. Mitral annular abnormalities:
1. *Annular dilatation from:*
   i. Dilated cardiomyopathy
   ii. Ischemic disease
   iii. Hypertension
2. *Mitral annular calcification:*
   i. Degenerative disorder   ii. Marfan syndrome
   iii. Hurler syndrome

III. Chordal abnormalities:
1. Chordal rupture—results in loss of leaflet support usually with myxomatous degeration
2. Rheumatic heart disease

IV. Papillary abnormalities:
1. Rupture due to myocardial infarction
2. Dysfunctional papillary muscle

Mitral Regurgitation (According to Severity)

I. Acute mitral regurgitation:
1. Acute myocardial infarction with papillary muscle rupture
2. Following blunt chest wall trauma

3. Infective endocarditis

   In acute MI

   Posteromedial papillary muscle is involved much more frequently than anterolateral papillary muscle because of its single blood supply.

4. Rupture of chordae—due to myxomatous degeneration of mitral valve apparatus.

II. Chronic mitral regurgitation (Fig. 1.11):
1. Rheumatic heart disease
2. Prolapsed mitral valve
3. Extensive mitral annular calcification
4. Congenital valve defect
5. HOCM
6. Dilated cardiomyopathy

Type I dysfunction: Here normal leaflet motion, but free edges of the leaflets are positioned 5 to 10 mm below the annulus. Here mitral regurgitation is due to annular dilatation, leaflet perforation or leaflet tear.

Type II dysfunction: Here the free edges of one or more leaflets override the plane of annulus during systole. Most common lesions are chordae or papillary muscles dysfunction or ruptures.

Type IIIa dysfunction: Here there are restricted motions of leaflets during systole or diastole. Most common lesions are leaflet thickening/retraction, chordae thickening/shortening/fusion, commissural fusion.

Type IIIb dysfunction: Here there is restricted leaflet motion during systole. The lesion is left ventricular enlargement leading to apico-lateral papillary muscle displacement and chordae tethering.

Left Atrial Compliances

I. In acute mitral regurgitation

Regurgitant volume is delivered into left atrium which is normal in size and normal or reduced compliance
↓
Left atrial pressure rises markedly for any increase in left atrial volume
↓
As a result pulmonary venous pressure is markedly elevated
↓
Increased pulmonary capillary wedge pressure
↓
Development of pulmonary edema

Characteristic of murmur:
   i. Due to rapid rise in left atrial pressure—murmur duration of mitral regurgitation is early in timing
   ii. Decrescendo in character due to rapidly progressive diminution of LV-LA pressure gradient.
   iii. Murmur ends well before 2nd heart sound.

II. In chronic mitral regurgitation:

Marked left atrial enlargement and increased left atrial compliance
↓
So there is little or no increase in left atrial pressure for any increase in left atrial volume
↓
No increase in pulmonary capillary wedge pressure
↓
No development in pulmonary edema.

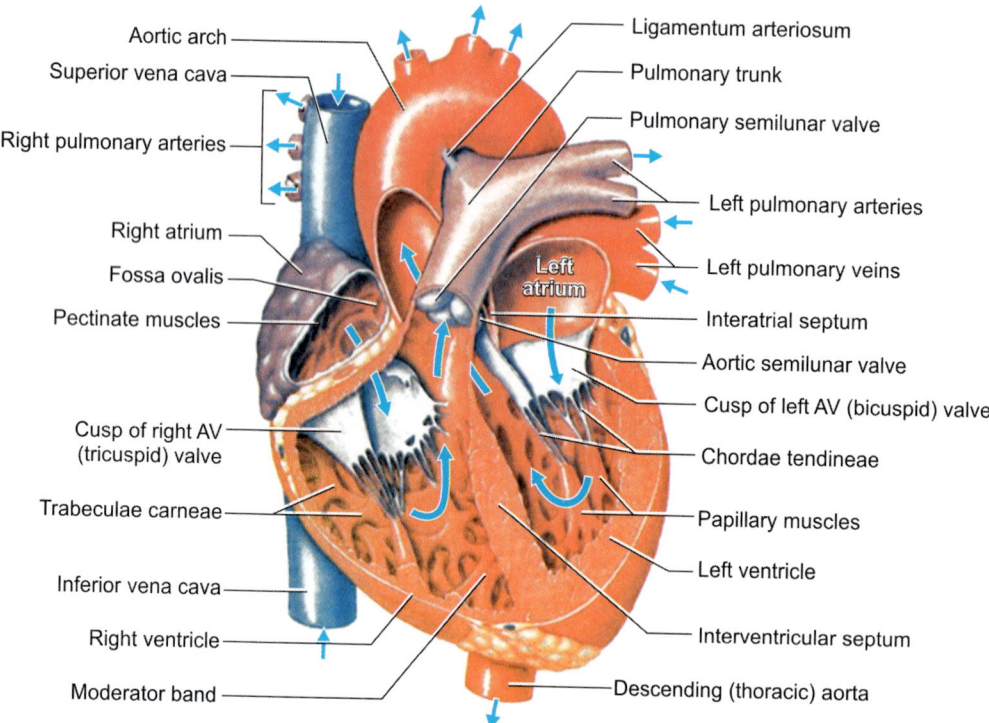

Fig. 1.9: Cross-section of normal heart

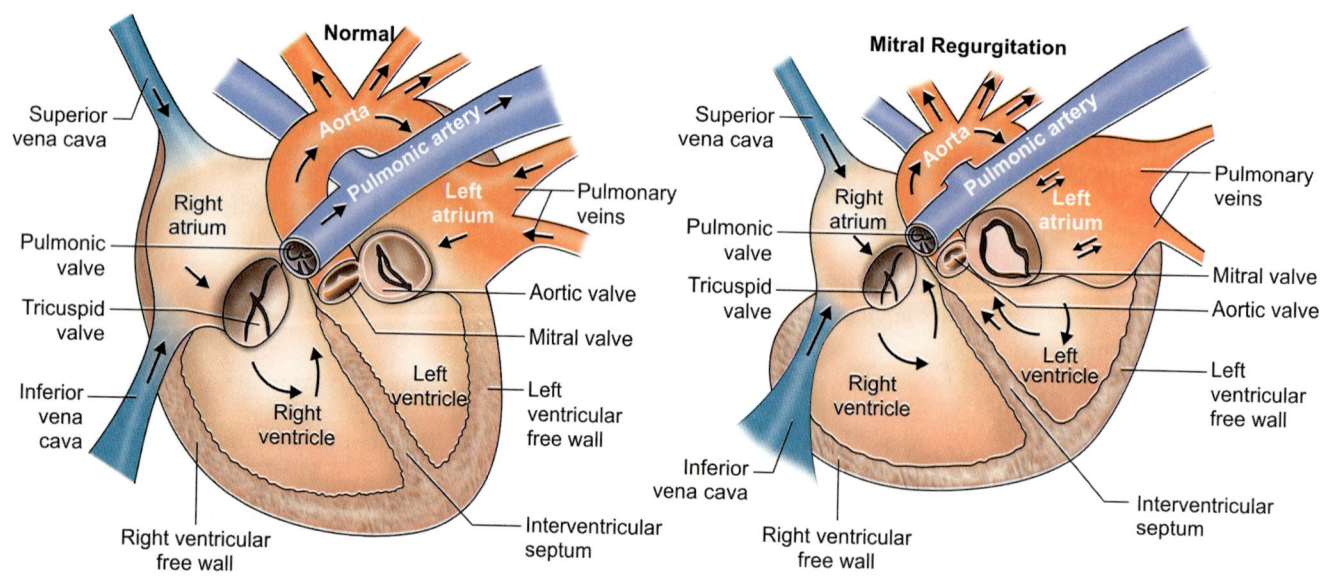

Fig. 1.10: Comparison of flow of blood in normal heart and heart having mitral regurgitation

Characteristic of murmur:
   i. Murmur of mitral regurgitation is holosystolic in timing and plateau in configuration.
       This is an indication of near constant LV-LA gradient.

Symptoms

I. In case of acute mitral regurgitation—due to abrupt pulmonary congestion.
   i. Dyspnea
   ii. Orthopnea
   iii. Cardiogenic shock

II. In case of chronic mitral regurgitation:
   i. Asymptomatic—usually
   ii. Exertional dyspnea, occurs in early phase, followed by orthopnea, paroxysmal exertional dyspnea
   iii. Fatigue—due to diminished cardiac output

III. In case of long-standing mitral regurgitation—due to pulmonary hypertension, patient may present with right-sided heart failure, e.g.
   i. Painful hepatic congestion
   ii. Ankle edema
   iii. Ascites

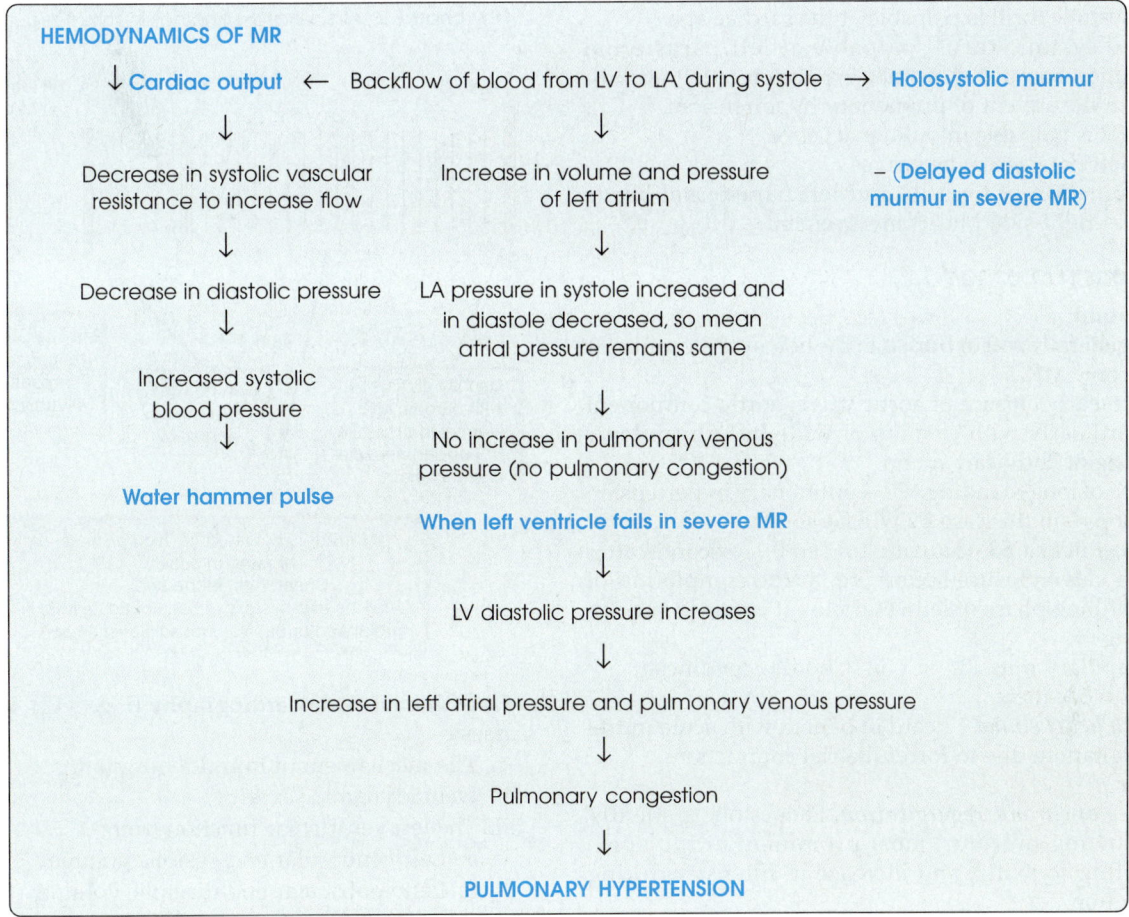

HEMODYNAMICS OF MR

↓ Cardiac output ← Backflow of blood from LV to LA during systole → Holosystolic murmur

↓ ↓

Decrease in systolic vascular resistance to increase flow | Increase in volume and pressure of left atrium | – (Delayed diastolic murmur in severe MR)

↓ ↓

Decrease in diastolic pressure | LA pressure in systole increased and in diastole decreased, so mean atrial pressure remains same

↓

Increased systolic blood pressure ↓

↓ No increase in pulmonary venous pressure (no pulmonary congestion)

Water hammer pulse

When left ventricle fails in severe MR

↓

LV diastolic pressure increases

↓

Increase in left atrial pressure and pulmonary venous pressure

↓

Pulmonary congestion

↓

PULMONARY HYPERTENSION

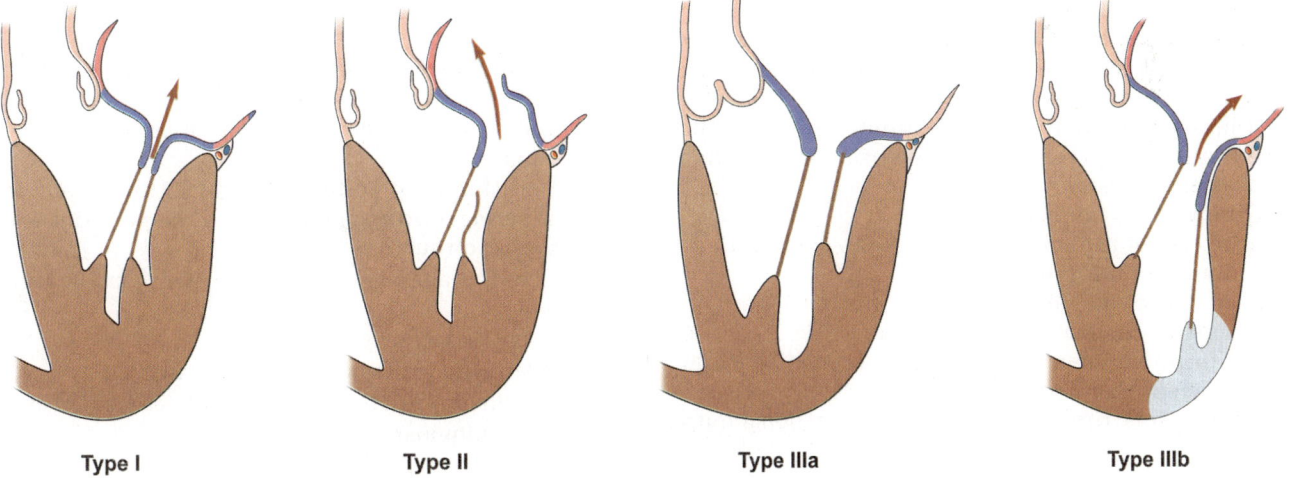

| Type I | Type II | Type IIIa | Type IIIb |

Fig. 1.11: Different types of mitral leaflet dysfunction in mitral regurgitation

Physical Findings

I. In patient with chronic severe mitral regurgitation:
  i. Arterial pressure is usually normal
  ii. Carotid arterial pulse is of low volume
  iii. In case of tricuspid regurgitation, large V wake in jugular venous wave
  iv. Engorged pulsatile neck vein in case of pulmonary hypertension with right-sided heart failure.

II. In patient with acute severe mitral regurgitation:
  i. Arterial pulse is reduced with narrow pulse press
  ii. Jugular venous pressure is increased and exaggera.
  iii. Basal crepitations due to pulmonary venous and capillary congestion.

III. Cardiac palpations:
  i. Cardiac apical impulse is hyperdynamic—it is pushed outwards.

ii. A systolic thrill is palpable at the cardiac apex
iii. Late systolic thrust palpable at left parasternal location because of systolic expansion of left atrium.
iv. With the advent of pulmonary hypertension:
    a. P2 is palpable in pulmonary area
    b. left parasternal be heave
Combination of loud P2 and left parasternal heave suggests—right-sided heart involvement.

Auscultations *(Flowchart 1.2)*

I. Heart sound:
  a. **S1**—generally soft or buried in the holosystolic murmur of chronic MR.
  b. Due to early closure of aortic valve, **aortic component** is heard early with creation of **wide but physiologic spitting** of 2nd heart sound.
  c. In case of long-standing MR—pulmonary hypertension develops—in this case **P2 will be loud**.
  d. *A low-pitched S3* occurring 0.12 to 0.17 seconds after aortic valve closure sound, i.e. at the completion of rapid filling phase of left ventricle—it is due to sudden tensing of:
    i. Papillary muscles   ii. Chordae tendineae
    iii. Valve leaflets.
  e. *Fourth heart sound*—heard in patient with acute mitral regurgitation, due to forceful atrial contraction.

II. Murmur
  a. *In case of chronic regurgitation:* Pansystolic grade III/VI blowing murmur, most prominent at the apex, radiating to axilla, and increase in intensity during expiration.
  b. *In case of acute regurgitation:* Harsh early systolic murmur heard at the apex, ends well before P2 component of 2nd sound.
  c. *In case of ruptured chordae*—or primary involvement of posterior mitral leaflet with prolapse, regurgitant jet is eccentric, directed anteriorly and strikes the left atrial wall adjacent to aortic root; as a result, systolic murmur is transmitted to base of heart confusing with murmur of aortic stenosis.
    Quality of this murmur:
    i. In case of ruptured chordate—systolic murmur has cooing or sea gull quality.
    ii. In case of flail leaflet—systolic murmur of musical quality. Systolic murmur of chronic MR is reduced during Valsalva maneuver, and intensified during isometric hand grip.
  d. Mid-diastolic rumbling occurs due to functional mitral stenosis.

Laboratory Investigations

A. ECG (Fig. 1.12):
  i. Nonspecific
  ii. Principal findings are:
    a. Left atrial enlargement in chronic MR produces negative P wave in V1 and/or a wide notched, bifid P wave in leads II,II or aVF.
    b. Atrial fibrillation
    c. Left ventricular hypertrophy
    d. Ischemia or infarction of inferior or posterior leads may be present when acute MR due to papillary muscle rupture.

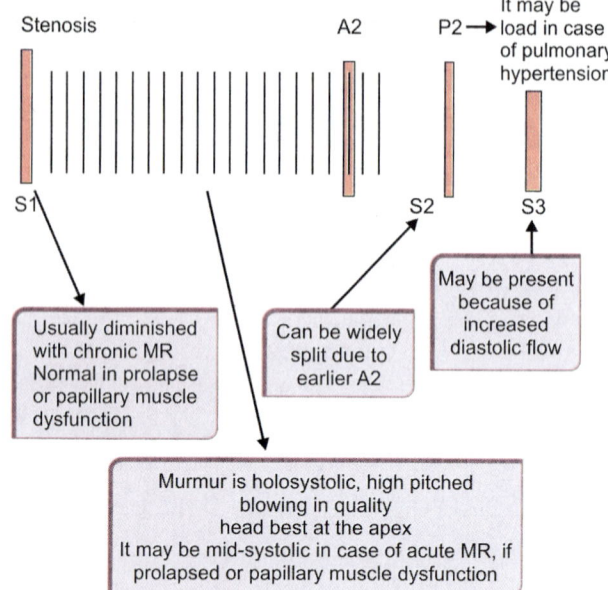

Flowchart 1.2: Auscultatory findings in mitral regurgitation.

B. Transthoracic echocardiography (Fig. 1.13). It is used to assess:
  i. The mechanism of mitral regurgitation
  ii. Hemodynamic severity
  iii. The left ventricular function from:
    a. Left ventricular end systolic volume
    b. Left ventricular end diastolic volume
    c. Ejection fraction
  iv. Left ventricular and left atrial size
  v. Annular calcification
  vi. Regional and global left ventricular wall motion
  European Society of Cardiology criteria for the definition of severe mitral regurgitation are:
  i. Flail leaflet/ruptured papillary muscles/large coaptation defect.
  ii. Very large color flow central jet or eccentric jet adhering, swirling and reaching the posterior wall of the left atrium.
  iii. Dense/triangular continuous wave signal or regurgitant jet.
  iv. Large flow convergence zone.

C. Doppler echocardiography. It demonstrates:
  i. Width or area of color flow of MR jet into left atrium
  ii. The pulmonary venous flow contour
  iii. The early peak mitral inflow velocity
  iv. Quantitative measurement of regurgitant volume
  v. Quantitative measurement of regurgitant fraction
  vi. Effective regurgitant surface area
  vii. Pulmonary artery pressure

D. Chest X-ray (Fig. 1.14)
  In acute regurgitation:
  i. Pulmonary venous congestion
  ii. Interstitial edema
  iii. Kerley's B lines
  iv. Asymmetric pulmonary edema, if regurgitant volume is directed predominantly towards the orifice of upper lobe pulmonary vein.

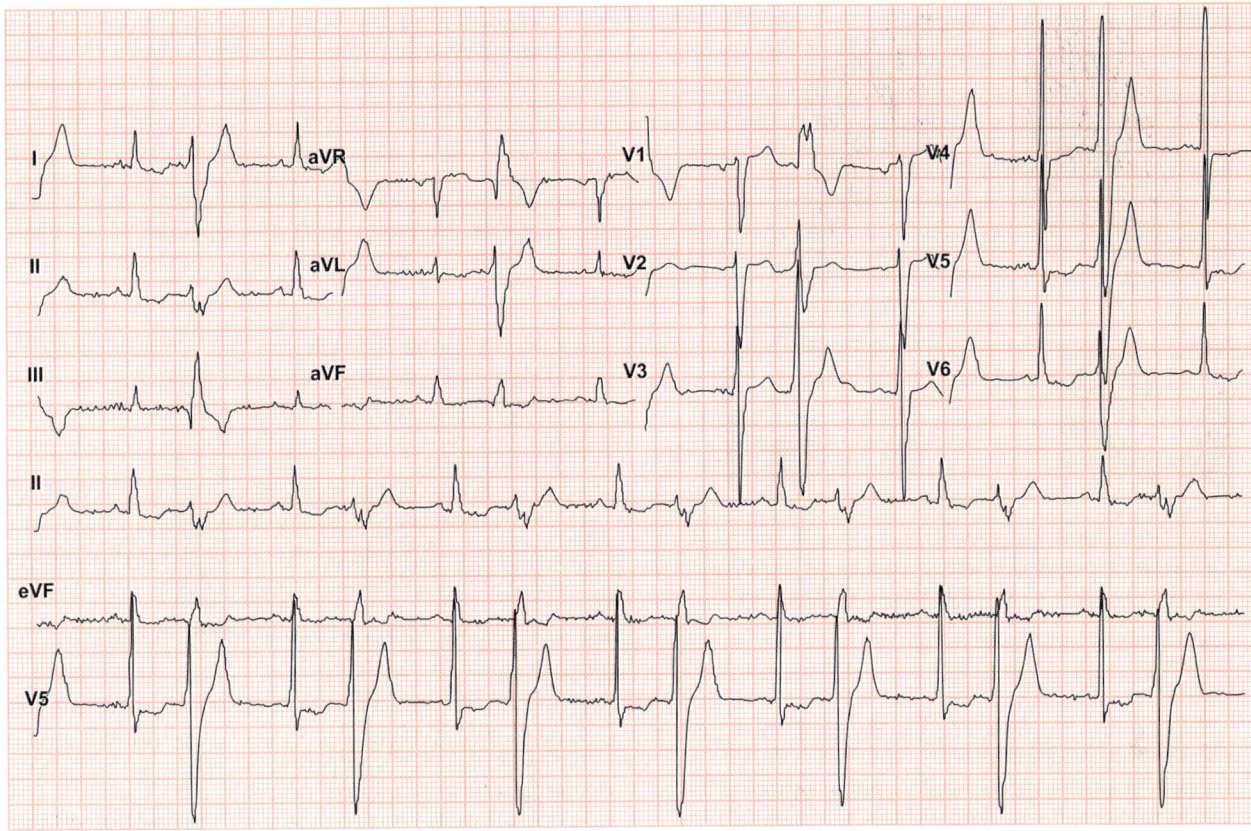

Fig. 1.12: ECG in mitral regurgitation

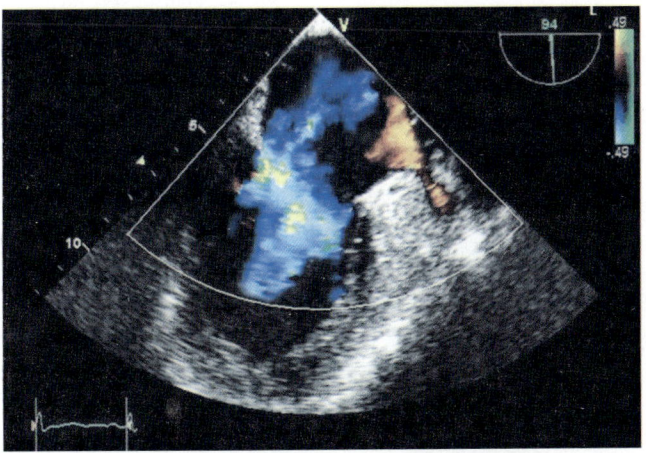

Fig. 1.13: Echocardiography in mitral regurgitation

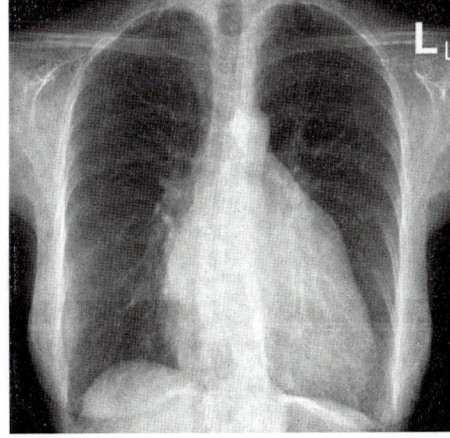

Fig. 1.14: Chest X-ray in mitral regurgitation

In chronic long-standing mitral regurgitation:

i. Left atrium and left ventricular enlargement

ii. In some cases—massive left atrial enlargement produces right border of the heart, producing double shadow in the right cardiac silhouette and straightening of the left cardiac border due to large left atrial appendages.

Therapy

I. In acute mitral regurgitation:

  A. *Medical therapy:*

    a. *Afterload reducing agents* (nitroprusside and nitroglycerin):

    1. They reduce the pulmonary venous pressure.
    2. They maximize the forward flow.
      If operative intervention is not required immediately.

    b. *Orally afterload reducing agents* can be administered. They are:

     i. Angiotensin-converting enzyme inhibitor
     ii. Directly acting vasodilator—hydralazine

    They:

     i. Maximize forward output
     ii. Reduce regurgitant fraction

  B. *Percutaneous therapy:* In hemodynamically compromised significant mitral regurgitation, producing **cardiogenic shock**—placement of an intra-aortic

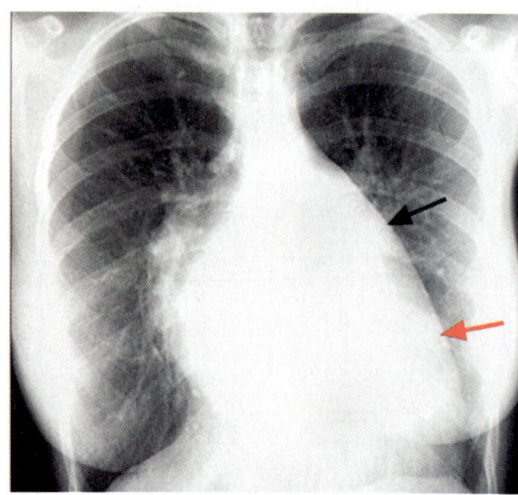

Fig. 1.15: Mitral regurgitation—This plain chest radiograph from a female with known mitral regurgitation demonstrates cardiomegaly with left atrial (black arrow) and left ventricular enlargement (red arrow), as well as mild pulmonary venous redistribution, all features characteristic of mitral regurgitation (*Courtesy:* Jonathan Kruskal, MD.)

balloon pump for temporary stabilizing measure till definite surgical repair.

   C. *Surgical repair:* Urgent surgical intervention.

II. Chronic mitral regurgitation:

1. Most patients with moderately severe to severe form mitral regurgitation and are symptomatic should be considered for surgical treatment. **Surgical treatment depends upon:**
   - a. Age of the patient
   - b. Likehood of valve repair
   - c. Comorbidities
   - d. Left ventricular function
2. When severe mitral regurgitation is **due to primarily valve involvement** (prolapsed, rheumatic heart disease, or congenital), surgical intervention should be done
3. When severe mitral regurgitation is **secondary to ventricular dysfunction** (ischemic heart disease or dilated cardiomyopathy)
   Initial treatment should be **after load reducing agents** followed by surgical interventions for refractory symptoms.
4. In **minimally symptomatic or asymptomatic patient**—with severe mitral regurgitation—surgical repair of valve should be advisable before left ventricular contractile function becomes irreversible.

Indications for Mitral Valve Surgery in MR (Fig. 1.16)

Class-I:

1. Symptomatic patient with acute mitral regurgitation.
2. Patient with chronic severe mitral regurgitation and NYHA class II, III, IV symptoms in absence of severe left ventricular dysfunction.
3. Asymptomatic patient with chronic severe MR mild to moderate LV dysfunction, ejection fraction 0.30 to 0.60 and end-systolic dimension $\geq$ 40 mm.

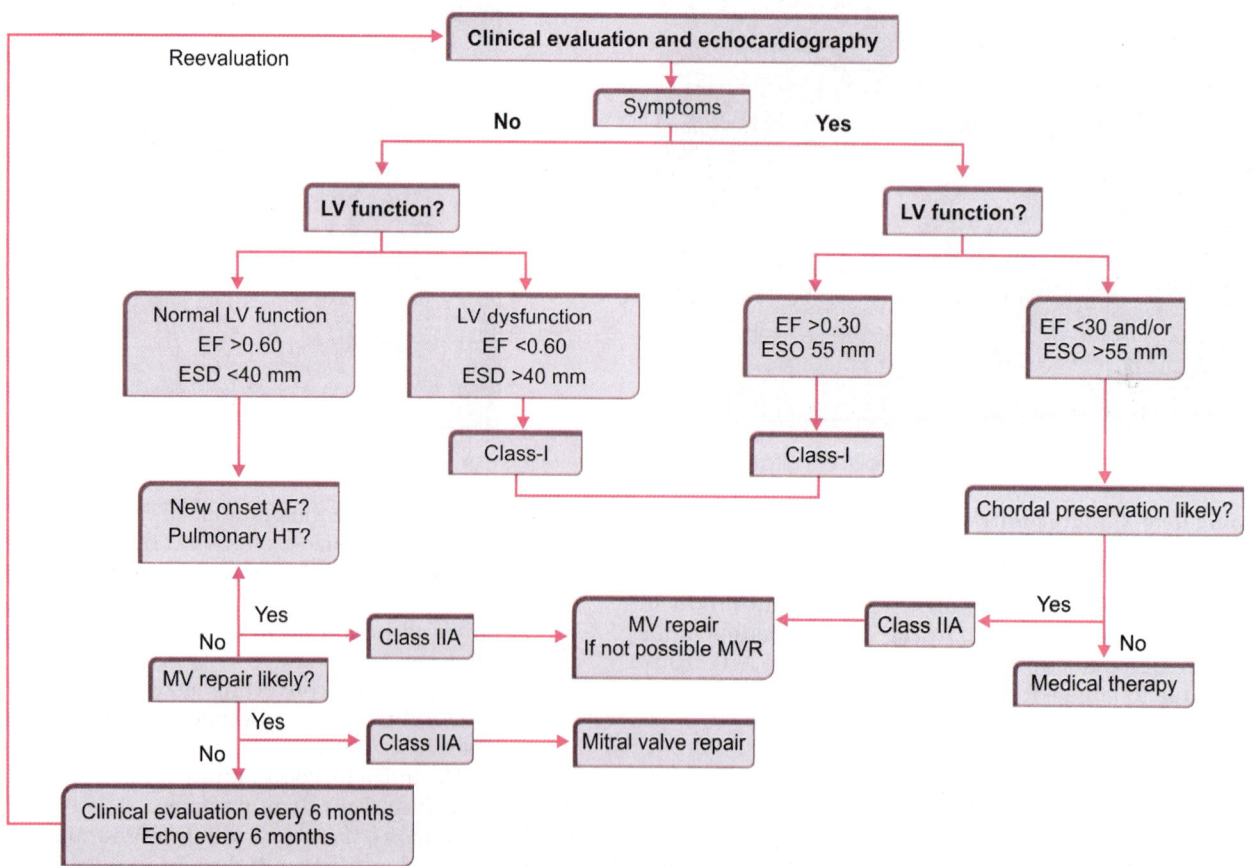

Fig. 1.16: Evaluation of mitral incompetence

Class-IIA:

1. Asymptomatic patient with chronic severe MR, preserved LV function (ejection fraction >0.6 and end systolic dimension <40 mm) is the candidate for repair.
2. Asymptomatic patient with chronic severe MR, preserved LV function, new on set atrial fibrillation.
3. Asymptomatic patient with chronic severe MR, preserved LV function, pulmonary hypertension (pulmonary artery systolic pressure >50 mmHg at rest, >60 mmHg with exercise.
4. Patient with chronic severe MR due to primary mitral valve apparatus, NYHA class-III and IV symptoms, severe left ventricular dysfunction (ejection fraction <0.30 and/or end systolic dimension >55 mm).

Class-IIB:

Mitral valve repair is indicated in: Patient with chronic severe MR, severe LV dysfunction (ejection fraction <0.30), persisting

NYHA class-III–IV symptoms despite optimal therapy, biventricular pains.

Class-III

Mitral valve surgery is not indicated in:

1. Asymptomatic patient with severe MR, preserved LV function (ejection fraction >0.60, end-systolic dimension <40 mm)
2. Mild to moderate MR.

Surgical Management for Ischemic MR (Fig. 1.17)

i. Simultaneous coronary revascularization
ii. Annuloplasty repair with an undersized ring for patient with moderate MR at the time of CABG.

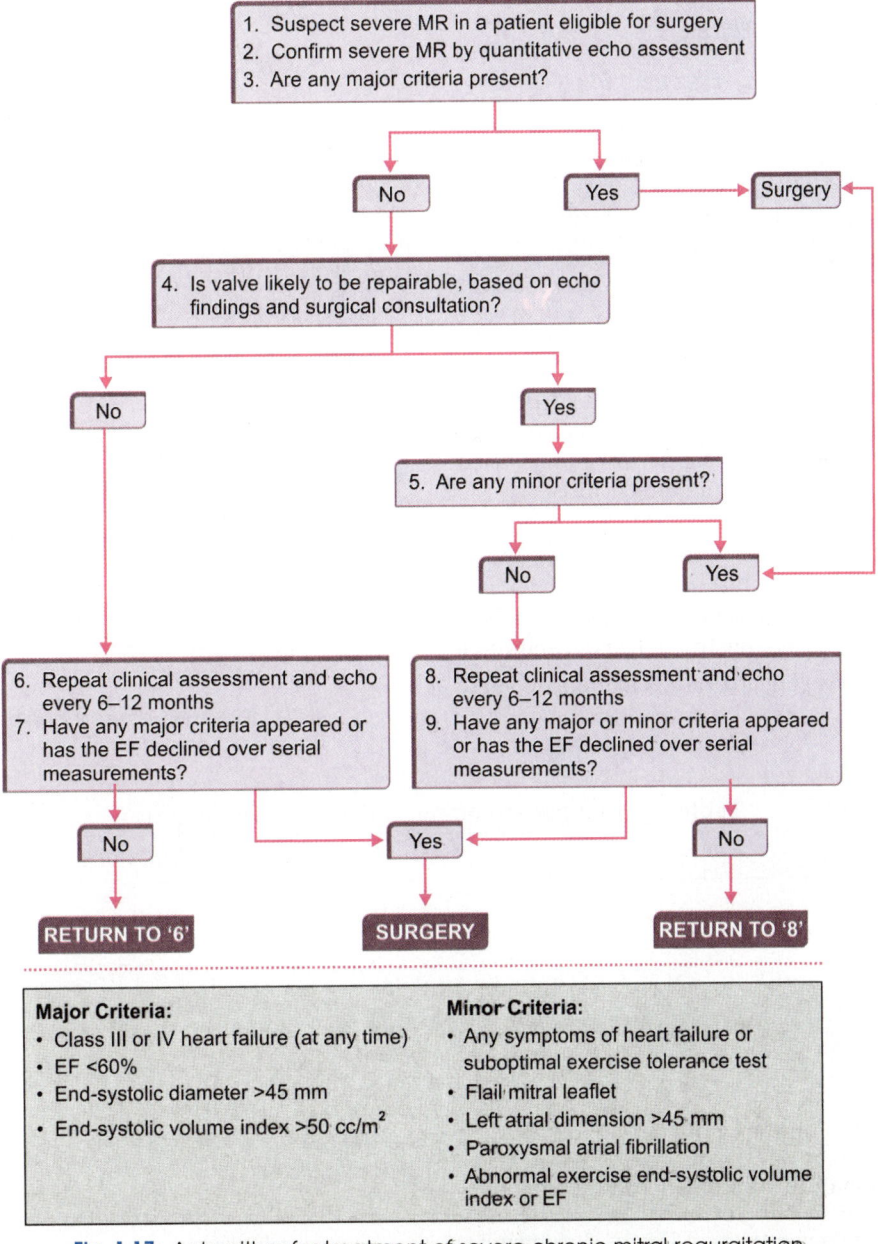

Fig. 1.17: Aalgorithm for treatment of severe chronic mitral regurgitation

Mitral regurgitation (Table 1.1):
1. Dyspnea or orthopnea
2. Characteristic apical systolic murmur
3. Color flow Doppler echocardiography shows evidence of systolic regurgitation into the left atrium.

Any maneuver that increases left ventricular volume will decrease the amount of mitral valve prolapse and decrease the amount of mitral regurgitation, thereby lessening the intensity of murmur.

Thus rapid squatting will diminish the murmur of mitral valve prolapse and move the timing of the click-murmur complex later in the systole.

Conversely, the maneuver that decreases the left ventricular volume, increases the intensity and duration of murmur of mitral valve prolapse.

Thus standing rapidly from squatting position, will make the murmur louder and move the click–murmur complex towards early systole.

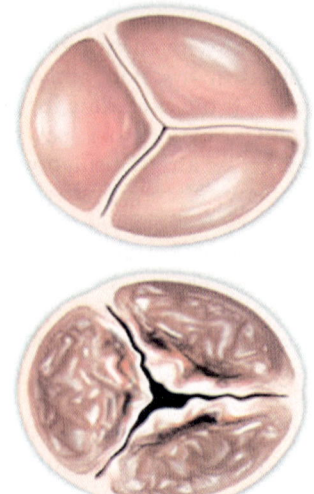

Fig. 1.18: Valvular aortic stenosis

AORTIC STENOSIS

Key points to diagnosis

1. **Symptoms:** Anginal pain, dyspnea, effort syncope.
2. **Signs:** Pulsus tardus, ejection click with ejection systolic murmur in neoaortic area, radiating to carotid.
3. **Echocardiographic evidence** of thickened immobile aortic valve leaflets.
4. **Doppler echocardiography** shows and quantities increased transvalvular pressure gradient across the reduced valvular area.
5. **Emerging role of BNP** as marker of early myocardial failure.

This is caused by progressive obstruction of the left ventricular out flow tract resulting in left ventricular hypertrophy due to pressure and classic symptoms tried including heart failure, syncope and angina pectoris.

Three types of stenosis:
1. Valvular aortic stenosis (Fig. 1.18).
2. Subvalvular aortic stenosis—obstruction below the valve
3. Supravalvular aortic stenosis—obstruction above the valve

Valvular aortic stenosis (Fig. 1.19): Normal aortic valve area is 3 to 4 cm^2

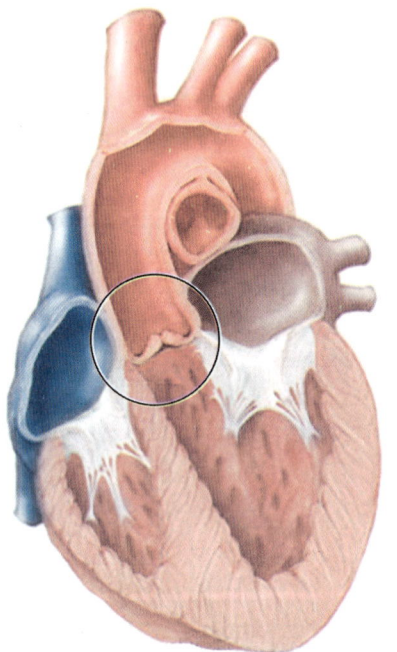

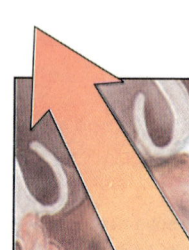

Normal aortic valve in the open position

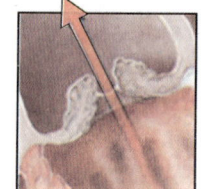

Stenotic aortic valve

Fig. 1.19: Valvular aortic stenosis

Table 1.1: Comparsion of murmur in different diseases							
Origin of murmur		*Flow*	*TR*	*AS*	*MR/VPD*	*MVP*	*HOCM*
1. Inspiration	→	- or ↑	↑	–	–	–	–
2. Standing	→	↓	–	–	–	↑	↑
3. Squat	→	↑	–	–	–	↓	↓
4. Valsalva	→	↓	↓	↓	↓	↑	↑
5. Hand gripping transient arterial occlusion	→	↓	–	–	↑	↑	↓
6. Post-premature ventricular contraction	→	↑	–	↑	–	–	↑

↑ Increased murmur intensity; ↓ Decreased murmur intensity; – No predictable change

Causes of Valvular Aortic Stenosis

1. **Degenerative**—most common in United States, age related, and calcific—deposition of calcium at the fusion lines of valve leaflet.

   In case of aortic sclerosis (caused by the calcification and thickening of aortic valve)—usually there is no pressure gradient.
2. **Bicuspid aortic valve**—produces features or aortic stenosis in 5th or 6th decade of life. It occurs due to fusion of right and left coronary cusps.
3. **Rheumatic etiology**—May coexists with mitral stenosis and aortic regurgitation.

Pathophysiology (Fig. 1.20)

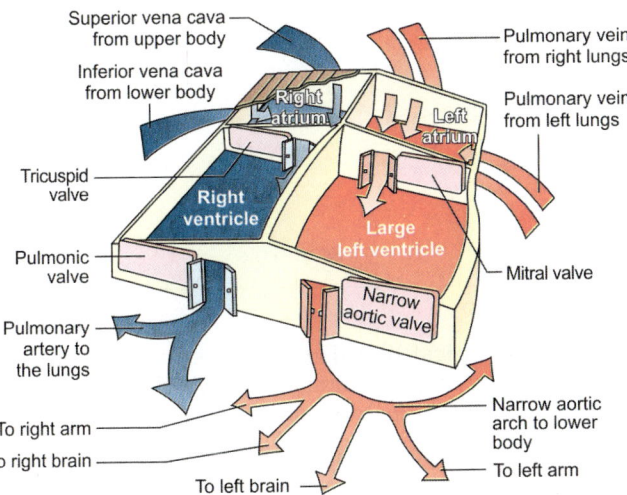

Fig. 1.20: Pathophysiology of aortic stenosis

In case of aortic stenosis due to resistance to systolic ejection, there is development of increased pressure gradient between left ventricle and aorta

↓

Left ventricle develops high systolic pressure to maintain normal cardiac output.

↓

Left ventricular wall will be in stress

↓

Left ventricular wall thickness increases by parallel replication of sarcomere producing

1. Left ventricular hypertrophy

↓

As a result, there is reduction in left ventricular compliance—during diastole.

↓

Passive left ventricular diastolic filling is reduced due to impaired left ventricular relaxation.

↓

2. Development of diastolic dysfunction.
In severe aortic stenosis, left ventricular diastolic filling depends upon forceful left atrial contraction.

↓

3. Development of atrial fibrillation

Myocardial subendocardial oxygen requirement will be increased due to:

1. Increased left ventricular muscle mass
2. Increased left ventricular systolic pressure.
3. Prolongation of systolic ejection time.

But in aortic stenosis:

1. **Coronary blood flow** may be normal when corrected for left ventricular muscle mass, but coronary reserve will be diminished.
2. Myocardial perfusion will be reduced due to:
   i. Declining the myocardial capillary bed
   ii. Reduced diastolic transmyocardial coronary perfusion due to left ventricular elevated diastolic pressure.

So angina pectoris develops due to:

1. **Increased oxygen demand** by hypertrophied left ventricular myocardium
2. **Diminished coronary blood flow** due to:
   i. Decreased diastolic perfusion pressure
   ii. Decreased coronary flow reserve
3. **Relative subendocardial ischemia.**

Symptoms and Related Pathophysiology

1. Asymptomatic for 10–20 years—during this time, left ventricular pressure gradient and left ventricular pressure loads gradually increase.
2. Exertional dyspnea—initial complaint may be due to exertion-related left ventricular diastolic and systolic dysfunction.
3. Exertional chest pain, light headedness, fatigability
4. **Ultimately patient develops clinical triad**
   a. *Angina*—chest pain—precipitated by exertion and relieved by rest.
   b. *Heart failure:* Symptoms—**dyspnea** at rest, orthopnea, paroxysmal nocturnal dyspnea may be due to:
      i. Systolic left ventricular dysfunction secondary to—mismatch after load, myocardial ischemia or separate cardiomyopathic process.
      ii. Diastolic dysfunction from left ventricular hypertrophy or myocardial ischemia.
   c. *Syncope:* It results from:
      1. *During exertion*-related systemic vasodilatation in the face of fixed cardiac output:
         i. Producing sudden decline in arterial systolic blood pressure.
         ii. Atrial tachyarrhythmia
         iii. Ventricular tachyarrhythmia
      2. *During rest*, it can occur secondary to:
         i. Ventricular tachyarrhythmia
         ii. Atrial fibrillation
         iii. Atrioventricular block
      3. *Vasodepressor syncope*—abnormal vasodepressor reflex. Secondary to increased left ventricular end-cavitary pressure.
      4. *Nitroglycerin-induced syncope:* It can occur in general population due to:
         i. Low cardiac output will be further decreased.
         ii. Particular hypersensitivity to nitrates

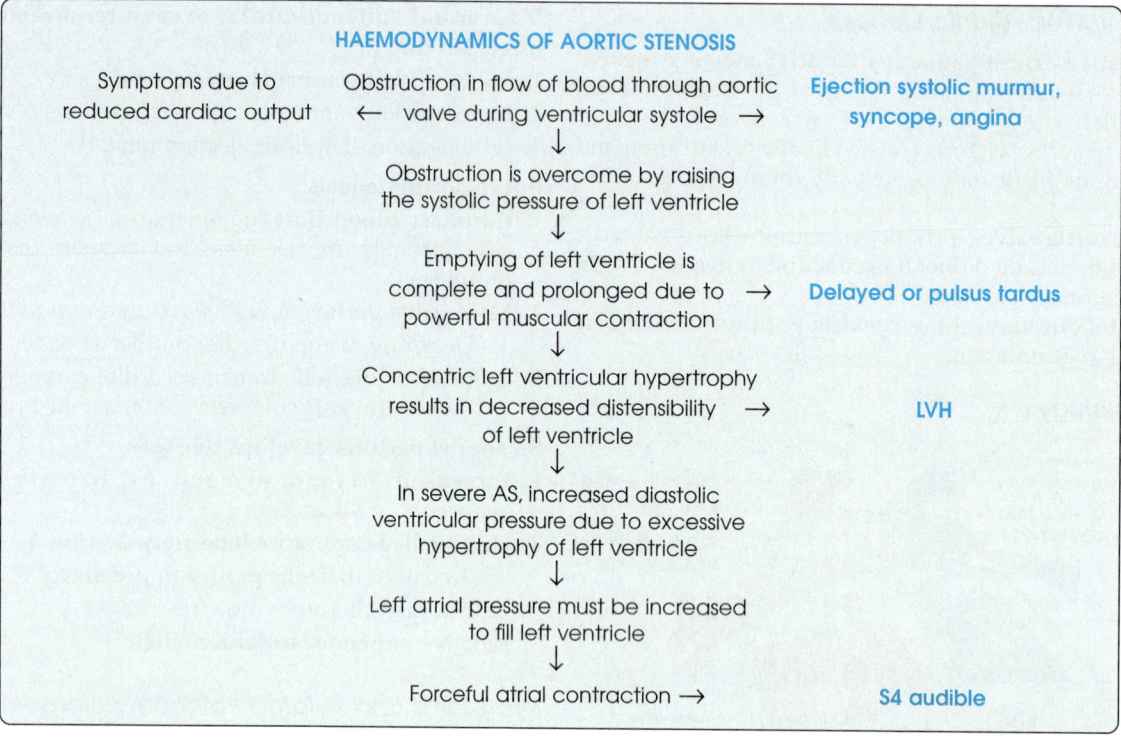

HAEMODYNAMICS OF AORTIC STENOSIS

Symptoms due to reduced cardiac output	← Obstruction in flow of blood through aortic valve during ventricular systole →	Ejection systolic murmur, syncope, angina
	↓	
	Obstruction is overcome by raising the systolic pressure of left ventricle	
	↓	
	Emptying of left ventricle is complete and prolonged due to → powerful muscular contraction	Delayed or pulsus tardus
	↓	
	Concentric left ventricular hypertrophy results in decreased distensibility → of left ventricle	LVH
	↓	
	In severe AS, increased diastolic ventricular pressure due to excessive hypertrophy of left ventricle	
	↓	
	Left atrial pressure must be increased to fill left ventricle	
	↓	
	Forceful atrial contraction →	S4 audible

Other Manifestations

I. Gastrointestinal bleeding due to angiodysplasia (Heyde syndrome) or other vascular malformation mainly in patient with calcific aortic stenosis.

II. Features of infective endocarditis—fever, fatigue, anorexia, back pain, weight loss—occurs mainly in younger patient with mild valvular deformity.

But it can occur at any age with hospital-acquired staphylococcal bacteria.

Physical Examinations

I. **Pulse**: In severe stenosis:
a. Carotid pulse has:
  i. Delayed and plateau peak
  ii. Decreased amplitude
  iii. Gradual downstroke (pulsus parvus et tardus)
b. Lag time present between apical impulse and carotid impulse.
c. Pulsus alternans—due to severe left ventricular dysfunction.

II. **Jugular vein**: Prominent 'a' wave reflecting reduced right ventricular compliance secondary to hypertrophy of interventricular septum.

III. **Blood pressure:**
a. If it is present in association with aortic stenosis, it is rarely >200 mmHg in severe aortic stenosis.
b. Pulse pressure will be reduced.

Palpation

I. **Apical impulse**:
a. Non-displaced, diffuse and sustained due to left ventricular hypertrophy and normal left ventricular cavity dimension.
b. But in case of left ventricular systolic dysfunction—apical impulse may be displaced laterally.

c. Double apical impulse—represents palpable S4—secondary to non-compliant left ventricle.

II. **Systolic thrill:** It is palpable in 2nd right intercostal space.

Auscultation *(Figs 1.21 and 1.22)*

I. **1st heart sound (S1):** Normal or soft, but intensity will be decreased as left ventricular function worsens.

II. **2nd heart sound (S2):**
a. *Aortic component (A2):* Usually diminished or absent because:
  i. Aortic valve is calcified and immobile.
  ii. Obscured, if aortic ejection is prolonged and obscured by prolonged systolic murmur.
b. *Normal or accentuated A2:* Always against severe aortic stenosis.

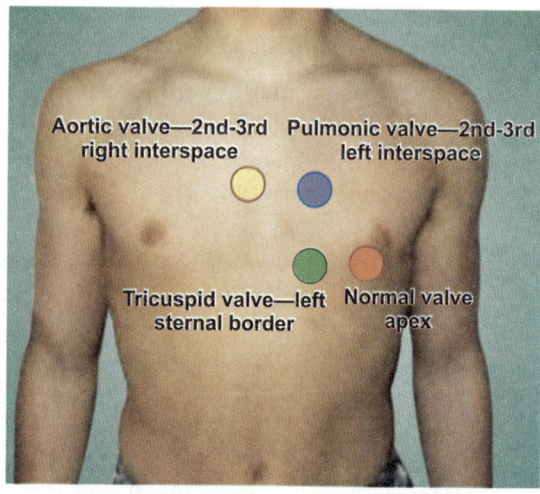

Fig. 1.21: Sites of auscultation

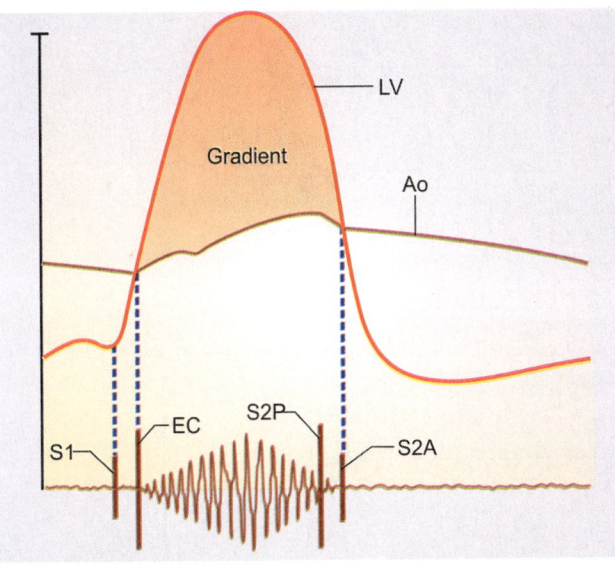

Fig. 1.22: Different parameters in aortic stenosis

c. *Pulmonary component (P₁)*—may be accentuated due to secondary pulmonary hypertension.

d. *Paradoxical splitting occurs*—due to late closure of A_2 secondary to prolonged systolic murmur.

III. Ejection systolic click:
1. It occurs in children and young adult with pliable aortic valve. It is absent in elderly person with calcific aortic stenosis.
2. This sound occurs 40–60 milliseconds after the onset of S1.
3. This may be transmitted occasionally to apex, making confusion with split S1.

IV. Fourth heart sound (S4): It can be headed due to forceful left atrial contraction into hypertrophied left ventricle in young patient, if signifies significant aortic stenosis.

V. Systolic murmur (Fig. 1.22):
i. It is crescendo–decrescendo systolic murmur—heard shortly after 1st heart sound.
ii. Intensity increases in mid-systole and ends just before 2nd heart sound.
iii. Character—rough, low-pitched sound—best heard in right 2nd intercostal space near right sternal border.
iv. It radiates to one or both carotid arteries.
v. In elderly person with calcific aortic stenosis, murmur may be prominent at the apex, because of radiation of high frequency components (Gallavardin phenomenon). This can be mis-diagnosed as murmur of mitral regurgitation.

Severity of stenosis can be determined by:
i. *Duration of murmur*—longer the duration of murmur—more severe will be the stenosis.
ii. *The peak of murmur* is towards end systole.

Variation of murmur can be altered by:
1. Murmur of valvular stenosis is augmented by—squatting and premature beat.
2. Murmur intensity can be reduced by—Valsalva maneuver.

In case of left ventricular failure:
i. Murmur of aortic stenosis becomes softer and barely audible.
ii. Atrial fibrillation with shorter R–R intervals decreases the murmur intensity.

Rare Presentation

1. Right ventricular failure, systemic venous congestion, hepatomegaly, pedal edema—due to bulging of inter-ventricular septum into right ventricle.
2. High-pitched diastolic blowing murmur—signifies there is associated aortic regurgitation.

Workup of Aortic Stenosis

Electrocardiography *(Fig. 1.23)*

i. Evidence of left ventricular hypertrophy
ii. Evidence of left atrial hypertrophy.
iii. Left axis deviation.
vi. Left atrial hypertrophy.
v. Conduction abnormalities due to calcification of conducting tissues (1st degree heart block, left bundle branch block).

Chest Radiography *(Fig. 1.24)*

i. Cardiac silhouette may be boot-shaped because of concentric left ventricular hypertrophy.
ii. Cardiomegaly:
  a. If there is left ventricular dysfunction
  b. If associated aortic regurgitation
iii. Valvular calcification or aortic root calcification in severe age-related calcific aortic stenosis
iv. Post-stenotic dilatation of aorta may be seen.

A. In older children and young adult:
Due to turbulent blood flow
↓
Post-stenotic dilatation of aorta
↓

Prominent ascending aorta (1): (2)Left ventricular heart configuration, which may be due to:
i. Normal-sized or enlarged left ventricle.
ii. Concentric hypertrophy of left ventricle producing relatively small left ventricular chamber with thick walls.

B. In adults more than 30 years:
Due to turbulent blood flow
↓
Post-stenotic dilatation of aorta
↓

Prominent ascending aorta (1); (2) Calcification of aortic valve (best seen in right anterior oblique view)—it indicates:
a. In females, hemodynamically significant aortic stenosis.
b. A gradient across the aortic valve >50 mmHg.
Calcification begins in bicuspid and rheumatic valv 4th decade but not until >65 years in tricuspid valve.

Echocardiography

Indications (ACC/AHA guideline):
1. Diagnosis and assessment of severity of aortic stenosis.

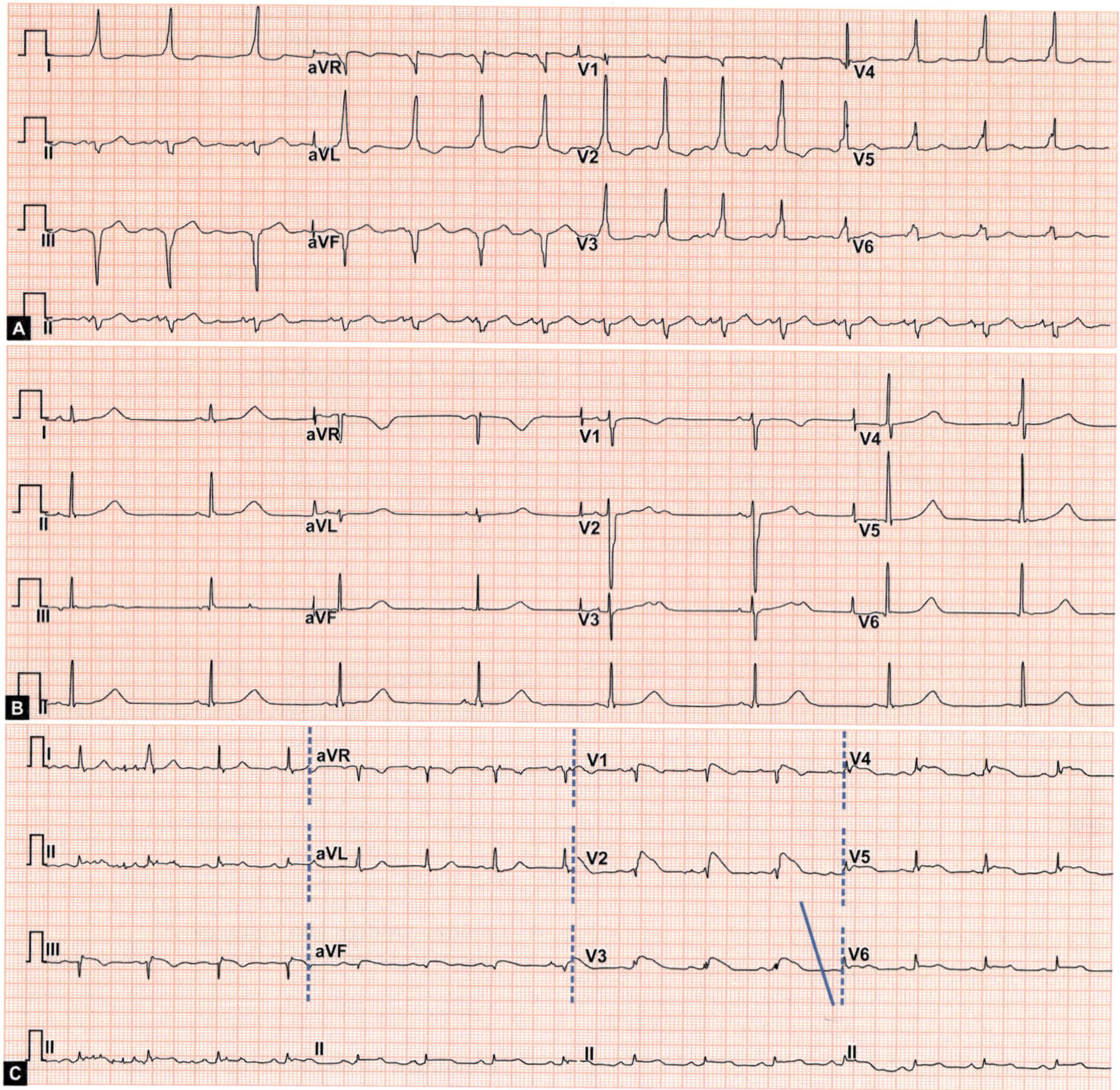

Fig. 1.23: ECG in aortic stenosis

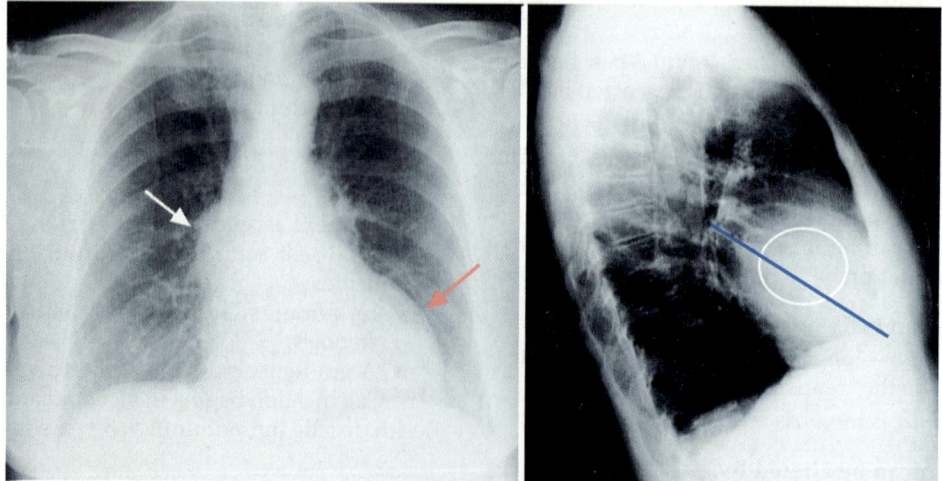

Fig. 1.24: White arrow indicates isolated enlargement or ascending or ascending aorta. Red arrow indicates left ventricular enlargement. In lateral view on right: Calcification in the region of aortic valve leaflets (circle). Aortic valve lies above a line drawn from the carinum to the junction of the diaphragm with the anterior chest wall.

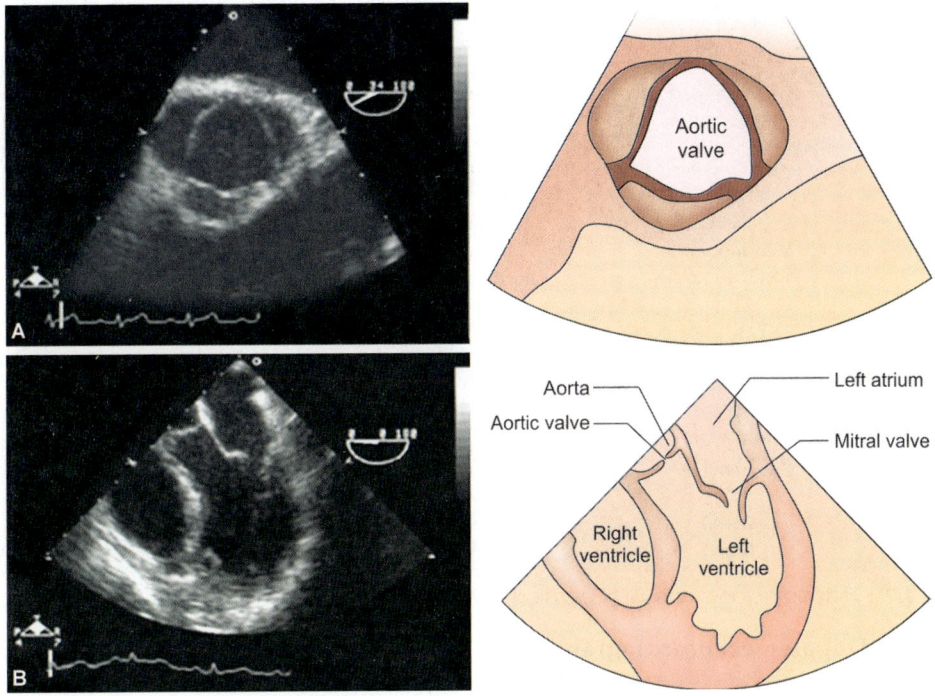

Fig. 1.25: Evidence of aortic stenosis in echocardiography

2. Assessment of left ventricular size, function and/or hemodynamics.
3. Reevaluation of patients with known aortic stenosis with changing symptoms and signs.
4. Assessment of changes is hemodynamic severity and ventricular function in patients with known aortic stenosis in pregnancy.
5. Reevaluation of asymptomatic patient with severe aortic stenosis.
6. Reevaluation of asymptomatic patients with mild to moderate aortic stenosis and evidence of left ventricular hypertrophy and dysfunction.

Echocardiographic findings (Fig. 1.25):
1. Thickened and calcified aortic valve with multiple dense cusp echoes throughout cardiac cycle (right > non-coronary > left coronary cusp).
2. Decreased separation of leaflets in systole with reduced opening orifice (13–14 mm = mild AS, 8–12 mm = moderate AS, <8 mm = severe AS).
3. ± doming in systole.
4. Dilated aortic root.
5. Increased thickness of left ventricular wall (= concentric left ventricular hypertrophy).
6. Hyperdynamic contraction of left ventricle (in compensated state).
7. Decreased mitral EF slope.
8. Left atrial enlargement.
9. Increased aortic valve gradient.
10. Decreased aortic valve area.

Following three echocardiographic findings are indicative of severe aortic stenosis (Figs 1.26 and 1.27).
1. Echo-dense aortic valve with no—cusp motion (may be unreliable in congenital or rheumatic valvular stenosis)

2. A decrease in the maximal aortic cusp separation (<8 mm in the adult)
3. Presence of otherwise left ventricular hypertrophy

Doppler Echocardiography

Xcellent tool for assessing the severity of aortic stenosis.

Criteria for determining severity of aortic stenosis

Severity	Mean gradient (mmHg)	Aortic valve area (cm²)
Mild	<25	>1.5
Moderate	25–40	1–1.5
Severe	>40	<1
Critical	>80	<0.5

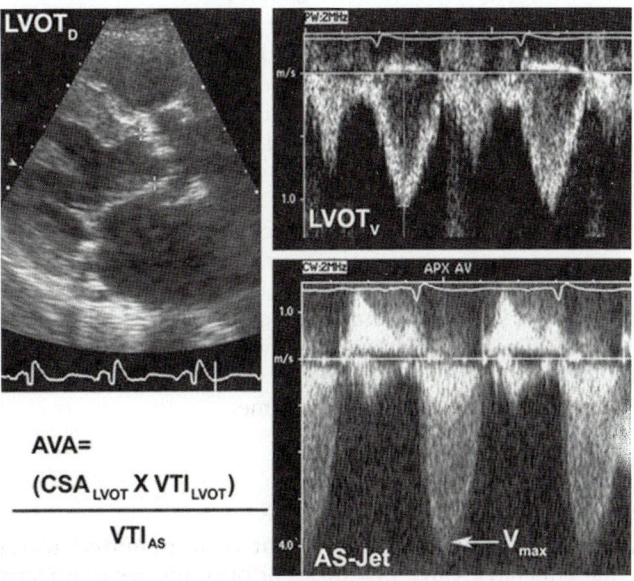

$$AVA = \frac{(CSA_{LVOT} \times VTI_{LVOT})}{VTI_{AS}}$$

Fig. 1.26: Echocardiographic findings in aortic stenosis

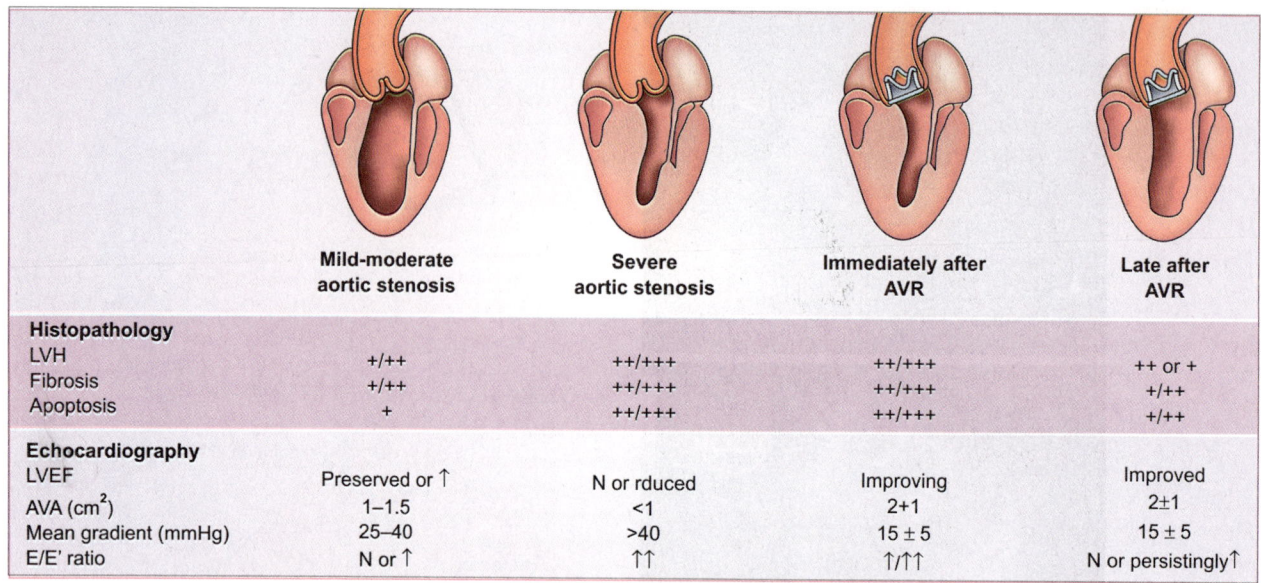

	Mild-moderate aortic stenosis	Severe aortic stenosis	Immediately after AVR	Late after AVR
Histopathology				
LVH	+/++	++/+++	++/+++	++ or +
Fibrosis	+/++	++/+++	++/+++	+/++
Apoptosis	+	++/+++	++/+++	+/++
Echocardiography				
LVEF	Preserved or ↑	N or rduced	Improving	Improved
AVA (cm^2)	1–1.5	<1	2+1	2±1
Mean gradient (mmHg)	25–40	>40	15 ± 5	15 ± 5
E/E' ratio	N or ↑	↑↑	↑/↑↑	N or persistingly↑

Fig. 1.27: Histopathologic and echocardiographic findings in different stages of aortic stenosis

Major limitation of Doppler echocardiography in assessing severity of stenosis.

Underestimation of gradient, if the beam is not parallel to the aortic stenosis velocity yet.

Overestimation of severity of aortic stenosis in following conditions:

1. Severe anemia (hemoglobin <8 gm/dl)
2. Small aortic root
3. Sequential stenosis in parallel (coexistent with left ventricular outflow tract and valvular obstruction)

Cardiac catheterization and coronary angiography

Indications:

1. Coronary angiography before aortic valve replacement, in patient with risk of IHD.
2. Assessment of severity of aortic stenosis in symptomatic patient who need aortic valve replacement.
3. Before valve replacement in patients whose coronary artery origin cannot be identified by non-invasive procedure.

Radionucleotide Ventriculography

To evaluate:

i. Myocardial perfusion at rest and during exertion.
ii. Left ventricular function—including:
   • Left ventricular ejection fraction
   • End-systolic volume • End-diastolic volume

B Type Natriuretic Peptide

i. Provide incremental prognostic information in predicting symptom onset in asymptomatic patient with severe aortic stenosis.
ii. Steady rising BNP may predict need for valve replacement in a symptomatic patient with severe aortic stenosis.
iii. Preoperative BNP provides prognostic information regarding postoperative outcome.

Therapy

Medical Therapy

1. **Antibiotic prophylaxis** is not recommended unless patients have valve prosthesis or prior history of infective endocarditis.

2. **In asymptomatic patient**—therapy is directed at prevention or coronary artery disease, maintenance of sinus rhythm and blood pressure control.

3. **In symptomatic patient:** Heart failure can be treated by relieving pulmonary congestion by:
   a. *Diuretics*—it can cause hypotension and hypvolemia.
   b. *Nitrate*—can cause cerebral hypoperfusion and syncope so it should be avoided or to be used with caution.
   c. *Digoxin* to control rate in case of atrial fibrillation
   d. *Moist oxygen inhalation*
   e. *Cardiac and oxymetry monitoring*
   f. *Morphine*—as needed and tolerated

4. **In patient with angina pectoris:**
   a. *Oxygen*
   b. *Morphine*
   c. *Nitrates*—cautiously
   d. *Cardiac and oxymetry monitoring*

Percutaneous Balloon Valvuloplasty

Valvuloplasty can be considered in cases of severe heart failure or cardiogenic shock in following patients:

1. Patients with other comorbid conditions with very short life expectancy.
2. Patient who refuses surgery
3. Patients with heart failure who need an urgent, major non-cardiac surgical procedure.
4. Pregnant patient with critical aortic stenosis.

Complications:

1. In critically ill patients—mortality 3–7%
2. Perforation
3. Myocardial infarction
4. Aortic regurgitation
5. In children, adolescents, young adult—mortality 1%
6. Restenosis—in patient with unicuspid aortic valves.

Median survival rate 3 years.

Aortic Valve Replacement

Indications for aortic valve replacement:
1. Symptomatic patients with severe aortic stenosis
2. Patients with severe aortic stenosis undergoing CABG
3. Patient with severe aortic stenosis undergoing surgery on the aorta or other heart valves
4. Patient with severe aortic stenosis and LVSD (ejection fraction (0.50)
5. Patient with aortic stenosis (moderate) undergoing CABG or surgery on the aorta or other heart valves.
6. Patient with mild aortic stenosis undergoing CABG when there is evidence that progression may be rapid, such as moderate to severe valve calcification.

Class I and II AHA/ACC Recommendation for Choice of Prosthetic Valve

Recommendations for valve replacement with mechanical prosthesis:

1. Patient with expected long lifespan	= class I
2. Patient with a mechanical valve already in place in a different position than the valve being replaced.	= class I
3. Patient with renal failure on hemodialysis or with hypercalcemia	= class II
4. Patient requiring anticoagulation due to risk factors for thromboembolism	= class IIa
5. Patients >65 years for AVR and <70 years for MVR	= class IIa

Recommendation for valve replacement with a bioprosthesis:

1. Patient who cannot and will not take warfarin treatment	= I
2. Patient >65 years needing AVR with no risk factors for thromboembolism	= I
3. Patients considered to have possible compliance problems with warfarin	= IIa

4. Patient >70 years needing MVR with no risk factors for thromboembolism	= IIa
5. Valve replacement for thrombosed mechanical valve	= IIb

Prosthetic Heart Valves

Types:
1. Mechanical:
   i. Ball and cage (Starr-Edwards)
   ii. Tilting disc (single leaflet—Medtronic-Hall, Bjork-Shiley, bileaflet—St. Jude Medical)
2. Bioprosthetic—porcine or bovine (carpentier-Edwards)
3. Homograft—preserved human valve

Mechanical valve:
1. Very durable >20 years
2. Thrombogenic—requiring lifelong warfarin therapy
3. Ball and cage is early model:
   i. Very durable
   ii. Very thrombogenic, requiring more intensive anti-coagulation
4. Tilting disc:
   i. Less thrombogenic—bileaflet is lesser thrombogenic than single thrombogenic

Tissue valve:
1. Not requiring long-term anticoagulation
2. Not as durable as mechanical valve
3. Mechanical valves tend to be placed in younger patients, bioprosthesis tends to be placed in older patients.

Assessment of Prosthetic Valve Function

1. **Clinically:** Each prosthetic valve has distinct sound. If there is new sound or change in sound character or volume, or arise of new murmur.
2. **Imaging:**
   a. *Fluoroscopy*—used to assess valve leaflet movement:
      i. Diminished motion—thrombosis
      ii. Excessive movement—dehiscence of valve

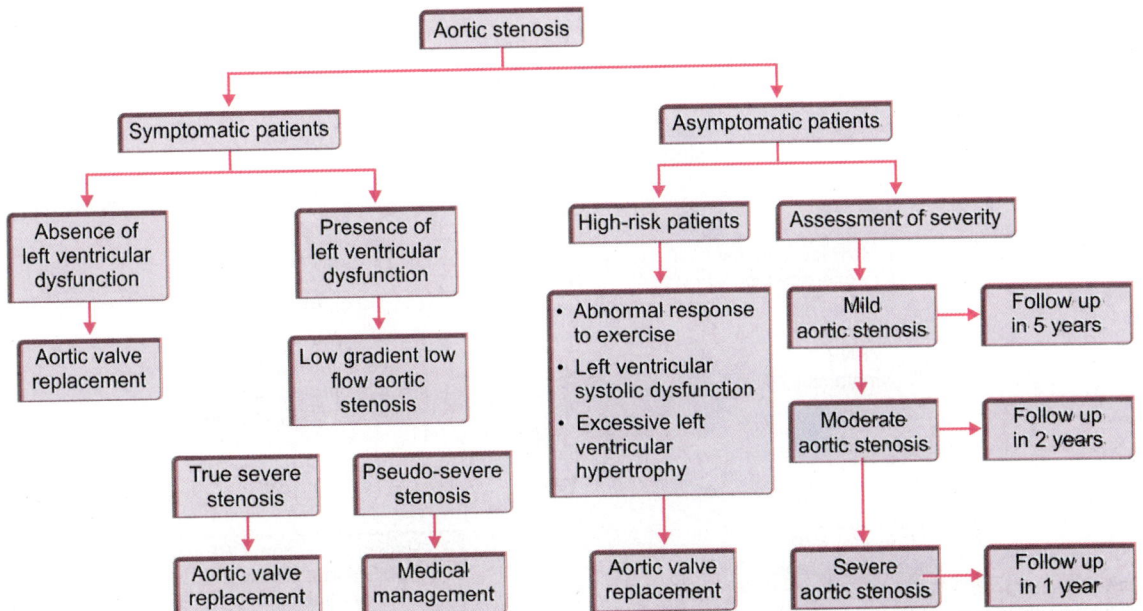

Fig. 1.28: Treatment algorithm in aortic stenosis

b. *Transthoracic echocardiography*—can be used to look at valve ring motion (mechanical valve), leaflet motion (tissue valve).

c. *Transesophageal echocardiography:* Useful for assessing mitral valve prosthesis.

d. *MRI* is safe for modern mechanical valves.

3. Cardiac catheterization: It can assess valve gradient and valve area.

Complication of heart valves:

a. Valve thrombosis   b. Embolization

c. Hemolysis   d. Endocarditis

Risk Factors for Late Death after Aortic Valve Replacement

1. High preoperative NYHA class
2. Left ventricular systolic dysfunction
3. Preoperative ventricular arrhythmias
4. Concomitant aortic regurgitation
5. Atrial fibrillation
6. CAD

Algorithm of management of aortic stenosis (Figs 1.28 to 1.31).

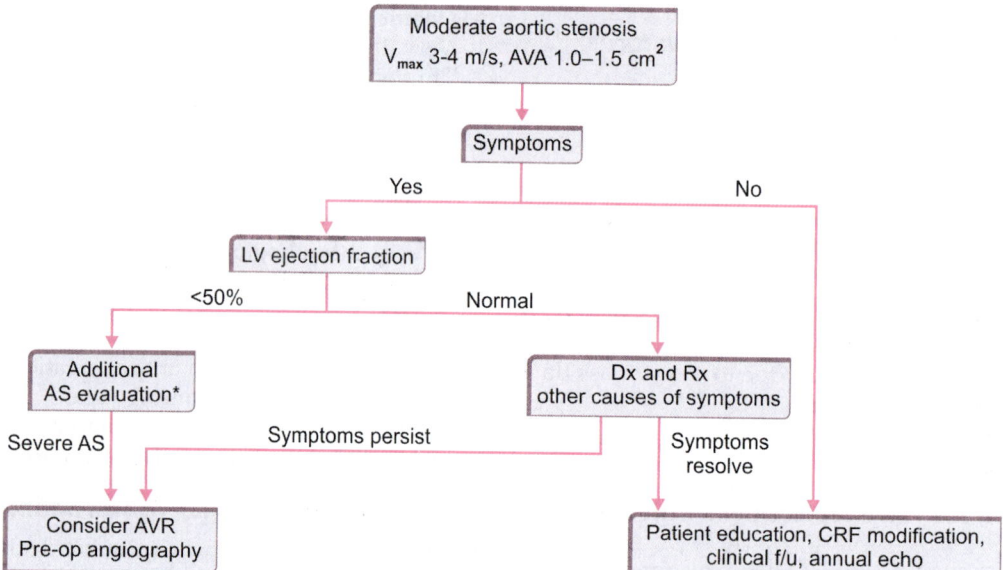

Fig. 1.29: Diagnostic algorithm in moderate aortic stenosis

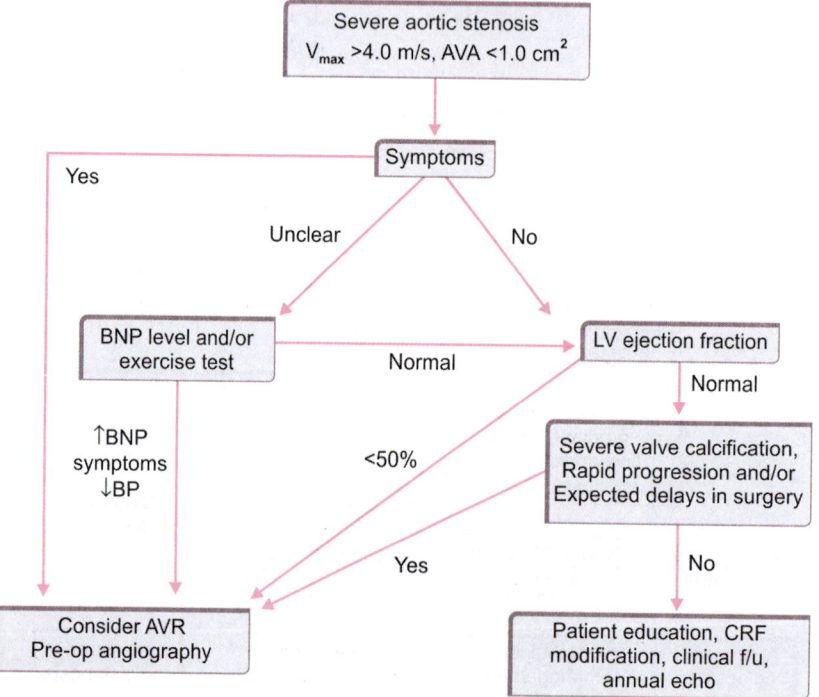

Fig. 1.30: Diagnostic algorithm in severe aortic stenosis

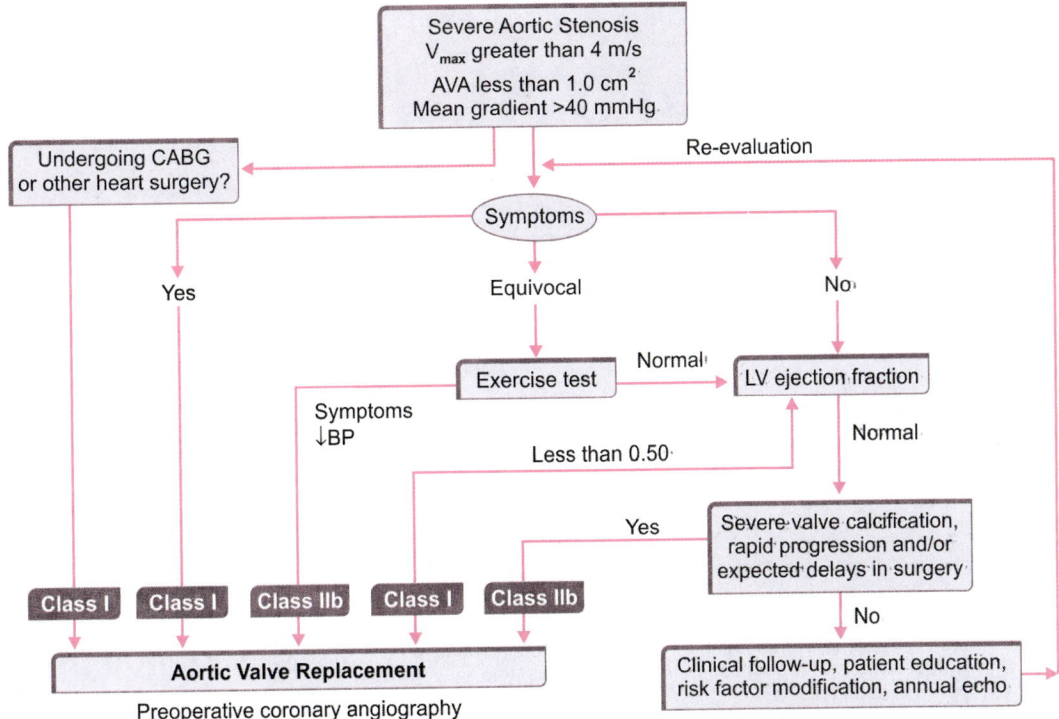

Fig. 1.31: Treatment algorithm in severe aortic stenosis

AORTIC REGURGITATION

Key Points to Diagnosis
1. **Symptoms:** Long asymptomatic period followed by evidence of heart failure symptoms.
2. **Peripheral signs:** (i) Wide pulse pressure, (ii) Taube sound and Duroziez signs. Quincke's sign.
3. Early diastolic decrescendo murmur at left sternal border.
4. **Chest X-ray:** Left ventricular dilatation and hypertrophy with preserved function of left ventricular function.
5. **Diagnosis** confirmed by Doppler echocardiography.
6. **Surgery is indicated** for symptoms, EF <55%, left ventricular end-systolic dimension >5–5.5 cm.

Etiology (Fig. 1.32)

I. Valvular:
   i. Congenital bicuspid aortic valve leaflet
   ii. Endocarditis
   iii. Rheumatic fever
   iv. Myxomatous (prolapsed) degeneration of aortic valve leaflet
   v. Traumatic
   vi. Syphilis
   vii. Ankylosing spondylosis.

II. Root disease:
   i. Aortic dissection
   ii. Cystic medial necrosis/degeneration:
      a. Turner syndrome
      b. Marfan syndrome
      c. Bicuspid aortic valve
      d. Osteogenesis imperfecta
   iii. Aortitis
   iv. Severe hypertension

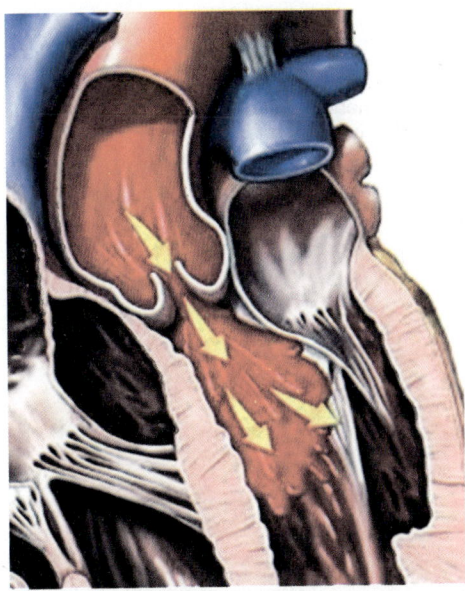

Fig. 1.32: Flow of blood in aortic regurgitation

Hemodynamics (Fig. 1.33)

In case of mitral regurgitation, left ventricular stroke volume is delivered into low pressure zone—left atrium, but **in case of aortic regurgitation,** left ventricular stroke volume is delivered into high pressure zone—aorta; so end-diastolic volume will be increased in aortic regurgitation—this is major hemodynamic compensation in AR (Flowchart 1.3).

In case of severe aortic regurgitation (Fig. 1.34), left ventricular EF slope will be normal with normal stroke volume together with increased LV end-diastolic pressure and volume.

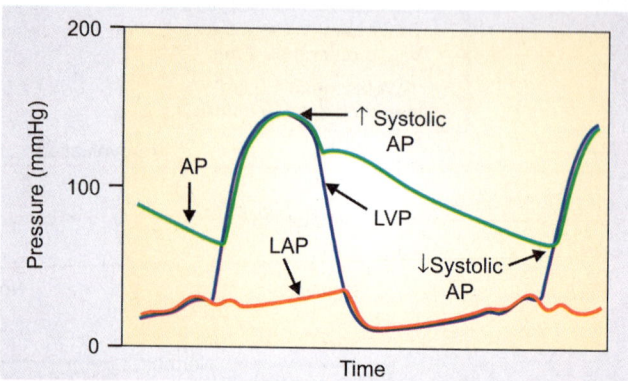

Fig. 1.33: Aortic valve regurgitation: During ventricular relaxation, blood flows backwards from aorta into the ventricle. Aortic systolic pressure increases, aortic diastolic pressure decreases, and pulse pressure increases; LAP increases (LAP, left atrial pressure; LVP, left ventricular pressure; AP, aortic pressure)

Flowchart 1.3: Hemodynamics and signs in AR

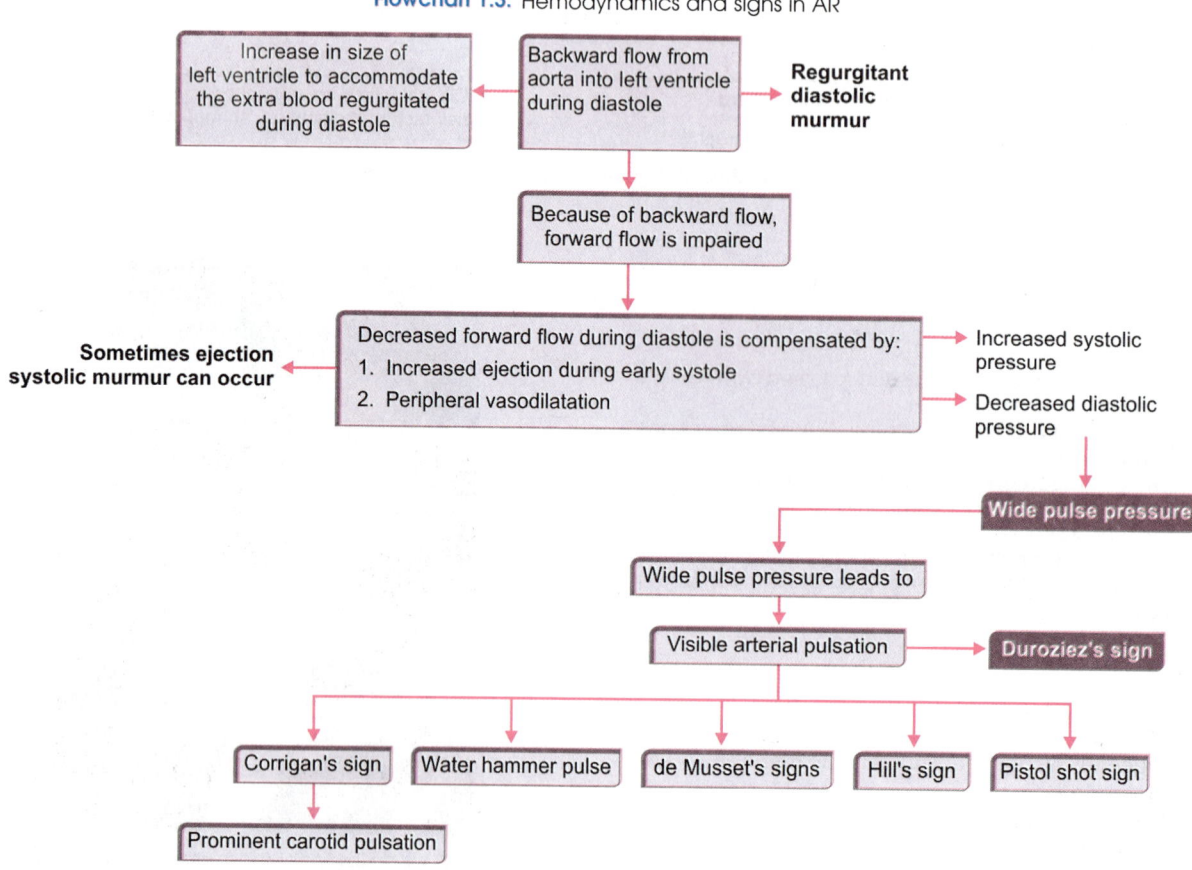

An LV function deteriorates—forward stroke volume diminishes and EF declines. As a result, LA pressure, PA pressure and wedge pressure are increased producing pulmonary congestion.

In case of chronic aortic regurgitation
↓
Forward cardiac output normal at rest but fails to rise during exercise
↓

There is reduction EF slope
↓
There is considerable increase in left atrial pressure
↓
Increase in pulmonary artery wedge pressure
↓
Pulmonary artery pressure will be increased
↓
Increase in right ventricular pressure

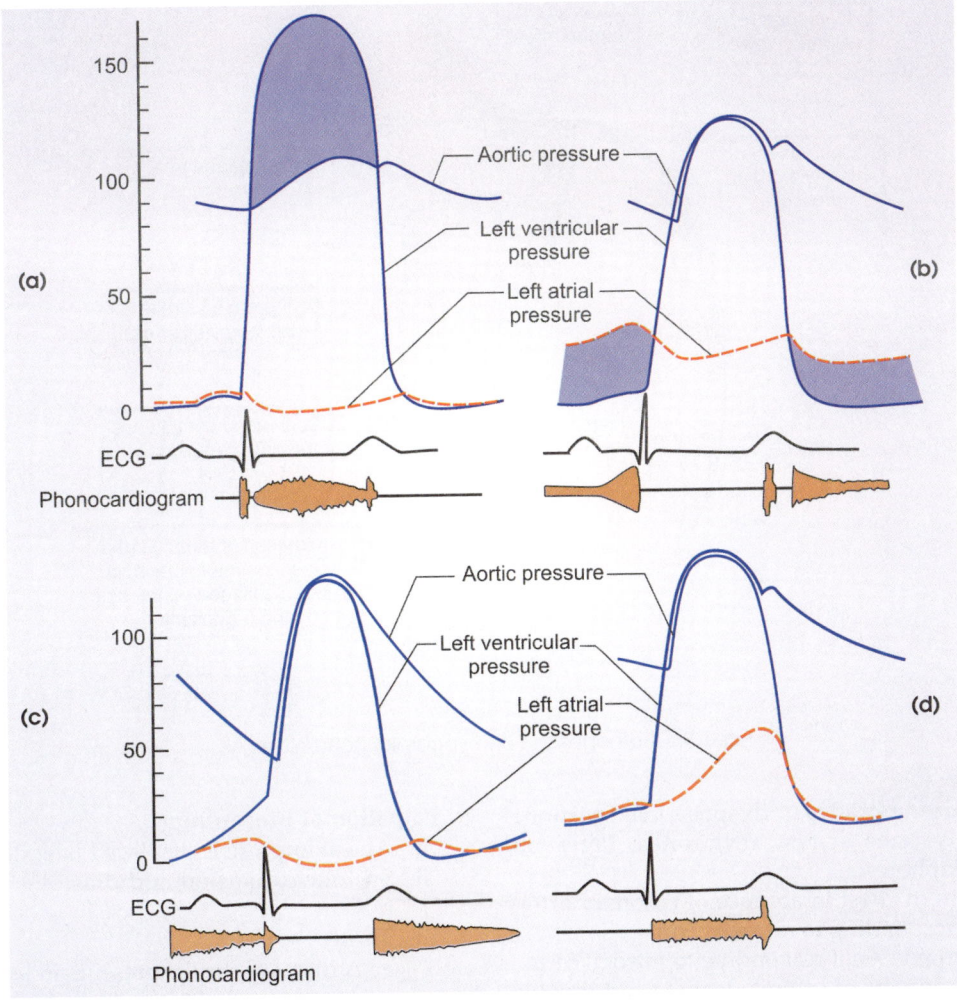

Fig. 1.34: (a) Aortic stenosis, (b) Mitral stenosis, (c) Aortic insufficiency, (d) Mitral insufficiency

So, in chronic aortic regurgitation:

Regurgitant volume of blood from aorta and the usual blood volume from left atrium during ventricular diastole produce cumulative rise in blood volume just before ventricular systole. As a result, both left ventricular force of contraction and stroke volume are increased, as—

Stroke volume = End-diastolic volume/end-systolic volume.

So, gradual rise in end-diastolic volume will lead to sarcomere replication, which in turn, will lead to hypertrophy of left ventricle. Later on, gradual left ventricular dilatation will occur. As, stroke volume is increased, pulse pressure will also increase, because

Pulse pressure = Stroke volume/aortic elasticity.

As a result, there will be wide pulse pressure, which will be responsible for peripheral signs of AR.

Myocardial Ischemia (Fig. 1.35)

In AR, myocardial oxygen requirement will be increased due to:

i. Left ventricular dilatation
ii. Left ventricular hypertrophy
iii. Elevated left ventricular systolic tension
iv. Compromised coronary blood flow.

Coronary blood flow occurs during diastole. But in AR— when arterial pressure will be low, **coronary perfusion will also be low**.

History

1. one-fourth of patients with predominant valvular AR are male. But in female, AR is of mainly rheumatic associated with MS.
2. History of infective endocarditis may be present in patients with rheumatic or congenital involvement of AR.
3. **Acute AR** may occur in:
   i. Infective endocarditis
   ii. Aortic dissection
   iii. Trauma.
   Patient may present with cough, dyspnea, orthopnea o PND or cardiogenic shock.
4. In case of **chronic AR:**
   i. Patient may be asymptomatic for 10–15 years.
   ii. Uncomfortable awareness of own heart beat specially on lying down position—may be early complaint.
   iii. Sinus tachycardia during exertion or emotion or premature ventricular contraction may be evidenced by uncomfortable palpitations and head pounding.

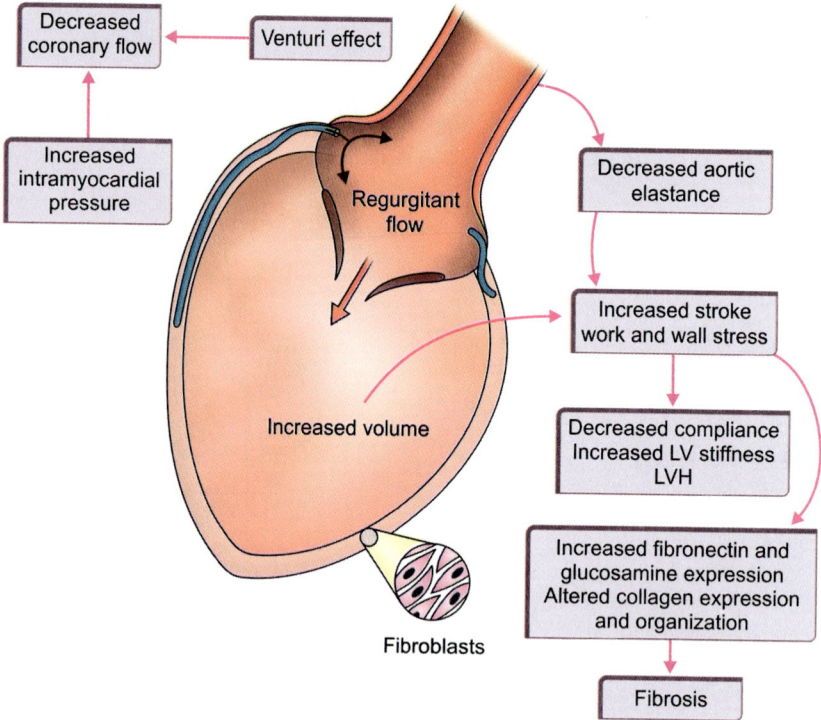

Fig. 1.35: Pathogenesis of myocardial ischemia in AR

iv. Later on varying grades of dyspnea like exertional dyspnea, dyspnea at rest, orthopnea, PND and excessive diaphoresis.

v. Anginal pain in chest in absence of coronary artery disease not responding to nitroglycerin.

vi. Nocturnal angina—not responding to nitroglycerin.

vii. Systemic symptoms of (ectopia lentis) heart involvement—ankle edema, right upper abdominal pain

Physical Signs

General Sign

1. Jarring of entire body and bobbing motion of the head with each heart beat.
2. Visible abrupt collapse of peripheral arteries.
3. Non-cardiac features of Marfan's syndrome (ectopia lentis) ankylosing spondylitis (skeletal features).
4. **Arterial pulse**
   i. Water hammer pulse—collapsing pulse (Corrigan pulse)
   ii. Capillary pulsation—alternate flushing and blanching of skin at the root of nail bed when pressure is applied to the tip of the nail bed (Quineke's pulse).
   iii. Booming pistol shot sound—over femoral arteries (Traube's sign).
   iv. To and fro murmur audible over femoral artery when pressure is applied over femoral artery with diaphragm of stethoscope (Duroziez's sign).
   v. Pulsus bisferiens—due to combined AR and AS.
5. **Blood pressure**
   i. Widened pulse pressure—due to both systolic hypertension and diastolic collapse
   ii. Systolic sounds are frequently heard while cuff is completely deflated.
   iii. In acute AR, slight widening of pulse pressure.

6. **Palpation of precordium**
   i. Apical impulse is displaced laterally and inferiorly.
   ii. Systolic expansion and diastolic retraction are prominent.
   iii. Thrill
      a. A diastolic thrill—presents in left sternal border
      b. A systolic thrill may be palpable in suprasternal notch with transmission along the carotid—it may be due to function AS or rheumatic AS.
7. **Auscultation**
   i. Heart sound:
      a. S1—may be diminished due to
         • Prolonged PR interval
         • Left ventricular dysfunction
         • Preclosure of mitral valve
      b. S2—A1 is soft or inaudible
         P2 is obscured by diastolic murmur
      c. S3—heard in presence of severe left ventricular dysfunction.
      d. S4—often heard—represents—left atrial contraction into poorly compliant LV.
   ii. Murmur (Fig. 1.36):
      Diastolic murmur: Blowing decrescendo murmur starts immediately after A2—best heard in the left upper sternal border in sitting posture and leaning forward in full expiration.

Variability of Duration of Murmur

i. **Early in course of disease**—murmur is typically short
ii. **As the disease progresses**—murmur becomes pandiastolic.
iii. **Late in the disease**—murmur will be shortened due to:
   a. Elevated left ventricular end-diastolic pressure
   b. Rapid equilibration of pressure in the aorta.

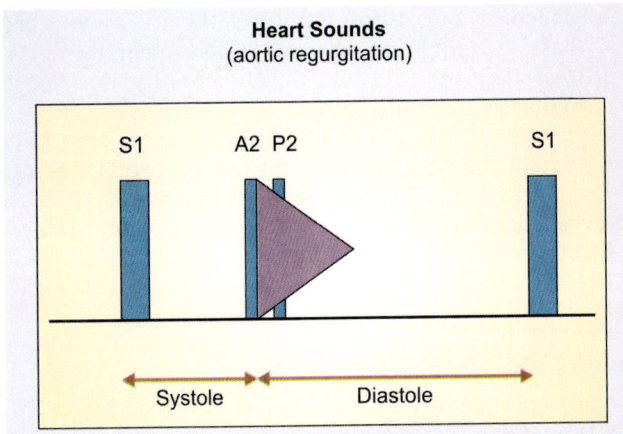

Fig. 1.36: Heart sounds in AR

Severity of aortic regurgitation depends upon duration of murmur not the intensity of murmur:

a. *Mid to late diastolic murmur:* It is audible at the apex in severe AR. This is caused by vibration of anterior leaflet of mitral valve struck by regurgitant jet in AR or by turbulence in mitral inflow from partial closure of mitral valve—this is **Austin Flint murmur.**

b. *Mid-systolic ejection murmur:* Audible at the base of heart radiating to neck—radiating to carotid arteries. It reflects:
  i. Increased ejection rate
  ii. Large stroke volume traversing aortic valve

c. *Sometimes aortic diastolic murmur* heard on right border of sternum—suggests aneurysmal dilatation of aortic root.

d. *Cooning or musical diastolic murmur*—suggests eversion of aortic cusp vibrating in an aneurysmal stream.

Acute aortic regurgitation: It is hemodynamically completely different and more severe from chronic AR. Acute AR produces more severe hemodynamic compromise—producing following signs and symptom:
  i. Hypotension
  ii. Pallor
  iii. Tachycardia
  iv. Cyanosis
  v. Diaphoresis
  vi. Cool extremities and
  vii. Pulmonary congestion

Peripheral Examination

1. Sign of hyperdynamic circulation is absent.
2. Heart size is normal.
3. Point of maximum intensity of apex beat is not displaced laterally.

Heart Sounds

1. S1 is diminished due to preclosure of mitral valve.
2. Increased P2 due to pulmonary hypertension.
3. S3—may be due to left ventricular dysfunction.

Murmur

1. Early diastolic murmur—shorter and lower in pitch.
2. In severe aortic regurgitation, murmur may not be audible.

Laboratory Abnormalities

A. **Hematological studies:**
  1. Complete blood count
  2. Prothrombin time
  3. APTT
  4. Electrolytes
  5. CPK-MB
  6. Cardiac troponin
  7. Lactate dehydrogenase
  8. Serological test to exclude rheumatological causes

B. **ECG:** Typical feature of chronic aortic regurgitation:
  1. Left ventricular hypertrophy with strain
  2. Left axis elevation
  3. Left atrial abnormality
  4. Conduction abnormalities

C. **Chest X-ray** (Fig. 1.37)
  In chronic aortic regurgitation:
  1. Cardiomegaly with displacement of apex inferiorly and leftward.
  2. In left anterior oblique view and lateral view—left ventricle displaced posteriorly and encroaching over spine.
  3. In case of primary disease of aortic root—primary dilatation of aortic root is seen and aorta may fill retrosternal space in lateral view.
  In acute aortic regurgitation:
  1. Minimal cardiac enlargement.
  2. Normal aortic root/arch.
  3. Increased pulmonary venous pattern.

D. **Echocardiogram** (Fig. 1.38):
  1. Left ventricular size is increased and myocardial function is normal until late stage, when decrease in EF slope and increased end-systolic dimension.
  2. Rapid high frequency diastolic fluttering of anterior mitral leaflet.
  3. Detection of cause:
      i. Dilatation of aortic root
      ii. Leaflet pathology
      iii. Aortic dissection

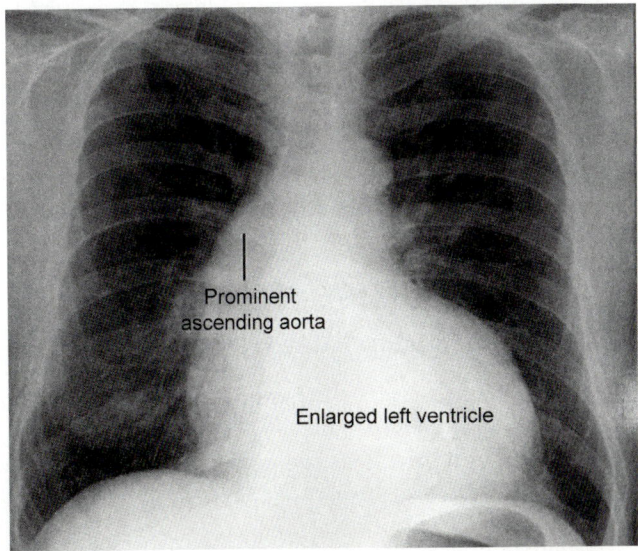

Fig. 1.37: Chest X-ray in AR

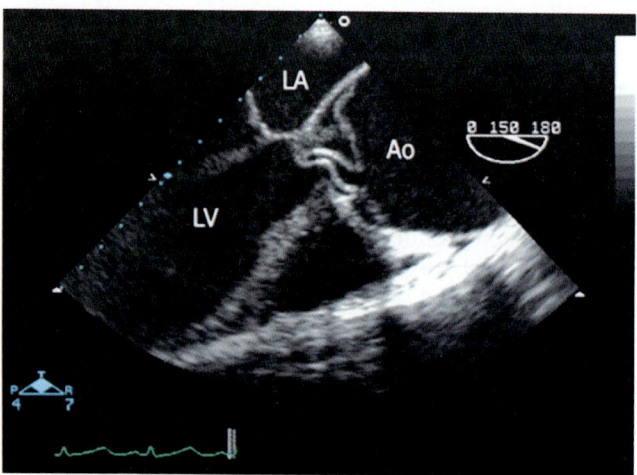

Fig. 1.38: Echocardiographic picture in AR

   vi. Aneurysm.
   v. Ectasia.
4. Aortic valve structure morphology—bileaflet, trileaflet, flail, thickening.
5. Presence of vegetations or nodules.
6. Regurgitant volume, fraction and orifice area.
7. Premature closure of mitral valve and opening of aortic valve (with severely elevated left ventricular end-diastolic pressure).
8. Ejection fraction and end-systolic dimension—surgery is recommended, if EF is ≤55% or end-systolic dimension ≥ 55 mm.

E. Doppler echocardiography (Fig. 1.39). Central jet width assessed by:
   i. Exceeds 65% of left ventricular out flow tract
   ii. Regurgitant volume is ≥60 ml/beat
   iii. Regurgitant fraction is >50%
   iv. Diastolic flow reversal in the proximal descending thoracic aorta.

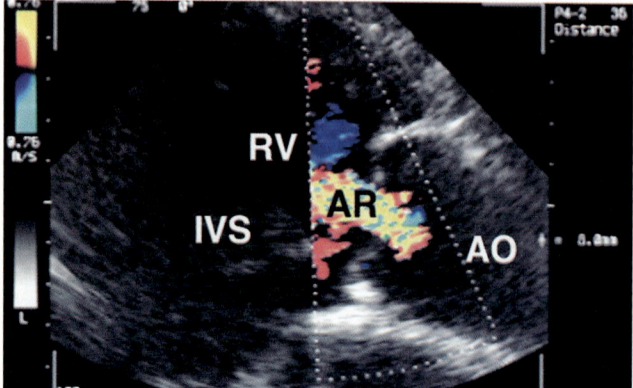

Fig. 1.39: Doppler echocardiography in AR

F. Radionuclide imaging: It detects the following:
1. AR regurgitant fraction
2. LV/RV stroke volume ratio. In absence of MR or TR, LV/RV ratio ≥2.5 denotes severe aortic regurgitation.

G. Aortic angiography: It can be performed during cardiac catheterization and provides the severity of AR. Grading is as follows:
1. *Mild (1+):* A small amount of contrast enters the LV during each diastole and clears with each systole.

2. *Moderate (2+):* Contrast enters the LV during each diastole, but LV chamber is less dense than the aorta.
3. *Moderately severe (3+):* LV chamber is equal in density to that of ascending aorta.
4. *Svere (4+):* Complete, dense opacification of left ventricular chamber occurs on the first beat and LV is more densely opacified than the ascending aorta.

   Surveillance by TTE is the cornerstone of follow-up of AR—in the form of:
   i. Detection of size of left ventricle
   ii. Detection of function of left ventricle

Medical Therapy in Chronic AR

A. Antihypertensive:
1. Vasodilator therapy is recommended in nonsurgical candidates with severe AR, who develop symptoms or LV dysfunction.
2. Vasodilator may be used as short-term therapy for improving hemodynamics in heart failure patient having left ventricular systolic dysfunction prior to aortic valve replacement.
3. In asymptomatic AR patient, long-term vasodilator therapy is recommended for those with normal LV systolic function.
4. Long-term vasodilator therapy is not recommended in asymptomatic patients with normal LV function by mild to moderate GNR.

The vasodilators are:
   i. ACE-I
   ii. Dihydropyridine
   iii. Calcium channel blocker
   iv. Hydralazine

When blood pressure is within target (systolic blood pressure <140 mmHg) in patient with AR, vasodilators are 1st line of choice.

Current guidelines regarding the vasodilator therapy:
1. Long-term treatment in patients with severe chronic AR and symptoms of left ventricular dysfunction but not the candidate for surgery.
2. It is reasonable for short-term therapy in patients in patients with severe left ventricular dysfunction and symptoms of heart failure in order to improve hemodynamic profile before surgery.
3. It is acceptable for long-term therapy in asymptomatic patients with severe AR and left ventricular dilatation with normal EF.

Under current guidelines, vasodilator therapy is not indicated for the following:
1. Long-term therapy in asymptomatic patients with less than severe AR and normal EF.
2. Long-term therapy in asymptomatic patients with LV dysfunction who are the candidates for surgery.
3. Long-term therapy in asymptomatic patients with severe LV dysfunction who are the candidates for surgery.

B. Treatment of cardiac arrhythmia—if present.
C. Treatment of infection is poorly tolerated in patient with severe AR, so it must be treated promptly and vigorously.
Indications for antibiotic prophylaxis:
1. Patients with prosthetic material in the heart like artificial valves.
2. Patients with prior infective endocarditis.

3. Following cardiac transplantation, have valve regurgitation due to abnormally structured valve.
4. Patients with congenital heart disease, who meet any of the following:
   a. Cyanotic CHD that have not been repaired or incompletely repaired.
   b. Repair of CHD with prosthetic material.
   c. Repaired CHD, but the patient is at risk for inhibited endothelialization.
D. **Patient with syphilitic aortitis** requires penicillin prophylaxis.
E. **In patient with Marfan syndrome**, beta blocker, ARBs, Losartan retards aortic root dilatation.
F. **Patient with severe aortic regurgitation, associated aortopathy**, should avoid isometric exercise.
G. **Beta-blockers** can lower hypertension in patient with AR

Surgical Treatment

To decide proper timing of treatment—**two points should be kept in mind:**
1. Patient with chronic severe AR becomes symptomatic after development of left ventricular dysfunction.
2. If treatment time will be delayed for >1 year after development of symptoms of left ventricular dysfunction, surgery will not restore the left ventricular function.
   Hence **6 monthly echocardiography** is necessary, if surgical treatment to be done at proper time, i.e. after the onset of LV dysfunction, but prior to development of symptoms (LVED—dimension <75 mm).

Indications of Surgical Treatment

Asymptomatic with severe aortic regurgitation and progressive left ventricular dysfunction defined by:
   i. Left ventricular ejection fraction <50%
  ii. Left ventricular end-systolic dimension >55 mm
 iii. Left ventricular end-systolic volume >55 ml/m^2
  iv. Left ventricular diastolic dimension >75 mm.
   A few circumstances in which the aortic valve surgery is reasonable:
1. Patient has moderate AR and is undergoing CABG or other surgery involving ascending aorta.
2. Patient with severe AR with no symptom, normal EF and less severe LV dilatation (LVESD >50 mm or LVEDD >70 mm), if this patient experiences:
   i. Progressive LV dilatation on serial imaging studies.
  ii. Deterioration of exercise tolerance.
 iii. Abnormal hemodynamic response to exercise.

Methods of Treatment

1. In case of AR due to rheumatic etiology—**valve replacement**
2. If valve leaflet is fenestrated due to infective endocarditis or form due to trauma—**primary surgical repair**
3. If AR is due to aneurysmal dilatation of root—or proximal ascending aorta—**narrowing the annulus or excision of a portion of aortic root.**

Types of valves:
1. *Mechanical valves:*
   i. More durable.
  ii. They require long-term anticoagulation.
 iii. They have increased risk of thrombosis.

2. *Bioprosthetic valves:*
   i. Avoid the need of anticoagulation.
  ii. They carry a greater risk of long-term deterioration and need for reoperation.
   Transcatheter aortic valve replacement has emerged as an important therapy for AS, but nowadays, it is being evaluated for patient of AR.

Postoperative mortality depends upon:
1. Time at which or stage at which operation is being carried out.
2. Condition of lest ventricle at the time of operation.

Prognosis

The prognosis for patients with severe AR depends on the presence or absence of LV dysfunction and symptoms. In asymptomatic patients with normal EF, the following has been found:
- Rate of progression to symptoms or LV dysfunction—less than 6% per year.
- Rate of progression to asymptomatic LV dysfunction—less than 3.5% per year.
- Rate of sudden death—less than 0.2% per year.

   In asymptomatic patients with decreased EF, the rate of progression to symptoms is greater than 25% per year, while in symptomatic patients, the mortality rate is over 10% per year.

Peripheral Signs of Aortic Regurgitation *(Fig. 1.40)*

A. **Pulse:**
   1. *Water hammer (collapsing) pulse:* Rapid upstroke followed by rapid descent.
   2. *Pulsus bisferiens:* This is characterized by two systolic peaks separated by distinct mid-systolic dip.
      Here percussion and tidal waves are equal or tidal wave is prominent.
B. **Blood pressure:**
   1. *Diastolic blood pressure* <40 mmHg: Pulse pressure >70 mmHg or ≥50% of systolic blood pressure
   2. *Hill sign:* Peak systolic pressure gradient between posterior tibial and radial arteries.
C. **Eye:**
   1. *Landolfi's sign:* Due to hyperemia of iris, there is contraction and dilatation of pupil in systole and diastole, respectively.
   2. *Becker's sign:* It is characterized by prominent retinal artery pulsation.
D. **Head and neck:**
   1. *De Musset's sign:* Synchronous nodding of head with heart beat.
   2. *Corrigan's sign:* Visible carotid pulsation (dancing carotid).
   3. *Muller's sign:* Pulsation of the uvula.
   4. *Minervini's sign:* Tongue depressor moves up and down when the tongue is lightly depressed.
   5. *Logue's sign:* It is the pulsation of sternoclavicular joint when AR is associated with aortic dissection.
E. **Upper limb:**
   1. *Locomotor brachialis:* Visible pulsation of the brachial artery.

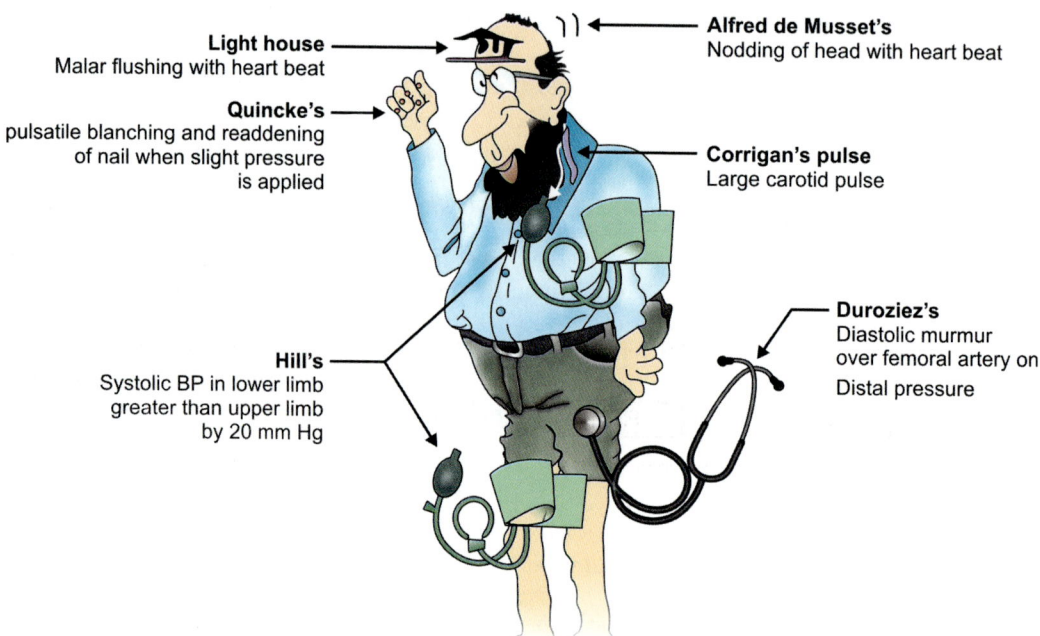

Fig. 1.40: Different signs in AR

2. *Quineke's pulse:* Visible capillary pulsation—alternate blanching and reddening in the nail bed can be visualized by transmitting light on patient's nail bed.
3. *Palfrey's sign:* Pistol shot sound heard over the radial artery.

F. Lower limb:
1. *Traube's sign:* Booming of systolic sound (pistol sound) heard over the femoral artery.
2. *Duroziez's sign:* Most specific of all peripheral signs of AR.
   Systolic murmur: Forward murmur perceived by pressing the femoral artery 2 cm above the stethoscope.
   Diastolic murmur: Backward murmur perceived by pressing femoral artery 2 cm below the stethoscope.

G. Abdomen:
1. *Rosenbach sign:* Pulsation in liver
2. *Gerhard's sign:* Pulsation in spleen
3. *Dennison's sign:* Pulsation in cervix in female.

MITRAL VALVE PROLAPSE

Synonym

Systolic click murmur syndrome, Barlow's syndrome, floppy valve syndrome, billowing mitral leaflet syndrome.

Pathophysiological Mechanism (Fig. 1.41)

Diverse pathologic mechanisms:
1. Excessive or redundant mitral leaflet tissue
2. Myxomatous degeneration of valve leaflets
3. Greatly increased concentration of certain glycos-aminoglycan

Prolapse can be caused by:
i. Papillary muscle dysfunction
ii. Elongated chordae tendineae
iii. Enlarged mitral annulus

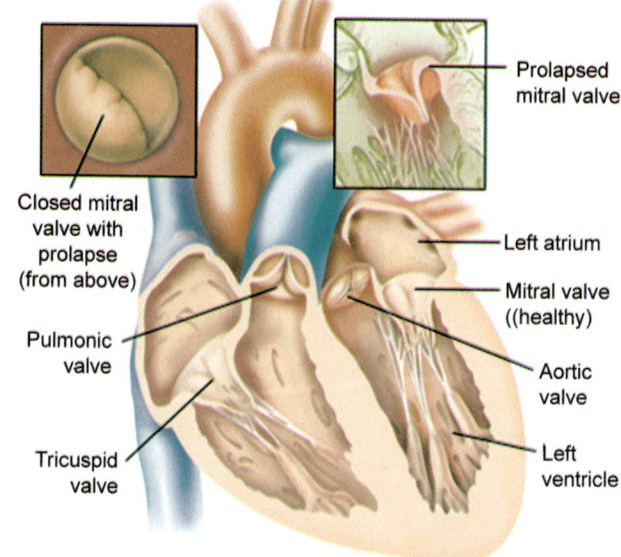

Fig. 1.41: Cross-section of heart showing prolapse of mitral valve

Mitral valve leaflet (usually posterior leaflet) porolapses into left atrium during ventricular systole.

Subclassification of mitral valve prolapse is given in Figs 1.42 and 1.43.

Etiology

1. Unknown
2. But it may be due to genetically determined collagen disorder here production of type III collagen has been increased.

Mitral valve prolapse is usually associated with congenital disorders.
i. Turner syndrome
ii. Ehlers-Danlos syndrome

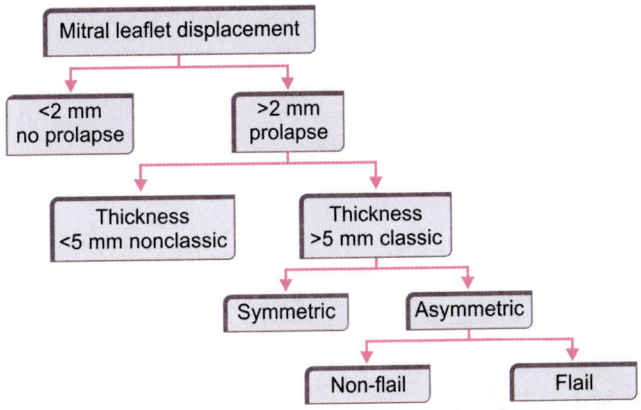

Fig. 1.42: Types of displacement of mitral valve

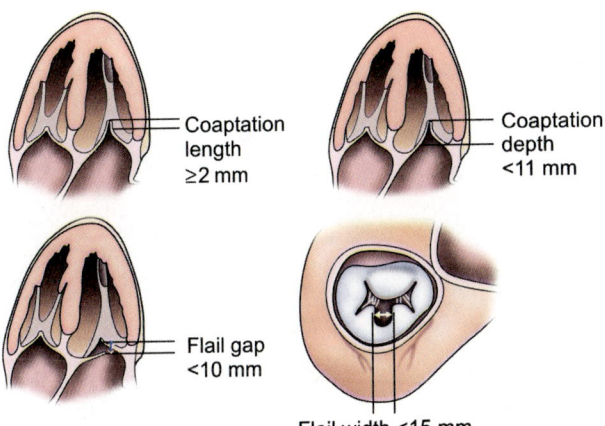

Fig. 1.43: Different measurements in mitral leaflets

iii. Thoracic skeletal deformities
iv. Straight back syndrome

MVP may occur:
  i. As a sequela of acute rheumatic fever
  ii. In ischemic heart disease
  iii. Various cardiomyopathies.
  iv. 20% patient with osteum secundum atrial septal defect.

Pathology

1. Myxomatous degeneration involves usually posterior leaflet of mitral valve.
2. Aortic and tricuspid valves may be involved.
3. Mitral valve annulus is dilated.

Epidemiology

1. Autosomal dominant with incomplete penetrance.
2. In age 15–30 years—females are mostly affected.
   In age >50 years—males are mostly affected and more severe, may require valve replacement.

Symptoms

1. Asymptomatic throughout the life
2. Palpitation, light headedness, syncope
3. Sudden death—it may be due to:
   a. Severe mitral regurgitation with depressed LV ejection fraction
   b. Flail leaflets

4. Chest pain—substernal, resemble angina pectoris
5. Cerebral ischemic attack secondary to emboli from mitral valve.

Auscultation

1. **Mid or late systolic click**—occurs 0.14 sec or move after S1—it occurs due to:
   a. Sudden tensing of slack of elongated chordae tendineae
   b. Prolapse of mitral valve—when it reaches maximum excursion
2. **Systolic click is followed by late systolic crescendo murmur (Fig. 1.44)**—which is occasionally whooping—heard best at the apex.

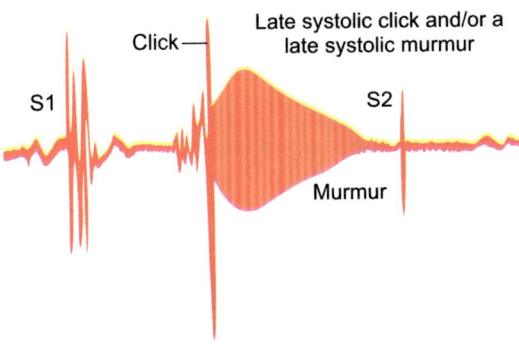

Fig. 1.44: Murmur with systolic click in mitral valve prolapse

3. **Murmur with click may be earlier** during:
   i. Standing
   ii. Strain phase of Valsalva maneuver
   iii. Any intervention that may decrease left ventricular volume (exposure to amyl nitrate) and propensity of mitral valve prolapsed
4. **Click and murmur will be delayed or may be absent during:**
   i. Squatting
   ii. Isometric exercise
   iii. Infusion of phenylephrine
   They increase LV size by decreasing venous returns, decrease contractility or increase systemic volume.
5. Sometimes murmur may be present without click or click may be present without murmur.

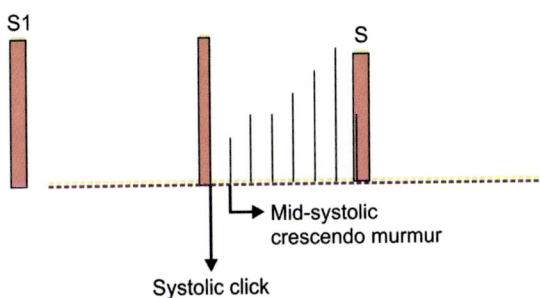

Laboratory Investigation

1. **ECG:**
   i. Inverted T in II, III, aVF
   ii. Supraventricular or ventricular premature beats
2. **Transthoracic echocardiography** (Fig. 1.45): Echocardiographic definition of MVP is systolic displacement of

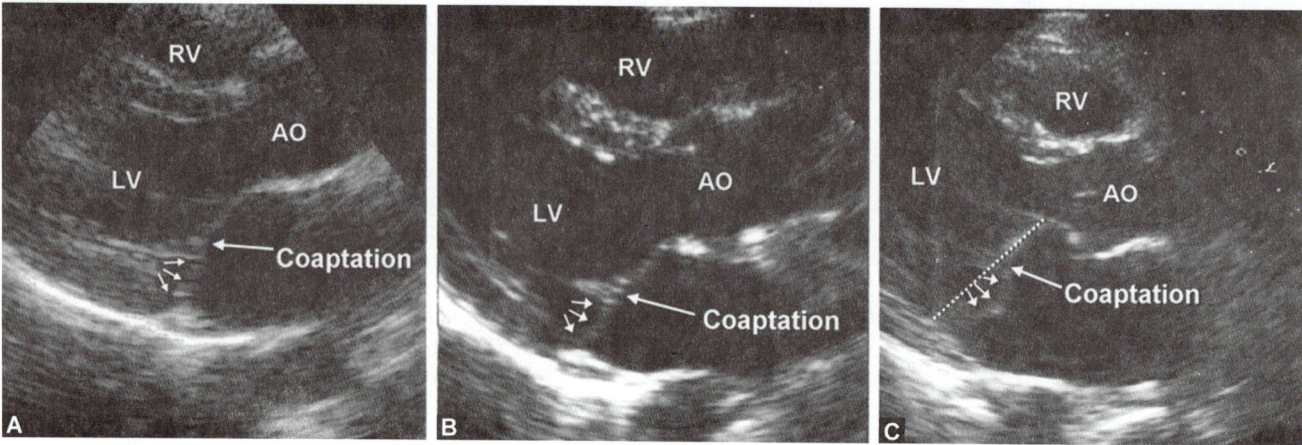

Fig. 1.45: Echocardiographic pictures in mitral valve prolapse

mitral valve leaflets by at least 2 mm into left atrium superior to the plane of mitral valve annulus.

3. **Doppler echocardiography** (Fig. 1.46)—estimate the severity of MR.
4. **Invasive ventriculography**—may show prolapse of posterior or sometimes both mitral valve leaflets.

Treatment (Fig. 1.47)

1. Prophylaxis of infective endocarditis in patient having past history of infective endocarditis.
2. Beta blockers prevent chest pain and palpitation.
3. Antiplatelet agents as aspirin should be given to patients with transient ischemic attack.
4. Warfarin—if atrial fibrillation supervenes.
5. If patient is symptomatic due to severe MR—valve repair or replacement.

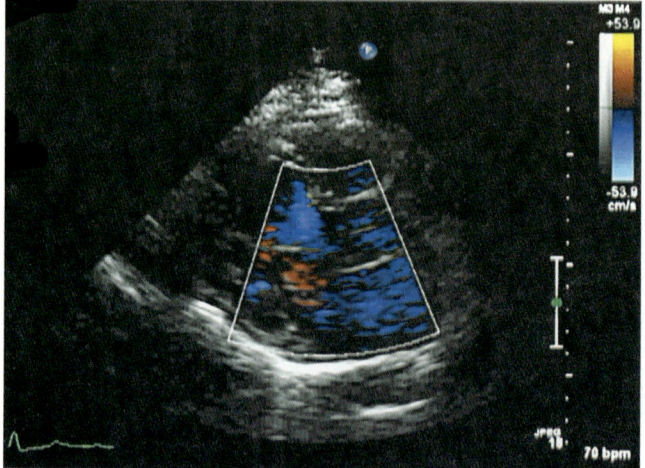

Fig. 1.46: Doppler echo to measure severity of MR

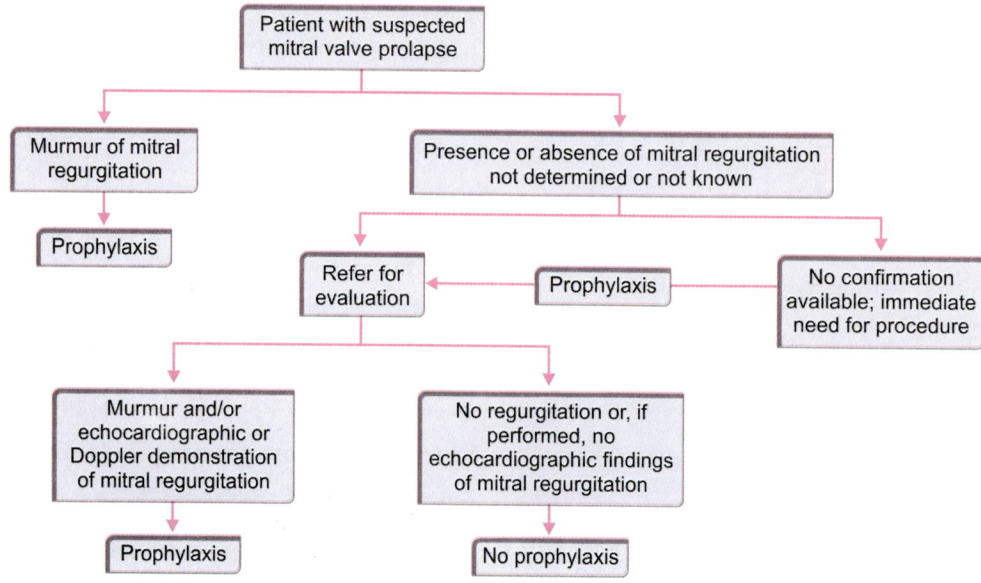

Fig. 1.47: Management algorithm in mitral valve prolapse

TRICUSPID REGURGITATION

Key points to diagnosis

1. Prominent 'v' wave in jugular venous pulse
2. Systolic murmur at lower left sternal border, that increases with inspiration.
3. Characteristic echocardiographic findings:
   i. Right ventricular volume overload:
      a. Right ventricular enlargement
      b. Paradoxical septal wall motion
      c. Diastolic fluttering of the interventricular septum.
   ii. Right atrial enlargement
4. Characteristics Doppler echocardiographic finding—systolic turbulence in the right atrium.

Etiologies of Tricuspid Regurgitation

Structural abnormalities responsible for tricuspid regurgitation (Fig. 1.48):

a. Rheumatic—it always coexists with initial valve involvement.
b. Infective endocarditis—it occurs primarily in—intravenous drug users, left to right shunts, burns and immune compromised states.
c. Congenital anomalies:
   i. Ebstein anomaly of tricuspid valve—here apical displacement of septal and posterior tricuspid leaflets (atrialization of variable portion of the right ventricle)
   ii. Downward displacement of tricuspid valve leaflets
d. Carcinoid tumors
e. Systemic lupus erythematosus—producing valvular thickening isolated tricuspid involvement, development of non-bacterial vegetations.
f. Catheter induced
g. Trauma
h. Tumors
i. Endomyocardial fibrosis
k. Antiphospholipid syndrome.

Clinical Presentations

I. **Symptoms:** The spectrum of clinical presentation depends upon the sites of involvement:
   a. In case of right-sided heart failure:
      i. Abdominal discomfort
      ii. Jaundice
      iii. Wasting
      iv. Inanimation
      v. Abdominal distension.
   b. In case of left heart involvement (associated with mitral valve involvement):
      i. Orthopnea
      ii. Paroxysmal nocturnal dyspnea.

II. **Signs:**
   a. Jugular venous distension with prominent 'v' waves (c-v waves) with rapid y descent.
      *Pulsation of earlobes
   b. Peripheral edema
   c. Pulse—tachycardia, low volume pulse irregular
   d. Cachexia
   e. Systemic examinations

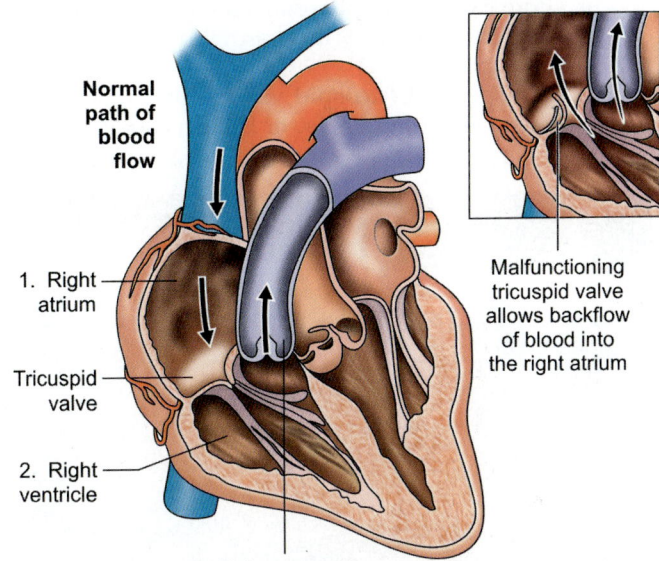

1. Right atrium
2. Right ventricle
3. Pulmonary artery
Tricuspid valve

Normal path of blood flow

Malfunctioning tricuspid valve allows backflow of blood into the right atrium

Fig. 1.48: Anatomy of tricuspid regurgitation

A. *Cardiovascular system:*
   i. Prominent pulsation at lower left sternal border—due to right ventricular volume overload.
   ii. Right parasternal heave—due to right ventricular enlargement.
   iii. S4—due to forceful right atrial contraction.
   iv. Murmur:
      1. In acute tricuspid regurgitation: murmur is decrescendo type.
      2. In chronic tricuspid regurgitation—holosystolic murmur is best heard at lower right or left sternal border, having inspiratory augmentation due to inspiratory increase in systemic venous flow and tricuspid valve flow. This murmur is not accompanied by thrill, and it has no radiation.
      3. In case of wide open tricuspid valve—there may be no murmur.

B. *Gastrointestinal examination:*
   i. Enlarged, pulsatile, tender liver
   ii. Ascites

Investigations

A. **Chest X-ray:**
   i. Marked cardiomegaly—due to right atrial and right ventricular enlargement.
   ii. Evidence of elevated right atrial pressure may include distension of the azygos vein and pleural effusions.
   iii. Ascites with diaphragmatic effusion may be present.
   iv. Dilated heart in absence of pulmonary congestion or pulmonary hypertension should suggest wither tricuspid valve disease or pericardial effusion.
   v. Massive right atrial enlargement suggest Ebstein anomaly.

B. **Echocardiography** (Fig. 1.49):
   a. *2D echocardiography:*
      i. Right ventricle is dilated.
      ii. Paradoxical motion of ventricular septum.

iii. Primary structure abnormalities of leaflets, chordae or from secondary myocardial dysfunction and dilatation.

iv. Prolapsed of tricuspid valve, endocarditis, and rheumatic heart disease or Ebstein anomaly.

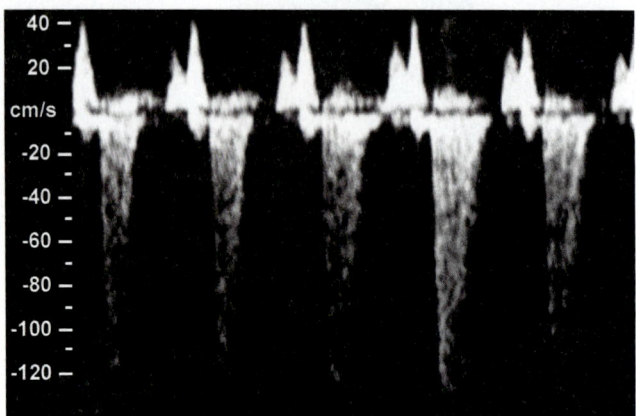

Fig. 1.49: Echocardiography showing the regurgitant jet

b. *Doppler studies:*

i. To visualize regurgitant blood

ii. To measure the flow velocities of the regurgitant jets

iii. To estimate accurately the right ventricular systolic pressure.

C. **Color Doppler studies** (Fig. 1.50): It is the mainstay for evaluating tricuspid regurgitation.

i. In trivial to mild regurgitation, it is central and narrow.

ii. In moderate to severe pulmonic regurgitation—the width of the jet increases as does the penetration of the jet into right atrium.

According to European Society of Cardiology, echocardiographic criteria for definition of severed tricuspid regurgitation include:

1. Abnormal/flail/large cooptation defect.

2. Very large color flow central jet or eccentric wall impinging jet.

3. Dense/triangular continuous wave signal with early peaking.

D. **Blood:**

i. ANA and dsDNA—for SLE

ii. Serum level of serotonin and urinary excretion of 5-hydroxyindoleacetic acid—carcinoid tumor.

iii. Blood culture—to exclude infective endocarditis

iv. Complete blood count—raised ESR, leukocytosis.

v. C-reactive protein—to exclude rheumatic etiology.

vi. Antiphospholipid antibodies—collagen vascular disease.

E. **Electrocardiography:**

i. Evidence of right atrial and right ventricular enlargement

ii. Right axis deviation

iii. Atrial fibrillation

iv. Incomplete right bundle branch block

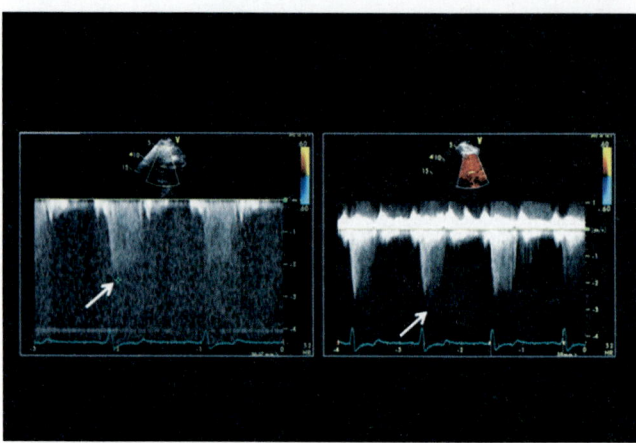

Fig. 1.50: Doppler study showing tricuspid regurgitation

F. **Cardiac catheterization:**

i. Opacification of right atrium following injection of radiographic contrasts into the right ventricle detects and estimates the severity of the regurgitation.

ii. Right atrial pressure becomes right ventriculorized as a result of 'c-v' wave and absent 'x' descent.

Treatment

Medical Treatment

1. When pulmonary arterial pressure increases, cardiac output falls—leading to right-sided heart failure. Treatment will be:

a. Restriction of sodium intake

b. Use of loop diuretics.

c. Angiotensin-converting enzyme inhibitors.

d. Angiotensin receptor antagonists.

All the above decrease the right arterial pressure.

2. To reduce pulmonary arterial pressure:

a. Nitric oxide donors

b. Phosphodiesterase inhibitors

c. Endothelin antagonists

d. Prostacycline analogues

3. To control heart rate in atrial fibrillation:

a. Cardiac glycosides

Causes of functional regurgitation: It occurs as a result of:

1. Diseases of left side of the heart:

i. Left ventricular dysfunction

ii. Mitral valve diseases

2. Pulmonary vascular and parenchymal disease

3. Right ventricular infarction

4. Arrhythmogenic right ventricular dysplasia

5. Congenital heart diseases

Surgical Treatment

a. It has to be decided that:

i. Whether the tricuspid regurgitation is functional or organic.

ii. If it is functional, the response of the pulmonary arterial pressure to the primary procedure.

iii. In patient with TR, whether this patient has severe right ventricular dysfunction.

b. If TR is due to annular dilatation with annular diameter >21 mm/m²—annuloplasty has been recommended.

c. In patients with chronic thromboembolic disease, pulmonary thromboendarterectomy dramatically reduces functional tricuspid regurgitation without any change in tricuspid annular diameter.

d. Tricuspid valve should be repaired than using prosthesis because; thrombosis is a more frequent problem with tricuspid rather than mitral prosthesis.

e. Selective plication of anterior and posterior annuli.

f. If prosthesis is required:
   i. Porcine prosthesis is of choice, because of low risk of thrombosis.
   ii. Recent change in mechanical prosthesis reduces the risk of thrombosis.
   iii. If anticoagulation is necessary for other reasons, St. Jude prosthesis is preferred, especially for younger patients.

Indications of surgery in patients with tricuspid valve infective endocarditis:

i. Uncontrollable infections
ii. Septic emboli
iii. Refractive congestive heart failure

TRICUSPID STENOSIS

Key Points to Diagnosis

1. Female preponderance
2. Jugular venous wave shows prominent 'a' wave and reduced 'Y' descent.
3. Mid-diastolic murmur in left lower sternum, increased with inspiration.
4. Characteristic echocardiographic findings includes: thickened tricuspid valve leaflets with restricted motion, right atrial enlargement.
5. Doppler echocardiographic sign includes: increased diastolic velocity across the tricuspid valve, >5 mmHg—indicates severe stenosis.

Tricuspid valve dysfunction results from morphological alterations in the valve leaflets (Fig. 1.48) or from functional aberrations of the myocardium.

Causes

1. Rheumatic fever—most common cause
2. Carcinoid heart disease
3. Congenital (Ebstein anomaly)
4. Systemic lupus erythematosus
5. Regional cardiac tamponade
6. Whipple's disease
7. Infective endocarditis
8. Endomyocardial fibrosis
9. Endomyocardial fibroelastosis
10. Methysergide therapy
11. Antiphospholipid syndrome

Pathophysiology

In rheumatic tricuspid stenosis, valve leaflets become thickened and sclerotic as the chordae tendineae become shortened.

Restricted valve opening
↓
It hampers blood flow into right ventricle
↓
Reduced blood flow to pulmonary vasculature
↓
Evidence of right atrial enlargement
↓
Obscured venous return to the right heart
↓
Congested and enlarged liver
↓
Appearance of pulmonary edema

In congenital leaflet stenosis:

i. Deformed leaflets
ii. Deformed chordae.
iii. Displacement of entire valve apparatus.

Epidemiology

i. General mortality rate is approximately 5%.
ii. It is more common in women than men, but in case of congenital form, there is male preponderance.

Clinical Presentation

Symptoms

1. Fatigue—due to low cardiac output.
2. Abdominal discomfort and swelling—due to systemic venous congestion—it may be gradual or rapid—if there is presence of atrial fibrillation or flutter.
3. When there is associated mitral stenosis, there is decrease in cardiac output from right ventricle to pulmonary vascular bed—leading to low incidence of dyspnea, orthopnea.
4. Patient may present with prominent pulsation in the neck.
5. History suggestive of rheumatic fever, carcinoid syndrome.
6. Wasting
7. In late case, there may be jaundice.

Signs

A. **General survey:**
   1. Jugular venous wave shown (Fig. 1.51)
      a. In normal sinus rhythm, prominent 'a' wave which may be confused with arterial pulse.
      b. In case of atrial fibrillation, 'a' wave may be absent.
   2. Peripheral edema.

B. **Cardiovascular system:**
   1. *Palpation:* Prominent right atrium may be palpable to the right of sternum.
   2. *Auscultation:*
      a. *First heart sound*—may be split widely.
      b. *Second heart sound:* It may be single—it may be due to inaudible closure of pulmonary valve which is the consequence of decreased blood flow through the stenotic tricuspid valve.
      c. *Murmur*—a mid-diastolic murmur can be heard along the left sternal border or at the xiphoid, which

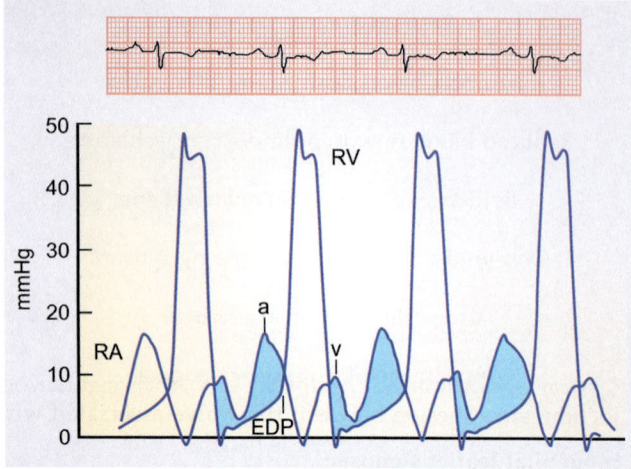

Fig. 1.51: Venous wave in TS

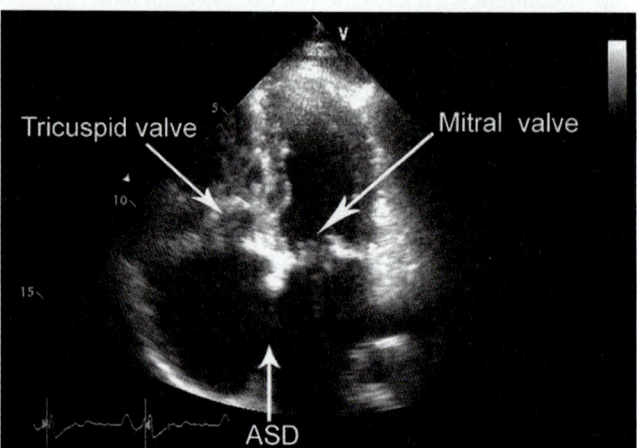

Fig. 1.52: Echocardiography

increases with inspiration and is reduced during expiration and Valsalva maneuver.

There is no presystolic accentuation in patient with sinus rhythm.

    d. *Opening snap* may be rarely heard approximately 0.06 seconds after pulmonary valve closure.

C. Gastrointestinal examination:
1. Presystolic hepatic pulsation—it may be due to reflux from atrial contraction.
2. Ascites

Laboratory Investigations

1. **Complete blood count:**
   a. If WBC count is raised, it indicates infection.
   b. If disproportional elevation of hemoglobin (poly-cythemia)—it indicates poor pulmonary blood flow.
2. **Complete chemistry profile**—it may defect certain metabolic abnormalities or inborn error of metabolism.
3. **Imaging studies:**
   a. *Chest X-ray:*
      i. Cardiac size may be normal.
      ii. Right atrial enlargement with prominent superior vena cava and azygos vein.
      iii. No enlargement of pulmonary artery with less evidence of pulmonary vascular congestion.
   b. *Echocardiography* (Fig. 1.52): Two-dimensional echocardiography can detect:
      i. Structural abnormalities of the tricuspid valve
      ii. Thickened leaflet
      iii. Decreased mobility
      iv. Compression of tricuspid annulus
      v. Prolapse of leaflet
      vi. Displacement of leaflets and vegetations
      vii. Other valve involvement
   c. *Doppler echocardiography* (Fig. 1.53) can detect:
      i. Pressure gradient between right atrium and ventricle
      ii. Associated other valvular abnormalities
4. **Electrocardiography**
   i. Right atrial hypertrophy with normal right ventricle
   ii. May be presence of atrial fibrillation

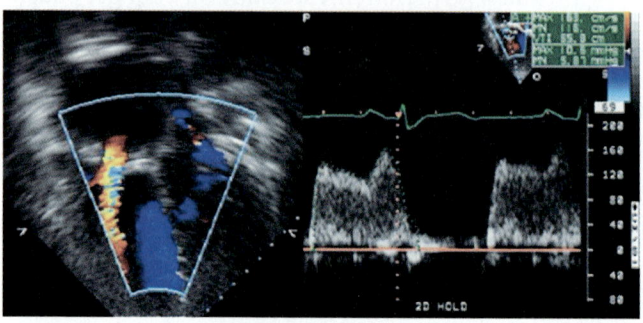

Fig. 1.53: Doppler study in TS

5. **Cardiac catheterization**
   i. This is usually required to assess the concomitant coronary artery disease.
   ii. It can determine the gradient across the valve and valve area (severity of stenosis).
   iii. it can assess the presence of associated congenital defects (septal defects, intracardiac shunts, anomalous veins)
   iv. It can assess aortic and mitral valves

Treatment

I. **Medical care:** It consists of assessment and treatment of the underlying cause of valvular etiology.
   i. Treatment of infective endocarditis with antibiotics according to the sensitivity of the organism.
   ii. Treatment of cardiac arrhythmias.
   iii. Decreasing right atrial volume overloads with diuretic treatment and salt restriction decrease symptoms and improve hepatic functions.
II. **Surgical cure:** It consists of—either commissurotomy or replacement of the valve in case of right heart failure or low cardiac output. Tricuspid valve repair is usually done associated with repair of mitral valve or aortic valve.

A few recommendations should be remembered:
1. For mechanical or bioprosthetic valve replacements, surgeon advises warfarin therapy to avoid risk of thrombosis.

2. If there is no associated regurgitation, percutaneous balloon valvoplasty is indicated.
3. Surgical therapy depends upon:
   i. Structure of the valve
   ii. Deformity of the valve

4. Intracardiac pathology like tumor, thrombus should be successfully treated.
5. Redundant portion of right atrium should be excised.
6. In a few patients with prior tricuspid valve surgery and significant stenosis of bioprosthetic valve, percutaneous tricuspid valve replacement is the only option.

CONGENITAL CARDIAC DISEASE

ATRIAL SEPTAL DEFECT

Key points to the diagnosis
1. Wide and fixed split of 2nd heart sound and a mid-diastolic murmur are characteristic.
2. In ECG—right bundle branch block—incomplete with vertical QRS axis (ostium secundum ASD), or superior QRS axis (ostium primum ASD)
3. On X-ray—prominent pulmonary arteries with right ventricular hypertrophy and increased pulmonary vascular markings.
4. On contrast and Doppler echocardiography:
   i. Right ventricular dilatation
   ii. Increased pulmonary artery flow velocity
   iii. Left to right heart shunt
5. Oxygen step up in right atrium
6. Right-sided catheter enters into left atrium across the defect.

It is one of the commonly recognized congenital cardiac abnormalities present in adult hood (Fig. 1.54). It is characterized by defect in the interatrial septum allowing oxygenated pulmonary venous blood return from left atrium to right atrium directly, responsible for spectrum of cardiac sequelae like right ventricular volume overload, pulmonary hypertension and atrial arrhythmias.

Frequency: Three major types of atrial septal defect account for 10% of all congenital heart disease (Fig. 1.55).

The types of ASD are the following:
1. *Ostium secundum*—most common type, accounting for 75% of ASD cases and 30–40% of all congenital heart disease in patients older than 40 years.
2. *Ostium primum:* 2nd most common type of ASD, 15–20% of all ASD cases—it is a form of atrioventricular septal defect and commonly associated with mitral valve abnormalities.
3. *Sinus venosus type:* It is least common, seen in 5–10% of cases. Defect is located along the superior aspect of atrial septum. It is associated with anomalous connection of right-sided pulmonary veins.

Sex: ASD occurs with female to male ratio 2:1.

Age:
i. ASD is usually asymptomatic in infancy.
ii. Commencement of symptoms depends upon degree of left to right heart shunt.
iii. Symptoms more common with advancing age: (>40 years)

Etiology
ASD occurs due to spontaneous malformation of interatrial septum (developmental defect).

A. **Ostium secundum ASD:** This type of ASD results from incomplete adhesion between flap valve associated with foramen ovale and septum secundum after birth.
   Patent foramen results from abnormal resorption of septum primum during formation of foramen secundum. Excessive resorption of septum primum results in a short septum primum, which does not close foramen ovale.
   Again large foramen ovale results from defective development of large ostium secundum.
   So ostium secundum results from:
   i. Excessive resorption of septum primum
   ii. Abnormally large foramen ovale
B. **Ostium primum ASD:** This is caused by incomplete fusion of septum primum with the endocardial cushion. This defect is close to atrioventricular valves, which may be absent or defective.
   It may be associated with displacement of anterior or septal leaflet of mitral valve.
   But tricuspid valve is usually not involved.
C. **Sinus venous type ASD:** This is caused by abnormal fusion between embryologic sinus venosus and atrium near the entry of superior vena cava. It may be associated with anomalous drainage of right superior pulmonary vein.
   In uncommon inferior type, there is association with anomalous drainage of right inferior pulmonary vein. Anomalous drainage may be into:
   1. Right atrium
   2. Superior vena cava
   3. Interior vena cava
D. **Coronary sinus type ASD:** Here the defect is characterized by:
   i. Unroofed coronary sinus
   ii. Persistent left superior vena cava, that drains into left atrium. As a result, there is right to left heart stunt.

Genetics
I. **Holt-Oram syndrome**—is characterized by:
   a. Autosomal dominant defect
   b. Deformities of upper limb (absent radii)
   c. Genetic defect TB × 5
II. **Ellis-van Creveld syndrome**—is characterized by:
   a. Autosomal recessive disorder
   b. Skeletal dysplasia:
      i. Short limbs
      ii. Short ribs
      iii. Postaxial polydactyly
      iv. Dysplastic nails and teeth
   c. Common atrium

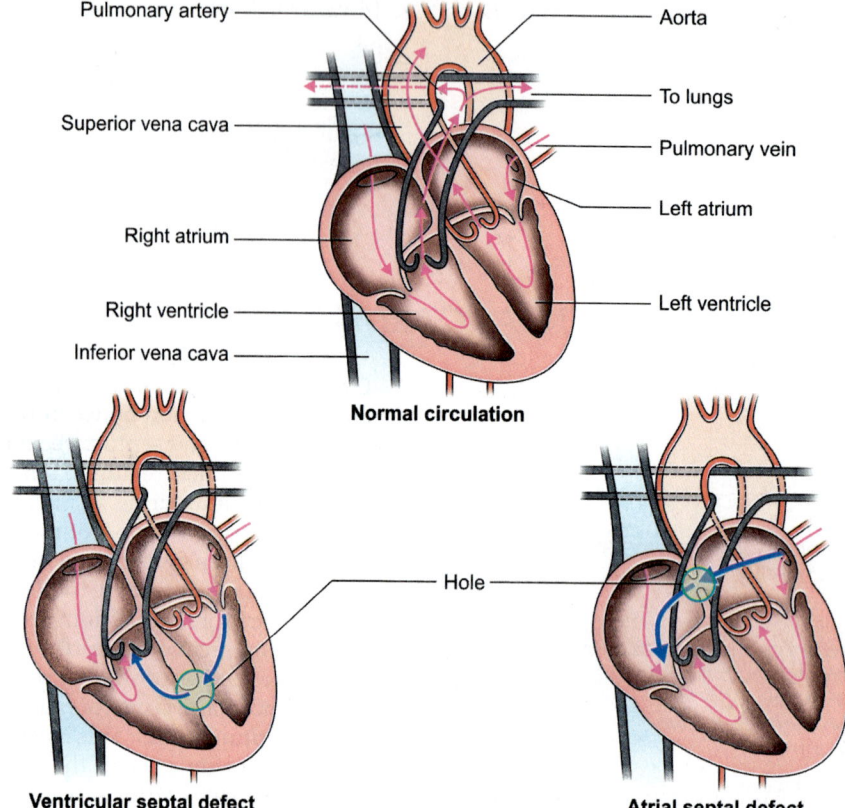

Fig. 1.54: Atrial septal defect

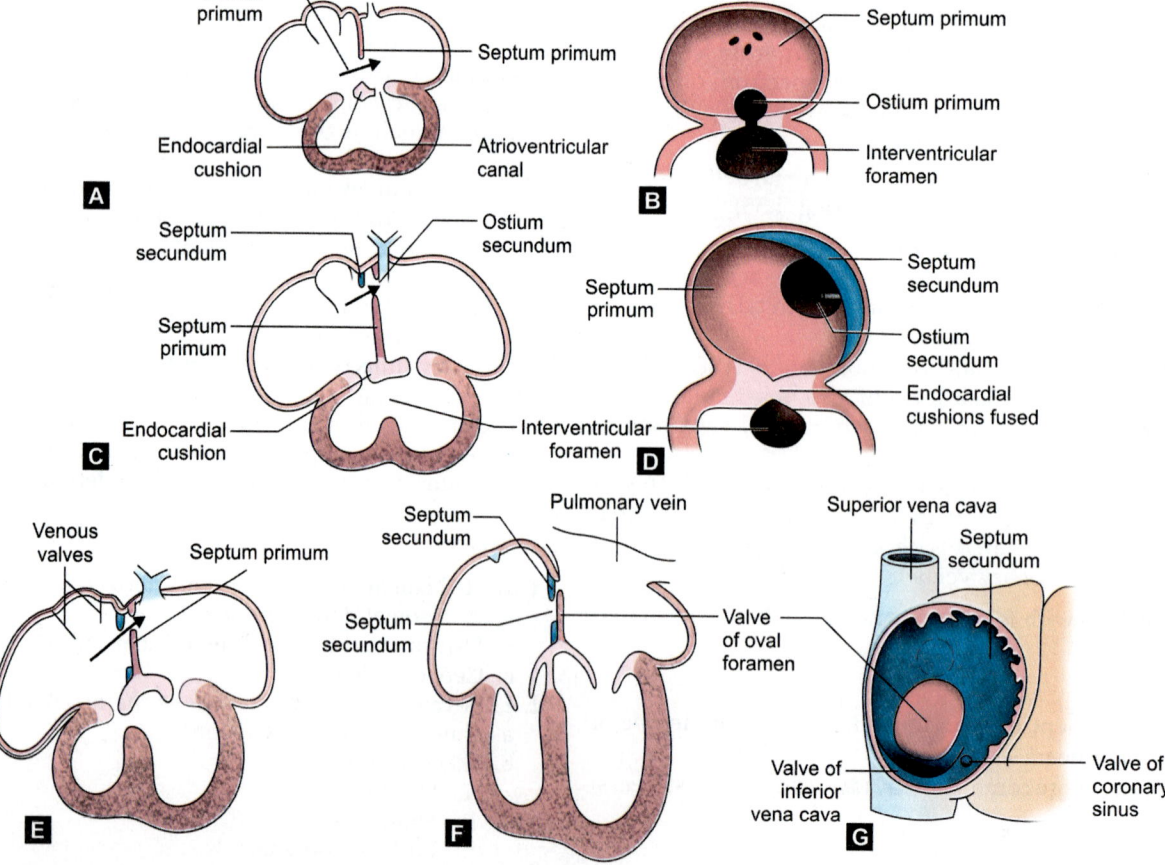

Fig. 1.55: Types of atrial septal defect: (A) and (B) Ostium primum, (C) Ostium secundum, (D) Large ostium secundum, (E) to (G) Sinus venosus

III. **Familial ASD associated with progressive atrioventricular block**—characterized by:
   a. Autosomal dominant with high degree of penetrance
   b. No associated skeletal abnormalities
IV. **Down syndrome** (trisomy 21)—is associated with spectrum of AV septal canal defect.

Classification of Atrial Septal Defect According to Locations

   i. Ostium secundum presents in the region of fossa ovalis.
   ii. Ostium primum presents in lower portion of the atrial septum.
   iii. Sinus venosus in the upper part of the septum near the entrance of the superior vena cava or inferior vena cava and unroofed coronary sinus (communication between the coronary sinus and left atrium).

Associated Abnormalities with Atrial Septal Defect

   i. Anomalous drainage of the right upper pulmonary vein into superior vena cava associated with a superior sinus venosus ASD.
   ii. Persistent left superior vena cava draining into coronary sinus with ostium secundum type ASD.
   iii. Cleft in anterior mitral leaflet and mitral regurgitation associated with ostium type ASD.

Sex Incidence

1. In ostium secundum—male: female = 1:2
2. In ostium primum and sinus venosus—ASD male: female—1:1

Pathophysiology

The amount of left to right heart shunt across the atrial septal defect depends on:
   i. Defect size
   ii. Compliance of the ventricles
   iii. Relative resistance in both pulmonary and systemic circulation

If the defect in ASD is small: Left atrial pressure exceeds the right atrial pressure by several mmHg—producing left to right shunt.

If the defect in ASD is large: Both the atrial pressures are mere or less equal.

The left-to-right shunt occurs predominantly in left ventricular systole and early diastole, and during atrial contraction some augmentation occurs.

But there may be small right-to-left heart shunt during respiratory periods of decreasing intrathoracic pressure, in absence of pulmonary hypertension.

In chronic left-to-right heart shunt:
   i. Increased blood flow through pulmonary artery.
   ii. Increased volume overload in right ventricle.

But resistance in the pulmonary vascular bed is normal until late age and right ventricular volume overload is well tolerated.

In older adult, due to coronary artery disease, systemic abnormalities, and aging producing left ventricular diastolic abnormalities, which ultimately culminates into right heart failure.

In older adult, pulmonary hypertension may develop—producing right ventricular pressure overload and right-to-left heart shunt and Eisenmenger syndrome.

Clinical Features

Symptoms

1. It may be undetected for decades due to subtle physical examinations and lack of symptoms.
2. In few cases, it can be accidentally detected during routine auscultation of heart.
3. In some cases, it may be detected after an abnormal finding observed during echocardiography.
4. Some patients may develop easy fatigability, recurrent respiratory tract infection or exertional dyspnea.
5. All patients with ASD are usually symptomatic after 6th decade. **The age-related deterioration occurs due to following facts:**
   i. Age-related decrease in left ventricular compliance augments left-to-right shunt.
   ii. Atrial arrhythmias are increased in 6th decade and can precipitate right heart failure.
   iii. In patient of more than 40 years of age, there will be mild to moderate pulmonary hypertension in presence of large left-to-right shunt.
   iv. There may be right ventricular volume and pressure over load.
6. In case of ostium premium type ASD, there may be mitral regurgitation—which leads to large volume overload in left atrium, which increases the amount of left-to-right shunt.
7. Most common presenting features are—dyspnea, easy fatigability, palpitation, syncope, stroke and/or heart failure.

Physical Findings

It depends upon:
1. Degree of left to right heart shunt
2. Its hemodynamic consequences depend on:
   i. Size of the defect
   ii. Dynamic properties of both ventricles
   iii. Relative resistance by pulmonary circulation.

The findings are the following:
a. First heart sound is split—second component is increased in intensity—due to:
   i. Forceful right ventricular contraction
   ii. Delayed closure of tricuspid leaflets
b. Second heart sound—fixed and wick split, due to reduced respiratory variation due to delayed pulmonary valve closure, in absence of pulmonary hypertensions.
c. Right ventricular hyperdynamic impulse producing left parasternal heaves—due to:
   i. Increased diastolic filling
   ii. Large stroke volume
d. Palpable pulmonary component of second heart sound—it may be due to dilated pulmonary artery.
e. Blood flow across the ASD usually does not cause any murmur at the site of shunt because of non-substantial pressure gradient between the atria.

But, if the shunt is moderate to large, large amount of blood will flow from left atrium to right atrium, as a result, large amount of blood will flow across the pulmonary outflow tract—produces crescendo–decrescendo systolic ejection murmur—to be heard at left 2nd intercostal space at left sternal border.

f. Patient with large left-to-right shunt, large volume of blood will flow actors the tricuspid valve producing mid-diastolic rumbling murmur to be heard at lower left sternal border.
So auscultatory finding resembles those of valvular or infundibular pulmonary stenosis and idiopathic dilatation of the pulmonary artery. But in these cases, there is:
   i. Absence of tricuspid flow murmur
   ii. Presence of pulmonary ejection click
   iii. Absence of fixed and wide split of S2
g. In case of ostium primum defect, and associated mitral valve cleft, there may be presence of apical systolic regurgitant murmur of mitral regurgitation.
h. In long-standing case of moderate to severe ASD, pulmonary hypertension develops, so:
   i. Midsystolic pulmonary murmur will be shorter and softer
   ii. Tricuspid flow murmur will be absent.
   iii. Splitting of 2nd heart sound will be narrower.
   iv. Pulmonary component of 2nd heart sound will be accentuated.
   v. Murmur of early diastolic pulmonary regurgitation may be present.
i. In severe pulmonary hypertension with ASD, the patient becomes cyanotic due to reversal of flow in ASD from right-to-left atrium—Eisenmenger syndrome.

Laboratory Workup

Laboratory Studies

Routine laboratory studies should be performnce of the patient is undergoing intervention for ASD.
a. Complete blood count
b. Type and screen
c. Serology
d. Coagulation profile
   i. Prothrombin time (PT)
   ii. Activated partial thromboplastin time (APTT)

Imaging Studies

1. **Chest radiography** (Fig. 1.56):
   i. Due to presence of significant left to right shunt, there may be cardiomegaly—mostly due to dilatation of right atrium and right ventricle.
   ii. If pulmonary artery is prominent, increased pulmonary vascular markings in the lung fields.
   iii. In case of sinus venosus defect, there will be proximal dilatation of pulmonary artery.
2. **Transthoracic echocardiography** (Fig. 1.57):
   i. Anomalies of systemic venous connections.
   ii. Right atrial and right ventricular enlargement without identification of cause.
   iii. Direct noninvasive visualization of most type of ASDs.
3. **Transesophageal echocardiography:**
   i. It can detect sinus venosus defect.
   ii. It provides excellent definition of atrial septum.
   iii. It is useful in guiding device placement during catheter ASD occlusion procedures.
   iv. It provides immediate intraoperative assurance of operative closure of the defect.
4. **Doppler echocardiography:** It demonstrates biphasic (systolic and diastolic) pattern with small right-to-left heart shunt at the beginning of systole.

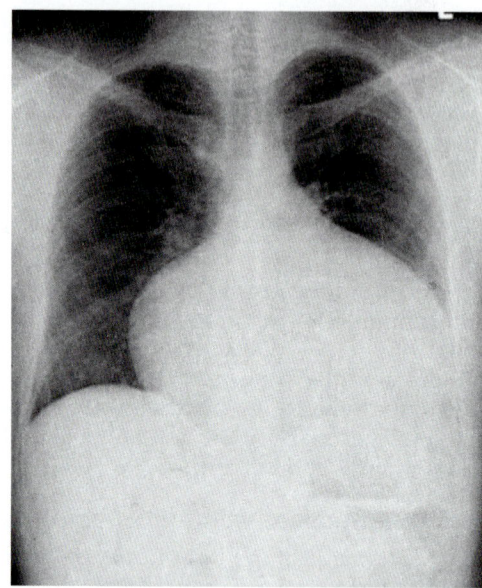

Fig. 1.56: Chest X-ray—ASD

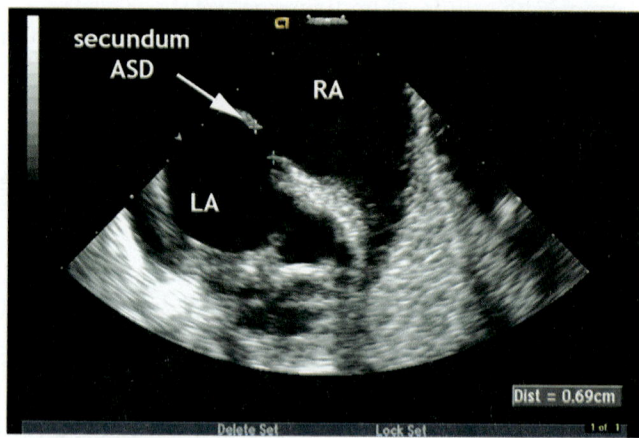

Fig. 1.57: Echocardiography

5. **Continuous wave Doppler echocardiography:**
   i. It estimates right ventricular (and pulmonary arterial pressure in absence of right ventricular outflow tract obstruction) systolic pressure in presence of tricuspid regurgitation.
   ii. It helps in evaluating the patient for obstruction to pulmonary venous return.
6. **Contrast echocardiography:**
   i. Right-to-left heart shunt can be detected by visualizing microcavitation bubbles in left atrium and left ventricle.
   ii. Left-to-right shunt can be detected as negative contrast wash out effect in the right atrium.

Electrocardiography

1. **In case of ostium secundum:**
   i. Normal sinus rhythm
   ii. Right axis deviation
   iii. rSR′ pattern in V_1—right bundle branch block
2. **In ostium primum defect:**
   i. Left axis deviation
   ii. rSR′ pattern in V_1
   iii. Interventricular conduction defect.

3. In sinus venosus defect:
  i. Loss of rSR's pattern in V1
  ii. Negative P wave.
4. In case of increased pulmonary hypertension:
  i. Loss of rSR's pattern in V_1
  ii. Tall monophonic R wave with deeply inverted T ware

Diagnostic Procedures

Cardiac catheterization
  i. In case of uncomplicated ASD in a child, routine cardiac catheterization is unnecessary.
  ii. It may be useful in following circumstances:
    a. If clinical data is inconsistent.
    b. If there is suspicion of clinical pulmonary hypertension.
    c. If there is suspicion of coronary artery disease in patient >40 years old.
    d. As an alternative for intervention for secundum ASD.

Following can be done through cardiac catheterization:
  i. Serial oxygen saturation measurement to confirm magnitude of shunt.
  ii. In young patient, right heart pressure is normal in spite of magnitude of the shunt.
  iii. If high oxygen saturation in SVC or cardiac catheter directly enters into right atrium, and pulmonary vein directly from right atrium, defect is sinus venosus type.
  iv. Partial anomalous pulmonary venus return is usually associated with sinus venosus defect.

Prognosis

A. In case of defect in ostium secundum:
  i. Patient may survive into adulthood, but, life expectancy is not normal. Mortality rate after the age of 40 is 6% per year.
  ii. Small ASD (Qp: Qs <1.5–2.1)—may produce following problem in patient with systemic hypertension and coronary artery disease:
    a. Increased left-to-right shunting
    b. Atrial arrhythmias
    c. Potential biventricular failure
    d. Intrinsic abnormalities in left ventricular diastolic dysfunction
  iii. In case of large ASD (Qp: Qs >2.1)—patient may develop severe pulmonary hypertension.
  iv. The other complications are:
    a. Paradoxical embolization
    b. Endocarditis is rare, hence prophylaxis is not recommended.
B. In case of sinus venosus defect:
  i. Similar to ostium secundum defect
  ii. May be associated with anomalous pulmonary venous drainage.
C. In case of ostium primum type ASD: Complications resulting from the consequences of mitral regurgitation.

Surgical Therapy

1. Ostium secundum defect:
  i. Small defect can be closed by using a direct continuous routine of 3.0–4.0 polypropylenes (prolene)
  ii. Large defect can be closed by:
    a. Autologous pericardium
    b. Synthetic patches made of polyester polymer (Dacron)

c. Polytetrafluoroethylene care must be taken to completely remove any air or debris from left atrium and ventricle before cardiopulmonary by-pass being discontinued.
2. In case of ostium primum defect:
  a. Patches must be attached to the septum at the junction of mitral valves and tricuspid valves.
  b. Repair of deft in mitral leaflet and annuloplasty
  c. Rarely mitral valve replacement
3. In case of sinus venosus defect: ASD must be patched in such a way that the anomalous pulmonary venous drainage is being diverted into the left atrium.

Complications

A. Following complications are associated with ASD:
  i. Congestive heart failure
  ii. Arrhythmias
  iii. Pulmonary hypertension
  iv. Cyanosis
  v. Paradoxical embolization
  vi. Stroke
  vi. Rarely infective endocarditis.
B. Following complications are associated with use of transcatheter occlusion devices:
  i. Device embolization and mal positioning.
  ii. Post-implantation arrhythmias
  iii. Thrombus formation
  iv. Cardiac perforation
  v. Device erosion
  vi. Increased level of cardiac troponin I
  vii. Residual stunts
  viii. Pericardial effusions
  ix. Transient ischemic attack
  x. Sudden death

Comorbidities in Atrial Septal Defect

  i. **Pulmonary hypertension:** PAP >20 mmHg (mean) or systolic PAP > 50 mmHg occurs 15–20% patient with ASD.
  ii. **Eisenmenger syndrome:** Rare complication of isolated secundum ASD—occurs due to reversal of shunt (right to left).
  iii. **Right-sided heart failure**—due to right ventricular volume overload as a result of right-to-left heart shunting.
  iv. **Atrial fibrillation or atrial flutter:** These are reported in 50–60% patients of >40 years.
  v. **Stroke:** It occurs in 5–10% of patients in long-term follow-up.

VENTRICULAR SEPTAL DEFECT

Key points to diagnosis of VSD

1. History of murmur appears just after birth.
2. Holosystolic murmur at lower left sternal border radiating to right.
3. Left atrial, right ventricular or biventricular enlargement.
4. In color Doppler study—high velocity color flow.
5. Enhanced pulmonary blood flow.

Ventricular septal defect (VSD) is a hole or a defect in the septum that divides the two ventricles of the heart, resulting in communication between the two ventricular cavities. It may occur—as a single component or wide variety of intracardiac anomalies including:

i. Tetralogy of Fallot
ii. Complete atrioventricular canal defect
iii. Transposition of great varieties
iv. Corrected transpositions.

Incidence

i. Isolated VSD occurs in approximately 2–6/1000 live births.
ii. It is more than 20% of all congenital heart diseases.
iii. After bicuspid aortic valves, VSDs are most common.

Developmental Anatomy (Fig. 1.58)

At 4–8 weeks of gestation, single ventricular chamber is effectively divided into two chambers. This division is accomplished with fusion of:

i. Membranous portion of interventricular septum
ii. Endocardial cushion
iii. Bulbus cordis (proximal portion of truncus arteriosus)

Muscular portion of interventricular septum grows cephalad along with the enlargement of ventricle.

↓

Ultimately meet right and left ridges of bulbus cordis

a. **Right ridge of bulbus cordis fuses with:**
   i. Tricuspid valve,   ii. Endocardial cushion
   Thus right ridge separates tricuspid valve from pulmonary valve.
b. **Left ridge of bulbus cordis fuses with** ridge of interventricular septum leaving aortic ring in continuity with mitral ring.
   Endocardial cushion finally fuses with bulbar ridges and muscular portion of interventricular septum.
   Fibrous tissue of membranous portion of septum makes the final closure and separates two ventricles.

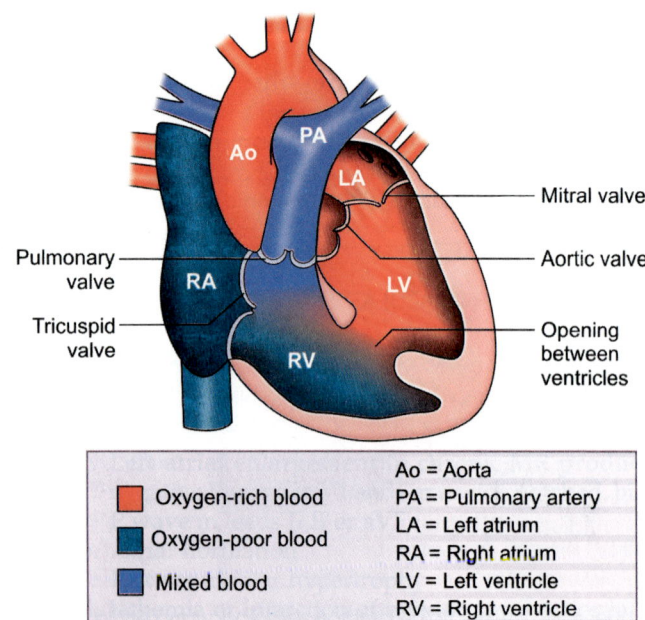

Ao = Aorta
PA = Pulmonary artery
LA = Left atrium
RA = Right atrium
LV = Left ventricle
RV = Right ventricle

■ Oxygen-rich blood
■ Oxygen-poor blood
■ Mixed blood

Fig.1.58: Anatomy of ventricular septal defect

Structure of Interventricular Septum

It is a curvilinear complex; it is divided into 4 zones on the basis of anatomic land marks in the right ventricle:

1. **Inlet septum:** This region extends from septal attachment of tricuspid valve to distal attachments of tricuspid tensor apparatus—it is called AV canal septum.
2. **Trabecular septum:** This apical trabecular zone separates the course trabeculations of the right ventricle from fine trabeculations seen in the left ventricle—it is also known as muscular septum or ventricular sinus septum.
3. **Outlet (infundibular) septum:** This smooth-walled region is separated from trabecular portion of right ventricle by septal band of the trabecular marginalis—it is known as distal conal septum.
4. **Membranous septum:** This is the last and smallest part of interventricular septum. It lies between anterior and septal tricuspid leaflets and below right and non-coronary cusps of aortic valve.

In normal heart, tricuspid and mitral valves are attached at different levels, so that septal leaflet of tricuspid valve is apically displaced relative to mitral valve attachment. As a result, a small portion of ventricular septum, called atrioventricular septum, lies between right atrium and left ventricle—this part consists of:

i. Membranous part anteriorly
ii. Muscular part posteriorly.

Classification of Ventricular Septal Defect

A. **Pars membranous VSD or infracristal or conoventricular type VSD:** It lies in the left ventricular out flow tract just below the aortic valve. Since it occurs in membranous part or adjacent muscular portion of septum—it is subclassified into:
   a. Perimembranous inlet
   b. Perimembranous outlet
   c. Perimembranous muscular
   This is most common type of VSD—80% of defects.
   Associated phenomenon: Perimembranous VSDs are associated with:
   i. Pouches or aneurysm of septal leaflet of tricuspid valve
   ii. Left ventricle to right atrial shunt
B. **Supracristal (conal septal, infundibular, subpulmonic):** This defect lies beneath the pulmonic valve and communicates with right ventricular outflow tract above the supraventricular crest.
   Associated phenomena: Aortic regurgitation secondary to prolapsed of right aortic cusp.
C. **Muscular VSD (trabecular):**
   i. This defect is entirely bounded by muscular septum.
   ii. This is multiple.
   iii. Sub-classification depends upon site of defect:
      a. Central muscular   b. Mid-muscular
      c. Apical muscular   d. Marginal muscular
D. **Posterior VSD (endocardial cushion type, canal type AV septum type):** It lies posterior to septal leaflet of tricuspid valve. This VSD constitutes 8–10% of total incidence of VSDs.

Other Anatomical Consideration

The relation of AV conduction bundle with VSD is most important in concern with surgical repair.

AV node occupies apex of triangle of Koch winch is bounded:
i. Posteriorly by tendon of Todaro
ii. Interiorly by coronary sinus ostium
iii. Superiorly by tricuspid valve annulus
    Bundle of His arises from AV node.
a. **In perimembranous defect:** Bundle of His lies in subendocardial position, during its courses along the posterior inferior margin of the defect.
b. **In inlet defect:** Bundle of His runs anterosuperiorly in relation to the defect.
c. **In muscular VSD and outlet defect:** Bundle is remote from the defect.

Pathophysiology (Fig. 1.59)

As a result of defect in interventricular septum, there is communication between systemic and pulmonary circulations. Blood flows from high pressure zone to low pressure zone, i.e. from left ventricle to right ventricle, till the commencement of change in pulmonary vasculature.

The key features of left-to-right heart shunt:
1. Increase in left ventricular volume over load.
2. Excessive pulmonary blood flow.
3. Reduced systemic cardiac output.

The pathophysiological consequences of left-to-right heart shunt:

Oxygenated blow flows from LV to RV through the defect.
↓
As blood is being shunted through VSD away from the aorta
↓
Cardiac output will be decreased
↓
Compensatory mechanisms come into play to maintain adequate organ perfusion through following mechanism:
i. Increased catecholamine secretion
ii. Salt and water retention through renin–angiotensin system.

Now left-to-right shunt depends upon two following factors:
a. **Anatomic factors**—size of VSD rather than position of VSD.
i. *If VSD is small:* Normal pressure difference between right ventricle and left ventricle—in normal heart, right ventricular pressure is 25–30% that of left ventricle. This type of defect is called restrictive VSD—because blood flow across the defect is somewhat restricted.

↓

As a result, this extra blood will be mixed with the normal deoxygenated blood flow from the superior and inferior vena cava.
↓
So, larger than the normal amount of blood will flow through lungs
↓
Large amount of blood enters the left atrium and ultimately to left ventricle.
↓
As a result of large left ventricular blood volume, there is left ventricular dilatation and left ventricular hypertrophy.
↓
There is increase in left atrial pressure
↓
There is rise in pulmonary venous pressure.
↓
There is increase in pulmonary capillary pressure
↓
There is leak of fluid into pulmonary interstitial tissue
↓
There is development of pulmonary edema

ii. *In large VSD:* There is more or less no restriction to blood flow from left ventricle to right ventricle, so the pressure differences between two ventricular chamber are no longer maintained. So this defect is called nonrestrictive VSD.
b. **Changes in pulmonary vasculature:** Pulmonary vascular resistance is a function of numerous factors:

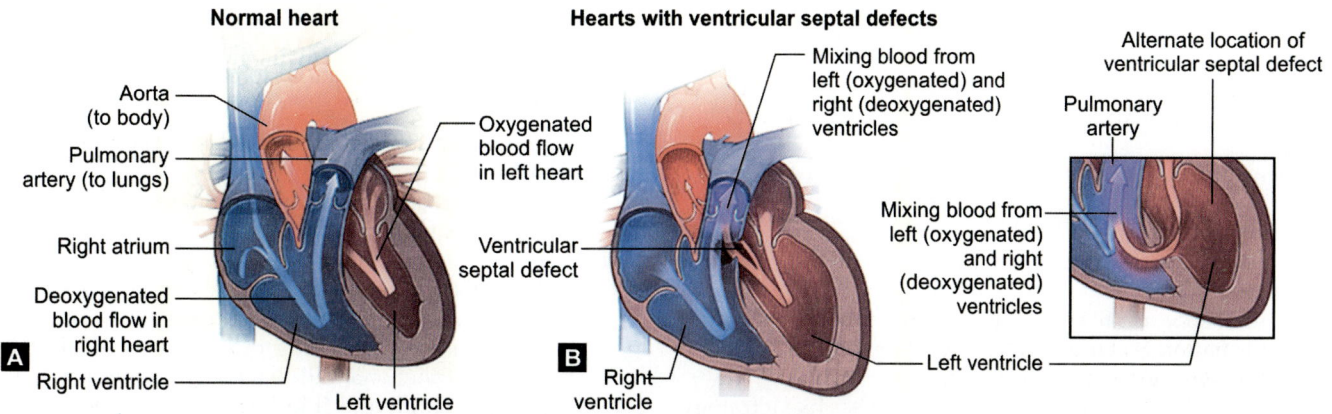

Fig. 1.59: Pathophysiology of VSD

i. Age
ii. Altitude
iii. Hematocrit
iv. Diameter of the pulmonary arterioles.

In neonates:

> Increase in media of pulmonary arterioles
> ↓
> This decreases the effective diameter of the arterioles
> ↓
> The resultant hypoxemia produces relative secondary polycythemia.
> ↓
> This elevated pulmonary vascular resistance declines to adult levels by 6–8 weeks.

But in case of large left-to-right shunt, there is increased pressure in pulmonary vascular circuit. In case of long duration of shunt, there is irreversible change in pulmonary vascular wall and development of pulmonary vascular resistance and secondary pulmonary hypertension.

Natural History of VSD

Spectrum of natural history of VSD ranges from spontaneous closure to congestive heart failure to death infancy.

Spontaneous closure mainly occurs in children by the age of 2 years, it is uncommon after the age of 4 years.

The following VSDs are liable to close:
 i. Muscular defects (80% cases)
 ii. Perimembranous defects (35–40%)
 iii. Outlet VSD—very low incidence of closure
 iv. Inlet VSD will never close.

Closure may occur in following processes:
 i. Hypertrophy of septum
 ii. Formation of fibrous tissue
 iii. Subaortic tags.
 iv. Opposition of septal leaflets of tricuspid valve
 v. Prolapse of a leaflet of the aortic valve
 During closure of perimembranous defect, an aneurysm of the interventricular septum my appear.

 Following pathological classifications allow the comparison of similar defects:
 i. Subarterial VSDs can be classified as abnormalities of ectomesenchymal tissue migration.
 ii. Perimembranous VSDs can be classified as abnormalities of intracardiac blood flow.
 iii. Muscular VSDs can be classified as abnormalities in cell death.
 iv. Type III inflow VSD can be classified as abnormalities of extracellular matrix and endocardial cushion defect.

Etiology

Etiologies are multifactorial:

1. **Maternal factors:** Material diabetes
2. **Genetic factors:**
 i. Incidence of VSD in siblings of patient with same malformation is about 3 times that of general population.
 ii. It is reported in identical twins.
 iii. It may be present in following diseases—like tetralogy of Fallot, truncus arteriosus.

Epidemiology

1. **Sex:**
 a. VSDs are more common in females than males.
 b. Subarterial VSDs are highest in boys.
2. **Race:** This defect is most common in Asian population.

Clinical Presentations in VSDs

Symptoms and signs of VSDs depend upon:
1. Size of the defect of VSD
2. Magnitude of the left to right shunt.

Symptoms

1. **In case of small VSDs:**
 i. There is usually mild or no symptoms.
 ii. It can be detected during routine cardiological examination—when murmur is being detected.
2. **In case of moderate VSDs:**
 i. Excessive fatigue during feeding
 ii. Excessive sweating during feeding due to consequences of increased sympathetic tone producing increase in cardiac output.
 iii. Inadequate growth due to:
 a. Increased calorie requirement
 b. Inadequate breast feeding
 iv. Diminished exercise tolerance.
3. **In case of large VSDs:** Symptoms may occur later because of a delayed decrease in pulmonary vascular pressures.
 i. Poor weight gain.
 ii. Frequent respiratory infection
 iii. Exertional dyspnea.
 iv. Atypical chest pain.
 v. Symptoms of right ventricular failure may occur due to:
 a. Pulmonary hypertension, or
 b. Long-standing volume overload.

Physical Examinations

1. **Small VSDs:**
 i. Normal vital signs
 ii. Physiologic splitting of 2nd heart sound.
 iii. Harsh holosystolic murmur at lower left sternal border.
 In smaller defects—murmur will be high pitched or squeaky noise.
 This murmur is usually detected at about 4–8 weeks of age after decrease in pulmonary vascular resistance.
2. **Moderate VSDs:**
 i. Infant has normal height but decreased weight; it may indicate congestive cardiac failure.
 ii. Mild tachycardia
 iii. Mild tachypnea
 iv. Enlarged tender liver—may be due to right-sided heart failure.
 v. Pulmonary component of second heart sound usually normal or slightly increased.
 vi. Murmur
 a. Holosystolic harsh murmur—will be heard of lower left sternal border, increased during expiration.
 b. Mid-diastolic rumbling murmur at mitral area— suggest functional mitral stenosis secondary to left-to-right shunt and it indicates surgical level shunt (pulmonary to systemic flow ratio >2:1)

3. **In case of large VSDs:**
   A. Cardinal signs are:
      a. Tachycardia   b. Tachypnea
      c. Hepatomegaly   d. Murmur
         i. Holosystolic harsh murmur at lower left sternal border, with radiation to right parasternal region
         ii. Diastolic rumbling murmur, at mitral area, secondary to functional mitral stenosis
         VSD is usually not associated with cyanosis, i.e. the patient is pink. So if patient with VSDs has cyanosis, there is always associated lesion.
   B. If pulmonary hypertension develops, P₂ will be accentuated.
   C. Signs of tricuspid inefficiency—may develop
      a. Prominent jugular venous wave 'v'
      b. Systolic murmur
   D. Signs of aortic insufficiency:
      a. Diastolic blowing murmur in upper right 2nd intercostal space
      b. Water hammer pulses.
      It indicates—VSD is of supracristal variety.
4. **Maladie de Roger**—small asymptomatic VSD with loud murmur.

Complications

   i. VSD with pulmonary hypertension producing right-to-left heart shunt—Eisenmenger complex
   ii. Irreversible and fixed pulmonary hypertension
   iii. Secondary aortic insufficiency due to prolapsed aortic valve leaflets—rare in children less than 2 years—it is more common is supracristal VSD than perimembranous VSDs.
   iv. AR in case of subarterial VSD—due to:
      a. Poorly supported right coronary cusp
      b. Venturi effect produced by VSD jet.
   v. Right ventricular out-flow tract obstruction—mainly due to obstruction at infundibular level.
   vi. Discrete fibrous subvalvular aortic stenosis—most often occurs in perimembranous VSDs.
   vii. Infective endocarditis—rare in children younger than 2 years. In VSDs, both systemic and pulmonary circulations may be affected, so vegetation manifest on both sides.
   viii. Embolization—may occur despite the size of vegetations.
   If vegetation is more than 10 mm in size and pedunculated, it indicates surgical intervention.

Investigations (Fig. 1.60)

Chest Radiograph

a. **In small VSDs:**
   i. Normal heart size
   ii. Normal pulmonary vascularity
b. **Moderate to large VSDs:**
   i. Increased cardiac silhouette
   ii. Increased pulmonary vascular markings with prominent main pulmonary artery segment.
   iii. Enlarged left atrium—visible on lateral radiograph
c. **In large VSDs:**
   i. Markedly increased pulmonary vascular resistance
   ii. Essentially normal size heart.

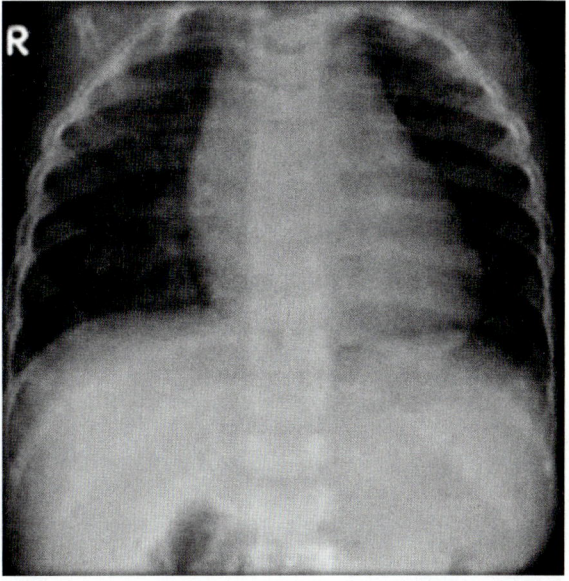

Fig. 1.60: Chest radiography in VSD

   iii. Right ventricular hypertrophy with cardiac apex rotated slightly upward and to the left, and posteriorly
   iv. Markedly prominent main pulmonary artery and adjacent vessels.
   v. Decreased pulmonary vascularity in outer third of lung fields—in case of pulmonary hypertension.

Echocardiography (Fig. 1.61)

a. **Two-dimensional echocardiography:** It detects:
   i. Size of the defect
   ii. Position of the defect
   The findings are:
   i. Left atrial and left ventricular dilation
   ii. Right atrium size is normal.
   iii. Main pulmonary artery is dilated.
   iv. Right ventricular hypertrophy—signifies:
      a. Associated pulmonary hypertension, or
      b. Associated pulmonary stenosis (presence right-to-left heart shunt and cyanosis)

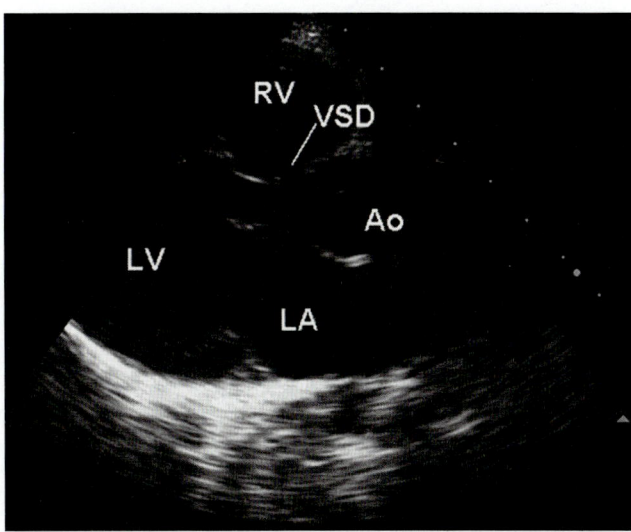

Fig. 1.61: Echocardiography

v. Ventricular septal aneurysm may be seen below the aortic valve in the inlet portion of septum near septal leaflet of tricuspid valve.

b. Color Doppler studies (Fig. 1.62): It shows:
i. High velocity systolic jet across the ventricular septum from LV to RV—it detects the position of defect.
ii. Jet from membranous VSD may be seen:
1. In the region of tricuspid valve (perimembranous), or
2. Towards pulmonary artery (doubly committed subarterial or supracristal)

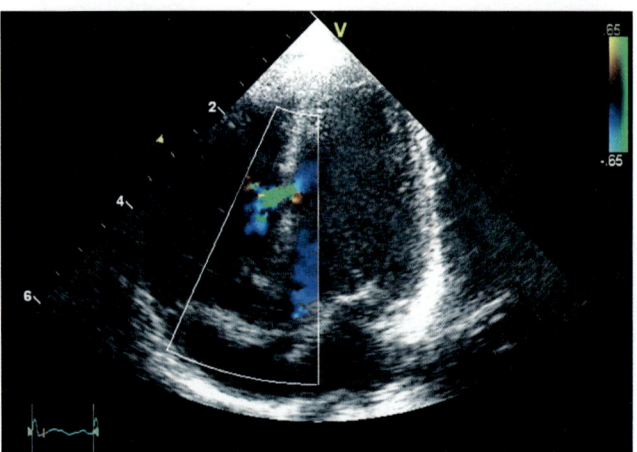

Fig. 1.62: Color Doppler study

c. Continuous wave Doppler studies:
i. It provides the peak systolic LV and RV gradient.
↓
ii. Subtracting this gradient from systolic blood pressure gives the peak RV systolic pressure.
iii. In absence of pressure gradient across the right ventricular outflow tract—right ventricular systolic pressure is equivalent to pulmonary artery systolic pressure.

Cardiac catheterization: Right heart catheterization with sequential measurement of oxygen saturation reveals step up of oxygen saturation in the body of right ventricle.

Left ventriculography: In cranial left anterior oblique position—reveals—the location of the defect as contrast enters the right ventricle.

Electrocardiography

i. Evidence of LVH
ii. Evidence of biventricular hypertrophy
iii. Evidence of left atrial enlargement as evidenced by biphasic p waves in lead 1, avR, and V_6 with prominent negative deflection in V_1.

Treatment

A. In children with small VSDs: Asymptomatic and medical and surgical therapies are not indicated.
Prophylactic antibiotic therapy against infective endocarditic is no longer indicated.

B. In children with moderate to large VSDs: Trial of medical therapy to manage symptomatic CCF.

Indications of Surgery

i. Uncontrolled chronic heart failure with growth failure and recurrent respiratory tract infection.
ii. Large asymptomatic defects associated with elevated pulmonary artery pressure when infants are younger than 1 year.
iii. Older asymptomatic children with normal pulmonary pressure, if pulmonary to systemic flow ratio >2:1.
iv. Prolapse of aortic valve cusp, even if VSD is small.

Medical Management of Congestive Heart Failure

i. Oral feeding with or without tube-feeding to raise calorie needs.
ii. Diuretics to relieve pulmonary congestion:
• Furosemide in the dose of 1–3 mg/kg/day in divided 2–3 doses.
• Long-term furosemide treatment results in hypercalcemia and electrolyte disturbances.
iii. Angiotensin-converting enzyme inhibitors (captopril and enalapril)—reduce both systemic and pulmonary pressure and reduce left to right shunt.
iv. Digoxin (5–10 mg/kg/day): This drug can be given, if diuresis and afterload reduction do not relieve symptoms.

Surgical Therapy

A. Surgical closure:
i. Most perimembranous and inlet VSDs are repaired by transatrial surgical approach.
ii. Outlet septa defects are approached through pulmonary valve.
iii. Multiple muscular defects are usually approached through apical left ventriculotomy and closing the defect with single patch.

B. Transcatheter closure

Complications of surgery:
i. Right bundle branch block
ii. Ventricular arrhythmias.
iii. Sudden death
iv. Complete heart block

TETRALOGY OF FALLOT

Key Points to Diagnosis

1. History of squatting in childhood
2. History of anoxic spells in infants.
3. Physical findings: Cyanosis, clubbing, right parasternal heave, murmur of pulmonary stenosis, absent P_2
4. Chest X-ray: Boot-shaped heart, post-stenotic pulmonary artery dilation.
   In milder cases—right-sided aortic arch
5. Echocardiography:
   i. RVH
   ii. Overriding of aorta
   iii. Large perimembranous ventricular septal defects,
   iv. Obstruction of right ventricular outflow tract (subvalvular, valvular, supravalvular or in pulmonary arterial branches)
6. Gradient across the pulmonary outflow tract.
   i. Normal pulmonary artery pressure.
   ii. Equalization of both ventricular pressure.

Definition

Tetralogy of Fallot, most common cyanotic heart disease, comprises of:

i. Right ventricular hypertrophy
ii. Right ventricular out flow tract obstruction (infundibular stenosis)
iii. Ventricular septal defect
iv. Aortic dextroposition.

Mortality

i. In case of untreated patient, mortality reaches 50% by the age of 6 years.
ii. In the era of successful cardiac surgery, patient enjoys good long-term survival and excellent quality of life.

Anatomical Consideration in Fallot's Tetralogy

1. **Right ventricular outflow tract obstruction:** Anterior displacement and associated rotation of infundibular septum produces variable degree of right ventricular outflow tract obstruction.

   If obstruction is adjacent to pulmonary valve, it produces additional obstruction.

2. **Pulmonary arteries:**
   i. They may vary in size and distribution—may be atretic or hypoplastic.
   ii. Rarely left pulmonary artery may be absent.
   iii. In some cases, varying degrees of stenosis of the pulmonary arteries.
   In case of pulmonary atresia:

   > No communication between right ventricle and main pulmonary artery.
   >
   > ↓
   >
   > Pulmonary blood flow is maintained through:
   > a. Patent ductus arteriosus, or
   > b. Collateral circulation through bronchial vessels

   iv. In case of minimal right ventricular tract obstruction, excessive pulmonary blood flow through left-to-right shunt or large aortopulmonary collaterals—ultimately produce secondary pulmonary vascular disease.
   v. In 75% of tetralogy of Fallot, some degree of pulmonary valve stenosis occurs due to leaflet tethering.

3. **Aorta:**
   a. Overriding of aorta to a varying degrees due to:
      i. True dextroposition
      ii. Abnormal rotation of aortic root.
   b. In 50% of cases, aorta may originate from right ventricle.
   c. In a few cases, right aortic arch occurs.

4. **Ventricular septal defect** associated malalignment of the census septum.

5. **Associated abnormalities:**
   i. In a few cases—co-existence of atrial septal defect—produces pentalogy of Fallot
   ii. Patent ductus arteriosus
   iii. Atrioventricular septal defect
   iv. Muscular type ventricular septal defect
   v. Anomalous pulmonary vascular return
   vi. Anomalous coronary arteries
   vii. Absent pulmonary valve
   viii. Aortopulmonary window
   ix. Aortic incompetence

Types of Coronary Artery Abnormalities

In 9% of cases, left anterior descending coronary (LAD) artery originates from proximal right coronary artery and crosses right ventricular outflow tract at variable distance from pulmonary valve annulus. As a result, placement of a patch across the pulmonary annulus will be risky.

In some cases, LAD is prone to injury during VSD repair.

Etiology

The etiology is unknown, but following possible etiologies are identified:

1. Genetic polymorphism
2. Prenatal factors:
   i. Maternal rubella during pregnancy
   ii. Poor prenatal nutrition
   iii. Maternal alcohol abuse
   iv. Maternal age more than 40 years.
   v. Maternal phenylketonuria
   vi. Birth defect
   vii. Diabetes
   viii. Children with Down syndrome
   ix. Fetal hydantoin syndrome
   x. Fetal carbamazepine syndrome

Tetralogy of Fallot may be associated with:
   i. CATCH22 (cardiac defects, abnormal facies, thymic hypoplasia, cleft palate, hypocalcemia, deletion of a segment of chromosome band $^{22}q^{11}$ (DiGeorge critical region).
   ii. DiGeorge syndrome
   iii. Brachial arch abnormalities.

Hemodynamic abnormalities: It depends upon:
i. Degree of right ventricular outflow tract obstruction
ii. Size of ventricular septal defect
   The VSD is non-restrictive—as a result there is equalization of right and left ventricular pressure.
   If right ventricular outflow tract obstruction is severe:
   a. There is right to left intracardiac shunt
   b. Pulmonary blood flow will be diminished.
   So, in these cases, blood flow depends upon:
   a. Patent ductus arteriosus
   b. Blood flow through bronchial collaterals.

Epidemiology

1. It represents 10% of total congenital heart disease.
2. It occurs 3–6 infants for every 10000 births.
3. It is most common congenital cyanotic heart disease.
4. It occurs more commonly in males than females.

Prognosis

1. In present era of reconstructive cardiac surgery, there is good long-term survival with excellent quality of life.
2. Without surgery:
   a. Mortality rates gradually increase, ranging from 30% at 2 years of age to 50% at 6 years of age.
   b. Mortality rate is highest in the 1st year, and then remains constant until 2nd decade.

c. Not more than 20% of patients expected to reach the age of 10 years.
d. 5–10% reaches the 2nd decade of life.
e. Most patients who survive more than 30 years, usually develop congestive cardiac failure:
    i. Stroke
    ii. Pulmonary embolism
    iii. Subacute bacterial endocarditis.

The causes of stroke in these patients may be due to:
  i. Thromboembolism
  ii. Prolonged hypotension
  iii. Anoxia
  iv. Secondary polycythemia

Clinical Presentation in Tetralogy of Fallot

1. Most patients (infants) present with failure to thrive and difficulty in feeding.
2. Infants with associated pulmonary atresia—became profoundly cyanotic as ductus arteriosus closes.
3. Occasionally, children with enough pulmonary blood flow remain asymptomatic, until they outgrow their pulmonary blood supply.
4. Hypoxia spells—infants during crying or feeding may become bluish pale skin—it is potentially lethal and unpredictable. It may occur in non-cyanotic Fallot also. The mechanisms may be:
   - Spasm of infundibular septum—it worsens the right ventricular outflow tract obstruction.
   These spells can be aborted by simple oxygenation and rest.
5. **Squatting**: Usually older children with TOF increase their pulmonary blood flow by their compensatory mechanism. The mechanism behind it is

Squatting
↓
Increases peripheral vascular resistance
↓
Decreases the magnitude of VSD (right-to-left shunt)

6. Exertional dyspnea worsens with age.
7. Hemoptysis—occasionally—may be due to rupture of bronchial collaterals—usually occurs in older child.
8. Cyanosis—it progresses with age and outgrowth of pulmonary vasculature. The following factors are responsible for worsening of cyanosis:
    i. Acidosis
    ii. Stress
    iii. Infection
    iv. Posture
    v. Exercise
    vi. Beta adrenergic agonists
    vii. Dehydration
    viii. Closure of ductus arteriosus

The Direction of Shunt

i. Normally predominant shunt is right to left through ventricular septal defect.
ii. If pulmonary stenosis is mild, usually there is bidirectional shunt.
iii. In some patients, infundibular stenosis is minimal, here the shunt is left to right—in this case it produces pink

tetralogy. They often have oxygen desaturation in systemic circulation.

Symptoms progression is mainly due to worsening of right ventricular outflow tract obstruction—which leads to right ventricular hypertrophy, right to left heart shunting and systemic hypoxemia.

Physical Examinations

1. **General survey** include:
    i. Central cyanosis
    ii. Clubbing
    iii. Smaller height as expected per age
    iv. Frequent squatting position.
    v. Scoliosis (common)
    vi. Retinal engorgement
    vii. Tachypnea
2. **Cardiac examination:**
    i. First heart sound is normal.
    ii. 2nd heart sound is single—because pulmonary closure sound is not heard.
    iii. A harsh systolic murmur is heard over pulmonary area and along left sternal border.
       If right ventricular outflow tract obstruction is moderate—murmur is muffled. So more severe the obstruction or aggravation of cyanosis, murmur will be absent.
       The murmur will be accompanied by systolic thrill.
    iv. If there is accompanying aortopulmonary collateral—continuous murmur over the chest.
    v. May have bulging left hemithorax.
    vi. Right parasternal heave—indicating right ventricular hypertrophy.
    vii. Aortic ejection click may be due to functional aortic stenosis.

Investigations for Tetralogy of Fallot

1. **Hematological investigations:**
    i. Hemoglobin and hematocrit values—elevated according to the degree of cyanosis—producing secondary polycythemia—as compensatory mechanism.
    ii. Decreased platelet count and clotting factors—may be responsible for bleeding.
    iii. Hyperviscosity and coagulopathy—producing:
       a. Diminished coagulation factors
       b. Diminished total fibrinogen.
       c. Prolonged prothrombin time
       d. Prolonged coagulation time.
2. **Arterial blood gases:** This is most useful in dark-skinned or anemic patient. The level of cyanosis should be measured in these patients by arterial blood gases.
    i. Varying degrees of oxygen saturation—according to level of right to left heart shunt
    ii. Blood pH is normal.
    iii. Partial pressure of carbon dioxide normal.
3. **Radiological studies:**
    a. *Echocardiography:* The findings are:
       i. Severe right ventricular hypertrophy
       ii. Thickened, malformed pulmonary valve.
       iii. There may be primary infundibular stenosis with marked hypertrophic narrowing of the right ventricular outflow tract.

iv. Systolic color flow signal and a continuous wave Doppler gradient across right ventricular outflow tract or across the pulmonary valve.
v. Two-dimensional echocardiography reveals perimembranous ventricular septal defect.
vi. Aortic root is variably enlarged and overrides VSD.
vii. In pulmonary atresia with ventricular septal defect, aortopulmonary collaterals from descending aorta can be seen by transthoracic echocardiography.
viii. Complications of tetralogy of Fallot can be detected by echocardiography. These are:
  • Residual outflow tract obstruction
  • Pulmonary valve regurgitation
  • Right ventricular outflow obstruction
  • VSD patch leak
b. *Radiography:* The hallmark finding is:
  i. Boot-shaped heart (Coeur en sabot)—when:
    • Pulmonary stenosis severe
    • Left ventricle is small
  ii. Post-stenotic pulmonary artery dilatation
  iii. Right-sided aortic arch.
c. *Magnetic resonance imaging:*
  i. It delineates:
    a. Aorta
    b. Right ventricular out flow tract obstruction
    c. Right ventricular hypertrophy
    d. Pulmonary artery
  ii. It can measure:
    a. Intracardiac pressure
    b. Intracardiac pressure gradients
    c. Direction of blood flow
    d. Ejection fraction
    e. Pulmonary regurgitant fraction
4. **Cardiac catheterization:** It reveals:
  i. Gradient across the pulmonary outflow tract.
  ii. Normal pulmonary artery pressure.
  iii. Equalization of right and left ventricular pressure.
5. **Angiography:** It can better define:
  i. Anatomy of RV outflow tract
  ii. Size of ventricular septal defect.
6. **Coronary angiography** may reveal anomalous origin of left coronary artery.

Electrocardiography

The typical findings are:
 i. Right bundle branch block
 ii. Varying form of heart block
 iii. Right ventricular hypertrophy.
    The ECG findings depend on the severity of pulmonary stenosis and degree of shunting.
 iv. QRS duration of >180 msec—correlates with significant right ventricular dilatation due to pulmonary regurgitation—after surgical repair—it can predict sudden cardiac death in postoperative TOF.

Management

Prehospital Management

a. Infants with central cyanosis or respiratory distress—inhalation of oxygen with cannula or tube.

b. Allow the baby to remain with parents. If skilled personnel for IV placement is not available, an interosseous insertion is immediate life saving.

Emergency Department Management

This usually aims at the management of hypercyanotic episode (Tet spell). Hypercyanotic episode is characterized by:
 i. Hyperapneic paroxysm
 ii. Prolonged crying
 iii. Intense cyanosis
 iv. Decreased intensity of murmur of pulmonary stenosis.

The mechanisms are:
 i. Secondary infundibular spasm
 ii. Decreased systemic vascular resistance
 iii. Increased right to left ventricular shunting through ventricular septal defect.

The net result is diminished pulmonary blood flow.

If the patient cannot be treated—it may result in:
 i. Syncope
 ii. Seizure
 iii. Stroke
 iv. Death

Treatment of acute setting of hypercapnea:
 i. Oxygen is of limited value, because, main abnormality is reduced pulmonary blood flow.
 ii. Morphine sulfate—0.1–0.2 mg/kg—intramuscularly—it:
    a. Reduces ventilatory drive
    b. Decreases systemic venous return
 iii. Phenylephrine (0.02 mg/IV): It increases systemic vascular resistance.
 iv. Dexamethasone—low dose 0.1–0.125 µ/kg/hour—then this dose can be increased, if required.
 v. Intravenous sodium bicarbonate reduces the stimulating effect of acidosis on respiratory centre.
  vi. Last resort is general anesthesia.

Medical Treatment

 i. Asymptomatic patients do not require any treatment.
 ii. In case of cyanotic heart disease: Preparation for surgery—infants with cyanotic episodes—placement of the patient in knee chest position in addition to administration of oxygen and intravenous morphine.
 iii. In severe cyanotic episodes—intravenous propranolol can be administered to relax infundibular muscle spasm.

Surgical Management

Current trend is to perform reconstructive surgery before the age of 1 year and preferably by the age of 2 years.

Recent recommendation for all pediatric surgeons—is to administer prostaglandin to:
 i. Maintain ductus in open state.
 ii. Decrease the need to perform urgent surgery.

This is important time for surgeon to:
 i. Delineate coronary artery anatomy
 ii. Choice the procedure of surgery

Primary repair:
 i. Avoids prolonged right ventricular outflow tract obstruction
 ii. Avoids subsequent right ventricular hypertrophy

iii. Avoids prolonged cyanosis
iv. Avoids postnatal angiogenesis.

Following factors increase the risk for early repair of tetralogy of Fallot:
  i. Low birth weight
  ii. Pulmonary atrery atresia
  iii. Major associated anomalies
  iv. Multiple previous surgeries
  v. Absent pulmonary valve syndrome
  vi. Young or old age
  vii. Severe annular hypoplasia
  viii. Small pulmonary arteries
  ix. High break right ventricle to left ventricular pressure ratio
  x. Multiple ventricular septal defects
  xi. Coexisting cardiac anomalies.

Following are the contraindications to primary repair:
  i. Presence of an anomalous coronary artery
  ii. Very low birth weight
  iii. Small pulmonary arteries
  iv. Multiple VSDs
  v. Multiple coexisting intracardiac malformations.

Palliative procedures: Primary goals are:
  i. Increase in pulmonary blood flow independent of ductal patency
  ii. Allow pulmonary artery growth
  iii. Total correction

The procedures are: Blalock-Taussig shunt: Gore-Tex graft between the subclavian artery and pulmonary artery.

Advantages:
  i. Preservation of subclavian artery
  ii. Suitability for use on either side
  iii. Good relief of cyanosis
  iv. Easier control and closure at time of primary repair
  v. Excellent patency rate
  vi. Decreased incidence of iatrogenic trauma

Complications of the procedure:
  i. Hypoplasia of the arm
  ii. Digital gangrene
  iii. Phrenic nerve injury
  iv. Pulmonary artery stenosis

Longevity of this shunt depends upon:
  i. Patients' aim at the time of surgery
  ii. Type of shunt

Primary correction procedure done under cardiopulmonary bypass:
  i. Closure of the ventricular septal defect
  ii. Resection of the area of infundibular stenosis
  iii. Relief of right ventricular outflow tract obstruction.

Postoperative mortality and morbidity depend upon: Ratio of right ventricular to left ventricular pressure. If it will remain increased—it suggests:
  i. Residual VSD
  ii. Residual pulmonary stenosis

Newer methods of cardiac operation:
  i. Hypothermia
  ii. Cardioplegia
  iii. Total circulatory arrest

Surgical complications: Early postoperative complications:
  i. Creation of heart block
  ii. Residual ventricular septal defect
  iii. Sudden death from ventricular arrhythmia

PATENT DUCTUS ARTERIOSUS

Definition

Patent ductus arteriosus is a persistent communication between descending thoracic aorta and the pulmonary artery, as a result of failure of physiologic closure of fetal ductus.

It is usually diagnosed in infants, but it can be delayed until childhood even adulthood.

Shunt is usually left to right and usually depends upon:
  i. Size of open communication
  ii. Pulmonary vascular resistance

Anatomy (Fig. 1.63)

  i. Ductus arteriosus is a remnant of distal sixth aortic arch.
  ii. It connects pulmonary artery at the junction of main pulmonary artery and left main pulmonary artery with the proximal descending thoracic aorta just after the origin of left subclavian artery.
  iii. It passes from the anterior aspect of the pulmonary artery to the posterior aspect of the aorta.
  iv. It has large aortic end and narrow pulmonary end due to its conical shape.

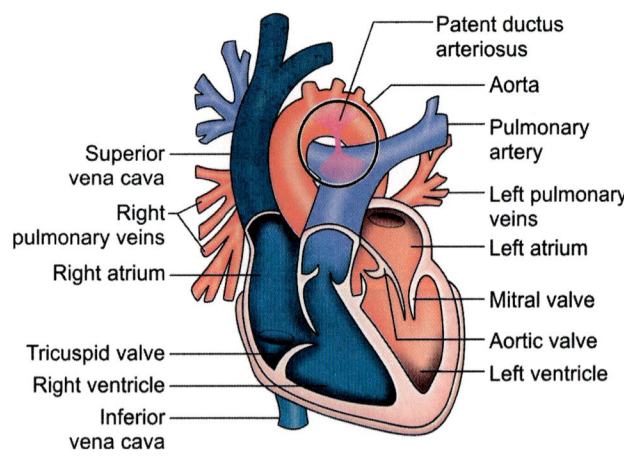

Fig. 1.63: Patent ductus arteriosus

Different shapes of ductus arteriosus according to Krichenko classification of PDA based on angiography:
1. Type A—conical
2. Type B—window
3. Type C—tubular
4. Type D—complex
5. Type E—elongated

Patent ductus arteriosus may be:
  i. Right-sided—it is usually associated with other congenital anomalies of cardiovascular system.
  ii. Left-sided—it is more common.
  iii. Both-sided—right or left.

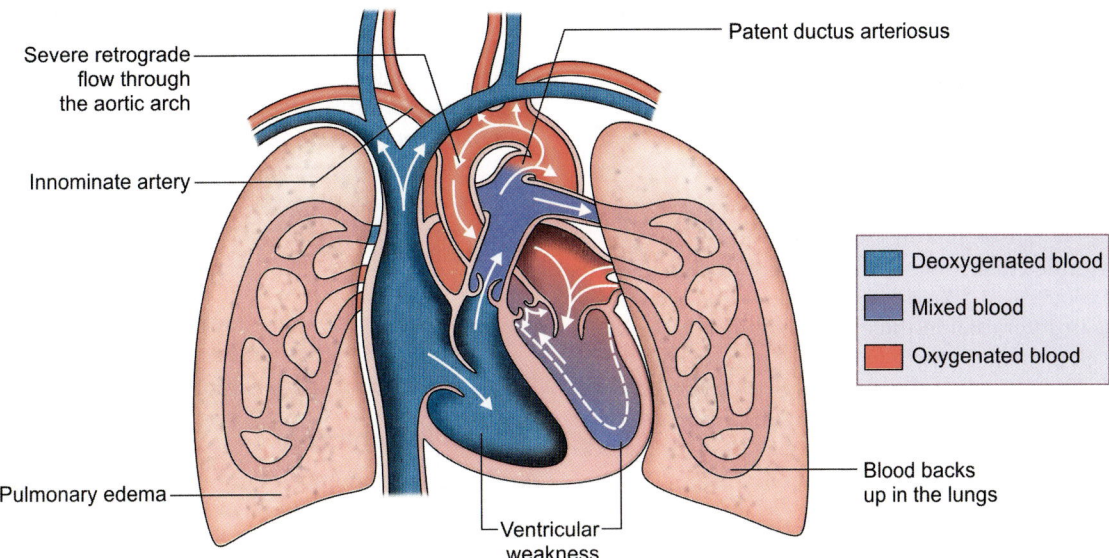

Fig. 1.64: Pathophysiology of PDA (arrows indicate direction of blood flow)

Pathophysiology (Fig. 1.64)

In fetal life from 6th weeks onwards, the ductus is responsible for most of the right ventricular outflow—contributing 60% of total cardiac output, supplying most of the fetal organs; only 5–10% of blood will go to lungs.

The patency of the ductus is promoted by PGE_2 produced by ductus itself. So prostaglandin antagonists, like NSAIDs, close the ductus and responsible for right-sided heart failure.

Just after birth, ductus arteriosus closes. So if the ductus will be patent, it produces left-to-right shunt.

So, large amount of blood will flow from systemic to pulmonary circulation producing pulmonary vascular engorgement and decrease in pulmonary compliance.

Magnitude of excess pulmonary blood flow depends on following factors:
  i. Larger the internal diameter of most narrow portion of ductus, larger the left-to-right shunt.
 ii. If the length of the narrow area is large, it decreases the magnitude of the shunt.
iii. Ratio of pulmonary vascular resistance to systemic vascular resistance (SVR):
   a. If ratio is larger—the flow will larger.
   b. If ratio is higher—the flow will lower.

The Pathways of Flow in PDA (Fig. 1.65)

PDA → pulmonary arteries → pulmonary capillaries → pulmonary vein → left atrium → left ventricle → aorta → PDA.

So in case of large left to right heart shunt, there is dilatation of pulmonary vein, left atrium, left ventricle, ascending aorta → it ultimately produces pulmonary hypertension.

Functional and Anatomic Closure

A. In fetus: Since pulmonary circulation is non-functional, hence oxygen tension is low. So patency of ductus arteriosus is maintained by high level of prostaglandin E_2—produced in:
  i. Pulmonary circulation
 ii. High level produced by placenta
B. At birth:
  i. Placenta is removed, eliminates a major source of prostaglandin production.

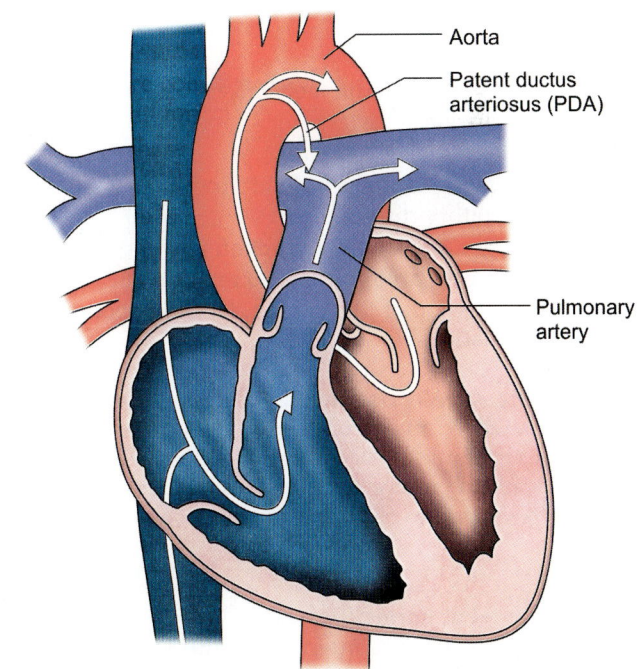

Fig. 1.65: Pathways of PDA

 ii. As the lung expands, activates the organ in which most prostaglandins are mobilized.
iii. With the onset of normal respiration, oxygen tension becomes normal in the blood.
 iv. Pulmonary vascular resistance will be decreased.
C. Closure of ductus: It occurs about 15 hours of life at term. It occurs due to:
  i. Abrupt closure of muscular wall
 ii. Increased partial pressure of oxygen
   So there is shift of blood flow occurs—blood moves directly from the right ventricle into lungs, away from ductus arteriosus.

Major factors responsible for relaxation of ductus:
1. High prostaglandin levels.
2. Hypoxemia
3. Nitric oxide production in ductus.

Major factors responsible for contraction of ductus:
1. Decreased prostaglandin levels
2. Increased oxygen tension
3. Increased endothelin-1
4. Acetylcholine
5. Norepinephrine
6. Bradykinin
7. Decreased prostaglandin E receptors

D. **True anatomic closure:** In this condition, ductus loses its ability to reopen—it takes several weeks—this occurs due to fibrous proliferation of the intima within 2–3 weeks.

If PDA is untreated, there is gradual increase in PVR—as a result, there is reversal of blood flow from left-to-right shunt to right-to-left shunt—producing 'Eisenmenger syndrome'. At this stage, correction of PDA is contraindicated as PVR is irreversible.

Failure of Ductus Arteriosus Contraction

a. Failure of ductus arteriosus contraction in neonates—due to poor prostaglandin metabolism because of immature lungs.
b. In full term neonates:
   1. Failure of prostaglandin metabolism due to:
      i. Hypoxemia
      ii. Asphyxia
      iii. Increased pulmonary blood flow
      iv. Respiratory disorders
   2. **Cyclooxygenase (Cox-2) induction and expression**
   3. **Activation of G protein-coupled receptors EP$_4$ by PGE$_2$.**
   Further progression of this disease depends upon volume and pressure relationship.

Volume = pressure/resistance: So high volume of blood produces increased pulmonary artery pressure, resulting endothelial and muscular changes in the vessel wall—this ultimately leads to pulmonary vascular obstructive disease—producing resistance to pulmonary blood flow.

Etiology

1. **Chromosomal abnormalities:**
   i. Congenital rubella infection in the 1st trimester of pregnancy, in 4th week of gestation.
   ii. Fetal alcohol syndrome.
   iii. Maternal amphetamine use
   iv. Maternal phenytoin use
2. Prematurity of infant at the time of delivery—the factors involved:
   i. Immaturity of smooth muscle within the structure
   ii. Inability of the immature lungs to clear the circulating prostaglandin.
3. Low oxygen tension in the blood: The factors are:
   i. Immature lungs
   ii. Co-existing congenital heart defect
   iii. High attitude
4. Other causes: Low birth weight.

Prognosis

1. If PDA closes—no further symptom develops and no further cardiac sequelae.

2. In premature infant with PDA—patient develops broncho-pulmonary dysplasia.
3. Spontaneous closure in older than 3 months is rare.
4. In adult, prognosis depends upon:
   i. The condition of pulmonary vasculature.
   ii. The status of myocardium, if congestive cardiomyopathy was present before ductal closure.

Morbidity

It is directly related to—flow volume through ductus arteriosus. In case of large patient ductus arteriosus, patient develops:
   i. Congestive cardiac failure.
   ii. Pulmonary hypertension.

Clinical Presentation

A. **Premature neonate** may develop life-threatening pulmonary overcirculation in 1st a few days of life; it depends on following factors:
   1. Size of patent ductus arteriosus
   2. Gestational age of the neonates
   3. Pulmonary vascular resistance
B. **Symptoms:**
   1. May be asymptomatic
   2. Decreased exercise tolerance
   3. Pulmonary congestion
   4. Three to six weeks old infant may present with:
      a. Tachypnea
      b. Diaphoresis
      c. Inability or difficulty in feeding
      d. Weight loss or no weight gain.
   5. In case of moderate to large left-to-right heart shunt:
      a. Hoarse cry
      b. Cough
      c. Lower respiratory tract infection
      d. Pneumonia
   6. With large defect
      a. History of feeding difficulties
      b. Poor growth during infancy
      c. Failure to thrive
      d. Symptoms of congestive cardiac failure
   7. In adult with undiagnosed PDA—they may present with:
      a. Symptoms of heart failure
      b. Atrial arrhythmia
      c. Differential cyanosis limited to lower extremities—it indicates shunting of deoxygenated blood from pulmonary to systemic circulation.
C. **Physical examinations:**
   1. *General examination:*
      a. Normal respiration
      b. Heart rate—normal
      c. Pulse pressure—widened
      d. Suprasternal pulsation—prominent
      e. Carotid pulsation—prominent
      f. Growth—stunted
      In case of pulmonary over circulation:
      a. Tachycardia
      b. Tachypnea
      c. Wide pulse pressure

2. *Cardiac assessment:*
   - *In case of neonates*—systolic murmur rather than continuous murmur in the first week of life mimicking benign systolic murmur.
   - *In adult, the cardiac findings are:*
     i. If left-to-right heart shunt is large—precordial activity is increased.
     ii. Apical impulse—displaced laterally
     iii. Thrill may be present in suprasternal notch or in left infraclavicular region.
     iv. First heart sound is normal
     v. Second heart sound is paradoxically split—due to:
        a. Premature closure of the pulmonary valve
        b. Prolonged ejection period across the aortic valve.
     vi. Murmur—it may be ejection systolic murmur or crescendo–decrescendo systolic murmur extending into diastole.
     vii. On auscultation—there may be numerous clicks or noises resembling bag of rocks.
        In 1898, Gibson described this classic murmur as machinery murmur—it is continuous, accentuated in systole, loudest at left upper chest.
     viii. If PVR: SVR is 2:1, there is apical flow rumble—due to high flow into the left ventricle.
   - *If the PDA is small*, amplitude of the murmur may be increased with inspiration (Fig. 1.66).

Diagnostic Workup

Electrocardiography

1. **With small PDA**—ECG is usually normal.
2. **With large PDA:**
   i. Left ventricular hypertrophy
   ii. Left atrial hypertrophy
   iii. In presence of pulmonary hypertension, there may be right ventricular hypertrophy.
3. **In neonates**, if premature with large PDA—T inversion with ST segment depression—due to:
   i. Increased myocardial work due to left-to-right shunt.
   ii. Pulmonary overcirculation in the face of low aortic and coronary diastolic blood pressure.

Chest Radiography

1. **In case of small PDA**—chest X-ray is usually normal.
2. **In case of large PDA**—there is enlargement of:
   i. Pulmonary arteries
   ii. Pulmonary veins
   iii. Left atrium
   iv. Left ventricle
   v. Ascending aorta
3. **In case pulmonary blood flow:**
   i. If pulmonary artery pressure and flow are increased—there is prominent pulmonary artery segment.
   ii. If marked pulmonary overcirculation—pulmonary edema may occur; accentuated peripheral pulmonary vascular markings, increased pulmonary venous markings.
4. **In case of elder individual**—calcified PDA

Echocardiography

a. **2D echocardiography:**
   i. Left atrial enlargement
   ii. Left ventricular enlargement. But imaging of the ductus itself is very difficult to detect.
b. **Color flow Doppler study:** It reveals continuous high velocity flow through pulmonary artery neon left breach (Figs 1.67 and 1.68).
   i. Aortic end of the ductus is localized first, followed by tracking back to find its other end in pulmonary trunk.
   ii. It can detect size, shape and coarse of the patent ductus arteriosus.

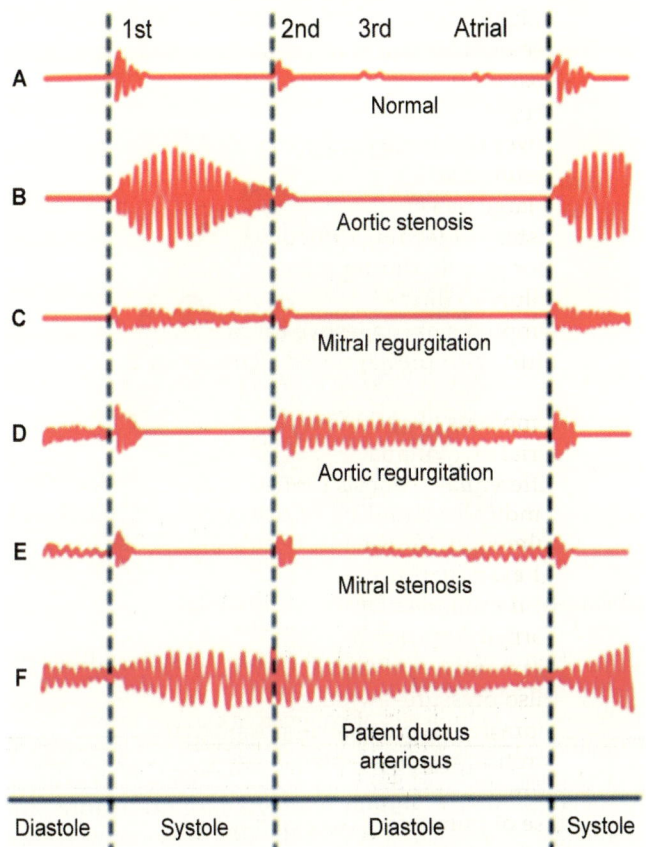

Fig. 1.66: Phonocardiograms from normal and abnormal heart sounds

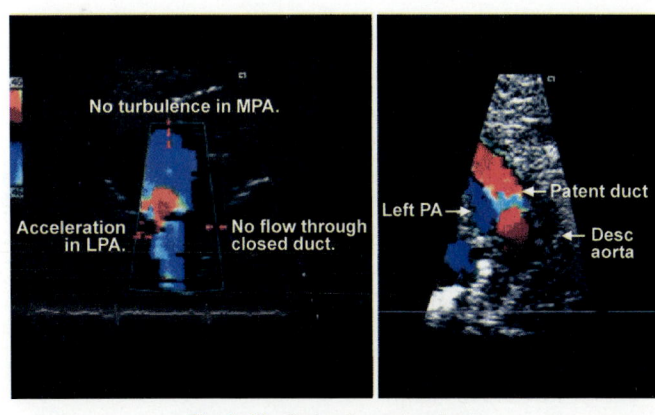

Fig. 1.67: Color-Doppler study

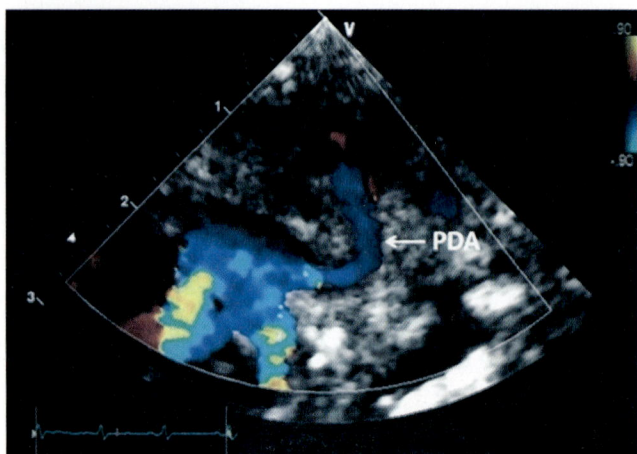

Fig. 1.68: Color-Doppler study

iii. Flow type is retrograde. It can differentiate aorto-pulmonary window, where the flow is retrograde.

Cardiac Catheterization

a. Right heart catheterization:
   i. Measures the pulmonary artery pressure
   ii. Measures pulmonary vascular resistance
   iii. Measures the flow ratio (Q_p–Q_s)
   iv. Oxygen step in the main pulmonary artery distal to ductus
   v. Catheter can be pushed through patent ductus into descending aorta.
   vi. Other co-existing cardiac abnormalities.
b. Selective angiography: It detects:
   i. Presence and size of the ductus.
   ii. Intracardiac anatomy whether any defect.

Histological Features in Severe Cases

i. The wall of ductus is composed of intima, media and adventitia.
ii. Medial layer is composed of:
   1. Longitudinal smooth muscle cells in the inner layer
   2. Circular muscle cells in outer layer.

Management

Conservative Management

A. Asymptomatic patient with patent ductus arteriosus:
   i. Administration of antibiotics during any instance of high exposure to bacteremia (instrumentation, dental extraction).
   ii. PDA closure at a suitable time.
   iii. Conservative standards include:
      a. Fluid restriction to 130 ml/kg/day beyond day 3.
      b. Adaptation of ventilation—by lowering of respiratory time and providing more positive pressure.
B. Infants presenting with congestive heart failure:
   i. Digoxin therapy
   ii. Diuretic therapy
   iii. Need surgical closure when:
      a. They are several years old and good candidates for ductal closure
      b. 'If medical treatment fails—urgent closure

Pharmacologic Management

1. Indomethacin:
   i. Intravenous indomethacin is efficacious in closure of PDA in premature infants. The duct may reopen days or weeks later.
   ii. Adverse effects: It has adverse renal effects, because renal perfusion and diuresis in early neonatal life are strongly influenced by circulating prostaglandin—it has dilating effect on renal afferent arteriole.
2. Ibuprofen:
   i. PDA closure is gestation dependent, cumulative closure rate being 65%. Prophylactic ibuprofen is used throughout the world.
   ii. Dose is 10 mg/kg bolus followed by 5 mg/kg for 2 additional days.
   iii. It has no oliguric effect on premature infants.

Indications for Surgery

i. Asymptomatic patient with mildly elevated pulmonary vascular resistance (<4 units)—result of operation is good.
ii. Infant with refractory CCF.

Methods of Surgical Closure

1. Gianturco spring occluding cells: It is most commonly used.
2. Amplatzer duct occluder: It is usually used for large defect. Major disadvantage is that aortic part of the device can protrude into the descending aorta partly obstructing the lumen.
3. Rashkind ductus occlusion device (Fig. 1.69): It is used either through transvenous or transarterial pathway.

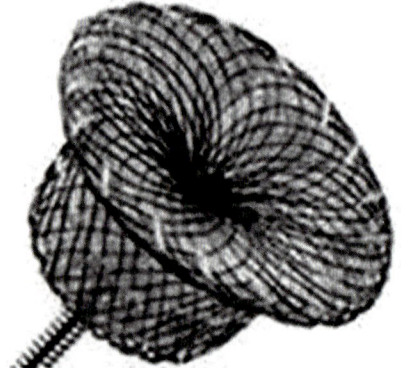

Fig. 1.69: Rashkind ductus occlusion device

Indications for surgical treatment include:
   i. Failure of indomethacin treatment.
   ii. Contraindication to medical therapy (renal insufficiency, thrombocytopenia).
   iii. Signs and symptoms of congestive cardiac failure.
   iv. In older infant with PDA.
   v. In infant found to have an asymptomatic PDA after the neonatal period, should undergo surgical ligation after the age of 1 year to prevent the development of complication.
   vi. To prevent cardiovascular complications like, subacute bacterial endocarditis, pulmonary hypertension.

Contraindications:
1. Pulmonary vascular disease—it is primary contraindications:
   a. Pulmonary artery hypoplasia
   b. Pulmonary atresia
2. Aortic valve stenosis
3. Mitral valve atresia with hypoplastic left ventricle
4. Severe coarctation of the aorta
5. Tricuspid atresia
6. Transposition of great vessels
7. Sepsis.
8. Inability of the patient to tolerate general anesthesia

Complications of Untreated PDA

1. Bacterial endocarditis
2. Late congestive cardiac failure
3. Pulmonary vascular obstructive disease
4. Circulatory or ventilator abnormalities:
   i. Aortic rupture
   ii. Eisenmenger physiology
   iii. Left heart failure
   iv. Myocardial ischemia
   v. Necrotizing enterocolitis
   vi. Pulmonary hypertension
   vii. Right heart failure

Complications of Surgical Treatment

i. Injury to the aorta
ii. Pulmonary artery injury
iii. Complications related to left lateral thoracotomy

Prognosis

a. If PDA is repaired after childhood, mortality and morbidity depend upon:
   i. Degree of pulmonary hypertension
   ii. Left ventricular overload
   iii. Calcification of the ductus

b. In the group of severe pulmonary vascular resistance (>10 MPa-s/m³), survival is poor.
c. If there is aneurysmal dilatation of ductus—there may be complication during surgery.

PULMONARY STENOSIS

Pulmonic stenosis is a congenital stenosis in 90% of cases. It is of three types:
1. Subvalvular lesions due to infundibular hypertrophy
2. Supravalvular (rare intracardiac tumors, congenital rubella syndrome).
3. Valvular lesions (Fig. 1.70):
   i. Due to fibrosis of the valve with thickening of leaflets—these leaflets dome into pulmonary trunk during systole, producing narrowing of central aperture.
   ii. Valvular leaflets are dysplastic and rubbery.
   iii. Bicuspid pulmonic valves
   iv. It may be associated phenomena in different congenital syndrome:
       a. Fallot's tetralogy (due to bicuspid pulmonary valve)
       b. Noonan syndrome
       c. Double outlet right ventricle
       d. Atrioventricular canal defect
       e. Leopard syndrome

Acquired causes of pulmonary valvular stenosis:
a. Carcinoid syndrome due to deposition of carcinoid plaque on the leaflets
b. Rheumatic

Symptoms

a. Patient is usually asymptomatic.
b. Symptoms of pulmonary valvular stenosis:
   i. History of heart murmur since birth.
   ii. Cyanosis
   iii. Dyspnea
   iv. Fatigue

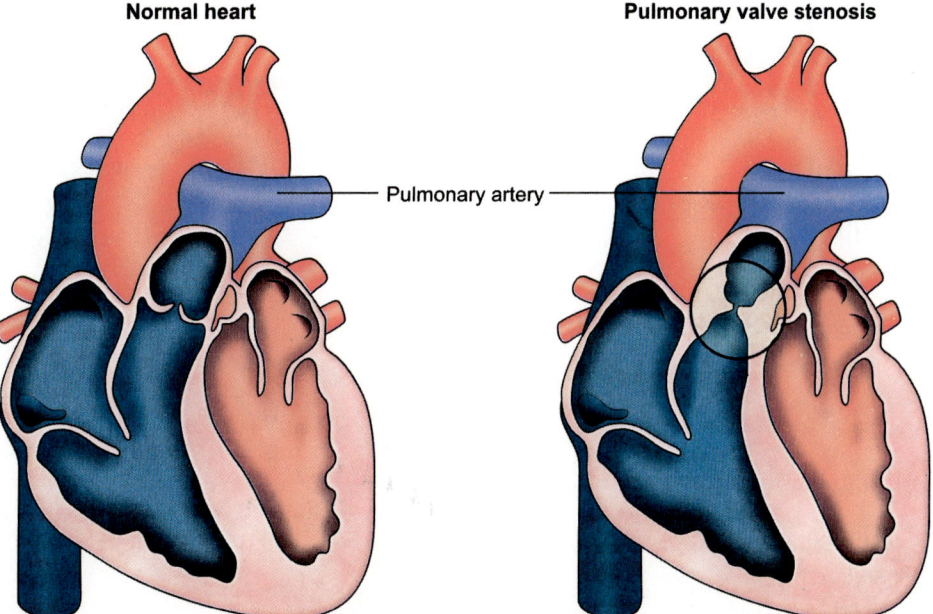

Fig. 1.70: Valvular aortic stenosis

v. Dizziness
vi. Syncope
vii. Chest pain
viii. Mental retardation or developmental disorder.

Signs

a. Jugular venous waveform—prominent jugular venous "a" wave in the setting of relatively normal central venous pressure.
b. Cyanosis
c. Tachycardia
d. Cardiovascular examination:
   i. Pulmonary component of 2nd heart sound is soft and split according to severity of stenosis.
   ii. Fourth heart sound is frequently appreciated in the left sternal border.
   iii. High frequency systolic click in upper left sternal border precedes the pulmonary systolic murmur, click becomes softer during inspiration due to enhanced late diastolic pulmonary valve opening with increase right ventricular filling.
   iv. There is palpable thrill in pulmonary area.
   v. Right ventricular impulse in left lower sternal border.
   vi. Grade 5/6 systolic ejection (crescendo–decrescendo) murmur audible at left upper sternal border, transmitting into the back and posterior lung fields.

The murmur is best heard in left 1st to 3rd intercostal spaces—it usually does not radiate to left sternal border.

Severity of murmur can be determined by (Fig. 1.71):
   i. Duration of murmur
   ii. Intensity of murmur

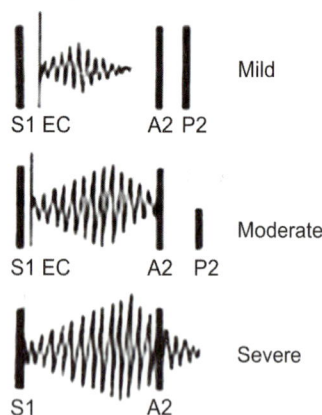

Fig. 1.71: Murmur of pulmonary stenosis

In severe stenosis:
   i. Murmur extends into diastole (beyond the 2nd heart sound)
   ii. Features of tricuspid regurgitation
   iii. Hepatosplenomegaly
   iv. Pulsatile liver
   v. Jugular venous pulsations
   vi. Hepatojugular reflux

Laboratory Workup

Oxymetry provides—information regarding right-to-left heart stenosis in borderline cyanotic lesion or in patients with anemia.

Imaging Studies

1. **Chest radiography:** It demonstrates (Figs 1.72 and 1.73):
   i. Prominent main pulmonary artery with normal heart size.
   ii. Pulmonary vascular sizes are usually normal, but may be decreased in severe pulmonary valvular stenosis.
   iii. In severe pulmonary valvular stenosis—cardiomegaly with right ventricular and right atrial enlargement.
2. **Electrocardiography:**
   i. Different degrees of right ventricular hypertrophy and deep 'S' wave in left (precordial leads and prominent 'R' in right precordial leads).
   ii. Right axis deviation with right ventricular hypertrophy—seen in moderate pulmonary valvular stenosis.

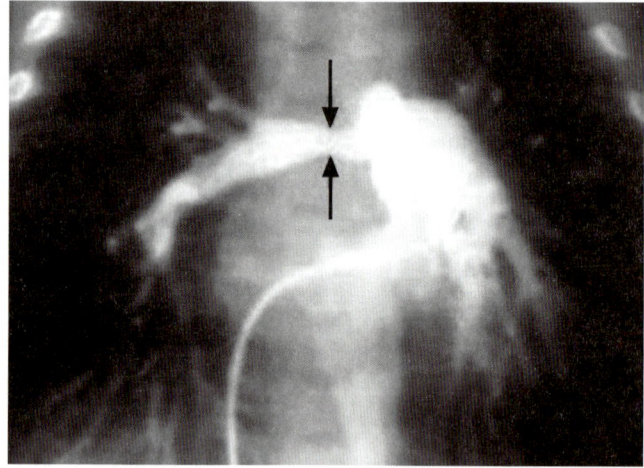

Fig. 1.72: Supravalvular pulmonary stenosis

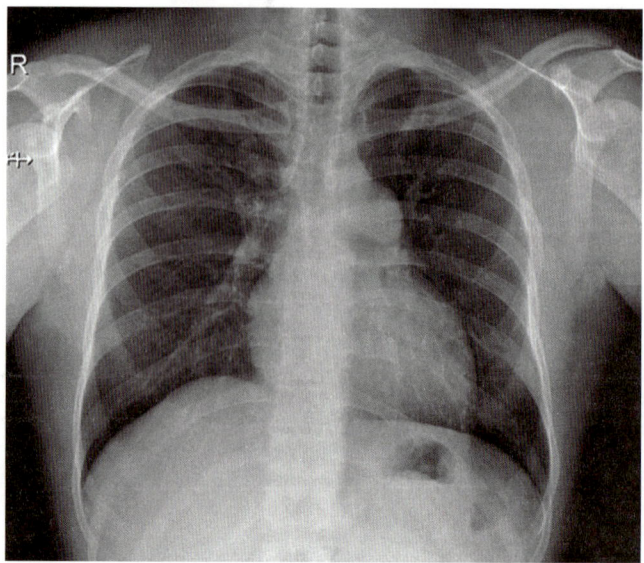

Fig. 1.73: Subvalvular pulmonary stenosis

iii. Tall 'R' wave in V1 >10 mm suggests severe stenosis.
iv. Increased incidence of arrhythmias.
v. Evidence of 'P' pulmonale in inferior leads (II, III, and aVF)

3. **Echocardiography** (Fig. 1.74):
   i. It detects sites of obstruction and other possible congenital abnormalities.
   ii. Thickened pulmonary valve with restricted systolic motion—called doming.
   iii. Main pulmonary artery distal to stenotic orifice is dilated.

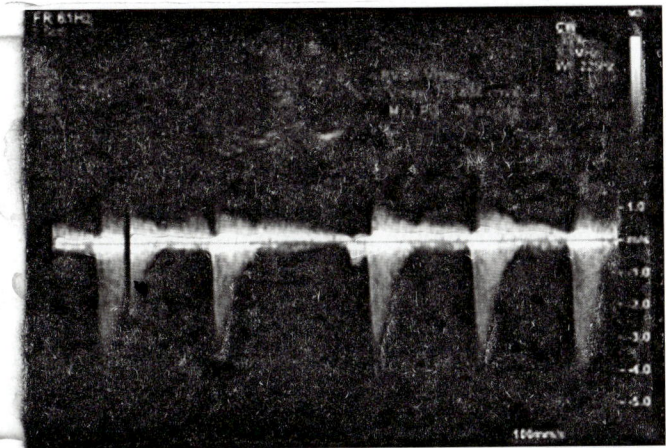

Fig. 1.74: Echocardiography of pulmonary stenosis

4. **Doppler echocardiography** (Fig. 1.75):
   i. It measures peak systolic gradients across the pulmonary valve—indicates disease severity.
   Gradient is calculated from 4 times the peak systolic velocity squared.
   $$\text{Pressure gradient} = 4 \times V^2$$
   ii. Multiple views and measurements increase the accuracy of the predicted peak systolic pressure gradient.

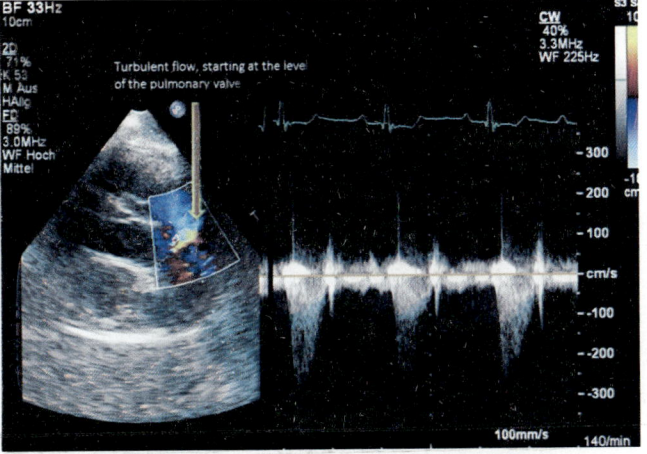

Fig. 1.75: Doppler study of pulmonary stenosis

5. **Cardiac catheterization**
   Indications:
   i. Where pulmonary stenosis is not properly evaluated by echocardiography.

ii. Cardiac catheterization with balloon valvoplasty is indicated, if pulmonary valvular pressure gradient is >50 mmHg.
iii. It can detect valvular pressure gradient, if the Doppler peak jet velocity is >3 meter per second and balloon valvoplasty infeasible.

Management

A. **Prehospital care:** If patient has large left-to-right shunt—and has respiratory distress:
   i. Diuresis to reduce cyanosis and pulmonary edema.
   ii. Use of oxygen to reduce pulmonary artery pressure in patients with reactive pulmonary vasculature and thus increasing pulmonary blood flow.

B. **Emergency department care:**
   i. Severe stenosis, peak gradient of 60 mmHg, emergency dilatation of valves by balloon valvotomy.
   ii. Patients with mild pulmonary valvular stenosis, usually do not require treatment.
   iii. Patients with severe or symptomatic infundibular, or supravalvular pulmonary stenosis require prompt intervention—valvotomy.
   iv. Cyanotic patients with respiratory distress and hypotensive shock—undergo workup of septic patients.
   v. Bacterial endocarditis prophylaxis.
   vi. Patients with severe dysplastic valves may not respond to balloon valvoplasty, may require valve replacement with porcine valve or pulmonary homograft.

CONGENITALLY CORRECTED TRANSPOSITION

Definition

It is a rare congenital heart defect associated with multiple cardiac morphological abnormalities and conduction defect.

Pathophysiology (Fig. 1.76)

During embryological development:
   i. Left-handed looping of the heart tube results in atrioventricular discordance.
   ii. Aortopulmonary septum fails to rotate 180° producing ventriculoarterial discordance.

As a result, the circulation will be in following direction:
Venus blood from all body areas enters into right atrium passes through mitral valve into left ventricle. From left ventricle, blood enters the lung via pulmonic valve into main pulmonary artery.

After circulation through lungs, blood flows into left atrium, then blood passes from left atrium through tricuspid valve into right ventricle from where it enters aorta through aortic valve.

Since aorta is anterior as well as to the left of pulmonary artery, hence ventricles are transposed.

Epidemiology

1. Ten years–survival rate ranges from 64–83% from the time of diagnosis—it depends on associated abnormalities.
2. Medium age of death is 40 years whether operated or not.

History

   i. Usually the patient is asymptomatic in early life—during this time it can be diagnosed by electrocardiography or chest X-ray—which may be done for other causes.

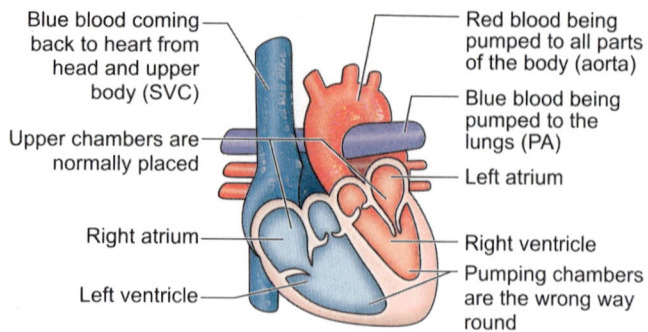

Blue blood coming back to heart from head and upper body (SVC)

Red blood being pumped to all parts of the body (aorta)

Upper chambers are normally placed

Blue blood being pumped to the lungs (PA)

Left atrium

Right atrium

Right ventricle

Left ventricle

Pumping chambers are the wrong way round

Fig.1.76: Pathophysiology in congenitally corrected transposition

ii. The patient is usually diagnosed late in childhood or in early adult life, during this time patients present with features of complete heart block or features of heart failure due to right heart decompensation or systemic tricuspid regurgitation.

iii. Most common presenting features are:
   a. Bradycardia—due to high degree AV block
   b. Single second heart sound heard left of sternum due to anteriorly positioned aortic valve.
   c. Heart murmur related to ventricular septal defect, pulmonary stenosis or tricuspid regurgitation.
   d. Cyanosis
   e. Heart failure
   f. Tachycardia

Associated Cardiac Abnormalities

1. Atrial situs—Atria is situs solitus:
2. Ventricular septal defect—it is most common. Defect is perimembranous, tends to be subpulmonary. Here, shunt is left to right.
3. Conduction system abnormalities—normal AV node cannot give rise to AV bundle.
   Here anomalous AV node is functional. AV conduction system is generally located beneath the opening of the right atrial appendages at the lateral margin between the pulmonic valve and mitral valve. So the node has an anterior position and gives rise to AV bundle immediately underneath the right anterior pulmonary valve leaflet. This accessory node may be hypoplastic or non-functional. Conduction disturbances may be:
   i. Complete heart block
   ii. Sick sinus syndrome
   iii. Atrial flutter
   iv. Reentrant AV tachycardia
   v. Ventricular tachycardia.
4. Coronary anatomy: Early entrapment of coronaries in fat or myocardium.
   a. Left ventricular outflow tract obstruction
   b. Coarctation of aorta
   c. Interruption of aortic arch
   d. Hypoplastic of one ventricle
   e. Abnormal tricuspid valve morphology.

Physical Findings

i. Hyperdynamic precordium due to large left-to-right shunt and consequent cardiac enlargement.
ii. In case of pulmonic stenosis, quiet precordium associated with cyanosis.

iii. Loud palpable single 2nd sound—heard at left sternal border—due to anterior and left ward position aorta.
iv. Systolic murmur of left AV (tricuspid) valve may confuse with murmur of ventricular septal defect—since it is heard at left lower sternal border rather than its apex.
v. Murmur of pulmonary stenosis is often heard at the pulmonary area—loudest in aortic area—due to interior and posterior displacement of pulmonary valve.

Laboratory Studies

Hematology

i. Complete blood count—raised MCV, hematocrit, hemoglobin, ESR low.
ii. Renal function test.
iii. Serum ferritin.
iv. Serum uric acid.

Imaging Studies

i. **Echocardiography** in utero or transthoracic or transesophageal imaging to confirm diagnosis.
ii. **Chest radiography** reveals (Fig. 1.77):
   a. Parallel blood vessels.
   b. Upper left border is formed by the aorta and appeared to straight.
   c. Pulmonary artery knob is absent because this artery is displaced posteriorly and rightward.
iii. **Transesophageal echocardiography** is required to assess:
   a. Ventricular function
   b. Atrioventricular valve regurgitation
   c. Pulmonary outflow tract
iv. **Truckar cardiology**—assesses ventricular function.
v. **Radionuclide angiography** better assesses right ventricular function.
vi. **Cardiac MRI** evaluates:
   a. Ventricular volumes
   b. Ventricular function
   c. Valvular function
   d. Conduit function

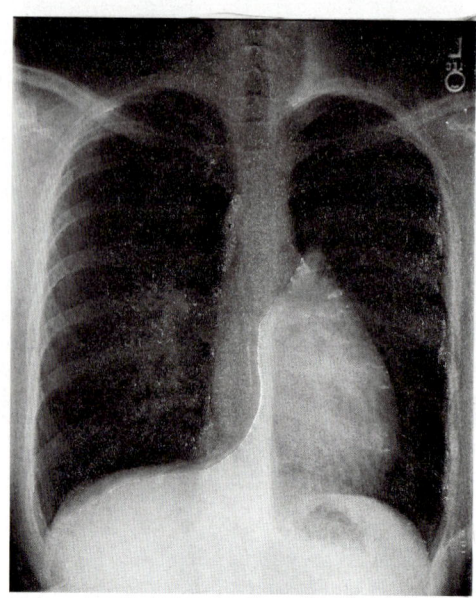

Fig. 1.77: Chest X-ray

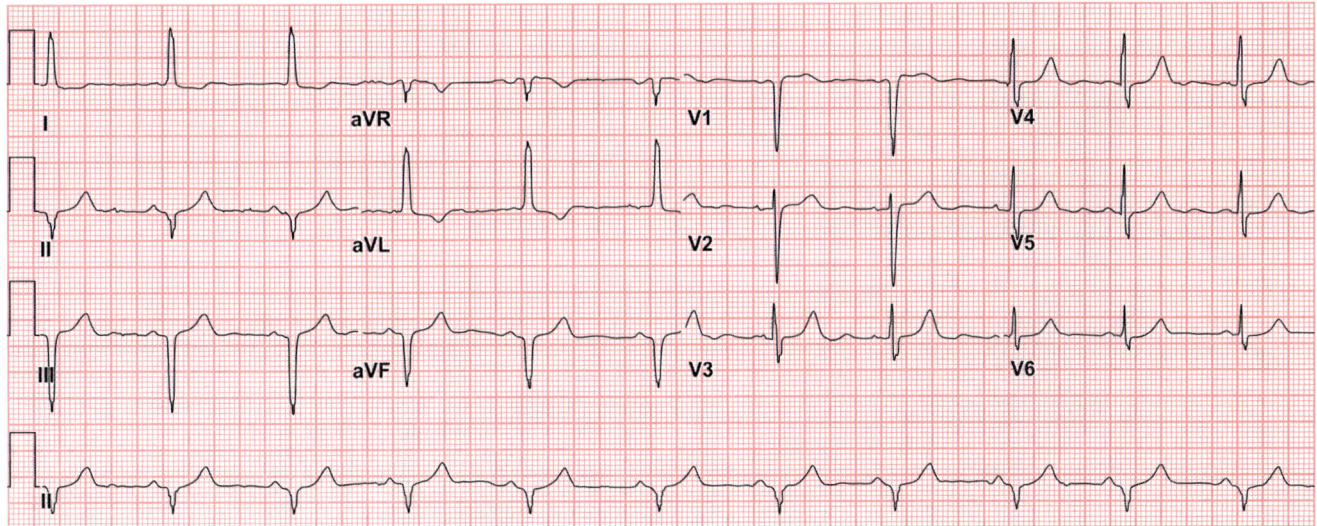

Fig. 1.78: ECG

viii. Electrocardiography (Fig. 1.78): It detects:
  a. AV block b. Atrial arrhythmias
  c. Abnormal initial ventricular activation due to disordered anatomy of conduction system.
  Due to ventricular inversion, ventricular bundle branches are also inverted. As a result, initial activation is oriented from right to left.
  The net result is as shown in ECG readings: Reversions of Q wave pattern seen in precordial leads, i.e. Q waves are present in right precordial leads but absent in left precordial leads.
viii. 24 to 72 hours Holter monitoring—to detect AV block or arrhythmias.
  ix. Cardiac catheterization:
  a. It is a risky procedure, because it induces transient or complete heart block since conduction system has just below pulmonary valve.
  b. Always balloon-tipped catheter should be introduced through pulmonary valve.
  c. It is used to assess the grade of pulmonary stenosis, shunt volume, pulmonary vascular resistance before and in response to therapy.

Treatment

Medical Treatment

a. Antibiotic prophylaxis is indicated according to the recommendation of American Heart Association.
b. Management of heart failure by diuretics, beta-blockers, angiotensin-converting enzyme inhibitors. This treatment does not improve the mortality.
c. Caution should be taken during administration of beta-blockers, because it may precipitate complete heart block in these patients with known conduction system abnormalities.

Surgical Treatment

  i. This treatment is recommended in symptomatic patients with associated other lesions, whose correction can symptomatically benefit the patient.
  ii. Right coronary artery divides into anterior descending and circumflex branches supplying morphological left

ventricle. So placement of conduit in these patients to relieve pulmonary stenosis may produce complication.
  iii. Correction of ventricular septal defect, if the patient is symptomatic—failure to thrive, fall to respond to medical therapy or if the pulmonary vascular pressure is progressively increasing.
  But it may exacerbate symptomatic AV valve regurgitation due to:
  a. Septal shift
  b. Distortion of AV valve annulus
  iv. In case of grade 2/4 tricuspid regurgitation, tricuspid valve must be replaced.
  v. Early pacemaker replacement is recommended in the setting of complete heart block either during or after surgical intervention or in case of any associated defects:
  a. Cardiomegaly
  b. Decreased right ventricular function
  c. Symptomatic bradycardia
  d. Heart failure

EISENMENGER SYNDROME

Definition

It refers to untreated congenital cardiac defect with intracardiac communications, which leads to pulmonary hypertension, reversal of flow and cyanosis (Fig. 1.79). Lesions in Eisenmenger syndrome, like large septal defects, are—high pulmonary artery pressure or increased pulmonary flow. It indicates:
  i. Pulmonary hypertension is irreversible.
  ii. Cardiac lesions are likely inoperable.
The congenital cardiac defects are:
  i. Ventricular septal defect
  ii. Atrioventricular canal defect
  iii. Atrial septal defect—ostium primum type
  iv. Aortopulmonary window
  v. Patent ductus arteriosus.

Pulmonary arterial hypertension: This can be defined as mean pulmonary artery pressure of more than 25 mmHg at rest or more than 30 mmHg during exercise.

Eisenmenger syndrome

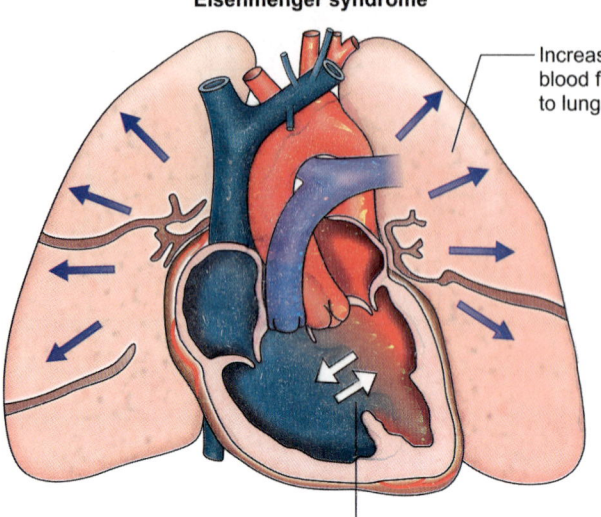

Fig. 1.79: Anatomical defect

Epidemiology

Eisenmenger syndrome usually develops before puberty, but it may occur in adolescence or in early adulthood.

Pathophysiology

This occurs in patients with large congenital cardiac or surgically created extracardiac left-to-right shunt. This type of shunt increases pulmonary blood flow.

According to Ohms Low

Blood flow (Q) is inversely related to resistance (R) of the arterial wall and directly related to pressure, i.e.

$$Q = \frac{P}{R}$$

So if blood flow through pulmonary artery increases, there is increase in pulmonary arterial pressure.

On the other hand, if pulmonary vascular resistance increases, as occurs in pulmonary vascular obstructive diseases, blood flow through the pulmonary artery decreases. There are spectrum of morphological and histological changes seen in pulmonary vasculature—which are reversible at first, but on progression it will become irreversible.

The histological changes are—inflammation, cellular proliferation, vasoconstriction and fibrosis.

Causes of Eisenmenger Syndrome

1. Non-restrictive patent ductus arteriosus
2. Large uncorrected cardiac shunt
3. Surgically created systemic pulmonary shunt for congenital heart disease.
4. Large non-restrictive VSD
5. Atrioventricular septal defect mainly large ostium primum ASD without any ventricular component
6. Aortopulmonary window.

Prognosis

1. Eisenmenger syndrome is uniformly fatal with life expectancy of 20–50 years, if the syndrome is diagnosed promptly and treated intensively.

2. This syndrome affects multiple organ systems in the body:
   i. Hematologic
   ii. Renal
   iii. Skeletal
   iv. Neurologic
3. Poor prognosis can be predicted by:
   i. Hypoxemia
   ii. Syncope
   iii. Elevated right-sided pressures.

Table 1.2: Occurrence of Eisenmenger syndrome

Parent disease	Duration of development	Percentage
1. Large non-restrictive VSD or PDA	Early childhood	50%
2. VSD, PDA or transposition of GV	1st year of life	40%
3. Large secundum ASD	Third decade of life	10%
4. Persistant truncus arteriosus with unrestricted pulmonary flow	2nd year of life	100%
5. Common atrio-ventricular canal	2nd year of life	100%
6. Surgically created SP shunt	Depends on size and anatomy	
7. Blalock-Taussig anastomosis	Not known	10%

Complications of Eisenmenger Syndrome

1. Hematologic—hyperviscosity syndrome secondary to secondary erythrocytosis.
2. Nervous system:
   i. Brain abscess
   ii. Transient cerebral ischemia
   iii. Thrombotic stroke
   iv. Intracerebral hemorrhage.
3. Hepatic—hyperbilirubinemia—liable to development of gallstones.
4. Metabolic—hyperuricemia—may develop nephrolithiasis and secondary gout.
5. Skeletal—hypertrophic osteoarthropathy—produces bone pain and tenderness.
6. Eye—vision loss—related to peripheral retinal microvascular abnormalities.
7. Cardiac:
   i. Congestive cardiac failure
   ii. Dysrrhythmias
   iii. Infective endocarditis
   iv. Syncope—because, systemic vascular bed is prone to develop vasodilatation and subsequent arterial hypotension.
   v. Sudden death

Most common terminating events of this syndrome is combination of hypoxemia and arrhythmia in pulmonary vascular resistance or progressive decrease in systemic vascular resistance.

Death commonly results from:
  i. Congestive heart failure
 ii. Massive hemoptysis
iii. Thromboembolism

Physical Symptoms (Fig. 1.80)

The symptoms of Eisenmenger syndrome are related to pulmonary hypertension itself or various multisystem complications.

A. Symptoms related to pulmonary hypertension:
   i. Breathlessness
   ii. Fatigue
   iii. Lethargy
   iv. Presyncope
   v. Syncope
   vi. Exceptionally reduced exercise tolerance.
B. Symptoms related to heart failure:
   i. Exertional dyspnea
   ii. Orthopnea
   iii. Paroxysmal nocturnal dyspnea
   iv. Edema
   v. Anorexia
   vi. Ascites
C. Symptoms related to erythrocytosis:
   i. Myalgia
   ii. Muscle weakness
   iii. Anorexia
   iv. Fatigue
   v. Lassitude
   vi. Tinnitus
   vii. Blurred vision
   viii. Scotoma
   ix. Headache
   x. Dizziness
   xi. Slowed mentation
   xii. Irritability.
D. Symptoms of tendency toward bleeding:
   i. Mild mucocuteneous bleeding
   ii. Epistaxis
   iii. Menorrhagia
   iv. Pulmonary hemorrhage
E. Symptoms related to vasodilatation:
   i. Presyncope
   ii. Syncope
F. Symptoms of cholelithiasis:
   i. Right upper quadrant pain
   ii. Biliary colic
   iii. Fever
   iv. Pale stools
   v. Jaundice
G. Symptoms related to nephrolithiasis:
   i. Renal colic
   ii. Secondary gout
   iii. Painful swelling of the joints.
H. Other symptoms are:
   i. Symptoms related to localized vascular insufficiency and end organ ischemia—due to paradoxical embolus.
   ii. Bone pain and tenderness due to hypertrophic osteoarthropathy.

1. **In 1st week of life**—with large ASD, VSD or PDA, when pulmonary vascular resistance falls towards adult level, patient usually presents with congestive cardiac failure due to large left to right shunt—during this period, patient may present with poor weight gain.
2. **Infants** with large ASD, VSD or PDA maintains high pulmonary vascular resistance with left-to-right intracardiac shunting and less pulmonary blood flow. During

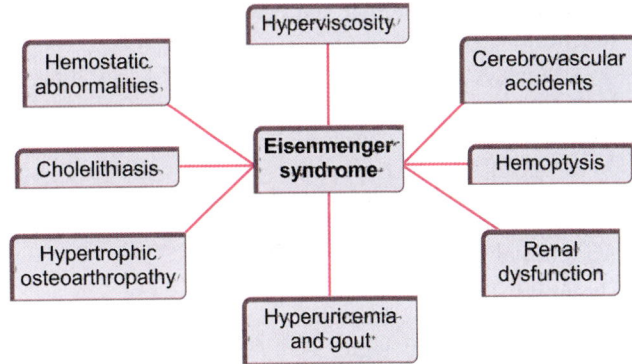

Fig. 1.80: Pathophysiology in Eisenmenger syndrome

this developing period of Eisenmenger syndrome, they are usually undetected because of lack of loud systolic murmur, and/or diastolic rumble and symptoms of heart failure.

During this time, clues to the diagnosis are:
   i. Exertional dyspnea
   ii. Exercise intolerance.

Physical Examinations

Cardiovascular Findings

   i. Central cyanosis, (differential cyanosis in case of PDA).
   ii. Clubbing (Fig. 1.81).
   iii. Jugular venous pulse shows:
      a. Dominant 'A' wave
      b. Prominent 'V' wave in case of tricuspid regurgitation
   iv. Elevated central venous pressure
   v. On precordial palpation:
      a. Left parasternal heave
      b. Palpable P2
   vi. On oscultation:
      a. Loud P2
      b. High-pitched early diastolic murmur of pulmonary regurgitation.
      c. Right-sided fourth heart sound
      d. Pulmonary ejection click
      e. Occasionally single S2.

With the progressive increase in pulmonary vascular resistance: Progressive shortening and softening of holosystolic murmur of VSD—firstly becoming early systolic followed by disappearance of murmur.

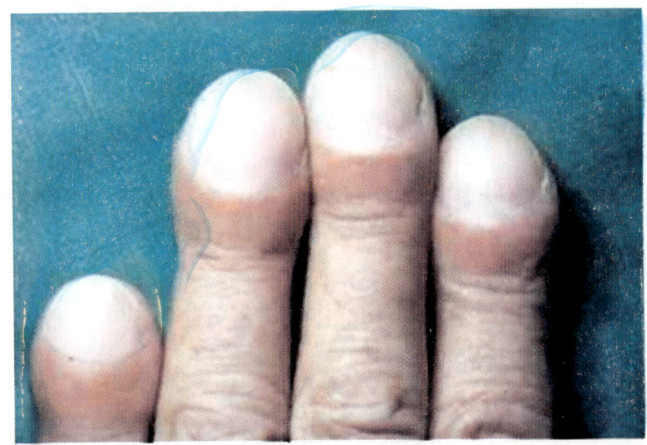

Fig. 1.81: Clubbing

Other signs of Eisenmenger syndrome include:
A. Respiratory signs:
   i. Cyanosis   ii. Tachypnea
B. Hematologic:
   i. Bruising
   ii. Bleeding
   iii. Other related fundoscopic findings—microaneurysm, papilledema, hemorrhages.
C. Abdominal signs:
   i. Jaundice
   ii. Right upper quadrant pain
   iii. Positive Murphy sign.
D. Vascular signs:
   i. Postural hypotension
   ii. Signs related to ischemia
E. Musculoskeletal signs:
   i. Clubbing
   ii. Tenderness of over metacarpal or metatarsal joints
   iii. Joint effusions
F. Cutaneous signs:
   i. Urate deposit—gouty topic
   ii. Different types of hemorrhages.
G. Ocular signs:
   i. Conjunctivitis
   ii. Rubeosis iridis
   iii. Symptoms related to hyperviscosity syndrome.

Clinical Signs in Progressing Disease

Examination findings vary according to the progression of the disease:
1. In infant, with large systemic to pulmonary communication and evidence of pulmonary over circulation, patient may present with signs or symptoms of heart failure, physical examinations show:
   a. Tachypnea   b. Tachycardia
   c. Nasal flaring   d. Chest retraction
   e. Grunting   f. Delayed capillary

   Auscultatory findings include:
   a. Hyperactive precordium
   b. Systolic flow murmur
   c. Diastolic rumble
   d. Hepatomegaly
2. As pulmonary vascular resistance increases, with gradual increase in pulmonary artery pressure, there is gradual decline in symptoms of congestive heart failure. But here, right ventricle becomes hypertrophied—producing left parasternal heave, palpable P2 and on auscultation, there is loud P2.
3. As pulmonary vascular resistance increases, left-to-right intracardiac shunts will be changed to bidirectional shunting followed by frank right-to-left heart shunting—when following symptoms and signs will occur:
   a. Central cyanosis
   b. Clubbing
   c. Polycythemia (ruddy appearance of the skin).

Laboratory Workup

A. Hematological investigations include:
   i. Raised hemoglobin and hematocrit due to erythrocytosis.
   ii. Increased red cell mass.
   iii. Bleeding time is raised due to platelet dysfunction.
B. Blood biochemistry shows:
   i. Raised bilirubin
   ii. Raised uric acid
   iii. Sometimes raised urea and creatinine
C. Urinalysis shows:
   i. Proteinuria.
   ii. Erythrocytic hypoglycemia—it means artifactually low blood glucose caused by increased in vitro glycolysis in presence of increased red cell mass.
D. Iron profile showed:
   i. Reduced serum ferrites level due to phlebotomy-related iron store reduction.
   ii. Increased iron binding capacity
E. Arterial blood gases:
   i. Reduced partial pressure of CO_2—due to resting tachypnea.
   ii. Reduced partial pressure of O_2—due to right-to-left heart shunting.
   iii. Mixed metabolic and respiratory acidosis.
F. Pulse oxymetry—cyanosis and decreased saturation.
G. Brain natriuretic peptide—it is the marker for prognosis in pulmonary hypertension.

Chest Radiography *(Fig. 1.82)*

A. In early stages:
   i. Typical appearance of increased pulmonary flow with right ventricular or biventricular enlargement.
   ii. Right or biatrial enlargement.
   iii. Pulmonary vascular plethora.
   iv. Enlarged main pulmonary artery.
B. In advancing pulmonary artery disease:
   i. Normal cardiac silhouette.
   ii. Dilated main pulmonary artery and its proximal branches.
   iii. No evidence of pulmonary over circulation.
C. In case of severe pulmonary disease:
   i. Normal size heart
   ii. Peripheral pruning pulmonary vasculature.
   iii. Pulmonary infarction.
   iv. Calcification of patent ductus arteriosus.

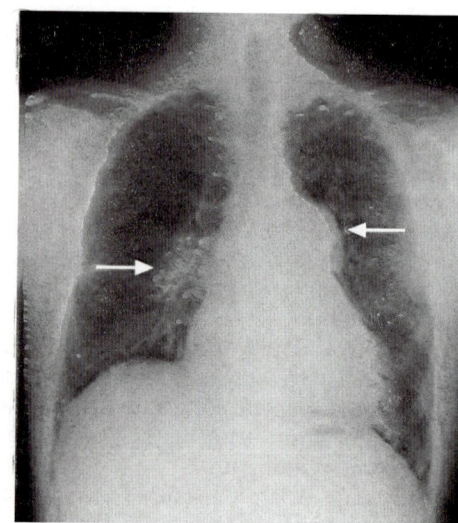

Fig. 1.82: Chest X-ray showing pulmonary vascular plethora

Magnetic Resonance Imaging

i. Estimation of magnitude of right-to-left heart shunt
ii. Anatomical delineation.

Echocardiography

A. Two-dimensional echocardiography reveals—structural abnormalities of heart or great vessels.
B. Color Doppler studies—demonstrate—direction of intra-cardiac blood flow.
C. Pulse and continuous wave Doppler measurement shows:
   i. Quantification of intracardiac shunt
   ii. Measurement of right ventricular pressure.
   iii. Estimation of pulmonary artery systolic/diastolic and mean pressure.

   Supine bicycle ergometry shows increased right-to-left shunting with exercise.

Electrocardiography

i. Evidence of right heart hypertrophy.
ii. Frontal plane QRS right axis deviation.
iii. Tall monophasic R wave in V_1, deep S wave in V_6, ± ST and T wave abnormalities.
iv. P pulmonale

Cardiac catheterization: It demonstrates the following:
i. Severity of pulmonary artery hypertension
ii. Patency of conduit and pressure gradient
iii. Co-existing coronary artery abnormalities
iv. Degree of shunting

Table 1.3: Difference between 6 minutes walk test versus cardiopulmonary exercise test

6 minutes walk test	Cardiopulmonary exercise test
1. Minimal equipment, simple test Subspecialty experience	1. More equipment, complex test More experience
2. Better tolerated in younger children, who will not comply with multiple leads, facemask	2. Not better tolerated in younger children who will not comply with multiple leads, facemask
3. It is effective in patient with walk distance of less than 300 meters	3. It is effective when distance is more than 300 meters

Treatment

Management depends upon:
i. Patient's age
ii. Degree or cyanosis
iii. Subsequent polycythemia

Patients with intracardiac right-to-left heart shunt have potential for the following:
i. Syncope
ii. Paradoxical embolus
iii. Stroke
iv. Brain abscess
v. Sudden death
vi. S/S of erythrocytosis:

a. Polycythemia
b. Hemoptysis
c. Pulmonary infarction
vii. Congestive cardiac failure
viii. Endocarditis

Line of Management

A. Fluid balance and climate control:
   i. Since dehydration increases right-to-left shunting—proper fluid intake.
   ii. Avoid humid or very hot conditions—because it exacerbates vasodilatation, syncope and increased right-to-left heart shunting.
B. Treatment of right-sided heart failure:
   i. Diuretics—cautiously used, since it is a preload-dependant condition. It is used to relief of congestion. Loop diuretic is usually used.
   ii. Digoxin

Treatment of CNS events: These occur due to:
i. Paradoxical embolus
ii. CNS venous thrombosis
iii. Intracranial hemorrhage
iv. Brain abscess, in presence of endocarditis

Treatment option:
i. Endocarditis prophylaxis
ii. Use of air fibers with all intravenous catheters
iii. Adequate management of hyperviscosity syndrome

Air travel precaution: During air travel, there is risk of:
i. Deep vein thrombosis
ii. Central cyanosis because of compromised oxygen delivery in high altitude.
   Treatment option—adequate hydration

Tobacco and alcohol use:
i. Tobacco is absolutely contraindicated because of its deleterious effects on heart, lung and blood vessels.
ii. Alcohol is absolutely contraindicated because it exacerbates:
   a. Myocardial dysfunction
   b. Hypovolemia
   c. Worsening of hyperviscosity
   d. Systemic hypotension
   e. Right-to-left heart shunt

Oxygen therapy:
i. It is controversial because it has no impact on exercise capacity, and survival of adult patient.
ii. It is beneficial as nocturnal supplementation.
iii. Supplemental oxygen during commercial air-travel.

   Pulmonary vasodilator therapy: There is always imbalance between endogenous vasoconstriction (endothelin, thromboxane) and vasodilators (prostacycline, nitric oxide). This imbalance leads to:
i. Vascular remodeling
ii. Intimal fibrosis

   So use of pulmonary artery vasodilators has been shown to be useful in the management of Eisenmenger syndrome.

Prostacycline: It is used to improve hemodynamics:
i. Mean pulmonary artery pressure
ii. Cardiac index
iii. Decreased pulmonary vascular resistance

The drugs are:

a. *Epoprostenol*—continuous intravenous infusion via central catheter, because of its short half life (5 min)

Caution:
 i. Patient must carry proton pump inhibitor
 ii. Keeping drug in cool temperature.

Effect: It improves:
 i. Pulmonary pressure
 ii. 6 minutes walking test
 iii. Oxygenation
 iv. Quality of life

b. *Treprostinil*—it is administered by continuous subcutaneous infusion.

c. *Iloprost:*
 i. It can be administered intermittently 6–9 times daily via nebulizer.
 ii. It is approved for adult PAH.
 iii. It can be used in children with PAH with cardiac lesions.

Endothelin receptor antagonists: It is second vasodilator to be used in PAH. Multiple trials have been done to show their efficacy. But data on its use in Eisenmenger syndrome have been limited.

Drugs—ambrisentan

Phosphodiesterase inhibitors:

i. It increases cyclic guanosine monophosphate and produces vasodilatation.
ii. It works synergistically with nitric oxide (inhaled)

Drugs—sildenafil

Nitric oxide replacement: It has been used in patient with pulmonary hypertension.

Endocarditis: They are at high risk of endocarditis, so prophylaxis for dental, oral, respiratory tract, esophagus, genitourinary, gastrointestinal procedures has been recommended by American Heart Association. Prophylaxis should be:

1. Good oral hygiene—mouthwash with H_2O_2 rinse, tooth brushing, rubber stimulator
2. Skin care:
 i. Use of non-abrasive cleanser
 ii. Avoidance of squeezing skin
3. Avoidance of nail biting.

Treatment of Erythrocytosis

Erythrocytosis is almost always accompanied by Eisenmenger syndrome. This erythrocytosis is responsible for hyperviscosity syndrome.

Treatment option: To manage erythrocytosis, dehydration must be ruled out, because it falsely increases the hematocrit level.

Then through venesection, 250–500 ml of blood has to be taken out and it will be replaced by equivalent amount of isotonic sodium chloride or in case of overt heart failure by 5% dextrose solution.

Effect of phlebotomy—patient develops iron deficiency anemia with normal hematocrit and low mean corpuscular volume.

Again iron deficient RBCs became less deformable hence there is chance of worsening of hyperviscosity, thus thrombotic and bleeding complication.

Thrombotic complication is due to hyperviscosity syndrome, whereas, bleeding complication is due to platelet dysfunctions. The above complications can be treated by fluid replacement and phlebotomy.

Use of anticoagulation: Since there is increased risk of thrombosis as well as increased risk of bleeding and pulmonary hemorrhage, hence routine anticoagulation is not recommended in Eisenmenger syndrome.

Pregnancy and Eisenmenger Syndrome

i. Fetal mortality is 25%.
ii. Maternal mortality is 50%.

Hence pregnancy should be avoided in woman with Eisenmenger syndrome and hence, tubal ligation is strongly recommended.

If patient refuses tubal ligation, hormone therapy (controlled release levonorgestrel or norethidrone and ethinyl estradiol) should be of choice.

Intrauterine devices have to be avoided because there is chance of menorrhagia.

The risk of congenital heart defect in offspring of women with Eisenmenger syndrome is 10%, so fetal echocardiographies are recommended in these patients.

Maternal consideration in pregnancy: Factors increasing the risk of peripartum death include:

1. Congestive heart failure
2. Bleeding/anemia
3. Hematocrit greater than 60%
4. Oxygen saturation less than 80%
5. Syncope
6. Sudden increase in pulmonary vascular resistance and decrease in systemic vascular resistance.

Treatment options:

1. To avoid excessive straining during 2nd stage of labor, assisted delivery should be of choice
2. Cesarean delivery—carries high mortality rate.
3. Since there is increased risk of clotting during pregnancy, anticoagulation may be given—heparin until 12 hours predelivery followed by warfarin for 48 hours postdelivery to the end of the puerperium.

Transplantation:

1. Heart lung transplantation is the procedure of choice, if underlying cardiac defect is not possible to correct in Eisenmenger syndrome.
2. Bilateral lung transplantation: Bilateral lung transplantation is considered as preferable procedure of choice, if cardiac defect is simple.

EBSTEIN ANOMALY

Definition

It is a congenital malformation of the heart which is characterized by apical displacement of the septal and posterior leaflet of the tricuspid valve resulting atrialization of the right ventricle with variable degrees of malformation and displacement of anterior leaflet (Fig. 1.83).

Background: Wilhelm Ebstein describes the cardiac defects typical of Ebstein anomaly in 1866.

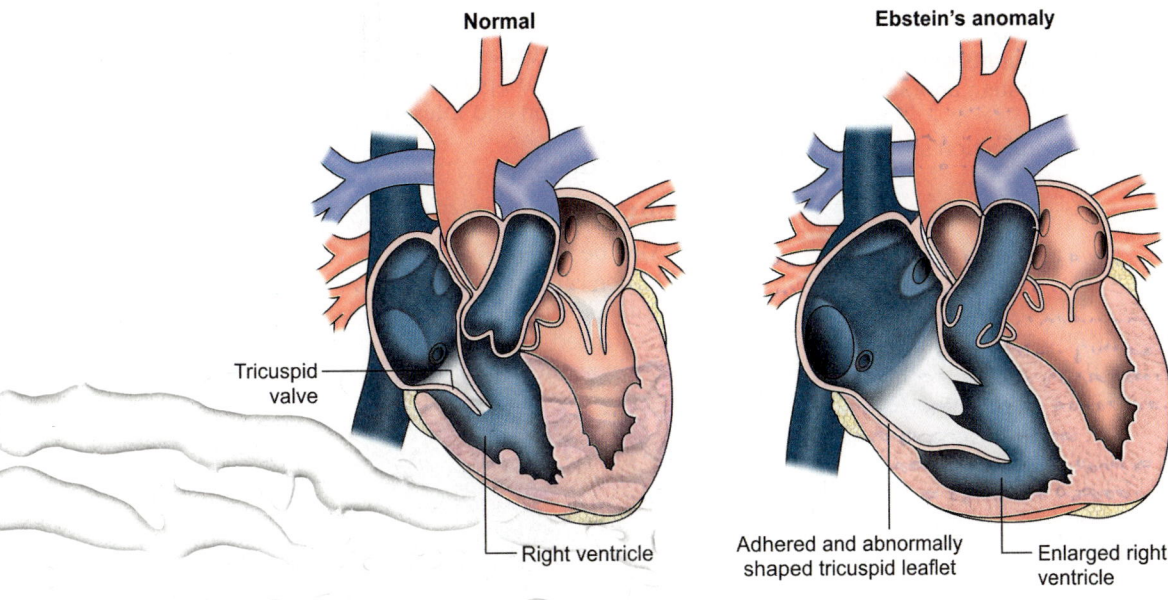

Normal | Ebstein's anomaly

Tricuspid valve

Right ventricle

Adhered and abnormally shaped tricuspid leaflet

Enlarged right ventricle

Fig. 1.83: Anatomy of Ebstein anomaly

Pathophysiology

1. Undermining of the right ventricular free wall is the key feature during embryological development of tricuspid valve leaflets and chordae. This undermining of right ventricle continues to the level of atrioventricular (AV) junction.

   But in Ebstein anomaly, this process of undermining is incomplete and falls short of AV junction.

2. Apical portion of valve tissue fails to be reabsorbed completely. As a result:
   i. There is distortion and displacement of tricuspid valve leaflets
   ii. Some portion of right ventricle becomes atrialized.

Ebstein anomaly may be associated with—congenital, structural or conduction system disease like valvular lesions, intracardiac shunt and accessory conduction pathways.

Hemodynamic Consequences *(Fig. 1.84)*

i. There is presence of tricuspid regurgitation—its severity depends upon extent of tricuspid leaflet displacement.

ii. Atrialized portion of right ventricle, though anatomically is a part of right atrium, contracts and relaxes with right ventricle. As a result, there is stagnation of blood in right atrium due to discordant right ventricular contraction.

During ventricular systole, atrialized portion of right ventricle contracts with the rest of right ventricle. As a result, there is backward flow of blood into right atrium and accentuation of the effect of tricuspid regurgitation.

Race: It is more common in children and white females.

Sex: There is no sex predilection.

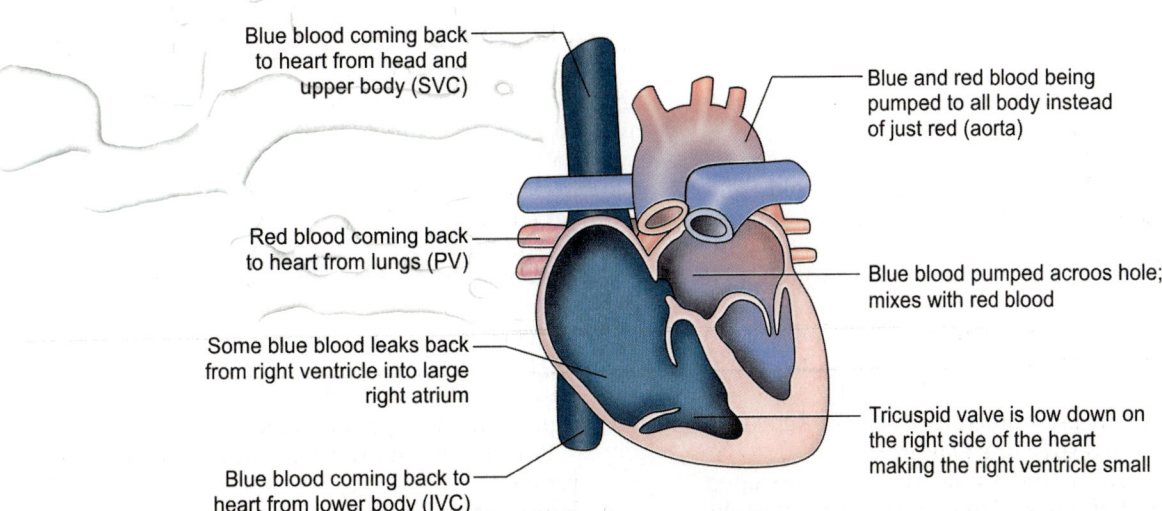

Blue blood coming back to heart from head and upper body (SVC)

Red blood coming back to heart from lungs (PV)

Some blue blood leaks back from right ventricle into large right atrium

Blue blood coming back to heart from lower body (IVC)

Blue and red blood being pumped to all body instead of just red (aorta)

Blue blood pumped across hole; mixes with red blood

Tricuspid valve is low down on the right side of the heart making the right ventricle small

Fig. 1.84: Hemodynamics in Ebstein anomaly

Clinical Presentation

The clinical presentation of the patients depends upon:
i. Anatomic abnormalities of Ebstein anomaly
ii. Their hemodynamic effects
iii. Associated structural and conduction system disease.

Symptoms

a. Cyanosis:
  i. Common—may be due to right-to-left heart shunt at atrial level or severe heart failure.
  ii. Transient in neonate and recurrence in adult.
  iii. May be for the first time in adult life.
  iv. Worsening of cyanosis in adult life due to paroxysmal arrhythmias.
  v. Once apparent, progressively worsens.
b. Fatigue: Due to poor cardiac output, as a result of:
  i. Right ventricular failure, or
  ii. Decreased left ventricular ejection fraction
c. Dyspnea:
  i. Due to right ventricular failure, or
  ii. Decreased left ventricular output
d. Palpitation and sudden cardiac death:
  i. Due to paroxysmal supraventricular tachycardia
  ii. Fatal ventricular arrhythmia—which may be due to presence of accessory pathways.
e. Ankle edema and ascites—due to right heart failure.
f. Other presenting symptoms:
  i. Brain absence due to right-to-left heart shunt
  ii. Bacterial endocarditis
  iii. Cerebrovascular accidents—may be due to paroxysmal embolism.

Signs

a. Central cyanosis
b. Clubbing
c. Jugular venous pulse:
  i. May be normal due to accommodation of large volume of blood and pressure transmitted from right ventricle to thin-walled right atrium through incompetent tricuspid valve.
  ii. Large 'a' and 'v' waves in due course as a result of right ventricular failure.
d. Arterial pulse:
  i. Usually normal
  ii. In due course, may be low due to:
   1. Severe right ventricular failure
   2. Decreased left ventricular ejection fraction
e. Heart sounds:
  i. First sound is widely split with loud tricuspid component due to delayed closure of elongated anterior mitral leaflet.
  ii. Mitral component may soft due to prolonged PR interval.
  iii. Second sound may be normal or widely split due to delay of pulmonary component as a result of right bundle branch block.
  iv. Third and fourth heart sounds are usually present even in absence of congestive heart failure.
    Summation of 3rd and 4th heart sound associated with prolonged PR interval may mimic early diastolic murmur.
  v. Murmur of tricuspid regurgitation—it is holosystolic maximum at lower left sternum, sometimes at the apex, due to displaced tricuspid valve. It is increased in duration and intensity during inspiration.

Investigation

Chest Radiograph (Fig. 1.85)

1. May be normal.
2. My be cardiomegaly.
3. Small aortic root and pulmonary artery.
4. Decreased pulmonary vasculature.
5. Right atrium will be enlarged.

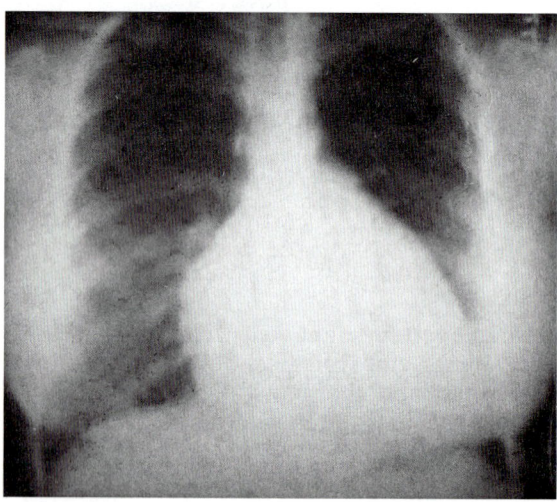

Fig. 1.85: Chest radiograph (adult) in Ebstein's anomaly—cardiomegaly

Echocardiography

1. M-mode echocardiography:
  i. Paradoxical septal motion
  ii. Dilated right ventricle and right atrium
  iii. Delayed closure of tricuspid valve more than 65 milliseconds after mitral valve closure
2. Two-dimensional echocardiography:
  i. Septal or tricuspid leaflet will be displaced apically by 8 mm/m^2—it is most specific sign.
  ii. Morphology and septal attachment of septal and anterior tricuspid leaflets are abnormal.
  iii. Eccentric leaflet coaptation.
  iv. Dilated right ventricle with decreased contractility.
  v. Dilated right atrium.
  vi. Different types of left heart structural abnormalities
3. Doppler studies (Fig. 1.86):
  i. Any stunt
  ii. Different degrees of tricuspid regurgitation.
  Assessment for surgical options and severity of abnormalities:
  i. Functional right ventricular area is less than 35% of total right ventricular area.
  ii. Ratio of arterialized right ventricle and functional right ventricle is greater than 0.5.
    Both of above are associated with unfavorable prognosis
  iii. Functional right ventricular size
  iv. Degree of displacement of septal leaflet.

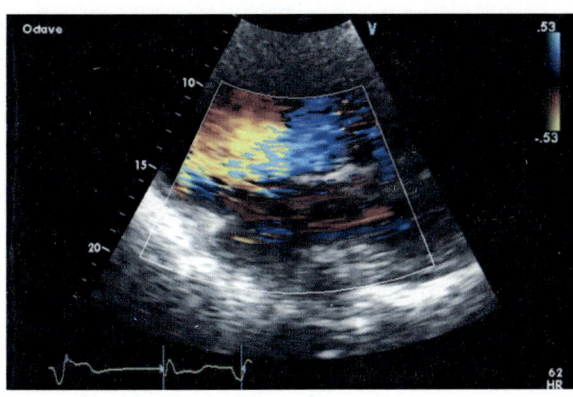

Fig. 1.86: Tricuspid regurgitation

v. Amount of leaflet tethering.
vi. Magnitude of leaflet deformity and dysplasia
vii. Ratio of right ventricular outflow tract to aortic root ratio >2.1 on parasternal short axis view
viii. Moderate to severe aortic regurgitation

Twelve-Lead ECG *(Fig. 1.87)*

1. **Rhythm:**
   i. Usually regular
   ii. May be irregular due to:
      a. Intermittent SVT
      b. Paroxysmal SVT
      c. Atrial flutter
      d. Atrial fibrillation
      e. Ventricular tachycardia
2. **Abnormal P wave**—consistent with right atrial enlargement

3. **PR interval:**
   i. May be prolonged
   ii. May be short due to conduction through accessory pathway.
4. **QRS complex:**
   i. Right bundle branch block
   ii. Low voltage complexes

Cardiac Catheterization

i. It confirms echocardiographic tracings.
ii. It can reveal right ventricular activity on the intracardiac ECG with simultaneous right atrial pressure and waveform.

Electrophysiological Studies

i. 25–30% have accessory pathways.
ii. 5–25% have evidence of preexitation on the surface ECG.
iii. Right-sided accessory pathways are more common.
iv. 50% patients have multiple pathways.

Treatment of Ebstein Anomaly

Treatment depends upon:
i. Severity of the disease
ii. The effect of accompanying congenital structural abnormalities.
iii. The effect of accompanying congenital electrical abnormalities.

Treatment Option

a. Treatment of heart failure:
   i. Angiotensin-converting enzyme (ACE) inhibitors
   ii. Diuretics   iii. Digoxin

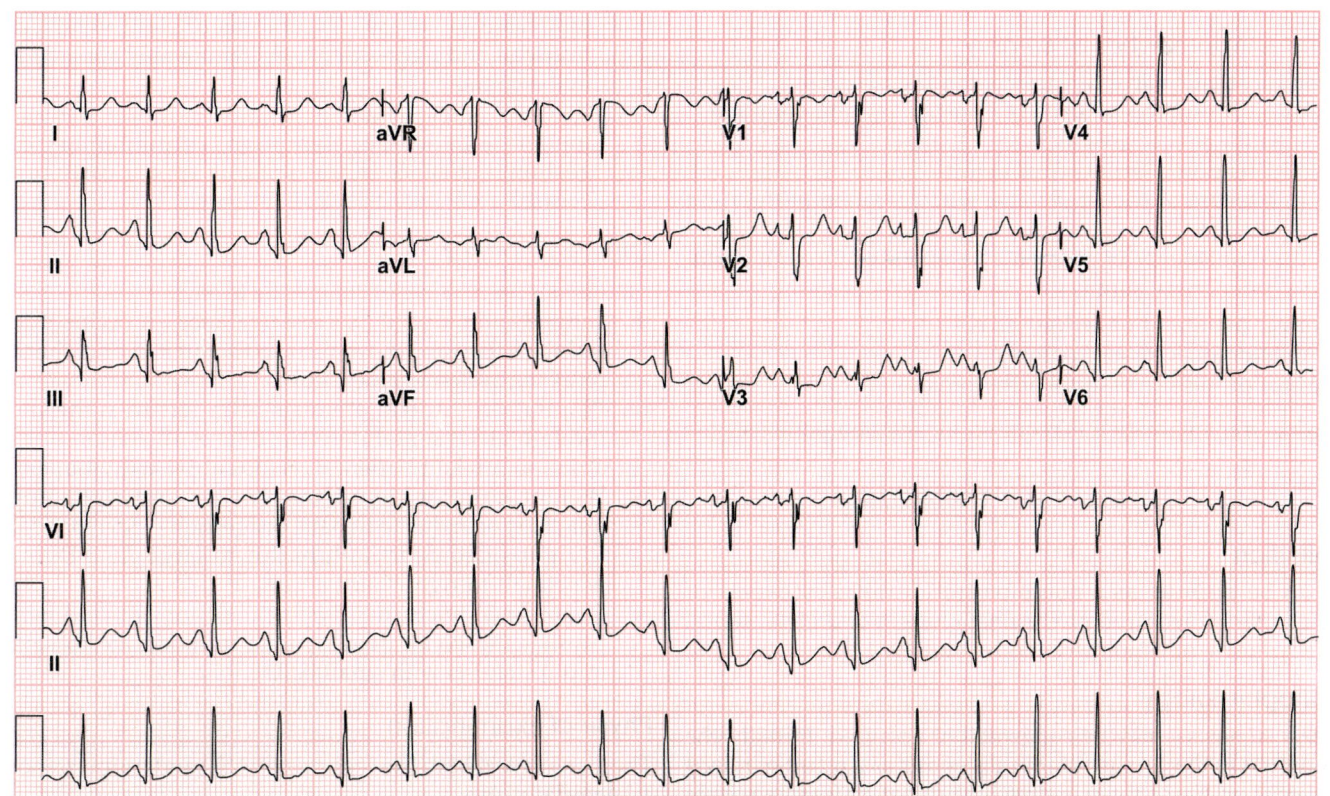

Fig. 1.87: ECG

b. Antibiotic prophylaxis—for infective endocarditis
c. Antiarrhythmic treatment:
   i. Medical treatment with antiarrhythmic drugs
   ii. Radiofrequency ablation of accessory pathways

Factors associated with lower rate of success are:
   i. Multiple accessory pathways
   ii. Complex geometry of the pathways
   iii. Accessory pathways located along the atrialized right ventricle
   iv. Abnormal morphology of the endocardial action potentials

Surgical Treatment

It includes:
   i. Correction of underlying tricuspid valve
   ii. Correction of right ventricular abnormalities
   iii. Correction of any associated intracardiac defect
   iv. Surgical treatment of associated arrhythmias

Prognosis

1. In symptomatic neonates, complete repair of Ebstein anomaly is associated with good early and late surgical and good functional status.
2. In patient of ≥ 50 years old, surgery is associated with good long-term survival and good functional status.

Indications for Surgery

1. NYHA Class I–II heart failure with worsening of symptoms with cardiothoracic ratio 0.65 or greater.
2. NYHA class III–IV heart failure
3. History of paradoxical embolism
4. Significant cyanosis with arterial O_2 saturation of 80%
5. Arrhythmias refractory to medical and radiofrequency ablation.

Various Approaches of Surgery

1. Bioprosthetic valve replacement in tricuspid area
2. Surgical resection of atrialized portion of right ventricle
3. Palliative procedures include:
   i. Creation of atrial septal defect
   ii. Closure of tricuspid valve with placation of the right atrium
   iii. Maintenance of pulmonary blood flow through aorto-pulmonary shunt.

Surgical treatment of arrhythmias:
1. Ablation of accessory pathways.
2. Maze procedure of atrial arrhythmias.

Cardiac transplantation is required for selected patients.

LUTEMBACHER SYNDROME

Definition

It can be defined as a combination of mitral stenosis of congenital or acquired of rheumatic origin and atrial septal defect mostly of ostium secundum variety.

Pathophysiology

Mitral stenosis—may be congenital or acquired. Initially the thought was that in case of mitral stenosis as a result of raised left atrial pressure, there is stretching of patent foramen ovale producing left-to-right atrial shunt. Nowadays, like mitral stenosis, ASD is also a congenital variety. But it may be acquired—may be intentional or the result of complication of percutaneous intervention procedure.

Hemodynamic effects of this syndrome are the result of interplay between the relative effect of ASD and mitral stenosis.

The direction of shunt depends upon the compliance of left and right ventricles, normally right ventricle is more complaint than the left one.

As a result, in presence of mitral stenosis, blood flows from left atrium to right atrium through ASD, instead of going backward towards pulmonary vein, hence pulmonary congestion is avoided.

The presence of large ASD and high atrial pressure due to mitral stenosis make less chance of development of Eisenmenger syndrome.

Reverse Lutembacher syndrome is a rare condition where there is right-to-left heart shunt due to severe tricuspid stenosis.

Age: It can be diagnosed at any age. Lutembacher's original case was a 61 years old woman, who became pregnant 7 times.

History

Symptoms in these patients depend upon:
   i. Size of atrial septal defect.
   ii. Severity of the stenosis
      a. If size of atrial septal defect is large—symptoms of typical isolated mitral stenosis (pulmonary congestion) does not appear until late stage of the disease.
      b. If the size of atrial septal defect is small, symptoms of mitral stenosis, like pulmonary congestion, appear early in the course.
      c. If size of ASD is large and grade of mitral stenosis is moderate to severe—symptoms of right ventricular overload and right-sided heart failure may appear early in the course.
      d. If size of ASD is small and grade of mitral stenosis is moderate to severe—symptoms of pulmonary congestion, typical of mitral stenosis appear early in the course.

Other Symptoms

   i. Patient has history of rheumatic fever.
   ii. Fatigue and reduced exercise tolerance—it occurs due to reduced forward flow into left ventricle and thereby reducing systemic blood flow.
   iii. Palpitation—mitral stenosis with left-to-right shunt through atrial septal defect produces dilatation of both atria—as a result patient develops atrial arrhythmias.
   iv. Weight gain, ankle edema, ascites and right upper quadrant pain due to hepatic congestion—developed due to right-sided heart failure due to large ASD through which left-to-right shunt occurs.
   v. Paroxysmal nocturnal dyspnea, orthopnea, and hemoptysis—these can develop due to moderate to severe mitral stenosis with small ASD.

Physical Examination

The signs reveal both the features of ASD and mitral stenosis.
1. **Arterial pulse:**
   a. Small volume due to low cardiac output

b. Irregular rhythm—due to atrial arrhythmia or atrial fibrillation.

2. **Jugular venous pulse:**
   a. Large 'a' wave in presence of sinus rhythm.
   b. Distended jugular vein—due to right ventricular overload and failure.
   c. Increased right ventricular pressure is more important determinant of the equalization of atrial pressures in increasing jugular venous pressure.

3. **Examination of precordium:**
   a. Tapping apex beat due to palpable loud 1st heart sound—if mitral stenosis is moderate to severe.
   b. Left parasternal heave—due to right ventricular hypertrophy.
   c. Palpable pulmonary sound due to pulmonary hypertension.
   d. Mid-diastolic thrill in mitral area—may be present.

4. **Heart sounds:**
   a. Features of typical mitral stenosis, like, loud 1st sound, mid-diastolic thrill, opening snap and mid-diastolic rumbling murmur—may be present.
      But following features may change the typical features of MS:
      i. Reduced transmitral pressure gradient due to decompression of left atrium through atrial septal defect and displacement of left ventricular apex due to large right ventricle change, the classic findings of mitral stenosis.
      ii. Increase in right and left atrial pressure may increase the transmitral pressure, development of pulmonary hypertension and further dilatation of right ventricle ultimately obscure the left ventricular apex.
   b. 2nd heart sound is widely split for two reasons:
      i. Increased flow through ASD produces large amount of blood flow through pulmonary orifice—as a result, there is late closure of pulmonary valve.
      ii. Decreased flow through aortic orifice produces early closure of aortic valve.
   c. Third and fourth heart sounds are of right ventricular origin—can be heard at left sternal border and louder in inspiration.
   d. Systolic murmur:
      i. In case of ASD, increased flow through pulmonary orifice produces flow murmur in upper left parasternal area.
      ii. Systolic regurgitant murmur in lower left sternal border due to displacement of tricuspid valve secondary to right ventricular dilatation.
      iii. Holosystolic murmur in left parasternal area increases in inspiration (Carvallo's sign). It is due to tricuspid regurgitation and can differentiate it from ASD and mitral regurgitation.
   e. Diastolic murmur:
      i. Mitral stenosis—murmur in apical area in left lateral position best head during expiration.
      ii. Increased flow across the tricuspid orifice best heard at left sternal border during inspiration.
   f. Continuous murmur: Heard at right sternal border due to continuous shunting of blood across the small ASD in presence of severe mitral stenosis.

5. **Examination of the abdomen:**
   a. Ascites
   b. Hepatomegaly
      These occur due to right-sided heart failure.

6. **Extremities:** Ankle edema—due to right-sided heart failure.

Investigations

A. **Chest radiograph:**
   i. Pulmonary plethora due to left to right shunt
   ii. Mild left atrial enlargement
   iii. Right ventricular enlargement
   iv. Enlargement of pulmonary artery
   v. Calcification of mitral valve may be present.
   vi. In case of small ASD with severe mitral stenosis—marked left atrial enlargement and pulmonary vascular congestion.

B. **Transthoracic or transesophageal echocardiography:**
   a. Two-dimensional echocardiography shows:
      i. Large left atrium
      ii. Large right atrium
      iii. Large right ventricle
      iv. Atrial septal defect
      v. Mitral valvular stenotic lesion

C. **Color Doppler studies** confirm:
   i. Severity of mitral stenosis
   ii. Size of ASD
   iii. Size of left-to-right shunt
   iv. Tricuspid regurgitation
   v. Pulmonary artery pressure

D. **Doppler pressure half time method:** Planimetry and Doppler continuity equation method give the accurate assessment of mitral valve area.

Treatment of Lutembacher Syndrome

A. **Symptomatic relief:**
   i. Right-sided heart failure—diuretics
   ii. Atrial arrhythmic—digoxin, beta-blocker, calcium channel blocker—for rate control
      Amiodarone—for rate control and conversion to sinus rhythm
      Subacute bacterial endocarditis—prophylaxis

B. **Surgical care:**
   i. Percutaneous closure of ASD
   ii. Mitral valvoplasty

Indications of surgery:
1. ASD with Qp/Qs—ratio >1.5
2. Moderate to severe mitral stenosis
3. Any degree of pulmonary hypertension except in individual with irreversible pulmonary hypertension.

SINUS OF VALSALVA ANEURYSM

Definition

It is a rare congenital anomaly, having wide range of spectrum, at one end of which patient is clinically silent, only diagnosed as mild asymptomatic dilatation detected in routine two-dimensional echocardiography, and at other end there is symptomatic presentation related to compression of adjacent structures or intracardiac shunting caused by rupture of sinus of Valsalva into right side of the heart.

Origin of Sinus of Valsalva Aneurysm

1. In 65 to 85% cases, it originates from right sinus.
2. In 10 to 30% cases, it originates from noncoronary sinus.
3. In <5 cases, it originates from left coronary sinus.

Pathophysiology

1. It is a congenital dilatation of any one sinus of Valsalva—produced as a result of deficiency of normal elastic tissue and abnormal development of bulbus cordis.
2. Disease processes involving aortic root:
   i. Atherosclerotic aneurysm
   ii. Syphilis
   iii. Endocarditis
   iv. Cystic medial neurosis
   v. Chest trauma
   In these cases, aneurysm involves multiple sinuses.
   Rupture of sinus usually occurs into:
   i. Right atrium (10%)
   ii. Right ventricle (80–90%)
   iii. Pericardial spaces—producing cardiac tamponade.

Epidemiology

i. Male: Female = 4:1
ii. Though there is no racial difference, but higher frequency.

Mortality

Rupture of sinus with progressive heart failure, left-to-right shunting, endocarditis, is the main cause of death before 20 years of age.

Associated Defects

More common:
i. Ventricular septal defect
ii. Bicuspid aortic valve
iii. Aortic regurgitation

Less commonly:
i. Pulmonary stenosis
ii. Coarctation
iii. Atrial septal defect

History

A. 25% cases are asymptomatic—detected by routine 2D echocardiography.
B. In rest 75% of cases—symptoms occur due to rupture, precipitated by:
   i. Exertion
   ii. Trauma
   iii. Cardiac catheterization
1. Rupture of SVA progresses in 3 stages:
   i. Acute chest or right upper quadrant pain
   ii. Subacute dyspnea on exertion or at rest
   iii. Progressively increasing cough, dyspnea, edema and oliguria.
2. It may present with infective endocarditis originating at the edges of the aneurysm.

3. Palpitation or syncope—due to obstruction of either right or left ventricular outflow tract
4. Most common is dyspnea.

Physical Signs

Specific signs of left-to-right heart shunting due to rupture of SVA are sometimes indistinguishable from coronary arteriovenous fistula.
   i. Loud, superficial "machine type" continuous murmur aggravated during diastole in 40% patients.
   ii. Palpable thrill along right or left lower sternal border.
   iii. Bounding pulses
   iv. There may be associated features of aortic regurgitation.

Causes of Sinus of Valsalva Aneurysm

1. Primary causes—congenital
2. Secondary causes:
   i. Atherosclerosis
   ii. Syphilis
   iii. Cystic medial necrosis
   iv. Infective endocarditis
   v. Blunt trauma

Laboratory Working

A. Two-dimensional echocardiography:
   i. Generalized single sinus enlargement
   ii. "Wind-sock" extension of sinus from body or apex of normal sinus when ruptured.
   iii. Lack of associated lesions such as ventricular septal defect.
B. Three-dimensional TIE—valuable especially in ruptured situation.
C. Transesophageal echocardiography—allows:
   i. Identification of structural abnormalities.
   ii. Shunt location for perioperative assessment.
D. Cine magnetic resonance imaging
E. Electrocardiography
   i. Sinus tachycardia
   ii. May be conduction defect

Management

A. Medical care: Perioperative assessment
B. Surgical closure: Transcatheter closure of ruptured sinus of Valsalva aneurysm using Amplatze devices.

Intracardiac shunting is the usual recommendation. Following associated abnormalities must be corrected using operation:
   i. Aortic root reconstruction or replacement
   ii. Aortic valve repair or replacement
   iii. Bentall procedure (valved conduit)
   iv. Ventricular septal defect repair
   v. Atrial septal defect repair
   vi. Primary suture closure (pledges), if rupture—patch closure.

ARRHYTHMIAS

SINUS NODE DYSFUNCTION

Sinus node dysfunction refers to:
1. Abnormalities in sinus node impulse formation:
   i. Sinus bradycardia
   ii. Sinus pause (Figs 1.88 and 1.89)
   iii. Sinus arrest
2. Abnormalities in impulse propagation:
   i. Chronotropic incompetence
   ii. Sinoatrial block (Fig. 1.90)
   Sinus node dysfunction occurs, if:
   i. Associated with supraventricular arrhythmias, like, atrial flutter or atrial fibrillation—it is called tachy-brady syndrome.
   ii. Associated with symptoms like syncope or dizziness— it is called sick sinus syndrome.

Physiology

1. Sinus node presents subpericardially in the right atrial wall, near the entrance of superior vena cava on the upper end of sulcus terminalis.
2. It is formed by cluster of cells which can spontaneously depolarize themselves.
3. These cells can depolarize faster than any other latent cardiac pacemaker of the heart.

   After formation of electrical impulse, it propagates outside the sinus node to other structures of the heart to depolarize other structures.

   Sinus node impulse formation is controlled by nervous system.

i. Parasympathetic nervous system stimulation produces decreased automaticity of sinus node, thus decreasing heart rate.
ii. Sympathetic nervous system stimulation increases automaticity of sinus node and increases heart rate.

Pathophysiology

Due to abnormalities in atrium and conducting system of the heart, there are abnormalities in impulse formation and impulse propagation.

As a result, there is slowing of ventricular rates or pause.

If the sinus node dysfunction is mild, the patient will be asymptomatic.

If the sinus node dysfunction is severe, the patient may develop signs of hypoperfusion and/or irregular pulse:

i. Dizziness   ii. Confusion
iii. Syncope   iv. Heart failure   v. Angina

Etiology

Exact etiology is not known, but it may be a combination of intrinsic or extrinsic factors.

Intrinsic Factors

1. Age-related changes:
   i. Fibrotic changes in the atrium and conduction system of the heart—responsible for tachy-brady syndrome, conducting system disease, inappropriate slowing of escape rhythm.

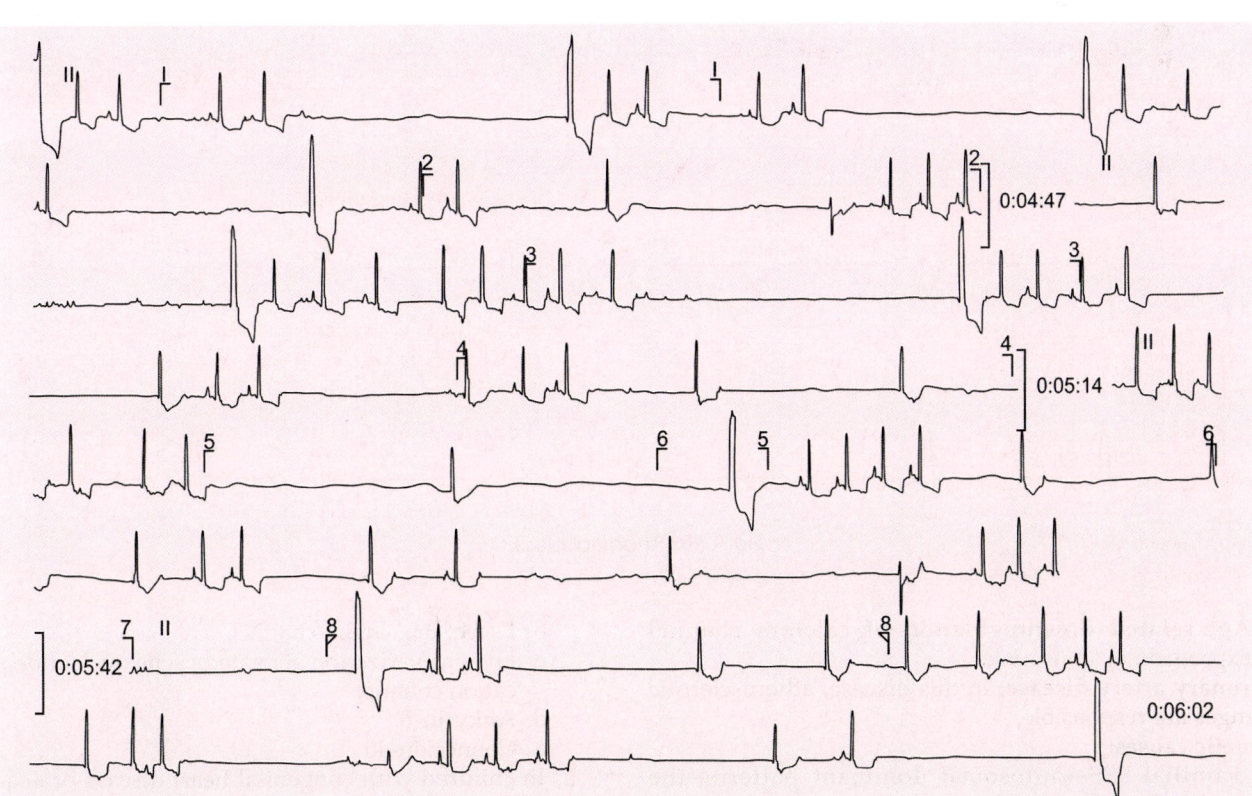

Fig. 1.88: Sinus pause

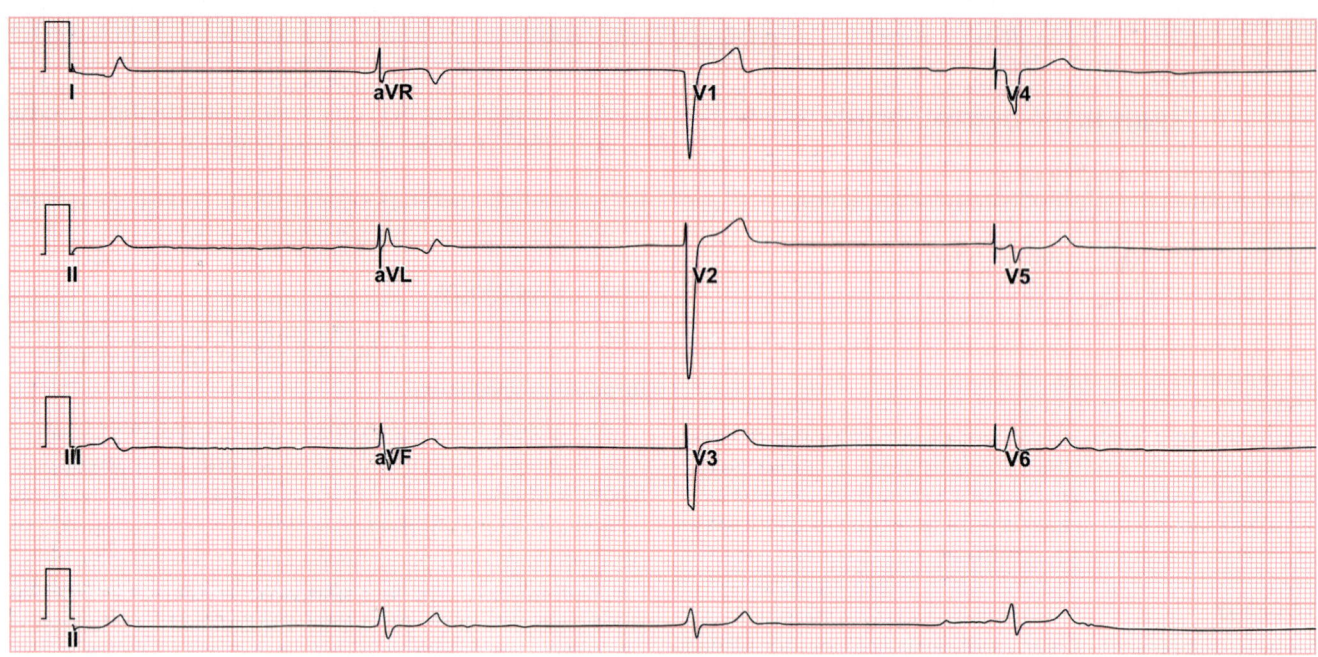

Fig. 1.89: Sinus pause

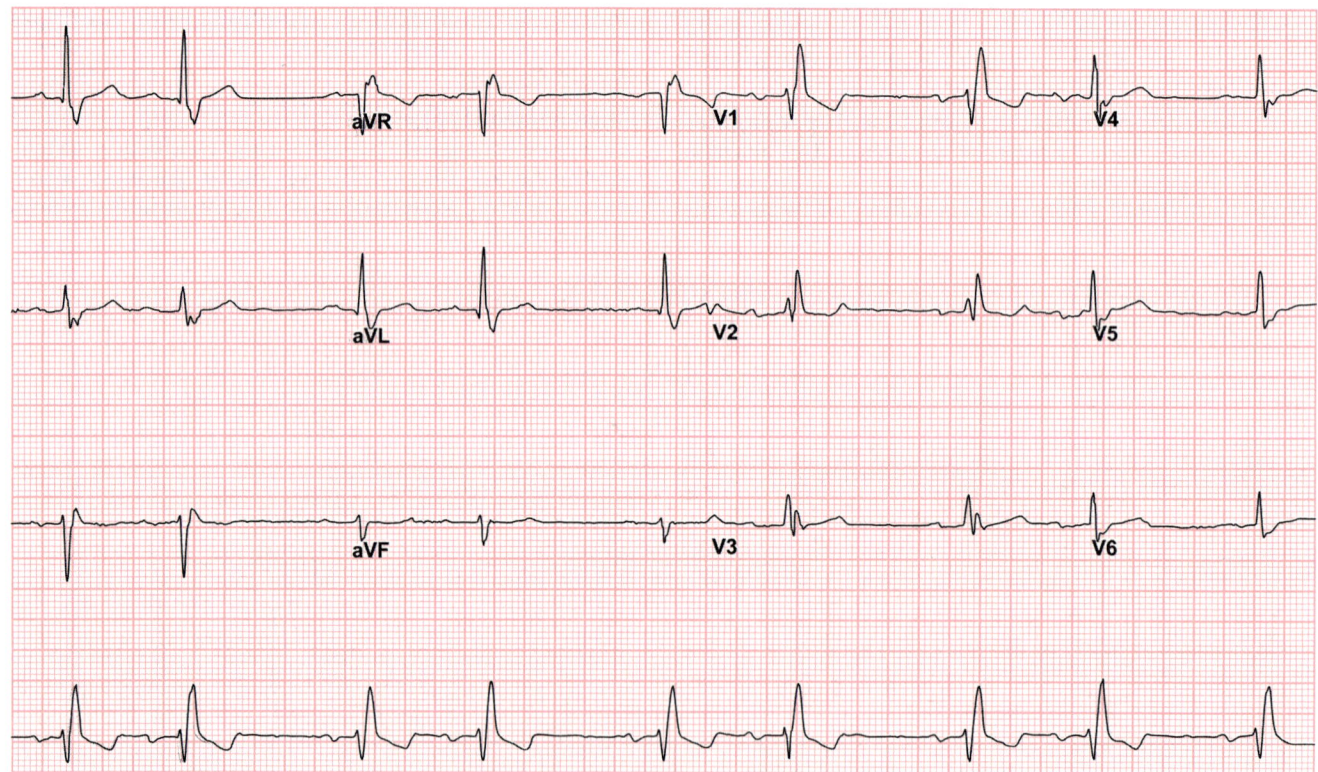

Fig. 1.90: Sinoatrial block

ii. Age-related downregulation of calcium channel expression in sinus node.

2. **Coronary artery disease:** In this disease, atherosclerotic changes are responsible.

3. **Genetic causes:**
   i. Familial SSS—autosomal dominant pattern—the molecular defects are:
      a. Defects in sodium channel
      b. Defect in calcium channel
      c. Hyperpolarization activated cyclic nucleotide gated cation channel
      d. Ankyrin-B
      e. Connecxin-40
   ii. In children with congenital heart disease or acquired heart disease or during correction of trauma to sinus nodal artery.

iii. Emery Dreifuss muscular dystrophy—X-linked muscular disorder—in this disease, AV conduction defect may be associated with SND which may produce sudden cardiac defect.

Hence, permanent pacing is required, if associated AV conduction defect is present.

4. **Congenital diseases:**
   a. Atrial septal defect
   b. Ebstein anomaly
   c. Heterotaxy syndrome particularly left atrial isomerism.

5. **Other uncommon causes of sinus node dysfunction:**
   a. Various cardiomyopathies.
   b. Myocarditis
   c. Pericarditis
   d. Collagen vascular disease—SLE, scleroderma
   e. Infiltrative heart disease—amyloidosis, hemochromatosis
   f. Neuromuscular

Extrinsic Sinus Node Dysfunction

1. **Medications:**
   i. Digitalis
   ii. Beta-blockers—propranolol
   iii. Calcium channel blocker—verapamil
   iv. Antiarrhythmic drugs—quinidine, procainamide, lidocaine, disopyramide.

2. **Autonomic dysfunction:**
   i. Carotid sinus hypersensitivity
   ii. Marked vagotonia—as in well-trained athletes.

3. **Surgical causes involving operation in right atrium**—Mustard, Senning and all varieties of Fontan operation. The congenital defects in heart whose operation may be responsible for SND:
   i. Repair of sinus venosus ASD
   ii. Surgery for endocardial cushion defect
   iii. Blalock-Hanlon atrial septectomy
   iv. Repair of partial anomalous pulmonary venus return or total anomalous pulmonary venous return
   v. Cannulation of superior vena cava during performing cardiopulmonary bypass.

4. **Other causes:**
   • Rheumatic fever
   • Increase in intracranial pressure with subsequent increase in parasympathetic tone.
   • Endocrine and metabolic diseases:
     i. Hypothyroidism
     ii. Hypothermia
     iii. Hypokalemia
     iv. Hypocalcemia

Epidemiology

It occurs 1 in 600 cardiac patients older than 65 years.
Age: Age of occurrence is 68 years.

Prognosis

Patient's mortality and morbidity depends upon:
i. Additional systemic ventricular dysfunction
ii. Degree of congestive heart failure

Complications of Sinus Node Dysfunctions

i. Sudden cardiac death
ii. Syncope
iii. Fall
iv. Congestive heart failure
v. Thromboembolic events
vi. Cardiac dysfunction due to bradycardia and loss of AV synchrony.
vii. Atrial dysrhythmias—atrial flutter and atrial fibrillation.

The patient having tachy—brady syndrome has high risk of sudden cardiac death and stroke.

Symptoms

Patients with sinus node dysfunction are usually asymptomatic, but if sinus node dysfunction progresses, it may produce moderate severe organ dysfunction.

The symptoms related to different organs:
1. Cerebral symptoms: Irritability, dizziness, slurred speech, syncope, black out, falls.
2. Cardiac symptoms: Angina, palpitations, sudden cardiac death.
3. Gastrointestinal symptoms—abdominal pain.
4. Genitourinary symptoms—oliguria
5. Transient ischemic attack—in case of tachy-brady syndrome.
6. Fatigue
7. Shortness of breath with or without palpitations.

Physical Examination

1. Heart rate—bradycardia
2. In patients with carotid sinus hypersensitivity—carotid sinus massage produce severe bradycardia, sinus pause and syncope.
3. In patients with structural heart disease may or may not be any symptom.
4. But patient with operation for transposition of great arteries may present with congestive cardiac failure.
5. Infant with sinus node dysfunction may present with congestive cardiac failure—showing—tachypnea, crepitations and hepatomegaly, central cyanosis.

Sinus Node Dysfunction Workup

Its diagnosis mainly relies on—non-invasive method rather than electrophysiological study. Most reliable non-invasive method is 24 hours Holter monitoring.

Laboratory Studies

To exclude electrolyte abnormalities—Na^+, K^+, Ca^{++}.

Echocardiography

i. This can identify the etiology of SND mainly valvular, congenital or ischemic heart disease and may suggest the diagnosis of amyloid in case of diffuse conducting system disease.
ii. It can evaluate ventricular dysfunction.
iii. It can evaluate and assess anatomic and hemodynamic abnormalities.

Electrocardiography

The ECG criteria include any one of the following:
1. Sinus bradycardia below the rate expected for following ages:
   i. In case of infant <100 beats/min
   ii. In case of preschool child <80 beats/min

iii. In case of school child <60 beats/min
iv. In case of adult <50 beats/min
2. Sinus pause or absence of expected P for more than 3 seconds—may be due to:
   i. Sinus arrest (failure of sinus node pacemaker cells)
   ii. Sinoatrial exit block (failure of conduction of depolarization of sinus node to atrium)
3. Slow escape rhythm originating from atrium, His bundle or ventricle.
4. Marked sinus arrhythmia with constant variation in P–P interval which is accompanied by sinus bradycardia.
5. Presence of bradyarrhythmias or tachyarrhythmias, i.e. sinus node tachycardia, atrial fibrillation.

Sinus pause: It can be defined as absence of 'P' wave on electrocardiogram for more than 2 seconds due to lack of sinus node activity.

The duration of sinus pause has no arithmetical relationship with the baseline sinus rate (PP interval should not be an interval of the pause).

Occasionally symptomatic sinus pause occurs in patients after termination of atrial fibrillation or atrial flutter.

If the sinus pause occurs for more than 3 seconds, the patient will be symptomatic. It commonly occurs under following conditions:
i. Sleep apnea
ii. Hypervagotonia
iii. Seizure activity

Sinoatrial block: There are three degrees of block:
1. *First degree block:* It refers to block of electrical propagation between sinus node and atrium, it cannot be recognized on regular electrocardiographic findings.
2. *Second degree sinoatrial block:* It refers to intermittent block in electrical propagation between sinus node and atrium. It has typical, classic and atypical subtypes. The classic subtypes can be recognized in electrocardiographic findings. Classical subtypes are the followings.
   i. *Type I (wenekebach type)* (Fig. 1.91): It refers to prolonged conduction of sinus node impulse through atrial tissue without any actual block in AV node (P wave precedes all QRS complexes). So there is progressive shortening of PP interval until block occurs, i.e. sinus impulse is not followed by P wave.

      In surface ECG—there is progressive shortening of PP interval until sinus node impulse is dropped.
   ii. *Type II sinoatrial block:* It refers to multiple pauses at the base line ECG (PP interval).

3. *Third degree sinoatrial block:* It refers to complete block in the propagation of impulses from sinus node to atrium. It cannot distinguish sinus arrest or sinus pause from third degree SA block. In case third degree SA block, escape rhythm (atrial, junctional or ventricular) will be present.

Escape rhythm: It usually originates from atrium, His-Purkinje fibers or ventricular muscles. These rates will be slower than sinus node rate:
i. Atrial escape rhythm—it may originate from right or left atrium or in multiple foci in the atria (wondering pacemaker)—in these cases, there will be change axis in P wave in surface ECG.
ii. Escape rhythm from His-Purkinje systems: Rate will be 60–80/min in infants and 50–70/min in children.
iii. Escape rhythm from ventricular muscles: The rate will be further slower.

Chronotropic incompetence: This can be defined as failure to achieve 85% of maximal predicted heart rate (maximal predicted heart rate = 220–age) or failure to achieve >100/min heart rate with exercise or, maximum heart rate with exercise less than 2 standard deviations below that of an age match control population.

Sinus node is under autonomic control, so exercise increases the heart rate in response to increased sympathetic tone. But in sinus node dysfunction, autonomic response will be blunted.

Tachy-brady syndrome: In this cases, tachyarrhythmia and bradyarrhythmia alternate. Bradyarrhythmia may originate in sinus node, atria, AV junction or ventricle. Tachyarrhythmia is usually caused by atrial flutter and fibrillation or supraventricular reentrant tachycardia.

Holter monitoring: 24–48 hours Holter monitoring is useful in assessment of sinoatrial dysfunction.

Specificity of direct observation of sinus node dysfunction is 100%, more than electrophysiological study, hence it may be a method of choice.

Pharmacologic stimulation test: Due to moderate sensitivity and specificity of this type of stimulation test for sinus node dysfunction, intrinsic heart rate, atropine stimulation tests are used as accessory tests for its diagnosis in selected patients.

The values of adenosine, isoproterenol, propranolol tests are more controversial.

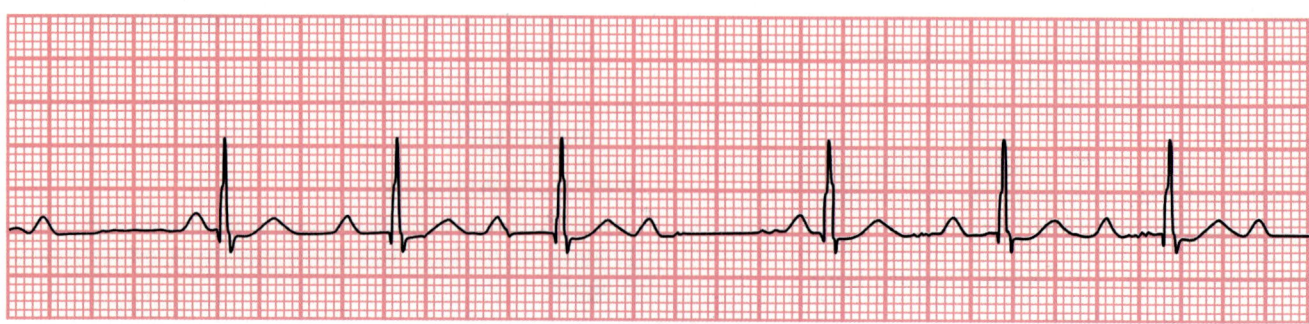

Fig. 1.91: Type I second degree block

Intrinsic Heart Rate

Atropine (0.04 mg/kg) and propranolol (0.2 mg/kg) pre-used to dennervate sinus node pharmacologically
↓
5–20 minutes later
↓
Evaluate the intrinsic heart rate (IHR).
Intrinsic heart rate of a healthy person is 117.2—(0.53 × age)

Intrinsic sinus node dysfunction is present, if sinus rate after medications is below the calculated intrinsic heart rate (IHR).

This test is helpful for—patients with sinus bradycardia due to suspected hypervagotonia to exclude sinus mode dysfunction, because the patient with hypervagotonia has normal intrinsic heart rate.

Atropine Test

Atropine is the most commonly used agent to know the degree of parasympathetic tone. Here, atropine 0.04 mg/kg is administered isolatedly.
1. Normal response: Increase in heart rate more than 90/min or 25% more than baseline sinus rate.
2. In case of symptomatic sinus node dysfunction, decrease in intrinsic heart rate.
3. In case of mild sinus node dysfunction—normal or exacerbated response to atropine.

Electrophysiological Studies

Classic electrophysiological (EP) studies criteria for sinus node dysfunction include the presence of one or more of the following:
  i. Corrected sinus node recovery time greater than 275 milliseconds
 ii. Sinoatrial conduction time greater than 200 milliseconds.
iii. SA node arrest
 iv. Sinoatrial block
  v. Sinus node reentry tachycardia.

Complications of EP studies: It is very rare, but may occur. These include:
1. Hematoma at the puncture site in groin or neck
2. Hemorrhage
3. Infection caused by manipulation of catheter inside the heart
4. Perforation during manipulation inside the heart. Right atrial appendages, right ventricular outflow tract.

Treatment

Baseline Approach

1. Only effective medical care is to treat the extrinsic causes responsible for SND.
2. Inspite of abnormal SNRT, usually no treatment is required for asymptomatic patients.
3. If patient is receiving bradyarrhythmias producing medications—these should be stopped, if possible.
4. In symptomatic patient, atropine (0.04 mg/kg IV every 2–4 hours) and/or isoproterenol (0.05—0.5 mg/kg/min) intravenously should be administered. In a few cases, intravenous temporary pacemaker may be given.
5. In case of tachy-brady syndrome, tachyarrhythmias may be controlled by digoxin, propranolol or quinidine. But patient should be constantly monitored by Holter monitoring to

prevent the development of symptomatic bradyarrhythmias. In that case, permanent pacemaker may be the only option.

Pacemaker Therapy

Since occurrence of sudden death in patient with SND is very low, pacemaker may be implanted to give the patient relief from symptoms rather than from death.

Indication of pacemaker implantation: According to 2008 ACC/AHA/HRS guidelines:
1. *Class-I indication:* In case of patient with documented sinus bradycardia, sinus pause, chronotropic incompetence—in this case SND due to medications, for which acceptable alternative exists.
2. *Class IIa indication:* Patients with symptomatic SND with sinus rate below 40 beats/min and here bradyarrhythmias cannot be documented.
3. *Class IIb indications:* In patients of unexplained syncope, when clinically significant abnormalities are observed in electrophysiology studies.
4. *Class IIIb indications:* Patients with minimal symptoms and chronic heart rate of <40 beats/minute during awaking.
5. *Class III indication:* Pacemaker is contraindicated in case of asymptomatic sinus node dysfunction or in case of medication-induced bradyarrhythmias, that are not essential.

Single versus dual chamber pacemakers:
1. In US—dual chamber pacemaker is preferred, because of advanced anticipation of dysfunction of conducting system.
2. In case of single chamber pacemaker, there is chance of atrial fibrillation than dual chamber pacemaker.
3. In respect of mortality, there is no difference.
4. In case of SND and normal AV and intraventricular conduction, single chamber with AAI mode is more acceptable.
5. Dual chamber has added expenses; there is chance of lid extraction.
6. In patients with SND with AV conduction abnormality (bundle branch block and bifascicular block)—dual chamber pacemaker is better option.

Chronic right ventricular pacing therapy is associated with—increased incidence of:
  i. Atrial fibrillation   ii. Stroke
iii. Heart failure   iv. Death

So it is better to avoid right ventricular pacing in case of SND.

Indications of EP Testing

  i. Assessment of SND in patient with syncope
 ii. Assessment and evaluation of syncope in patients with structural heart disease.
iii. To rule out other etiologies of syncope—such as, ventricular tachyarrhythmias and AV conduction block.

Method of Assessment of SA Node Function

1. **Sinus node recovery time (SNRT):** It can be defined as longer pause after cessation of overdrive packing of right atrium near SA node.
   Normal value is <1500 ms.
   Corrected for sinus cycle length is <550 ms.

2. **Sinoatrial conduction time (SACT):** This can be defined as one-half of the difference between the intrinsic sinus cycle length and a noncompensatory pause after a premature atrial stimulus (normal <125 ms)

So, the combination of 1. abnormal SNRT, 2. abnormal SACT, 3. Low intrinsic heart rate—specific for sinus node dysfunction.

Beta-blocker and calcium channel blocker increase sinus node recovery time.

Class I and III antiarrhythmic drugs produce sinus node exit block.

So these drugs should be discontinued.

Some pharmacologic therapy may improve sinus node functions:

i. Digitalis shortened SNRT
ii. Isoproterenol, atropine increase the heart rate.
iii. Theophyline can be used in SND to increase the heart rate, but in case of tachy-brady syndrome, it may produce severe ventricular arrhythmias.

In patient with inferior wall or posterior wall myocardial infarction, sinus bradycardia is common and it will be aggravated by morphine. Again ischemia in SA nodal artery may occur in acute coronary syndrome, but it will be transient.

ATRIAL FLUTTER

Definition

It can be defined as a type of cardiac arrhythmia, where atrial rate is 240–400/min with some degrees of atrioventricular node conduction block.

Type 1 atrial flutter: It is typical or classical atrial flutter. It involves a single reentrant circuit with circus activation around tricuspid valve annulus in right atrium. It travels in counterclockwise direction.

Type 2 atrial flutter: It is an atypical type of atrial flutter, which follows different circuits, and it may involve right or left atrium.

Pathophysiology of Atrial Flutter

In type 1 atrial flutter, there is single reentrant circuit with circus activation around tricuspid valve annulus in right atrium in counterclockwise direction, with an area of slow conduction located between tricuspid valve annulus and coronary sinus ostium (subeustachian isthmus). This flutter is often referred to as isthmus-dependent flutter.

The orifice of inferior and superior venae cavae, the Eustachian ridge, the coronary sinus orifice and tricuspid annulus complete the barrier for reentry circuit.

ECG shows negative saw-toothed wave in L-II, L-III and NF.

In some type I atrial flutter, there is clockwise activation around tricuspid valve annulus. ECG shows positive saw toothed wave or sinusoidal wave in leads II, III and AVF. It is sometimes called reverse typical atrial flutter.

Type 2 atrial flutter: This atypical atrial flutter may originate from:

i. Right atrium in surgical scar (incisional re-entry)
ii. Left atrium, specifically the pulmonary veins (focal reentry)

iii. Mitral valve annulus
iv. In left atrium after incomplete left atrial linear ablation.

Etiology

A. From cardiac diseases:

i. Coronary artery diseases	30% cases
ii. Hypertensive heart disease	30% cases
iii. No underlying cause	30% cause
iv. Rheumatic heart diseases	
v. Congenital heart disease	
vi. Cardiomyopathy	

B. From non-cardiac diseases:

i. Hypoxia
ii. Chronic obstructive pulmonary diseases
iii. Pulmonary embolism
iv. Hyperthyroid disease
v. Pheochromocytoma
vi. Diabetes
vii. Electrolyte imbalance
viii. Alcohol consumption
ix. Obesity
x. Digitoxin toxicity
xi. Myotonic dystrophy

C. Genetic: Genome-wide association studies have identified genes associated with atrial flutter.

PITx2 (paired-like homeodomain 2) gene on chromosome locus 4q25—may play major role in development of atrial flutter.

Prognosis

1. Prognosis in patients with atrial flutter depends upon their underlying medical condition. Since prolonged arrhythmia may induce tachycardia-induced cardiomyopathy, hence control of ventricular rate or reversion of rhythm to sinus rhythm is essential.

   Thromboembolic complications also have been described.

2. In atrial flutter, because of the conduction properties of AV node, there is rapid ventricular response than those with atrial fibrillation.

3. In case of atrial fibrillation, ventricular response is difficult to control because of concealed conduction, in case of atrial flutter, ventricular rate can be controlled easily.

4. In patient with atrial flutter with WPW syndrome, there may be life-threatening ventricular response which can be corrected by catheter ablation because there is choice of 1:1 conduction of flutter waves, which can terminate into VF.

5. In some patients, after catheter ablation treatment of atrial flutter, result of type 1 is excellent, but in a few cases, atrial fibrillation may occur, which is responsive to antiarrhythmic agents.

6. In patients with AF, during treatment with class IC antiarrhythmic agents, it can be converted to atrial flutter with rapid ventricular response—which can be corrected by AV node blocking agents.

History Related to Atrial Flutter

Symptoms in atrial flutter occurs due to low cardiac output due to rapid ventricular rate. The symptoms are:

i. Palpitations
ii. Fatigue
iii. Poor exercise tolerance
iv. Presyncope
v. Mild dyspnea.

Results from compromised left ventricular function:
i. Profound dyspnea
ii. Syncope
iii. Angina symptoms due to non-cardiac causes:
   a. Features of hyperthyroidism
   b. Symptoms of pulmonary disease

The precipitating factors are:
i. Alcohol
ii. Caffeine
iii. Medical conditions:
   a. Pneumonia
   b. Myocardial infarction
iv. Surgical procedures
v. Stimulant drugs:
   a. Ginseng
   b. Cocaine
   c. Ephedra
   d. Methamphetamine

History of onset or duration of symptoms is critical. If atrial flutter lasts for more than 48 hours, preoperative transesophageal echocardiography to rule out thrombus or treatment with anticoagulant is essential.

Physical Examination

Patient's initial cardiopulmonary evaluation and monitoring of signs of cardiac and pulmonary failure guide the management.

Primary attention to be paid to heart rate, blood pressure and oxygen saturation

Heart rate: Tachycardia may or may not be present depending on degree of AV block.

Block may be 2:1—producing ventricular rate 150/min. There may be variable block—producing irregular pulse (Fig. 1.92).

Blood pressure: It may be normal, or there may be hypotension.

Other signs are:
i. Neck—gland palpation to exclude goiter.
ii. Evaluation of the neck for jugular venous distension.
iii. Auscultation of lung to evaluate crackles, if any.
iv. Auscultation of the heart to evaluate extra sounds or murmur, if any.
v. Evaluation of point of maximum impulse on the chest wall.
vi. Lower limb assessment to elicit edema or impaired perfusion.
vii. Features of embolization—in brain, peripheral limb
viii. Severe bradycardia
ix. Congestive cardiac failure
x. Myocardial ischemia.

Workup for Atrial Flutter

Non-Cardiac Workup

1. Complete blood count, if:
   a. Anemia is being suspected.
   b. If there is history of blood transfusion.
2. Serum electrolytes and digoxin level.
3. Pulmonary function test—in pulmonary disease.
4. Blood gas measurement to diagnose:
   a. Hypoxia
   b. Carbon monoxide intoxication.
5. Chest radiography to evaluate:
   a. Lung disease
   b. Pulmonary edema in subacute cases.

Cardiac Workup

Electrocardiography:
1. Type 1 flutter:
   a. Anticlockwise reentry
      i. Negative flutter waves in leads II, III, and aVF
      ii. Positive flutter wave in V1.
   b. Clockwise reentry:
      i. Negative flutter waves in V1.
      ii. Positive flutter waves in Leads II, III and aVF

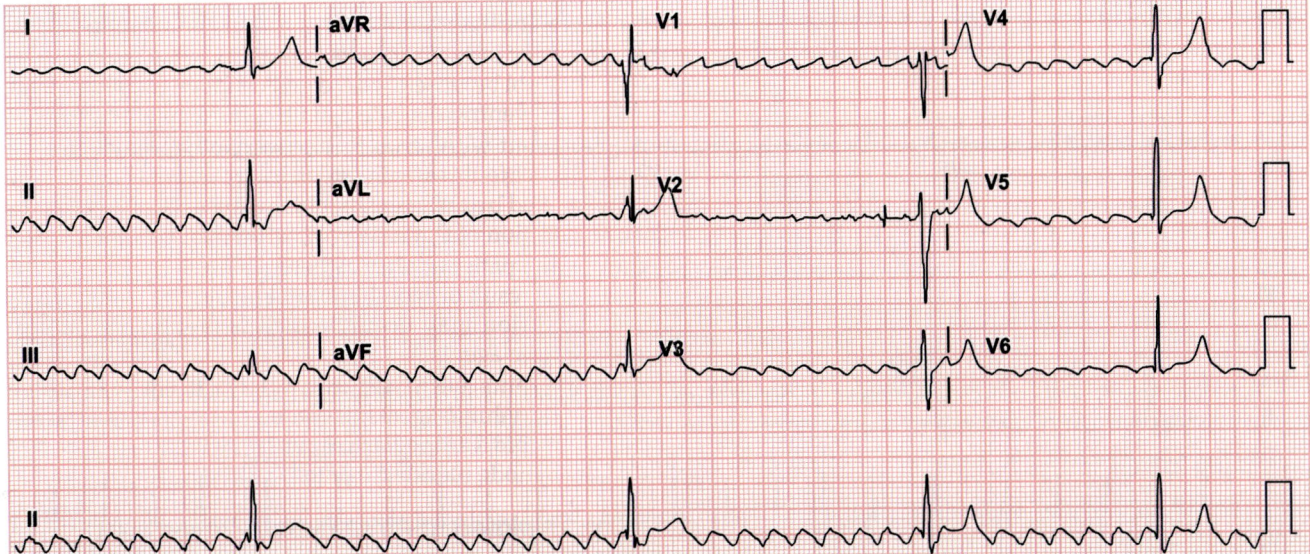

Fig. 1.92: Atrial flutter with varying block

2. A typical atrial flutter: It does not fulfill the criteria of any other above types of typical atrial flutter.

Other Common Regular Features *(Fig. 1.93)*

i. Atrial rate is 250–350 beat/minute in typical atrial flutter. In case of atypical atrial flutter, atrial rate will be 350–450/min.

ii. Ventricular rate is usually regular with 2:1 AV block producing ventricular rate 150/min.

iii. QRS morphology in <120 ms, unless there is pre-existing AV block, accessory pathway or rate-related aberrant conduction.

iv. If the AV block is variable (2:1, or 3:1), rate will be irregular.

v. Absence of isoelectric baseline.

vi. In patient with atrial flutter and pre-excitation syndrome:
1. There is short PR interval
2. No delta wave

Diagnostic Aids

I. Vagal maneuver can differentiate atrial flutter from sinus tachycardia.
In atrial flutter, this maneuver produces rapid decrease in rate revealing flutter way to be seen more easily.

II. Flutter wave may be more easily seen by turning ECG upside down.

III. Measurement of 'R-R' interval: In atrial flutter, with variable block, R-R distance will be multiplies of each other.
In atrial fibrillation, no such relationship exists.

IV. Exercise testing can be done to identify:
i. Exercise-induced atrial fibrillation
ii. Ischemic heart disease.

V. Holter monitoring: It can be done to identify:
i. Arrhythmias in patient with non-specific symptom.
ii. Triggers.
iii. Associated atrial arrhythmias.

Echocardiography

Transthoracic echocardiography evaluates:
i. Atrial flutter
ii. Right and left atrial size
iii. Size and functions of both ventricles.

So it can facilitate diagnosis of:
i. Valvular heart disease
ii. Left ventricular hypertrophy
iii. Pericardial disease

Management of Atrial Flutter

Main approaches to treat atrial flutter are:
1. Control of rapid ventricular response
2. Conversion to sinus rhythm
3. Prevention of recurrent episodes or reduction of their frequency or duration.
4. Prevention and/or treatment of thromboembolic complication.
5. Minimization of adverse effects from therapy.

But the above goals can be modified according to condition of patients.

The main difference between treatment of atrial flutter and atrial fibrillation is that atrial flutter can be cured by radiofrequency ablation rather than administration of rate control and rhythm control strategies with antiarrhythmic drugs and this approach is superior to medical therapy.

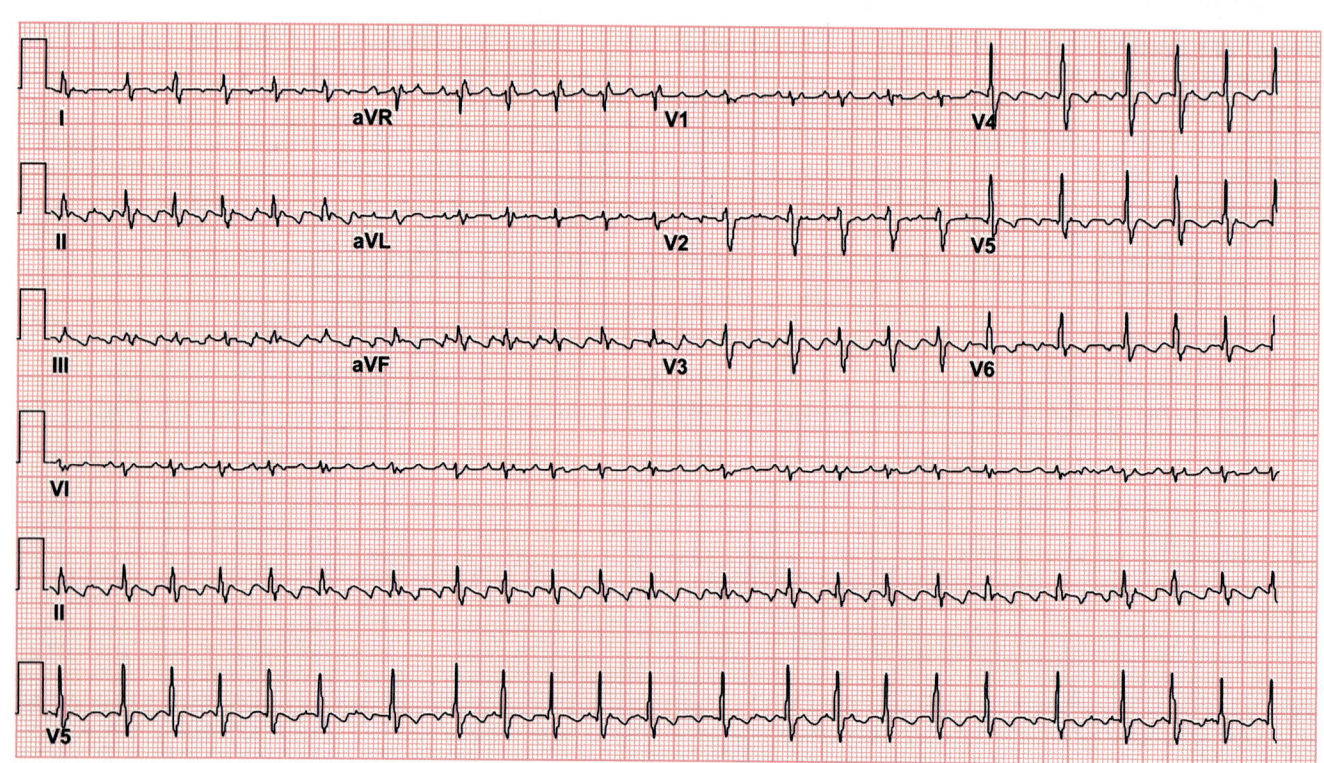

Fig. 1.93: Atrial flutter with varying block

Successful ablation may reduce the need for long-term anticoagulation and antiarrhythmic therapies.

1. **For atrial flutter of less than 48 hours**—electrical cardioversion is to be done as soon as possible. But postconversion, anticoagulant therapy should be given for a few days, because, blood flow velocities in the left atrial appendages is low immediately after cardioversion.

2. **For atrial flutter of more than 48 hours duration**, perform transesophageal echocardiography to see the presence of thrombus or not.

   a. *If there is no thrombus*, and urgent cardioversion is needed, start anticoagulant like intravenous heparin and perform cardioversion and continue anticoagulation up to 4 weeks.

   b. *If presence of thrombus* in left atrial appendages, continue rate control and anticoagulation therapies up to 4 weeks followed by cardioversion.

2. **If the patient is not a candidate for catheter-induced ablation procedure**, antiarrhythmic drugs, like, ibutilide, sotalol, and dofetilide should be initiated, though chance of proarrhythmia is greater during first 24–48 hours after initiation of antiarrhythmic drugs.

3. **Drugs that slow ventricular rate include** beta blockers (atenolol, metoprolol, and prenolol) and calcium channel blocker (verapamil, diltiazem) can be initiated. These drugs to be added in patients who are taking class 1A and 1C antiarrhythmic drugs. Anticoagulation therapy should be started and to be continued until sinus rhythm is maintained, in the patient with atrial flutter of >48 hours duration.

   The aim is to maintain INR to 2–3 during anticoagulation therapy and should be continued for 3 weeks preconversion and 4 weeks after conversion to sinus rhythm. **This is the guideline for atrial flutter for >48 hours duration.**

Ventricular Rate Control

Rapid ventricular response can be treated by AV nodal blocking agents like IV calcium channel blocker or beta-blocker. But, before the initiation of these drugs, we have to exclude the presence of WPW syndrome; otherwise these drugs may initiative ventricular tachycardia or VF.

Electrical Cardioversion

The factors included in electrical cardioversion are:
 i. Proper sedation
 ii. Electrode position
 iii. Proper energy—it is less than AF, 50 Jules may be needed.

If cardioversion is not successful in one electrode position, another electrode position may be necessary.

Points to be remembered regarding electrical cardioversion:
 i. A wide electrode separation is necessary—one in right anterior and another in left posterior position.
 ii. Application of pressure on paddles to reduce thoracic impedance.
 iii. In women, placement of electrode patches under or lateral to breast.

Pharmacological cardioversion:
 i. Dofetilide—it should be stared as in-patient setting.
 ii. Ibutilide: It converts atrial flutter to sinus rhythm in 63% cases. Because it may produce QT prolongation and torsade

de pontes, hence continuous electrocardiographic monitoring is indicated for at least 4 hours after infusion.

Contraindication:
 i. Severe chronic heart failure
 ii. Hypokalemia
 iii. Baseline prolongation of 'QT'

Prevention of Thromboembolic Complication

As compared to general population, risk of thromboembolic complications is high is atrial flutter, hence adequate anti-coagulation must be initiated in patient with atrial flutter of >48 hours. Anticoagulation is recommended for 4 weeks to reduce the incidence of thromboembolic complication in postconversion phase. At the same time, INR should be maintained 2–3 times of normal to prevent the risk of bleeding.

Unlike AF, atrial flutter has regular phase of atrial contraction. **But patient with atrial fibrillation unlike atrial flutter:**
 i. Has decreased left atrial appendage function
 ii. Has more spontaneous echo contrast.
 iii. Has larger left atria and accompanying appendages

In non-rheumatic atrial flutter, following are the risk factors:
 i. Hypertension
 ii. Structural heart disease
 iii. Left ventricular dysfunction
 iv. Diabetes mellitus.

$CHA2DS_2$ score act as predictors of risk of thromboembolism.
1. Congestive heart failure
2. Hypertension
3. Age 65–74 years
4. Diabetes
5. Previous stroke
6. Vascular disease
7. Female sex.

Post-conversion embolic event occurs within 10 days after cardioversion—but to a lesser degree in atrial flutter than atrial fibrillation.

Radiofrequency Ablation

 i. It is the first-line of therapy to convert atrial flutter to sinus rhythm.
 ii. In case of chronic or recurrent atrial flutter, which is isthmus-dependent, success rate is 95% with current technology.
 iii. Quality of life will be high.
 iv. Recurrent admission in cardiology emergency department will be reduced.

A few patients after RFA of atrial flutter can develop AF. But in patients with obstructive sleep apnea syndrome, administration of continuous positive airway pressure may reduce the incidence of atrial fibrillation after RFA for atrial flutter.

In type 1 atrial flutter—catheter ablation is an out patient procedure, atrial mapping is not required.

A line of conduction block is required to interrupt the circuit.

In type 2 atrial flutter (non-isthmus dependent), mapping of left atrium is required.

Success depends upon localization circuit and creating a line of block that includes electrically inert anatomic structure (mitral valve annulus).

Recurrence is more common than type I flutter and necessitates the initiation of antiarrhythmic therapy.

Antiarrhythmic Therapy

Data on the use of antiarrhythmic therapy on atrial flutter is limited, **but the choice of medication according to following cardiac pathology:**

1. **No structural disease,** class IC agent can be used safely, but class III agents are more effective.
2. **LVH without ischemia or conduction delay,** class III agents, specially, amiodarone.
3. **Ischemic heart disease**—sotalol or amiodarone can be used, but class IC agent must be avoided.
4. **Significant systolic dysfunction**—Amiodarone, or do dofetilide may be used, but class IC agents must be avoided.

ATRIAL FIBRILLATION

Introduction

i. It is most common sustained arrhythmia.
ii. Incidence and prevalence of atrial fibrillation is gradually increasing.
iii. Lifetime risk over the age of 40 years is 25%.
iv. It is characterized by disorganized atrial activity and contraction.

Classification

According to guidelines from an American College of Cardiology (ACC)/American Heart Association (AHA)/European Society of Cardiology (ESC) committee of experts, atrial fibrillation has been classified into 3 patterns:

a. **Paroxysmal atrial fibrillation:** Atrial fibrillation has been considered recurrent when patient has 2 or more episodes of atrial fibrillation. If recurrent AF terminates spontaneously within 7 days, it is described as paroxysmal.
   i. These patients are younger.
   ii. The foci are usually found within pulmonary veins.
   iii. These patients generally have many atrial premature beats—detected in Holter monitoring.
   iv. Elimination of these foci can eliminate triggering to paroxysmal AF.
   v. It may progress into permanent AF.

b. **Persistent atrial fibrillation:** If the episodes of atrial fibrillation persist for more than 7 days and may require either pharmacologic or electrical interventions to terminate it, it is called persistant atrial fibrillation.
   i. These patients tend to be older.
   ii. This type of AF occurs secondary to diseases that affect atria—like congestive cardiac failure, hypertensive heart disease, rheumatic heart disease, and coronary artery disease.
   iii. Persistent AF with uncontrolled rapid ventricular response can lead to dilated cardiomyopathy or electrical remodeling of atria (atrial cardiomyopathy).
   iv. Atrioventricular nodal ablation and permanent pacemaker implantation can control ventricular rate and also improve ventricular function.

c. **Permanent atrial fibrillation:** If atrial fibrillation persists for more than 1 year either because of failure of electrical cardioversion or non-attempt of cardioversion, it is called as permanent atrial fibrillation.
   i. Here the main aim is, rate control and prophylactic anticoagulation.

   Lone atrial fibrillation:
   i. It is usually identified in younger patients.
   ii. There is no structural heart disease.
   iii. There is lower risk of thromboembolism.
   iv. It is generally referred to paroxysmal, persistent or permanent AF in younger patients.

Etiology

Atrial fibrillation is associated with following risk factors:

a. **Hemodynamic stress:** Increased intra-atrial pressure may lead to electrical as well as structural remodeling which may predispose to atrial fibrillation. The causes are:
   i. Mitral or tricuspid stenosis or regurgitation.
   ii. Pulmonary or systemic hypertension.
   iii. Intracardiac tumors.
   iv. Intracardiac thrombus.

b. **Atrial ischemia:**
   i. Coronary artery disease directly leads to atrial ischemia.
   ii. Severe ventricular ischemia may lead to increased intra-atrial pressure and it may lead to AF.

c. **Inflammation:** Myocarditis or pericarditis may be idiopathic or collagen vascular disease related, viral, bacterial or traumatic.

d. **Non-cardiovascular:**
   1. Respiratory cause:
      i. Pulmonary embolism
      ii. Pneumonia
      iii. Lung cancer
      iv. Hypothermia
   2. Drugs and alcohol abuse:
      i. Stimulants
      ii. Acute or chronic alcohol abuse, alcoholic cardiomyopathy.
      iii. Illicit drug use—methamphetamine, cocaine.
   3. Endocrine disorder:
      i. Hyperthyroidism
      ii. Diabetes
      iii. Pheochromocytoma
   4. Neurologic disorders:
      i. Intracranial hemorrhage
      ii. Stroke
   5. Advanced age:
      i. 4% individuals more than 60 years old.
      ii. 8% individuals more than 80 years old.
   6. **Familial atrial fibrillation**—due to ion channel, mainly sodium channel abnormalities.

Pathophysiology (Fig. 1.94)

The exact mechanisms by which cardiovascular risk factors may be responsible for the development of AF are not fully understood. But this is under investigation. But catecholamine excess, haemodynamic stress, atrial ischemia, atrial inflammation, metabolic stress and neurohumoral cascade activation may promote AF.

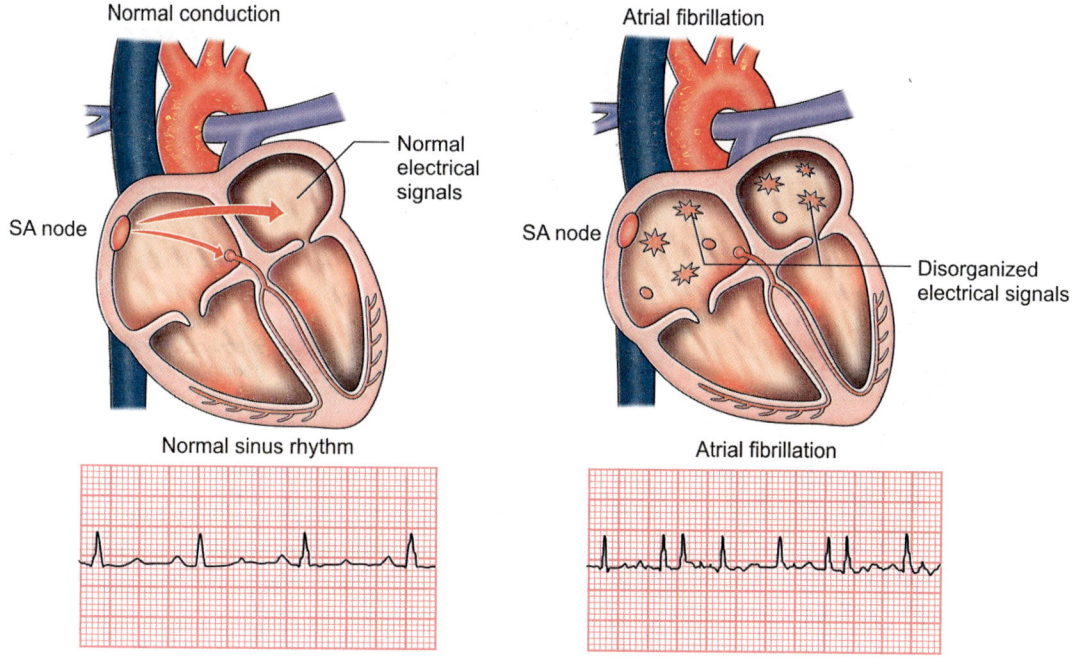

Fig. 1.94: Mechanism of atrial fibrillation

Atrial fibrillation requires both initiating event and permissive atrial substrate. The following mechanisms are responsible for development of AF:

i. Multiple wavelets
ii. Mother waves
iii. Fixed and moving rotors
iv. Macro re-entry circuits.

A. Automatic focus: Pulmonary veins appear to be most frequent source of these autonomic foci. But it may be from other areas of atria.

Cardiac muscles in the pulmonary vein appear to have active electrical properties identical to those of atrial myocytes. This electrical conduction around pulmonary veins promotes re-entry and sustained AF.

B. Multiple wave left: This hypothesis proposes the fractionation of the wave fronts propagating through the atria results in formation of self propagating "daughter wavelets". The number of wavelets is determined by:

i. Amount of atrial mass
ii. Refractory period
iii. Conduction velocity

Increased atrial mass, shortened refractory period and delayed intra-atrial conduction velocity result in formation of increased number of wavelets which lead to persistent atrial fibrillation.

Again, atrial structure and electrical remodeling is responsible for maintenance of atrial fibrillation—hence it is said "atrial fibrillation begets atrial fibrillation."

Symptoms of Atrial Fibrillation

There is a wide spectrum of presentation in atrial fibrillation—which ranges from asymptomatic atrial fibrillation (90% of cases) to symptomatic atrial fibrillation producing cardiogenic shock or devastating cerebrovascular events (CVA). Cardiogenic shock may require direct cardioversion. The unstable patients requiring direct cardioversion are:

i. Patients with decompensated congestive cardiac failure
ii. Patients with hypotension
iii. In uncontrolled angina/ischemia

Less severe symptoms are:

i. Palpitations
ii. Dyspnea
iii. Fatigue
iv. Presyncope or syncope
v. Decompensated heart failure.

Other symptom is—features of cerebral thromboembolism.

The following questions should be asked to identify precipitating factors:

i. Hydration status
ii. Infection
iii. Alcohol use
iv. Presence of any heart disease
v. History of pharmacology or electric intervention.

To identify the types of atrial fibrillation (paroxysmal, persistent or permanent), following documentation history should be taken:

i. Assessment of type, duration or frequency of symptoms.
ii. Assessment of precipitating factors like sleep, caffeine, alcohol.
iii. Assessment of mode of termination vagal maneuvers.
iv. Documentation of prior use of antiarrhythmic agents or rate controlling drugs.
v. Assessment of prior cardiac disease
vi. Documentation of prior surgical or percuteneous ablation procedures.

Physical Examinations (Fig. 1.95)

It begins with airway, breathing and circulation (ABC) support and maintenance of vital signs followed by searching for the signs to identify the etiology.

A. Heart rate: It is irregularly irregular, tachycardia with rate between 110 and 140/minutes

In following cases—there may be bradycardia:

a. Hypothermia.
b. Cardiac drug toxicity.

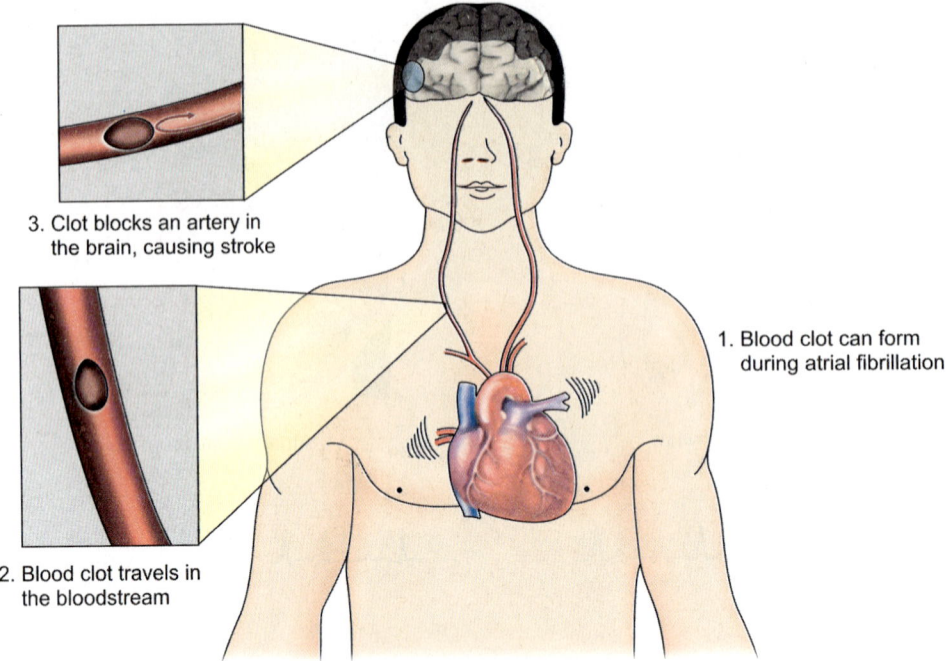

3. Clot blocks an artery in the brain, causing stroke

2. Blood clot travels in the bloodstream

1. Blood clot can form during atrial fibrillation

Fig. 1.95: Mechanism of stroke in AF

B. Examination of neck and head:
  i. Jugular venous wave—absent 'a' wave
  ii. Elevated jugular venous pressure
  iii. Exophthalmos
  iv. Thyromegaly
  v. Cyanosis
  vi. Carotid artery bruit—detects peripheral arterial disease.
C. Pulmonary:
  i. Crepitations or pleural effusion—evidence of heart failure
  ii. Diminished breath sounds, rhonchi suggest underlying pulmonary disease.
D. Cardiac:
  i. Displacement of apical impulse—suggests ventricular enlargement or elevated left ventricular pressure.
  ii. Loud P2 suggests pulmonary hypertension.
  iii. Different types of murmur suggest its etiology regarding cardiac disease.
E. Abdomen:
  i. Tender hepatomegaly suggests right ventricular failure.
  ii. Ascites suggests right ventricular failure.
  iii. Left upper quadrant tenderness—splenic infarction from peripheral embolization.
F. Lower limb:
  i. Cyanosis
  ii. Clubbing
  iii. Edema
  iv. Cool or cold extremities—suggest peripheral embolization.
  v. Assessment of peripheral arterial pulses
  vi. Warm and moist extremities—hyperthyroidism
G. Neurology:
  i. Signs of transient ischemic attack or cerebrovascular accident.

  ii. Prior history of cerebrovascular accident.
  iii. Increased reflexes—hyperthyroidism.

Investigations of Atrial Fibrillation

A. ECG features of atrial fibrillation:
  i. Irregularly irregular rhythm
  ii. No P wave
  iii. Absence of isoelectric baseline
  iv. Variable ventricular rate.
  v. QRS complex is casually <120 ms, unless there is presence of:
    a. Pre-existing bundle branch block.
    b. Accessory pathway.
    c. Rate-related aberrant conduction.
  vi. Fibrillatory waves may be fine (amplitude <0.5 mm) or coarse (amplitude >0.5 mm)

Other features
i. *Ashman's phenomenon*—presence of aberrantly conducted beats of right bundle branch block due to long refractory period as evidenced by preceding RR interval.
ii. *Ventricular response*—depends upon:
    a. Vagal tone
    b. AV node function
    c. Refractory period
    d. Other pacemaker foci
    e. Medications
Ventricular is usually between 110 and 160/minute.
So atrial fibrillation with rapid ventricular response when ventricular rate is >100/min (Fig. 1.96).
Atrial fibrillation with slow ventricular response when ventricular rate is <60/min (Figs 1.97 and 1.98).
B. Laboratory studies to diagnose different conditions:
  i. Complete blood count—for anemia, infection.
  ii. Serum electrolytes—electrolyte disturbances, renal failure.

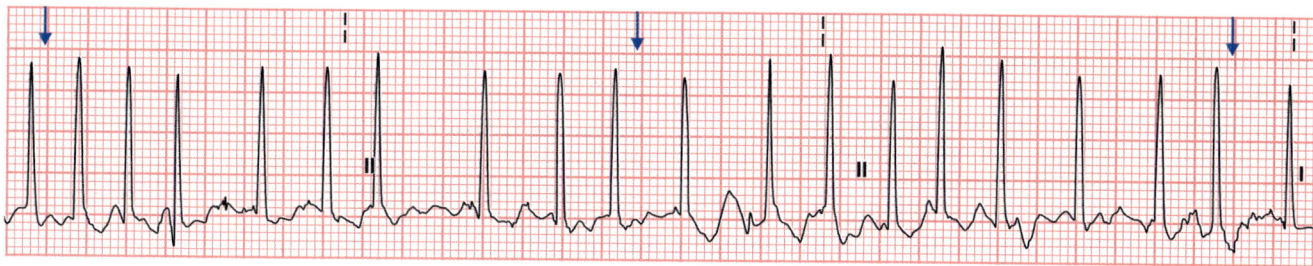

Fig. 1.96: AF with rapid ventricular response

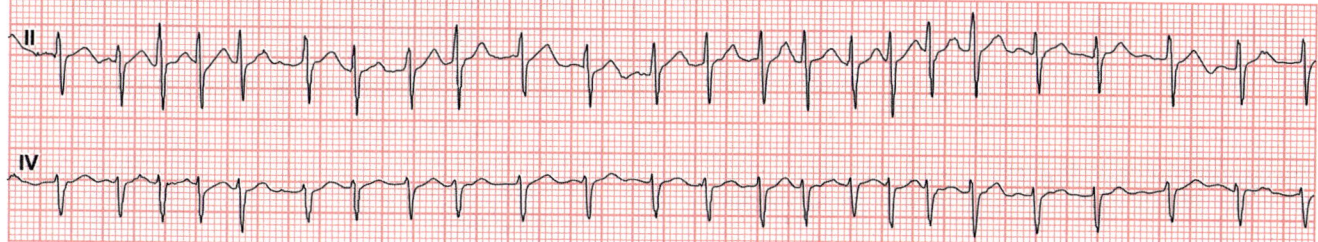

Fig. 1.97: AF with normal ventricular response

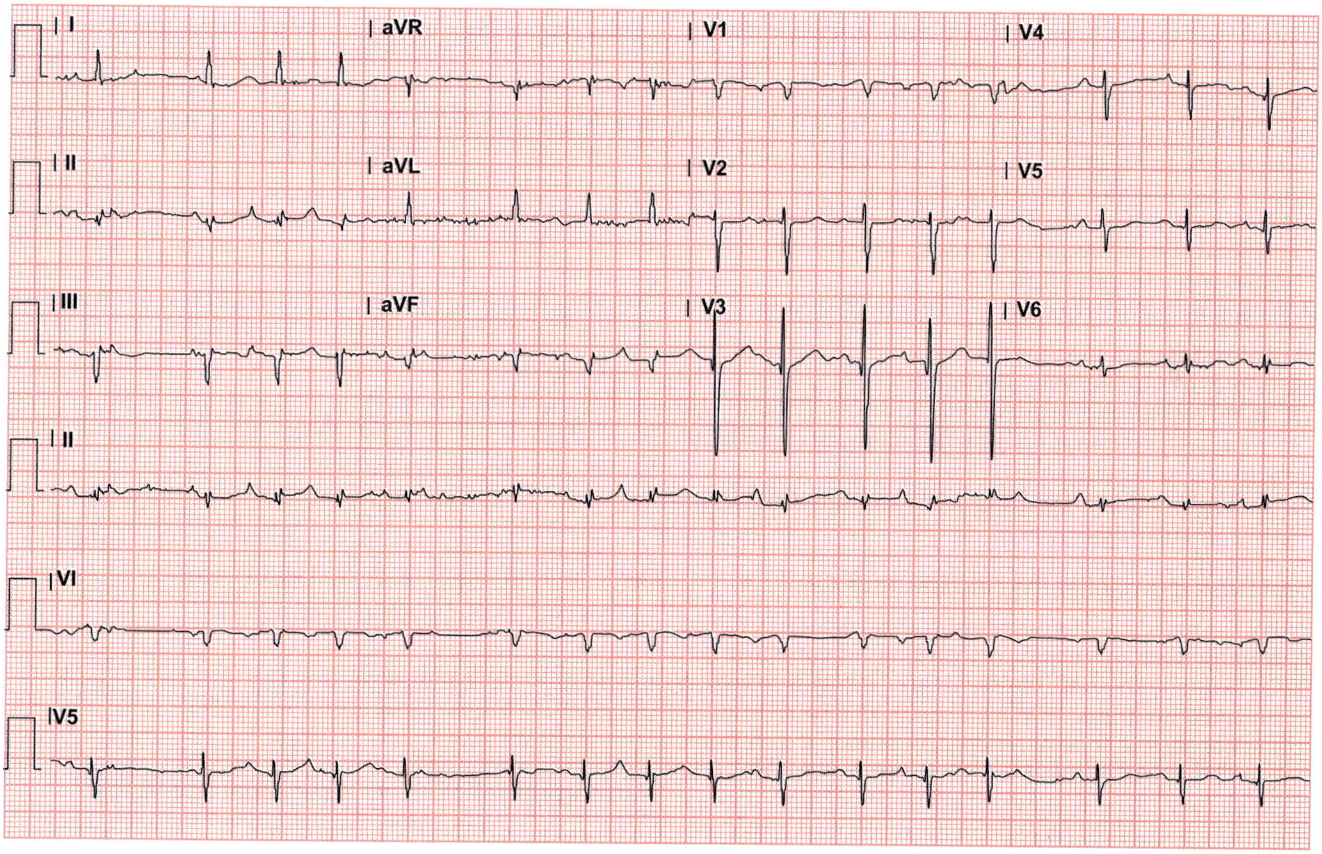

Fig. 1.98: Multifocal atrial tachycardia

iii. Cardiac enzymes—CPK MB, troponin level—to diagnose myocardial infarction as primary or secondary event.

iv. BNP—to diagnose congestive heart failure

v. Thyroid function studies—to exclude thyrotoxicosis

vi. Toxicology level or ethanol level

C. Echocardiography: Transthoracic echocardiography is helpful in following conditions:

i. Evaluation of valvular heart disease.

ii. Evaluation of atrial and ventricular chamber wall dimensions

iii. Estimation of ventricular function.

iv. Evaluation of ventricular thrombi

v. Estimation of pulmonary systolic pressure (pulmonary hypertension)

vi. Evaluation of pericardial disease

vii. Evaluation of left atrial thrombus

viii. To guide cardioversion procedures.

D. Chest X-ray:
   i. Evidence of congestive cardiac failure
   ii. Vascular pathology—pulmonary embolism
   iii. Pulmonary pathology—pneumonia

E. Six-minute walk test: It can assess the adequate rate control (e.g. largest heart rate of 110/mm or less during six minute walk).

F. Exercise test: It can exclude ischemia prior to treatment of patients with class, i.e. antiarrhythmic drugs.

G. Holter monitoring:
   i. It can establish the diagnosis (e.g. in case of paroxysmal atrial fibrillation which is not evident on presentation)
   ii. It can evaluate rate control (target heart rate ≤100/minute).

H. Electrophysiologic study:
   i. It can identify the mechanism of wide QRS—tachycardia.
   ii. AV node

Treatment of Atrial Fibrillation

The cornerstones of management of atrial fibrillation are:
a. Rate control and anticoagulation
b. Rhythm control for those symptomatically limited by atrial fibrillation.

Decision for use of above treatment strategies requires an integrated consideration of several factors:
   i. Degree of symptoms
   ii. Likelihood of successful cardioversion
   iii. Presence of comorbidities.
   iv. Candidates for AF oblation.

Effects of restoration to sinus rhythm:
   i. It improves cardiac hemodynamics.
   ii. It improves exercise tolerance.
   iii. It improves the symptoms of heart failure by increasing effective cardiac output.
   iv. It shows, in some cases, reversal of atrial dilatation and left ventricular dysfunction.

Newer Development in the Treatment of AF

A. MAZE procedure: Reduction of critical mass of atria through either surgical or catheter based compartmentalization of atria direct the fibrillatory wavelets to collide with fixed anatomic obstacles, such as suture lines or complete lines of ablation, and thus reduces or terminates the development of sustained AF to permanent AF.

   Drawback: Due to severe hypocontractility of atria, there is high chance of development of thrombus and consequent risk of embolic stroke.

B. Simple electrical isolation of the origin of pulmonary veins—is 80% successful in reducing the duration and frequency of AF.

Risk Management

Commonest complication of AF is stroke of embolic origin. Known risk factors for stroke in patients with atrial fibrillation are:
   i. Make sex
   ii. Rheumatic valvular disease

iii. Heart failure

iv. Hypertension

v. Diabetes

Other risk factors are:
   i. Advanced age
   ii. Prior history of stroke
   iii. Diabetes
   iv. Hypertension

Mainstay of treatment in these patients is anticoagulation therapy. For each anticoagulant, benefit of stroke reduction must be weighed against the risk of serious bleeding.

So several risk factor assessment algorhythms have been developed which helped the clinician to take decisions for anticoagulation treatment. **This is called CHADS$_2$.**

C = Congestive cardiac failure	-	1 point
H = Hypertension	-	1 point
A = Age >75 years	-	1 points
D = Diabetes	-	1 points
S = Stroke/Tia	-	2 points

Low risk = 0 point. Moderate risk =1 point, High risk = 2 points.

Recommendations on anticoagulation for patients with non-valvular atrial fibrillation are based on 2006, American College of Cardiology (ACC), American Heart Association (AHA), European Society of Cardiology (ESC) guidelines on the management of patients with AF.

1. No risk factors	- Aspirin—81–325 mg/day
2. One moderate risk factor	- Aspirin—81–325 mg/day or warfarin to maintain INR 2–3.
3. High risk factor or more than 1 moderate risk factor	- Warfarin to maintain INR 2–3

High-risk factors include:
   i. Prior stroke
   ii. Systemic thromboembolism

Moderate-risk factors include:
   i. Age >75 years
   ii. Hypertension
   iii. Heart failure
   iv. Left ventricular functional mass <35%

Risk factors of unknown significance:
   i. Female sex
   ii. Age 65–74 years
   iii. Coronary artery disease
   iv. Thyrotoxicosis.

Management of New Onset Atrial Fibrillation

According to ARFIRM study and ACC/AHA/ESC 2006 guidelines:

Initial rate control is "reasonable" for asymptomatic and minimally symptomatic older patients with hypertension or comorbid heart disease.

Whereas, for young individuals without significant co-morbid cardiovascular disease, rhythm control therapy is better approach.

a. Beta-blocker or calcium channel blockers are the 1st line agent for rate control in AF. These can be given orally or intravenously, effective at rest or in exertion.
   Contraindication: Airway obstructive disease.

b. Metoprolol - 5 mg over 3–5 min × 3 doses (loading dose)
↓
  1.25–5 mg 6 hourly (maintenance dose)

c. Verapamil - 5–10 mg over 3–5 minutes (loading dose)
↓
  2.5–10 mg/hour (maintenance dose)

Orally:

1. Metoprolol   25–100 mg   6 hourly
2. Verapamil   80–120 mg   6–8 hourly
3. Diltiazem   30–60 mg   6 hourly

Route of administration depends upon:

i. Clinical status of the patient.
ii. Ventricular rate.

a. **Digoxin:** It can be used in acute setting; but has little control over ventricular rates so it is rarely used as monotherapy.
   Caution: i. In elderly patient
          ii. In renal failure
   Dose **(intravenous):** 0.25 mg 2 hourly until total dose is 1 mg (loading)
          0.125–0.25 mg/day (maintenance dose)
   Orally: 0.125–0.25 mg/day

b. **Amiodarone:** It is used as rate controlling agent for the patients who are intolerant or unresponsive to other above agents.

Caution: It should be exercised in those who are not receiving anticoagulation, as amiodarone can promote cardioversion.

Atrial Fibrillation with WPW Syndrome

1. AF can occur in 20% of patients with WPW syndrome.
2. This pathway allows for rapid conduction directly to the ventricles bypassing AV node.
3. Rapid ventricular rate can terminate ventricular tachycardia or ventricular fibrillation.

ECG feature of AF in WPW syndrome:

i. Rate >200/min
ii. Irregular rhythm
iii. Wide QRS complexes due to abnormal ventricular depolarization via accessory pathway.
iv. Change is shape in QRS morphology.

Treatment: β-blocker, calcium channel blocker, amiodarone are contraindicated in these patients, because they block the AV mode, and impulses traverse through accessory pathways, resulting VT or VF.

SU treatment option is—procainamide, or ibutilide or DC cardioversion.

Anticoagulation: Risk of thromboembolism is high in:
i. Acute cardioversion
ii. Pharmacologic or electrical cardioversion
iii. Patient with AF, where it is present more than 48 hours.

If no thrombus is detected in left atrial appendages by echocardiography, there is low risk of stroke.

The Mode of Treatment

1. In patient with newly diagnosed AF, awaiting cardioversion, IV heparin (APTT—45–60 seconds) or low molecular weight heparin (1 mg/kg/twice daily).

2. Patient can be started with warfarin while waiting at the same time for INR value (2–3 times). Later on serial INR should be done.

   Oral direct thrombin inhibitors may be an alternative to warfarin in high-risk population with non-valvular AF.

3. *Dabigatran*—new oral anticoagulant:
   i. It is as effective as warfarin.
   ii. It is safe.
   iii. It does not require serial INR measurement.
   iv. It is not significantly affected by almost any medication or vitamin.

   Several scoring systems have been developed to estimate the risk benefit ratio for warfarin use in AF.

4. *Rivaroxaban*—direct factor Xa inhibitor with oral bio-availability and rapid onset of action—it was approved by FDA in 2011.

5. *Apixaban*—it is approved by FDA in 2012.

Cardioversion

It can be performed as elective basis or emergent basis.

Indication: Where AF is responsible for hypotension, tachycardia or angina.

It is most successful, if it can be initiated within 7 days after the onset of AF.

Pharmacologic agents can be used to cardiovert the patient.

Advantages: It does not require sedation or anesthesia.

Disadvantages: Risk of ventricular tachycardia or other serious arrhythmias.

Direct Current Cardioversion

i. Patient must be anticoagulated with warfarin for at least 3 weeks with INR confirmed to be >1.8 for last two consecutive occasions before the attempt of cardioversion.

ii. If the condition is warrant or emergent, under short-acting anesthesia 200-J biphasic shock to be delivered synchronously with the QRS complex typically > 90%.

Indications of Pharmacotherapy

To prevent recurrent AF unresponsive to both blockades, a trial of antiarrhythmic therapy should be warranted, if AF is associated with rapid rate or symptomatic.

Selected antiarrhythmic drugs should be given to the following patient:
i. Presence of CAD
ii. Depressed LV functions not attributable to a reversible tachycardia-induced cardiomyopathy.
iii. Severe hypertension with left ventricular hypertrophy.

In case of structural heart disease, the following drugs should be prescribed:
• Sotalol
• Amiodarone
• Dofetilide
• Dronedarone.

In case of severe LV function with heart failure, dronedarone should be prescribed.

In absence of structural heart disease, hypertensive heart disease, without any evidence of severe hypertrophy, Class IC antiarrhythmic drugs—the flecainide or propafenone are well tolerated and without any significant proarrhythmic risk.

Long-term management of AF: Its aim is:

i. Reducing the likehood of AF recurrence

ii. Reduce AF-related symptoms

iii. Controlling of ventricular rate

iv. Reducing the stroke risk.

Anticoagulation: Anticoagulation therapy with warfarin is significantly more effective than antiplatelet therapy.

Here INR adjustment is necessary:

i. The goal in AF is to maintain INR at 2 to 3.

ii. In patient with stroke (artificial valve, rheumatic valve disease, recurrent prior stroke) INR should by 2.5 to 3.5.

iii. Lower INR 1.8–2 in elderly patient with high risk of fall.

Major adverse effect of anticoagulation with warfarin is bleeding.

Factors that increase the risk:

i. History of bleeding

ii. Age >75 years

iii. Liver disease

iv. Renal disease

v. Malignancy

vi. Thrombocytopenia or aspirin use

vii. Hypertension

viii. Diabetes mellitus

ix. Anemia

x. Prior stroke

xi. Risk of fall

xii. Genetic predisposition

xiii. Supratherapeutic INR

ACCF/AHP Guidance Recommendation

Dabigatran—can be used as an alternative to warfarin for prevention of stroke and systemic thromboembolism in patient with paroxysmal to permanent AF.

Contraindication:

i. Prosthetic heart valves

ii. Hemodynamically significant valve disease

iii. Renal failure (creatinine clearance <15 ml/min)

iv. Advanced liver disease.

Indications of chronic rate control therapy: Older patient with comorbid cardiovascular disease who has less likehood of successful long-term rhythm control, adequate rate control should be tested both at rest and in exertion.

Adequate rate control definition by ACCF/AHA/HRS in 2011: <80/min at rest and <110/min after 6-minute walk and lenient rate control <110/min at rest.

Strict rate control in patient with stable ventricular function is no longer recommended.

Drugs are: AV node blocking agents—β-blockers, calcium channel blocker, digoxin.

Generally, combination of β-blockers and CCB is reserved for patient refractory to single agent.

Class 1C antiarrhythmic agents may produce life-threatening atrial flutter with 1:1 AV conduction.

Therefore, administration of β-blocker or CCB is recommended before administration of class 1C antiarrhythmic agents.

In presence of tachycardia-mediated cardiomyopathy or inadequate control of ventricular rate despite of drug therapy, AV nodal ablation or pacemaker implantation must be considered.

Rhythm Control

Proper treatment of underlying disorders (thyrotoxicosis) should be treated to prevent triggering of AF.

The drugs used are:

a. **Amiodarone**: This is the drug of choice in patients with cardiac disease like:

   i. Coronary artery disease

   ii. Systolic or diastolic failure.

   Amiodarone decreases the proarrhythmic effects.

b. According the 2011 updated guidelines by ACCF/HA/HRS—it is reasonable to **use dronedarone** because, it reduces probability of hospitalization of patients with paroxysmal AF or after conversion of persistent AF.

c. **Sotalol**: It can be used for long-term maintenance of sinus rhythm.

Caution:

i. Close monitoring is required because it may produce QT prolongation and torsade de pontes.

ii. In patient with congestive heart failure, there may be greater chance of proarrhythmic effect.

iii. Serum electrolytes should be measured; because in presence of hypokalemia, there may be chance of prolongation of 'QT' interval.

Catheter ablation, as recommended by 2011 guidelines by ACCF/AHA/HRS—for following indications:

i. It is used as an alternative to pharmacologic therapy to prevent recurrent paroxysmal AF in significantly symptomatic patient with no or little structural heart disease.

ii. Symptomatic persistent AF.

iii. Symptomatic paroxysmal AF with structural heart disease.

Surgical ablation is also an option in patients where pharmacologic or contraindicated.

Atrial fibrillation ablation is superior to AV nodal ablation and biventricular pacing in heart failure patients, but it is technically difficult and demanding.

Newer medical rhythm control therapies:

i. Renin—angiotensin—system antagonists.

ii. HMG CoA—reductase inhibitions (statins).

The above drugs reduce the chances AF as they help in successful cardioversion

Newer device controlled therapies:

i. Single or dual—site atrial pacemakers

ii. Atrial defibrillators

They rapidly restore the sinus rhythm.

Invasive (surgical and catheter-based) therapies:

i. It compartmentalizes the atria.

ii. Localized focal triggers (in the pulmonary veins) are being evaluated and refined.

Cardioversion

1. Electrical cardioversion

Indications:
a. In unstable patient:
   i. Sever dyspnea
   ii. Severe chest pain
   iii. Pre-exited atrial fibrillation
b. In stable patient:
   i. If rate control treatment does not elicit response.
   ii. If echocardiography does not reveal any valvular or functional abnormality of the heart.

Method:
i. DC cardioversion means the delivery of electric current to synchronize QRS complexes.
ii. It can be in monophasic or biphasic waveform.
iii. Energy requirement is usually 100J–200J for monophasic waveform and less for biphasic waveforms.
iv. Sedation is required.
v. Success rate is 75% in patient with AF of short duration.

Complication:
i. Thrombus formation even in patient with sinus rhythm.
   Hence transesophageal electrocardiography is required to exclude thrombus and anticoagulation should be started 4 weeks before the commencement of the procedure.
ii. Pulmonary edema
iii. Hypotension
iv. Myocardial dysfunction
v. Skin burns
vi. Serious ventricular arrhythmias, which can be avoided by synchronization.
   Skin burns can be avoided by use of steroid cream and proper technique.
vii. Elevation of serum cardiac biomarkers.

Paddle should be placed in anterolaterally (ventricular apex and right infraclavicular), and anteroposteriorly (sternum and left scapular).

Energy escalation during the procedures:
1. 70, 120, 150, 170 Jules for biphasic waveforms
2. 100, 200, 300, 360 Jules for monophasic waveforms.

2. Pharmacologic cardioversion

Indications:
i. It can be used as 1st line strategy
ii. It can be used when DC cardioversion fails.
iii. It can be used followed by repeat DC cardioversion.

Pretreatment with amiodarone, flecainide, ibutilide, propafenone or sotalol increases the success rate of DC cardioversion.

ACC/AHA/ESC guideline regarding pharmacologic conversion:
1. For conversion of AF of less than 7 days duration—effective drugs include dofetilide, flecainide, ibutilide, propafenone, effective to lesser degree include amiodarone, and quinidine, less effective or incompletely studied drugs are procainamide, digoxin and sotalol.

2. For conversion of AF lasting for 7–90 days—drugs with proven efficacy are dofetilide, amiodarone, ibutilide, flecainide, propafenone and quinidine, less effective or incompletely studied include procainamide, sotalol and digoxin.
3. For conversion of AF of >90 days duration, propafenone, amiodarone, and dofetilide have been shown to be effective to covert AF to normal sinus rhythm.

Postoperative Atrial Fibrillation

a. It can be prevented by:
   1. Recommendation of perioperative-blocker—in patient undergoing cardiac surgery.
   2. Preoperative administration of amiodarone or sotalol in patients undergoing cardiac surgery
b. It can be treated by landiolol hydrochloride—mechanism of action:
   i. Amelioration of ischemia
   ii. Anti-inflammatory effect
   iii. Inhibition of sympathetic hypertonia
   In this treatment—hypotension and bradycardia do not develop.

Catheter and Surgical Ablation

Goal of catheter ablation:
i. To disconnect the triggers
ii. To modify the substrate for AF

Paroxysmal AF is produced by ectopic trigger activity in pulmonary veins—so ablation wound the veins may terminate AF.

In persistent AF: Triggering foci and reentry circuit are both present in atrial tissue, it requires more extensive mapping to terminate AF.

Compartmentalization of the Atria

There are two approaches:
1. **Surgical compartmentalization of atria (MAZE procedure).** This procedure involves a series of small endocardial incisions in right and left atria. It isolates pulmonary veins and interrupts reentrant pathways, which is required for maintenance of AF.
2. **Compartmentalization of atria with continuous ablation lines of blockage:** It includes MAZE procedure along with suture lines with radiofrequency lesions.
   Result is disappointing and it can start left atrial reentrant tachycardia and left atrial flutters.

Catheter Ablation of Focal Triggers of AF

Combined procedures include—individual pulmonary vein isolation and left atrial ablation (encircling pulmonary veins pairs, connecting right and left pairs along the left atrial roof and connection to mitral valve annulus).

Radiofrequency ablation is an option in patients with persistant AF.

Complications

i. Cardiac perforation
ii. Pericardial effusion
iii. Cardiac tamponade
iv. Vascular access complications
v. Pulmonary vein stenosis

vi Thromboembolism
vii. Atrio-oesophageal fistula
viii. Left atrial flutter
ix. Pulmonary vein stenosis in 6% patients may produce dyspnea, chest pain, cough and hemoptysis.

AV Nodal Ablation and Permanent Pacemaker

It is usually done in patients with AF with uncontrolled ventricular response despite medical therapy.

Because of permanent AV block, a permanent ventricular pacemaker is required—which governs ventricular rate.

There is risk of thromboembolism—hence prior anti-coagulation is required.

ACCELERATED IDIOVENTRICULAR RHYTHM

Definition

This can be defined as enhanced ectopic ventricular rhythm with at least 3 consecutive beats, which is faster than normal intrinsic escape ventricular rhythm (≤40 beats/minute) but slower than ventricular tachycardia (100–120 beats per minute).

But to diagnose accelerated idioventricular rhythm, one cannot depend upon ventricular rate. The characteristics of AIVR are:
i. It is transient rhythm.
ii. It rarely produces hemodynamic instability.
iii. It rarely requires treatment.
iv. It can be misdiagnosed as slow ventricular tachycardia or complete heart block, whose treatment may lead to potential complications.

Pathophysiology

Main mechanisms of AIVR are:
i. Enhanced automaticity of His-Purkinje fibers and/or myocardium
ii. Decreased vagal access

iii. Decreased sympathetic activity
↓
Triggering factors are: Ischemia, reperfusion, hypoxia, drugs and electrolyte abnormalities.
↓
Accelerate phase 4 depolarization rates in His-Purkinje fibers and myocardium
↓
Faster spontaneous cell depolarization (enhanced automaticity)
↓
When suppresses the rate of sinus node
AVR becomes the dominant rhythm of the heart

Focus of AVR may be single or multiple. Ventricular rate of AVR is between 40 and 100/minute.

In case of myocardial infarction, AVR may be responsible hemodynamic instability, because it may liable to produce ventricular asynchrony leading to ventricular tachycardia and ventricular fibrillation.

In ST segment elevated myocardial infarction:

i. It occurs in single or multiple foci of His-Purkinje system or ventricular myocardium.
ii. It may be an indicator of coronary artery reopening. But it is not a marker of complete reperfusion.

Symptoms for AIVR

1. Chest pain, breathing discomfort—related to myocardial ischemia.
2. There may be history coronary artery reperfusion related to myocardial infarction.
3. There may be shortness of breath, cyanosis, clubbing, peripheral edema related to cardiomyopathy, myocarditis.
4. There may be history of intake of drugs, like, digoxin, illicit drugs intake.
5. There may be no history.

Signs

1. Pulse:
    a. Rate:
        i. Tachycardia with rate >100 beats/minute.
        ii. Bradycardia with rate <55 beats/minute.
    b. Rhythm: Regularly irregular—due to presence of sinus rhythm in between junctional rhythm
2. Venous wave: Cannon wave
3. Heart sound—variable
4. Blood pressure—hypotension due to AV synchrony

Causes of AIVR

1. Most common cause is coronary artery reperfusion in case of acute myocardial infarction.
2. Other causes are:
    i. Congenital cyanotic heart disease
    ii. Myocarditis
    iii. Drugs:
        a. Digoxin
        b. Illicit drug—cocaine
        c. Anesthetic drugs
    iv. Dilated cardiomyopathy
    v. Post-resuscitation
    vi. Buerger disease

Laboratory Studies

A. **Blood tests:**
    i. Troponin, CPK and CPK—MB to diagnose myocardial infarction.
    ii. Blood urea nitrogen, creatinine—to assess renal function.
    iii. Blood potassium—to exclude digoxin—toxicity
    iv. Blood digoxin levels.

B. **Electrocardiography** (Figs 1.99, 1.100)
    i. Three or more ventricular complexes at a rate >40/min and <120/min.
    ii. It is of gradual onset and offset and more variability in cycle length.
    iii. It should be differentiated from complete heart block

    In complete heart block, 'P' waves are present preceding QRS complex, but fail to conduct to the ventricle.

C. **Telemetry monitoring**

D. **Holter monitoring**

E. **Loop recorder**

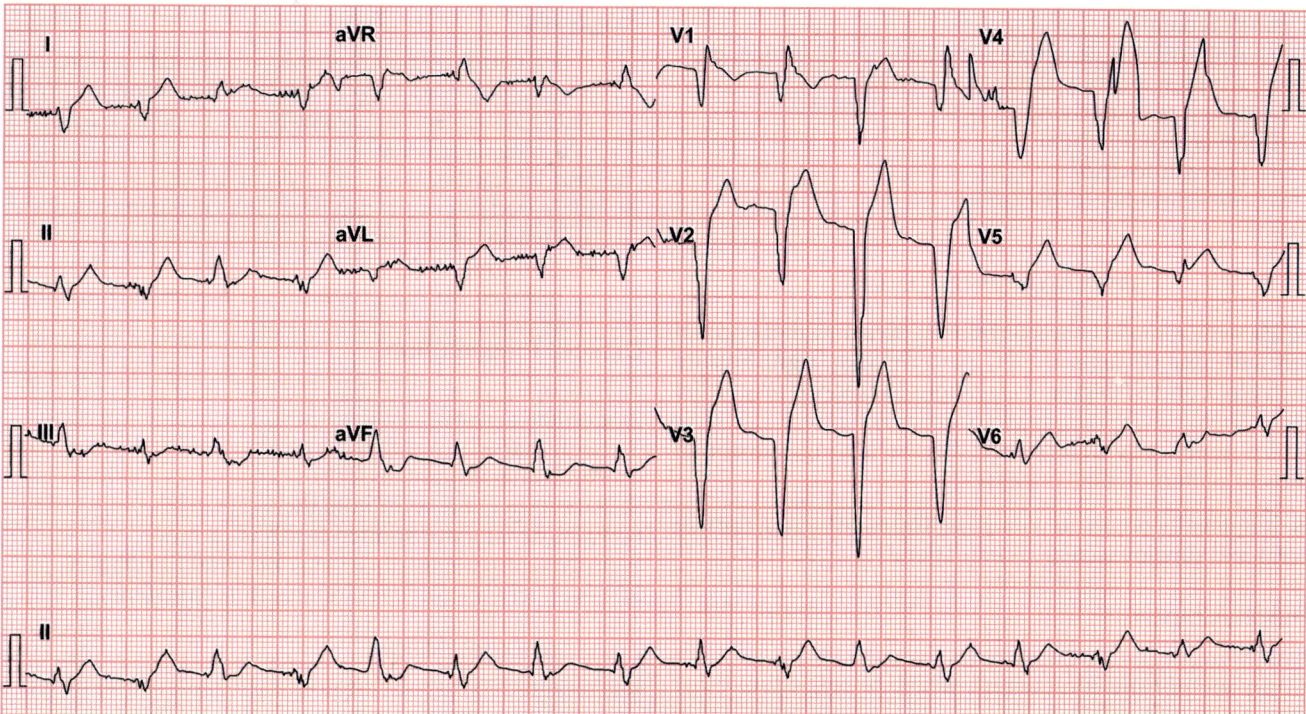

Fig. 1.99: Accelerated idioventricular rhythm

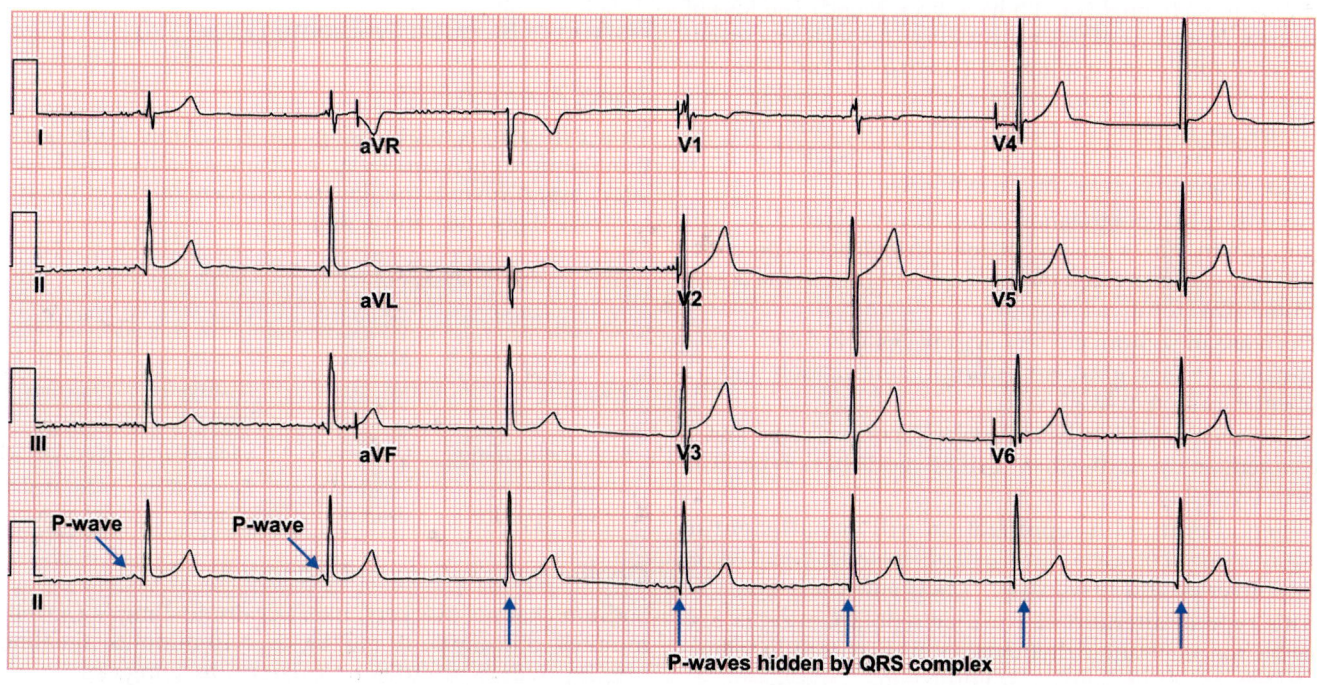

Fig. 1.100: Idioventricular rhythm

F. Imaging studies:

i. Echocardiogram—it can detect structural myocardial disease.

ii. Nuclear perfusion scan—it can evaluate myocardial ischemia

iii. Coronary angiogram: It can evaluate coronary artery patency.

Treatment

Most important treatment of AIVR is to treat underlying etiology.

I. AIVR is usually self-limited and hemodynamically tolerated—hence it does not require any treatment.

II. In a few cases, AIVR is not tolerated because:

i. There may be atrial ventricular asynchrony

ii. Relatively rapid ventricular rate

iii. AIVR may generate to VT or VF

In above conditions, atropine may be used to increase sinus rate and to inhibit AIVR.

III. Other treatments include:

i. Isoproterenol

ii. Verapamil
iii. Antiarrhythmic drugs—lidocaine, amiodarone, and
iv. Atrial overdrive pacing.
IV. Treatment of underlying causes:
  i. Myocardial ischemia
  ii. Digoxin toxicity
  iii. Structural heart disease

BRUGADA SYNDROME

Brugada syndrome is characterized by occurrence of sudden death with one or several ECG patterns like, right bundle branch block and ST segment elevations in anterior precordial leads.

It is a genetically determined disease having autosomal dominant pattern in 50% of cases.

Sex: It usually occurs in young healthy male having normal general and cardiovascular examination.

Pathophysiology

It is an example of channelopathies—caused by alteration in the transmembrane ion current which is responsible for cardiac action potential.

Mutation of SCN5A gene, which encodes cardiac voltage-gated sodium channel Na_v 1.5 have been found. The loss of functional mutations of this gene reduces the sodium current (I_{Na}) available during phase 0 (upstroke) and 1 (early repolarization) of action potential of cardiac muscle. This decrease in I_{Na} affects right ventricular endocardium differently from epicardium. It is responsible for ECG manifestations as well as clinical syndrome.

According to repolarization defect theory—epicardial cells of epicardium show a prominent notch in their action potential due to transient increased outward current (I_{PO}) to the action potential waveform.

Decrease in sodium current aggravates this difference—producing voltage gradient during repolarization and ST segment elevation in ECG.

When relative durations of repolarization are same and T waves remain up right—there will be saddleback type ECG pattern (type 2 or 3).

When alteration in repolrization will be sufficient to produce reversal of normal gradient of repolarization, T wave will be inverted and coved (type 1) ECG pattern.

This type of alteration in cardiac repolarization is responsible for reentrant arrhythmias—this may lead to ventricular tachycardia or ventricular fibrillation.

Etiology

1. Mutation of SCN5A gene
2. Genes coding alpha 1—and beta2b subunits of L type calcium channel (CACNA 1C and CACNB2).
3. Mutation in genes GPD1-L and SCN1B in familial cases.

In few cases, mutation of SCN5A gene cannot be demonstrated due to:
  i. Mutation of other genes
  ii. Other unidentified genes.
    These genes are located in the region of coding sequences or promoter region of SCN5A gene.

Prognosis

i. It is a cause of polymorphic ventricular tachycardia—which may lead to ventricular fibrillation and cardiac arrest. As a result of cardiac arrest, hypoxia may produce neurologic sequelae.
ii. Sudden cardiac death may occur in 8.2% of patients.
iii. Increased risk of sudden death may occur in patients with:
  a. History of syncope
  b. Abnormal ECG
  c. Induced during programmed electrical stimulation.

Clinical Presentation

1. Syncope
2. Cardiac arrest
3. Nightmares
4. Thrashing at night
5. Patient may be asymptomatic.
6. Family history of sudden death is common.
7. In 20% of patient—there may be atrial fibrillation.
8. Fever occasionally precipitates this syndrome.

Physical Examination

It is required to rule out the noncardiogenic causes of syncope and also other cardiac causes of cardiac arrest or syncope in otherwise healthy patients.

Workup of Brugada Syndrome (Table 1.4)

Signal Average ECG

This can differentiate Brugada syndrome from arrhythmogenic right ventricular cardiomyopathy—because in later case, it reveals the fibrofatty degeneration of the right ventricle (Figs 1.101 and 1.102).

Table 1.4: ECG pattern in Brugada syndrome

Characteristics	Type 1	Type 2	Type 3
J wave amplitude	≥2 mm	≥2 mm	>2 mm
T wave	Negative	Positive or biphasic	Positive
ST-T configuration	Cove type	Saddleback	Saddleback
ST segment terminal portion	Gradually descending	Elevated by ≥1 mm	Elevated by <1 mm

Challenge with Sodium Channel Blocker

Sodium channel blockers, like, flecainide 2 mg/kg, over 10 minutes, procainide 10 mg/kg over 10 minutes, ajmaline 1 mg/kg over 5 minutes or pilsicinide 1 mg/kg over 10 minutes—may show in positive cases—generate J wave with an absolute amplitude of ≥2 mm in leads V1, V2 and/or V3 with or without IBBB.
The above drugs should be stopped in following conditions:
1. When ventricular arrhythmia occurs
2. When the result will be positive
3. ≥30% duration of widened QRS complex.

Isoproterenol and sodium lactate act as antidotes, if the above drugs (sodium channel blockers) induce arrhythmia.

Contraindication: In type 1 Brugada syndrome.

Recommendation: Type 2 and 3 Brugada syndrome can be tested by Na-channel blockers.

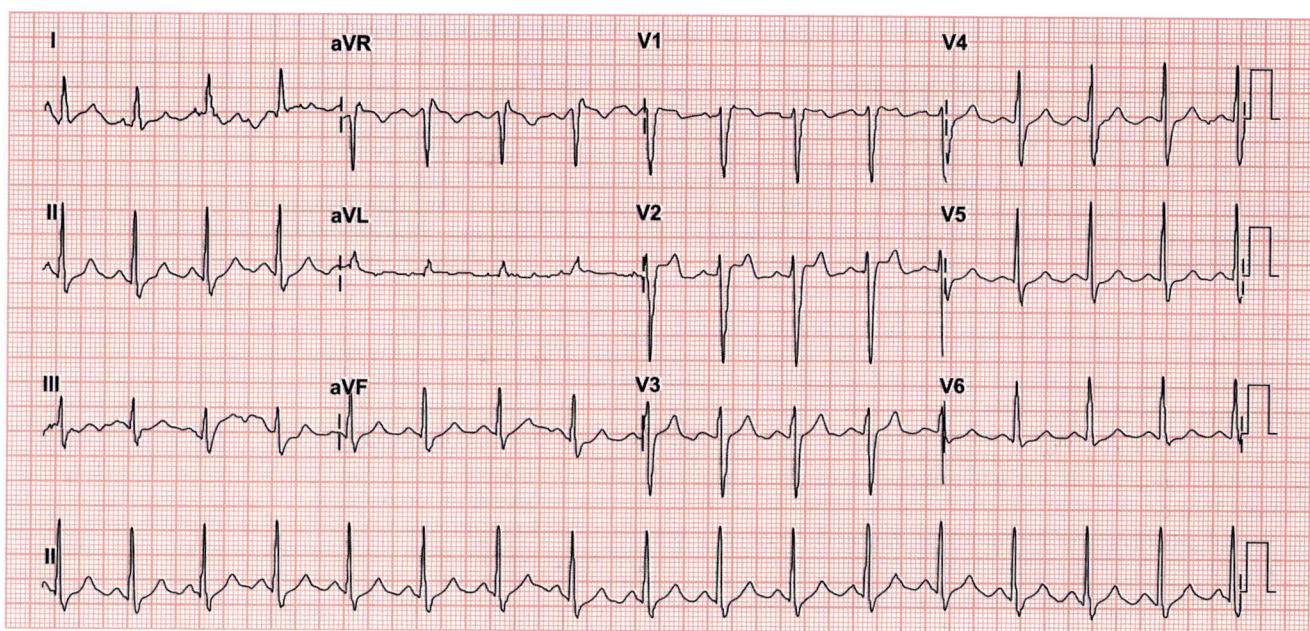

Fig. 1.101: Type 2 Brugada syndrome

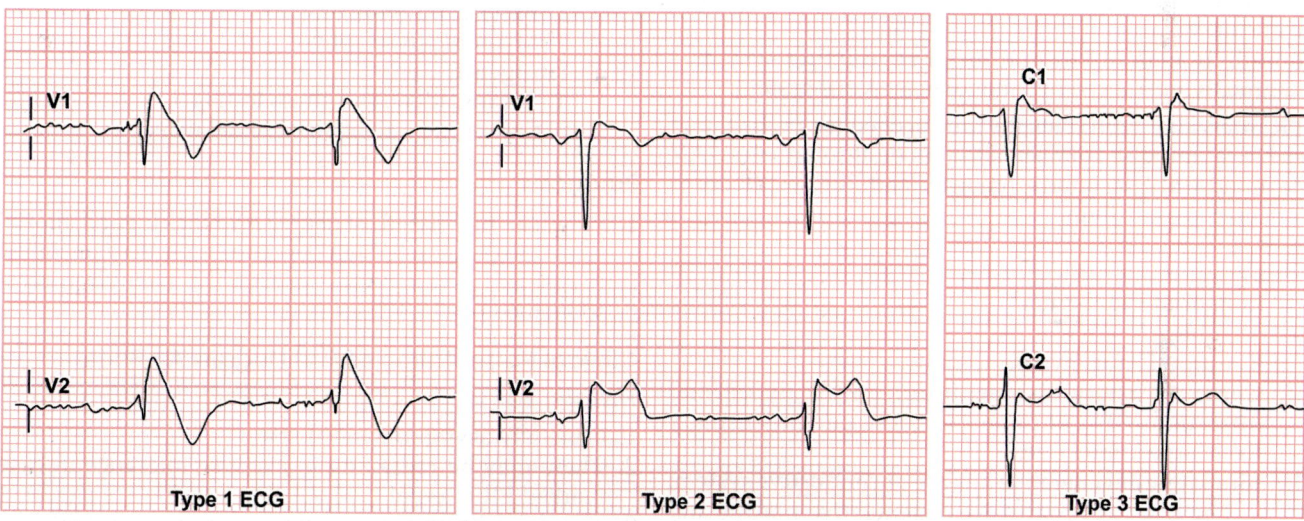

Fig. 1.102: Types 1, 2, and 3 Brugada syndrome

Electrophysiological study: This study is used to determine the inducibility of arrhythmias.

Hematological Test

1. Serum potassium and calcium levels should be checked in patient with elevated ST segment in precordial lead, because hyperkalemia and hypercalcemia may show similar ECG pattern.
2. CPK, CPK—MB and TropI should be checked in patients with symptoms similar to that of acute coronary syndrome.

Genetic Testing

Genetic test to look for the mutation of SCN5A—it codes for α subunits Na_v 1.5 of sodium channel.

Management

Implantable automatic cardiac defibrillator (ICD)—is proven effective in:

i. VT   ii. AF

iii. Presenting sudden death in patient with Brugada syndrome.

ATRIOVENTRICULAR CONDUCTION DISEASE

Anatomy of AV Node

Atrioventricular conduction axis is composed of atria, ventricles and AV node. It is a subendocardial oval or elliptical structure, 7–8 mm in anteroposterior axis and 3 mm in vertical axis and 1 mm in transverse axis.

Superior, medial and posterior atrionodal bundle converge into AV node.

AV node is situated at the apex of triangle of Koch which is composed of:

1. Coronary sinus ostium posteriorly.
2. Septal tricuspid valve annulus anteriorly.
3. Tendon of Todaro superiorly.

AV node continues as penetrating AV bundle traverses the central fibrous body in close proximity to aortic, mitral and tricuspid valve annuli, hence it is liable to injury during operation.

The penetrating bundle continues through annulus fibrosus and emerges along the ventricular septum adjacent to membranous part of it as bundle of His. From the distal AV bundle—right bundle branch traverses the right ventricle as band—it is known as moderator band.

Left bundle branch emerges on septal part of left ventricle as a sheet of tissue.

From right and left bundle branches, Purkinje fibers arise and ramify extensively along the right and left ventricles.

Blood Supply

1. Penetrating AV bundle:
   i. AV nodal artery 90%.
   ii. First septal perforator of left anterior descending artery.
2. Bundle branch:
   i. Septal perforator of left anterior descending coronary artery
   ii. Branches of posterior descending coronary artery.

Nerve Supply

1. AV node—postganglionic parasympathetic and sympathetic nerves.
2. Bundle branch of His and distal conducting system—minimally influenced by autonomic nervous system.

PR interval: It represents the time needed for propagation of electrical impulse from sinoatrial node through atria, AV node, bundle of His, bundle branches and Purkinje fibers to ventricular myocardium.

Etiology

 I. **Enhanced vagal tone:**
   i. Athlete
   ii. Carotid sinus hypersensitivity
 II. **Coronary artery disease:** Inferior wall myocardial infarction—15% of patients—these patients usually have large infarct size.
 III. **Idiopathic degenerative disease of conductive system:**
   i. Lev disease: Progressive degenerative fibrosis and calcification of neighboring cardiac structures (mitral valve annulus, central fibrous body, membranous septum, base of the aorta, crest of ventricular septum).
   ii. Lenegre disease—idiopathic degenerative disease, restricted to Purkinje system.
 IV. **Drugs commonly responsible for 1st degree block:**
   1. Class Ia antiarrhythmic drugs—quinidine, procainamide
   2. Class Ic antiarrhythmic drugs—flecainide, encainide
   3. Class II antiarrhythmic drugs—β blockers
   4. Class III antiarrhythmic drugs—Amiodarone, sotalol
   5. Class IV antiarrhythmic drugs—calcium channel blocker
   6. Digoxin and other cardiac glycosides
   7. Magnesium
 V. **Metabolic/endocrine:**
   1. Hyperkalemia
   2. Hypermagnesemia
   3. Hypothyroidism
 VI. **Infectious diseases:**
   1. Endocarditis
   2. Diphtheria
   3. Rheumatic fever
   4. Chagas disease
   5. Lyme's disease
 VII. **Collagen vascular disease:**
   1. Systemic lupus erythematosus
   2. Rheumatoid arthritis
   3. Mixed connective tissue disease
   4. Scleroderma.
 VIII. **Infiltrative diseases:**
   1. Amyloidosis
   2. Sarcoidosis
   3. Hemochromatosis
 IX. **Malignant:**
   1. Mesothelioma
   2. Lymphoma
   3. Radiation
   4. Melanoma
 X. **Traumatic:** Catheter ablation
 XI. **Congenital:**
   1. Congenital heart disease
   2. Facioscapulohumeral
   3. Myotonic dystrophy
 XII. **Iatrogenic:**
   i. During adenosine stress testing
   ii. During closure of atrial septal defect

Prognosis

1. Prognosis of isolated 1st degree AV block is good, mortality is nil. Progression to high degree block is very uncommon.
2. In case of Lyme carditis—heart bock in children recover spontaneously in 3 days.

Clinical Presentation of First Degree AV Bock

History

1. Generally asymptomatic at rest.
2. There may be reduction in exercise tolerance in case of marked PR interval.
3. There may be syncope—mainly occurs in case of infranodal block with wide QRS complexes.

Relevant Past History

   i. Myocarditis
   ii. Myocardial infarction
   iii. Trained athlete
   iv. Intake of drugs producing slow conduction through atrioventricular node.
   v. Lyme carditis mostly in children older than 10 years of age, arthralgia.
   vi. History of long-standing SLE may be a clue to significant cardiac disease.
   vii. History of undergone mitral valve replacement or mitral valve annuloplasty.

Physical Examinations

1. No significant findings in physical examination.
2. Intensity of 1st heart sound is softened.
3. There may be soft blowing diastolic murmur not due to mitral regurgitation because its peak reaches before the onset of regurgitation.

It is due to slow antegrade flow of blood through closing mitral valve leaflets.

This murmur will be absent, if in this patient atropine will be administered.

Complications

i. First degree AV block may progress to Mobiz type 1 2nd degree block or high degree AV block. This can occur in patients with myocardial infarction, myocarditis or drug over dose.
ii. Pace maker syndrome
iii. Reduction in left ventricular stroke volume and cardiac output.

Laboratory Workup

First degree AV block is an accidental finding in ECG. So, routine evaluation is not usually required.

But electrolyte and drug screen should be done to search for etiology.

Electrocardiography (Fig. 1.103)

1. PR interval will be more than 200 msec
2. All P waves are followed by normal QRS complexes.

His bundle electrocardiography: This is necessary, if the first degree AV block is followed by wide QRS complexes—this indicates bundle branch block.

Management

1. Usually no treatment is required for 1st degree AV block.
2. Patient with severe bradycardia and marked 1st degree AV block (PR interval > 300 msec)—may require medications (atropine, isoproterenol) in the anticipation of insertion of cardiac pacemaker.
3. Treatment of underlying cardiac conditions, like, myocardial infarction
4. Treatment of underlying other condition, e.g. digitalis interactions, electrolyte abnormalities.

Pacemaker Implantation

According AHA/ACC/HRS—the indications are:
1. First degree AV block with or without symptoms when it may be associated with:
   a. Myotonic muscular dystrophy
   b. Erb dystrophy (limb–girdle muscular dystrophy).
   c. Peroneal muscular atrophy
   Because, these patients may experience unpredictable progression of AV conduction disease (class IIb recommendation, level of evidence, B)
2. Symptoms similar to pacemaker syndrome or hemodynamic compromise (class IIa recommendation; level of evidence B)
   Pacemaker is not indicated in asymptomatic AV block (clas III recommendation, level of evidence B).

Second Degree Atrioventricular Block

Definition

It can be defined as disturbance, delay or interruption of atrial impulse propagation through atrioventricular node to ventricular muscles. This block may be transient or permanent—it depends upon anatomic or functional disorganization of the tissue.

Classification

This block can be classified based on electrocardiographic criteria into two types:
1. **Mobitz 1 second degree block** (Fig. 1.04): It is characterized by progressive lengthening of PR interval followed by loss of propagation of atrial impulse, as evidenced by absence of P wave as well as QRS. So in the 1st beat of cycle, PR interval will be shorted and in the last beat of cycle, PR interval will be longest.
2. **Mobitz 2 second degree AV block** (Fig. 1.105): It is characterized by sudden and non-conducted atrial impulse, as well as absence of QRS wave-Here:
   i. There is no progressive lengthening of PR interval
   ii. PR interval and PR interval between the conducted beats will be constant.

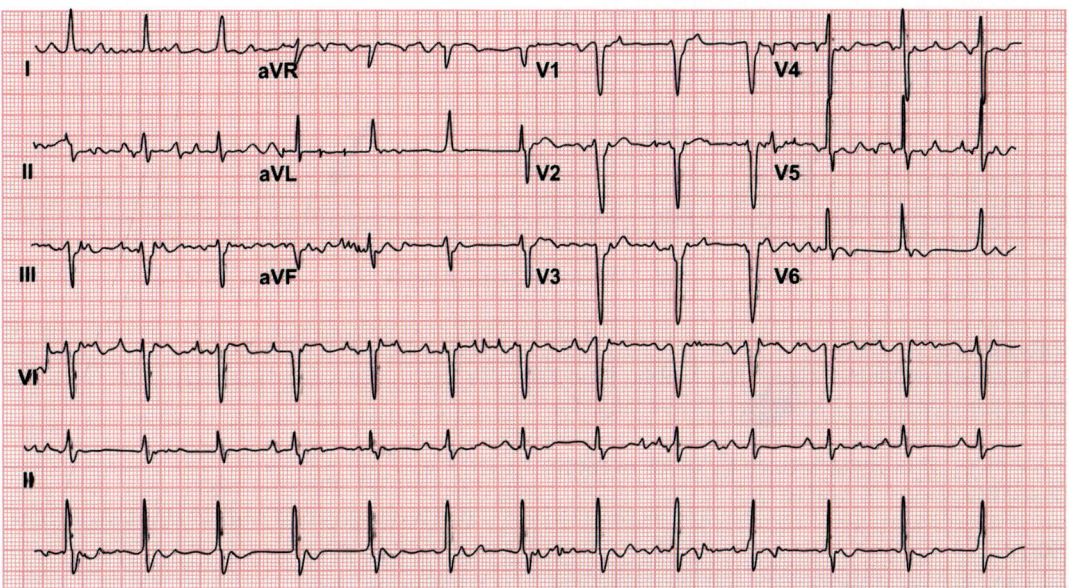

Fig. 1.103: 1st degree AV block

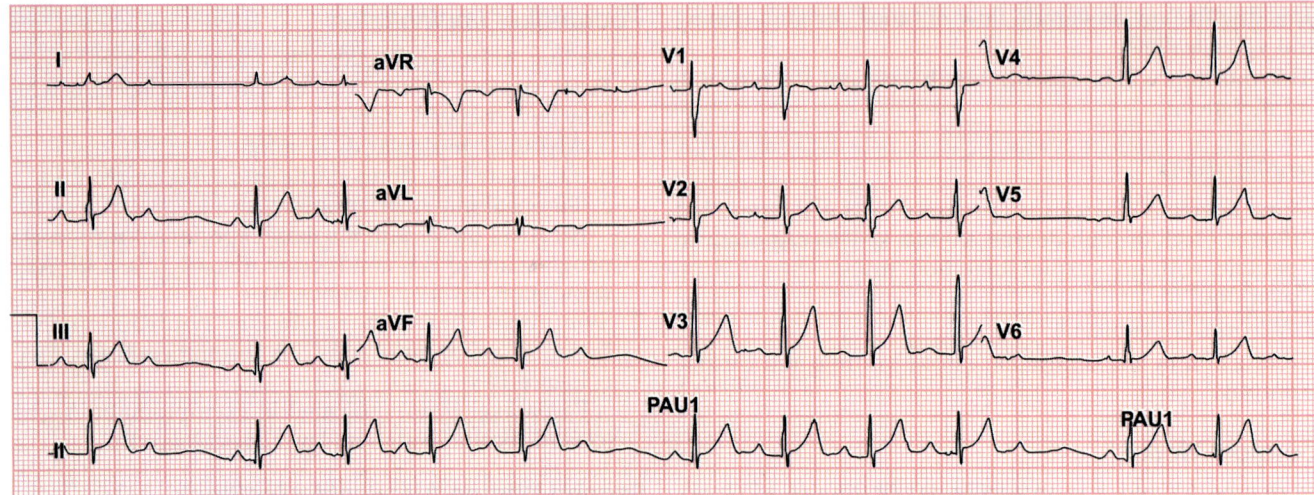

Fig. 1.104: Mobitz type 1 block

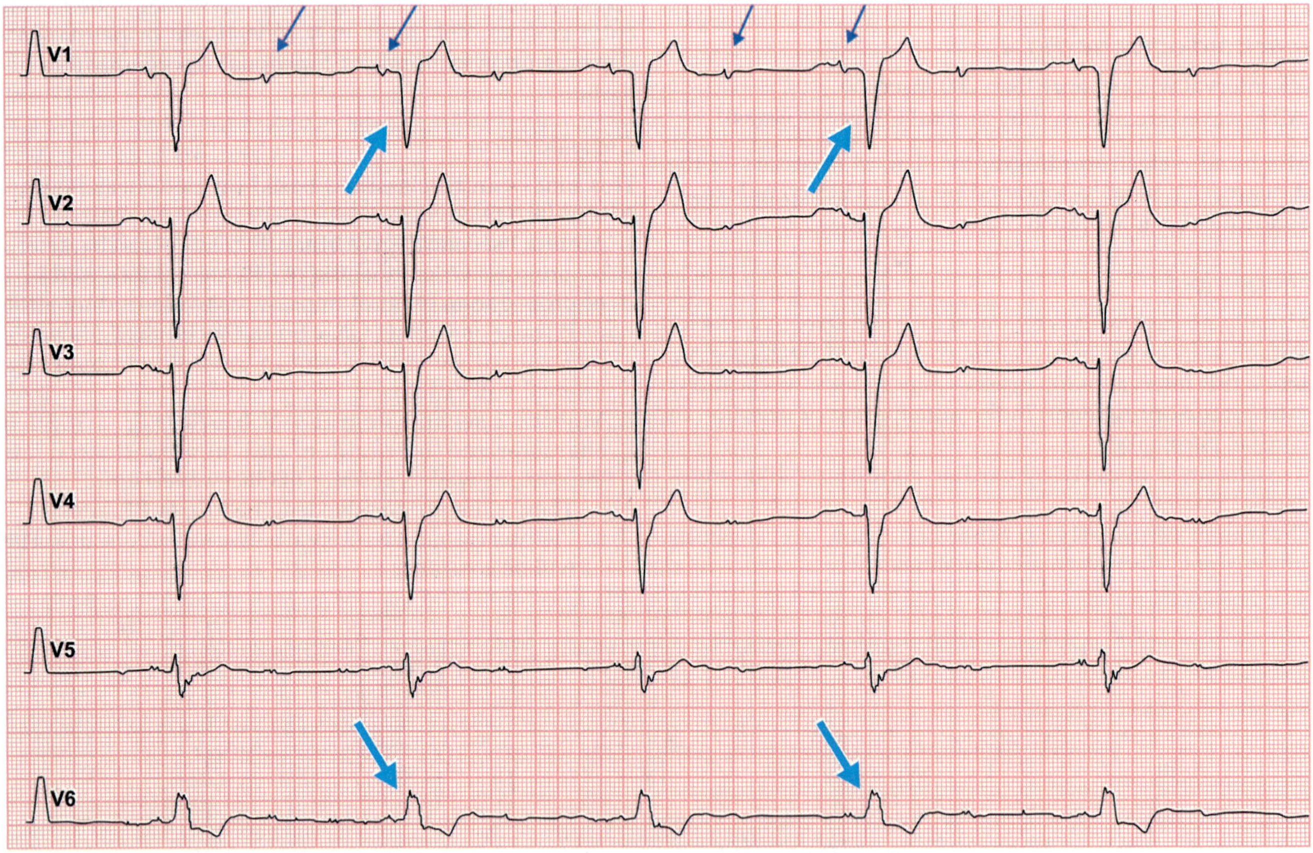

Fig. 1.105: Mobitz type 2 block

Other classifications are:

i. 2:1 AV block: It is neither Mobitz type 1 nor Mobitz type 2 blocks; because, here, only one PR interval is available for analysis.

ii. High grade AV block: It is characterized by block of more than two consecutive sinus 'P' waves.

Pathophysiology

In Mobitz type 1 block—conduction delay mostly occurs in AV node (70% cases) and intranodal region (30% cases).

If it occurs in AV node:

i. QRS complex width is narrow.

ii. No underlying cardiac disease.

iii. It is usually vagally mediated.

a. Carotid sinus massage

b. Hypersensitive carotid sinus syndrome

c. Athlete at rest

d. During sleep

e. Digitalis excess

If it occurs distal to AV node (bundle of His):
  i. QRS width will be wide.
 ii. There is associated cardiac disease.
iii. Baseline PR interval is shorter with smaller PR increments preceding block.
 iv. It carries worst prognosis.

In Mobitz type 2 blocks:
  i. Block usually occurs infranodally.
 ii. QRS complex is usually wide.
iii. Infranodal block carries worse prognosis.

To differentiate Mobitz 1 from 2 block, at least three consecutive P tracing must be present in ECG tracing.

Etiology

   I. **Inflammatory disease:**
      1. Endocarditis
      2. Myocarditis
      3. Lyme disease
      4. Acute rheumatic fever
  II. **Infiltrative disease:**
      1. Hemochromatosis
      2. Sarcoidosis
      3. Amyloidosis
      AV conduction abnormality may be the first sign.
 III. **Infiltrative malignancies:**
      1. Hodgkin and non-Hodgkin lymphoma
      2. Multiple myeloma
  IV. **Metabolic causes:**
      1. Hyperkalemia
      2. Hypermagnesemia
   V. **Endocrine disorders:**
      1. Hyperthyroidism
      2. Addison disease
      3. Myxedema
      4. Thyrotoxic periodic paralysis.
  VI. **Collagen vascular disease:**
      1. Rheumatoid arthritis
      2. Scleroderma
      3. SLE
      4. Ankylosing spondylitis.
 VII. **Other cardiac condition:**
      1. Cardiac tumors
      2. Cardiac trauma
      3. Myocardial bridging
      4. Progressive fibrosis of cardiac skeleton
      5. AMI
VIII. **Procedures related:**
      1. Ethanol septal reduction
      2. Transcortical ablation of septal hypertrophy in the treatment of HOCM
      3. Corrective congenital cardiac surgery, near septum
      4. Transcatheter closure of ASD and VSD
  IX. **Non-cardiac causes:**
      1. Obstructive sleep apnea
      2. Muscular dystrophies
      3. Acute ethanol poisoning
   X. **Drugs producing heart block:**
      1. Drugs responsible for negative ionotropic effect on AV node:
          i. Digoxin
         ii. β-blocker
        iii. Calcium channel blocker
      2. Antiarrhythmic drugs responsible for block in His-Purkinje system
          i. Procainamide—sodium channel blocker
         ii. Adenosine
      3. Other drugs are:
          i. Lithium carbonate at toxic levels
         ii. Benzathine penicillin
        iii. Presynapic alpha agonist—clonidine
  XI. **Genetic causes:**
      1. Several mutations in SCN5A—responsible for familiar AV block
      2. Long QT syndrome
      3. Brugada syndrome

Prognosis

1. Vagally mediated AV nodal block is typically benign.
2. Mobitz type 1 block in the background of myocardial infarction has poor prognosis.
3. Infranodal type 1 or type 2 blocks may progress to complete block and have poor prognosis.
4. AV nodal block usually does not progress to Mobitz type 2 block or complete heart block.
5. Mobitz type 2 block progresses to complete heart block and is associated with increased mortality.

Clinical Presentation

In case of Mobitz type 1 block—there is wide spectrum of clinical presentations like:
  i. Asymptomatic in case of trained athlete or without structural heart disease.
 ii. Recurrent syncope, presyncope in patient with heart disease.
iii. Chest pain—in patient with myocardial ischemia or myocarditis.

In patient with Mobitz type 2 block:
  i. Light headedness
 ii. Dizziness
iii. Syncope or
 iv. Asymptomatic.
  v. Chest pain—in patients with myocarditis or ischemia

Signs:
 i. Regularly irregular heart beat.
ii. There may be bradycardia.

Workup for 2nd Degree AV Block

Blood level:
  i. Electrolytes—K, Ca, Na—magnesium
 ii. Digoxin
iii. Cardiac biomarkers in suspected case of myocardial ischemia.
 iv. To search for etiology of myocarditis:
      a. Lyme titers
      b. HIV serology
      c. Enterovirus polymerase chain reaction PCR.
      d. Adenovirus PCR
      e. Chagas titers
  v. Thyroid function test
 vi. Cortisol level

Electrocardiography:

In type 1 AV block:

i. Progressive increase in PR interval followed by block in atrial impulse.

ii. Greater PR increment typically occurs between 1st and 2nd beats of the cycle.

iii. Shortening of PR interval occurs after the blocked sinus impulse, provided P wave is propagated to the ventricles.

iv. Pause after blocked P wave is less than the sum of the 2 beats before the block.

v. In very long sequences (typically 6:5), PR interval prolongation may be minimal until last beat of the cycle.

vi. Post-block PR interval shortening is the cornerstone of the diagnosis of Mobitz type 1 block.

In Mobitz 2 block:

i. Consecutively conducted beats having same PR interval is followed by blocked sinus P wave

ii. PR interval just after blocked sinus wave is same as that of previous beat before block.

iii. Pause surrounding the blocked P wave = 2 × sinus cycle length.

iv. Since this block is associated with underlying cardiac disease, hence QRS complex will be wide with normal PR interval.

But narrow QRS complex with prolonged PR interval cannot exclude type 2 block, because nodal lesion may be associated with infranodal lesion.

Electrophysiological testing:

Indications:

1. To evaluate the site of block.
2. To evaluate the necessity of permanent pacemaker.
3. To whom block at His-Purkinje system is suspected.
   i. Mobitz type 1 block with wide QRS complex but asymptomatic.
   ii. In asymptomatic patient having 2:1 2nd degree AV block and wide QRS complexes.
   iii. History of syncope in patient with Mobitz 1 block.
   iv. If symptoms is suspected to be related with another arrhythmia in patient having 2nd or 3rd degree block.

Management

1. No specific therapy is usually required for asymptomatic patient with Mobitz type 1 block, if it does not progress to complete heart block.
2. In patient with Mobitz type 2 block, there is nearly always association of myocardial disease hence, it should be treated with anti-ischemic drugs.
3. In these patient with AV nodal affection, drugs like digoxin, calcium channel blockers, beta blocker should be avoided.
4. In symptomatic patient, advanced life care support is usually given to treat severe bradycardia (use of atropine and/or transvenous pacemaker).

Acute management of Mobitz type 1 AV block:

i. Patient with acute myocardial ischemia or acute myocardial infarction should be admitted in a unit having facility of transcutaneous pacing.

ii. Symptomatic patient should be treated with intravenous atropine or transcutaneous pacing.
   a. Atropine should be cautiously administered in patient with myocardial ischemia because there is chance of ventricular dysrrhythmia.
   b. Atropine is effective in case of AV nodal blocks. Atropine is not useful in following:
      i. Patients with intranodal block
      ii. In patient with denervated heart (cardiac transplant patient)

Acute management in Mobitz type 2 block:

i. Admit all the patients with Mobitz type 2 block in ICU with facility for transcutaneous pacing.

ii. In all asymptomatic or symptomatic patients, transcutaneous pacing pads are applied to evaluate the progression to complete block.

iii. Transcutaneous pacemaker should be tested to ensure its capture. If it cannot capture, transvenous pacemaker should be applied to capture.

iv. Urgent cardiac consultation is required where transcutaneous pacing is unable to capture in symptomatic or asymptomatic patients.

v. According to some schools, in all patients of Mobitz 2 block, transvenous pacemaker should be given at the beginning.

vi. In absence of cardiologist, in case of hemodynamically unstable patients, urgent temporary transvenous pacing wire should be implanted under radiological screening in emergency department.

Guideline for implantation of permanent pacemaker:

1. Second degree heart block with symptoms like severe bradycardia, heart failure or asystole for more than 3 seconds.
2. Second degree atrioventricular block in patient with neuromuscular diseases like Erbs muscular dystrophy, myotonic dystrophy, peroneal muscular dystrophy.
3. Wide QRS complexes in patient with Mobitz type 2 block.
4. Mobitz type 1 block in intra- or infra-His bundle region in asymptomatic patient.
5. In patient with acute anterior wall myocardial infarction with high degree AV block, even if transient.
6. Post-cardiac surgery, persistent 2nd degree block.
7. Post-myocardial infarction, persistant symptomatic 2nd degree bundle branch block.

In following conditions, pacemaker may not be required:

1. Transient and symptomatic 2nd degree AV block—in post-MI patient.
2. 2nd degree AV block in patient with drug toxicity, Lyme disease or hypoxia in sleep.
3. When correction of underlying pathology will correct 2nd degree AV block.

Third Degree AV Block or Complete AV Block

This is also called complete heart block. This is characterized by disorder in the conduction system of the heart, where there is no evidence of propagation of impulses through the AV node. As a result, there is complete dissociation of atrial and ventricular activity.

Here this is to be emphasized that in complete heart block, there is complete dissociation of atrial and ventricular activity, but in not all cases of AV dissociation; complete heart block is present.

Pathophysiology

In complete heart block (Fig. 1.106):
  i. No P wave is followed by QRS complexes.
  ii. Number of P waves is more than number of QRS complexes.
  iii. There is no relation between P and QRS waves.

The levels of block are in the following areas:
  i. In 61% of case, below the bundle of His.
  ii. In 20% of case, block at the level of AV node.
  iii. In 20% of cases, block at the His bundle.

Morphology of QRS complexes depends upon the site of block:
  i. Block above the His bundle—narrow QRS complexes.
  ii. Block below the His bundle—wide QRS complexes.

Rate of escape thythm varies according to site of block:
  i. If the block is at the level of AV node—impulse will be generated from junctional pacemaker and the rate will be 45–60 beats/minute, patient will be stable.
  ii. If the bock is below the level of AV node—impulse will be generated from His bundle or bundle branch Purkinje system and the rate will be <45 beats/minute. The patient will be hemodynamically unstable.

Etiology

I. **Congenital** form of complete AV block—in it, the block will be in AV node.

In absence of any major structural abnormalities, it is often associated with maternal antibodies to SS-A (Ro) and SS-B (La).

II. **Acquired:**
  1. *Drugs:*
  2. *Degenerative diseases:*
      i. Lenegre disease (sclera-degenerative process of cardiac conduction system).
      ii. Lev disease (calcification of the conduction system and valves).
      iii. Nail patella syndrome
      iv. Mitochondrial myopathy.
  3. *Infectious causes:*
      i. Lyme disease (Borreliosis)
      ii. Trypanosoma cruzi
      iii. Rheumatic myocarditis
      iv. Chagas disease
      v. Aspergillus myocarditis
      vi. Varicella zoster virus
  4. *Rheumatic diseases:*
      i. Ankylosing spondylitis
      ii. Scleroderma
      iii. Rheumatoid arthritis
      iv. Reiter syndrome
      v. Relapsing polychondritis
  5. *Infiltrative diseases:*
      a. Non-malignant
          i. Amyloidosis
          ii. Sarcoidosis
      b. Malignant
          i. Tumors
          ii. Multiple myeloma
          iii. Hodgkin's lymphoma
  6. *Neuromuscular diseases:*
      i. Myotonic dystrophy
      ii. Becker muscular dystrophy.

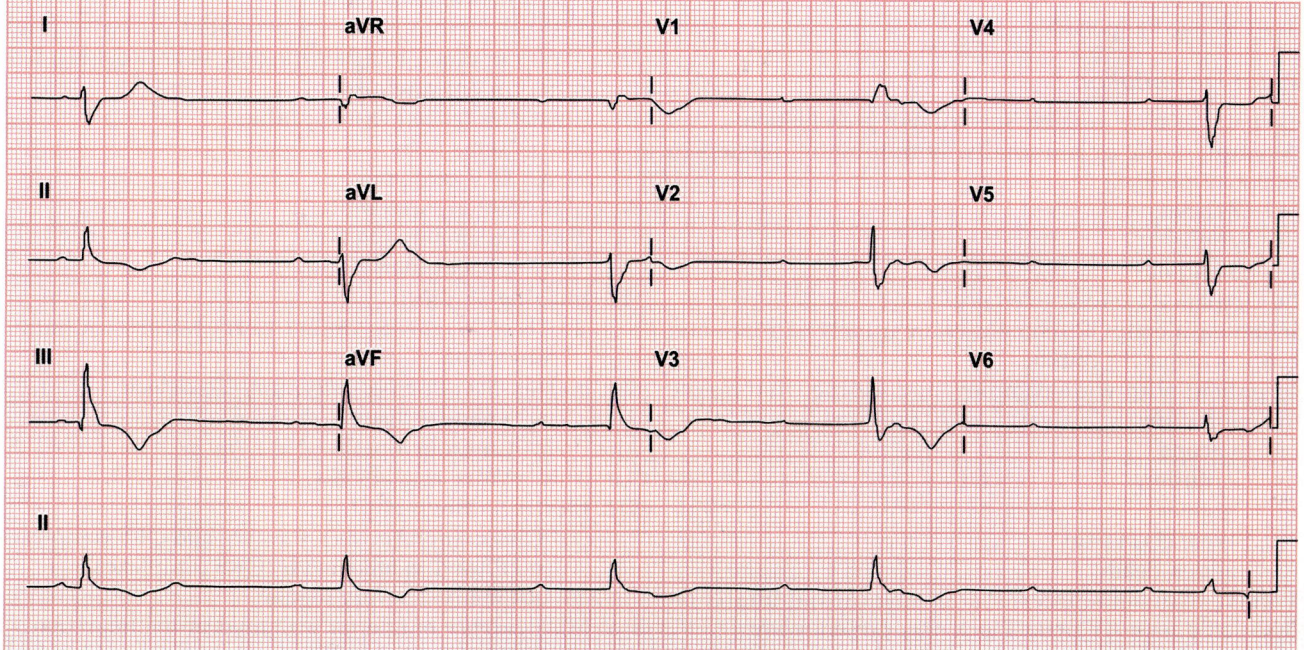

Fig. 1.106: Complete heart block

7. *Ischemic:*
   i. In inferior wall MI—AV node affected
   ii. In anterior wall MI—His-Purkinje system will be affected.
8. *Metabolic causes:*
   i. Hypoxia
   ii. Hyperkalemia
9. *Endocrine causes:* Hypothyroidism
10. *Toxin:*
    i. "Mad" Honey (gray anotoxin)
    ii. Cardiac glycosides (oleandrin).
11. *Phase IV block*—bradycardia related block.
12. *Iatrogenic causes:*
    i. Aortic valve surgery
    ii. Septal alcohol ablation
    iii. Percutaneous coronary intervention to the anterior descending artery.

Prognosis

Patient with CHB is hemodynamically unstable, and he may develop:
   i. Syncope
   ii. Presyncope
   iii. Hypotension
   iv. Cardiovascular collapse, and
   v. Death
   In these patients, sudden cardiac death occurs due to:
      i. Tachyarrhythmias—produced by secondary changes in ventricular repolarization (QT prolongation)
      ii. In some patients, polymorphic ventricular tachycardia due to prolongation of repolarization with extremely slow rates.
      iii. Atropine-induced ventricular arrhythmias.

Complications related to pacemaker insertion:
   i. Arterial injury
   ii. Hemithorax
   iii. Pneumothorax
   iv. Cardiac tamponade

Clinical Presentation

These patients have variable spectrum of presentation:
1. Asymptomatic or minimally symptomatic, related to hypotension like:
   i. Dizziness
   ii. Fatigue
   iii. Chest pain
   iv. Impaired exercise tolerance.
   In these patients, QRS complexes are usually narrow—and block is above the bundle.
2. In patient with wide complex, and escape rhythm, the symptoms are:
   i. Syncope
   ii. Confusion
   iii. Dyspnea
   iv. Severe chest pain
   v. Sudden death
3. Patient with acute interior wall myocardial infarction associated with AV nodal block may present with:
   i. Chest pain
   ii. Dyspnea
   iii. Nausea or vomiting
   iv. Diaphoresis
4. History of intake of medication that alter the conduction system of the heart—β blockers, digitalis, CCB
5. History of cardiac surgery.

Physical Examination

1. Pulse—severe bradycardia.
2. Neck vein—evidence of canon 'a' waves.
3. Heart sound—variable intensity of first heart sound
4. Arousal of new murmur or gallop—may indicate cardio-myopathies, mitral calcification, aortic calcification or endocarditis.
5. If patient has heat failure as evidence by:
   i. Tachypnea
   ii. Peripheral edema
   iii. Crepitations
   iv. Jugular venous distension
   v. S3 gallop
   vi. Tender hepatomegaly
6. In patients with endocarditis—different peripheral signs—Osler nodes, janeway lesion, and splinter hemorrhage.
7. Patient may present with evidence of hypoperfusion:
   i. Altered mental status
   ii. Hypotension
   iii. Lethargy
8. In patients with acute myocardial infarction:
   i. Tachypnea
   ii. Diaphoresis
   iii. Pale complexion
9. In case of digitalis toxicity: Regularized atrial fibrillation is the classic sign
I. **Laboratory studies:**
   a. Complete blood count—to detect anemia, infection
   b. Raised ESR and leukocytosis may direct the physician for blood culture.
   c. Serum potassium, magnesium—to detect metabolic imbalance, renal failure.
   d. Prothrombin time and activated partial thrombo-plastin time—to titrate the dose of anticoagulant.
   e. Serum digoxin level
   f. Studies related to myocarditis:
      i. Lyme titers
      ii. HIV serotypes
      iii. Enterovirus PCR
      iv. Adenovirus PCR
      v. Chagas titer
II. **Imaging studies:**
   a. *Chest X-ray*—to detect heart failure, pulmonary congestion
   b. *Transthoracic echocardiography:* To detect:
      i. Valvular disease
      ii. Cardiomyopathy
      iii. Valve ring abscess.
III. **Electrocardiography**
   i. Dissociation between P waves and QRS complexes—no P wave is followed by QRS complexes.
   ii. RR interval is very regular.
   iii. Evidence of inferior wall myocardial infarction.
   iv. If QRS complexes are narrow—indicate block at AV node (<120 msec.)

v. If QRS complexes are wide—indicate block below the His bundle (>120 msec).

IV. Diagnostic electrophysiological studies: They can detect site of block.

Management

1. Withdrawal of the offending drug—can resolve the block
2. Asymptomatic patient with inferior wall MI with complete heart block at AV node and rate of 35/mm are at less risk.
3. Patient with acute anterior wall MI with distal high grade block requires urgent pacing because there is chance of development of asystole, though the heart rate is 90 beats/min.
4. If patient develops CHB due to calcium channel blocker—treatment should be:
   i. Intravenous fluid
   ii. Calcium
   iii. Glucagon
   iv. Vasopressor
   v. High dose of insulin

   Similar treatment should be given in case of β-blocker toxicity except high dose insulin (hyperinsulinemic euglycemia therapy)
5. In absence of ischemia, AV node block can be treated by vagolytic therapy.
6. Most patients with acquired complete heart block can be treated by:
   i. Permanent pacemaker, or
   ii. Implantable cardioverter defibrillator.

Indications of transvenous/transcutaneous temporary pacing: In patients with complete heart block associated with:
   i. Repeated pauses
   ii. Inadequate escape rhythm
   iii. Block below atrioventricular node

Method of assessing the capture: By palpation of pulse, rather than looking for capture in monitor. Transvenous pacemaker should be applied when:
   i. Fully trained personnel are available.
   ii. Equipment for placing is available.

Place of temporary placing placement:
   i. In case of hemodynamically stable patient—ICU or telemetry unit.
   ii. In case of hemodynamically unstable patient—emergency department

In case of AV nodal block: Atropine intravenously, improves conduction through AV node by reducing vagal tone via receptor blockade; as a result ventricular rate will be improved.

But if the block is below AV node, atropine will increase the atrial rate and block will be increased with more slowing of ventricular rate.

Again, in case of acute myocardial infarction, atropine produces vagolysis, with unopposed sympathetic stimulation, which in turn, ultimately leads to severe ventricular dysrrhythmias.

Indications of Implantation of Permanent Pacemaker

Class I Recommendations:

A. Third degree and advanced 2nd degree AV block at any anatomic level:
   i. Associated with bradycardia with symptoms (including heart failure) or ventricular arrhythmias presumed to be due to AV block.
   ii. Associated with arrhythmia and other medical conditions requiring drug therapy that result in symptomatic bradycardia.
   iii. In awake, symptom free patients in sinus rhythm with documented periods of asystole for 3 seconds or longer or any escape beat at a rate less than 40 beats/minute or escape rhythm from below the AV node.
   iv. In awake, symptom free patients with atrial fibrillation and bradycardia with 1 or more pause having duration of 5 seconds or longer.
   v. After catheter ablation of the AV junction.
   vi. Associated with postoperative AV block that is not expected to be resolved after cardiac surgery.
   vii. Associated with neuromuscular disease with AV block, such as myotonic muscular dystrophy, Keams-Sayre syndrome, Erb dystrophy (limb girdle muscular dystrophy), period muscular atrophy, with or without symptoms.

B. For 2nd degree AV block with associated symptomatic bradycardia, regardless the type of block.

C. For asymptomatic persistent third degree AV block at any anatomic site with average ventricular rate of 40 beats per minute or faster if cardiomegaly or left ventricular failure is present or if the site of block is below AV node.

D. For 2nd degree AV bock or 3rd degree AV block during exercise in absence of myocardial ischemia.

Class IIa Recommendations: Permanent pacemaker implantation is reasonable for:

A. Persistent 3rd degree AV block with escape rate faster than 40 beats/minute in asymptomatic adult patients without cardiomegaly.

B. Asymptomatic 2nd degree AV block at intra- or infra- His levels found in electrophysiological study.

C. 1st or 2nd degree AV block with symptoms similar to those of pacemaker syndrome or hemodynamic compromise.

D. Asymptomatic Mobitz 2nd degree AV block with narrow QRS.

   But Mobitz 2nd degree AV block with wide QRS, including isolated right bundle branch block becomes a Class I recommendation.

Class IIb Recommendations: Permanent pacemaker implantation may be considered for:

A. Neuromuscular diseases with any degree of AV block including 1st degree AV block, with or without symptoms, because there may be unpredictable progression of AV conduction disease.

B. AV block in the setting of drug use and/or drug toxicity when the block is expected to recur even after withdrawal of drugs.

Class III Recommendation: Permanent pacemaker implantation is not indicated for:
A. Asymptomatic AV block
B. Asymptomatic Mobitz 1 2nd degree AV block at supra His (AVN) level or which is not known to be intra or intra His.
C. AV block that is expected to resolve and is unlikely to recur (e.g. drug toxicity, Lyme disease, transient increase in vagal tone or during hypoxia in sleep apnea syndrome in the absence of symptoms).

Indication of Pacemaker Implantation in Chronic Bifascicular or Trifascicular Block

Class I Recommendations: Permanent pacemaker implantation is indicated for:
A. Advanced 2nd degree AV block or intermittent third degree AV block.
B. Mobitz II 2nd degree AV block
C. Alternating bundle branch block.

Class IIa Recommendations: Permanent pacemaker is reasonable for:
A. Syncope not demonstrated to be due to AV block when other likely causes have been excluded, especially VT.
B. Incidental finding at electrophysiologic study of a markedly prolonged HV interval (>100 msec) in asymptomatic patients.
C. Incidental finding at electrophysiological study of pacing induced infra-His block, that is not physiological.

Class IIb Recommendations: Permanent pacemakers may be considered in neuromuscular diseases with bifascicular block or any block with or without symptoms.

Class III Recommendations: Permanent pacemaker is not indicated for:
A. Fascicular block without AV block or symptoms.
B. Fascicular block with 1st degree AV block without symptoms.

Selection of Pacing Mode

Pacing made, who maintains AV synchrony, may reduce following complications like:
i. Pacemaker syndrome
ii. Pacemaker-mediated tachycardia.

This is particularly common in younger patients. Some studies showed physiologic pacing may decrease the risk of chronic atrial fibrillation and stroke.

In patients with sinus rhythm and AV block—dual chamber pacing is better than single chamber pacing to avoid the risk of possible complications.

CAROTID SINUS HYPERSENSITIVITY

Definition

Carotid sinus hypersensitivity (CAH) can be defined as exaggerated response to carotid sinus baroceptor stimulation resulting presyncope or syncope due to cerebral hypoperfusion.

Anatomy

Carotid sinus baroceptor is present at the bifurcation of common carotid artery (Figs 1.107 and 1.108).

Physiology

1. Baroceptor in heart, carotid sinus, aortic arch and other blood vessels detects changes in stretch and transmural pressure.
2. Afferent impulses are transmitted via glossopharyngeal and vagus nerves to the nuclei of tractus solitarius and paramedian nucleus in the brainstem.
3. Efferent impulses pass through sympathetic and vagus nerves to the heart and great vessels and control heart rate and blood pressures.

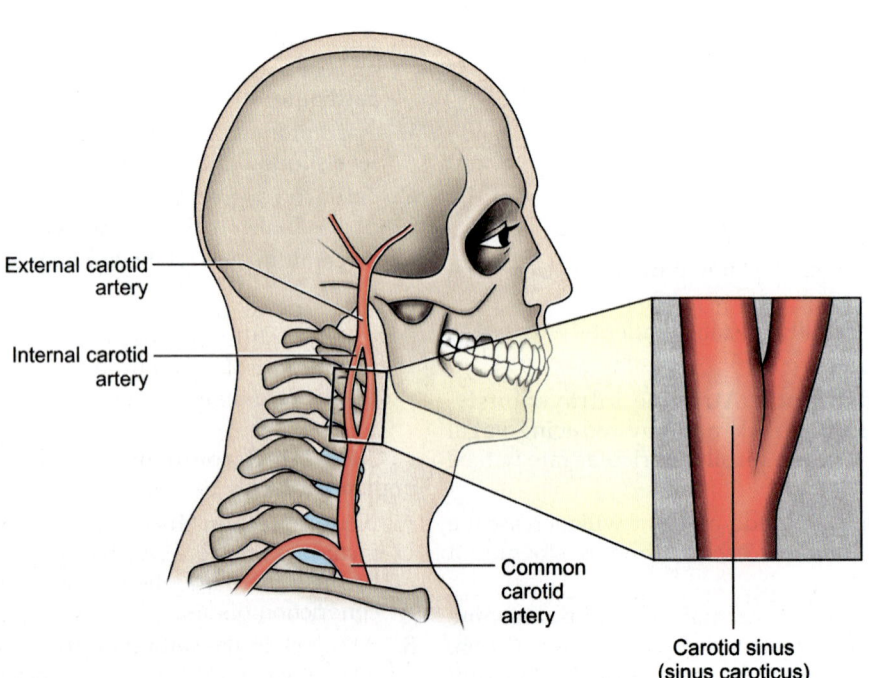

External carotid artery

Internal carotid artery

Common carotid artery

Carotid sinus (sinus caroticus)

Fig. 1.107: Anatomy of carotid sinus

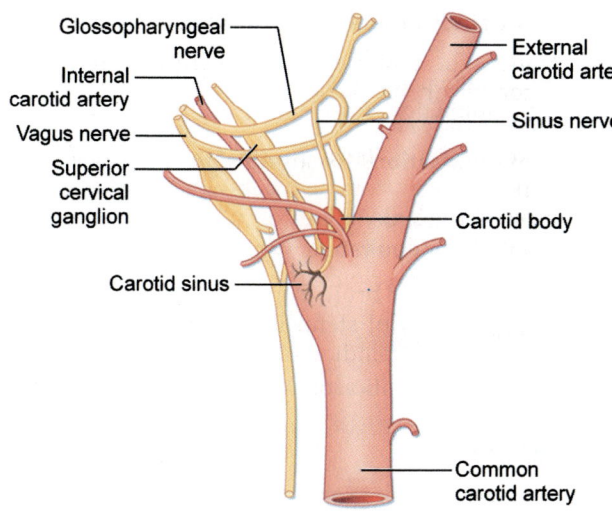

Fig. 1.108: Anatomy of carotid sinus

Pathophysiology

Hemodynamic changes following carotid sinus hyper-stimulation are:

i. Initially changes in cardiac output driven by heart rate.

ii. Later on, fall in total peripheral resistance.

It has been shown that accumulation of hyperphos-phorylated tau or alpha-synuclein in the neuron in medulla leading to neuronal degeneration, which in turn, leads to impairment of central regulation of barorecepter reflex responses mainly in elderly patient—producing carotid sinus hypersensitivity.

However, exact mechanism of CAH is unknown, but it may be due to changes in any part of reflex arc or the target organs.

Types of Carotid Sinus Hypersensitivity

1. **Cardioinhibitory response** (70–75% cases): In this type—there is decrease in heart rate which may lead to:
   a. Sinus bradycardia
   b. Atrioventricular block
   c. Sinus asystole.
   Mechanism: Vagal inhibition on sinus and atrioven-tricular nodes.
   This can be abolished by atropine injection.

2. **Vasopressor response** (5–10% cases): In this type, there is drop in blood pressure without any change in heart rate.
   Mechanism: Imbalance between sympathetic and parasympathetic effects on blood vessels.
   This response cannot be abolished by atropine injection.

3. **Mixed type:** (20–25% of cases): In this type, both decrease in heart rate and vasopressor response occur.
   But according to recent view—all CAH are of mixed types, i.e. both vasodepressor and cardioinhibition types.
   There are two terms have been introduced to categorize the patients with CAH:

   a. **Spontaneous carotid sinus syndrome:**
      i. It occurs in 1% of cases, so very rare.
      ii. In this type, symptoms are attributed to history of mechanical manipulation of carotid sinus like shaving, palpation for carotid impulse.
      iii. This can be reproduced by carotid sinus massage.

   b. **Induced carotid sinus syndrome:**
      i. In this type, there is no history of carotid sinus mani-pulation or no positive result from workup of syncope.
      ii. There is hypersensitivity response to carotid sinus massage.
      iii. It is more prevalent than spontaneous carotid sinus syndrome.

Epidemiology

Sex: It is more common in females than males.

Clinical Presentation of Carotid Sinus Hypersensitivity

Most of the patients are asymptomatic. But in case of symptomatic patients—following are the symptoms:

1. Recurrent dizziness or syncope
2. Pre-syncope
3. Fall without any explanation
4. Sudden dizziness or syncope triggered by some maneuvers—head turning, wearing garments or tight-fitting collars.
5. Extensive scarring secondary to radical dissection or radiation fibrosis.
6. Neck tumor
7. Neck trauma
8. Symptoms of dizziness or presyncope produced during pulse examination or neck surgery.

Physical Signs

i. Hypertension
ii. Bradycardia
iii. Asystole
iv. Auscultation for bruit in carotid artery prior to carotid sinus massage.

Causes

i. Advanced age
ii. Hypertension
iii. Coronary artery disease
iv. Orthostatic hypotension
v. Vasovagal syncope
vi. Alzheimer disease
vii. Parkinson disease
viii. Lewy body in case of dementia
ix. On medication like digitalis, beta blockers, methyldopa.

Workup of Carotid Sinus Hypersensitivity

Differential diagnoses are: Exclusion of following diagnoses:

1. Vasovagal syncope
2. Orthostatic hypotension
3. Sick sinus syndrome
4. Heart block
5. Situational syncope
6. Neutropenic syncope
7. Metabolic syncope
8. Psychogenic syncope.

Prelaboratory evaluation:
 i. Proper and meticulous history
 ii. Thorough physical examination
 iii. ECG

Procedures

Carotid sinus massage is the diagnostic procedure of choice—though it is not standardized till now.

The method includes:
a. Patient should be in supine position with neck extended for 5 minutes, before the commencement of carotid sinus massage.
b. Place of massage—should be over the point of maximum carotid impulse, medial to sternocleidomastoid muscle, at the upper border of thyroid cartilage.
c. Carotid sinus massage should be continued for 5–10 seconds on each side, having gap of a minute between each massages.
d. Since CSH is more prominent on right side, it should be preferably applied on right side.
e. ECG, blood pressure should be monitored continuously. Phasic, non-invasive, beat-to-beat blood pressure is usually preferred.

'Carotid sinus hypersensitivity is positive, when any of the following criteria are met:
 i. Asystole of more than 3 seconds (cardioinhibitory CSA)
 ii. Lowering of systolic blood pressure more than 50 mmHg, irrespective of heart rate (vasodepressor CSH).
 iii. Combination of above (mixed CSH)

It has been shown that, carotid sinus massage in an upright position is highly sensitive showing high diagnostic accuracy (Fig. 1.109).

Absolute contraindication to carotid sinus massage:
1. Stroke
2. Transient ischemic attack
3. Myocardial infarction

Relative contraindications to carotid sinus massage:
1. History of VT
2. Ventricular fibrillation
3. Carotid bruit on auscultation.

In patient with carotid bruit, Doppler ultrasound should be done to detect amount of stenosis—if it is more than 70%, carotid massage is contraindicated.

Neurological complication of carotid sinus massage is 0.2%.

Complications

 i. Neurological complications
 ii. Coronary artery spasm
 iii. Ventricular and atrial arrhythmias

Medical Care

It depends upon:
 i. Frequency of symptom
 ii. Severity of symptoms
 iii. Consequences of symptoms

Main treatment is:
 i. Proper education
 ii. Life style changes
 iii. Life expectancy

Pharmacotherapy can be done in case of symptomatic conditions.

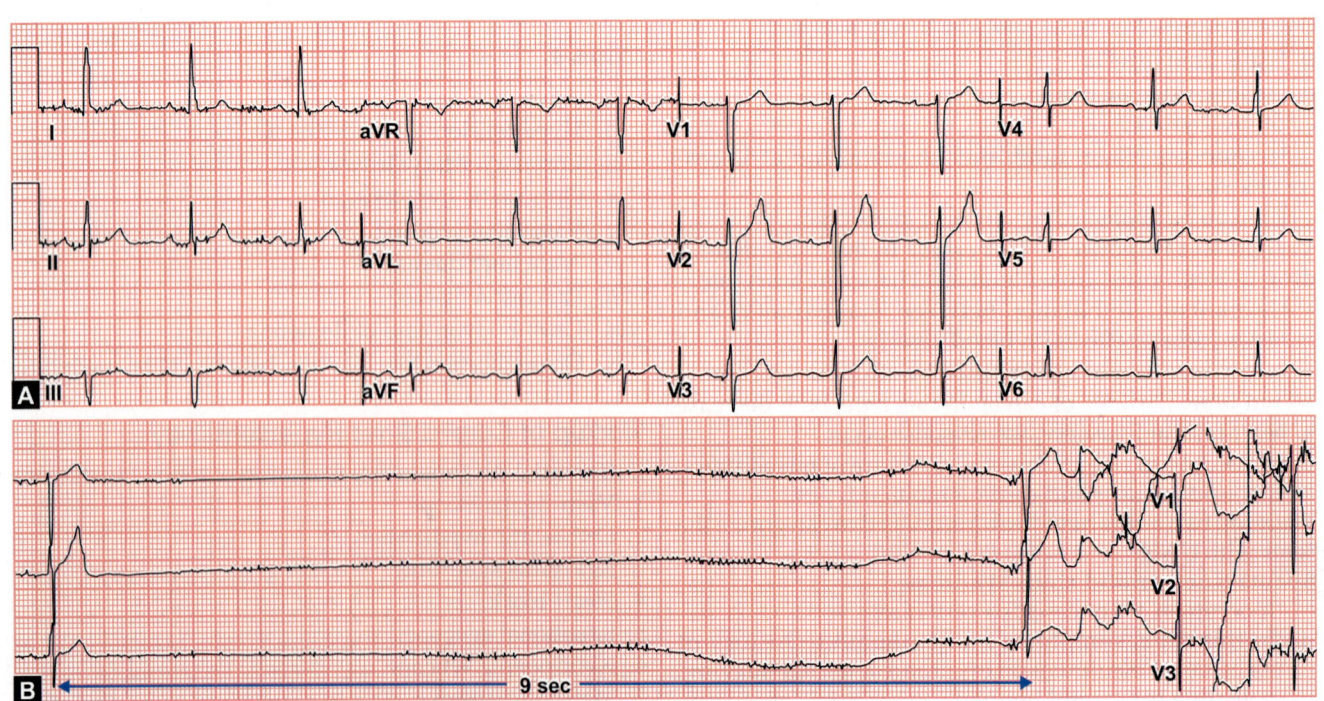

Fig. 1.109: Effect of carotid sinus massage

Pacemaker is considered in:
 i. Cardioinhibitory CSH
 ii. Mixed form CSH

ACC/AHA Guidelines for Permanent Pacemakers

I. Class I indication:
Permanent pacemaker is indicated (Class I) in patient with recurrent syncope caused by carotid sinus stimulation in absence of any drug that depresses the sinus node or atrioventricular conduction.

   Permanent pacemaker is considered (Class IIa indication) in patient with recurrent syncope without clear, provocative events and with a hypersensitive cardioinhibitory response.

   Permanent pacemaker is discouraged (Class III) in patients with hypersensitive cardioinhibitory response to carotid sinus stimulation in absence of symptoms.

Type of pacemaker:
1. Dual chamber pacemaker (DDD, DVI, DDI)
2. VVI mode is also effective.

Permanent pacemaker:
 i. Has no or little effect on vasodepressor type of CAH.
 ii. It may not reduce frequency of falls.
 iii. It may diminish but cannot eliminate symptoms of CSH.

VENTRICULAR TACHYCARDIA

Definition
Ventricular tachycardia refers to any rhythm faster than 100/minute with 3 or more irregular consecutive beats in a row, arising from distal to bundle of His, like distal conduction system or ventricular myocardium.

Pathophysiology (Fig. 1.110)
Cardiac output is reduced in ventricular tachycardia due to:
 i. Rapid heart rate
 ii. Lack of properly timed atrial contraction
 iii. Incoordinated atrial contractions
 iv. Myocardial ischemia
 v. Mitral insufficiency
 vi. Ventricular dysfunction

As a result of diminished cardiac output:
 i. Diminished myocardial perfusion.
 ii. Worsening of ionotropic response.
 iii. Degeneration to ventricular fibrillation

The net result may be sudden death.
The following heart diseases are at risk of developing **monomorphic ventricular tachycardia which leads to ventricular fibrillation:**
 i. Ischemic cardiomyopathy
 ii. Dilated cardiomyopathy
 iii. Hypertrophic cardiomyopathy
 iv. Chagas disease.
 v. Right ventricular dysplasia.

Ventricular tachycardia can degenerate into:
 i. Ventricular fibrillation
 ii. Congestive cardiac failure
 iii. Severe hemodynamic compromise producing sudden death

Etiology
A. Structural heart diseases
B. Electrolyte disturbances:
   i. Hypokalemia
   ii. Hypomagnesemia
   iii. Hypocalcemia
C. Systemic diseases affecting myocardium:
   i. Sarcoidosis
   ii. Systemic lupus erythematosus
   iii. Hemochromatosis
   iv. Rheumatoid arthritis
D. Congenital cyanotic heart disease—tetralogy of Fallot.
E. Drugs—digitalis toxicity
F. Use of sympathomimetic agents:
   i. Methamphetamine
   ii. Cocaine
G. Inherited channelopathies
H. Drugs prolonging QT complexes:
   i. Type 1 antiarrhythmic drug
   ii. Droperidol.

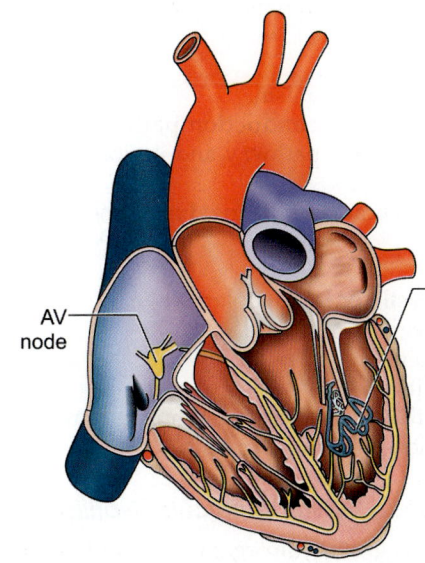

AV node

Abnormal electrical impulses in the ventricles may occur as isolated extra beats, brief runs of extra beats, or long runs of rapid and often dangerous arrhythmias. Ventricular arrhythmias may occur because the tissue is damaged, scarred or inflamed

Fig. 1.110: Pathophysiology of VT

Monomorphic Ventricular Tachycardia
 i. Here it originates from a single focus with identical QRS complexes.
 ii. Regular rhythm
 iii. Produces uniform QRS complexes within each lead—each QRS is identical except fusion beat/captured beat.

Polymorphic Ventricular Tachycardia (Fig. 1.111)
 i. Rhythm is irregular
 ii. Varying QRS complexes of different morphology.

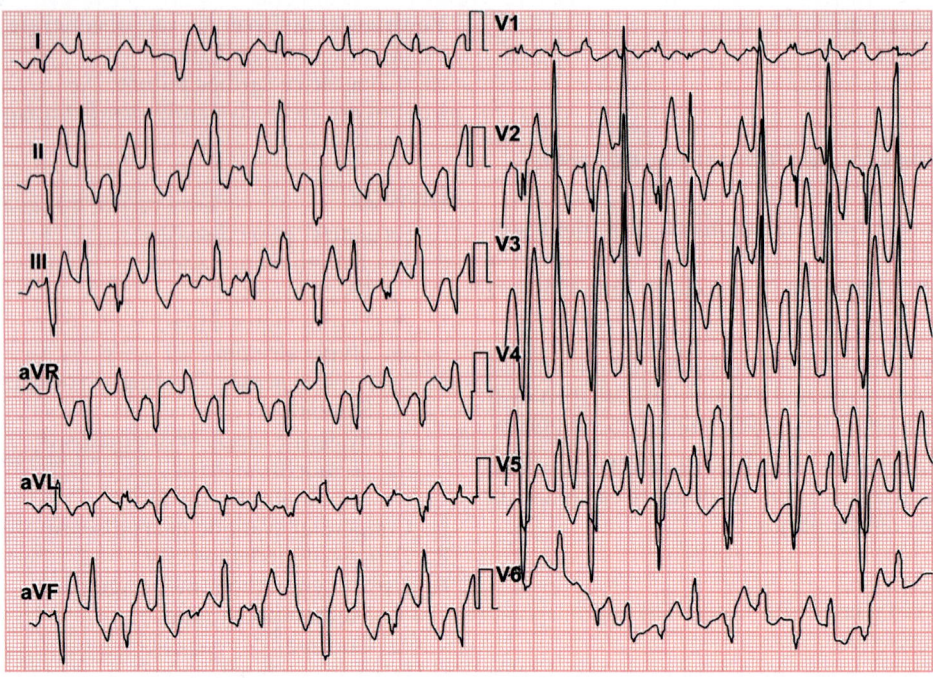

Fig. 1.111: Polymorphic VT

Mechanism of Ventricular Tachycardia

There are three mechanisms for initiation and propagation of ventricular tachycardia

1. **Re-entry mechanism:**
   i. It is the commonest mechanism.
   ii. It requires two distinct conduction pathways with conduction block in one pathway and region of slow conduction in the other.
   iii. It occurs due to myocardial scarring due to ischemia or infarction.
2. **Triggered activity:**
   i. It occurs due to easily or late depolarization
   ii. Examples include:
      a. Torsades de pointes
      b. Digitalis toxicity
3. **Abnormal automaticity:** Accelerated abnormal impulse generation by a region of ventricular cells.

Ventricular Tachycardia Versus Ventricular Fibrillation

Ventricular fibrillation is grossly disorganized, rapid ventricular rhythm which varies in interval and waveform.

Atrioventricular Dissociation

In this type of conduction, sinus node is depolarizing the atria at a rate which is slower than the pathologic ventricular rate. So 'P' waves can be visualized in between QRS complexes or embedded in QRS complexes. Here Atria and ventricles have their own independent rates.

Fusion Beat

In this type, there is mixed morphology due to normal AV node/His-Purkinje conduction occurring simultaneously with abnormal (wide QRS complexes) ventricular depolarization.

One normally conducted impulse passes along the normal pathway, crosses AV node and complete with impulses originates from abnormal ventricular focus outside normal conduction pathway (wide QRS). These two complexes fuse to forms mixed (fused) QRS.

Captured Beats

In this type, atrial impulse reaches AV node at a time, when AV node just has been recovered from refractory period. Because due to retrograde conduction of rapid ventricular impulse, AV node is frequently in refractory period, so if atrial impulse passes through normal AV node in between the refractory period and proceeds normally through AV node/His-Purkinje system and captures the ventricles, leading to normal and narrow complexes in between wide ventricular complexes.

There may be retrograde conduction of ventricular impulses to the atria through AV node. This is not AV dissociation, it is just 1:1 correlation between wide QRS complex and inverted P ware followed by QRS complex.

Monomorphic ventricular tachycardia: It mostly occurs in structural heart diseases producing scar and/or fibrillary disarray.

Re-entrant Tachycardia

In this type, electrical wave front passes through the zone of slow conduction (scar tissue) allowing the rest of the circuit to become repolarized. Then the wavefront breaks of the scar, activates the ventricle and again re-enters the zone of slow conduction.

The QRS morphology during VT can be used to predict the exit site from the zone of slow conduction.

This type of monomorphic VT can occur in normal heart (idiopathic VT), they are often exercise dependent.

Monomorphic VT is typically named according to the site of origin—the sites are:

i. Right ventricular outflow tract
ii. Left ventricular outflow tract
iii. Left ventricular septum
iv. Aortic root.

Though the monomorphic ventricular tachycardia is classically benign, but sudden death can occur.

Polymorphic Ventricular Tachycardia

When QRS complex varies from beat-to-beat due to variable electrical activation sequence—it is called polymorphic ventricular tachycardia. Torsade de pointes is a type of polymorphic VT—this name suggest "Twisting of the points of the QRS complexes from time to time".

In torsades de pointes; there is unusual shifting axis of QRS complexes appearing in ECG.

The causes are:
i. Type 1A antiarrhythmic drugs
ii. Hypomagnesemia
iii. Droperidol

It may occur in presence or absence of myocardial ischemia or infarction.

Torsades de pointes produces prolonged QT interval. The following potassium channel blockers producing prolonged QT interval:
i. Quinidine
ii. Erythromycin
iii. Haloperidol

Sustained ventricular tachycardia: It is monomorphic VT results from ventricular scar due to prior myocardial infarction—which is responsible for slow conduction followed by associated re-entrant mechanism.

Non-sustained ventricular tachycardia: This occurs from abnormal automaticity mechanisms due to areas of acute myocardial ischemia.

Idioventricular rhythm: Second variant of VT is accelerated idioventricular rhythm, sometimes called slow ventricular tachycardia having ventricular rate of 60–100 beats/minute.
i. It occurs in structural heart disease.
ii. It is transient.
iii. It is associated with hemodynamic collapse.

Inherited dysrhythmias: These are:
i. Brugada syndrome
ii. Congenital long and short QT syndrome
iii. Catecholaminergic polymorphic VT.

Mechanism: Inherited abnormal ion transport across the cardiac cellular membrane, leading to abnormalities in cardiac repolarisation which in turn produces cardiac dysrrhythmias.

Supraventricular tachycardia: Wide complex conduction during supraventricular tachycardia may mimic ventricular tachycardia. Two most common forms are:
1. AV re-entrant tachycardia (AVRT)
2. AV nodal re-entrant tachycardia with aberrant conduction (AVNRT)

AVRT may be orthodromic or antidromic depending upon direction of conduction through AV node.

All antidromic AVRT produces wide complex tachycardia due to activation of ventricle outside the His-Purkinje system.

Some orthodromic AVRT produces wide complex due to pre-existing or functional bundle branch block or intraventricular conduction delay.

Risk Factors for Ventricular Tachycardia

1. Electrolyte abnormalities:
   a. Hypokalemia
   b. Hypomagnesemia
2. Ischemia
3. Inflammation—myocarditis
4. Sleep apnea syndrome
5. Genetic abnormalities:
   a. Brugada syndrome
   b. Right ventricular dysplasia
6. Right ventricular cardiomyopathy
7. Hypertrophic cardiomyopathy

Sex Predilection

i. It is more frequently found in men, because in them, ischemic heart disease is more common.
ii. Females with congenital or acquired prolonged 'QT' syndrome are at risk of sudden death
iii. Twofold male predominance in right ventricular dysplasia and 8-fold increase in Brugada syndrome.

Age Predilection

Incidence of VT is more common in middle decades of life, because incidence of structural heart disease is more common is this age group.

Mortality and Morbidity

i. It occurs due to spontaneous degeneration of VT into VF.
ii. In patient with ischemic cardiomyopathy and non-sustained VT, sudden death is 30% in 2 years.

Morbidity in resuscitated survivors includes:
a. Ischemic cardiomyopathy
b. Acute renal insufficiency
c. Transient ventricular dysfunction
d. Aspiration pneumonitis
e. Trauma during resuscitation procedure.

Prognosis

It depends upon—left ventricular function. In idiopathic VT, prognosis is excellent, but major risk is recurrent "syncope" spells.

But exceptions are:
1. Hypertrophic cardiomyopathy
2. Prolonged QT syndrome
3. Right ventricular dysplasia

Here left ventricular function is well preserved.

History of Ventricular Tachycardia

Main symptoms are:
i. Palpitation
ii. Light headedness
iii. Syncope due to diminished cerebral perfusion or structural heart disease

iv. Chest pain—due to ischemia or abnormalities in rhythm.
v. Neck fullness—may be due to increased central venous pressure or cannon 'a' wave—due to right atrial contraction against closed tricuspid valve.
vi. Dyspnea—due to:
   a. Increased pulmonary venous pressures
   b. Left atrial contraction against closed mitral valve
vii. Recurrent syncope in athlete.
viii. Strong family history of sudden death below the age of 40 years—should be evaluated for genetic arrhythmic syndrome:
   a. Brugada syndrome
   b. Long QT syndrome
   c. Short QT syndrome
   d. Arrhythmogenic right ventricular dysplasia
   e. Catecholaminergic polymorphic VT
   f. Hypertrophic cardiomyopathy.

Physical Examinations

Findings of VT depend upon degree of hemodynamic instability.

A. During ventricular tachycardia:
   i. Tachycardia
   ii. Tachypnea
   iii. Hypotension
   iv. Signs of diminished perfusion—as evidenced by:
      a. Pallor
      b. Diminished level of consciousness
      c. Diaphoresis.
   v. Raised jugular venous pressure and cannon 'w' wave
   vi. Varying intensity of 1st heart sound due to loss of AV synchrony.

B. During sinus rhythm following conversion:
   i. Evidence of structural heart disease as evidenced by:
      a. Displacement of point of maximal impulse.
      b. Murmur related to valvular heart disease.
      c. Murmur related to hypertrophic cardiomyopathy
      d. S3 gallop
   ii. Chest examination—rales due to congestive cardiac failure
   iii. Sinus rhythm may be interrupted by ventricular extrasystoles.

C. Mental status changes:
   i. Anxiety
   ii. Agitation
   iii. Lethargy
   iv. Coma

D. Sudden death

Workup of Ventricular Tachycardia

In patient with ventricular tachycardia with hemodynamic compromise, 1st, patient should be stabilized with direct cardioversion or defibrillation under retardation, **then workup of VT can be done.**

A. Assessment of electrolytes: Serum calcium magnesium, phosphorus.

B. Estimation of drug level—digoxin.

C. Evaluation of myocardial ischemic or infarction by measurement of Troponin I or T levels or other biomarkers.

Ventricular Tachycardia in Acute Presentation

a. In case of VT with unconsciousness or hemodynamic instability—patient should be stabilized first by direct cardioversion followed by workup.
b. In case VT with stability—long ECG strip and electrolytes measurement should be done followed by cardioversion.
   1. Serum levels of the follow electrolytes must be measured:
      i. Calcium
      ii. Magnesium
      iii. Phosphate
      In case of calcium, ionized calcium level is preferred over total serum calcium.
   2. Serum level of drugs—digoxin
   3. Evaluation of myocardial ischemia:
      i. Troponin I
      ii. Troponin T
      iii. Other cardiac biomarkers.

According to ACC/AHA/ESC–2006, Quinidine–serum phosphate level should be maintained above 4 mmol/L in case of acute myocardial infarction.

Post-Conversion in Case of VT

After conversion to sinus rhythm, evaluation to be done in the following lines:
   i. Acute or chronic infarction
   ii. Presence of scar
   iii. Ventricular preexitation
   iv. Conduction disease
   v. Hypertrophy
   vi. QT prolongation
   vii. Any other repolarization abnormalities
   viii. Evaluation of electrolytes—because according to **ACC/AHA/ESC 2006 guidelines**—administration of potassium or magnesium is necessary in the patient taking diuretics.
   ix. Toxicology screening includes:
      a. Tricyclic antidepressants
      b. Cocaine metabolites—should be done according to patients clinical history
   x. Genetic studies in patient with spontaneous polymorphic VT.

Adenosine in VT

In case of wide QRS tachycardia, one should not give adenosine as this arrhythmia involves atrial fibrillation in presence of accessory pathway. Because, administration of adenosine may allows conduction through accessory pathway to produce rapid intolerable ventricular rate.

Electrocardiography (Figs 1.112 and 1.113)

1. Single averaged electrocardiography often produces abnormal results in patients with VT related to prior infarct or right ventricular dysplasia.
2. Simultaneous 3 channel recordings are more helpful than rhythm strips, which can analyze dysrhythmias.
3. Features common to any broad complex tachycardia:
   i. Rapid heart rate (>100/min)
   ii. Broad QRS complexes (>120 msec)
4. Features suggestive of ventricular tachycardia:
   i. Very broad complexes (>160 ms)
   ii. Absence of typical RBBB or LBBB morphology

iii. Extreme axis deviation (North West axis)—QRS is positive in AVR and negative in 1 and AVF.

iv. AV dissociation, i.e. P and QRS ratio are different.

v. Positive or negative concordance throughout chest leads, i.e. all the chest leads show entirely positive or negative complexes.

vi. Brugada's sign: Distance between the onset of QRS complex to the nadir of S wave is >100 msec.

vii. Josephson's sign: Notching near nadir of S wave

viii. rSR' pattern—it can be differentiated from RBBB
  a. In VT—left rabbit ear is fallen
  b. In RBBB—right rabbit ear is fuller.

Additional Morphological Criteria in Monomorphic VT

i. Regular rhythm.

ii. Produces uniform complexes within each lead—each QRS in identical (except in case of capture beat or fusion beat)

iii. Very broad QRS complexes (≥ 200) msec)

iv. Indeterminate axis

v. Josephson's sign

Chest radiography: It is indicated, if there is possibility of congestive cardiac failure.

CT Scan and MRI

i. It is required for quantification of ventricular function.

ii. Cardiac MRI is helpful for diagnosis of some uncommon myocardial infiltrative diseases, e.g. sarcoidosis, amyloidosis.

iii. For evaluation of arrhythmogenic right ventricular dysplasia.

Right ventriculography: It is used on right ventricular arrhythmogenic dysplasia.

Holter monitoring: It is indicated in recurrent syncope or palpitation. It has a low yield.

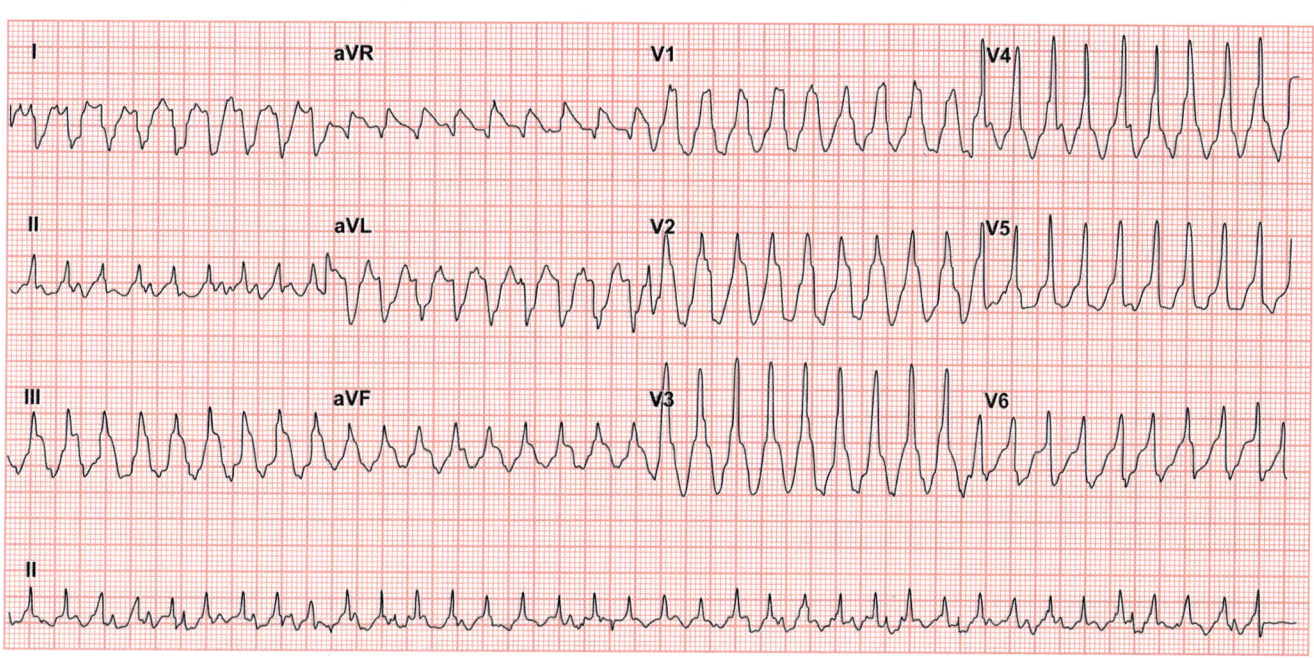

Fig. 1.112: ECG of VT

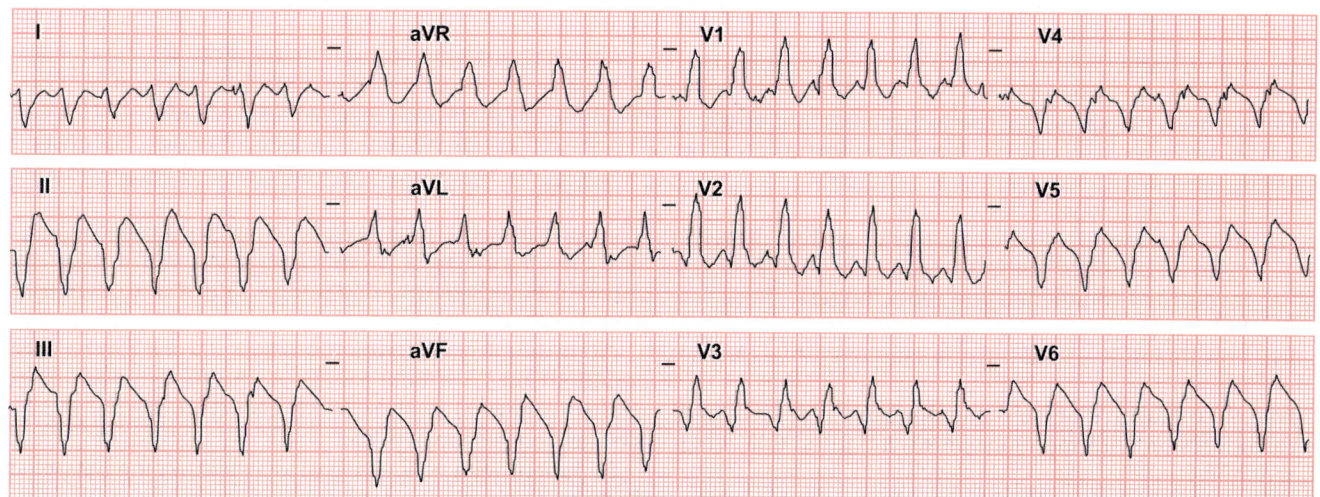

Fig. 1.113: ECG of VT

The goal is to demonstrate the rhythm in 24 to 72 hours during occurrence of symptoms.

Electrophysiologic Study

This requires placement of electrode catheter in the ventricle, followed by programmed electrical stimulation by progressive pacing protocols.

Indications: According to ACC/AHA/ESC 2006 guidelines:
  i. Diagnostic assessment of patients with remote MI.
  ii. Diagnostic assessment of patients' symptoms related to ventricular tachyarrhythmias lies palpitation, presyncope, syncope.
  iii. In patient with CHD to guide and measure the efficacy of VT ablations.
  iv. In patients at high risk of sudden death due to severe structural heart disease.
  v. To detect the substrate for sustained VT in patients presenting with symptoms related to VT.

In EPS, premature ventricular beats are induced by conditioning pacing drive and to look for reentrant arrhythmias.

Management of Ventricular Tachycardia

According to ACC/AHA/ESC-2006 guidelines—coronary revascularization is urgently needed for patient who is at risk of sudden cardiac death having VT in the background of myocardial ischemia.

In case of sustained ventricular tachycardia, it should be addressed properly as it may produce significant hemodynamic collapse.

Prehospital Care

Emergency medical service personnel should provide adequate attention to the patient in the following forms:
i. 'ABC'—Airway, breathing, circulation
   ECG rhythm strip
   Vascular access
   Supplemental oxygen

Acute Ventricular Tachycardia

1. **Symptomatic VT like hypotension, unconsciousness,** immediate biphasic cardioversion with 100–200 Jules. Using standard ACLS protocols.
2. **In case of stable VT (monomorphic VT with adequate end organ perfusion)** having no hemodynamic compromise, no coronary ischemia or infarction, rhythm can be converted to normal by intravenous medication or cardioversion.
   Antiarrhythmic medications include:
     i. **Amiodarone**—it should not be the 1st line of treatment because of its gradual onset of effects on myocardial conduction and refractoriness.
     ii. **Lidocaine**
     iii. **Procainamide**—it may precipitate congestive cardiac failure.
3. **In case of failure of medical therapy,** synchronized cardioversion with monophasic 90–200 Jules, following sedation.
4. **According to ACC/AHA/ESC—2006 guidelines,** the drugs those increase QT interval should not be used in those patients with polymorphic VT with prolonged 'QT' interval—so these drugs should be avoided.
5. **Hypokalemia** should be corrected to avoid arrhythmia.
6. **Administration of magnesium** is indicated in patient with prolonged QT interval, but magnesium is not effective in patients with normal QT interval.
7. **In patient with myocardial ischemia,** lidocaine is the primary antiarrhythmic drug of choice.
8. **In patients with polymorphic VT and hemodynamic compromise,** cardioversion with sedation is required.
9. **If there is any doubt about rhythm diagnosis**—whether it is VT or SVT with aberrant conduction, the safest strategy is to treat undiagnosed rhythm as VT.
10. **In case of tachycardia-induced cardiomyopathy** due to prolonged exposure to nonsustained VT—medical therapy or ablative therapy is indicated.

Treatment of Pulseless Ventricular Tachycardia

The treatment of choice is defibrillation—with high energy unsynchronized defibrillator.
a. Biphasic defibrillator with energy 150–200 Jules at initial shock followed by equal or higher energy shock.
b. Monophasic defibrillator with initial shock energy of 360 Jules.

The above shock is followed by:
  i. Chest compression
  ii. Airway management
  iii. Supplemental oxygen
  iv. Vascular access—for administration of vasopressor agents—which include:
    1. Epinephrine—1 mg/IV, every 3–5 minutes
    2. Vasopressin—40 units IV as one time dose.

Post-Conversion Follow-up Treatment

Following conversion to sinus rhythm, we have to determine:
  i. The severity of heart disease
  ii. Prognosis
  iii. Follow-up treatment.

In **case of structural heart disease,** combination therapies include medications, ICD implantation and catheter ablation.

In case of monomorphic VT with normal heart, since there is little risk of sudden death, medication or ablation is of choice.

Class ± antiarrhythmic drugs actually increase the mortality—because they slow the propagation and reduce the exicitity through sodium channel blockade.

Class III antiarrhythmic drugs is of choice, because, they prolong the myocardial repolarization through potassium channel blockade.

Amiodarone, though is class III antiarrhythmic agent, has side effects of class I, II and IV agents. But unlike class I antiarrhythmic agent, amiodarone is safe in case of ventricular dysfunctions.

According to 2006 guidelines, amiodarone can be used in combination with beta blockers—because amiodarone is useful in patient with post-MI LV dysfunction and beta-blocker non-responsive VT.

In patient with congestive cardiac failure, the beta-blocker drugs to be used are—carvidolol, metoprolol, and bisoprolol

The other drugs are ACE inhibitors, aldosterone antagonist.

VENTRICULAR FIBRILLATION

Definition

It is the most commonly occurred arrhythmia, occurred in patient with sudden cardiac arrest as evidenced by severe derangement in heart beat which can end the sufferer unless proper prompt corrective measures will be taken.

Pathophysiology

Sudden cardiac death due to ventricular fibrillation (VF) occurs during early morning—which may be related to increased platelet aggregability—use of aspirin and clopidogrel reduces this type of mortality now. Again spike of SCD occurs during winter month due to same reasons.

Following conditions are responsible for VF:
  i. Administration of antiarrhythmic drugs.
 ii. Hypoxia.
iii. Ischemia.
 iv. Atrial fibrillation.
  v. Very rapid ventricular rate in pre-exitation syndrome.
 vi. Electric shock administered during cardioversion.
vii. Competitive ventricular pacing to laminate VT.

60–85% patients of cardiac arrest have VF as initial rhythm during contact.

20–30% of patients of cardiac arrest have asystole as terminating event from massive myocyte necrosis, pump failure from progression of VF to asystole.

70–100% patients present with VT which precedes VF, which occurs in patients with ischemic heart disease.

The interplay among myocardial ischemia, left ventricular (LV) dysfunction and transient inciting events (worsened ischemic, hypoxemic, acidosis, drugs, and metabolic disturbances).

Epidemiology

1. Race: Blacks are mostly suffered from SCDs than whites.
2. Sex: Males have higher incidence of SCD than women (3:1).
3. Age: Peak age of incidence is 45–75 years.

Risk Factors for VF

Forty-five percent of patient having VF have been noted to visit their physician within 4 weeks before death. **Following are the common risk factors:**
  i. Left ventricular function impairment with left ventricular ejection fraction <30–35%, this is the single and most important risk factor.
 ii. Coronary artery disease and subsequent myocardial infarction.
iii. Family history of premature coronary artery disease.
 iv. Smoking, dyslipidemias
  v. Hypertension
 vi. Diabetes
vii. Obesity
viii. Sedentary lifestyle.

Other specific considerations are:
a. Coronary artery disease:
   i. Previous cardiac arrest
  ii. Prior myocardial infarction within 6 months
 iii. Syncope

 iv. Left ventricular ejection traction 30–35%
  v. Premature ventricular ectopic >10/hour.
 vi. Drop in systolic blood pressure or ventricular ectopic upon stress testing.
b. Dilated cardiomyopathy—from any cause:
   i. Previous cardiac arrest
  ii. Syncope or presyncope
 iii. Left ventricular ejection fraction 30–35%.
 iv. Use of ionotropic medication in patients with decompensated heart failure or acute myocardial ischemia.
c. Hypertrophic obstructive cardiomyopathy:
   i. Previous cardiac arrest
  ii. Presyncope or syncope
 iii. Family history of coronary artery disease
 iv. Drop of systolic blood pressure or appearance of ventricular ectopic on stress testing.
  v. Palpitations
d. Valvular heart disease:
   i. Severe uncorrected MS or AS.
  ii. Severe MI or AI.
 iii. Valve replacement within 6 months.
 iv. Syncope
  v. History of frequent ventricular ectopy.
e. Myocarditis:
   i. LVEF <30%
  ii. Symptoms of decompensated heart failure
 iii. Previous cardiac arrest
 iv. Syncope or presyncope
f. Congenital heart disease:
   i. Functional cause
  ii. Autonomic nervous system
 iii. Metabolic imbalance
 iv. Electrolyte imbalance.
g. Long QT syndrome:
   i. Family history of long QT syndrome
  ii. Medications that prolong QT interval
h. Wolf-Parkinson-White syndrome: Atrial flutter or atrial fibrillation with rapid ventricular rate.
   a. Brugada syndrome
   b. Arrhythmogenic right ventricular dysplasia

Physical Examination

Cardiac arrest, developed by Thompson and McCullough can be used for patients suffered from cardiac arrest can be defined by following criteria:
  i. ED systolic blood pressure >90 mmHg = 1 point
 ii. ED systolic blood pressure <90 mmHg = 0 point
iii. Time to ROSC less than 25 minutes = 1 point
 iv. Time to ROSC >25 minutes = 0 point.
  v. Neurologically responsive =1 point
 vi. Comatose = 0 point
    Maximum scope = 3 points

Patients with score of 3 points have a chance of 80% neurologic recovery and 82% chances of survival to discharge.

Even in the setting of ST elevation, early invasive management with primary angioplasty and intra-aortic balloon pump insertion, the patient with low scores is unlikely to survive.

Causes

Ischemic Heart Disease

VF may occur in chronic scar or acute or chronic ischemic area. This scar may act as a focus for re-entrant arrhythmia, may occur shortly or years later:

1. **Coronary artery abnormalities:** Coronary vasospasm—it exposes the myocardium to both ischemic or reperfusion insult, which occurs during thrombolysis or direct angioplasty as a result there is transient electrical instability by several unknown mechanism. These are:
    a. α-adrenergic activity
    b. Vagal activity
    c. Vessel susceptibility
    d. Humoral factors—platelet activation and aggregation.
2. **Atherosclerotic abnormalities of coronary arteries.**
3. **Non-atherosclerotic abnormalities of coronary arteries:**
    i. Congenital lesion
    ii. Coronary artery embolism
    iii. Coronary arteritis
    iv. Mechanical abnormalities of coronary artery.

Non-Ischemic Heart Disease

a. **Dilated cardiomyopathy:** Factors contribute to the risk of VF in these patients:
    i. Increase in end diastolic pressure
    ii. Subsequent wall tension
    iii. Increased sympathetic tone
    iv. Neurohumoral activation
    v. Electrolyte abnormalities
    vi. Drugs like antiarrhythmic agents, inotropic agents, diuretics—may provoke arrhythmias.
b. **Hypertrophic cardiomyopathy:** The mechanism of VF is not clearly understood. The possible mechanisms which may worsen the outflow tract gradient and induce cardiac ischemia and subsequent malignant arrhythmias are:
    i. Post-exertional drop in blood pressure
    ii. Shunting of blood to extracardiac tissues.
    This cycle does not revert spontaneously. It poorly responds to resuscitation.
c. **Arrhythmogenic right ventricular dysplasia:** Here right ventricular wall is being replaced by fibrous tissue. There may be involvement of interventricular septum. This scar is responsible for development of reentrant arrhythmias.
d. **Vascular heart disease:**
    1. In aortic stenosis, mechanism of VF is unknown. But incidence of VF after aortic valve surgery is highest in 1st 3 weeks after the procedure.
    2. In aortic insufficiency—reentrant or automatic ventricular foci may be responsible for VF.
    3. Incidence of VF in mitral valve prolapse is low.

Congenital Heart Disease (Fig. 1.114)

A. **Primary electrophysiologic abnormalities:** In these abnormalities, no apparent structural heart disease.

ECG is the only clue to the diagnosis:
a. Congenital long QT syndrome
b. Acquired QT syndrome

Diagnosis of congenital long QT syndrome requires the presence of 2 major criteria or 1 major criterion.

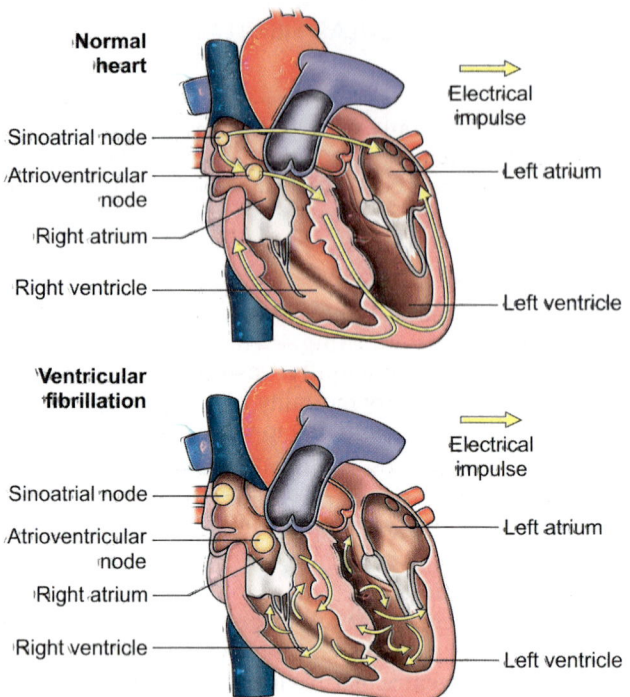

Fig. 1.114: Mechanism of ventricular fibrillation

Major criteria include:
1. Long QT interval (QTc >420 ms in females and >450 ms in males)
2. Stress-induced syncope
3. Family history of long QT syndrome
Minor criteria:
1. Congenital deafness
2. T-wave alternans
3. Bradycardia (children)
c. WPW syndrome
d. Brugada syndrome
e. Primary ventricular fibrillation
f. Right ventricular outflow tract tachycardia
g. Lower-Ganong-Levine syndrome

B. **Pulmonary embolism**—risk factors include:
    i. Personal or family history of DVT
    ii. Malignancy
    iii. Hypercoagulable states
    iv. Recent mechanical trauma
    Here mechanism of VF is:
    i. Hemodynamic collapse
    ii. Severe hypoxia

C. **Aortic dissection or aneurysmal rupture**

Workup of Ventricular Fibrillation

Laboratory Studies

a. *Cardiac enzymes:* Creative kinase, myoglobin, troponin—increased in ischemia and myocardial infarction. Extent of elevation of cardiac enzymes correlates with extent of cardiac damage.
b. Electrolytes, calcium, magnesium, potassium, an ion gap—because metabolic acidosis, hypokalemia, hyperkalemia,

hypocalcemia, hypomagnesemia—increase the risk of arrhythmia and SCD.

c. Quantitative measurement of quinidine, procainamide, TCA, digoxin—if these drug levels are higher than their therapeutic index, they may be proarrhythmic.

d. Toxicology screen: Blood level of cocaine (it can produce vasospasm-induced ischemia) should be measured.

e. Thyroid-stimulating hormone—hyperthyroidism can lead to tachyarrhythmias—it can lead to heart failure.

f. β-type natriuretic peptide (BNP)—it is specific and sensitive for diagnosis of decompensated heart failure when elevated left ventricular end-diastolic pressure is responsible for increased myocardial oxygen consumption and decreased cardiac output, leading to abnormal myocardial substrate accumulation which in turn, lead to the development of VF.

Imaging Studies

a. **Chest X-ray:**
   i. Left ventricular hypertrophy
   ii. Right ventricular hypertrophy
   iii. Features of pulmonary hypertension

b. **Echocardiography:**
   i. Left ventricular wall motion abnormalities—in MI.
   ii. Decrease in ejection fraction.
   iii. Worsening of wall motion abnormalities upon exercise echocardiography.

c. **Nuclear imaging studies:** Resting thallium (TI) or technetium (Tc-99m) scintigraphy. It can detect the extent of myocardial damage.

d. **Exercise nuclear scintigraphy:** It is very sensitive in detecting presence, extent and location of myocardial ischemia.

Other Tests: ECG (Fig. 1.115)

i. Evidence of MI	ii. Prolonged QT interval
iii. Epsilon sign	iv. Brugada sign
v. Short PR	vi. WPW pattern.

Procedures

a. **Coronary angiography:**
   i. It can assess the state of ventricular function.
   ii. It can assess the severity and extent of CAD.
   iii. It can detect number of vessels with severe obstruction.
   iv. It can detect coronary anomalies and other forms of congenital heart diseases.

b. **Electrophysiological studies:** They play diagnostic, prognostic and therapeutic roles.

   i. It should be performed after ischemic or structural heart disease has been diagnosed.
   Contraindications: In patient with VF within 1st 24–48 hours of AMI unless the patient had a history of previous VF events.

   ii. It can identify inducible sustained VT and VF, when the patient is on antiarrhythmic medications, this patient is at risk of sudden death—rather than non-inducible sustained VT.

   iii. It can detect inducible bundle branch block in patient with dilated cardiomyopathy and in postoperative period after valve replacement.

   iv. It can detect inducible VT in 20% of hypertrophic cardiomyopathy.

   v. It can identify accessory pathway.

   vi. EPS are performed the following in mind:
      1. Ablation VT foci.
      2. Internal coronary defibrillator.

Ventricular Fibrillation—Treatment and Management

Medical Care

1. **Advanced cardiac life support**—it must be done in case of cardiac arrest.

2. **Defibrillation:** External defibrillator—is the most successful way of medical treatment.

   In this method—a shock is delivered to the heart to depolarize simultaneously and uniformly the critical cardiac mass of excitable myocardium.

   Thus it can interfere with re-entrant arrhythmia, and allows the cardiac intrinsic pacemaker to assume the role of pacemaker.

Successful defibrillation depends on:
1. Duration between onset of VF and defibrillation
2. Metabolic conditions of the myocardium

   VF waveform starts with high amplitude and frequency, then it degenerates to smaller and smaller wave form until asystole after approximately 15 minutes; possible due to progressive depletion of cardiac reserves. Hence early defibrillation is vital.

   Success rate of defibrillation gradually decreases by 5–10% after the onset of VF.

   Factors that increase the energy required for successful defibrillation:
   i. Time before defibrillation begins
   ii. Paddle size
   iii. Paddle to myocardium distance (obesity, mechanical ventilation)

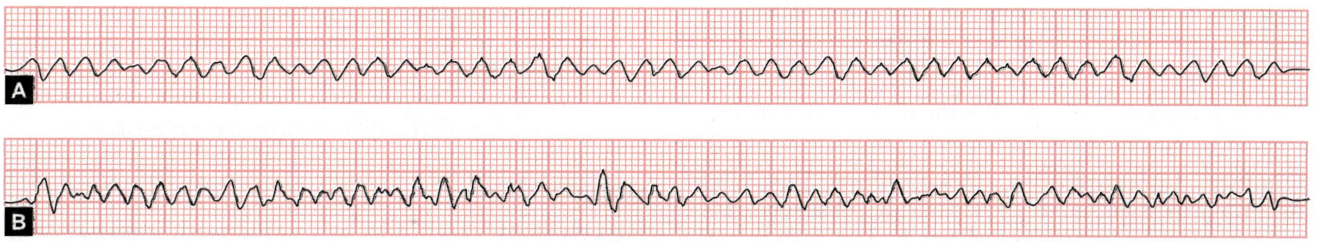

Fig. 1.115: Bizarre pattern in ECG

iv. Use of conduction fluid (e.g. disposable pad, electrode jelly)
v. Contact pressure
vi. Elimination of strong conductive pathways (electrode jelly bridges on the skin)
vii. Previous shocks—which decreases defibrillation threshold.
 1. The goal is to use minimal energy required to overcome the threshold of defibrillation.
 2. Paddle size 8–12.5 cm for adult, 8–10 cm for child.
 3. For artificial pacemaker, anteroposterior paddle placement is required.
 4. Before any defibrillation, all patches or ointments from the chest must be removed to avoid risk of fire or explosion.
 5. Patient must be dry, has no metallic contact.
 6. Following defibrillation, a period of low cardiac output followed by recovery of normal cardiac output.
 7. Defibrillation causes serum creatine kinase to increase proportionate to the amount of energy delivered. But the proportion of myocardial fraction (CK-MB) should remain within reference range except in myocardial infraction.

Algorithm:

Activation of emergency response system and retrieve automatic defibrillator.
↓
Open airway, if patient is pulseless. Initiate CPR giving 30 chest compressions and 2 breaths—until AED arrive. Chest compression—must be hard and fast at a rate of 100/minute
↓
Connect AED and check for shockable rhythm
↓
Deliver 1 shock to patient (AED, by specific, monophasic, adult—200 Joules, child—2 Joules/kg)
↓
Start CPR immediately—3 cycles of CPR
↓
Check rhythm
↓
If patient is in asystole—and CPR has been given for 5 cycles, search for IV access; give vasopressor, in the form of epinephrine or vasopressin **as per asystole/pulseless electrical activity advanced cardiac life support algorithm.**
↓
If shockable rhythm is present, continue CPR till defibrillator is charging.
↓
Deliver 1 shock and start CPR immediately after shock.
↓
Administer vasopressor during CPR (before or after shock) at a dose of epinephrine 1 mg/IV and repeat it every 3–5 minutes.

Or
Intravenous vasopressin 40 units to replace 1st or 2nd dose of epinephrine.
↓
Administer 5 cycles of CPR and check rhythm

If rhythm is not shockable, go to asystole algorithm   **if rhythm is shockable,** continue CPR, when defibrillator is charging

Give 1 shock as before, and then resume CPR (before and after shock) with intravenous drugs at the following doses:

1. Amiodarone—300 mg IV once, then consider additional 150 mg IV once
 Or
 Lidocaine—1–1.5 mg/kg IV 1st dose, then 0.5–0.75 mg/kg IV, maximum 3 doses or 3 mg/kg
2. Consider magnesium sulphate—loading dose 1–2 mg IV for torsades de pointes.
↓
Repeat algorithm as before, if the patient is pulseless without spontaneous rhythm.

Treatment of underlying provocative factors for VF:
 i. Myocardial infarction
 ii. Hypovolemia
 iii. Hemorrhagic shock
 iv. Anoxia
 v. Pneumothorax
 vi. Hemothorax
 vii. Hypercalcemia
 viii. Drug overdose (narcotic, tricyclic antidepressant—cocaine, barbiturates
 ix. Carbon monoxide poisoning
 x. Hyperkalemia.

Treatment of refractory publication:
i. If there is lack of response to standard defibrillation, supplementation of magnesium or procainamide may be effective.
ii. It amiodarone has not been used earlier, add—loading dose of amiodarone (15 mg/min for 10 minutes), followed by 1 mg/min for 6 hours, then 0.5 mg/min for 18 hours.

Post-resuscitative Care

i. Continue antiarrhythmic drugs—lidocaine at 1–4 mg/min or amiodarone at 0.5 mg/min.
ii. Maintain hemodynamic stability.
iii. Vasopressin can be added.
 Post-resuscitative arrhythmias (commonly AV block) may be related to amount of energy used during defibrillation.
iv. Concomitant treatment of myocardial ischemia, heart failure, electrolyte disturbances should be done.

Surgical Care

Survivors of VF should be treated with internal cardiac defibrillator (ICD).

Radiofrequency ablation: Indications are the followings:
 i. AV bypass tract
 ii. Bundle branch block VT
 iii. Right ventricular outflow tract tachycardia
 iv. Idiopathic left ventricular tachycardia
 v. Automatic foci VT

ICD therapy:
 i. It is beneficial for antiarrhythmic refractory patients.
 ii. Newer ICD have pacing capabilities, can address bradyarrhythmias complicating VT or VF.
 iii. Currently, transvenous method of implantation of ICD is well accepted.

Cardiac surgery can be primary treatment for VF via variety of strategies:
1. Surgical treatment of VF and IHD is CABG. It can only prevent VF if ejection fraction is normal and ischemia is the cause of arrest. In these patients, ICD can be implanted even after CABG.
2. In case of non-ischemic heart disease, the method of treatment may be:
 i. Excisions of VT foci, after endocardial mapping
 ii. Excision of left ventricular aneurysm.
3. Aortic valve and mitral valve replacement can improve the outcome of aortic stenosis and mitral valve prolapsed syndrome respectively.
4. Orthotopic heart transplantation is indicated in refractory heart failure with evidence of significant improvement.
5. Patients with long QT syndrome not responding beta blocker are the candidates for ICD placement or high thoracic left sympathectomy.

WOLF-PARKINSON-WHITE SYNDROME

Definition

WPW syndrome can be defined as congenital abnormality which involves abnormal conduction pathways between atria and ventricles in patient with supraventricular tachycardia without any involvement of atrioventricular node hence it is also called preexitation syndrome.

Fate of WPW Syndrome

1. Some patients have increased risk of ventricular arrhythmias due to extremely rapid conduction through accessory pathway, if they have atrial flatter or atrial fibrillation.
2. In some patients, in spite of presence of concealed bypass tract, they do not show antegrade conduction, hence their ECG does not show any abnormality.
3. Less than one percent of patients are at risk of sudden death.

Pathophysiology

Accessory pathways are the anomalous embryonic myocardial tissue bridging the fibrous tissue between two chambers, as a result, the impulse travels from atria to ventricle through this pathway bypassing atrioventricular node. So the normal delay that usually occurs in AV node does not occur during conduction through this pathway, as a result, tachyarrhythmias occur.

There are several by pass tracts—these are:

 i. Atrioventricular
 ii. Fasciculoventricular
 iii. Nodofascicular
 iv. Nodoventricular

The most common pathway is atrioventricular, also known as "bundle of Kent", which is the characteristic of WPW syndrome.

The single distinguishing feature which can differentiate from other accessory pathways is—conduction through this pathway is either antegrade (atrial to ventricle) or retrograde (ventricle to atrium).

Re-entrant tachycardia is the main mechanism in patient with W-P-W syndrome. This involves the presence of dual conducting pathways—between atria and ventricles:
 i. Normal AV node, bundle of His tract
 ii. One or more accessory fibers (bundle of Kent, Mahaim fibers)

These pathways have different conduction properties and refractory periods. The effective refractory period (the time necessary for the electrical recovery which is needed for conduction of the next impulse) of the accessory tract is often longer than the effective refractory period of AV node bundle of His tract.

The degree of pre-excitation in ECG of WPW syndrome can be estimated by:
 i. Width of QRS
 ii. Length of QRS interval

Wider QRS with short PR interval and absent or nearly absent isoelectric component means that most of the ventricular depolarization passes through accessory pathways rather than AV nodal/His-Purkinje system.

But in case of tachycardia, QRS width becomes narrower due to rapid heart rate and catecholamine allows the AV node to accept more and more number of conduction through AV node.

There are several types of supraventricular tachycardia—these are:
1. Orthodromic tachycardia:
 i. Antegrade conduction through AV nodal Purkinje system
 ii. Retrograde conduction through accessory pathway.
2. Orthodromic tachycardia with concealed accessory pathway—here retrograde conduction occurs only.
3. Antedromic tachycardia:
 i. Antegrade conduction through accessory pathway.
 ii. Retrograde conduction through AV nodal pathway.

In patients with WPW syndrome:
 i. 95% of SVT is orthodromic tachycardia.
 ii. 5% of SVT is antedromic tachycardia.

Lown-Ganong-Levine Syndrome

This is also a pre-excitation syndrome where accessory pathway is James fibers; it connects atria to lower portion of AV node or bundle of His.

This leads to accelerated conduction from atria to ventricle without QRS widening—because, the distal pathway is the Purkinje system.

Etiology

a. It is a congenital phenomenon, where there is failure of maturation of insulating tissue within the AV ring—but the symptoms appear in late age.
b. It may have genetic component, may be inherited as a familial trait with or without congenital trait. Inheritance may be:
   1. Mendelian dominant
   2. Mitochondrial inheritance
c. It may be associated with cardiac or non-cardiac defect like atrial septal defect, familial hypokalemic periodic paralysis and tuberous sclerosis, familial hypertrophic cardio-myopathy.
d. The mutation in gamma 2 subunits of adenosine mono-phosphate-activated protein kinase produces disruption of annulus fibrosus by accumulation of glycogen within myocytes—leading to pre-excitation. This mutation can also produce:
   1. Ventricular hypertrophy
   2. AV block
   3. Progressive degenerative conduction system disease. This mutation can occur in following congenital diseases:
      i. Pompe disease
      ii. Danon disease
      iii. Other glycogen storage disease
e. Ebstein anomaly—due to presence of multiple accessory bypass tract mostly on the right, in the posterior part of the septum.

Epidemiology

Its incidence is 0.1–3 cases/1000 population in USA. The locations of accessory pathways in descending order of frequency are:
   i. 54% left free wall
   ii. 36% posteroseptal wall
   iii. 8% right free wall
   iv. 3% anteroseptal
1. 80% of patients with WPW syndrome have reciprocating tachycardia.
2. 15–30% develop atrial fibrillation.
3. 5% patients develop atrial flutter.
4. VT is rather uncommon.

Age-related incidence: It is found in all ages having first peak in infancy and second peak at school age children and adolescents.

The prevalence of WPW syndrome decreases with age due to apparent attenuation of conduction speed through AP.

Sex-related incidence: WPW syndrome occurs more commonly in males than females.

Prognosis

1. Once treated, WPD syndrome has excellent prognosis.
2. Asymptomatic patient with ECG evidence of WPW syndrome has excellent prognosis.
3. Patients with family history of sudden cardiac death or significant symptoms of tachyarrhythmia have worst prognosis.

Mortality in WPW Syndrome

It is rare but sudden cardiac death may occur.

Risk Factors Related to Mortality

   i. Medical therapy with digoxin may increase in case of atrial flutter or atrial fibrillation.
   ii. Presence of multiple bypass tracts.
   iii. Short accessory pathway refractory period (<240 ms).
   iv. Atrial fibrillation
   v. Atrial flutter
   vi. Family history of premature sudden cardiac death.
   vii. Risk factors for the development of atrial fibrillation in the setting of WPW syndrome:
      a. Advancing age (2 peak ages for AF, one at 30 years and the other at 50 years)
      b. Male gender
      c. History of syncope.
   viii. Factors that increase the likelihood of VF—including rapidly conducting accessory pathways and multiple pathways.

Symptoms and Signs of WPW Syndrome

A. Infants with WPW syndrome:
   i. Irritability
   ii. Intolerant to feedings
   iii. Evidence of congestive cardiac failure
   iv. Intercurrent febrile illness
   v. Improper behavior for 1–2 days.
B. Child with WPW syndrome may present with:
   i. Chest pain
   ii. Palpitation
   iii. Breathlessness
C. Older children and adult with WPW syndrome may present with:
   i. Sudden and accidental onset of pounding heart beat.
   ii. Pulse is too rapid to count.
   iii. Intolerance to activity.
   iv. Sudden discovery of concurrent tachyarrhythmia in electrocardiography.
D. Other symptoms are:
   i. Light headedness or presyncope—in patients who have paroxysmal supraventricular tachycardia or atrial fibrillation with AV nodal re-entry.
   ii. Syncope—as a result of inadequate cerebral circulation due to:
      a. Rapid ventricular rate, or
      b. Tachycardia by depressing sinus pacemaker pro-duces a period of asystole at the point of tachycardia termination.
   iii. Polyuria—due to atrial dilatation and release of atrial natriuretic factor.

Physical Examinations

A. In majority of cases, normal cardiac findings
B. Few patients during symptoms—may be cool, diaphoretic and hypotensive.
C. Due to pulmonary congestion as a result of congestive cardiac failure, there are crackles in the lung.
D. In minimally symptomatic patients (palpitation weakness and dizziness)—inspite of very rapid heart rate.
E. In infants with WPW syndrome:
   i. Tachypnea
   ii. Irritable
   iii. Pallor

iv. Low volume and rapid pulse
v. Low blood pressure
vi. Ventricular rate 200–250 beat/minute.

If untreated for several hours, this patient shows the evidence of:
i. Congestive cardiac failure
ii. Tender hepatomegaly
iii. Tachypnea with tachycardia

The associated cardiac defects are:
a. Cardiomyopathy
b. Ebstein anomaly—10% of these patients involving tricuspid valve have more than one accessory on the right side.

Patient with corrected transposition of great veins and left-sided Ebstein anomaly may have accessory pathways on left side or septal wall.

These patients usually present with—cyanosis tachypnea, signs of congestive cardiac failure.
c. Hypertrophic cardiomyopathy (AMPK mutation).
d. Ventricular septal defect.
e. Coronary sinus diverticula

The other associated non-cardiac cause—glycogen storage diseases—symptoms and signs of muscle weakness, increased muscle bulk, macroglossia, hepatomegaly. The diseases are:
i. Pompe disease.
ii. Danon disease with mental retardation.

WPW Syndromes—Workup

In severely symptomatic patient, i.e. patient with cardiogenic shock or unconsciousness, direct cardioversion must be given to restore the sinus rhythm when this patient become hemodynamically stable, following batteries of investigation should be started.

Laboratory Studies

1. Complete blood count—to identity intercurrent infection
2. Serum electrolyte:
   i. Potassium
   ii. Magnesium
   iii. Calcium
3. Serum lactate level
4. Serum renal profile to see renal status
5. Liver function test
6. Thyroid panel—FT4, TSH
7. Blood level of lidocaine, procainamide, and digoxin.

Digoxin should be avoided in patient with WPW syndrome, because it decreases or nodal conduction.

Echocardiographic Studies

i. Proper evaluation of left ventricular function and/or motion abnormalities.
ii. To rule out following cardiac defects:
   1. Ebstein anomaly
   2. Hypertrophic cardiomyopathies
   3. L—transposition of great vessels.

Electrocardiographic Study

Classical ECG findings include:
i. Shortened PR interval.
ii. Slurries and slow rise of initial upstroke of QRS complex (delta wave)
iii. Widened QRS complex (total duration >0.12 seconds)
iv. ST segment—T wave changes

In orthodromic tachycardia:
i. Delta weve is absent.
ii. Normal duration of QRS complex.
iii. Typically inverted P waves in inferior and lateral leads.

In orthodromic tachycardia with concealed accessory pathways: This is very difficult to distinguish from AV nodal reentrant tachycardia.

But heart rate if >200 beats/minute—the presence of the following may support above diagnosis:
i. QRS alternans
ii. Retrograde P wave is visible in ST segment (long R-P tachycardia) following QRS complex.

In antedromic tachycardia: Wide QRS—reflecting exaggeration of delta wave during sinus rhythm (wide QRS tachycardia). QRS complex is widened because, ventricles are initially activated through accessory pathway, producing early, albeit, and relatively slow initial progression of depolarization through ventricular tissue—as a result, delta wave is generated. Due to presence of this delta wave, there is widened QRS complex and shortened PR interval.

There are two types of WPW syndrome—depending on the presence of delta waves/QRS complex in precordial leads.
1. Type A WPW syndrome:
   i. Upright positive delta wave in all precordial leads
   ii. Amplitude of R ware is greater than S wave in V1.
2. Type B WPW syndrome:
   i. Negative delta wave in V1 and V2.
   ii. Negative QRS complex in V1 and V2.

In Lown-Ganong-Levine syndrome:
i. Shortened PR interval—it is due to presence of accessory pathway by passing AV node.
ii. Normal QRS morphology—it is due direct connection of accessory fibers (James fibers) with this bundle so the electrical impulse depolarizes via His-Purkinje system, not directly ventricular muscles.

In a few cases of WPW syndrome: Simultaneous electrical impulses pass through normal conducting pathways and via accessory pathway. In this case, pre-exitation is absent and ECG is normal. It depends upon the speed of excitation. But if the rate exceeds, the refractory period of AV node evidence of pre-exitation occurs in ECG.

Explanation of concealed accessory pathway: This type of concealed accessory pathway is used only during retrograde conduction (circus movement tachycardia). So, it is not detectable in normal surface ECG, because ventricle is not preexcitated. So, if there is normal QRS complex with retrograde P wave after completion of QRS complex on ST segment, or even on the T wave, thin concealed conduction can be considered.

Differentiation between WPW syndrome and PSVT—when ventricular rate is more than 220/min, it is WPW syndrome or VT. If the rate <220/min, it is PSVT.

Location of accessory pathways: Usually negative delta wave signals the site of accessory pathways.
   i. Negative delta wave in left-sided lead such as L1, avL—indicative of left-sided accessory pathway.
   ii. Negative delta wave in right sided lead such as V1—indicates right-sided accessory pathway.
   iii. Isoelectric delta wave in V1 predicts anteroseptal AP.
   iv. Negative delta wave in inferior leads (L1, L2 and aVF)—indicates posterolateral AP.
   v. Positive wave in interior leads—indicates anteroseptal AP.

   Specific algorithm for location of AP: It is based on the polarity of delta wave or first 40 ms of QRS.
1. Left lateral wall:
   i. Negative delta wave on L1 and aVL
   ii. Positive or isoelectric delta wave in L1, L2 and aVF and V1–4
   iii. Negative or isoelectric delta wave in V5–6.
2. Left posterior free wall:
   i. Positive delta wave in L1 and aVL.
   ii. Negative delta wave in L2, L3 and aVF.
   iii. Positive delta wave in V1–5.
   iv. Negative or isoelectric delta wave in V6.
3. Posterolateral wall:
   i. Positive delta wave in L1 and aVL
   ii. Negative delta wave in L2, L3 and aVF.
   iii. Isoelectric or positive delta waves in V1.
   iv. Positive delta wave in V2–6.
4. Right ventricular free wall:
   i. Positive delta wave in L1 and L2.
   ii. Negative delta wave in aVR
   iii. Isoelectric or negative delta wave in aVF.
   iv. Isoelectric delta wave in V1.
   v. Isoelectric or positive delta waves V2—V3.
   vi. Positive delta wave in V4–6.
5. Left anteroseptal:
   i. Positive delta wave in L1 and L2 and aVF
   ii. Negative delta wave in aVR
   iii. Isoelectric or positive delta wave in V1.
   iv. Positive delta wave in V2–6.
6. Right anteroseptal:
   i. Positive delta wave in L1 and L2, aVF
   ii. Negative delta wave in aVR
   iii. Isoelectric or negative delta wave in V1–3.
   iv. Positive delta waves in V4–6.

Stress Testing

This is used in following indications:
   i. To reproduce transient paroxysmal dysrhythmia.
   ii. To document the relationship between exercise and onset of tachycardia.
   iii. To evaluate the efficacy of antiarrhythmic drugs.

   Stress testing may reveal refractory periods of accessory pathways, in patients with WPW syndrome.

   Exercise alters the competitive conduction properties of AV node and favors the conduction of accessory pathways over AV node in use of septal or left-sided AP.

Electrophysiological Study

This study is performed to assess:
   i. Behavior of accessory pathway
   ii. Inducibility of supraventricular tachycardia
   iii. To evaluate the response to drug.
   This study can be performed in outpatient department only with sedation.

   Invasive EP study can be done in patient undergoing radio-frequency ablation.

   It is usually done with multipolar catheter electrode, collecting recordings from many intracardiac sites simultaneously.

   It can delineate the sequence of depolarization and impulse conduction from atria, AV junction and ventricle.

   It is used to determine the following:
   i. Mechanism of clinical dysrhythmia.
   ii. Electrophysiological properties of accessory pathways, normal AV nodal and His-Purkinje system.
   iii. Number and location of accessory pathways. (Because it is urgent for catheter ablation).
   iv. Response to pharmacotherapy or ablation procedure.

   Features of preexitation: Electrical impulses pass through normal AV-nodal pathway and through bundle of Kent (AP). In case of conduction through normal pathway, there will be physiological delay, whereas, in case of accessory pathway (Kent bundles), there will not be any delay during passage of impulse firm atria to ventricle.

   As a result of dual path mechanism, there will be a fusion beat with a delta wave due to passage of impulse through accessory path. The degree of delta depends upon:
   i. Distance between bypass tract and AV node
   ii. Speed of conduction through AV node and His Purkinjee system.
   Followings are the extent to which the wavefront over each route contribute to ventricular depolarization:
   i. In case of delay in AV nodal conduction occurs through rapid atrial pacing or premature atrial complex, the accessory pathway conduct the impulses to greater proportion of ventricles; hence QRS complex becomes more pre excited.
   ii. It the distance between sinus node and bypass tract is large or AV nodal conduction is rapid, large proportions of impulses are carried through normal pathways, hence pre-exitation will be less.
   iii. Normal fusion beat during sinus rhythm has short or negative HV interval.
   iv. Analysis of delta wave can localize the potential site of pathway for radiofrequency ablation.
      In patient with WPW syndrome, in case of normal sinus rhythm, deflection of His bundle at the beginning of QRS deflection—means negative HV interval.
      But in case of pre-excitation, HV deflection will be towards end of QRS complex.

Recognition and location of accessory pathways:
   i. When retrograde atrial activation during tachycardia occurs through accessory pathway connecting left atrium to left ventricle, earlier retrograde activity will be recorded from left atrial electrode presents in coronary sinus—indicates lateral pathway.
   ii. When retrograde activation during tachycardia occurs through AP connecting right atrium to right ventricle,

earliest retrograde activation will be recorded from electrode placed in right lateral wall—indicates right ventricular free wall pathway.

iii. Earliest retrograde activation will be recorded from an electrode placed in low right atrium—situated near the septum anteriorly or posteriorly.

Activation mapping using three-dimensional electro-anatomical mapping systems may improve pathway localization—specially when the bypass tract is anteroseptal or midseptal.

Risk assessment by EP study: During induction of AF during either intraesophageal or intracardiac study, if the shortest PR interval during 2 consecutive studies is less than 220 ms, the risk of sudden death due to AF is very high.

Treatment of WPW Syndrome

Initial Management

1. Patient with cardiac arrest or hemodynamic compromise
   i. ABC (A—airway, B—breathing, C—circulation)
   ii. Defibrillator
   iii. Appropriate monitoring
   iv. Direct cardioversion
2. In stable patient, various vagal maneuvers:
   i. In infants—bag of ice scrubbing to the face
   ii. Older children or adult:
      a. Carotid sinus massage—unilateral
      b. Ocular compression
      c. Valsalva maneuver

When conservative measures failed, intravenous access should be of choice followed by medicines:

i.	IV adenosine	6–12 mg via large bore line
ii.	IV verapamil	5–10 mg
iii.	IV diltiazem	10 mg

The above vagal maneuvers and pharmacotherapy can be applied in narrow complex AV reentrant tachycardia and AV nodal reentrant tachycardia.

In case of atrial flutter or atrial fibrillation or wide complex tachycardia:
   i. IV procainamide or amiodarone
   ii. Ibutilide

In hemodynamical sustainable tachycardia, the initial treatment of choice is—direct current synchronized electrical biphasic cardioversion:

i. A level of 100 Jules (monophasic or lower biphasic) initially.
ii. If necessary, second shock with energy of 200 or 360 Jules.

Pharmacotherapy

A. Agents acting on atrioventricular node:
   1. Verapamil and diltiazem (calcium channel blocker), metoprolol and atenolol (beta blocker) and digitalis— these drugs:
      i. Prolong the refractoriness of AV node.
      ii. Prolong conduction time
      Verapamil and digitalis are not recommended for the patients with WPW syndrome, because they do not affect conduction of AV bypass tract (except Mahaim fibers or atriofascicular pathway), on the other hand,

they accelerate the ventricular response in patient with atrial fibrillation.
   2. Adenosine slows the conduction through AV node, producing transient AV block, but it does not affect conduction of bypass tract, hence it should not be used in these patients.

B. Drugs acting on accessory pathway:
   1. Class IA drug (quinidine) or class IC drugs (flecainide, propafenone)
      i. Slow the conduction of bypass tract
      ii. Increase the refractory period of bypass tract
   2. Amiodarone, dofetilide and sotalol: They prolong refractoriness of myocardial tissue and bypass tract.

Complications of cardioversion:
   i. Dysrhythmia—due to inadequate synchronization.
   ii. Shock occurring during ST segment of T wave charges— post-cardioversion arrhythmia is transient and it usually does not require any treatment.
   iii. Embolic episode during conversion of atrial fibrillation to sinus rhythm.

Hence anticoagulant is usually required prior to cardioversion.

Further measures:
1. Continuous telemetry monitoring to look:
   a. Reappearance of tachyarrhythmia
   b. Degree of control of ventricular rate in patient with atrial fibrillation.
2. Initiation, dosing and maintenance of long-term antiarrhythmic drugs to prevent recurrent arrhythmias.
3. Laboratory studies to evaluate metabolic, electrolyte imbalance.
4. Careful evaluation of proarrhythmic drugs like, quinidine, amiodarone, sotalol, and dofetilide.

Radiofrequency Ablation (RF)

Indications:
   i. Patient with symptomatic AV nodal reentrant tachycardia.
   ii. Patient with atrial flutter or atrial fibrillation with rapid ventricular response via accessory pathway.
   iii. Patient with AVRT or AF with rapid ventricular response found accidentally during electrophysiological study for untreated dysrhythmias, if shortest RR interval during AF is less than 250 ms.
   iv. Patient with WPW syndrome having family history of sudden cardiac death.
   v. Asymptomatic patient with ventricular pre-excitation who is likely to be influenced by unpredictable tachyarrhythmias.

Identification of accessory pathway site before ablation prerequisite:
1. One has to be determined that AP is the part of reentrant tachycardia.
2. One has to locate the site of ablation—it may on the right or left free wall, in 5–10% patient—multiple pathways are present.

i. Ventricular insertion site is indicated by—earliest onset of ventricular electrocardiogram in relation to delta wave during sinus rhythm or atrial pacing.

ii. Atrial insertion site is indicated by region of the shortest VA interval during orthodromic tachycardia or ventricular pacing.

During ablation procedure, tip temperature requires 50°C for permanent elimination of accessory pathway conduction.

Success rate: Success rate of RF ablation is 90%, except anteroseptal or midseptal pathways, it is due to difficulty in achieving safe site for ablation due to nearby AV node and His bundle.

Complications: Complication rate is 1%. The adverse consequences are:
i. Bleeding complication
ii. Pericardial effusion
iii. Chest pain
iv. Stroke
v. Myocardial infarction
vi. AV node block

Surgical Treatment

Though radiofrequency ablation procedure may cure WPW syndrome in most of the patient, but surgery may be required in following patients:

i. Failure of radiofrequency ablation
ii. Where requirement of concomitant cardiac surgery.
iii. Where AP is due to involvement of multiple pathways.

Long-Term Antiarrhythmic Therapy

Oral medication is the main story of therapy in patients with radiofrequency ablation—the choice includes:
i. Class IA (Procainamide) + Verapamil—dual therapy
ii. Class IC drugs (Flecainide, propafenone) used with AV nodal blocking agent.
iii. Class III drugs (Amiodarone, sotalol)
iv. In case of pregnant patient—sotalol or class IC drug (flecainide).

Long-term follow-up: Follow-up visit is required for:
i. Recurrence of dysrhythmia
ii. Effectiveness of antiarrhythmic therapy
iii. Adverse effect of the drugs
iv. Follow-up ECG or Holter monitoring to assess:
   a. Changes in QT duration
   b. Recurrence of dysrhythmias
   c. Proarrhythmias
v. If patient is taking amiodarone, following careful monitorinrs are required:
   a. Thyroid function test
   b. Hepatic function test
   c. Pulmonary function test
d. Hepatic function test.

COARCTATION OF AORTA

It is a common, 5.8% of all congenital heart defect.

Pathologic Anatomy

This is a constricted aortic segment—produced by localized medical thickening with some intending of the medial and superimposed neointimal tissue.

Types

It may be:
i. Shelf-like structure with eccentric opening of aorta.
ii. Membranous curtain-like structure with central or eccentric opening of aorta.
   In the past, it was classified as (Fig. 1.116):
   1. Preductal (infantile)—when coarctation segment was proximal to ductus arteriosus, or
   2. Postductal (or adult)—when coarctation segment was distal to ductus arteriosus.
   But really, the coarctation segment is juxtraductal.

Shape

i. It may discrete.
ii. It may involve long segment.

Classical Site of Coarctation

1. It is usually located in thoracic aorta distal to the origin of left subclavian artery at the level of ductal structure.
2. It may be in distal thoracic aorta.
3. It may be in abdominal aorta.

Condition of Aorta

1. Distal to coarctation of aorta, descending aorta is dilated (post-stenotic dilatation).
2. A Jet lesion on the aortic wall distal to coarctation is present.
3. Hypoplasia of isthmus of the aorta in thoracic coarctation—site is the portion of aorta between the origin of left subclavian artery and ductus arteriosus.
   i. It may be significant—in neonates and infants
   ii. It may be mild—in children and adults
4. Transverse aortic arch (the arch between right in nominate artery and left subclavian artery) may be hypoplastic in infants and neonates.
5. Collateral vessels connect arteries from upper part of the body to the vessels in lower part of the body below the levels of coarctation.

Associated Conditions

i. Patent ductus arteriosus
ii. Ventricular septal defect
iii. Aortic stenosis
iv. Bicuspid aortic valve—in two-thirds of infants with coarctation of aorta. Sometimes, coarctation may be the complicating feature of more complex cyanotic heart disease, like:
   a. Transposition of great vessels
   b. Taussig-Bing anomaly
   c. Double inlet left ventricle
   d. Tricuspid atresia
   e. Hypoplastic left heart syndrome.

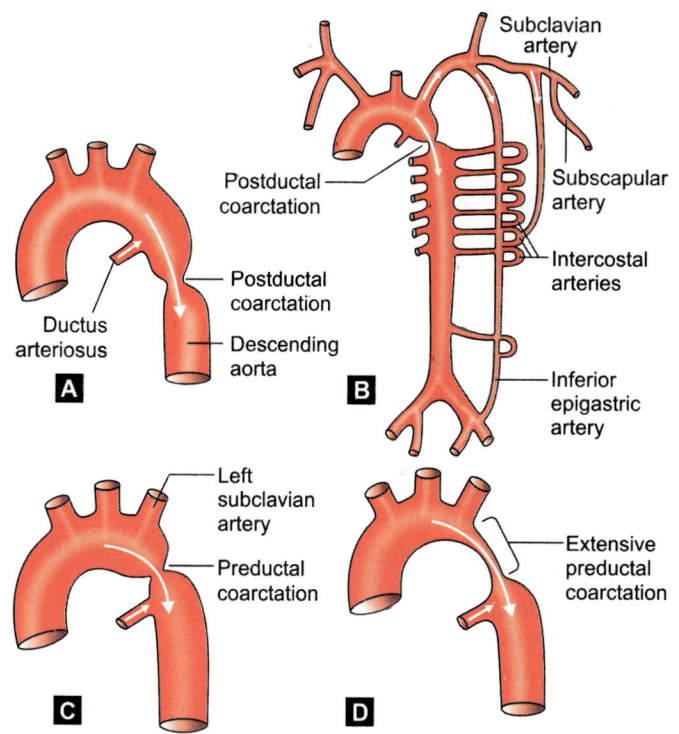

Fig. 1.116: Preductal and post-ductal coarctation of aorta

Pathogenesis

There are two theories—regarding production of coarctation of aorta.

1. Hemodynamic theory

> Abnormal preductal flow
> Or
> Abnormal angle between the ductus and the aorta
> ↓
> Increases right to left ductal flow
> ↓
> Decreases isthmic flow
> ↓
> Helps to produce coarctation of aorta

2. Ductal tissue theories: Abnormal extension of ductal tissue into the aorta (ectopic ductal tissue)—probably produces shelf of coarctation.

Pathophysiology

Coarctation of the aorta imposes significant after load on the left ventricle, producing increased muscle wall stress followed by left ventricular hypertrophy.

a. If ductus closes acutely at its aortic end

> ↓
> Left ventricular afterload increases acutely
> ↓
> Increase in left ventricular (systolic and diastolic) pressure
> ↓
> There is elevation of left atrial pressure

(Contd.)

(Contd.)

If foramen ovale opens	If the foramen ovale does not open
↓	↓
Dilatation of right atrium and right ventricles	Rise in pulmonary venous pressure
	↓
	Rise in pulmonary artery pressure
	↓
	Right ventricular dilatation

b. In children with less severe coarctation: Blood will flow through arterial collaterals from upper parts of the body to lower parts by passing obstruction. So they are asymptomatic until the development of hypertension. The development of hypertension may be due to:
  i. Postulated renin–angiotensin-mediated humeral mechanism.
  ii. Activation of central sympathetic nervous systems.

c. Ventricular septal defect exacerbates the associated left to right shunt.

d. Other associated conditions like, aortic stenosis or subaortic stenosis may aggravate LV afterload.

> As a result of activation of sympathetic nervous system
> ↓
> Increase in heart rate and blood pressure
> Coarctation of aorta produces low cardiac output
> Decrease in renal perfusion
> ↓
> Activation of renin–angiotensin system
> ↓
> Vasoconstriction   Cell hypertrophy   Release of aldosterone
> In congestive cardiac failure
> ↓
> Vasopressin is increased
> ↓
> It affects free water retention   Vasoconstrictive properties
> ↓   ↓
> Hyponatremia   Elevate blood pressure in coarctation

Epidemiology

1. **Race:** No definitive racial difference.
2. **Sex:** Male: Female = 2:1, except in abdominal coarctation, which predominantly affects female.
3. **Age:** In early life—it presents as congestive cardiac failure. In later life, it may present with hypertension.

Symptoms

The presentation of coarctation of aorta may be of two types:

Early Presentation

This type of presentation depends upon:
  i. Extent of patency of ductus arteriosus
  ii. Presence of associated defects
  iii. Presence of aortic arch abnormalities.
  iv. Rapidity of closure of ductus arteriosus
  v. Level of pulmonary vascular resistance

The above factors may determine:

i. Timing of clinical presentation
ii. Severity of symptoms

Infants and neonates may present with:

a. Poor feeding
b. Tachypnea
c. Lethargy
d. Congestive heart failure
e. Shock

In case of acute closure, the symptom may be acute. The symptoms of failure may be accelerated by associated cardiac abnormalities like VSD.

Late Presentation

i. In this case, the patient may present with hypertension, but usually does not develop overt congestive cardiac failure—due to presence of arterial collateral vessels.
ii. Other presenting symptoms may be:
   a. Headache
   b. Chest pain
   c. Fatigue
   d. Life-threatening intracranial hemorrhage
   e. Intermittent claudication of lower legs.
iii. Asymptomatic, these patients can be detected by primary care physician.

Physical Examinations

This physical signs may be separated into two groups—early and late presentation.

Early Presentation

1. **Neonate** may present with—tachypnea, tachycardia, increased work of breathing. Key to diagnosis is:
   a. Discrepancies in blood pressure between upper and lower extremities.
   b. Reduced or absent pulses on lower extremity.
2. **In infant** with severe heart failure—all pulses are diminished. But on treatment, prominent brachial pulses and nonpalpable femoral pulses may be discerned.
3. **If right subclavian artery** originates from aorta distal to obstruction—discrepancies in limb blood pressure will not be present; in that case comparison should be done between brachial and carotid pulses.
4. **Differential cyanosis:**
   i. Pink upper extremities and cyanotic lower extremities—it may occur due to right to left heart shunt across the patent ductus arteriosus producing deoxygenated blood flow to lower extremities.
   ii. Coarctation with left-to-right shunt through ventricular septal defect produces pulmonary arterial saturation more or less similar to aortic saturations—as a result, differential oximetric findings are less obvious.
   iii. Reverse differential cyanosis: Cyanosis of upper body and normal lower body oxygen saturation—occurs with transportation of great vessels, patent ductus arteriosus and pulmonary hypertension, resulting right-to-left heart shunt through ductus.
5. **Murmur:**
   a. Systolic in the left infraclavicular area and under the scapula.

b. Other murmur may be due to associated abnormalities like, VSD, valvular stenosis.

Late Presentation

1. **Older children and infants** may present with hypertension comparison of blood pressure in all four limbs—to be done:
   a. If origin of left subclavian artery is involved in co-arctation—blood pressure in left arm is lower than that of right arm.
   b. If right innominate artery originates from below the level of coarctation—may produce decreased or absent right brachial pulse.

   The pressure difference of more than 20 mmHg in favor of arms is considered evidence of coarctation of aorta.
2. **Murmur:**
   i. Systolic murmur—can be heard in left infraclavicular area under the left scapula.
   ii. Murmur may be continuous in presence of multiple collateral vessels.
   iii. Ejection click—in presence of aortic stenosis.
   iv. Murmur of aortic insufficiency.
3. **Other findings are:**
   i. Abnormal retinal blood vessels.
   ii. Prominent pulsation in suprasternal notch.
   iii. Abdominal bruit in presence of abdominal coarctation of aorta

Laboratory Workup

Laboratory Studies

a. **Neonates presenting with shock:**
   1. Blood, urine, cerebrospinal fluid cultures
   2. Electrolytes
   3. Blood urea nitrogen
   4. Glucose concentration in blood
   5. Arterial blood gases
   6. Serum lactate levels
b. **In older patient with hypertension:**
   1. Urinalysis
   2. Electrolyte levels
   3. Blood urea
   4. Creatinine
   5. Serum glucose

Imaging Studies

a. **Chest radiography:**
   i. In early onset of coarctation of aorta:
      1. Cardiomegaly
      2. Pulmonary edema
      3. Other signs of congestive cardiac failure.
   ii. In patient with late onset of coarctation of the aorta:
      a. Cardiomegaly (Fig. 1.117)
      b. Inverted '3' sign of the barium filled esophagus
      c. '3' signs on highly penetrated chest radiograph (front view) (Fig. 1.118)
      d. Rib nothing secondary to collateral vessels (Fig. 1.119)
b. **Echocardiography:** It delineates intracardiac anatomy, assessment of associated intracardiac anomalies:
   i. Suprasternal notch in 2-D echocardiography

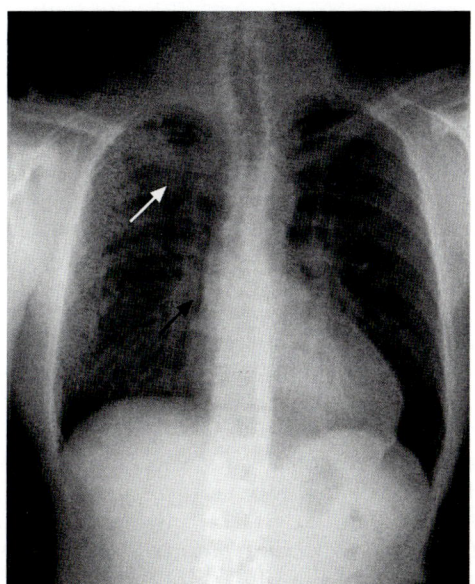

Fig. 1.117: Dilated ascending aorta, cardiomegaly

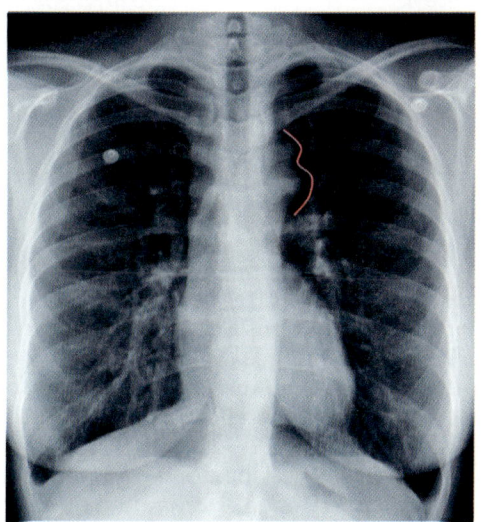

Fig. 1.118: Inverted 3 sign

The evaluation of aortic arch helps to assess:
i. Transverse aortic arch
ii. Isthmus
iii. Severity of coarctation

c. **Doppler echocardiography:**
   i. It measures the gradient at the site of coarctation.
   ii. It identifies the pattern of diastolic run off in case of severe obstruction
   iii. Peak pressure gradient across the coarctation area—it can be estimated with modified Bernoulli equation

$$\triangle p = 4\ (V_2{}^2 — V_1{}^2)$$

$\triangle p$ is the peak instantaneous gradient across the coarctation area
V_2 = peak flow velocities in the descending aorta distal to co-arctation.
V_1 = peak flow velocities in the descending aorta proximal to coarctation.
  This calculated gradient overestimates the measured blood pressure.

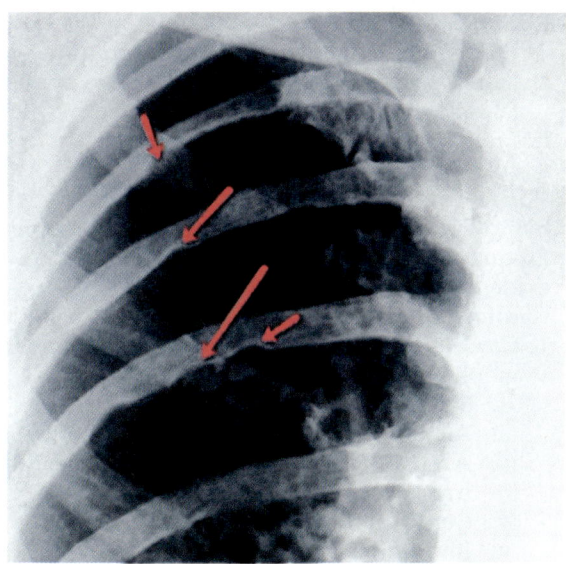

Fig. 1.119: Rib notching

Pan diastolic flow across the gradient indicates significant obstruction.
  The accuracy of the gradient calculation can be improved by duration related Doppler flow parameters.
d. **MRI or CT scan:** These help to assess:
   i. Residual arch obstruction (Fig. 1.120)
   ii. Arch hypoplasia
   iii. Formation of aneurysm
e. **Ultrafast CT scanning** is preferable, if:
   i. There is presence of multiple surgical clips or stent in the area of coarctation.

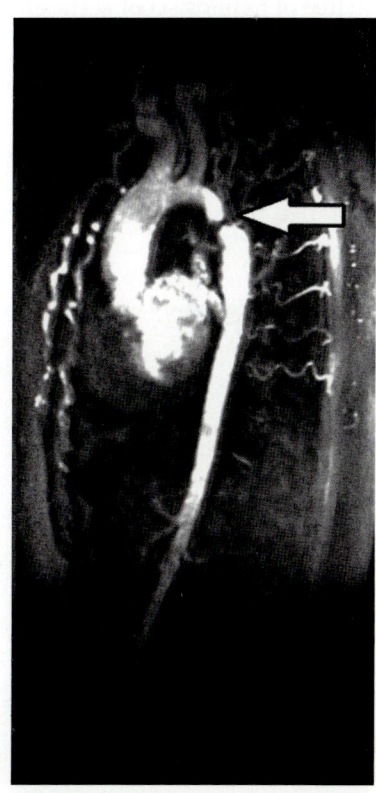

Fig. 1.120: MRI showing coarctation

f. **Electrocardiography:**
   i. *In neonates*—right ventricular hypertrophy—rather than left ventricular involvement due to presence of left-to-right shunt.
   ii. *In adult*—with late onset coarctation—left ventricular hypertrophy with strain.
   In few cases, increased amplitude S waves in V5—V6 indicate posterobasal left ventricular hypertrophy.
g. **Preductal and postductal pulse oxymetry**—shows evidence of right-to-left heart shunting.
h. **Cardiac catheterization:**
   1. Cardiac catheterization and selective cineangiography evaluate:
      i. Severity of coarctation (Fig. 1.121)
      ii. Anatomic nature of obstruction of aorta
      iii. Arch anatomy—hypoplasia of isthmus or transverse arch.
      iv. Confirms the echocardiographic findings.
      v. Intracardiac anatomy
   2. It is a prerequisite for intervention—in the form of balloon angioplasty.
   3. Elevation of left ventricular, ascending aortic pressure.
   4. Peak-to-peak systolic pressure gradient across the coarctation of aorta should be evaluated. If it is >20 mmHg—indicates significant obstruction.
   5. Selective aortic root or aortic arch angiography—shows aortic narrowing.
   6. Aortography demonstrates:
      i. Types of obstruction (diffuse, long segment, aortic kinking)
      ii. Extent of collateral circulation.
      iii. Size of ductus arteriosus—if patient
      iv. Presence of hypoplasia of aortic arch
      v. Degree of hypoplasia of aortic arch
      vi. Abdominal aortography demonstrates abdominal coarctation.
i. **Histological findings:**
   i. Marked ridge-like thickening of the media of the aortic wall opposite the insertion of PDA or ligamentum arteriosum.
   ii. Intima started thickening overtime.

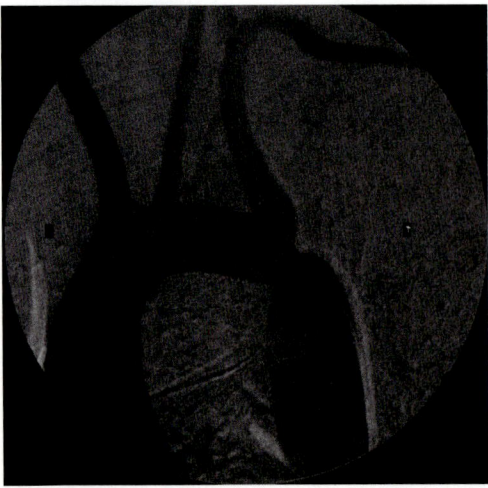

Fig. 1.121: Aortography showing coarctation

Treatment of Coarctation of Aorta

Medical Care

A. **Early presentation of coarctation of aorta:**
   1. Treatment of patient with congestive heart failure—with diuretics and inotropic drugs.
   2. Opening of ductus arteriosus by—intravenous infusion of prostaglandin E_1 (0.05–0.15 µg/kg/minute).
   3. To increase the work of breathing—ventilation is required.
   4. To monitor infusion and to prevent fluid overload, maintain intake output chart.
   5. To monitor urine output, Foley's catheter to be inserted.
   6. To prevent metabolic acidosis—arterial blood gases.
   7. To assess the response to prostaglandin infusion, because it is responsible for lower body blood flow.
   8. After improvement by above intervention, patient should undergo surgical or catheter intervention.
   9. If the patient with coarctation of aorta has associated defects:
      i. He or she should be assessed by echo-Doppler, cardiac catheterization or angiographic studies.
      ii. If coarctation has significant adverse effect on the associated defects, it should be treated first by surgery or balloon angioplasty.
      ↓
      Then the patient must be reassessed for associated defects.
      ↓
      If required should be intervened.

B. **Late presentation of coarctation of aorta:**
   1. Preoperative hypertension should be treated by beta-blocker—with the goal to reduce upper extremity hypertension. But vigorous attempt should not be done to reduce the upper extremity blood pressure because it may reduce lower body—perfusion.
   2. Postoperative hypertension—can be treated by—sodium nitroprusside, intravenous beta-blockers, esmolol.
   3. If long-term anti-hypertensive therapy is required, beta-blocker therapy should be of choice.
   4. If no-residual arch obstruction exist, ACE inhibitors or angiotensin II antagonists may be added in case of persistant hypertension despite beta-blocker therapy.
   5. Evaluate associated abnormalities such as aortic stenosis or mitral valve disease.

Surgical Care

Techniques are:
1. Surgery of aortic obstruction.
2. Catheter-induced interventional technique—balloon angioplasty and stents.

In symptomatic neonates and infants—urgent intervention has to be done.

In asymptomatic infants, children, adolescents and adults, elective procedure is of choice.

Any one procedure should be done in asymptomatic infants aged 2–5 years.

But if operation will be done after the age of 5 years, residual hypertension may persist.

Various surgical techniques are:
i. Resection and end-to-end anastomosis
ii. Patch aortoplasty.
iii. Left subclavian flap aortoplasty.
iv. Tubular bypass grafts.

Operative mortality:
i. In infants and neonates—are high (4.50%)
ii. In older children—are low (0–5%)

Complications:
a. In all types of repair:
   i. Significant recoarctation
   ii. Formation of aneurysm
b. In case of left subclavian flap repair:
   i. Paraplegia
   ii. Paradoxical hypertension
   iii. Vascular complication

Indications of balloon angioplasty:
i. Coarctation involving long segment of the aorta.
ii. Coarctations that are completely or almost completely occluded, so that catheter or guidewire cannot be passed through the narrowed segment.
iii. When coarctation is associated with VSD, PDA—which may require prompt surgical intervention for primary cardiac problem.

Results
A. Short-term results:
   i. Reduction in pressure across the coarctation segment
   ii. Increase in size of coarcted segment
   iii. Prompt diminution of collateral vessels
   iv. Femoral pulse become palpable, and increase in volume.
   v. Infant with heart failure should be weaned off the ventilator support.
   vi. Most infants and children are discharged from the hospital within 24 hours after balloon angioplasty.

B. Intermediate results:
   i. Incidence of recoarctation is higher in infants and neonates.
   ii. Aneurysm
C. Long-term follow up results:
   i. Events free survival following initial ballon angioplasty.
   ii. In most children, arm blood pressure remainds normal
   Major determinant of long-term survival following repair of aortic coarctation are:
   i. Presence of associated lesions
   ii. Age at operation
   Causes of cardiovascular death in order of frequency:
   i. Coronary artery disease
   ii. Sudden death
   iii. Aortic regurgitation and heart failure
   iv. Heart failure with hypertension
   v. Cerebrovascular accidents

Complications of stent implantation have been classified into three categories:
a. *Technical:*
   i. Stent migration
   ii. Stent fracture
   iii. Balloon ruptures
   iv. Overlap of the brachiocephalic vessels
b. *Aortic:*
   i. Intimal tear
   ii. Intimal dissection
   iii. Aortic aneurysm formation
c. *Peripheral vascular:*
   i. Cerebrovascular accidents
   ii. Peripheral embolization
   iii. Injury to access vessels
   Compared with surgical therapy, endovascular stenting has a similar mortality and morbidity, because of higher incidence of:
   i. Recoarctation—which needs reconstruction
   ii. Persistant hypertension

CARDIOMYOPATHIES

Types and Definitions (Fig. 1.122)

I. Genetic:

   A. Hypertrophic (HOCM): 1. Septal thickness; 2. Increased thickness of the posterior wall.

   B. Arrhythmogenic right ventricle—fibrofatty tissue replacement of the right ventricular myocardium.

   C. LV noncompaction—spongy left ventricular cavity (apical).

   D. Glycogen storage disease—Danon disease. PRKAG2

   E. Ion channelopathies—conduction defect, Brugada syndrome.

II. Mixed:
   A. Dilated cardiomyopathies:
      1. Increased end diastolic volume
      2. Increased end systolic volume
      3. Low ejection fraction
   B. Restrictive cardiomyopathies:
      1. Increased end diastolic volume
      2. Increased left ventricular filling pressure
      3. Normal ejection fraction

III. Acquired:
   A. Myocarditis—inflammatory.
   B. Stress-induced—left ventricular dysfunction (reversible)

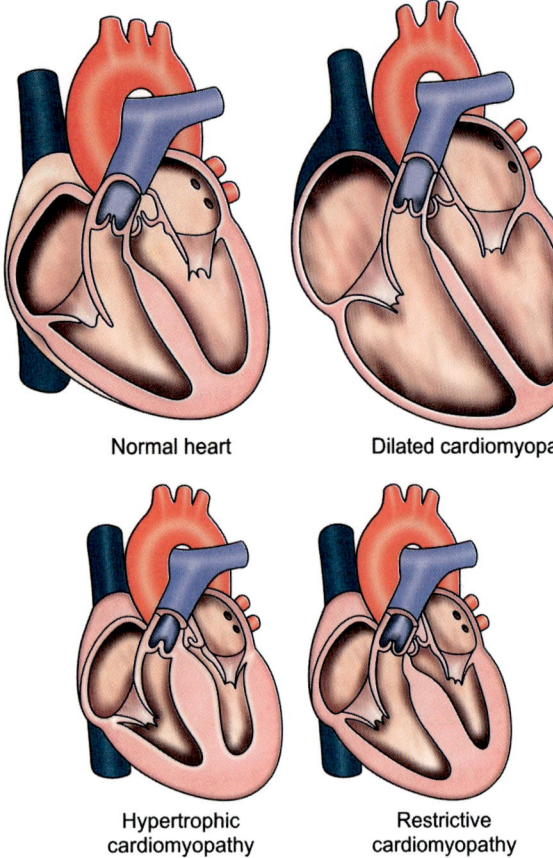

Normal heart   Dilated cardiomyopathy

Hypertrophic cardiomyopathy   Restrictive cardiomyopathy

Fig. 1.122: Types of cardiomyopathy

C. Peripartum—third trimester of pregnancy.
D. Tachycardia induced—following prolonged period of SVT and VT.
E. Insulin dependent.

DILATED CARDIOMYOPATHY

Definition

This can be defined as impaired left ventricular or both ventricular systolic dysfunction in absence of: i) Coronary artery disease, ii) valvular heart disease, iii) pericardial disease.

Types of Dilated Cardiomyopathy

1. **Idiopathic**.
2. **Toxin:**
    i. Alcohol
    ii. Chemotherapeutic agents—doxorubicin, daunorubicin
    iii. Antiviral agent—zidovudine, zalcitabine
    iv. Phenothiazine
    v. Carbon monoxide
    vi. Cocaine.
    vii. Mercury.
3. **Metabolic abnormalities:**
    i. Nutritional deficiency—thiamin, selenium.
    ii. Endocrine disorders—hypothyroidism, acromegaly, thyrotoxicosis, Cushing's disease, pheochromocytoma.

iii. Electrolyte disturbances—hypomagnesemia, hypophosphatemia.
4. **Infections:**
    i. Viral—coxasackie virus, HIV, cytomegaly
    ii. Bacterial—Mycobacterium
    iii. Fungal
5. **Autoimmune:**
    i. SLE
    ii. Polyarteritis nodosa
    iii. Dermatomyositis
    iv. Kawasaki disease
6. **Systemic diseases:**
    i. Amyloidosis   ii. Sarcoidosis
7. **Endomyocardial fibrosis**
8. **Peripartum or postpartum cardiomyopathies**.
9. **Neuromuscular dystrophies:**
    i. Becker or Duchenne muscular dystrophy
    ii. Fascioscapulohumeral type
    iii. Myotonic dystrophy
10. **Friedreich ataxia**
11. **Mitochondrial cardiomyopathies**.
12. **Keshan cardiomyopathies**.

Incidence

1. In Western, African and Asian population—it affects both gender and all ages.
2. In North America, Europe—incidence 2 and 38 per 100,000 populations respectively.

Causes

1. **Familial diseases** in 25% of cases. 10–20% have mild abnormalities of left ventricular performance, of which one third may develop DCM in future.
2. **Autosomal dominant** with incomplete penetrance—which is age dependant:
    i. 10%—in <20 years
    ii. 34%—in young adult
    iii. 60%—in 30–40 years
    iv. 90%—in <40 years
3. **Genetic causes:** Mutation of the following genes:
    i. Dystrophin (causes childhood—Duchenne and adult—Becker form)
    ii. Taffazin (Barth syndrome)
    iii. Metavinculin.
    iv. Cardiac actin (autosomal dominant).
    v. Desmin (may cause conduction disease)
    vi. Troponin C and T.
    vii. B myosin heavy chain.
    viii. Lamin A/C—(produce—Emery-Dreifuss, and limb girdle muscular dystrophy)

Criteria for Diagnosis of Familial DCM

1. **Major criteria:**
    i. Reduced EF of left ventricle <45% and/or fractional shortening (<25%) as assessed by echocardiography, radio-nuclide scanning or angiography.
    ii. Increased left ventricular end diastolic diameter corresponding to >117% of predictive value corrected for age and body surface area.
2. **Minor criteria:**
    i. Unexplained supraventricular or ventricular arrhythmia.

ii. Ventricular dilatation (>12% of predictive value).

iii. Conduction defect.

iv. Intermediate impairment of left ventricular dysfunction.

v. Segmental wall motion abnormalities in absence of—IHD and intraventricular conduction defect.

vi. Unexplained sudden death of its degree relative or stroke before 50 years of age.

Pattern of the Disease

i. Slow over decades—conduction defect may be late complication.

ii. In case of DCM, due to mutation of lamin A/C—in early stage—progressive conduction disease, in late stage—left ventricular dilation and impairment.

iii. In DCM due to mutation of dystrophin gene, it develops in the later stage—may be associated with:

a. Skeletal myopathy.

b. Sensory—neural hearing loss since childhood.

Pathology (Fig. 1.123)

Macroscopically

1. Dilated cardiac chamber
2. Normal extra and intramural coronary arteries
3. Mural thrombi
4. Platelet aggregates
5. Increased myocardial mass
6. Ventricular wall thickness may be normal or reduced

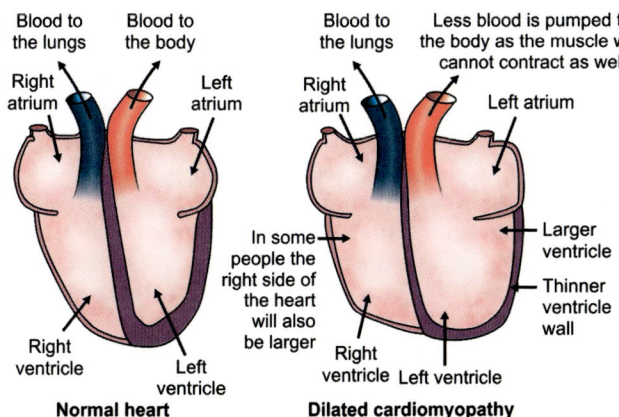

Fig. 1.123: Morphology of dilated cardiomyopathy

Microscopically

1. Patchy perimyocyte and interstitial fibrosis.
2. Various stages of myocardial cell death.
3. Vacuolation of myocytes.
4. T lymphocytic and macrophage infiltrates.

Two Theories Responsible for Production of DCM

1. Common channel pathway hypothesis—DCM is a degenerative state resulting from various stimuli—like genetic mutation, viral infection, toxin and volume overload.
2. Alternate pathway—dictates DCM is the result of remodeling stimulated by distinct independent pathways.

Clinical Features

Presentation

1. May present with symptoms of heart failure—like fatigue, breathlessness, and decreased exercise tolerance.
2. May present with symptoms of arrhythmia—irregular pulse, palpitation and syncope.
3. May be diagnosed as incidental finding of echocardiographic and radiographic abnormality.

Physical Examination

1. Pulse —a. low volume; b. Pulsus alternans—in case of severe left ventricular failure.
2. Blood pressure—low, narrow pulse pressure.
3. Jugular vein—prominent V wave—reflecting tricuspid regurgitation.
4. Precordial examination:

a. Apex displaced laterally—due to ventricular dilation.

b. Diffuse and dyskinetic left ventricular impulse.

c. Right parasternal heave—due to right ventricular hypertrophy.

d. First heart sound muffled due to left ventricular dilatation.

e. Second heart sound:

i. P2 component may be accentuated due to evidence of pulmonary hypertension.

ii. May be paradoxical splitting—due to LBBB (15% of cases).

f. Fourth heart sound (presystolic gallop)—in case of impending heart failure.

g. Third heart sound or ventricular gallop—in case of cardiac decompensation.

h. In few cases—systolic murmur of mitral regurgitation in case of extensive left ventricular dilation.

i. In case of congestive cardiac failure—there may be:

1. Pedal edema, 2. Enlarged tender liver, 3. Ascites.

Prognosis

a. Usually the symptoms will present as late manifestation of the disease and disease is obvious.

b. Precipitating factors may be:

1. Upper respiratory infection.
2. Fluid overload.
3. Salt overload.

c. Symptoms will be obvious when:

1. LV filling pressure is increased.
2. LV stroke volume is decreased.

d. Prognosis is poor when left ventricular function starts impairing, it depends upon:

1. Degree of left ventricular dilatation.
2. Impaired contractile activity.

e. This disease requires early diagnosis and treatment.

f. Estimated mortality is 4%, cause may be sudden death.

Arrhythmias

a. Atrial fibrillation:

1. Commonly associated with symptoms of left ventricular dysfunction.
2. May cause gradual deterioration of left ventricular dysfunction—producing resembling dilated cardiomyopathies (tachycardiopathies).

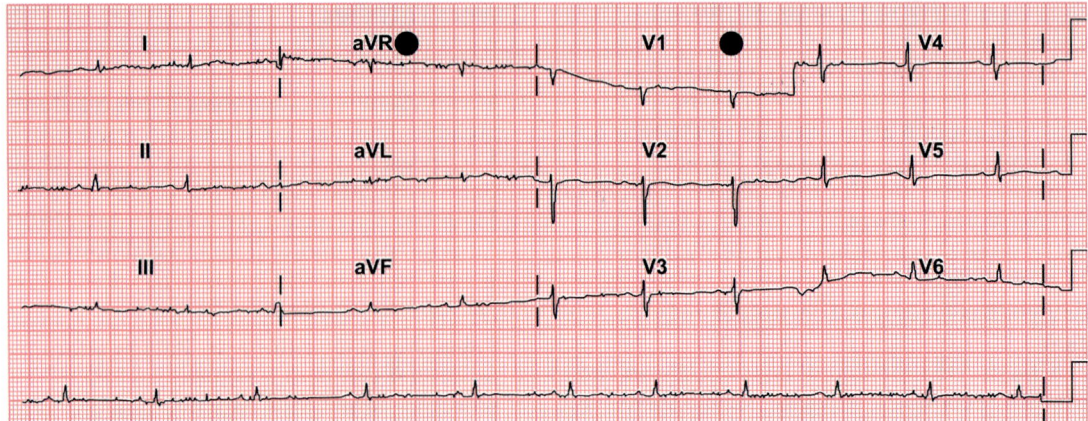

Fig. 1.124: Low voltage wave in DCM

b. Ventricular tachycardia—may be:
1. Asymptomatic
2. Mildly symptomatic.
3. Severely symptomatic.
4. It may be a marker of sudden death. It may occur in severe disease (NYHA Class III or IV)—may be preceded by syncope.

Investigation

Electrocardiography (Fig. 1.124): The following findings may be present:
1. Sinus tachycardia—particularly in children and infants.
2. Non-specific ST-T wave changes—commonly in inferior and lateral leads.
3. Pathological Q wave—in septal leads associated with extensive left ventricular fibrosis.
4. All types of atrioventricular block raise the suspicion of mutation of Lamin A/C gene.
5. Features of left atrial enlargement.

Chest X-ray (Figs 1.125, 1.126): Usually abnormal except viral myocarditis.
I. Increased cardiothoracic ratio (>0.5)—indicates left ventricular and left atrial enlargement.

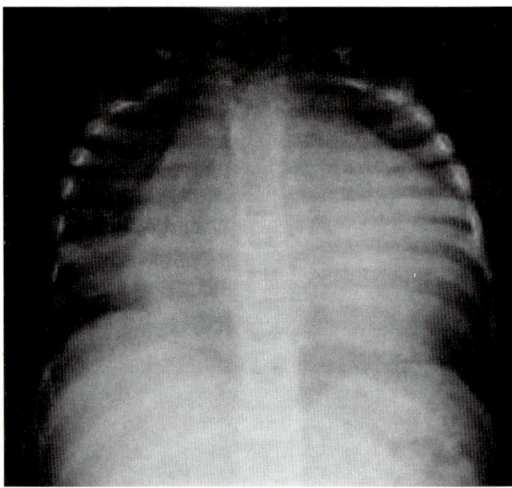

Fig. 1.126: Pediatric dilated cardiomyopathy

II. Increased pulmonary vascular markings.
III. Evidence of plural effusion.

Echocardiography (Fig. 1.127): The following findings are important:
I. Presence of left ventricular end diastolic dimension (EDD).
II. Fractional shortening less than 25%.
III. Intracavitary thrombus in left ventricle.
IV. Color Doppler study shows:

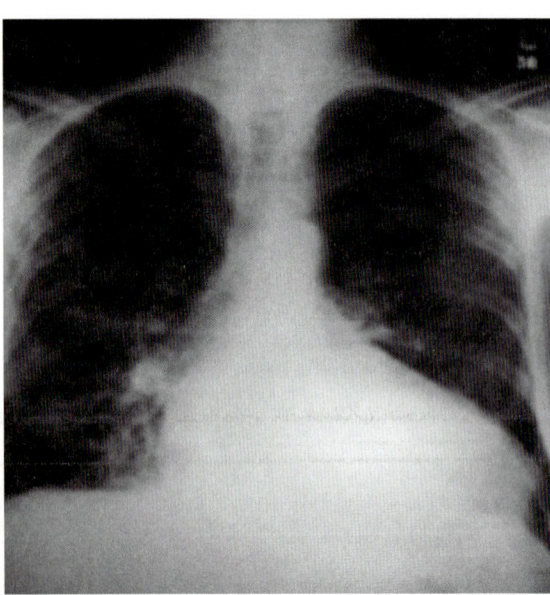

Fig. 1.125: Dilated cardiomyopathy

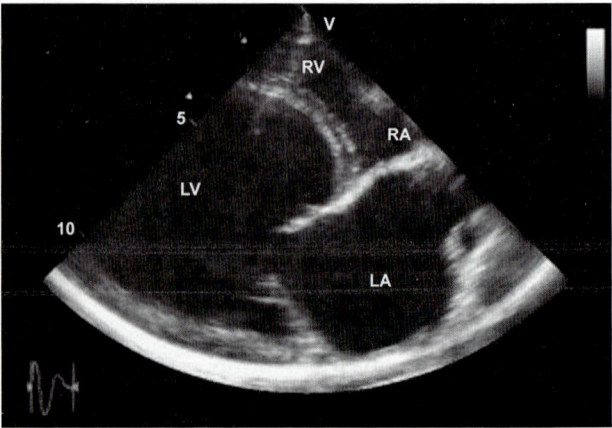

Fig. 1.127: Echocardiography

1. Presence, quantify the severity of mitral and/or tricuspid regurgitation.
2. Pulse wave Doppler and continuous wave Doppler can be used to estimate pulmonary artery pressure.
3. Abnormal diastolic left ventricular function.

Cardiac Biomarkers

I. Serum creatine kinase—should be done in all patients to get clue to the etiology (muscular dystrophy, Lamin A/C defect).
II. Troponin I and troponin T may be elevated.
III. Plasma natriuretic peptide—elevated in chronic heart failure.
IV. Biochemical markers:
   1. Serum phosphorus (hyperphosphatemia).
   2. Serum calcium (hypocalcemia).
   3. Serum urea and creatinine (uremia).
   4. Thyroid function test (hypothyroidism).
   5. Serum iron and ferritin (hemochromatosis).
V. Immunological markers.
VI. Exercise testing:
   1. Symptoms limited treadmill test combined with respiratory gas analysis—can evaluate the disease progression.
   2. Detection of respiratory markers during metabolic exercise—suggests—mitochondrial or other metabolic causes or dilated cardiomyopathy.
VII. Cardiac catheterization:
   1. Exclude coronary artery disease—to detect impaired systolic function.
   2. Hemodynamic assessment of left ventricular end diastolic and pulmonary artery pressure—it is diastolic and pulmonary artery pressure—it is usually required for cardiac transplant work up.
   3. Endomyocardial biopsy. To detect mitochondrial, metabolic cardiomyopathy.
VIII. Cardiac MRI—it is useful alternative imaging technique.
IX. Gadolinium contrast enhancement—it detects fibrosis.
X. Electrophysiologic testing—it is of limited clinical value in identification of high-risk patients:
   1. Polymorphic ventricular tachycardia—can be induced in 30% of cases.
   2. Monomorphic ventricular tachycardia (sustained)—approximately one-third may die suddenly.

   This tachycardia is the result of bundle branch reentry—uses macroreentry circuit, involves His Purkinje system.

Management

The aims are:
a. To improve symptoms.
b. To attenuate disease progression.
c. To prevent arrhythmia, stroke and sudden death. The treatment may be pharmacological or non-pharmacological.

Pharmacological Treatment

Diuretics:
1. Loop diuretics or thiazide diuretic:
   a. To reduce fluid retention.
   b. To achieve euvolemic state.

They should never be used as monotherapy—because they exacerbate neurohumoral activation and working the disease progression.
2. Potassium sparing diuretic—It reduces risk of death by 30% in adult with severe heart failure NYHA class IV, ejection fraction >35%.
3. ACE inhibitor and ARBS: Background—activation of renin–angiotensin system is the main pathological basis of cardiac failure, regardless of underlying etiology. ACEI:
   a. Improves symptom
   b. Reduces hospitalization
   c. Reduces cardiovascular mortality
   d. Reduces rate of disease progression in asymptomatic patient.

In first three—in symptomatic patient, these drugs are well tolerated, side effects are mainly—cough and symptomatic hypotension.

ARB (angiotensin receptor blocker): This can be used:
  i. In combination with ACE inhibitor.
  ii. Who is intolerant to ACE inhibitor.

β-blocker—basis—sympathetic activity is the basis of heart failure.

The drugs used are—carvidolol, metoprolol and bisoprolol.

Aim—it reduces mortality (sudden death, death from progressive heart failure) in NYHA—class II and III heart failure.

Side effects—mainly bradycardia, hypotension.

Contraindication—bronchial asthma, decompensated heart failure.

Digoxin: It is used:
1. Symptomatic patient in spite of treatment with ACEI, ARB, β blocker and diuretic.
2. To control heart rate in patient with atrial fibrillation.
   Its use has no survival benefit.
   High serum level is associated with increased mortality.

Anticoagulation: Basis—Presence of intraluminal thrombus and systemic thrombo embolism ranges from 3–50%—incidence varies between 1.5 and 3.5% per year.

Drug—warfarin
Indication:
1. H/O thromboembolism.
2. Echocardiographic identification of intraluminal thrombus.
3. Severe left ventricular dilation.
4. Moderate to severe systolic impairment

Treatment of arrhythmia: Commonly prescribed arrhythmic agents should be avoided, because of:
1. Negative inotrophic effect.
2. Proarrhythmic effect.

Amioderone has no beneficial effect on survival when compared with implantable cardiac defibrillator.

Non-Pharmacological Treatment

Pacemaker implantation: It improves two abnormalities.
A. Marked prolongation in PR interval secondary to AV nodal disease. Dual chamber pacing:
   1. It reduces diastolic ventricular filling time.
   2. Develops end diastolic mitral and tricuspid regurgitation.
B. Marked intraventricular conduction delay (LBBB >150 ms) produces:

1. Asynchronous contraction of left ventricular free wall and interventricular septum—produces decrease in ejection fraction.
2. Late activation of anterolateral papillary muscle—increases functional mitral regurgitation.
   This can be corrected by biventricular or left ventricular pacing—via coronary sinus.
C. Surgical procedure:
   1. Surgical removal of nonviable myocardium to reduce left ventricular volume.
   2. Partial left ventriculotomy—it has no role.
D. Cardiac transplantation: It can be done in patient with progressive deterioration.
E. Left ventricular assisted devices.
F. Artificial heart technology.

HYPERTROPHIC OBSTRUCTIVE CARDIOMYOPATHY

This can be defined as increased myocardial thickness in absence of loading conditions (systemic hypertension, valvular heart disease).

This should be separated from myocardial hypertrophy due to amyloidosis, glycogen storage disease—in which there is interstitial infiltration and/or intracellular accumulation of metabolic substrates.

Causes

Inheritance is autosomal dominant. Pedigree analysis showed 40–50% are familial. Again 60% familial HOCM have: Mutation of genes encoding proteins of cardiac sarcomere:
1. Cardiac beta myosin heavy chain.
2. Cardiac myosin binding protein C.
3. Essential and refractory myosin light chain.
4. Alfa–tropomyosin.
5. Cardiac troponin I and T.
6. Cardiac actin and alfa myosin.

Most mutations involve a single pair change in exons encoding highly conservative regions by substituting amino acid.

A beta myosin heavy chain mutation with full penetration is associated with sudden death.

Troponin T mutation is associated with a few symptoms that may produce sudden death.

Pathology (Fig. 1.128)

This includes:
1. Asymmetric septal hypertrophy—involving anterior and posterior parts of septum and left ventricular free wall.
2. Symmetric left ventricular hypertrophy in 30% of patients.
3. Structural abnormalities of mitral valve include:
   a. Increased leaflet area.
   b. Increased leaflet length.
   c. Malposition or anomalous insertion of papillary muscles.
4. Patchy endocardial thickening due to contact of septum with anterior mitral valve leaflet in patient with dynamic left ventricular outflow tract obstruction.

Histological Findings (Fig. 1.129)

1. Fibrosis with gross disorganization of muscle bundles—resulting characteristic "Whorled" pattern.
2. Disorganization of myofibrillar architecture.
3. Broad, short, bizarre-shaped myocardial cells present in the midst of hypertrophied muscle cells.

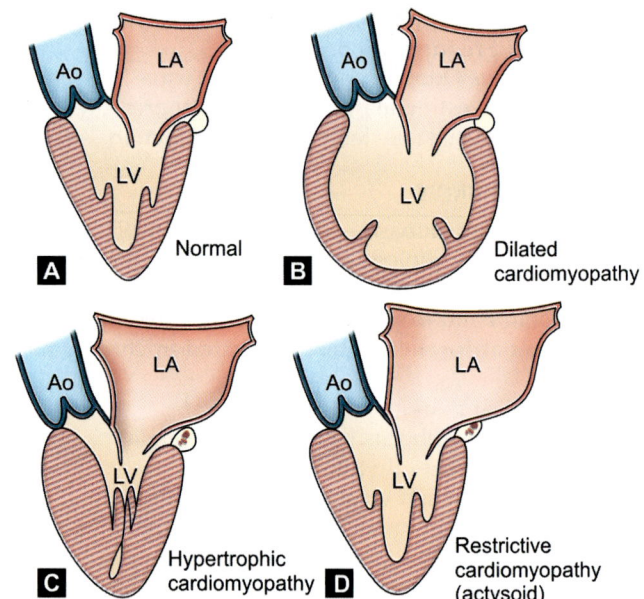

Fig. 1.128: Pathology of hypertrophic cardiomyopathy

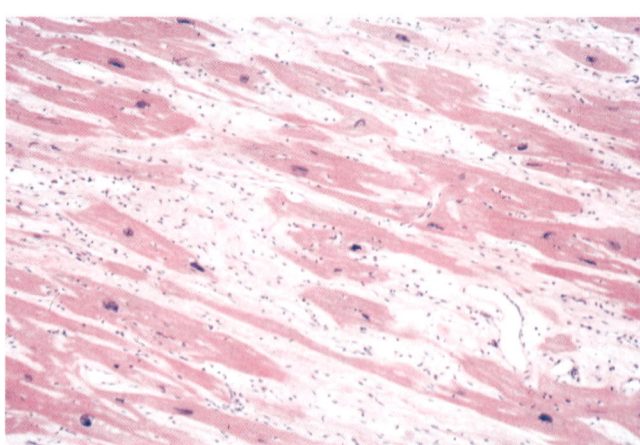

Fig. 1.129: Histology of HOCM

Pathophysiology

1. **Diastolic dysfunction:** Causes are:
   a. Myocardial hypertrophy.
   b. Myocardial ischemia.
   c. Myocyte disarray.
   d. Myocardial fibrosis.
   Effects:
   a. Abnormal left ventricular end diastolic filling and reduced compliance
      Increased left ventricular end diastolic pressure
      Increased left atrial pressure
   b. Isovolumic relaxation time is increased.
   c. Proportional filling volume as a result of atrial contraction will be increased.
2. **Systolic dysfunction:**
   a. Increased ejection fraction results from near complete ventricular emptying.
   b. In end stage HOCM—severe impairment of cardiac contractile performance, restrictive left ventricle—producing symptoms related to heart failure.

It occurs at any age, from childhood to adulthood. But the time span between the onset of symptom to severe form of symptoms is usually 10–14 years.

3. **Dynamic out flow tract obstruction:**
   a. 30% of patients has gradient between the body of ventricle and outflow tract at rest.
   b. 20% of patients have this gradient:
      i. During maneuvers that increase myocardial contractility.
      ii. Reduction of ventricular after load.
      iii. Reduction in venous return.

Presence and magnitude of gradient is determined by:
   a. Outflow tract size.
   b. Outflow tract geometry.
      This is determined by:
      • Severity of septal hypertrophy.
      • Mitral valve morphology.
      • Papillary muscle size and position.

4. **Myocardial ischemia:** In HOCM, there is reduced coronary flow—produces myocardial ischemia—may trigger ventricular arrhythmia. But detection of ischemia is challenging in clinical practice, because conventional markers of ischemia, e.g. ST segment change and reversible perfusion abnormalities correlate poorly with more objective biomarkers.

Diagnosis

Annual incidence is 0–3 to 0–5 per 100,000 population.

Myocardial hypertrophy can be defined as wall thickness measurement exceeding two standard deviation for genders and age.

In clinical practice, in case of adult of normal size, left ventricular wall thickness >1.5 cm is diagnostic.

In case of patient with hypertension—myocardial hypertrophy is partially influenced by racial origin, e.g. in African—Caribbean individual.

So, in this case, left ventricular wall thickness >1.5 cm with ECG evidence of repolarization abnormalities are diagnostic.

In case of trained athlete due to both isotonic and isometric activities—left ventricular wall is thickened. So case of trained athlete, if left ventricular wall thickness >1.6 cm in males and >1.4 cm in females, having family history of HOCM and sudden death and marked repolarization abnormalities.

Major and Minor Criteria of Diagnosis of HOCM

A. Major criteria:
   1. *Echocardiography:*
      a. Left ventricular wall thickness:
         >1.3 cm in the anterior septum or posterior wall or >1.5 cm in the posterior septum or free wall.
      b. Severe septal-leaflet contact (SAM)
   2. *Electrocardiography:*
      a. Left ventricular hypertrophy and repolarization changes.
      b. T wave inversion in lead I and aVL (>3 mm), with (QRS-T wave axis difference >30°), V3 –V6(>3 mm) or II or III and aVF (>3 mm).
      c. Abnormal Q (>40 ms or >25% R wave) in at least two leads from II, III, aVF (in absence of anterior hemiblock)
   3. *Chemical*—there is no clinical major criteria.

B. Minor criteria:
   1. *Echocardiography:*
      a. Left ventricular wall thickness of 12 mm in the anterior septum or posterior wall or 14 mm in the posterior septum or free wall.
      b. Moderate SAM (septal-leaflet contact).
      c. Redundant mitral valve leaflet.
   2. *Electrocardiography:*
      a. Complete bundle branch block or interventricular conduction defect (in LV lead).
      b. Minor repolarization changes in LV leads.
      c. Deep S in V2 (>25 mm).
   3. *Clinical*—unexplained chest pain, dyspnea or syncope.
      Criteria are fulfilled if: a. One major echocardiographic or b. Two minor echocardiographic or c. One minor echocardiographic plus two minor electrographic abnormalities are seen.

Clinical Features

History: In children and adolescents—diagnosis often made during screening of siblings and offsprings.

50% of adult present with symptoms.

In 50% of adults—diagnosis is made during family screening.

Symptoms are:
a. Dyspnea is due to elevated left atrial pressure and pulmonary capillary wedge pressure—resulting impaired left ventricular relaxation and filling.
b. 50% of patients have chest pain—atypical—it may follow exercise or anxiety related tachycardia.
c. 15–25% patients develop syncope—may be due to arrhythmia or conduction defect.
d. PND.
e. Peripheral edema.
f. Sudden death.

Physical Examination

a. **Pulse**—rapid upstroke—reflecting dynamic left ventricular emptying.
b. JVP—prominent "a" wave—reflects diminished right ventricular compliance, secondary to right ventricular hypertrophy.
c. Forceful left ventricular cardiac impulse—best palpated during full expiration and in left lateral position.
d. Palpable atrial pulse—secondary to forceful atrial contraction.
e. **Heart sound:**
   1. 1st and 2nd heart sounds are normal except in atrial fibrillation—where Ist heart sound is absent.
   2. Loud 4th heart sound due to forceful atrial contraction in non-compliant ventricle.
f. **Murmur:**
   1. *Ejection systolic murmur*—starts well after 1st heart sound and ends before 2nd sound, best heard in left sternal border, radiates to aortic and mitral areas. Intensity varies with left ventricular volume.
      Murmur is increased by physiological (standing, Valsalva) or pharmacological (amyl nitrate) maneuvers that decreases the afterload or venous return.
      Murmur is decreased by maneuvers that increase afterload and venous return (squatting, phenylephrine).

2. Murmur of mitral regurgitation—difficult to distinguish during clinical examination—detected by Doppler examination—it reveals that it starts just before the onset of gradient and continuous throughout the duration of systole. It can radiate to axilla.
3. Mid-diastolic rumbling murmur—due to transmitral flow in severe mitral regurgitation.
4. Early diastolic murmur of aortic regurgitation—following myotomy or myomectomy or infective endocarditis involving aortic valve. It occurs due to traction of non-coronary cusp of aortic valve by ventricular septum.
5. In ejection systolic murmur in the pulmonary area reflecting right ventricular outflow tract obstruction.

Prognosis

Annual mortality rate 1–2%.
Myocardial fibrosis and severe reduction in left ventricular performance

$$\downarrow$$

1. Progressive left ventricular wall thinning
$$\downarrow$$
Symptoms of left ventricular failure
$$\downarrow$$
Gross enlarged left atrium
2. Increased pulmonary capillary wedge pressure
$$\downarrow$$
Right heart failure
Development of systolic failure—suggests poor prognosis.
Rapid progression from the onset to death or heart transplantation is 11% per year.

3. Atrial dilatation followed development of atrial fibrillation or atrial flutter and may produce:
i. Acute or chronic cardiac deterioration.
ii. Embolic stroke.
iii. If early onset, it is an ominous sign.
iv. Left ventricular hypertrophy—occurs during childhood or adolescence—not progressive in adult.

Investigations

1. **Electrocardiography** (Fig. 1.130):
   a. There is no ECG specific to HOCM.
   b. Non-specific ST-T wave changes are the most common, may be associated with voltage changes of left ventricular hypertrophy or deep S wave in lead II, III and aVF, less commonly V1–V3 leads.
   c. P wave abnormalities related to right or left atrial hypertrophy.
   d. Short PR interval may be associated with slurred up strokes of QRS resembling WPW syndrome.
   e. Arrhythmia—atrial fibrillation—5–10% cases, 20% left axis deviation, complete right or left bundle branch block.
2. **24–48 hours Holter monitoring:**
   a. Non-sustained ventricular tachycardia—asymptomatic, associated with incidence of sudden death.
   b. Sustained ventricular tachycardia—may be associated with ventricular aneurysm. Ventricular arrhythmia may be associated with myocardial fibrosis.
   c. Non-sustained supraventricular arrhythmia—occurs in adult, may be associated with thromboembolism—they are poorly tolerated.

   d. In children and adolescent—there is sinus rhythm.
   e. Supraventricular arghythmia may be due to:
      i. Increased left atrial diameter.
      ii. Increased left atrial diastolic pressure.
3. **Chest X-ray** (Fig. 1.131):
   a. Left ventricular enlargement.
   b. Left and/or right atrial enlargement.
   c. In case chronically elevated left atrial pressure, redistribution of blood flow to upper lung zones.
   d. Mitral valve annulus calcification, especially in elder patient.
4. **Echocardiography** (Fig. 1.132):
   a. Symmetric or asymmetric both septal and free wall of left ventricle with sparing of posterior wall.
   b. Isolated apical hypertrophy—common in Japan.
   c. Hypertrophy—maximal in distal ventricle from the level of papillary muscles down to apex (10% of patients).
   d. In one-third of patients, hypertrophy of right ventricular free wall—it is strongly related to severity of left ventricular hypertrophy.
   e. Reduced left ventricular end diastolic and end systolic dimension.
   f. Increased left atrial dimension.
5. **Color Doppler studies:** It can detect:
   a. Left ventricular outflow tract turbulence.
   b. When combined with continuous wave Doppler, it can calculate or detect:
      i. Peak velocity of left ventricular blood flow.
      ii. Left ventricular outflow tract gradient.
      iii. Systolic anterior motion of mitral valve is present. Calculated outflow tract gradient is >30 mmHg.
      iv. Early closure or fluttering of aortic valve leaflet.
      v. Posteriorly directed mitral regurgitant jet is seen and related to magnitude of outflow tract gradient.
      vi. Anterior regurgitant jet in absence of obstruction—detects the coexistence of mitral regurgitation.
6. **MRI:** It is useful to assess the right ventricular, apical and left ventricular involvement.
7. **Cardiac catheterization:** It has been replaced by echocardiography and color Doppler studies. Now cardiac catheterization is indicated in:
   i. Refractory symptoms.
   ii. Direct measurement of cardiac pressures.
   Coronary angiography is necessary to exclude coexistent coronary artery disease.
8. **Angiography:** It detects:
   i. Left coronary artery is of large caliber.
   ii. Left anterior descending artery and septal perforators demonstrate narrowing during systole.
   iii. Left ventricular angiography recognizes abnormal shaped ventricle, which usually ejects at least 75% of its content in association with MR.
9. **Exercise testing:**
   i. Oxygen consumption at peak exercise is moderately reduced.
   ii. Continuous measurement of blood pressure during treadmill testing in younger patients (<40 years) shows:
      a. Drop of more than 10 mmHg, from peak recording.
      b. Failure to rise by 20 mmHg, or more in spite of increase in cardiac out put.

It may be—asymptomatic or associated with sudden death.

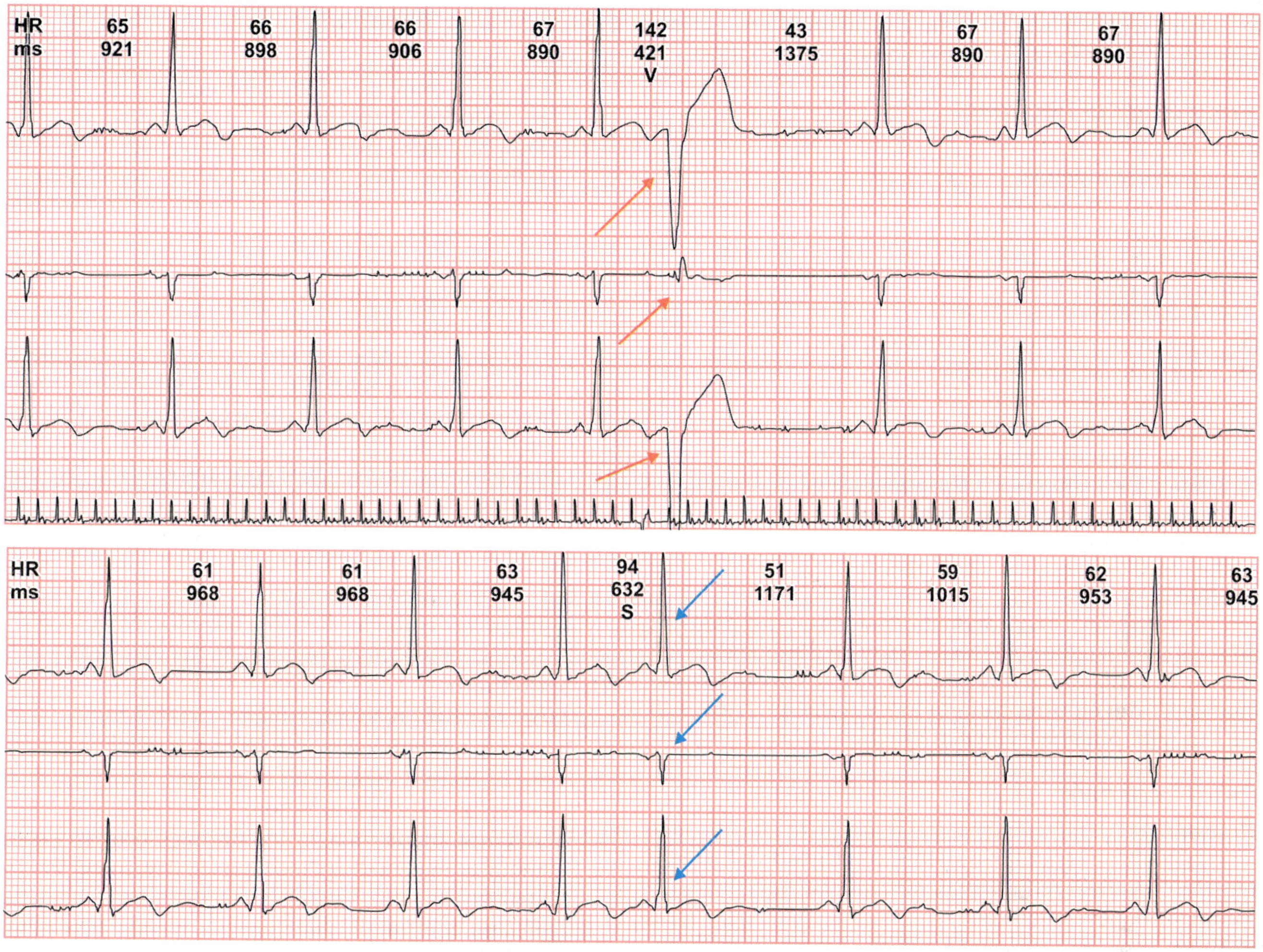

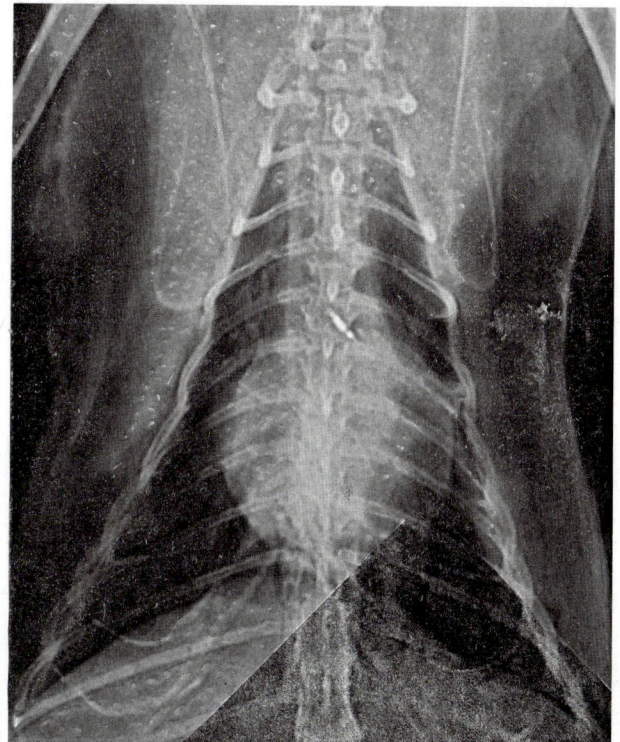

Fig. 1.130: ECG of HOCM

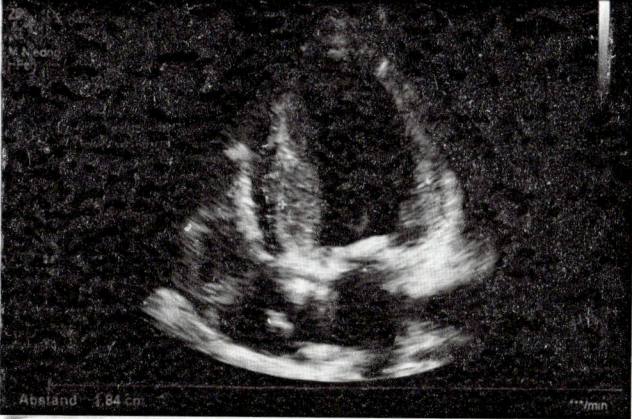

Fig. 1.131: X-ray picture of HOCM

Fig. 1.132: Echocardiography of HOCM

10. **Electrophysiologic studies:** It may be necessary in rapid palpitation to identify:
   a. Accessory pathways.
   b. Ventricular tachycardia and its management.

Management

Screening of the Asymptomatic Patient

1. In children or adolescents, with sarcomere protein gene mutation—screening should be done during growth.

2. In patient with myosin binding C gene mutation—unexplained LVH does not occur—so no need of screening.

Pharmacological Treatment

Indication:
1. To improve symptoms.
2. To prevent complication.

The drugs recommended are:
1. Beta blocker—Propranolol.
2. Calcium channel blocker.

The actions of above drugs are:
1. Decrease myocardial oxygen consumption.
2. Blunting of heart rate response.
3. Increase the time of ventricular filling.
4. Negative inotropic effect:
   a. Reduce hyperdynamic systolic function.
   b. Reduce left ventricular pressure gradient.
   c. Improve the diastolic function.
   d. Verapamil—improves relaxation.
   e. Beta blocker—increases compliance.

Side effects:
1. In case of pre-existing conduction disease—supplement effect of verapamil on AV node—may be detrimental.
2. Due to vasodilatory and negative inotripic effects, there is chance of developing pulmonary edema and death in patient with pulmonary hypertension.

Surgical Treatment

Indication:
1. Resting left ventricular outflow tract gradient of >50 mmHg. In patient refractory to medical therapy.
2. Mitral valve abnormalities.

Operation:
1. Removal of segment of upper anterior septum via transaortic approach or transventricular approach—but later approach may precipitate cardiac failure.
2. Mitral valve repair and papillary muscle remodeling.
3. Occasionally mitral valve replacement.
   Periperative mortality—1% or less.

Alcohol Septal Ablation

Indication: Older patients refractory to medical therapy.
   Method: Injection of alcohol into septal artery, supplying septal muscle—nonpharmacological, percutaneous approach.

Pacing

Indications:
1. Refractory to medical treatment.
2. In whom, surgery is not acceptable or approachable.
3. In erderly patient with localized septal hypertrophy without significant free wall involvement.
4. Patient with mitral regurgitation.

Methods:
1. Pacing the right ventricular apex results:
   a. Reduction of gradient.
   b. Reduction of filling pressure.
   c. Improve symptoms.
2. Atrioventricular pacing:
   a. Symptomatic improvement.
   b. Reduction of gradient.
   c. No change in exercise capacity.

Symptom-wise Treatment

I. Dyspnea:
1. Dyspnea with slow filling throughout the diastole—beta-blocker, verapamil.
2. Dyspnea with rapid early filling—benefit from relative tachycardia without negative chronotropic agent.
3. Dyspnea with significant obstruction—at least 505 of stroke volume remain in the ventricle—at the onset of gradient:
   a. Beta-blocker, disopyramide.
   b. Myotomy/myomectomy.
      Disopyramide should be given in maximal tolerated dose (anticholenergic properties limit higher dose).
4. Dyspnea with mitral regurgitation—mitral valve replacement.

II. Chest pain: Exertional chest pain, responds to verapamil, propranolol.
   In refractory cases—dose of propranolol—480 mg/day.
   Dose of verapamil—720 mg/day.
   Short-acting nitrate, verapamil:
1. Improves coronary flow to subendocardial layers.
2. Reducing the filling pressure in the ventricle.

III. Arrhythmia:
Atrial fibrillation—symptomatic—treated by:
1. Anticoagulant, verapamil or propranolol:
   a. To control ventricular response.
   b. To prevent embolization.
2. Asymptomatic—diagnosed during electrophysiologic monitoring—nodular tachycardia (treatment or above treatment).
3. In case of atrial fibrillation—whose atrial contribution to filling volume is small. Electrical cardioversion by amiodarone (300 mg/day).

IV. Sudden death: It is a common termination in HOCM. This is triggered by:
1. Hemodynamic manifestation.
2. Myocardial ischemia.
3. Arrhythmias:
   a. Atrial fibrillation.
   b. AV block.
   c. Rapid conduction of supraventricular arrhythmias.

Risk Factors of Sudden Death

1. Family history of sudden death (≥ premature, less than 40 years, sudden death).
2. Unexplained syncope in previous years.
3. Abnormal exercise blood pressure response.
4. Non-sustained ventricular tachycardia (≥3 beats at ≥120 beats/min).
5. Severe ventricular hypertrophy (>3 cm).
6. Severe left ventricular outflow tract obstruction (>90 mmHg).
7. Cardiac arrest or sustained ventricular tachycardia.

RESTRICTIVE CARDIOMYOPATHY

Increased stiffness of myocardium produces precipitous rise of intraventricular pressure with slight increase in ventricular volume, but thickness of the ventricular wall be same.

Causes

Familial—associated with:
a. Autosomal dominant with skeletal abnormality.
b. Autosomal recessive musculoskeletal abnormalities.
c. Noonan's syndrome.

Genes responsible are:
a. Mutation of gene encoding Desmin.
b. Mutation of gene encoding troponin.
c. Mutation of other sarcomeric protein genes.

Pathology (Fig. 1.133)

Macroscopically:
a. Normal heart weight.
b. Small ventricular weight.
c. No left ventricular hypertrophy.

Histologically:
a. Non-specific with patchy interstitial fibrosis.
b. Myocyte disarray.

In endomyocardial fibrosis:
a. Endocardial fibrosis.
b. Thrombosis involving inflow tract and apices sparing outflow tract of both ventricles.

There are three stages:
a. *Necrotic stages:* There is active inflammation—associated with eosinophilic abscess, arteritis and necrosis.
b. *Thrombotic stage:* This is evidenced by
   i. Endocardial thrombus formation.
   ii. Massive intracavitary thrombosis—producing restriction to left ventricular filling and low cardiac output.
c. *Fibrosis:* In survived patient, the inflammation is healed by fibrosis.

Clinical Features

a. Left-sided disease may present with evidence of pulmonary congestion and mitral regurgitation.
b. Right-sided disease may present with tricuspid regurgitation, raised JVP, enlarged tender liver, edema and ascites.

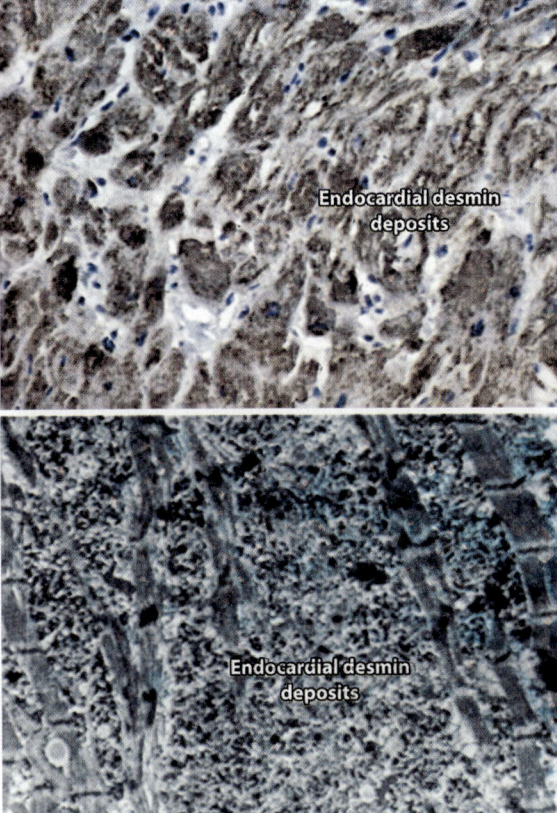

Fig. 1.133: Histology in restrictive cardiomyopathy

Investigations

Radiological Features

a. Enlarged cardiac size.
b. Pumonary infiltration.
c. Enlarged left atrium.

ECG (Fig. 1.134):
a. Evidence of left and right atrial pressure.
b. Left ventricular hypertrophy.

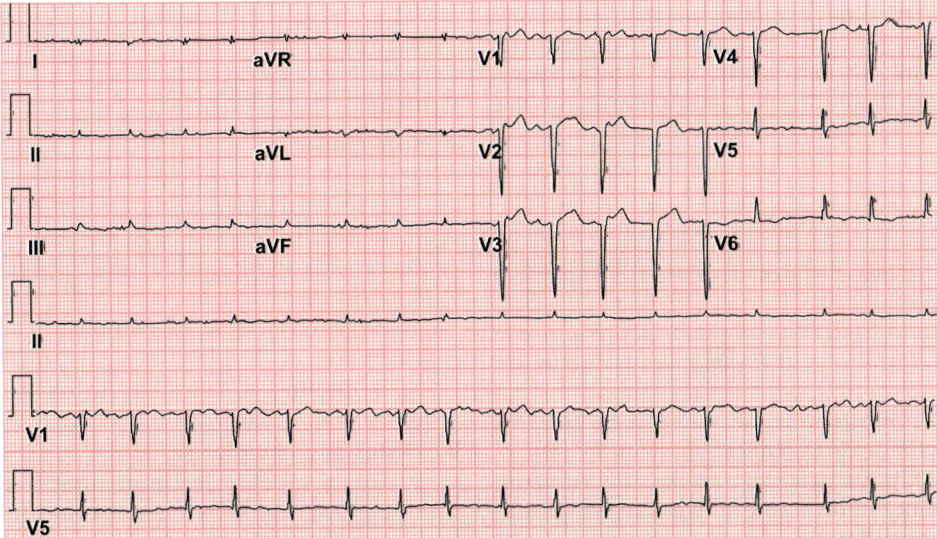

Fig. 1.134: ECG in restrictive cardiomyopathy

c. Cardiomegaly.

d. Non-specific repolarization changes.

Two-dimensional echocardiographic changes (Fig. 1.135):

a. Structural abnormalities of endocardium or AV valves.

b. Presence of intracavitary thrombus.

c. Apical cavity obliteration.

d. Bright echos from endocardium of right or left ventricle with tethering of chordae.

e. Reduced excursion of posterior mitral leaflet.

f. Ventricular wall thickness is normal.

g. Both atria are grossly enlarged.

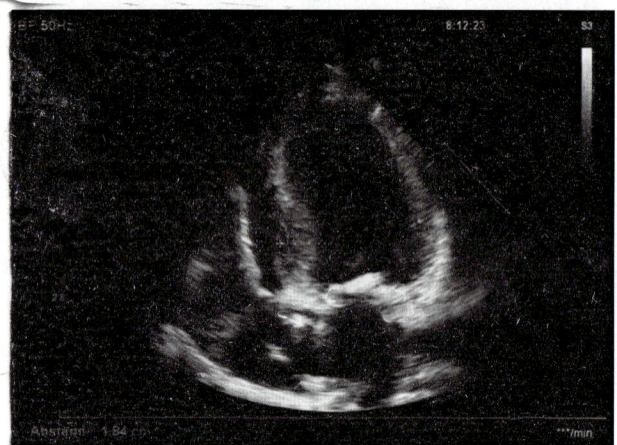

Fig. 1.135: Echocardiography in HOCM

Hemodynamic consequences:

a. Early diastolic pressure is normal.

b. Rapid mid-diastolic rise which plateaus and not associated with impaired systolic performances.

Similar hemodynamic abnormalities can be seen in pericardial constriction.

The difference is—end diastolic pressure is equal in the both ventricles in constrictive pericarditis, but these pressures are unequal in EMF.

Angiography reveals:

a. Evidence of tricuspid or mitral regurgitation.

b. Both ventricles are abnormal in shape with obliteration of apices—more marked in right ventricle and infundibulum.

c. Fibrotic process results in smoothening of internal endocardial structure of ventricle with loss of trabeculae.

d. Evidence of intracardiac thrombi—may mimic cardiac tumors.

Management

Medical

a. In case of advanced disease—no obvious medical treatment and prognosis is poor.

b. Congestive symptoms from raised right atrial pressure can be minimized by diuretics, but it produces reduction in cardiac output.

c. Arrhythmias, if asymptomatic, should not be treated, because anti-arrhythmic drugs may slow the heart rate.

d. Digoxin reduces the ventricular rate in case of atrial fibrillation, but cannot improve the congestive symptoms.

e. Anticoagulants/antiplatelet drugs prevent venous thrombosis or systemic embolism.

Surgery

Mitral and/or tricuspid valve replacement with or without decortications of endocardium—may be curative, but associated with significant perioperative mortality.

MYOCARDITIS

Inflammation of the myocardial tissue is called myocarditis. It affects young people, average age is 42 years. No obvious sex predilection.

True incidence is unknown, although autopsy studies give incidence of 3%. 10% of patients with influenza infection have ECG abnormalities.

In Europe and North America, patient with myocarditis may present with congestive cardiac failure of unknown cause.

Usually, the patient gives history of flu-like prodrome followed by symptoms of cardiac decompensation, e.g. fatigue, breathlessness and cough, chest pain in minority of patient. A few patients present with ventricular tachyarrhythmia with minimal or no dilatation.

Duration of symptoms may be less than 1 month to less than 1 year.

Clinical features show the features of acute left-sided heart failure or congestive cardiac failure.

ECG shows (Figs 1.136a, 11.136b)—conduction defect, arrhythmias, and ST-T wave changes.

Echocardiography reveals four chamber dilatations, reduced contractility.

Cardiac scintigraphy with Indium 111 antimyosin antibodies—detect myocarditis.

Single photon emission computerized tomography detects myocarditis.

Contrast enhanced MRI—assessment of regional myocardial involvement.

Coronary angiography shows no or minimal abnormalities.

Creatine phosphokinase—MB fraction will be elevated.

Viral titer is rarely useful in the diagnosis of viral myocarditis because:

1. Many viruses have been implicated as etiological agent of myocarditis.

2. Sometimes the time between viral prodrome and cardiac symptoms may be too long to diagnose it as viral myocarditis.

Causes

A. Infections:

1. Viral—adenovirus, arbovirus, coxackie virus (A and B), cytomegalovirus, echovirus, EB virus, mumps virus, rabies virus.

2. Bacteria—spirochaetes and bacteria like.

3. Rickettsia.

4. Protozoa—*Entamoeba histolytica, Toxoplasma gondii, T. cruzi*

5. Helminths—Cysticercus, Echynococcus, Toxocara.

6. Fungal

B. Drugs and chemicals:

1. Toxicity—amphetamine, interferon, arsenic, animal poison, catecholamines, cocaine, lithium, paracetamol.

2. Hypersensitivity—aminophylline, digoxin, methyldopa, penicillin, tetracycline, TCA, frusemide.

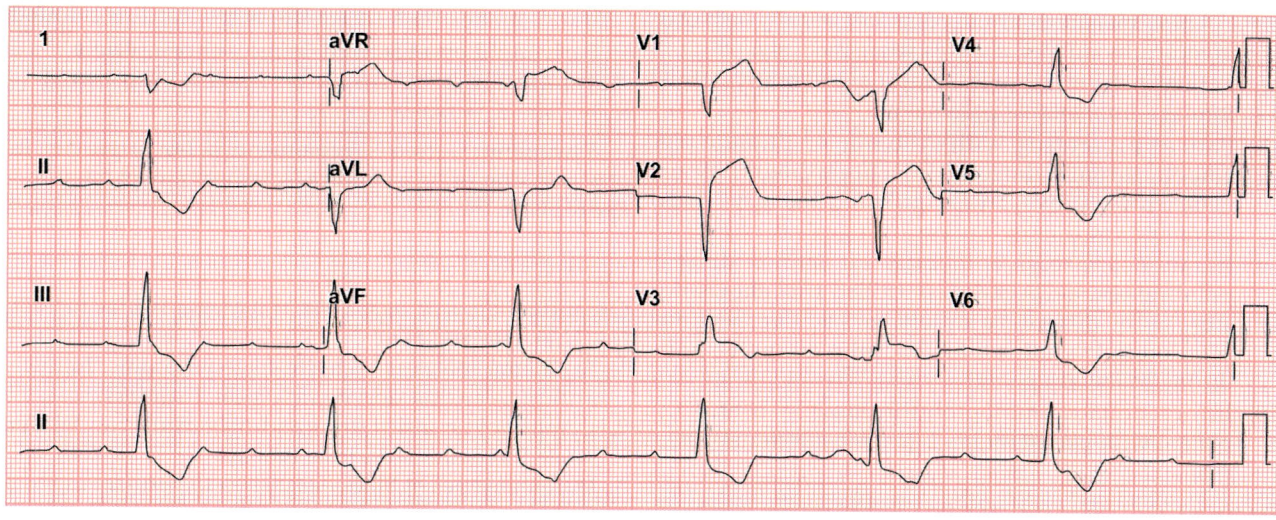

Fig. 1.136a: ECG changes in myocarditis showing ST-T wave changes.

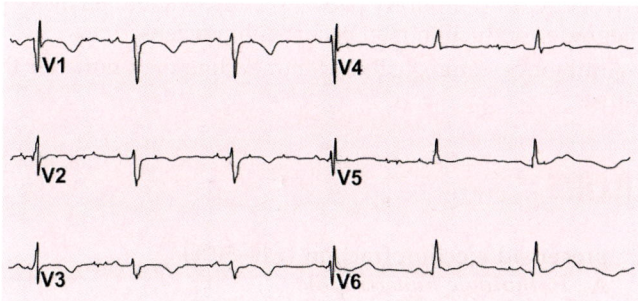

Fig. 1.136b: ECG changes in myocarditis

3. Autoimmunity—antigenic mimicry, cardiac myosin, cytokines, Dressler syndrome, post-cardiotomy syndrome, post-infectious, post-radiation.

Relation with dilated cardiomyopathy:
1. Myocarditis with any viral prodrome raises the possibility of virus as etiological agent of DCM.
2. Endomyocardial biopsy timing (Fig. 1.137)—it may not show any lymphocytic infiltrate, if the duration of symptom is longer.
3. Presence of virus genomic material in some of the negative biopsies may clue to the etiology of DCM.

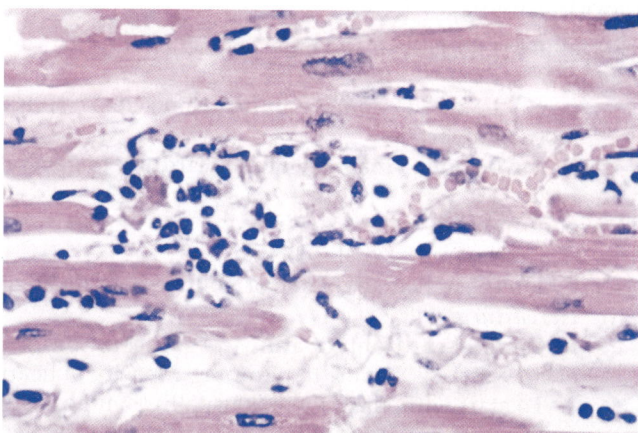

Fig. 1.137: Biopsy in myocarditis

4. Immunomodulatory therapy may improve cardiac function in patient with DCM.

Management

Patient should be hospitalized for close monitoring of:
1. Worsening of congestive heart failure.
2. Arrhythmias.
3. Conduction disturbances.
4. Presence of emboli.

  I. Bed rest must be essential.
 II. Activities that increase cardiac workload should be discouraged.
III. Tobacco and alcohol must be prohibited.
IV. Oxygen to prevent hypoxia, decrease cardiac output or arrhythmias.
 V. Drugs:
  1. Antipyretics other than NSAIDs in febrile patient.
  2. Analgesics are helpful in case of pleuropericarditis.
  3. Correction of anemia, if present.
  4. Patient with congestive heart failure should be treated by:
    a. Diuretics.
    b. Angiotensin-converting enzyme inhibitor.
    c. Angiotensin receptor blocker.
    d. Beta-blockers.
    e. Spironolactone.
  5. Patient presenting with cardiogenic shock:
    a. Intravenous vasodilator.
    b. Inotropic agent—dobutamine or milrinone.
    c. Refractory to conservative measure:
      • Mechanical circulatory support—it acts as "bridge to recovery".
      • Intra-aortic balloon counter-pulsation.
      • Ventricular assist devices.
      • Cardiac transplantation, as a last resort.
  6. Patient presenting with tachyarrhythmia, ventricular arrhythmia:
    a. Avoid negative inotropic drugs.
    b. Amiodarone.
    c. Cardiac defibrillator.

These measures are used as last resort, because myocarditis usually resolves spontaneously.

7. Patient presenting with symptomatic bradyarrhythmias—implantable pacemaker.
8. Patient presenting with systemic or pulmonary emboli, thrombi detected in echocardiography or ventriculography—anticoagulation therapy—it is contraindicated in case of coexisting pericarditis.
9. Immunosuppressive therapy—it shows disappointing results, because controlled trial shows no significant difference in left ventricular ejection fraction, left ventricular diastolic diameter and during follow-up period.
10. Intravenous immunoglobulin may be useful in patient with persistant viral genome interferon-beta.

PERIPARTUM CARDIOMYOPATHY

DCM developing during last trimester of pregnancy or within 6 months of delivery is known as peripartum or postpartum cardiomyopathy.

If heart failure develops very early—first few weeks after delivery—features of myocarditis may be found in endomyocardial biopsy.

If it is of late onset, no feature of myocarditis is found.

Early rapid onset is likely to recover completely.

Spontaneous resolution is common, but in few cases, recurrent heart failure is very common.

Treatment: Steroid is recommended, but unproven. In case of worsening of heart failure—cardiac transplantation is the appropriate therapy.

LYME CARDITIS

Organism—*Borrelia burgdorferi*, following Ixodes tick bite. It is characterized by:
1. Erythema migrans rash, flu-like symptoms, followed by arthritis, carditis, and neurological disorders.
2. Lymphocytic infiltration and bacterium can be demonstrated in endomyocardial biopsy.
3. Different types of block—transient to permanent block can occur.
4. Site of block—usually in AV node in most of the cases, block in the bundle was also reported.

Treatment—temporary pacing is sufficient, but recovery of antegrade conduction may occur within weeks.

Antibiotics—amoxycillin or tetracycline may not alter the course.

HEART FAILURE

Definition

It is a clinical syndrome in which patients having inherited or acquired abnormality in cardiac structure and/or function comprising of—constellation of clinical symptoms (dyspnea and fatigue) and signs (edema and rales) leading to frequent hospitalization, and/or death.

Epidemiology

1. Incidence is lower in women than men. Because the life expectancy increases in women nowadays, incidences are also higher.
2. Overall prevalence of HF increases with age, because current therapy for myocardial infarction or arrhythmia increases the life expectancy of the patients.

Etiologies of Heart Failure

I. **Depressed ejection fraction <40%**
   A. *Coronary artery disease:*
      i. Myocardial ischemia, ii. Myocardial infarction
   B. *Chronic pressure overload:*
      i. Hypertension
      ii. Obstructive valvular disease
   C. *Chronic valvular overload:*
      i. Regurgitant valvular disease
      ii. Intracardiac (left to right) shunting
      iii. Extracardiac shunting
   D. *Non-ischemic dilated cardiomyopathy:*
      i. Infiltrative disorders
      ii. Familial disorders
   E. *Toxic/drugs-induced damage:*
      i. Viral
      ii. Metabolic disorder
   F. *Chronic tachyarrhythmias*

II. **preserved ejection fraction (>40–50%)**
   A. *Pathologic hypertrophy:*
      i. Primary (hypertrophic cardiomyopathy)
      ii. Secondary (hypertension)
   B. *Aging:*
   C. *Restrictive cardiomyopathy:*
      i. Infiltrative disorder
      ii. Storage disorders

III. **Pulmonary heart disease:**
   A. Cor pulmonale
   B. Pulmonary vascular disorder

IV. **High output states:**
   A. Metabolic disorders
   B. Thyrotoxicosis
   C. Systemic arteriovenous fistula
   D. Chronic anemia

Pathophysiology

Heart failure is initiated by an index event.
a. **Type:**
   i. It may be **due to damage in heart muscle**—results in loose of myocytes
   ii. It may be due to **inability of myocardium to generate force**.
b. **Onset of index event:**
   i. *Acute*—in myocardial ischemia
   ii. *Gradual*—in hemodynamic or volume overloading.
   iii. *Hereditary*
      a. **Genetic cardiomyopathies:** As a result of index event—there is decline in pumping capacity of heart:
      • **To start with,** the patient is usually asymptomatic.
      • **But with increasing decline** in pumping capacity, patients become symptomatic.

- **A number of compensatory mechanisms** became activated during initial declining in cardiac pumping function. These are:
  - **i. Activation of renin–angiotensin–aldosterone axis**—responsible for retention of salt and water.
  - **ii. Increased myocardial contractility.**

The factors offsetting the excessive peripheral vaso-constriction:
  i. Atrial natriuretic peptide (ANP)
  ii. Brain natriuretic peptide (BNP)
  iii. Prostaglandin (PGE, PGI_2)
  iv. Nitric oxide

The factors may influence the compensatory mechanism and are able to modulate LV function:
  i. Genetic background
  ii. Sex
  iii. Age
  iv. Environment.

But at some point, patients come symptomatic overtly. The exact mechanism for this transition is not known, but neuro-humoral, adrenergic and cytokine systems are responsible for series of **adaptive changes** in left ventricle. **The changes are** (Fig. 1.38):
1. **Myocyte hypertrophy**
2. Alteration in contractile properties of the myocyte
3. **Progressive loss of myocyte**—through:
   i. Necrosis
   ii. Apoptosis
   iii. Autophagy
   iv. β adrenergic desensitization
   v. Abnormal myocardial energetics and metabolism
   vi. Recognition of extracellular matrix with dissolution of structural collogen.

Forms of Heart Failure

Acute Versus Chronic Heart Failure

1. **Acute heart failure:** This is often used to describe a patient with acute onset:
   i. Dyspnea
   ii. Pulmonary edema

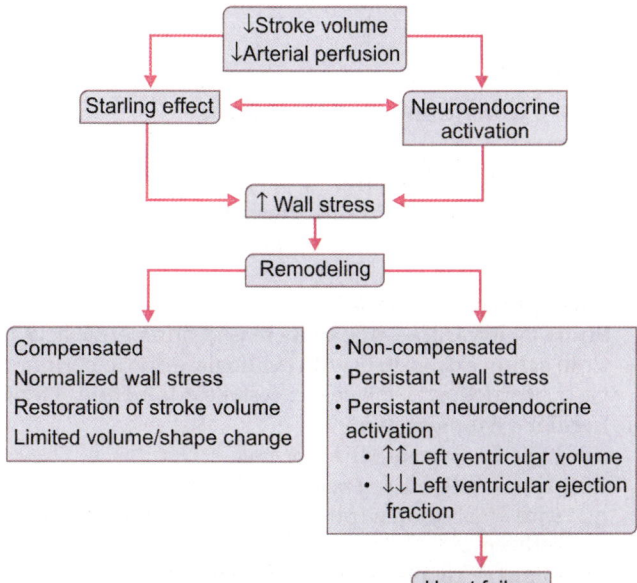

Fig. 1.138: Mechanism of heart failure

iii. Cardiogenic shock producing hypotension and oliguria
It may be the consequence of:
   i. Myocardial infarction
   ii. Arrhythmia
   iii. Acute valvular dysfunction
2. **Chronic heart failure:** This is used to describe a patient with gradual onset of:
   i. Pedal edema
   ii. Ascites
   iii. Tender enlarged liver
   iv. Cardiac cachexia
   v. Malabsorption

Systolic Versus Diastolic Heart Failure

1. **Systolic heart failure**—where there is inability to pump the blood by contractile left ventricle.
2. **Diastolic heart failure:**
   i. Where there is slowed myocardial relaxation
   ii. As there is left ventricular compliance is reduced → Left ventricular filling is delayed and left ventricular end diastolic pressure remains elevated at end of diastole.

↓
Increase in heart rate shortens the diastolic refilling time disproportionately
↓
It may lead to elevated left ventricular end diastolic filling pressure
↓
Increase in pulmonary capillary pressure
↓
Dyspnea

Right-Sided Versus Left-Sided Heart Failure

1. **Right-sided heart failure:** This patient presents with features of systemic venous congestion
2. **Left-sided heart failure:** This patient presents with feature of pulmonary venous congestion.

High-Output Versus Low-Output Failure

1. **High-output failure:** This patient presents with:
   a. Warm extremities.
   b. Normal or widened pulse pressure. The causes are:
      i. Thyrotoxicosis
      ii. Beriberi
      iii. Anemia
      iv. Paget's disease
2. **Low-output failure:** This patient presents with:
   i. Cool peripheral extremities
   ii. Cyanosis due to systemic vasoconstriction
   iii. Low pulse volume

Arterial—mixed venous oxygen saturation is abnormally high in low output states, low in high output states.

A patient having compensated heart failure may **develop acute decompensation**—due to emergence of precipitating factors. **These are:**
1. **Inappropriate reduction in antihypertensive therapy:** Self discontinuation of antihypertensive medications.
2. **Cardiac arrhythmia:** Any type of tachyarrhythmia reduces left ventricular filling, stroke volume and exacerbate ischemia.

3. **Myocardial ischemia or infarction:** It may exacerbate left ventricular dysfunction, may worsens mitral regurgitation due to ischemia of papillary muscles.
4. **Infection:** Respiratory infection or sepsis can precipitate:
    i. Direct myocardial depressions from inflammatory cytokines
    ii. Fever
    iii. Sinus tachycardia
5. **Anemia**—It may precipitate heart failure by:
    i. Increasing myocardial ischemia
    ii. Sinus tachycardia
6. **Concomitant dry therapy:**
    a. *Drugs those produce myocardial depression:*
        i. Calcium antagonists, verapamil, diltiazem
        ii. Many antiarrhythmic drugs
        iii. β blockers
        iv. Anesthetics
    b. *Drugs assessing salt and water retention:*
        i. NSAIDs
        ii. Estrogen
        iii. Steroid
7. **Alcohol:** It precipitates in following manner:
    i. Directly toxic to myocardium
    ii. Excess amount produces myocardial depression
    iii. Precipitation of arrhythmia
8. **Pulmonary embolism**: Its risk increases in immobile patient in:
    i. Low output states   ii. Atrial fibrillation

New York Heart Association Classification of Heart Failure

1. **Class-1**   No limitation in physical activity
2. **Class-2**   Slight limitation in physical activity. They are comfortable at rest. Ordinary physical activity results in fatigue, palpitation, dyspnea or angina pain.
3. **Class-3**   Marked limitation in physical activity.
            They are comfortable at rest. Less than ordinary activity causes fatigue, palpitation, dyspnea, or angina pain.
4. **Class-4**   Inability to carry out any physical activity without discomfort. Symptoms of antianginal syndrome may be present at rest.

Clinical Symptoms

1. **Dyspnea:**
    i. To start with dyspnea on exertion
    ii. As the disease progresses—dyspnea with less strenuous activity, ultimately dyspnea occurs in rest.
    The pathophysiological mechanisms are:
    i. Activation of J receptors by—accumulation of interstitial and intra-alveolar fluid.
    ii. Reduction in pulmonary compliance
    iii. Increased airway resistance
    iv. Respiratory muscle fatigue or diaphragmatic fatigue
    v. Anemia
        Dyspnea occurs with left ventricular failure, not with right ventricular failure.
2. **Orthopnea** Dyspnea occurring in recumbent position, relieved by sitting position.

The pathophysiological mechanism

Redistribution of fluid from splanchnic circulation and lower extremities to central circulation during recumbency
↓
Increased pulmonary capillary wedge pressure
↓
Orthopnea

3. **Paroxysmal exertional dyspnea:** This means—acute episodes of severe shortness of breath and coughing, occurring at night awakens the patient from sleep (usually 1–3 hours after going to sleep)
    The pathophysiological mechanisms:
    i. Increased pressure in bronchial arteries leading to airway compression.
    ii. Interstitial pulmonary edema leading to increased airway resistance.
4. **Cheyne-Stokes respiration:** It occurs in 40% patients with heart failure—usually associated with low cardiac output.
    Pathophysiological mechanisms: There are two phases of Cheyne-Stokes respiration:
    i. In apneic phase—there is fall in PO_2 and rise in PCO_2
    ii. In hyperpneic phase or hyperventilation phase—raised PCO_2 stimulates respiratory center—as a result PO_2 rises and PCO_2 falls.
5. **Other symptoms**
    I. *Gastrointestinal symptoms:*
        i. Anorexia
        ii. Satiety
        iii. Nausea
        iv. Abdominal pain and fullness
    Causes:
        i. Edema of bowel wall
        ii. Congestion in liver due to stretching of capsule surrounding liver.
    II. *Cerebral symptoms:*
        i. Confusion   ii. Disorientation
        iii. Sleep disturbances   iv. Mood disturbances

    Causes: Reduced cerebral perfusion

Physical Signs
General Examination and Vital Signs

1. **Position**—orthopnea with labored breathing
2. **Systolic blood pressure:**
    i. Normal or high in early heart failure.
    ii. Low in late phase of heart failure due to LV dysfunction
3. **Pulse pressure**: Diminished
4. **Sinus tachycardia**—due to increased adrenergic activity
5. **Cold calmy extremities with cyanosis**—due to peripheral vasoconstriction as a result excessive adrenergic activity.
6. **Jugular venous system:**
    i. In early stage of HF—normal
    ii. Abnormally raised with sustained (≥1 minute) pressure on abdomen (positive abdominal hepatojugular reflux)
    iii. Giant V waves—indicate presence of tricuspid regurgitation.
7. **Pulsus alternans**—sign of advanced heart failure

8. **Pulmonary examination:**
   i. *Pulmonary crackles*—due to transudation of fluid from intravascular spaces into alveoli
   ii. *Crackles* may be accompanied by wheezing (cardiac asthma)
   iii. *Crackles* are absent in chronic heart failure even when left ventricular filling pressure is elevated because of increased lymphatic drainage of alveolar fluid
   iv. *Pleural effusion*—due to elevation of pleural capillary pressure—producing transudation of fluid into pleural spaces.
      Pleural effusion occurs due to biventricular failure because: pleural veins drain into systemic and pulmonary veins.
      Pleural effusion is usually bilateral but may be unilateral (right pleural space).

9. **Cardiac examination:**
   i. Point of maximal impulse is displaced below 5th intercostal space and/or lateral to mid-clavicular line—*in case of cardiomegaly.*
   ii. Point of maximal impulse is sustained *in case of severe left ventricular hypertrophy*
   iii. *Third heart sound* most commonly presents in case of volume overload having tachycardia and tachypnea—heard at apex.
   iv. *Fourth heart second* (S4)—heard in patient with diastolic dysfunction.
   v. *Left parasternal heaves* may be present in case of right ventricular hypertrophy.
   vi. *Murmur of mitral or tricuspid regurgitation,* if present.

10. **Abdominal examination:**
    i. *Enlarged tender liver*—occasionally pulsatile, it is usually systolic—due to tricuspid regurgitation.
    ii. *Ascites:* It is late sign—occurs due to:
       a. Increased pressure in hepatic veins
       b. Increased pressure in the veins of peritoneum.
    iii. *Jaundice:* It occurs as a consequence of:
       a. Hepatic congestion
       b. Hepatocellular hypoxemia

11. **Peripheral examination:**
    Edema: It is usually symmetrical, predominantly:
    i. In ankle in case of ambulatory patient
    ii. In sacral area in case of bed-ridden patient (presacral edema), long-standing edema may be associated with indurated and pigmented skin.

12. **Cardiac cachexia**
    Cachexia and weight loss—is due to following factors:
    i. Elevation of resting metabolic rate
    ii. Anorexia, nausea, vomiting—due to:
       a. Congestive hepatomegaly
       b. Abdominal fullness
    iii. Impairment of intestinal absorption due to congestion of intestinal veins

Diagnosis

Blood

a. **Routine laboratory testing:**
   i. Complete blood count
   ii. Serum electrolytes
   iii. Blood urea nitrogen
   iv. Serum creatinine
   v. LFT
   vi. Urinalysis
   vii. Lipid profile
   viii. Fasting serum glucose
   ix. Thyroid function tests

b. **Biomarkers:**
   1. *BNP and pro-BNP*—BNP level <100 pg/ml and pro-BNP <123 pg/ml, if age <75 years
      The factors—which determine the BNP and pro-BNP level:
      i. Age—BNP and pro-BNP levels increase with age.
      ii. Sex—more elevated in women
      iii. Medical therapy
      iv. Body mass index
      v. Perioperative status
      vi. Concomitant disease (thyroid disease)
         BNP level falsely low in obese patient
         Hence BNP is not recommended as a guide to heart failure therapy.
   2. *Troponin T and troponin I*
   3. *C-reactive receptor*
   4. *TNF*
   5. *Uric acid*
      All the above are elevated in heart failure.

Complete blood count:
1. *Hb%* to rule out anemia
2. *Leukocytosis*—as to diagnose infection or sepsis
3. *Thyroid function test*—to rule out:
   i. Thyrotoxicosis
   ii. Myxedema

Electrolytes:
1. *Hypokalemia and hypomagnesemia and metabolic alkalosis*—diuretic abuse
2. *Hyperkalemia*—due to drugs inhibiting renin–angiotensin activating system
3. *Hyponatremia*—signifies fluid retention advanced heart failure
   Urea and creatinine: To measure renal function abnormality
   Liver function test: It occurs as a consequence of right sided heart failure.
   Lipid level and fasting blood glucose—to rule out hyperlipedemia, diabetes mellitus.

Electrocardiography

1. **Signs of:**
   i. Myocardial infarction
   ii. Chamber abnormalities
   iii. Left ventricular or right ventricular hypertrophy
   iv. Heart block (iatrogenic or infiltrative disease)
   v. Arrhythmia
   vi. Pericardial effusion (voltage <5 mm in frontal leads, <10 mm in precordial leads)
2. **Holter monitoring**—helpful in identifying arrhythmias

Chest Radiograph

1. **Enlargement of heart**—left ventricular or biventricular failure.
2. **Pulmonary or hilar congestion**—in acute left ventricular failure.

3. **Other findings of acute heart failure:**
   i. Kerley's B line
   ii. Frank pulmonary edema
   iii. Pleural effusion

Left Ventricular Assessment

1. **2D echocardiography/Doppler echocardiography:**
   It provides:
   i. Semiquantitative assessment of left ventricular size and function.
   ii. Presence or absence of valvular and regional wall motional abnormalities (indicative of poor myocardial infarction).
   iii. Presence of left atrial dilatation
   iv. Presence of left ventricular hypertrophy
   v. Estimation of left ventricular diastolic filling
   vi. Estimation of ejection fraction (EF)
   vii. Assessing the right ventricular size and pulmonary pressure
2. **Magnetic resonance imaging:** It is the gold standard:
   i. For assessing left ventricular size and volume, mass.
   ii. For evaluating cause of heart failure and assessing left ventricular structure.
   Most useful index of left ventricular function is ejection fraction

$$EF = \frac{\text{Stroke volume}}{\text{End diastolic volume}}$$

EF is influenced by alteration in preload or afterload.
EF normal ≥ 50% systolic function is adequate.
EF <30–40% contractility is depressed.

Framingham Criteria for Diagnosis of Heart Failure

Major Criteria

1. Paroxysmal nocturnal dyspnea
2. Raised JVP, distended neck vein
3. Crepitations in lung fields
4. Cardiomegaly in chest X-ray

5. Acute pulmonary edema
6. S3 gallop rhythm
7. Hepatojugular reflux.
8. Weight loss >4.5 kg in 5 days in response to treatment of heart failure.

Minor Criteria

1. Bilateral ankle edema
2. Nocturnal cough
3. Dyspnea on ordinary exertion
4. Hepatomegaly
5. Pleural effusion
6. Tachycardia rate >120/min
7. Decrease in vital capacity by one-third.

Minor criteria is only acceptable, if they are not attributed to another medical disorder.
Two major or 1 major and 2 minor criteria are required for diagnosis of heart failure (Fig. 1.139).

Treatment of Heart Failure

Heart failure should be viewed as a continuous process which is composed of 4 stages:

Stage-A: Patient at high risk of developing heart failure **does not have structural heart disease or symptoms of hart failure** (patient with diabetes mellitus and hypertension).

Stage-B: Patient **has structural heart disease** but does not have symptoms of heart failure (patient has previous myocardial infarction and asymptomatic left ventricular dysfunction).

Stage-C: Patient has **structural heart disease and developed symptoms of heart failure** (patient with previous myocardial infarction with dyspnea and fatigue).

Stage-D: Patient **with refractory heart failure** requiring special interventions (cardiac transplantations)

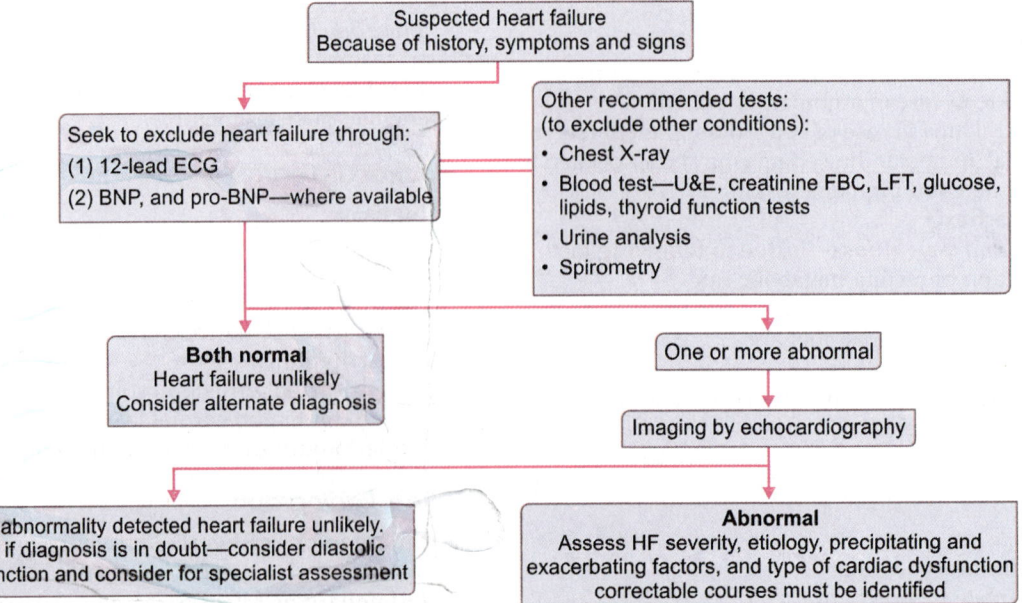

Fig. 1.139: Algorithm of diagnosis of heart failure

So aim of treatment is:
1. Treatment of preventable cause (stage-A)
2. Treating the stage B and stage-C with drugs
3. Symptomatic management of stage-D.

Therapeutic Strategy for Patient with Heart Failure

1. **Patient asymptomatic but having left ventricular dysfunction (Class-1):** Slow the disease progression by blowing the neurohormonal systems.
2. **Patient with class-II to IV**—primary goal:
   i. To alleviate fluid retention
   ii. To lessen disability
   iii. To reduce the risk of further disease progression and death.

Management of Heart Failure with Depressed Ejection Fractions

I. General measure:
   1. *Treatment of co-morbid conditions:*
      i. Hypertension
      ii. Coronary artery disease
      iii. Diabetes mellitus
      iv. Anemia
      v. Sleep disordered breathing
   2. *Alcohol consumption:*
      i. Two standard drinks per day for men
      ii. One standard drink per day for women
      iii. In case of alcoholic cardiomyopathy—complete abstinence
   3. *Avoidance of physical exertion in extreme temperature:*
   4. *Certain drugs to be avoided:*
      i. NSAID
      ii. β-blockers
      iii. Calcium antagonists.
      iv. Anti-arrhythmic agents (class-I agents)
      v. Anti-TNF antibodies
   5. *Immunization with influenza vaccine and pneumococcal vaccine*

II. Activity:
   i. *Routine modest exercise:* Beneficial in patient with NYHA Class I–III HF
   ii. *For euvolemic patient:* Regular isotonic exercise, walking, riding, stationary bicycle ergometer.

III. Diet:
   1. *Sodium restriction:*
      i. 2–3 gm/day—in patient with HF and preserved or depressed EF
      ii. <2 gm/day—in patients with moderate to severe HF
   2. *Fluid restriction:* <2 litre/day—considered:
      a. In hyponatremic patient
      b. Fluid retention difficult to control despite high dose of diuretics.
   3. *Calorie supplementation* in patient with cardiac cachexia.

Pharmacological Therapy for Heart Failure

Diuretics: Aim to maintain normal volume status in patient with congestive symptoms (dyspnea, orthopnea, and edema) or signs or elevated filling pressure (JVP raised).

Drugs are:
1. *Loop diuretics* (furosemide, torsemide, bumetanide)—act—at loop of Henle—by reversibly inhibiting the reabsorption of Na^+, K^+ and Cl in thick ascending limb of loop.
2. *Thiazide and metolazone*—inhibit or reduce the reabsorption of Na^+, and Cl in the first half of DCT.
3. *Potassium sparing diuretic*—spironolactone—acts at the level of collecting duct.

Doses:
- *Furosemide*—20–40 mg twice to 4 times daily
- *Torsemide*—10–20 mg twice daily
- *Bumetanide*—0.5–1 kg twice daily
- *Metolazone*—2.5 mg–5 mg twice or 4 time daily.

Instructions:
1. Direction to be started at low dose and then carefully titrated upward to relieve symptoms of fluid overload
2. Typically multiple daily doses are required
3. Intravenous loop diuretic can be administered to alleviate the symptoms of congestion, respiratory distress.
   Once the patient is relieved from his symptoms—oral dose should be commenced to maintain a steady state.
4. In patient with renal efficiency (creatinine >2.5 mg/dl)—thiazide diuretic should be avoided.

Refractory to diuretic therapy represents:
i. Patient non-adherence
ii. Progression of HF

In case of refractoriness to loop diuretics:
i. Metolazone or thiazide diuretics can be added as once or twice daily doses.
   But chronic daily use of metolazone should be avoided to avoid dyselectrolytemia
ii. Short-term dialysis or ultrafiltration

Adverse effect:
1. Electrolyte imbalance
2. Volume depletion
3. Worsening of azotemia
4. Worsening of neurohormonal activation and disease progression
5. Hypokalemia (loop diuretics, thiazide) or hyperkalemia (spironolactone) leading to life-threatening arrhythmia.

Angiotensin-converting enzyme inhibitors:

Drugs	Starting dose	Target dose
1. Captopril	6.25 mg thrice daily	50–100 mg thrice daily
2. Enalapril	2.5 mg twice daily	10–20 mg twice daily
3. Lisinopril	2.5–5 mg area once daily	20–35 mg once daily
4. Ramipril	1.25–2.5 mg twice daily	5 mg twice daily 10 mg once daily

Mode of action:
1. They inhibit the enzyme responsible for conversion of angiotensin I to angiotensin II.
2. They inhibit kininase II—leading to upregulation of bradykinin

Effect: ACE inhibitors:
  i. Stabilize LV remodeling
 ii. Improve symptoms
iii. Reduce hospitalization
 iv. Prolong life

Fluid retention can attenuate the effects of ACE inhibitors—so it is preferable to optimize dose of diuretic before starting the ACE inhibitors.

Method of administration:
  i. To be started with low dose
 ii. Double the dose at not less than 2 weeks interval
 ii. Aim for target dose

Adverse effect:
1. *Symptomatic hypotension:*
  i. If dizziness, light headedness—discontinue calcium channel blocker, nitrates and other vasodilators.
 ii. If no symptom of congestion—consider reduction of diuretic dose.
2. *Cough*—may be due to:
  i. Smoking related lung disease
 ii. Pulmonary edema—it should be under D/D when new or worsening of cough develops
iii. Enalapril—it should be discontinued.
3. *Worsening of renal function:*
  i. Little rise in urea, creatinine and K^+ are to be expected after initiation of ACE inhibitor—it is acceptable, if the rise is small.
 ii. An increase of K^+ up to ≤5.9 is acceptable; if patient is taking potassium sparing diuretic.
iii. If K^+ >6 mmol/L or creatinine >350 μmol/L, the dose of ACE inhibitor must be stopped.
4. *Angioedema:* If develops after ACE inhibitor; alternate therapy with ARB can be started.

Angiotensin receptor blocker: These drugs are used in patients intolerant to ACE inhibitor, because of cough, skin rash and angioedema.

Indication:
i. HF with EF <40%
ii. Intolerant to ACE-I

Mechanism of action:
These drugs block the effects of angiotensin-II on angiotensin type II receptor.

Drugs	Starting dose	Target dose
1. Valsartan	40 mg twice daily	160 mg twice daily
2. Losartan	12.5 mg qd	30 mg qd
3. Candesartan	4 mg qd	32 mg qd

Combination: Combination with β blockers—ARB:
  i. Reverses the process of left ventricular remodeling
 ii. Improves patient's symptoms
iii. Prevents hospitalization
 iv. Prolongs life

Adverse effects:
  i. Hypotension
 ii. Worsening of renal function
iii. Hyperkalemia

β-adrenergic receptor blocker: Most of deleterious effect of adrenergic activation are mediated by β1 receptor activation—so β-blocker interferes with harmful effects of sustained activation of adrenergic nervous system by competitive inhibition of these receptor.

Indication: β-blockers are given in patient with symptomatic or asymptomatic HF with decreased EF <40%.

Drugs	First dose	Increments	Target dose
1. Carvidolol	3.125 mg twice daily	6.25; 12.5; 25; 50	50 mg daily
2. Bisoprolol	1.25 mg once daily	2.5; 3.75; 5; 7.5; 10	19 mg daily
3. Metoprolol	12.5 mg daily	25, 50, 100, 200	200 mg daily

Combination: With ACE inhibitor:
  i. Reverses the process of LV remodeling.
 ii. Improves patient's symptoms.
iii. Prevents hospitalization.
 iv. Prolongs life.

Dose adjustment: Dose should be increased at 2 weeks interval, because rapid increasing the dose of these agents may lead to worsening of fluid retention as a consequence of withdrawal of adrenergic support to the heart and circulation.

So it is prudent to optimize the dose of diuretic to prevent fluid retention before starting the therapy with β-blocker.

Adverse effect:
1. Bradycardia (<50/min)
2. 2nd to 3rd degree AV block

Contraindication:
1. Bronchial asthma
2. Diabetes mellitus
   In above two cases—dose of β-blocker must be halved
3. Hypotension:
  i. If symptomatic (dizziness, light headedness confusion)—discontinue vasodilators, nitrates and calcium channel blocker.
 ii. If asymptomatic—consider reduction of diuretic dose.

Aldosterone receptor antagonist: ACE-I transiently inhibits aldosterone secretion—but chronic therapy with ACE-I, ultimately aldosterone level comes to pretreatment level.

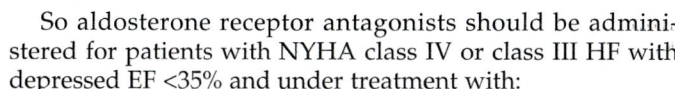

So aldosterone receptor antagonists should be administered for patients with NYHA class IV or class III HF with depressed EF <35% and under treatment with:

i. ACE-I
ii. Diuretics
iii. β-blockers.

Dose: Spironolactone—12.5—25 mg daily up to 50 mg daily.

Adverse effect:

1. Hyperkalemia—in patients who are also receiving potassium supplements:
   i. It should not be recommended when:
      a. Serum creatinine level >2.5 mg/dl or
      b. Creatinine clearance <30 ml/min
   ii. Serum K⁺ >5 mmol/L
2. Gynecomastia (painful)

Cardiac arrhythmia: Atrial fibrillation occurs in 15–30% of patients with heart failure.

Amiodarone: Class III antiarrhythmic agent having few or no negative inotropic effects—so it is effective against supraventricular arrhythmias. It is effective for maintaining:

a. Sinus rhythm
b. Success of electrocardioversion in patient with HF.

Amiodarone increases the level of phenytoin and digoxin, and prolongs INR in patients taking warfarin.

Hence the dose of all above drugs to be reduced as much as to 50%.

Adverse effect of amiodarone:

i. Hyperthyroidism
ii. Hypothyroidism
iii. Pulmonary fibrosis
iv. Hepatitis

Cardiac glycosides: It reduces the ventricular rate in patient with atrial fibrillation with chronic heart failure.

Contraindication:

i. Significant bradycardia
ii. Heart block
iii. WPW syndrome

Vasodilator therapy:

1. They are not effective in improving natural history of chronic heart failure, but useful in patient intolerant of both ACE-I and ARBS.
2. *Nitrate is usually venodilator*, but effective coronary vasodilator, so they are useful in ischemic heart failure.
3. *Isosorbide dinitrate:*
   i. Increases exercise tolerance
   ii. In combination with hydralazine improve survival
4. In class-II heart failure—enalapril is superior to hydralazine and isosorbide dinitrate.
5. *Nesisitide* (human brain natriuretic peptide):
   i. Improves hemodynamics and clinical status in decompensated heart failure
   ii. Lesses arrhythmogenic
   iii. Subcutaneous injection in chronic heart failure

6. *Natural endopeptidase inhibitor* with or without intrinsic ACE-I activity:
   i. Prevents the inactivation of BNP or ANP.
   ii. Useful in treatment of chronic heart failure.

Phosphodiesterase inhibitor: The agents are:
i. Milrinone
ii. Enoximone

Effect: In case of decompensated heart failure—intravenous administration produces sustained vasodilator.

Positive inotropic support: Intravenous dobutamine:
i. Acts on severe episodes of heart failure.
ii. Acts as bridge to transplantation in end stage heart failure.

Antiplatelet agents and anticoagulants:

1. NSAID must be avoided because of its fluid retention properties and nephrotoxic properties.
2. In ischemic heart failure—aspirin is of choice.
3. Warfarin is indicated—in:
   i. Heart failure with atrial fibrillation.
   ii. Heart failure with left atrial thrombus.
   iii. Very large left ventricular cavity where there is risk of developing thrombus.

Other drugs in heart failure:

i. Colchicines followed by allopurinol in acute gout.
ii. Correction of anemia with iron and erythropoietin prevents the risk of heart failure.

Device Therapy in Heart Failure

Patients fulfilling the indication of permanent pacemaker can accept this device therapy.

Implantable cardiac defibrillators

Indications:

1. Mild to moderate HF (NYHA class II and class III) to prevent or reduce the incidence of sudden death.
2. NYHA class II to class III heart failure with depressed EF <35%.

Management of Acute Heart Failure (Decompensated)

Therapeutic Goals

1. To stabilize the hemodynamic derangements responsible for symptoms and hospital administration.
2. To identify and correct reversible factors responsible for decompensation.
3. To establish effective out patient medical regimen that prevents disease progression and relapse.

Two primary determinants of acute decompensated heart failure:

1. Elevated left ventricular filling pressure
2. Depressed cardiac output—this results neurohumoral activation and followed by increased systemic vascular resistance.

Patients with acute heart failure usually present with one of the four hemodynamic profiles:

1. *Profile A*—normal left ventricular filling pressure with normal perfusion.
2. *Profile B*—elevated left ventricular filling pressure with normal perfusion.
3. *Profile C*—elevated left ventricular filling pressure with decreased perfusion.
4. *Profile L*—normal or decreased left ventricular filling pressure with decreased perfusion.

Elevated LV filling pressure?

	No	*Yes*	
No	Profile A	Profile B	↓ Cardiac output?
	Warm and dry	Warm and wet	
Yes	Profile L	Profile C	↓ Systemic vascular
	Cold and dry	Cold and wet	resistance?

Above profiles are made on the basis of brief bedside examination—including examination of:
i. Neck vein,   ii. Peripheral extremities,   iii. Lungs

Aim is to revert back and to maintain a patient in profile A. Patient with elevated left ventricular filling pressure—may have signs—rales, elevated neck veins and peripheral edema—**referred to as wet.**

Patient with depressed cardiac output and increased systolic vascular resistance may manifest as cold calmy extremities—**referred to as cold.**

So patient with normal LV filling pressure and no congestion—referred to **as dry and warm.** In these patients, acute presentation of symptoms may be due to other than heart failure, e.g. pulmonary disease, liver disease and transient myocardial ischemia.

If patients present with **congestive symptoms, normal perfusion and elevated LV filling pressure**—these patients can be treated with vasodilators and diuretics.

If patients present with elevated systemic vascular resistance low cardiac output **(profile C)**—they should be treated with **inotropic agent with vasodilatory action** (dobutamine, low dose dopamine, milrinone)—acts by:
i. Augment cardiac output—by increasing myocardial contractility
ii. Functionally unloading the heart.

Patients in profile L—should be investigated with right heart catheterization to investigate occult left ventricular filling pressure (by seeing pulmonary capillary wedge pressure <12 mmHg).

If this low—fluid repletion is required.

Pharmacological Management of Heart Failure

Vasodilators

Mode of action: It stimulates guanylyl cyclase within smooth muscle cells—and exerts—dilating effect on arterial resistance and venous capacitance vessels. **As a result—there is:**
i. Lowering of left ventricular filling pressure
ii. Reduction in mitral regurgitation

iii. Improved forward propulsion of cardiac output without increasing cardiac arrhythmias and heart rate.

The drugs are:
1. *Nitroglycerin*—intravenous—20 mg/min increase the dose in 20 µg increment until:
   i. Patient's symptom is improved.
   ii. Pulmonary capillary wedge pressure decreases to <16 mmHg.
   Without reducing systolic blood pressure below 80 mmHg.
   Side effects—headache—can be relieved by analgesic.
2. *Nitroprusside:* Intravenous 10 µg/min—increase the dose 10–20 mg every 10–20 minutes.
   Side effects: Cyanide toxicity—involving gastrointestinal and central nervous system—most likely to occur in patient receiving dose 250 µg/min over 48 hours.
3. *Nesiritide:* Recombinant form of brain type natriuretic peptide.
   Dose: Bolus dose—2 µg/kg followed by fixed dose infusion—0.01—0.03 µg/kg/min
   Side effect: In bolus dose, it has adverse effect on renal function.

Inotropic agents

Mode of action: Stimulate the cardiac contractility and produce peripheral vasodilatation.
1. *Dobutamine:* It stimulates β_1, β_2 receptors, little effect on $\propto 1$ receptors.

   Dose:
   • Continuous infusion 1–2 µg/kg/min
   • Higher dose >5 µg/kg/min required for severe hypo perfusion
   • No or little benefit from ≥ 10 µg/kg/min
2. *Milrinone:* Phosphodiesterase III inhibitor—it leads to increased cyclic AMP by inhibiting its breakdown.

   Dose Bolus dose—50 µg/kg/min followed by continuous infusion 0.1—0.75 µg/kg/min.

   Milrinone is more effective than dobutamine in reducing LV filling pressure.

   Milrinone has an additive effect when given with β adrenergic agonists.

The ionotropic drugs are used in following indications:
1. In patients where vasodilators and diuretics are not helpful.
2. In patient with poor systemic perfusion.
3. Patient with cardiogenic shock.
4. In patient requiring short-term hemodynamic support after acute myocardial infarction or surgery.
5. For patient awaiting for cardiac transplantation.
6. As palliative care in patient with advanced heart failure.

Vasoconstrictors

1. *Dopamine:* It is used where modest inotropic action and pressure support are usually required.

   Mode of actions: It is an endogenous catecholamine, that stimulate β, $\propto$, and dopaminergic receptors—both DA_1 and DA_2—present in heart and circulation.

   Action and receptor action is dose dependent:
   i. **At low dose** (<2 mg/kg/min)—stimulates DA_1 and DA_2 receptors—produces renal and splanchnic vasodilatation.

ii. At **moderate dose** (2–4 μg/kg/min)—stimulates β₁ receptors, increases cardiac output with little or no change in heart rate or systemic vascular resistance.

iii. **At higher dose** (>5 μg/kg/min)—stimulates ∝ receptors—it overwhelm dopaminergic receptors—leading to systemic vasoconstriction and increase in systemic vascular resistance, heart rate.

2. *Additional inotropic drugs:*
   a. Epinephrine
   b. Phenylephrine
   c. Vasopressin

Vasopressin antagonist: In patients having acute heart failure often vasopressin levels are often elevated—and may be responsible for hyponatremia:

Vasopressin antagonists:
   i. Reduce edema
   ii. Reduce body weight

iii. Normalize the serum sodium but they do not improve acute decompensated heart failure

The drugs are:
1. Tolvaptan (oral)
2. Conivaptan (intravenous)

These drugs are now recommended for hyponatremia but yet not approved for heart failure.

Mechanical and Surgical Intervention

If pharmacologic therapy fails to stabilize the patient with refractory heart failure, following interventions may be effective in maintaining circulator support:
1. Intra-aortic balloon counter-pulsation
2. Percutaneous and surgically implanted LV assist devices
3. Cardiac transplantation

INFECTIVE ENDOCARDITIS

Introduction

It is an infection of cardiac endothelium, macroscopically seen as vegetations—this is prototypic lesions in endocarditis.

Vegetation is a mass of:
   i. Platelet
   ii. Fibrin
   iii. Microcolonies of microorganisms
   iv. Scanty inflammatory cells

Endocarditis may be classified according to:
   i. Temporal evolution of disease
   ii. The site of infection
   iii. Predisposing risk factors, e.g. intravenous drug use.

Acute endocarditis is:
   i. Hectically febrile illness
   ii. Rapidly damaging cardiac structures
   iii. Hematogenous seeding to extracardiac tissues
   iv. If untreated, progresses to death within weeks

Subacute endocarditis:
   i. Follows indolent course
   ii. Produces structural damages very slowly
   iii. Rarely metastasizes and is gradually progressive unless complicated by mycotic aneurysm or major embolic event.

Incidence

2.6–7 cases per 100,000 population per year, which has been relatively stable during recent decades.

Etiology

Organisms can be subdivided according to portal of entry:
1. Oral cavity—*Streptococcus viridans*
2. Skin—staphylococci
3. Upper respiratory tract—HACEK organisms (*Haemophillus, Actinobacilus, Cardiobacterium, Eikenella, Kingella*).
4. Gastrointestinal tract—*Streptococcus gallolyticus (S. bovis)* (associated with polyps and colonic tumors)
5. Genitourinary tract—*Enterococcus*

Organisms can be isolated according to type of persons involved and type of valves

1. **Heath care worker associated with normal valve endocarditis:** By both nosocomial route and community acquired:
   i. *Staphylococcus aureus*
   ii. Coagulase negative staphylococci
   iii. Enterococci

2. **Patient having in dwelling catheter**—*Staphylococcus aureus*

3. **Prosthetic valve endocarditis within 2 months of valve surgery**—usually through nosocomial route by two methods:
   a. Intraoperative bacterial contamination
   b. Postoperative unrelated bacteremia
   The organisms are:
   i. *Staphylococcus aureus*
   ii. Coagulase negative staphylococci
   iii. Facultative gram-negative bacilli
   iv. Diphtheroids
   v. Fungi

4. **Prosthetic valve endocarditis occurring >12 months after surgery**—is usually community acquired.
   Coagulase negative staphylococci—which produce nosocomially acquired prosthetic valve endocarditis 2–12 months after surgery commonly resistant to methicillin.

5. **Transvenous pacemaker or implanter defibrillator associated endocarditis,** usually nosocomial organisms are:
   i. *Staphylococcus aureus*
   ii. Coagulase negative staphylococci
   Both are methicillin resistant.

6. **In case of intravenous drug users**—commonly involves tricuspid valve:
   i. Organism is methicillin resistant *Staphylococcus aureus*
   ii. Polymicrobial infection
7. **Infective endocarditis with negative blood cultures:**
   i. Due to prior antibiotic exposure
   ii. May be due to fastidious organisms—nutritionally variant organism, *Coxiella burnetii*, *Bartonella* species, HACEK organisms.

Pathogenesis (Fig. 1.140)

Main pathogenic factor is damaged endothelium due to:
   i. Impact of high velocity blood yet
   ii. Low pressure side of cardiac structural lesion

The conditions are:
   i. Mitral regurgitation
   ii. Aortic stenosis
   iii. Aortic regurgitation
   iv. Ventricular septal defect
   v. Complex congenital heart diseases.

Organism involves the endocardium by:
   i. Direct invasion by virulent organism (*Staphylococcus aureus*)
   ii. Development of an uninfected platelet fibrin thrombus—called non-bacterial thrombotic endocarditis—acts as nidus for bacterial attachment during transient bacteremia.

This non-bacterial thrombotic endocarditis also results from:
   i. Hypercoagulable state—this results in development of marantic endocarditis (uninfected vegetations occur in: a. chronic disease, b. malignancy)
   ii. Bland vegetations—resulting as a complication of SLE and antiphospholipid antibody syndrome.

Organisms enter the bloodstream from mucosal surface, skin, or from site of focal infection

↓

Adhere to the site of non-bacterial thrombotic endocarditis (NBTE)

↓ If resistant to antimicrobial activity in serum and microbial peptides released by platelets.

Organisms proliferate

Eliciting tissue factor from monocytes (*S. aureus*) ←— eliciting tissue factor from endothelium

↓

Induce platelet deposition and a procoagulant state at this site

↓

Fibrin deposition combines with platelet aggregation +microorganism proliferation

↓

Generate infected vegetations

↓ ←— Aided by adhesin molecules of microbial surfaces

Adheres to NBTE sites and/or injured endothelium

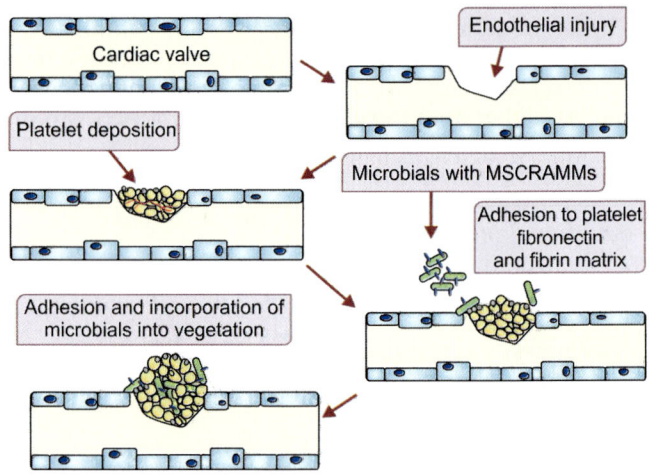

Fig. 1.140: Pathogenesis of infective endocarditis

Adhesin molecules are:
   i. Fibronectin binding protein present on many Gram positive bacteria.
   ii. Clumping factors in *Staphylococcus aureus*
   iii. Glucans on streptococci.

In absence of host defenses: Organisms embedded in platelet rich thrombi preliterate continuously to form dense colonies, at the same time organisms deep in the vegetations become:
   i. Metabolically inactive
   ii. Relatively resistant to killing by microbial agents

   Only surface organisms will be shaded continuous in bloodstream.

Pathophysiological consequences of endocarditis are:
   i. Damage of intracardiac structure
   ii. Deposition of vegetative fragments producing infection and infarction of tissue.
   iii. During bacteremia hematogenous infection of tissue
   iv. Deposition of immune complexes in the tissue producing injury of tissue
   v. Immune responses to deposited bacterial antigens.

Clinical Manifestations

Course of the Disease

It may be:
1. **Acute coarse**—organisms responsible:
   i. β-haemolytic *Streptococcus*
   ii. *Staphylococcus aureus*
   iii. *Pneumococcus*
   iv. Enterococci
   v. Coagulase negative staphylococci.
2. **Subacute course:** Organisms responsible:
   i. *Streptococcus viridans*
   ii. Enterococci
   iii. HACEK growth
3. **Indolent course:**
   i. *Bartonella* species
   ii. *Tinea whipplei*
   iii. *Coxiella burnetii*

Non-Specific Clinical Manifestations

1. Fever:
   i. Low grade rarely 103°F–104°F—suggests subacute course
   ii. High grade 103°–104°F—suggests acute course.
   iii. May be blunted or absent in elderly and severely debilitated persons, patient with renal failure.
2. Anorexia
3. Weight loss
4. Malaise
5. Arthralgia
6. Myalgia
7. Back pain
8. Clubbing

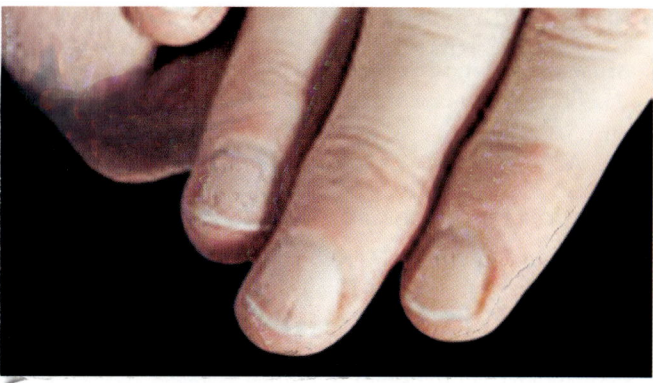

Fig. 1.141: Splinter hemorrhage

Cardiac Manifestations

Presence of murmur is not indicative of infective endocarditis rather appearance of new regurgitant murmur is suggestive.
1. **In acute endocarditis due to involvement of normal valve**—murmur may be absent initially, but later on it should be present in 85% of cases.
2. **Congestive heart failure** in 30–40% cases due to:
   a. Valvular dysfunction
   b. Endocarditis associated with myocarditis
   c. Intracardiac fistula

   In case of valvular dysfunction: Mitral valve dysfunction progresses less rapidly than aortic valve dysfunction.

   Extension of infection beyond the valvular leaflet into myocardial tissue—producing intracardiac abscess (perivalvular abscess)—which leads to intracardiac fistulae with appearance of new murmur.
3. **Extension of intracardiac abscess**
   i. Intracardiac fistulae
   ii. Abscess may burrow from aortic valve through pericardium—producing pericarditis.
   iii. Abscess extends into upper ventricular septum may interfere with conduction system—leading to varying degree of heart block.
   iv. Abscess from mitral valve area rarely interrupts the conduction pathway, atrioventricular node.
4. **Embolism in coronary artery** in 2% of patient produces myocardial infarction.

Symptoms and Signs due to Immune Complex Deposition

1. **Skin** (Fig. 1.141):
   i. Petechiae (most common)
   ii. Splinter hemorrhage (subungual dark linear streak)
   iii. Osler nodes (painful tender erythematous nodules on the pads of fingers and toes) persist for hours to days due to infection with *Staphylococcus aureus*, endocarditis.
   iii. Janeway lesions (non-tender erythematous and/or hemorrhage areas on the palm and soles).
   iv. Septic emboli
2. **Eyes:**
   i. Roth spots (oval retinal hemorrhages with pale center located near optic disk).
   ii. Conjunctival splinter hemorrhages
   iii. Retinal flame-shaped hemorrhages

3. **Renal manifestation:**
   i. Microscopic hematuria
   ii. Immune complex deposition on the glomerular basement membrane producing diffuse glomerulonephritis—producing microscopic hematuria.
   iii. Embolic renal infarction causes flank pain and hematuria
4. **CNS manifestations:**
   i. Cerebrovascular emboli present with stroke or encephalopathy—it may precede endocarditis
   ii. Aseptic or purulent meningitis
   iii. Intracranial hemorrhage due to hemorrhagic infarct or ruptured mycotic aneurysm
   iv. Seizures.
   Mycotic aneurysm (Fig. 1.142): This is characterized by focal dilatation of arteries occurring at the points in the arteries that have been weakened by infection in the vasa vasorum or where septic emboli have been lodged.

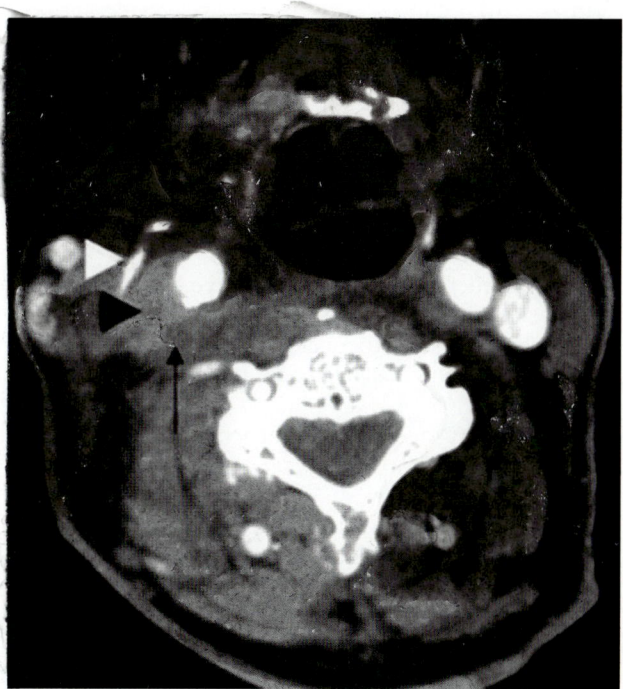

Fig. 1.142: Mycotic aneurysm in brain

v. Microabscess in brain and meninges occurring due to *Staphylococcus endocarditis*.

5. **Musculoskeletal involvement:**
   i. Focal metastatic infections (spondylodiscitis)
   ii. Arthralgia
   iii. Arthritis

Manifestations of Specific Predisposing Condition

1. **50% of endocarditis cases** are associated with injection of drug users—limited to tricuspid valve, present with fever.
2. **In 75% of cases**—septic emboli—cause (i) cough, (ii) pluritic chest pain, (iii) nodular pulmonary infiltrate, occasionally (v) pyopneumothorax.
3. **Infection of aortic and mitral valve** produces typical features of endocarditis.
4. **Transvenous pacemaker or implanted defibrillator device associated endocarditis**—is associated with cryptic generator pocket infection—resulting fever, minimal murmur and pulmonary symptoms.
5. **In case of prosthetic valve endocarditis:**
   i. If it is early onset infective endocarditis (within 60 days of valve surgery), typical symptoms may be masked by associated co morbidity.
   ii. But if it is late onset endocarditis—paravalvular infection is common, results in:
      a. Valve dehiscence
      b. Regurgitant murmur
      c. Congestive heart failure
      d. Conduction disturbances

Diagnosis

Diagnosis can be established with certainty when vegetations are examined histologically.

So Duke criteria have been developed on the basis of:
   i. Clinical
   ii. Laboratory
   iii. Echocardiographic findings

Diagnosis of infective endocarditis is certain when:
   i. Two major criteria, or
   ii. One major criteria and three minor criteria, or
   iii. Five minor criteria are present.

Major Criteria

1. **Positive blood culture:**
   • Typical microorganism for infective endocarditis from two separate blood cultures
      Viridans streptococci, *Streptococcus gallolyticus*, HACEK group, *Staphylococcus aureus*
   Or
      Community acquired enterococci in absence of a primary focus.
   Or
   • Persistently positive blood culture, defined as recovery of a microorganism consistent with infective endocarditis from:
      Blood cultures drawn >12 hours apart
   Or
      All of 3 or, a majority of ≥4 separate blood cultures, with first and last drawn at least 1 hour apart.

• Single positive blood culture for *Coxiella burnetii* or phase 1 IgG antibody titer of >1:800.

2. **Evidence of endocardial involvement:** Positive echocardiogram: Oscillating intracardiac mass on valve or supporting structures or in the path of regurgitant jets or in implanted material, in absence of an alternative anatomic explanation
   Or
   Abscess
   Or
   New partial dehiscence of positive valves
   Or
   New valvular regurgitation (increase or change in pre-existing murmur not sufficient)

Minor Criteria

1. **Predisposition:** Predisposing heart condition or injection drug use.
2. **Fever** ≥ 38°C (≥100.4°F)
3. **Vascular phenomena:**
   • Major arterial emboli
   • Septic pulmonary infarcts
   • Mycotic aneurysm
   • Intracranial hemorrhage.
   • Conjunctival hemorrhage
   • Janeway lesions.
4. **Immunologic phenomena:**
   • Glomerulonephritis
   • Osler's node
   • Roth's spots
   • Rheumatoid factor
5. **Microbiologic evidence:** Positive blood culture, but not meeting major criterion as noted previously, or, serologic evidence of active infection with organism consistent with infective endocarditis.

Diagnosis of infective endocarditis is rejected:
1. If alternative diagnosis is established.
2. If symptoms resolve and did not recur with ≤4 days of antimicrobial therapy.
3. If surgery or autopsy after ≤4 days of antimicrobial therapy yields no histological evidence of endocarditis.

Exclusion Criteria in Culture

Exclude
• Single positive blood cultures for coagulase negative staphylococci and Diphtheroids—who are the common contaminants.
• Organisms that do not cause endocarditis frequently—such as Gram-negative bacilli.

Laboratory Investigation

1. Full blood count: i. Normochromic normocytic anemia
                           ii. Neutrophil leukocytosis
                           iii. May be thrombocytopenia
2. LFT: May be deranged, especially with an increase in ALP and Y GT
3. ESR—raised
4. CRP—raised
5. Urine analysis   Microscopic hematuria ± proteinuria
6. Immunology   Polyclonal elevation of serum IgG, complement

7. Blood culture: In absence of prior antimicrobial therapy, three two-bottle blood culture sets:
   i. Separated from one another by at least 1 hour

   ii. Should be obtained from different venipuncture sites over 24 hours

   ↓← if negative after 48–72 hours

   i. Two to three additional blood culture sets should be obtained
   ii. Laboratory should be consulted for advice regarding optimum culture technique

In hemodynamically stable patient, empiric antibiotic therapy should be withheld till culture results, if patient already received antibiotic therapy within preceding weeks	If patient is not hemodynamically stable, he must be treated with antibiotics immediately after 3 sets of blood cultures one obtained.

8. Non-blood culture tests: Serologic tests are usually done where the organisms are difficult to recover from blood culture.

The methods are:
   i. *Coxiella burnetii, Brucella, Bartonella, Legionella, Chlamydophila psittaci*—can be identified in vegetations by culture.
   ii. Periodic acid-Schiff stain for *Tinea whipplei*.
   iii. Direct fluorescence antibody technique and by using polymerase chain reaction to recover microbial DNA or 16S rRNA

Echocardiography (Fig. 1.143)

It allows:
1. Anatomic confirmation of infective endocarditis
2. Sizing vegetations
3. Detection of intracardiac complications
4. Assessment of cardiac functions

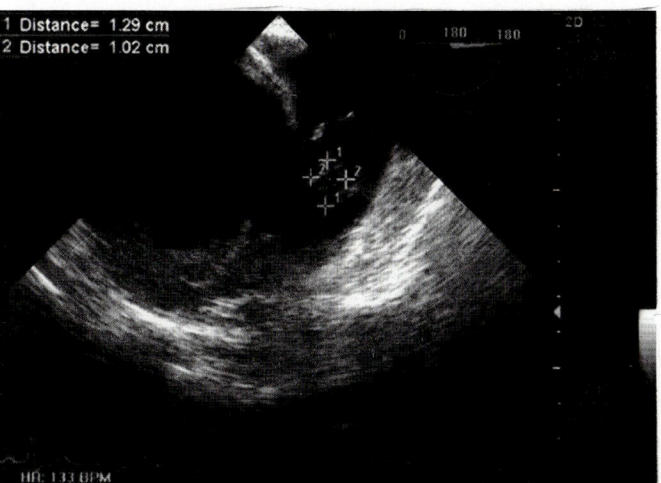

Fig. 1.143: Vegetation

Transthoracic echocardiography: It is optimal method of diagnosis for:
1. Prosthetic valve endocarditis
2. Myocardial abscess
3. Valve perforation
4. Intracardiac fistulae

Drawback:
i. TTE cannot detect vegetation <2 mm in diameter.
ii. TTE is difficult in obese patient and patient with emphysema:
   • TTE can defect vegetation in more than 90% of cases with definite endocarditis
   • Negative TTE cannot exclude the diagnosis of endocarditis rather warrants repetition of study in 7–10 days.

Cardiac Catheterization

It is required in older individuals who many under go surgery for infective endocarditic.

Treatment

Streptococci

1. **Penicillin susceptable streptococci**
   • **Penicillin** G—2–3 mU IV 4 hourly × 4 weeks
   • **Ceftriaxone**—2 gm/day IV as single dose × 4 weeks
   • **Vancomycin**—15 mg/kg IV 12 hourly × 4 weeks
     [Vancomycin in patients with severe or immediate β lactum allergy]
   • **Penicillin** G—2–3 mU IV, 4 hourly Or, **Ceftriaxone** 2 gm IV, 6 hourly } 2 weeks
     +
   • **Gentamicin**—3 mg/kg IV as a single dose or in divided doses, 8 hourly × 2 weeks

2. **Relatively penicillin—resistant streptococci**
   • Penicillin G—4 mU, 4 hourly, IV Or, ceftriaxone 2 gm, 4 times daily IV } 4 weeks
     +
   Gentamicin—3 mg/kg IV as single dose or in divided doses, 8 hourly × 2 weeks
   • Vancomycin—15 mg/kg IV 12 hourly × 4 weeks
     [Penicillin at this dose for 6 weeks or with gentamicin during initial 2 weeks for prosthetic valve endocarditis.]

3. **Moderate penicillin resistant streptococci or *Gemella morbillorum***
   • Penicillin G—4–5 mU IV 4 hourly) Or, Ceftriaxone—2 gm 6 hourly } × 6 weeks
     +
   Gentamicin—3 mg/kg IV as a single dose or in divided doses, 8 hourly × 6 weeks
   • Vancomycin—15 mg/kg IV, 12 hourly × 4 weeks

Enterococci
   • Penicillin G—4–5 mU 4 hourly IV
     +
   Gentamicin—1 mg/kg IV, 8 hourly } × 4–6 weeks

- Ampicillin—2 gm IV 4 hourly
    +
  Gentamicin—1 mg/kg IV 8 hourly $\Big\}$ × 4–6 weeks
- Vancomycin—15 gm IV, 12 hourly
    +
  Gentamicin—1 mg/kg IV, 8 hourly $\Big\}$ × 4–6 weeks

Staphylococci

1. **Methicillin-sensitive infecting native valves (no foreign devices)**
   - Nafcillin or oxacillin (2 gm IV, 4 hourly) × 4–6 weeks
   - Cefazolin (2 gm IV, 8 hourly) × 4–6 weeks
   - Vancomycin (15 mg/kg IV, 12 hourly) × 4–6 weeks
2. **Methicillin-resistant infecting native valves (no foreign devices)**
   - Vancomycin (15 mg/kg IV 12 hourly) × 4–6 weeks
3. **Methicillin-susceptible infecting prosthetic valves**
   - Nafcillin or oxacillin (2 gm IV, 4 hourly) × 6–8 weeks
        +
     Gentamicin (1 mg/kg IV, 8 hourly) × 2 weeks
        +
     Rifampin (300 mg orally, 8 hourly) × 6–8 weeks
4. **Methicillin-resistant infecting prosthetic valves**
   - Vancomycin (15 mg/kg IV, 12 hourly) × 6–8 weeks
        +
     Gentamicin (1 mg/kg IV, 8 hourly) × 2 weeks
        +
     Rifampin (300 mg orally, 8 hourly) × 6–8 weeks
   - Ceftriaxone (2 gm IV as a single dose) × 4 weeks
   - Ampicillin/sulbactam (3 gm IV, 6 hourly) × 4 weeks

Netilmicin (4 mg/kg 6 hourly) IV as a single dose can be used in lieu of gentamicin.

HACEK Species

1. Native valve endocarditis: IV cephalosporin (e.g. ceftriaxone) for 4 weeks
2. Prosthetic valve endocarditis: Ceftriaxone IV × 6 weeks

Streptococcus Pneumoniae

1. Penicillin MIC ≤ 1 µg/ml:
   - Penicillin G—4 mU IV 4 hourly
   - Ceftriaxone 2 gm IV daily $\Big\}$ × 4 weeks
   - Cefotaxim
2. Penicillin MIC ≥ 2 µg/ml:
   - Vancomycin IV × 4–6 weeks
3. If concurrent meningitis is suspected:
   - Vancomycin IV + ceftriaxone 2 gm IV daily × 4–6 weeks.

Pseudomonas aeruginosa

- Antipseudomonal penicillin (ticarcillin or pipercillin)
    +
  Tobramycin (8 mg/kg/day in divided doses)

Corynobacterium endocarditis

Penicillin + Aminoglycosides (if organism is susceptable to aminoglycosides)
   Or, Vancomycin

Candida endocarditis

Amphotericin B + Flucytosine and early surgery.
   On sporadic cases—Capsofungin treatment.

Empirical Therapy

Aim is:
1. Without culture data:
   i. Before culture results
   ii. Whose culture is negative
2. Clinical clues:
   i. Site of infection
   ii. Patient's predisposition
3. Epidemiological dues

Clinical presentation	Drugs to be given
1. Acute endocarditis in drug user and cover MRSA and gm –ve bacilli	– Vancomycin + Gentamicin
2. Culture –ve episode, marantic endocarditis to be excluded	– Ampicillin—sulbactum—12 gm/24 hours in divided doses Or, Ceftriaxone + Gentamicin + Doxycycline (100 mg twice daily (for Bartonella coverage)
3. Prosthetic valves in place ≤1 year	– Vancomycin, gentamicin, rifampin, cefopime
4. Prosthetic valves in phase ≥1 year	– Like culture –ve episode
5. IVB. drug user	– Vancomycin
6. Gradual onset	– Benzyl penicillin + Gentamicin

Right-Sided Endocarditis

1. Flucloxacillin (2 weeks) + aminoglycosides (2 weeks)
2. Ciprofloxacin (4 weeks) + Rifampin (3 weeks)
3. If MRSA—Vancomycin (4 weeks) + Rifampicin (4 weeks)

Monitoring treatment: Clinical monitoring should be done during and several months after the infections. Reappearance of features suggests infective endocarditis and should be investigated thoroughly.

A. Clinical features:
   1. *Signs of continued infection:*
      i. Persistent pyrexia
      ii. Persistence of systemic symptoms
      Persistent fever may be due to:
      i. Drug resistance
      ii. Concomitant infection:
         a. Central line   b. Urine   c. Chest
         d. Septic embolism   e. Lung or abdomen

iii. Allergy—a. Eosinophilia   b. Leukopenia
    c. Proteinuria—common with penicillin
Here antibiotic should be changed or stopped.
2. *Change in any cardiac murmur*
3. *Signs and symptoms of heart failure*
4. *Development of new embolic phenomena*
B. *Echocardiography* (Fig. 1.144): Regular weekly echo (TTE) may identify:
  i. Clinically silent, progressive valve destruction
  ii. Development of intracardiac abscess or vegetation
  iii. Type of long-standing central line may develop sterile fibrinous strands
     Here change the line and send the tip for culture.

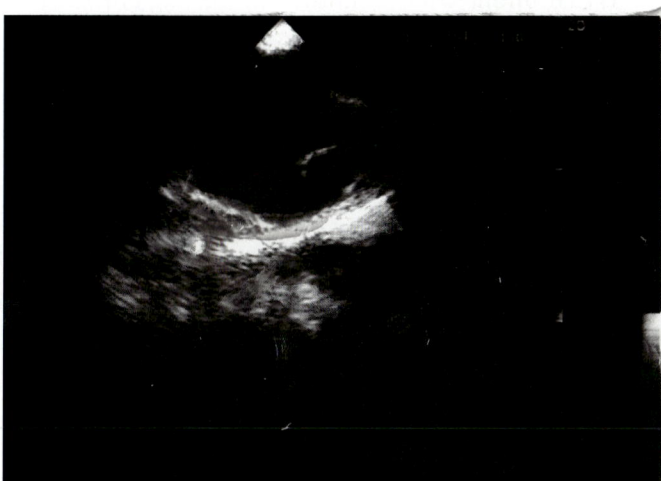

Fig. 1.144: Vegetation in valve

C. *ECG:* Features of AV block or other conduction abnormalities—suggesting intracardiac extension of infection.
D. *Microbiology:*
  i. Repeated blood culture—in case of continued fever
  ii. Regular vancomycin and aminoglycoside blood levels (presence of therapeutic level and avoidance of toxic levels)
  iii. Back titration to ensure MIC value being achieved.
E. *Laboratory indices:*
  i. Regular daily urinalysis
  ii. Regular urea and electrolytes, liver function tests
  iii. Regular CRP (ESR every 2 weeks)
  iv. Full blood count:
    • Rising hemoglobin + falling WBC
    • Watch for beta lactam associated neutropenia
  v. Serum magnesium (if patient is on gentamicin)

Causes of culture negative endocarditis:
1. Previous antibiotic therapy
2. Fastidious organism:
  i. Nutritionally deficient various *Streptococcus viridans:*
    a. *Brucella*
    b. *Legionella*
    c. *Neisseria*
  ii. *Mycobacterium*
  iii. HACEK
  iv. Cell wall deficient bacteria and anaerobes

3. Cell dependent organism
  i. *Chlamydia*
  ii. *Rickettsiae*
4. Fungi

Causes of vegetations on echocardiography:
1. Infective endocarditis
2. Sterile thrombotic vegetations:
  i. Libman-Sacks endocarditis (SLE)
  ii. Primary antiphospholipid syndrome
  iii. Marantic endocarditis (adenocarcinoma)
3. Myxomatous degeneration of valves (commonly mitral)
4. Ruptured mitral chordae
5. Exuberant rheumatic vegetations (Black—Africans)
6. Thrombus (pannus) on a prosthetic valve
7. A stitch or residual calcium after valve replacement.

Right-Sided Endocarditis

1. Always consider in case of IV drug user.
2. Endocarditis on endocardial permanent pacemaker leads is rare, but must be recognized cause.
3. Most commonly staphylococcal infection.
4. Patient requires immediate therapy and surgical intervention.
5. Lesions have to be sterilized with antibiotics.
6. Surgery to be indicated in:
  i. Resistant organism (*S. aureus, Pseudomonas, Candida* and polymicrobial infection)
  ii. Increase in vegetation size in spite of therapy
  iii. Infection in pacemaker leads
  iv. Recurrent mycotic emboli

Surgery

Indications

A. **Surgery required for optimum outcome:**
  i. Moderate to severe heart failure secondary to valve regurgitation
  ii. Unstable prosthesis
  iii. Uncontrolled infection, persistent bacteremia, in spite of antimicrobial therapy {infective endocarditis secondary to fungi, brucella, *Pseudomonas aeruginosa* (especially aortic and mitral valve)}
  iv. *Staphylococcus aureus* valve endocarditis with intracardiac complications.
B. **Surgery to be strongly considered for improved outcome:**
  i. Perivalvular extension of infection
  ii. Poor response to *Staphylococcus aureus* endocarditis involving aortic and mitral valve.
  iii. Relapse after adequate treatment
  iv. Large (>10 mm) hypermobile vegetations with increased risk of embolism.
  v. Persistent unexplained fever (>10 days) in culture negative endocarditis.
  vi. poor responsive or relapsed endocarditis due to highly antibiotic resistant enterococci or Gram-negative bacilli.
    • *Surgical intervention* is necessary during active infection or because of degree of valve destruction.
    Optimal timing depends upon:
    1. Hemodynamic tolerance of lesion
    2. Outcome of infection
    3. Presence of complications

- *Intraoperative specimen should be sent for:*
  i. Culture and sensitivity
  ii. Staining
  iii. Immunological testing
  iv. PCR depending on suspected organism
- *Duration of antimicrobial treatment depends on clinical presentation:*
  i. *Culture negative operative specimen:*
     a. 2–3 weeks for valve infection
     b. 3–4 weeks for abscess
  ii. *Culture positive operative specimen:*
     a. 3–4 weeks for valve infection
     b. 4–6 weeks for abscess
- *Timing is dictated by clinical picture:* In patient with neurological injury, surgery should be delayed to avoid intracranial hemorrhage:
  i. Embolic infarct delay—10–14 days
  ii. Hemorrhage delay—21–28 days

Timing of Cardiac Surgical Intervention in Patient with Endocarditis

I. **Emergent (same day):**
  1. Acute aortic regurgitation
     +
  Preclosure of mitral valve
  2. Sinus of Valsalva abscess ruptured into right heart
  3. Rupture into pericardial sac
II. **Urgent (within 1–2 days):**
  1. Valve obstruction by vegetations
  2. Unstable prosthesis
  3. Acute aortic or mitral regurgitation with heart failure (NYHA—Class III or IV)
  4. Septa perforation
  5. Perivalvular extension of infection with/without new electrocardiographic conduction system changes
  6. Lack of effective antibiotic therapy

III. **Elective:**
  1. Progressive paravalvular prosthetic regurgitation.
  2. Valve destruction + persistent infections after ≥ 7–10 days of antimicrobial therapy
  3. Fungal endocarditis

Antibiotic Regimen Prophylaxis in Adult with High Risk Cardiac Lesions

1. Standard oral regimen: Amoxicillin—2 gm orally 1 hour before procedure
2. Inability to take oral medication: Amoxicillin—2 gm IV or IM 1 hour before procedure
3. Penicillin allergy:
   i. Clarithromycin or azithromycin 500 mg orally 1 hour before procedure
   ii. Cephalexin: 2 gm orally 1 hour before procedure
   iii. Clindamycin—600 mg orally 1 hour before procedure
4. Penicillin allergy, inability to take oral medication:
   i. Ceftriaxone—1 gm IV or IM 30 minutes before procedure
   ii. Clindamycin—600 mg IV or IM 1 hour before procedure.

High-risk cardiac lesions, for which endocarditis prophylaxis is required:
1. Prosthetic heart valves
2. Prior endocarditis
3. Unrepaired congenital cyanotic heart disease—including palliative shunts
4. Completely repaired congenital heart defects during 6 months after repair.
5. Incompletely repaired congenital heart disease with residual defects adjacent to prosthetic material
6. Valvopathy developing after cardiac transplantation.

ACUTE CORONARY SYNDROME (ACS)

Acute coronary syndrome is the operational term used to describe constellation of symptoms resulting from myocardial ischemia

ACS includes the diagnosis of:
1. Unstable angina pectoris
2. ST elevated myocardial infarction (STEMI)
3. Non-ST elevated myocardial infarction (non-STEMI)

Current nomenclature divides ACS into two major groups:
1. *ST-elevated myocardial infarction (STEMI):* This group of patients must undergo reperfusion therapy as early as possible.
2. *Non-ST-elevated myocardial infarction (Non-STEMI):* This group of patients may present with chest discomfort, transient or permanent non-ST elevation ECG change.

   This group can be subdivided into two sub-categories:
   i. Biochemical evidence of myocardial injury + non-ST elevation ischemic changes in ECG—**diagnosis of non-STEMI.**

ii. No biochemical evidence of myocardial injury but non-ST elevation ischemic changes in ECG—**diagnosis of unstable angina.**

The above two subgroups are not treated with thrombolysis.

Initial Management of ACS

1. Patient should be admitted in environment having facilities of continuous ECG monitoring and defibrillation facility.
2. Oral aspirin 300 mg should be given, if no contraindication.
3. Intramuscular injection should be avoided, because it may raise total CK and there may be risk of bleeding, if the patient was being thrombolysed and under anticoagulant medication.

Immediate assessment should include:
1. Rapid examination to exclude:
   i. Hypertension
   ii. Presence of murmur
2. To identify and treat pulmonary edema
3. IV access

4. 12-lead ECG
5. Provide:
   i. Oxygen 2–4 litres/minute
   ii. Diamorphine 2.5–10 mg IV, if required for pain relief.
   iii. Metoclopramide or ondansetron IV to relief nausea.
   iv. GTN—2 puff if patient is not hypotensive.
6. ***Blood examination for:***
   i. Full blood count, urea, electrolytes—supplementation of K$^+$ to keep it at 4–5 mmol/L
   ii. Glucose—rise acutely in post-MI in absence of diabetes
    - Reflect stress-induced catecholamine response, resolves without treatment
   iii. Biochemical markers of cardiac injury:
    (a) CPK, (b) CPK—MB, (c) Troponin T, I, (d) SGOT, (e) LDH
   iv. Lipid profile: Total cholesterol—LDL, HDL, triglyceride
    Serum cholesterol remains close to baseline for 24–48 hours, falls thereafter then takes >8 weeks to return to baseline.
   v. Portable chest X-ray—to assess:
    a. Cardiac size   b. Pulmonary edema
    c. Mediastinal enlargement
   vi. General examinations include:
    a. Peripheral pulses   b. Fundoscopy
    c. Abdominal examination for organomegaly.
    d. Aortic aneurysm.

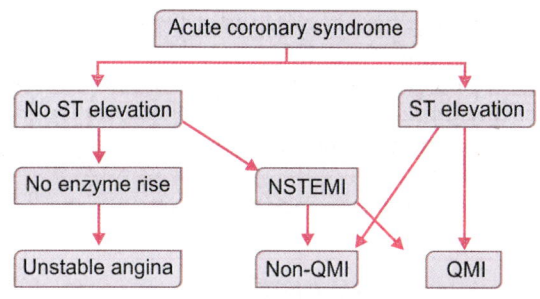

Fig. 1.145: Classification of ACS

Guidelines for Identification of Acute Coronary Syndrome

Unstable Angina Pectoris and Non-STEMI

1. **Angina pectoris:** It is characterized by chest or arm discomfort that may not be described as pain, but it is associated with—physical exertion or stress and relieved within 5–10 minutes by rest and/or sublingual nitroglycerin.
2. **Unstable angina:** It is characterized by angina pectoris or equivalent ischemic chest discomfort having at least one of the following three features:
   i. It occurs at rest (or with minimal exertion), usually lasting more than 10 minutes.

Table 1.5: Features of ACS in relation to risk in ACS			
Features	*High risk (at least 1 of the following features must be present*	*Intermediate risk (no high-risk features but must have 1 of the following)*	*Low risk (no high- or intermediate-risk features, but may have any one of the following)*
History	Accelerating tempo of ischemic symptoms in preceding 48 hours.	Prior MI, peripheral or cerebrovascular disease or CABG, prior aspirin use	—
Character of pain	Prolonged ongoing (>20 minutes), rest pain	Prolonged (>20 min) rest angina now resolved, with moderate of high liklihood of CAD. Rest angina (<20 min) or relieved with rest or sublingual NTG.	New onset or progressive ACS class-III or IV angina in the past two weeks without prolonged (>20 min) rest pain but with moderate or high likelihood of CAD
ECG	Angina at rest with transient ST segment changes >0.05 mv. Bundle branch block, new or presumed new. Sustained VT	T-wave inversion >0.2 mV Pathological Q waves	Normal or unchanged ECG during an episode of chest discomfort
Clinical findings	Pulmonary edema, most likely due to ischemia New or worsening of MR, S3 or New/worsening rales Hypotension, bradycardia, Tachycardia Age >75 years	Age >70 years	—
Cardiac markers	Elevated (Trop-T or Trop-I >0.1 ng/ml)	Slightly elevated (Trop-T >0.01 <0.01 ng/ml)	Normal

ii. It is severe and of new onset (i.e. within prior 4–6 weeks) and/or

iii. It occurs with a crescendo pattern (distinctly more severe, prolonged and frequent than previously)

3. **Non-ST segment elevation myocardial infarction:** It can be defined as:
   i. Clinical features of unstable angina
   ii. Elevated biomarkers of cardiac muscle injury

Pathophysiology of UA/NSTEMI

UA/NSTEMI is mostly caused by:

a. Reduction in oxygen supply to cardiac muscles and/or

b. Increased oxygen demand superimposed on coronary atherosclerosis

Four pathophysiological mechanisms are involved for development of UA/NSTEMI:

a. **Plaque rupture or erosion with an superimposed nonocclusive thrombus**—it is most common cause.

   In this case, **NSTEMI occurs** due to downstream embolization with platelet rich thrombi.

b. **Dynamic obstruction**—coronary spasm—**Prinzmetal angina.**

c. **Progressive coronary obstruction**—advancing coronary atherosclerosis, or re stenosis following percutaneous coronary interventions (PCI).

d. **UA** due to increased oxygen demand and/or decreased oxygen supply—tachycardia, anemia

More than one process may be involved in UA/NSTEMI (Fig. 1.146): These patients studied by coronary angiography:

   i.   5% in left main coronary artery.
   ii. 15% have three vessel diseases.
   iii. 30% have two vessel diseases.
   iv. 40% have single vessel disease.
   v.   10% have no apparent epicardial coronary artery stenosis.

Angioscopy have reported:

   i. White (platelet rich) thrombi
   ii. Red (fibrin rich) thrombi—more common in STEMI

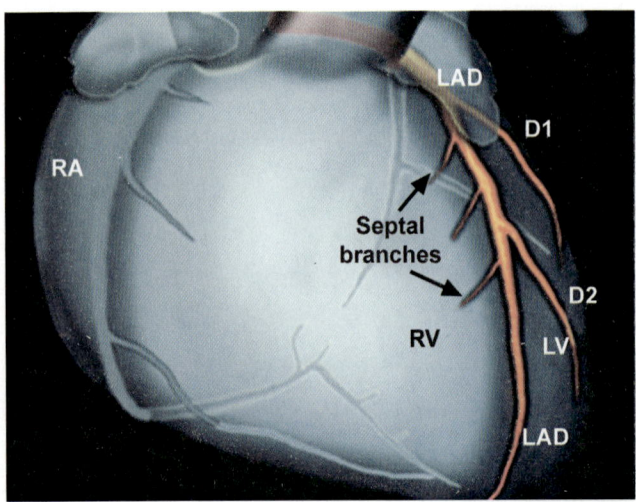

Fig. 1.146: Coronary artery anatomy

Clinical Presentation of UA/NSTEMI

Symptoms

1. Chest pain:
   i.   Substernal, sometimes in epigastrium
   ii. Radiation to neck, left shoulder or left arm.
   iii. Epigastric discomfort
   iv. It lasts for >10 minutes.
2. Epigastric discomfort
3. Dyspnea.

Physical Examination

1. In patient with unstable or stable angina—no obvious physical finding.
2. In patient with large area non-STEMI:
   i.   Sinus tachycardia
   ii. Pale and cool skin
   iii. Third and/or fourth heart sound
   iv. Basal crepitations
   v.   Sometimes hypotension

ECG: In unstable angina:

   i.   ST segment depression >0.05 mV—specific for myocardial ischemia
   ii. ST segment elevation and/or
   iii. T wave inversion >0.3 mV—deep and new—specific for NSTEMI

Serial biomarkers: This is useful:

   i. To differentiate between NSTEMI and UA
   ii. To determine the prognosis

   Measurement of biomarkers to be done 6, 12, 24 and 48 hours after the last episode of pain.

   ECG changes with positive biomarkers—suggestive of NSTEMI

   ECG changes with negative biomarkers—suggest UA

Minor troponin elevation occurs in:

   i.   Congestive cardiac failure
   ii. Myocarditis
   iii. Pulmonary embolism

   Troponin level: It is raised within 3 hours of infarction persists up to 10–14 days (troponin T) and 7–10 days (Troponin I)

   CPK level: It is usually raised in many other conditions, hence it is of little value in diagnosis of NSTEMI

   CPK-MB: It has low specificity and sensitivity.

   CPK-MB isoforms improves sensitivity

$$CPK—MB2 >1 \ U/L$$
$$Or$$
$$CPK-MB2/CPK-MB1 \ ratio >1.5$$

   Myoglobin: It is not cardiac specific. It is increased in as early as 2 hours after onset of symptoms.

   Negative test rule out myocardial necrosis.

Risk Stratification in UA/NSTEMI

Risk stratification should begin on initial evaluation and continuous throughout the hospital stay (Fig. 1.147).

There are two forms of risk stratification:

I. Early risk stratification: This stage starts from initial evaluation at presentation. It involves:
  i. Clinical features
  ii. ECG changes
  iii. Estimation of biomarkers of cardiac injury.

Patients are divided into two risk groups:

a. *High-risk groups:* They should be admitted in ICCU followed by invasive strategy. **They can be managed by:**
  i. Aspirin
  ii. Clopidogrel
  iii. Low molecular weight heparin
  iv. IIb/IIIa
  v. Anti-ischemic therapy—β-blockers (first line), GTN
  vi. Early invasive strategy—in patient catheterization and percutaneous coronary intervention within 48 hours of admission

b. *Intermediate/low risk:* Patient should be admitted in stepdown unit and undergo risk stratification.

Once their symptoms settled to determine timing of invasive investigations, initial management should include:
  i. Aspirin
  ii. Clopidogrel
  iii. Low molecular weight heparin
  iv. Anti-ischemic therapy—β-blocker—first line, GTN.
  v. Undergo late risk stratifications in 48–72 hours from Admission

II. Late risk stratifications: It involves—a number of non-invasive tests to determine: Optional timing for invasive investigations in intermediate/low risk patients.

But **intermediate/low risk patient** develops recurrent pain and/or ischemic ECG changes at any time during his admission or develops heart failure—he should be regarded as high-risk patient—(start IIb/IIIa and early invasive strategy).

Late risk stratification is based on one of the following non-invasive investigations:

A. Exercises ECG test:
  1. *Horizontal/down sloping ST depression with:*
    i. Onset at HR <120/min
    ii. Magnitude of >2.0 mm
    iii. Post-exercise duration of changes >6 min.
    iv. Depression in multiple leads reflecting multiple coronary distributions.
  2. *Abnormal systolic BP response:*
    • Sustained decrease of BP >10 mmHg
    • Flat BP response with abnormal ECG
  3. *Others:*
    i. Exercise-induced ST segment elevation
    ii. Ventricular tachycardia
    iii. Prolonged elevation of heart rate

B. Stress radionuclide myocardial perfusion imaging:
  1. Abnormal tracer distribution in more than one territory
  2. Cardiac enlargement

C. Left ventricular imaging:
  1. Stress echocardiography
    i. Rest EF <35%
    ii. Wall motion score index of >1
  2. Stress radionuclide ventriculography
    i. Rest EF < 35%
    ii. Fall in EF > 10%

Medical Management of NSTEMI/UA

Complete bed rest with continues ECG monitoring for ST segment deviation and cardiac arrhythmia

Ambulation is permitted, if:
  i. Patient shows no recurrence of ischemia
  ii. Patient does not develop biomarkers of necrosis for 12–24 hours

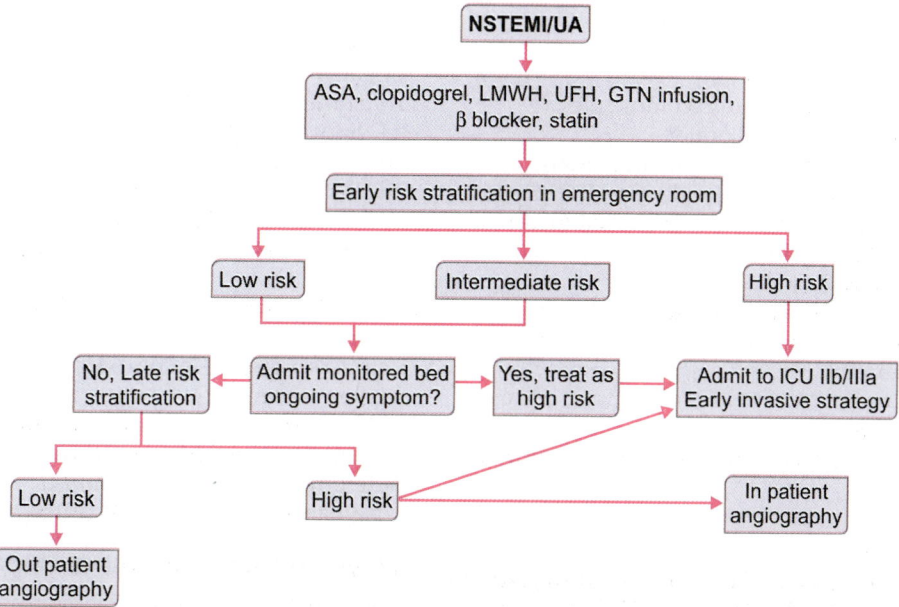

Fig. 1.147: Algorithm of risk stratification in NSTEMI/UA

Therapy should be divided into following categories

Anti-Ischemic Treatment

1. **Nitrates:** 1st to be given sublingually or buccal spray (0.3–0.6 mg)

   ↓

   If patient experiences persistence of pain after 3 doses given 5 min apart.

   ↓

   IV nitroglycerin (5–10 µg/min). Rate of infusion should be increased by 10 µg/min every 3–5 min until
   - i. Relief of pain
   Or   ii. SBP ≤100 mmHg

   ↓

   If pain is relieved, oral nitrates (for 12–24 hours)

   Contraindications:
   i. Patient is hypotensive
   ii. Use of sildenafil or other drugs in that class within previous 24–48 hours
   Side effects: i. Headache   ii. Hypotension

2. **Analgesics:** *Diamorphine* (2.5–5 mg) IV, with antiemetic therapy—acts:
   a. As anxiolytic
   b. Reduce pain and blood pressure through:
      • Venodilatation
      • Reduction in sympathetic arteriolar constriction

   Side effect: Respiratory depression—can be reverted by naloxone—400 µg to 2 mg IV

3. **β-blockers** to be started with

   Metoprolol (12.5–100 mg) thrice daily orally if well tolerated

   ↓

   Converted to atenolol (25–100 mg) once daily

   Rapid β blockade can be achieved by IV metoprolol to maintain heart rate 50–60/min.
   i. If there is overt heart failure—β-blocker is contraindicated.
   ii. Persistent or recurrence of symptoms after full dose of nitrate and β-blocker treatment.

4. **Calcium channel blockers**—having heart rate slowing capacity (verapamil, diltiazem) are recommended.
   Dose of diltiazem   60–360 mg orally
   Verapamil   40–120 mg thrice daily orally
   Calcium channel antagonist alone does not appear to reduce mortality in patient UA. But when combined with nitrate and/or β-blocker—they are effective in reducing symptomatic and silent episodes.

5. **Statin (HMG–CoA reductase inhibitor)**
   Atrovastatin—40 mg—once daily—it:
   i. Reduces the mortality
   ii. Reduces recurrence of MI. Statin is effective in primary and secondary prevention.

6. **ACE inhibitors:** It is effective in primary and secondary prevention

Antiplatelet Therapy

1. **Aspirin:** Initial dose is 325 mg/day—continued till symptomatic improvement followed by 75–150 mg/day to be continued indefinitely

   Side effect:
   i. Gastrointestinal tolerance
   ii. Hypersensitivity
   In that case clopidogrel can be used.

2. **Thienopyridine:** *Clopidogrel*—inactive prodrug—converted into active metabolite—which blocks platelet $P2Y_{12}$ component or adenosine diphosphate receptor.
   Initial treatment dose 300 mg followed by 75 mg orally daily for 9 months
   Clopidogrel better than ticlopidine because:
   i. Its rapid onset of action
   ii. Better safety profile
   Clopidogrel should be avoided in patient requiring CABG for 5–7 days to reduce hemorrhagic complication.
   Prasugrel:
   i. More rapid onset of action
   ii. Higher level of platelet inhibition
   Indication—Following angiography in whom PCI is planned, 60 mg loading dose followed by 10 mg/day for 15 months.

3. **Glycoprotein IIb/IIIa antagonists:**
   i. There are multiple short-acting and long-acting molecules.
   ii. They should be used with aspirin, clopidogrel, LMWH.
   iii. Eptifibatide and tirofiban are the drugs
      Eptifibatide—180 µg/kg IV bolus followed by infusion of 2 mg/kg/min for 72–96 hours
      Tirofiban—0.4 µg/kg/min for 30 mm followed by infusion of 0.1 mg/kg/min for 48 to 96 hours.
   Indication for administration:
   1. High-risk patient with ongoing ischemia and elevated troponin in whom invasive management strategy is not planned.
   2. In patient with early invasive strategy.

Antithrombotic Therapy

1. **Low molecular weight heparin (LMWH):** It is more effective in short-term reduction of death, myocardial infarction, and revascularization in patient with NSTEMI/UA, than unfractionated heparin.
   They should be used in conjunction with aspirin and clopidogrel and continued for 2–5 days after last episodes of pain and ischemic ECG pattern.
   Advantages over UFH:
   i. Subcutaneous administration
   ii. Lack of monitoring
   iii. Reduced resistance
   iv. Reduced incidence of thrombocytopenia

2. **Unfractionated heparin:** It reduces the risk of death in NSTEMI/UA. It is to be continued with aspirin and clopidogrel for 2–5 days or till pain relief or lack of ECG changes.
   Initial bolus 60–70 unit/kg IV followed by 12–15 unit/kg/hr. maximum 1000 unit/hour
   Monitor—APTT value 1.5–2 times normal control.
   Complications: Excessive bleeding is the most important side effect of all antithrombotic agents including anticoagulants and antiplatelet drugs.

Invasive Versus Conservative Strategy

Multiple trial showed that early invasive strategy benefits in high risk patient, e.g.

i. Have multiple risk factors.
ii. ST segment deviations
iii. Positive biomarkers:
  a. Recurrent angina   b. Elevated troponin T or I
  c. New ST segment depression
  d. Positive stress test
  e. EK <0.40   f. Decreased BP
  g. Sustained VT   h. PCI <6 months, prior CABG

In this strategy

Treatment with anti-ischemic, antithrombotic agents
↓
Coronary angiography within 48 hours
↓
Coronary vascularization or coronary or artery bypass grafting (It depends upon coronary anatomy).

Mortality

1. Early (30 days) mortality rate in AMI—30% more than half of these patients die **before reaching in the hospital**.
2. **Mortality rate after admission** decreased by 30%.
3. In past two decades, mortality is 4-fold higher in elderly individual than younger patient.

Pathophysiology of STEMI

Acute Plaque Rupture

Main cause is acute and abrupt decrease in blood through coronary artery due to thrombotic occlusion of that artery already previously affected by atherosclerosis.

Slow steady decrease in coronary blood never produces STEMI because of development of rich collateral circulation overtime.

Provocating factors:
  i. Smoking   ii. Diabetes   iii. Hyperlipedemia

Pathways Leading to Development of STEMI

1. Atherosclerotic plaque (having rich lipid core and thin fibrous disruption cap are prone to early risk of rupture)
↓
Platelet monolayer forms at the site of ruptured plaque
↓
Various agonists (ADP collagen, epinephrine, serotonin) are stimulated and come into play
↓

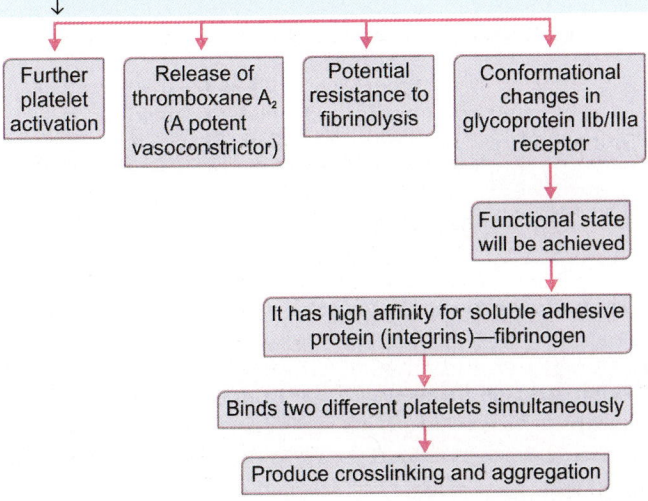

2. **Coagulation cascade will be activated** on exposure of tissue factors of damaged endothelial cell at the site of disruption
↓
Factor VII and factor X are activated
↓
Prothrombin → thrombin
↓
Fibrinogen → fibrin
Fluid phase and clot bound thrombin—participate in auto-amplification
↓
Further activation of co-agulation cascade

So coronary artery becomes occluded by—thrombus containing platelet aggregates and fibrin strands.

Amount of Myocardial Damage Caused by Coronary Artery

Occlusion depends upon following factors:
1. Territory supplied by affected vessels.
2. Whether the vessel is completely occluded or not
3. Duration of coronary artery occlusion
4. Emergence of collateral circulation or not
5. Amount of blood supplied to the affected tissue by collateral vessels
6. Oxygen demand of the affected myocardial tissue.
7. Presence or absence of endogenous factors—which can produce early spontaneous lysis of occlusive thrombus.
8. Adequacy of myocardial perfusion in infarct zone, when the flow is restored by reopening of epicardial coronary artery.

Less common medical conditions predispose to development of STEMI are:
  i. Hypercoagulability
 ii. Cocaine abuse
iii. Collagen vascular disease
 iv. Intracardiac thrombi

Clinical Presentations of STEMI

Precipitating factors:
1. Physical exercise
2. Emotional stress
3. Medical illness
4. Surgical illness

Pain

1. Site—central portion of chest and/or epigastrium
2. Radiation—radiation to arms—most common—less commonly to abdomen, back, lower jaw, and neck
3. Type of pain—heavy, squeezing, crushing, stabbing or burning
4. It usually occurs at rest, not relieved by sublingual nitroglycerin
5. Pain radiates as high as occiput but never below umbilicus
6. Pain may be accompanied by—sweating, nausea, vomiting, sense of impending doom

Important exclusion in diagnosis: Radiation of discomfort to trapezius—suggests pericarditis

Painless STEMI:
1. Diabetes mellitus
2. Elderly

In these conditions—patient may present with sudden onset of breathlessness, with progression to pulmonary edema.

Other less common presentation:
1. Sudden loss of consciousness
2. Confusional state
3. Sensation of profound weakness
4. Appearance of arrhythmia
5. Unexplained drop in blood pressure

Physical Findings

i. Patient becomes restless, unsuccessful moving on the bed to get rid of pain.
ii. Sweating, cool and clammy extremities
iii. In 1st hour of STEM—patients have normal pulse rate, and blood pressure.

But, ¼th of patients with anterior myocardial infarction have manifestation of sympathetic overactivity (tachycardia, hypertension).

Half of patients with inferior myocardial infarction have manifestation of parasympathetic overactivity (bradycardia, hypotension).

Signs in precordium:
1. In anterior myocardial infarction—abnormal systolic pulsation heard in periapical area within first a few days then resolve. This is caused by dyskinetic bulging of infracted myocardium.
2. Third heart sound due to ventricular dysfunction
3. Fourth heart sound
4. Paradoxical splitting of 2nd heart sound
5. A transient midsystolic or late systolic apical murmur due to dysfunction of mitral valve apparatus.
6. Pericardial friction rub—heard in case of transmural infarction

Signs in peripheral areas:
1. Carotid pulse—decrease in volume—due to reduced stroke volume
2. Systolic pulse pressure declines 10–15 mmHg from preinfarction state.

3. Temperature elevation up to 38°C—may be present in 1st week of STEMI.

Laboratory Investigations

Myocardial infarction progresses through three temporal stages:
1. Acute (first a few hours to 7th day) phase
2. Healing (8th day to 28th day) phase
3. Healed phase (≥ 29th day)

Laboratory investigations can be subdivided into 4 groups:
   i. ECG
   ii. Cardiac biomarkers
   iii. Non-specific

Electrocardiogram (Figs 1.148 to 1.152)

ST segment elevation: It occurs within minutes and may last for up to 2 weeks.
a. *Thrombolysis criteria are:*
   i. ST elevation ≥ 2 mm on adjacent chest leads
   ii. ST segment elevation ≥ 1 mm in limb leads
b. *Persistant ST segment elevation after 1 month:* Left ventricular aneurysm
c. *Infarction site can be diagnosed from ECG changes:*
   i. Anterior wall—ST elevation and/or Q waves in V1–V4/V5.
   ii. Anteroseptal wall—ST elevation and/or Q waves in V1–V3.
   iii. Anterolateral wall—ST elevation and/or Q waves in V1–V6 and L1 and aVL.

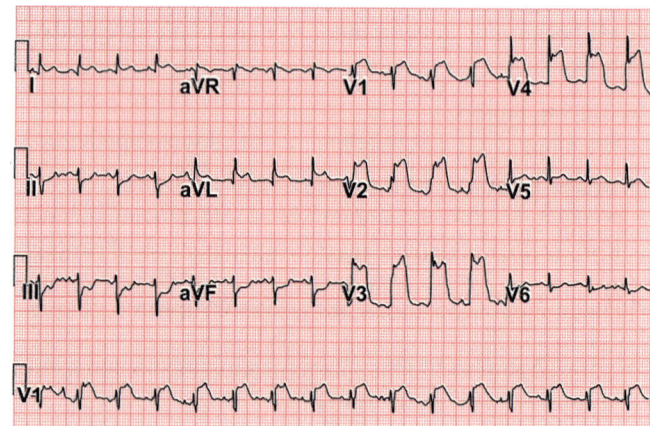

Fig. 1.148: Acute anterior wall myocardial infarction

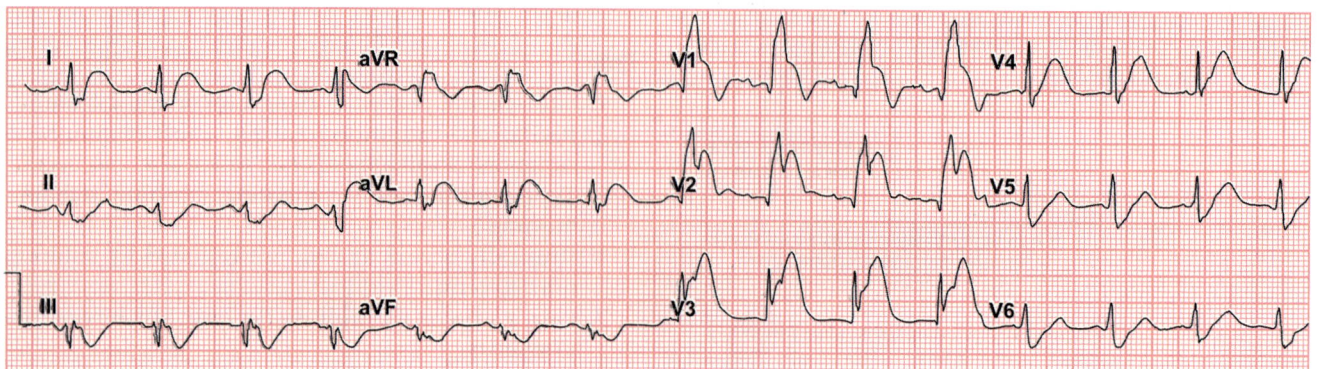

Fig. 1.149: Septal infarction

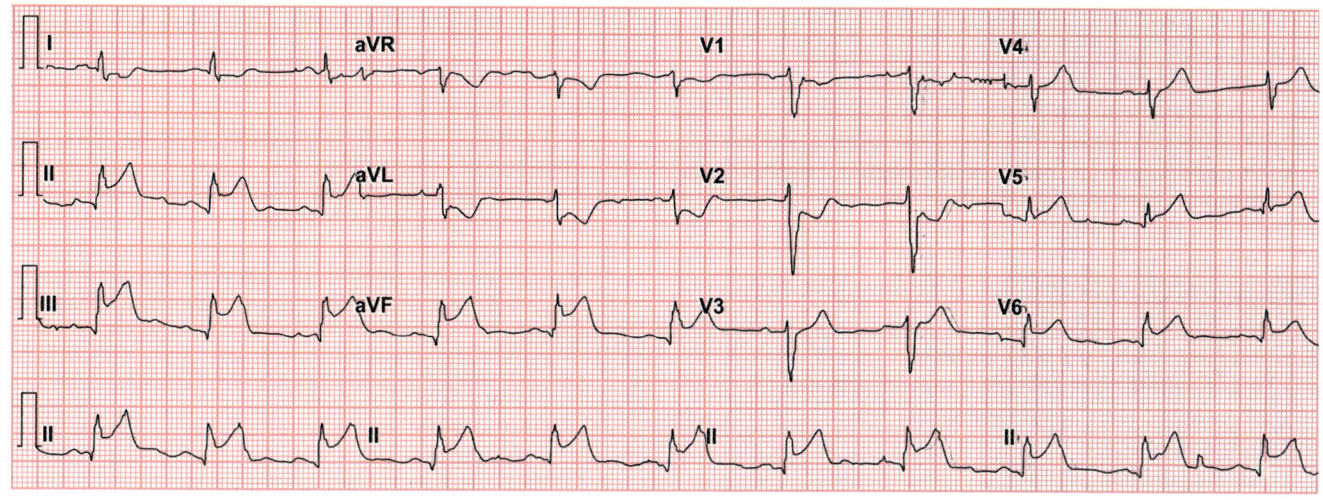

Fig. 1.150: Inferior wall myocardial infarction

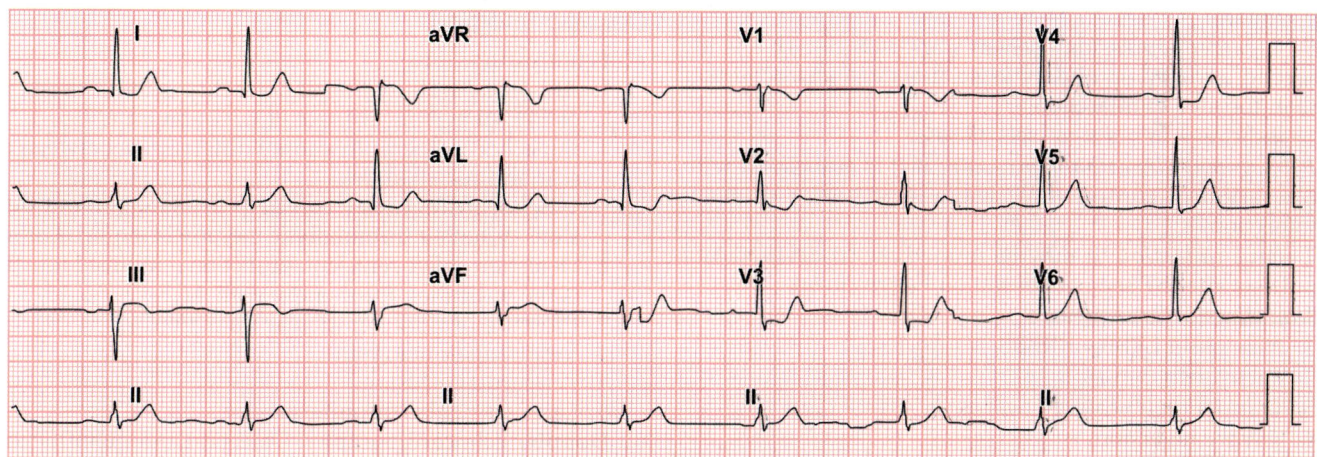

Fig. 1.151: Posterior wall myocardial infarction

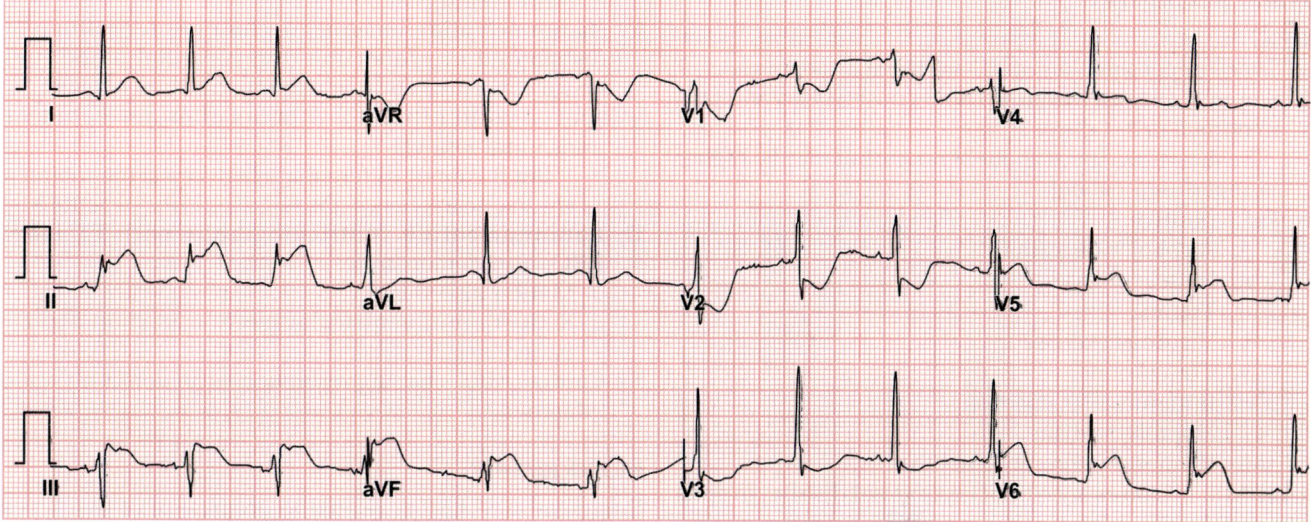

Fig. 1.152: Lateral wall myocardial infarction

iv. Lateral—ST segment elevation and/or Q waves in V5–V6 and T wave inversion/ST segment elevation—L1 and aVL

v. Inferolateral—ST segment elevation and/or Q waves—in L2, L3, aVF, V5–V6.

vi. Inferior wall—ST segment elevation and/or Q waves in L2 L3, aVF

vii. Inferoseptal—ST segment elevation and/or Q wave in L2, L3, aVF, V1–V3.

viii. True posterior:
- Tall R waves in V1–V2
- ST segment depression in V1–V3
- T waves remain upright in V1–V2
- This can be confirmed with an esophageal lead

ix. Right ventricular infarction: ST segment elevation in right precordial leads V_{1R}–V_{4R}

It is usually present with inferior wall myocardial infarction

d. *Pathological Q waves:* It indicates transmural infarction—and hours or days to develop.

Identification of pathological Q waves:
i. Q weave should be >25% of R wave having duration of 0.04 seconds, with negative T wave
ii. In precordial leads
   a. In V4 >0.4 mV
   b. In V6 >0.2 mV

In absence of LBBB (QRS width <0.1 sec or 3 small square)

e. *ST segment depression* (ischemia at distance): This is the second territory, secondary to ischemia in a territory other than the area of infarction.

Indicative of multi-vessels disease.

f. *PR segment elevation/depression:* If it is associated with alteration in contour of P wave—indicative of atrial infarction.

g. *T wave inversion:* It may be immediate or delayed and persists after ST segment elevation has resolved.

h. *Non-diagnostic changes:*
1. New onset LBBB, or RBBB
2. Tachyarrhythmias.
3. Transient tall peaked T waves
4. T wave inversion
5. Axis shift

Cardiac Biomarkers

a. **CPK:**
1. Twice upper limit of normal are taken as abnormal.
2. Serum level rises within 4–8 hours post-STEMI and falls to normal in 3–4 days.

   Peak level occurs at about 24 hours; but may be higher in reperfused patient.
3. False positive:
   i. Alcohol intoxication
   ii. Muscle disease
   iii. Trauma
   iv. Vigorous exercise
   v. Convulsions
   vi. Intramuscular injection
   vii. Hypothyroidism
   viii. Pulmonary thromboembolism

b. **CPK-MB:** It is more specific of myocardial disease, in spite of normal CPK.

CPK-MB is also present in small quantities in other tissues:
   i. Skeletal muscle
   ii. Tongue
   iii. Diaphragm
   iv. Uterus
   v. Prostate

False positive test—occurs in:
   i. Trauma   ii. Surgery
So cardiac troponin must be measured.

c. **Cardiac troponin:**
i. Both trop T and trop I are highly sensitive and specific markers of cardiac injury
ii. Serum levels start to rise by 3 hours post-STEMI. It may persists up to 7–14 days
iii. In the event of normal CPK—MB level, suspected non-cardiac sources of CPK, troponin level can be used.
iv. It is >20 times higher than normal in patient with STEMI.
v. Cardiac troponin can also be elevated in:
   a. Myocarditis
   b. Cardiomyopathy
   c. Pericarditis
   d. AST—rise in 18–36 hours post-MI
   e. LDH—rise in 24–36 hours post-MI

Cardiac Imaging

A. **Echocardiography:**
1. Abnormal wall motion abnormality is the earliest sign of STEMI even in absence of ECG abnormality.
   But echocardiography cannot differentiate between old scar and recent attack.

   Echocardiography can help in management decision—whether thrombolytic therapy is required or not.
2. Detection of left ventricular function—reduced function is the indication for therapy with ACE-I
3. Presence of right ventricular infarction
4. Ventricular aneurysm
5. Pericardial effusion
6. Left ventricular thrombus

B. **Doppler echocardiography:** Detection and quantification of:
   i. Ventricular septal defect
   ii. Mitral regurgitation

C. **Radionucleotide imagineg technique:** Technitium[99]—is distributed in proportion to myocardial blood flow—hence concentrated in viable myocardium—detect "cold spot"—within first a few hours after development of transmural infarct.

   But it cannot differentiate between acute infarct and chronic scar—hence it is not diagnostic of acute MI.

D. **Radionucleotide ventriculography with T[99] labeled RBC**—can demonstrate:
   i. Motion disorder
   ii. Reduction in ventricular ejection fraction in STEMI patient.

E. **Cardiac MRI**—having resolution—can detect myocardial infarction.

Management

Prognosis of STEMI is related to occurrence of two types of complications

i. Electrical complication (arrhythmia)
ii. Mechanical complication (pump failure)

Commonest complication in NSTEMI is ventricular fibrillation—which occurs within 24 hours of symptoms, half of them within 1 hour. **So major elements in prehospital care include:**

i. Recognition of symptoms by patients and seek medical advices.
ii. Rapid deployment of medical emergency team, capable of performing resuscitative maneuvers including fibrillation also.
iii. Urgent transportation of patient to proper cardiac care hospital
iv. Implementation of reperfusion therapy.

Management in Emergency Department

The goal of management is:
1. Control of discomfort
2. Rapid identification of patient, who are the candidates of reperfusion therapy.
3. Shifting of low-risk patient to proper location in hospital
4. Avoidance of inappropriate discharge from the hospital.

In emergency department:
i. **Aspirin**—325 mg to be given orally to be chewed in emergency room.
It inhibits cyclooxygenase–1 in platelets followed by reduction of thromboxane A_2 level. This is followed by daily 75 mg orally.
ii. **Supplemental oxygen**—to be given by face mask (2–4 L/min) for 6–12 hours after infarction.

Control of Discomfort

1. **Sublingual nitroglycerin:** Three doses of 0.4 mg each to be administered at 5 minutes intervals.
   Effect: It abolish chest discomfort in:
   i. Decreasing myocardial oxygen demand (lowering preload)
   ii. Dilating infarct related coronary vessels or collateral vessels—increasing oxygen supply to myocardium.
   If patient responds to sublingual nitroglycerin and return of discomfort after stoppage of sublingual nitroglycerin, then intravenous nitroglycerin should be started.

   Contraindication:
   i. Patient with systolic arterial pressure <90 mmHg
   ii. In patient with inferior wall infarction associated with right ventricular infarction—having features of elevated jugular venous pressure, clear lungs and hypotension.
   iii. In patient taking phosphodiesterase-5 inhibitor, sildenafil, preceding 24 hours—because it may potentiate action of nitrates.

   Idiosyncratic reaction: Sudden hypotension—can be recovered completely by administration of intravenous atropine.

2. **Morphine:** Dose is intravenous injection of 2–4 mg rather than subcutaneous administration of large doses.
   Effect: It reduces sympathetically mediated arteriolar and venular constriction—resulting venous pooling and reduces cardiac output and arterial pressure.
   This hemodynamic compromise can be reversed by:
   i. Elevation of legs
   ii. Volume expansion by IV saline

   Toxicity: Vagotonic effect—producing bradycardia and heart block—whilst can be revered by intravenous atropine.

3. **Beta-blocker:**
   Mode of action:
   i. Diminishes myocardial oxygen demand
   ii. It reduces the risk of reinfarction
   iii. It reduces the risk of ventricular fibrillation.
   Oral beta-blocker should be initiated in patient who does not have any of the following:
   a. Sign of heart failure
   b. Evidence of low output
   c. Evidence of cardiogenic shock

   Contraindication to beta-blocker:
   i. Prolonged PR interval
   ii. Second or third degree block
   iii. Bronchial asthma

   Dose: Metoprolol—5 mg every 2–5 minutes for a total 3 doses in patient having:
   i. Heart rate >60/min
   ii. Systolic blood pressure >100 mmHg
   iii. PR interval <24 seconds.
   iv. Rales not higher than 10 cm up from the diaphragm
   Oral dose:
   i. It should be started 15 minutes after the last intravenous dose.
   ii. 50 mg every 6 hours for 48 hours followed by 100 mg every 12 hours.

Measurement Strategies

Primary tool for screening the patient and making decision for PCI or reperfusion therapy is: ST segment elevation of at least 2 mm in 2 contiguous precordial leads and 1 mm in 2 adjacent limb leads.

Limitation of infarct size: In myocardial infarction:
i. Central zone of the infarct contains necrotic tissue which is irreversibly lost.
ii. Peripheral ischemic zone can be recovered by following methods
   a. Timely restoration of coronary perfusion
   b. Reduction of myocardial oxygen demand
   c. Prevention of accumulation of noxious metabolites
   d. Blunting the effect of mediators of reperfusion injury (calcium overload, oxygen derived free radicals)
One-third of patient may achieve spontaneous reperfusion of infarct related coronary artery.

In rest of the patients, reperfusion can be achieved by either fibrinolysis or primary percutaneous intervention.

Timely restoration flow to epicardial coronary artery (infarct related) combined with downstream zone perfusion, results in limitation of infarct size.

Glucocorticoid and NSAID should be avoided in patient with STEMI because:
i. It impairs the would healing
ii. Increased risk of myocardial rupture
iii. Development of large scar

Primary Percutaneous Coronary Perfusion

a. It means—angioplasty and/or stenting without preceding fibrinolysis.
b. It should be done within 1st a few hours of MI.

c. **It is more effective than fibrinolysis in opening occluded coronary arteries when:**
  i. Performed by experienced operators (>75 PCI cases/year)
  ii. Done in dedicated medical centers (≥ 36 PCI cases/year)

Primary PCI is generally preferred than fibrinolysis because:
  i. When diagnosis is in doubt.
  ii. Patient is in cardiogenic shock.
  iii. Bleeding risk is increased.
  iv. Symptoms have been present for at least 2–3 hours.
  v. Clot is mature.
  vi. Less easily lysed by fibrinolytic drugs.

Fibrinolysis

Fibrinolytic agents are:
1. Tissue plasminogen activator
2. Streptokinase
3. Tenecteplase (TNK)
4. Reteplase (rPA)

Mode of action: All the drugs promote the conversion of plasminogen to plasmin—which subsequently lyses fibrin thrombi.

Bolus fibrinolytics are TNK and rPA—because their administrations do not require prolonged intravenous infusions.

Angiographic assessment of culprit coronary artery described as **thrombolysis in myocardial infarction (TIMI) grading system (qualitative scale):**

Grade 0: Complete occlusion of infarct related artery.
Grade 1: Some penetration of contrast material beyond the point of obstruction but without perfusion of distal coronary bed
Grade 2: Perfusion of entries infarct vessel into distal bed, but flow is delayed as compared to normal coronary artery.
Grade 3: Full perfusion of infarct related vessel with normal flow.

Later is the goal of reperfusion therapy because full reperfusion of infarct related coronary artery:
  i. Limits the infarct size
  ii. Maintains left ventricular function
  iii. Reduction of both short- and long-term mortality rate by preventing serious complications:
    a. Septal rupture
    b. Cardiogenic shock
    c. Malignant ventricular arrhythmias.

So timing of reperfusion therapy is of extreme importance for salvaging injured myocardium and preventing complication, e.g.:
a. Best salvage in 1–2 hours of therapy
b. Therapy remains of benefit, if within 3–6 hours
c. Some benefit is within 12 hours.

Fibrinolysis is preferred than PCI in those cases where:
  i. Transport of patient to PCI center takes >1 hours.
  ii. Patients <70 years achieve greater relative reduction in mortality rate.

IPA, TNK and rPA are more effective than streptokinase in restoring full perfusion (TIMI grade 3 flow).

Current recommended doses of fibrinolytic drugs:
1. 1-PA—15 mg bolus followed by 50 mg intravenously over first 30 minutes followed by 35 mg over next 60 minutes.
2. Streptokinase: 1.5 MU intravenously over 1 hour.
3. rPA—10 MU bolus given over 2–3 minutes, followed by second 10 MU bolus 30 minutes later.
4. TNK—Bolus 0.53 mg/kg over 10 seconds.

Alternative pharmacologic regimen for reperfusion: Intravenous administration of glycoprotein IIb/IIIa inhibitor + reduced dose of fibrinolytic agents.

Above combination produces the following effective improvement: Facilitate the rate and extent of fibrinolysis by:
  a. Inhibiting platelet aggregation
  b. Weakening of clot structure
  c. Allowing the fibrinolytic agent to enter deep into clot
But contraindications:
  i. Age > 75 years
  ii. Risk of bleeding

Clear contraindication to use of fibrinolytic agents:
1. Histry of cerebrovascular hemorrhage at any time
2. Histry of non-hemorrhagic stroke or cerebrovascular events in last 1 year.
3. Marked hypertension (SBP >180 mmHg and DP >110 mmHg at any time during their acute presentation).
4. Suspicion of aortic dissection
5. Active bleeding from any site (excluding menses)
6. In elderly person, since there is chance of hemorrhagic complications—it should not be given except incase of large myocardial wall jeopardy.

Relative contraindications: This requires assessment of risk: benefit ratio—including:
  i. Current use of anticoagulant (INR—≥ 2)
  ii. Recent (<2 weeks) invasive or surgical procedure
  iii. Prolonged (>10 minute) cardiopulmonary resuscitation.
  iv. Known bleeding diathesis
  v. Pregnancy
  vi. Hemorrhagic ophthalmic condition
  vii. Peptic ulcer disease
  viii. History of recently controlled severe hypertension

Complications

Allergic Reactions

It occurs in 2% of patient with streptokinase therapy—ranging from mild hypotension to severe reaction.

Hemorrhagic Manifestation

From any sites—it may require blood transfusion. So unnecessary venous or arterial intervention should be avoided.

Hemorrhagic stroke occurs in 0.5 to 0.9%, mainly in >70 years. Incidence increases with advancing age.

Percutaneous coronary intervention is required in following cases:
1. Failure of reperfusion (persistant chest pain and ST segment elevation >90 minutes)
2. Coronary artery reocclusion (re-elevation of ST segment and/or recurrent chest pain)
3. Development of recurrent ischemia (chest pain, recurrent angina)

Clinical determination of successful reperfusion: Resolution of chest pain is an inaccurate measure of reperfusion because it may be blunted by narcotic analgesic administration.

Complete resolution of chest pain associated with electrocardiographic changes (>70% resolution of ST segment elevation) accompanied by accelerated idioventricular rhythm.

Hospital Phase Management

Admission in coronary care unit—patient should be monitored by electrocardiographic monitor, with provision of ventilator, defibrillator, respirator, non-invasive intrathoracic pacemaker.

Patient should be transferred out of the unit:
i. When the symptoms are well controlled by oral therapy.
ii. If the patient is at low risk (no prior infarction, no persistent chest discomfort, hypotension, congestive cardiac failure).

Activity:
1. First 12 hours—complete bed rest
2. Next 24 hours—he should be allowed to put his limbs by the side of bed dangling.
3. In absence of hypotension or other complication—he will be allowed to ambulate in his room. He may use showers or stand at the risk for bath.
4. By third day, infarction—patient should by gradually increasingly ambulant—the goal will be 600 ft/day.

Diet:
i. Because of risk of emesis or aspiration soon after STEMI, patient should receive nothing or clear liquid for 12 hours.
ii. If there is no complication—then patient can take solid food.

Cardiac diet usually contains:
i. >30% of total calories as fat
ii. Cholesterol content ≤300 mg
iii. 50–55% of total calories—complex carbohydrates.
iv. Dietary portion should not be unusually large.
v. Diet contains—high potassium, magnesium, and fiber but low in sodium
vi. Diabetes and hypertriglyceridemia—should be managed by restriction of sweets in diet.

Bowel movement: As narcotic analgesic is responsible for constipation, following methods are used to avoid constipation:
1. Regular use of bedside commode
2. Diet rich in bulk
3. Routine use of stool softener—Dioctyl sodium sulphosuccinante 200 mg/day
4. Use of laxative, if constipation persists.

Sedation: Diazepam 5 mg or oxazepam (15–30 mg) or lorazepam (0.5–2 mg) to be given 3–4 times daily.

But continuous vigilance in coronary care unit during first few days may interfere with sleep. Hence quiet surrounding is also necessary for proper sleep of patient.

Pharmacotherapy

Antithrombotic agents
Primary goal: To maintain patency in infarct related artery in conjunction with reperfusion strategy.

Secondary goal: To reduce the patient's tendency to develop rethrombosis, deep vein thrombosis and pulmonary embolization.

a. **P2Y12 receptor inhibitor:** Clopidogrel—it inhibits P2Y12 ADP receptors and prevents activation and aggregation of platelets.

If it is added to the treatment with aspirin in STEMI patient—it:
i. Reduces the risk of death, reinfarction, stroke
ii. Prevents reocclusion of successfully reperfused artery.
Newer agents—Prasugrel and ticagrelor—are more effective than clopidogrel in preventing PCI complications in STEMI patient undergoing PCI, but increased risk of bleeding

b. **Unfractionated heparin**—If it is added to the regimen containing aspirin and thrombolytic agents—mortality rate will be reduced (5 live saved/1000 patients treated).

It helps to maintain the patency of the vessels (infarct related artery) with small risk of bleeding.

Recommended dose: Initial bolus—60 U/kg (maximum 4000 units) intravenously followed by initial infusion of 12 U/kg per hour (maximum 1000 U/kg)
The target APTT should be 1.5–2 times the target value.

c. **Low molecular weight heparin**
Advantages:
i. High bioavailability
ii. Permitting administration subcutaneously
iii. No monitoring is required
iv. Greater anti-Xa: IIa activity
Enoxaparin has been shown to reduce significantly the composite end points of death/non-fatal MI.

The drug is fondaparinux—it should not be used alone in PCI because there is chance of catheter thrombosis. So it should used with other anticoagulant.

The other drug is bivalirudin—it has direct antithrombnin activity.

Beta adrenergic blocker: This drug can be given—acutely during MI can be continued in long term as secondary prevention after infarction.

Acute intravenous beta blockade:
i. Improves myocardial oxygen supply—demand relationship
ii. Decreases pain
iii. Reduces infarct size
iv. Decreases the incidence of serious ventricular arrhythmias
v. Decreases the incidence of recurrent ischemia and reinfarction.

β-blocker therapy is contraindicated in:
i. Heart failure
ii. Severe compromised left ventricular function
iii. Heart block
iv. Orthostatic hypotension
v. Bronchial asthma

It should not be used in patient with excellent long-term prognosis, defined as:
1. Expected mortality rate <1%/year
2. Patient <55 years
3. No previous myocardial infarction
4. Normal ventricular function
5. No complex ventricular ectopy
6. No angina

Inhibition of renin–angiotensin–aldosterone system: It reduces mortality when it will be added with Beta-blockers and aspirin.

Maximum benefit seen when used in following high-risk patient:
 i. Elderly patients
 ii. Anterior wall infarction
 iii. History of prior infarction
 iv. Globally depressed left ventricular function

The mechanism is:
1. Reduction in remodeling after infarction
2. Subsequent reduction in risk of congestive heart failure. Rate of recurrent infarction is lower in patient with ACE-1.

ACE-I should be continued indefinitely in following patients:
 i. Who have clinically evident congestive heart failure.
 ii. In whom imaging study shows reduction in global left ventricular function.
 iii. In whom large regional wall motional abnormality
 iv. Those are hypertensive.

Angiotensin receptor blocker should be administered to STEMI patient:
i. Who are intolerant to ACE inhibitor.
ii. Who have clinical and radiological sign of heart failure.

Long-term aldosterone blockade should be prescribed in patients with STEMI:
 i. Without significant renal dysfunction (creatinine ≥ 2.5 mg/dl in men, ≥ 2 mg/dl, in women
 ii. Without hyperkalemic (potassium ≥ 5.0 mEq/L)
 iii. Who have LV ejection fraction ≤40% and diabetic or symptomatic heart failure.

Other agents:
Intravenous nitroglycerin: 5–10 mg/min initial dose—up to 200 mg/min (as long as hemodynamic stability is maintained) for 24–48 hours after the onset of infarction.

Complications

Ventricular Dysfunction

There are series of changes in size, shape and thickness of infracted and non-infracted related left ventricular wall leading to discordant motion of ventricular wall.

Pathophysiology:

After STEMI, left ventricle begins to dilate due to expansion of infracted area of left ventricle
↓
Disproportionate thinning and elongation of infracted zone
↓

(Contd.)

(Contd.)

Disproportionate lengthening of non-infarcted segments
↓
As a result, there is gross dilatation of left ventricular wall and apex in relation to size and location of infarct
↓
Gross hemodynamic impairment
↓
Left ventricular failure or congestive cardiac failure (months to years after infarction)

Prognosis is poor

Treatment:
 i. ACE inhibitor
 ii. Other vasodilators (nitrates)
 iii. In patient with LVEF <40% with or without heart failure ACE-I or ARBs should be prescribed.

Pump Failure

Left ventricular dysfunction correlates with size of infarct area. Patients with small infarct have regional wall motion abnormality and normal left ventricular function, because of compensatory hyperkinesis of remaining normal ventricular wall.

Risk Factors for Cardiogenic Shock

 i. Prior myocardial infarction
 ii. Older age
 iii. Female sex
 iv. Diabetes
 v. Anterior infarction

Classification originally proposed by Killip divides patients into 4 groups:
a. **Class-I:** No sign of pulmonary or venous congestion
b. **Class-II:** Moderate heart failure evidence by rales at lung bases S3 gallop tachypnea, or sign of failure of right side of the heart including hepatic and venous congestion.
c. **Class-III:** Severe heart failure. Pulmonary edema
d. **Class-IV:** Shock with systolic pressure <90 mmHg evidence of peripheral vasoconstriction peripheral cyanosis, mental confusion, oliguria

Causes

1. Complication of acute myocardial infarction:
    i. Extensive left or right ventricular infarction
    ii. Ventricular septal rupture
    iii. Acute severe mitral regurgitation
    iv. Cardiac tamponade with or without free wall rupture
2. Other causes:
    i. Myocarditis
    ii. Aortic dissection
    iii. Massive pulmonary embolism
    iv. Critical valvular stenosis
    v. Acute mitral or aortic regurgitation.

Clinical Presentation

Symptoms:
  i. Respiratory distress
  ii. Diaphoresis
  iii. Cool and clammy extremities
  iv. Orthopnea
  v. Oliguria
  vi. Confusion

Signs:
  i. Dyskinetic ventricular impulse palpable
  ii. S3 gallop
  iii. Evidence of mitral regurgitation, if present.

Diagnosis

1. Combination of clinical and physiological measures
2. Clinical:
   i. Persistent hypotension >30 minutes
   ii. Systolic blood pressure <80–90 mmHg
3. Physiological—low cardiac index <1.8L/mm/m^2 with elevated left ventricular filling pressure (pulmonary capillary wedge pressure >18 mmHg)

Management

1. **Correction of reversible factors:**
   a. Arrhythmia—aim to restore sinus rhythm
   b. Acid-base, electrolyte abnormalities
   c. Ventilation abnormalities
2. **Rapid hemodynamic evaluation:** Adequate monitoring and access:
   a. Central venous access
   b. Swan-Ganz arterial line
   c. Urinary catheter
3. **Rapid echocardiographic evaluation:**
   a. Assess left ventricular systolic function
   b. Exclusion of mechanical lesion
      i. Mitral regurgitation
      ii. Ventricular septal defect
      iii. Ventricular aneurysm/pseudoaneurysm
4. **Rapid angiographic evaluation:**
   a. Systolic blood pressure ≥ 90 mmHg guided by
      i. Physical signs and
      ii. Left ventricular filling pressure
   b. PCWP <15 mmHg—cautious IV fluids (colloids) in 100–200 ml aliquots
   c. PCWP >15 mmHg—inotropic support and diuretic therapy, if pulmonary.
5. **Inotropic agent:**
   a. It should be avoided in STEMI patient, if at all possible.
   Aim:
      i. Rapidly restore the coronary artery flow
      ii. Decrease load of LV
   b. If hemodynamic status will not improve after revascularization—inotropic drugs should be used. Choice of agents should be guided by following manner:
      i. If patient is hypotensive (± pulmonary edema) Start with dopamine (up to 15 µg/kg/min), if ineffective Substitution with dobutamine and norepinephrine
      ii. If patient has adequate blood pressure (± pulmonary edema)—dobutamine to increase cardiac output (starting with 2.5–3 µg/kg/min and increase up to 20 mg/kg/min) till hemodynamic improvement. Norepinephrine can be added.
      iii. Diuretics, thrombolysis, GP IIb/IIIa antagonists: LMWA/UFH should be followed in original guideline

Bradyarrhythmias

1st degree AV block:
1. Common, therapy is not required
2. Significant PR prolongation—it is contraindication to beta blockade.
   2nd degree AV block: It occurs when conduction system will be affected due to large area of infarction. Types are:
1. *Mobitz type-1:*
   i. Self-limiting
   ii. No symptoms
   iii. If requires no specific treatment
   iv. If it will progress to complete heart block, if needs temporary pacing.
2. *Mobitz type-2:* It is always be treated by temporary pacing.

Third degree block:
1. In case of inferior wall MI, temporary pacemaker is not usually required unless:
   i. It is associated with hemodynamic abnormality or
   ii. Escape rhythm <40/min.
2. In case of anterior wall myocardial infarction—temporary pacing is always required.

Tachyarrhythmias

Supraventricular Tachyarrhythmia

It usually occurs, secondary to:
  i. Anemia
  ii. Fever
  iii. Heart failure
  iv. Metabolic derangement

Treatment:
1. Primary problem should be treated first
2. If tachyarrhythmia is due to sympathetic overstimulation—treatment with β-blocker.
   • IV 1 mg over 1 minute, repeated every 2 minutes up to maximum 10 mg.
   • Orally 10–40 mg—3–4 times/day
3. In case of atrial flutter or atrial fibrillation, secondary to left ventricular failure

> Digoxin—is the drug of choice
> • Loading IV—0.75–1 mg in 50 ml saline over 1–2 hours
> • Orally—0.5 mg—12 hourly × 2 days
> ↓
> 0.25 mg—12 hourly × 2 days
> Then maintenance dose—0.25 mg—daily or on alternate day

4. In absence of hart failure, beta blocker, verapamil or diltiazem is the drug of choice.
5. If abnormal rhythm persists >2 hours, ventricular rate >120/min.
   Or

If tachycardia includes congestive cardiac failure, shock, ischemia—(recurrent ischemic pain, and ECG changes)—synchronized electroshock (100–200 J monophasic wave form).

Accelerated Idioventricular Rhythm

It occurs is posteroinferior wall myocardial infarction—digitalis excess must be ruled out.

Treatment should be:
i. Right atrial pacing, or
ii. Coronary sinus pacing

Ventricular Premature Beats

i. It is common and not related to incidence of sustained ventricular tachycardia/ventricular fibrillation
ii. It is frequent, multifocal, early diastolic.
iii. Generally treated conservatively and aim to correct acid base and electrolyte abnormalities (aim K >4. 0 mmol/L)
iv. Pre-infarction beta blockade reduces ventricular premature beat.

Ventricular Tachycardia

Sustained Ventricular Tachycardia

Treatment
1. Correction of acid-base abnormalities or electrolyte imbalance
2. Intravenous administration

Amiodarone (bolus of 150 mg over 10 minutes followed by infusion of 1 mg/min for 6 hour → then 0.5 mg/min)
Or
Procainamide (bolus 15 mg/kg over 20–30 minutes, then infusion of 1–4 mg/min)
↓
If ventricular tachycardia continues
↓
Electrocardioversion (unsynchronized discharge of 200–300 Jules)
↓
If patient is refractory to electrocardioversion
↓
Epinephrine 1 mg IV or 10 ml of 1:10,000 solutions via intracardiac route.
Or
Amiodarone—75–150 mg bolus.

Torsades de Pointes

It is polymorphic ventricular tachycardia, occurs as a consequence of:
i. Hypoxemia
ii. Hypokalaemia
iii. Hypomagnesemia
iv. Other electrolyte imbalance
v. Toxic effects of digoxin, quinidine

Treatment:
i. Magnesium is the drug of choic—1–2 gm over 30–60 seconds
ii. Overdrive pacing.

Ventricular Fibrillation

In patient with STEMI, predisposing factors are:
1. Congestive heart failure
2. Shock
3. Bundle branch block
4. Ventricular aneurysm

The patient who develops VF or VT after first 48 hours of admission, mortality is high in long-term follow-up.

Such patient should be treated with implantation of defibrillator/cardioverter.

Right Ventricular Infarction

One-third of patients with inferior wall myocardial infarction may develop right ventricular necrosis and right ventricular infarction.

This may occur with inferoposterior left ventricular infarction.

Clinical presentation:
1. Jugular venous distension
2. Kussmaul's sign
3. Hepatosplenomegaly
4. With or without systemic hypotension

ECG manifestation: ST segment elevation in right precordial leads (V4R–V6R)

Echocardiographic presentation:
i. Right ventricular dilatation
ii. Right ventricular wall motion abnormalities

Management:
1. Aims to maintain high right ventricular preload:
    i. Volume expansion
    ii. Nitrates and diuretics should be avoided, because it may reduce preload and worsen hypotension.
    iii. In some patients, AV synchronous pacing to maintain normal cardiac output
    iv. Cardioversion in case of any arrhythmia.
2. Reduce afterload:
    i. This is particularly important, if there is concomitant LV dysfunction.
    ii. Arterial vasodilators can be used with caution (sodium nitroprusside, hydralazine) or ACE inhibitors.
3. Avoidance of inotropic drugs, but can be used if all other measures fail tor restore hemodynamic status.
4. Reperfusion of right coronary artery.

Ventricular Septal Rupture (Fig. 1.153)

It occurs within 24 hours to 10 days post-MI, affects 2–4% patients.

Clinical features: Low-cardiac output with harsh pansystolic murmur at left lower sternal edge, poor perfusion and pulmonary edema.

Diagnosis

i. Two-dimensional and Doppler echocardiography demonstrate the presence of left-to-right heart shunt.

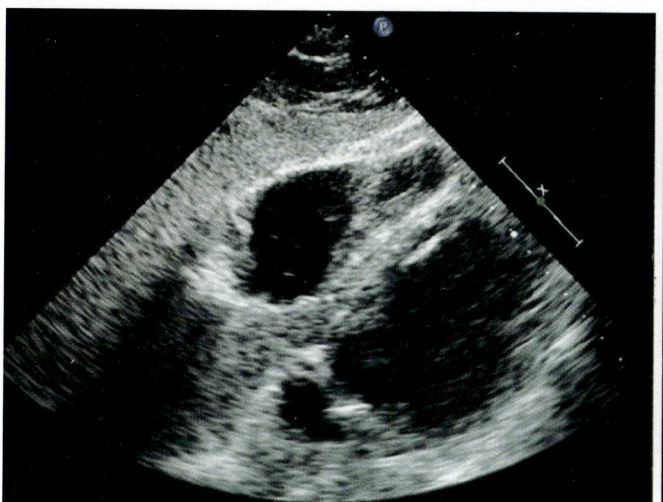 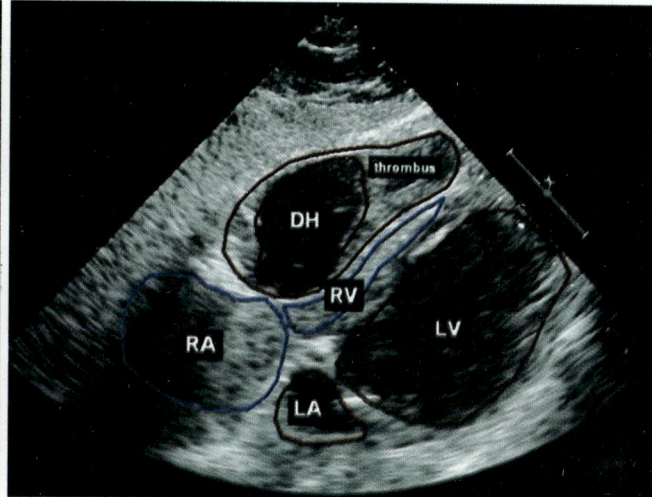

Fig. 1.153: *Septal rupture*

ii. In case of anterior wall myocardial infarction rupture occurs at apex.

iii. In case of interior wall myocardial infarction rupture occurs at base.

iv. Failure to demonstrate shunt on Echo does not exclude VSD.

Management:

1. *Stabilization* of the patient:

   a. Right atrial and pulmonary artery pressure dictate—fluid administration and diuretic use.

      Cardiac output, mean arterial pressure and arterial resistance determine the need for vasodilator therapy.

   b. If SBP >100 mmHg, vasodilator—**nitroprusside** will lower the:

      i. Systemic vascular resistance

      ii. Reduce the magnitude of shunt.

      Nitrate should be avoided because this venodilator increases the shunt.

   c. *Inotropes*—increases the systemic pressure, so should be avoided.

   d. In most cases, **intra-arterial balloon counter-pulsation** may reduce the shunt.

   Surgical: For high-risk patient; early surgical repair—combined with CABG ± mitral avalve replacement/repair.

Left Ventricular Aneurysm (Fig. 1.154)

It can be defined as dyskinesia or local expansile paradoxical wall motion of left ventricle.

In this case, normal myocardial fibers contract more, if cardiac output and stroke volume are to be maintained in patient with ventricular aneurysm.

True aneurysm is composed of scar tissue, so neither predisposes nor is associated with cardiac rupture.

This occurs weeks to months after STEMI.

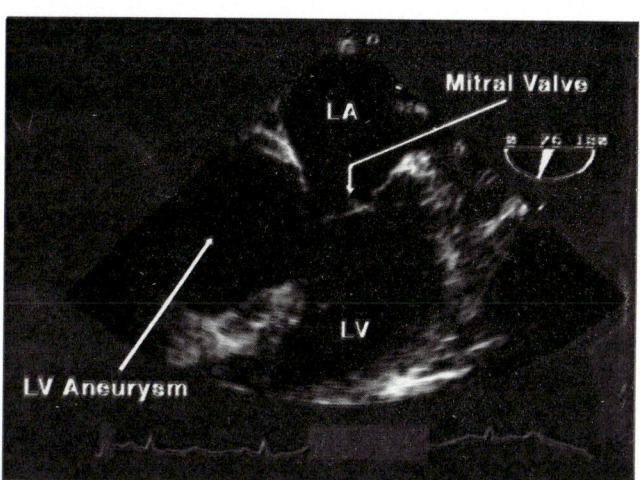

Fig. 1.154: *Left ventricular aneurysm*

Complication of ventricular aneurysm:

i. Congestive cardiac failure

ii. Arterial embolization

iii. Ventricular arrhythmias

Apical aneurysm is most common. It can present with—double, diffused, displaced apical impulse.

Echocardiography can demonstrate:

i. Apical aneurysm

ii. Thrombus

Myocardial Pseudoaneurysm

Sometimes myocardial rupture is contained by local area of pericardium along with organizing thrombus and hematoma—this is called pseudoaneurysm.

Later on, it communicates with left ventricle through a narrow neck.

Complication: Spontaneous rupture.

Treatment: Surgical repair.

Myocardial Infarction (Fig. 1.155)

Complications: Complications of acute myocardial infarction is depicted in Fig. 1.156.

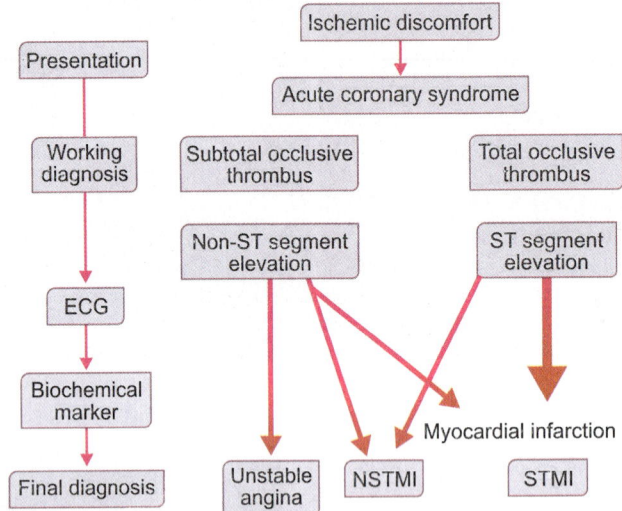

Fig. 155: ST elevated myocardial infarction

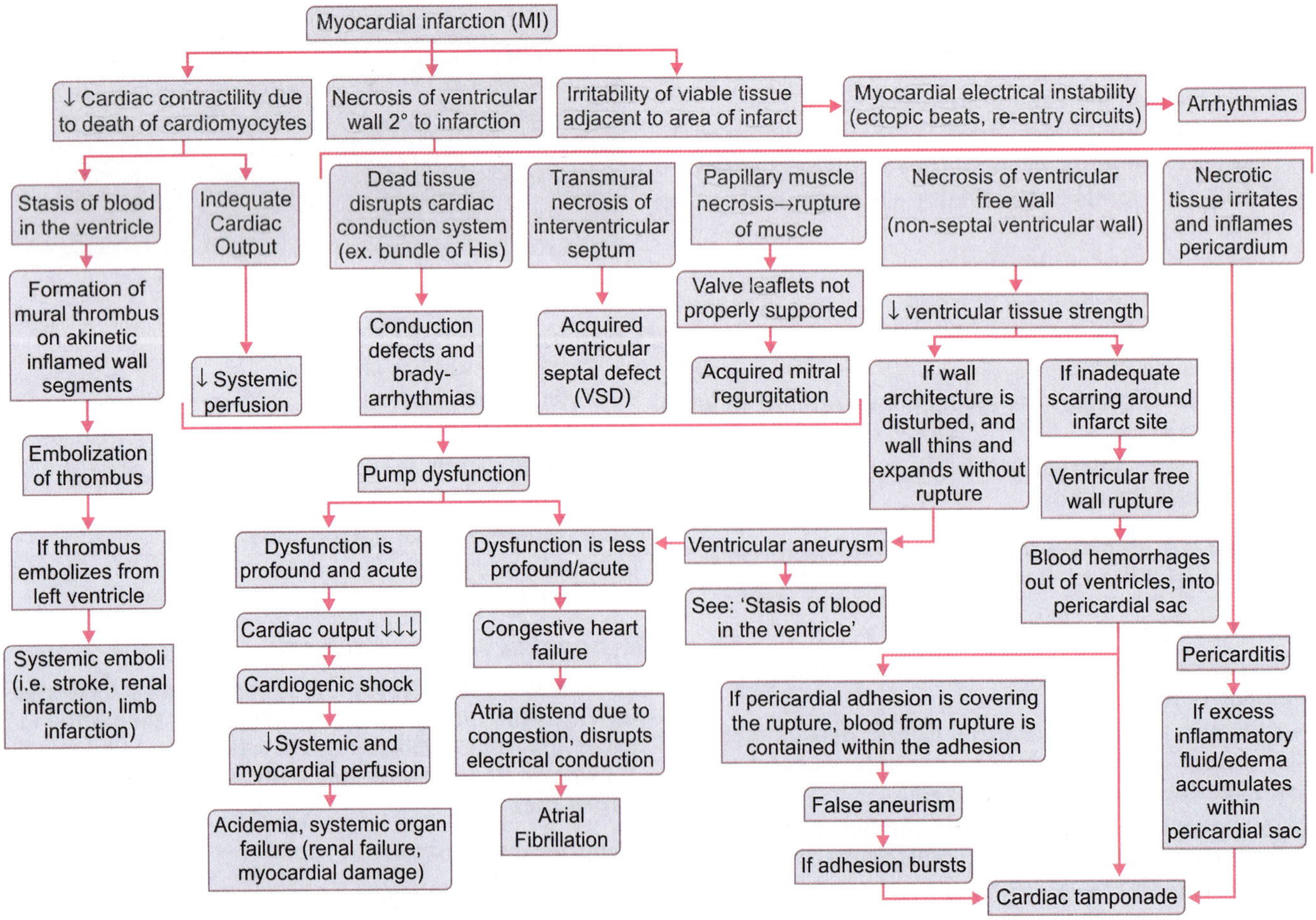

Fig. 156: Algorithm of complication of acute myocardial infarction

LOWN-GANONG-LEVINE SYNDROME

It is a pre-excitation syndrome consists of:
  i. WPW syndrome
 ii. LGL syndrome
iii. Mahaim type pre-exitation

An LGL syndrome has short PR interval and normal QRS complex. No single structural abnormality has been detected as a cause of LGL syndrome, but several structural abnormalities have been proposed—which include presence of James fiber, Mahaim fibers, Brechenmacher type fiber, or anatomically under developed small AV node.

According to modern view, electrophysiological studies, and histopathological studies have identified several underlying mechanism as a cause of short PR interval and normal QRS. These are:

  i. Enhanced AV nodal conduction
 ii. Several types of fibers that bypass all or part of AV node
iii. Anatomically small AV node.

Age: Average age of onset is 33.5 years.

History

  i. Palpitations
 ii. Light headedness
iii. Shortness of breath

Episodes of tachycardia may induce:

  i. Cardiac stress producing angina
 ii. Hypotension
iii. Other hemodynamic instability.

Physical Signs

During paroxysm:
a. Tachycardia
b. Accentuated 1st heart sound

Etiology: Not known

Workup

I. Laboratory studies:
  i. Serum electrolytes
 ii. Thyroid profile
iii. Complete blood count to exclude anemia, infection.

II. ECG:
  i. Short PR interval
 ii. Normal QRS complex. Presence of delta wave excludes the diagnosis of LGL.

III. Holter monitoring: It may diagnose paroxysms.
IV. Procedures:
  i. If tachycardia is present—Valsalva maneuvers can determine the cause.
 ii. In stable patient with no history of angina, pre-syncope, carotid sinus massage during 12-lead rhythm strip monitoring—it may terminate tachycardia or may produce transient AV block.
iii. Trial of intravenous adenosine to terminate tachycardia with simultaneous rhythm strip recording.

But it should not be administered, if there is any evidence of pre-excitation on surface ECG.

Management

1. **Medical care:** Treatment should be based on the cause of tachycardia, rather than tachycardia itself.

   But in outpatient setting—empiric therapies for recurrent RSVT like, beta blocker, calcium channel blocker, and digoxin can be instituted.
2. **Surgical therapy:** In rare cases, where medical therapy fails and in whom recurrent intolerable symptoms are continued, in such cases—pacemaker implantation followed by radiofrequency ablation of AV node or bundle of His can be considered.

PERICARDIAL DISEASE

Normal pericardium is double-layered sac (Fig. 1.157)—consisting of:

1. Visceral pericardium—serous membrane
2. Fibrous parietal pericardium

Two above layers are separated by an ultrafiltrate of plasma of 15–50 ml.

Function:
  i. It prevents sudden dilatation of cardiac chambers especially right atrium and right ventricle.
 ii. It restricts the anatomic position of the heart.
iii. It minimizes friction between heart and surrounding structures.
 iv. It prevents kinking of great vessels.
  v. It retards the progression of infection from lung and pleural cavities to the heart.

Acute Pericarditis

This is a clinical syndrome caused by inflammation of pericardium characterized by:

  i. Chest pain
 ii. Friction rub
iii. Characteristic electrocardiographic abnormalities.

It is common in adult male—aged between 20 and 50 years.

Classifications

Clinical classification
  I. *Acute pericarditis* (<6 weeks):
   A. Fibrinous
   B. Effusive (serous or serosanguinous)
 II. *Subacute pericarditis* (6 weeks to 6 months):
   A. Effusive—constrictive
   B. Constrictive

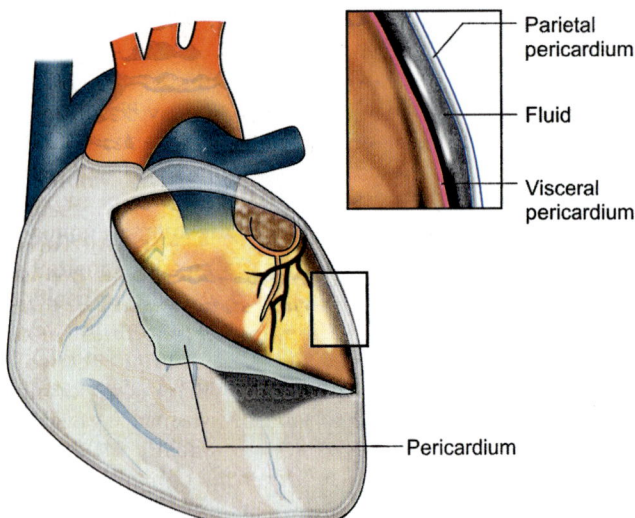

Parietal pericardium
Fluid
Visceral pericardium
Pericardium

Fig. 1.157: Anatomy of pericardium

III. Chronic pericarditis (>6 months):
  A. Constrictive   B. Effusive
  C. Adhesive (nonconstrictive)

Etiological classifications:
  I. Infectious pericarditis:
  A. Viral (coxasackie virus A and B, echovirus, mumps, adenovirus, HIV)
  B. Bacterial (Pneumococcus, Streptococcus, Staphylococcus, Neisseria)
  C. Tuberculous
  D. Fungal (Histoplasma, coccidioidomycosis, candida)
  E. Other infections (syphilitic, protozoal, parasitic)
  II. Non-infectious pericarditis:
  A. Acute myocardial infarction
  B. Uremia
  C. Neoplasia—i. Primary tumor (benign or malignant)
       ii. Tumor metastasis to pericardium
  D. Myxedema
  E. Cholesterol
  F. Trauma—i. Penetrating   ii. Nonpenetrating
  G. Aortic dissection—with leakage to pericardial sac.
  H. Post-irradiation—familial pericarditis
  I. Acute idiopathic sarcoidosis
  III. Autoimmune pericarditis:
  A. Rheumatic fever
  B. Collagen vascular disease (SLE, rheumatoid arthritis, ankylosing spondylitis, scleroderma, Wegener's granulomatosis)
  C. Drug-induced:
    i. Procainamide
    ii. Hydralazine
    iii. Phenytoin
    iv. Minoxidil
    v. Isoniazid
    vi. Methysergide
  D. Post-cardiac injury:
    i. Post-myocardial infarction
    ii. Post-pericardiotomy
    iii. Post-traumatic

Clinical Features

A. Chest pain: This symptom has spectrum of presentation:
  i. It may be absent in:
    a. Tuberculous
    b. Post-irradiation
    c. Neoplastic, and
    d. Uremic pericarditis
  ii. It may be severe, retrosternal and left precordial and referred to neck, arm and left shoulder.
  iii. Sometimes steady, constricting pain radiating to either arm or both arms—resembles that of acute myocardial ischemia (AMI)

Pericardial pain:
  i. May be relieved by sitting up and leaning forward
  ii. Intensified by lying supine position.
Serum biomarkers may be modestly elevated if there is involvement of epicardium along with pericardium. The biomarkers are:
  i. Creatine kinase
  ii. Troponin

B. Pericardial friction rub: It is heard in 85% of patient. It can be described as:
  i. High-pitched, rasping, scratching sound—can be elicitated when diaphragm of stethoscope is applied firmly to the chest wall at the left lower sternal border—it is heard at the end of expiration with upright position and leaning forward.
  ii. Loud, to and fro, leathery sound disappears within few hours and may reappear next day.

Difference between pleural rub and pericardial rub:
  i. Pericardial rub is usually heard in both phase of respiration. Pleural rub disappears when respiration is suspended.
  ii. Pericardial rub is lathery sound but pleural rub is gritty in character.
  iii. Pleural rub is intensified when diaphragm of the stethoscope is pressed over the affected areas but there is no change in character of pericardial rub.

C. Electrocardiographic abnormalities: This finding in absence of massive effusions—occurs due to acute subepicardial changes.

This evolves through four stages:
  1. Wide-spread elevation in ST segments with concavity upwards—in 2 to 3 standard leads and V2 to V6, with reciprocal depression in avR and V1
  2. In stage 2—after several drugs, ST segments returns to normal
  3. Stage-3—T waves become inverted
  4. Stage-4—weeks to months after—ECG returns to normal

In contrast in AMI:
  i. ST segment elevation with convexity upwards
  ii. More prominent reciprocal depression
  iii. Significant change in QRS complex
    a. Development of Q waves
    b. Nothing or loss of R wave amplitude
    c. T wave inversion is usually seen within hours before ST segment becomes isoelectric.

Comparison with early repolarization syndrome:
- T wave is usually tall and ST/T ratio is <0.25
- In acute pericarditis ST/T ratio is >0.25

D. Other features: Constitutional symptoms—depending upon the course:
  i. In purulent pericarditis—high fever, shaking chills, and night sweats.
  ii. In tuberculous pericarditis—fever, chills and night sweat.

Laboratory Abnormalities

1. **Chest X-ray**—may reveal cardiomegaly and yield important information in support of tuberculous and neoplastic process.
2. **Blood culture**—explore purulent or tuberculous pericarditis.
3. **Sputum to diagnosis infections etiology**—bacteria or tuberculosis.
4. **Pericardial biopsy** to diagnose tuberculosis.
5. **Blood test:**
   i. Leukocytosis
   ii. Raised ESR
   iii. Modest elevation of CPK-MB, troponin levels, creatinine suggests involvement of epicardium.
6. **Echocardiography:** Pericarditis is not an echocardiographic diagnosis. Its symptoms last longer than a week, echocardiography is essential to evaluate hemodynamic abnormalities.
7. **ECG.**

Treatment

Most of acute pericarditis is **self-limited**.

First line of therapy is NSAIDs with addition of colchicines in some cases.

NSAIDs:
  i. Ibuprofen—400–600 mg thrice daily
  ii. Indomethacin—25–50 mg thrice daily
  iii. Colchicine—0.6 mg twice daily

Steroid: Glucocorticoid can be administered in case of recurrent pericarditis with persistent symptoms despite NSAIDs and colchicine therapy, and exclude purulent pericarditis.

Dose: 1–1.5 mg/kg/day for at least 1 month.

After patient becomes asymptomatic for about a week, gradual tapering of dose of NSAID is usually required.

Colchicine and glucocorticoid are useful for recurrences. In spite of treatment with above drugs, if patient is symptomatic, pericardiotomy is necessary to terminate the illness.

Complications

1. **Recurrent pericarditis:** It occurs after:
   i. An episode of idiopathic pericarditis
   ii. Open heart surgery
   iii. Cardiac trauma
   iv. Dressler's syndrome
      It occurs in 20–30% of patients
      Clinical presentation similar to acute pericarditis.

Therapy:
  i. *Prednisolone* (1–1.5 mg/kg/day) for 1 month then tapered slowly. If there is recurrence on cessation of steroid
  ii. *Pericardiotomy*
2. **Cardiac tamponade:** It commonly occurs after cardiac surgery or neoplasm.
3. **Constrictive pericarditis**—9% of patients develop mild constrictive pericarditis—thin usually resolve after 3 months.
4. **Effusive constrictive pericarditis**—This is subacute term having both effusion and pericardial thickening.
   It may progress to constrictive pericarditis.

Pericardial Effusion

Accumulation fluid in pericardial sac is called pericardial effusion.

Etiology

Similar to acute pericarditis. But large effusions are mainly:
  i. Neoplastic   ii. Tuberculosis
  iii. Uremia   iv. Myxedema

Symptoms and Signs

Symptoms depend upon:
  i. Volume of fluid accumulated.
  ii. Rate of accumulation
  iii. Characteristics of fluid.

Patient having large pericardial effusion may be asymptomatic, again rapid accumulation of fluid may be severely symptomatic.

Unstretched pericardium may accumulate only 80–200 ml of fluid, but large pericardial effusion contains as much as 1.2 litre of fluid—but may be asymptomatic.

Clinical Presentation

  i. Slowly developing pericardial effusion with no elevation of intrapericardial pressure is asymptomatic.
  ii. May present with constant dull aching sensation or pressure on the chest.
  iii. May present with compressive symptoms:
      a. Dysphagia from esophageal compression.
      b. Dyspnea from lung compression or atelectasis.
      c. Hiccup from compression of phrenic nerve.
      d. Nausea, vomiting, abdominal distension from pressure on adjacent abdominal organs.

Signs:
  i. Sinus tachycardia
  ii. Hypertension—from hemodynamic compromise
  iii. Disappearance of friction rub
  iv. Non-palpable apex beat
  v. Heart sound on auscultation is usually distant.
  vi. Ewart's sign: Dullness on percussion, bronchial breath sounds and egophony below the angle of left scapula—due to compression of base of the lung.
  vii. If patient develops cardiac tamponade:
      a. Pulsus paradoxus greater than 10 mmHg
      b. Jugular venous distension with 'X' decent is typically predominant waveform
      c. Beck's triad:
        1. Jugular venous distension
        2. Distant heart sound   3. Hypotension

Laboratory Investigations

ECG abnormalities:

i. Sinus tachycardia
ii. Low voltage QRS complexes with non-specific ST-T wave changes
iii. Electric alternans—suggests massive pericardial effusion
iv. Total electrical alternans (P-QRS-T) pathognomonic of cardiac tamponade.

Chest X-ray (Fig. 1.158): Water bottle configuration of the cardiac silhouette.

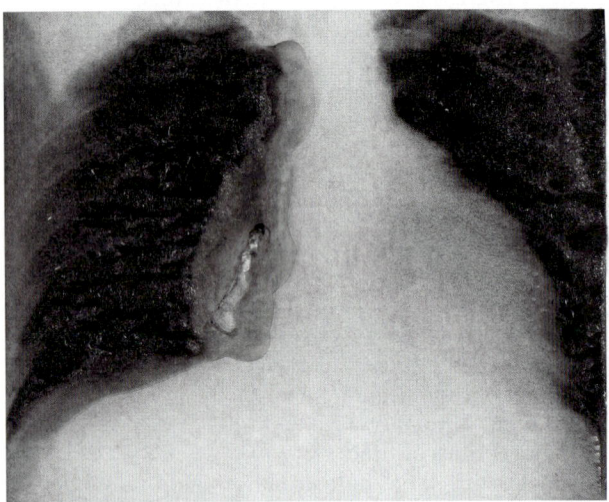

Fig. 1.158: Water bottle configuration of the cardiac silhouette

Echocardiography (Fig. 1.159):

i. *In case of small effusion:* A relatively echo free space between posterior pericardium and left ventricular epicardium.

ii. *In case of large effusion:* An echofree space between anterior right ventricle and parietal pericardium just beneath anterior chest wall.

Following features are more common in patients with marked inflammatory or malignant pericardial effusion:

a. Soft tissue density masses
b. Thickening of visceral pericardium
c. Presence of fibrinous strands.

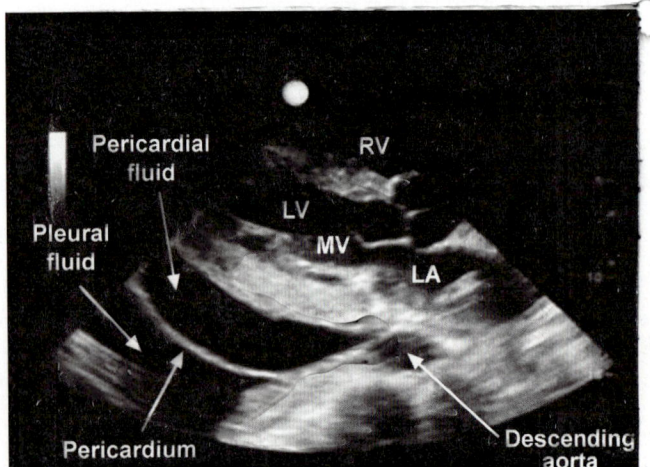

Fig. 1.159: Echocardiograophic demonstration of pericardial fluid

Cardiac catheterization: It can establish the diagnosis and severity of cardiac tamponade, but rarely necessary. **The important findings are:**

i. Equilibration of right atrial, right ventricular end diastolic and mean capillary wedge pressure
ii. Rapid 'x' descent or right atrial pressure waveform
iii. Pulsus paradoxus

Management

i. When effusion does not cause any hemodynamic impairment and cause is known (uremia, myxedema)—treatment of underlying cause.
ii. If the cause is unknown—**pericardiocentesis** and aspiration of pericardial fluid to clench the diagnosis, nature of effusion (exudative or transudative). The fluid has to be sent for culture and sensitivity (both aerobic and anaerobic), bactec culture for tuberculosis.
iii. **Surgical drainage** is necessary for:
   a. Purulent pericarditis
   b. Hemopericardium

Cardiac Tamponade

Definition

The accumulation of fluid in pericardial space in a quantity sufficient to cause serious obstruction to the inflow of blood into the ventricles results in cardiac tamponade.

Causes

Three most common causes of cardiac tamponade are:

i. Neoplastic cause
ii. Renal failure
iii. Idiopathic pericarditis

The other causes: Bleeding into pericardial space with cardiac tamponade occurs in:

i. Trauma
ii. Cardiac operations
iii. Treatment with anticoagulants
iv. CRF patients on MHD.

Clinical Features

a. Three principal features of cardiac tamponade (Beck's triad):
   i. Hypotension
   ii. Soft or absent heart sounds
   iii. Jugular venous distension with prominent 'x' descent and Absenty descent

   The quantity of fluid necessary to develop cardiac tamponade may be as small as 200 ml when it develops rapidly or >2000 ml in slowly developing effusion.

b. Pulsus paradoxus: >10 mmHg of inspiratory decline in systolic arterial pressure—it may be detected by palpation of peripheral pulse disappearance during inspiration.

   Low pressure tamponade: Here intrapericardial pressure is increased from slightly subatmospheric pressure to +5 to +10 mmHg associated with hypovolemia.

Here:

i. Central venous pressure is normal or slightly elevated
ii. Arterial pressure is unaffected.
iii. No pulsus paradoxus

The patients are usually asymptomatic or complains of mild dyspnea.

Diagnosis

Echocardiography—same as pericardial effusion.

Treatment

Clinical and hemodynamic improvement occurs after pericardiocentesis

Doppler ultrasound in cardiac tamponade:
i. Tricuspid and pulmonary valve flow velocities increase markedly during inspiration.
ii. Pulmonary vein, mitral and aortic flow velocities are diminished.
iii. Right ventricular cavity is reduced in diameter.
v. May be late diastolic inward motion of right ventricular free wall and right atrium.

Pericardiocentesis is the treatment of choice for cardiac tamponade. Post-pericardiocentesis pericardial fluid is examined for: Bloody fluid:

- Neoplasm in developed world
- Post-myocardial infarction
- Anemia
- Tuberculosis
- Post-cardiac injury
- Dialysis

Pericardial fluid should be analyzed for:
i. RBC
ii. WBC
iii. Cytogenic study for cancer
iv. Microscopic studies
v. Culture
vi. Presence of ADA >30 UIL and presence of DNA of *Mycobacterium tuberculosis*—as determined by PCR—supports the diagnosis of tuberculous pericarditis.

Treatment of the etiology of pericardial effusion to be done according to the nature of the fluid and the result of culture and sensitivity of the fluid.

Constrictive Pericarditis
Evolution of Chronic Pericarditis

i. During healing of acute serofibrinous or fibrinous pericarditis or
ii. Resorption of chronic pericardial effusion

↓

Followed by obliteration of pericardial cavity with formation of granulation tissue

↓

The granulation tissue contracts to form scar

↓

Calcification scar results in encasement of heart in a rigid pericardium

↓

This may interfere with filling of both ventricles

Common Causes of Constrictive Pericarditis

I. Idiopathic:
1. Infectious diseases
2. Tuberculous
3. Bacterial
4. Viral
5. Fungal
6. Parasitic
II. Trauma (post-cardiac surgery)
III. Radiation
IV. Inflammatory:
1. Rheumatoid arthritis
2. SLE
3. Scleroderma
4. Sarcoidosis
V. Neoplastic disease:
1. Breast cancer
2. Lung cancer
3. Lymphoma
4. Mesothelioma
VI. Chronic renal failure

Pathophysiology

i. In constrictive pericarditis, ventricular filling is unimpeded during early diastole, but as the elastic limit of rigid pericardium is reached, diastolic filling is reduced abruptly whereas, in case of cardiac tamponade; ventricular filling is impeded throughout the diastole.
ii. In both conditions ventricular end-diastolic volumes and stroke volumes are reduced.
   End diastolic pressure, in both ventricles, mean pressure in atria, pulmonary vein, systemic vein are all elevated to similar level (within 5 mmHg of one another)
iii. Fibrotic process may extend into myocardium—producing myocardial scarring and atrophy.
iv. Venous congestion—is due to both:
   a. Pericardial lesions
   b. Myocardial lesions

In constrictive pericarditis:
A. Left and right atrial pressure pulse shows:
   - **An M-shaped contour with prominent X and Y descent.**
   - Y descent is absent in cardiac tamponade but prominent in constrictive pericarditis, because it reflects rapid early filling of the ventricles. But Y descent is interrupted by rigid pericardium which impedes 'rapid early filling of ventricles and produces rapid rise in atrial pressure.
   This characteristic change is reflected in jugular vein -0 which can be seen.
B. Ventricular pressure pulse of both ventricle show '√ square root signs during diastole.

Clinical Features

1. Weakness
2. Fatigue
3. Weight gain
4. Increased abdominal girth
5. A protuberant abdomen
6. Edema

In late cases:
1. Anasarca
2. Skeletal muscle wasting
3. Cachexia
4. Exertional dyspnea is common. Negative history includes—no left ventricular failure.

Signs
1. *Jugular veins:*
   a. Prominent X and Y descent
   b. Jugular vein distended—reflects elevated right-sided pressure.
   c. Kushmaul's sign—inspiratory increase in venous distension—This is not pathognomonic, because it may occur in right ventricular infarction or right ventricular hypertrophy and tricuspid stenosis.
2. *Pulsus paradoxus*
3. *Congestive hepatomegaly*—may produce hepatic dysfunction and jaundice
4. *Apical impulse* reduced and retracts in systole (Broadbent's sign)
5. *Distant heart sound*
6. *Third heart sound* (pericardial knock) heard at cardiac apex 0.09–0.12 seconds after aortic valve closure—it occurs due to abrupt cessation of ventricular filling
7. *Systolic murmur* of tricuspid regurgitation
8. *Peripheral edema*
9. *In pulmonary area,* sudden instantaneous widened splitting of 2nd heard sound—occurs following 1st heart beat of inspiration (Vogelpoel-Beck sign)

ECG

i. Lowe voltage QRS complexes
ii. Wide flattening and inversion of T waves
iii. Atrial fibrillation common in 1/3rd of cases

Chest X-ray (Figs 1.160, 1.161)

1. Near normal cardiac size, in presence of marked venous distension or heart failure—suggestive of constrictive pericarditis or restrictive cardiomyopathy.
2. Pericardial calcification

Echocardiography

1. Pericardial thickening
2. Dilatation of inferior vena cava and hepatic veins
3. Sharp halt in ventricular filling in early diastole with normal ventricular systolic function

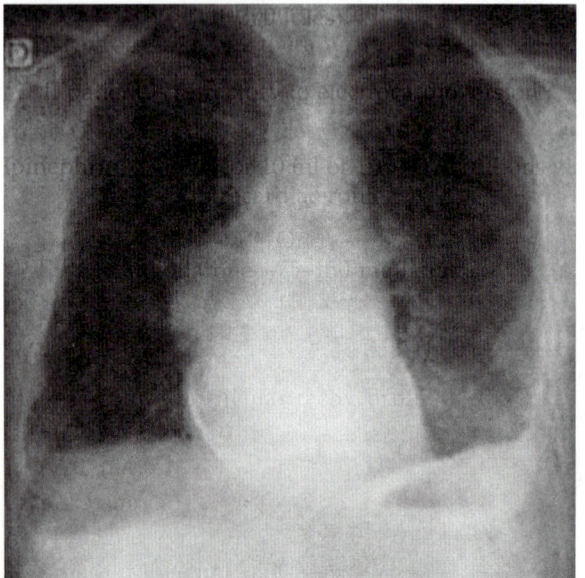

Fig. 1.160: Constrictive pericarditis

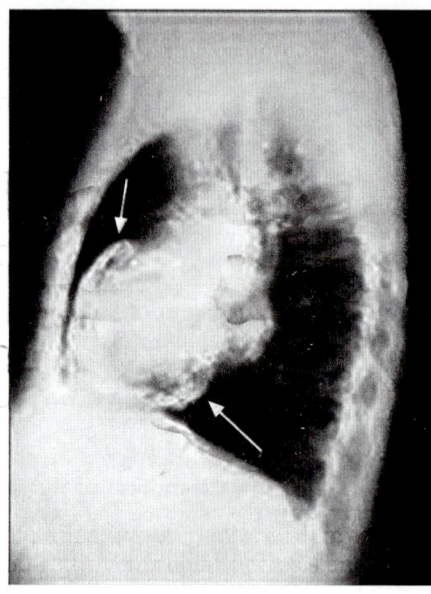

Fig. 1.161: Pericardial calcium: This lateral chest radiograph demonstrates coarse calcification involving the entire pericardium (arrows) in this patient who has a history of prior hemopericardium. (Photo courtesy of Jonathan Kruskal, MD)

4. Flattening of left ventricular posterior wall
5. Atrial enlargement in long-standing cases.

Doppler Echocardiography

Flow velocity observation
1. **During inspiration:**
   i. Exaggerated reduction in blood flow velocity in pulmonary veins and across the mitral valve.
   ii. Exaggerated increase in diastolic blood flow velocity into right atrium and across the tricuspid valve.
2. **During expiration,** opposite flow velocity occurs.

MRI Screening

It confirms thickened pericardium and pericardial calcification. But isolated presence of above finding does not confirm constrictive pericarditis, because it must be associated with impaired left ventricular filling.

Differential Diagnosis

A. **Cor pulmonale**
   Point in favor of diagnosis:
   i. May be associated with systemic hypertension
   ii. Little pulmonary congestion
   iii. Heart is not usually enlarged
   iv. Evidence of advanced pulmonary disease
   v. Exacerbated fall in venous pressure during inspiration (negative Kushmaul's sign)
   vi. Ascites absent
B. **Tricuspid stenosis:** Hepatomegaly, splenomegaly, ascites, and edema present.
   Point in favor of diagnosis: Murmur of tricuspid stenosis, and associated murmur of mitral stenosis are usually present.
C. **Restrictive cardiomyopathy**—points in favor of diagnosis:
   i. Well-defined apex best
   ii. Cardiac enlargement

iii. Pronounced orthopnea with attacks of acute left ventricular failaure
iv. Left ventricular hypertrophy
v. Gallop rhythm
vi. ECG findings—bundle branch block, abnormal Q wave
vii. Echocardiography—thickened ventricular wall, no calcification on thickening of pericardium.

Above are required for differential diagnosis in bedside clinics.

Treatment

Preoperative evaluation:
i. Coronary angiography in >50 years of age—exclude unsuspected coronary artery disease.
ii. Dietary sodium restriction and diuretics to reduce congestion and dyspnea.

Definitive treatment: Pericardial resection

The risk of operation depends upon:
i. Extent of penetration of myocardium by fibrous tissue and calcification process.
ii. Severity of myocardial atrophy
iii. Extent of secondary impairment of hepatic and renal function.
iv. Patient's comorbid condition.

Operative mortality: 5–10%
So operative treatment should be carried out in early course.

Tuberculous Pericardial Effusion

Pathophysiology

1. Commonest mode of presentation with or without tamponade.
2. Effusion is blood stained in 95% of cases.
3. It may be associated with parenchymal lung disease (30% of cases) or hilar lymphadenopathy—in this case—direct spread from hilar node to pericardium occurs.

Clinical Presentation

Symptoms may be variable by similar to that of pericardial effusion with fever, night sweat, weight loss.

Chest X-ray

i. Enlarged globular heart
ii. Pleural effusion one or both sides
iii. Evidence of pulmonary tuberculosis in 30% of cases.

Echocardiography

Features of pericardial effusion is typically associated with:
a. Soft tissue density masses
b. Thickening visceral pericardium
c. Fibrinous strands.

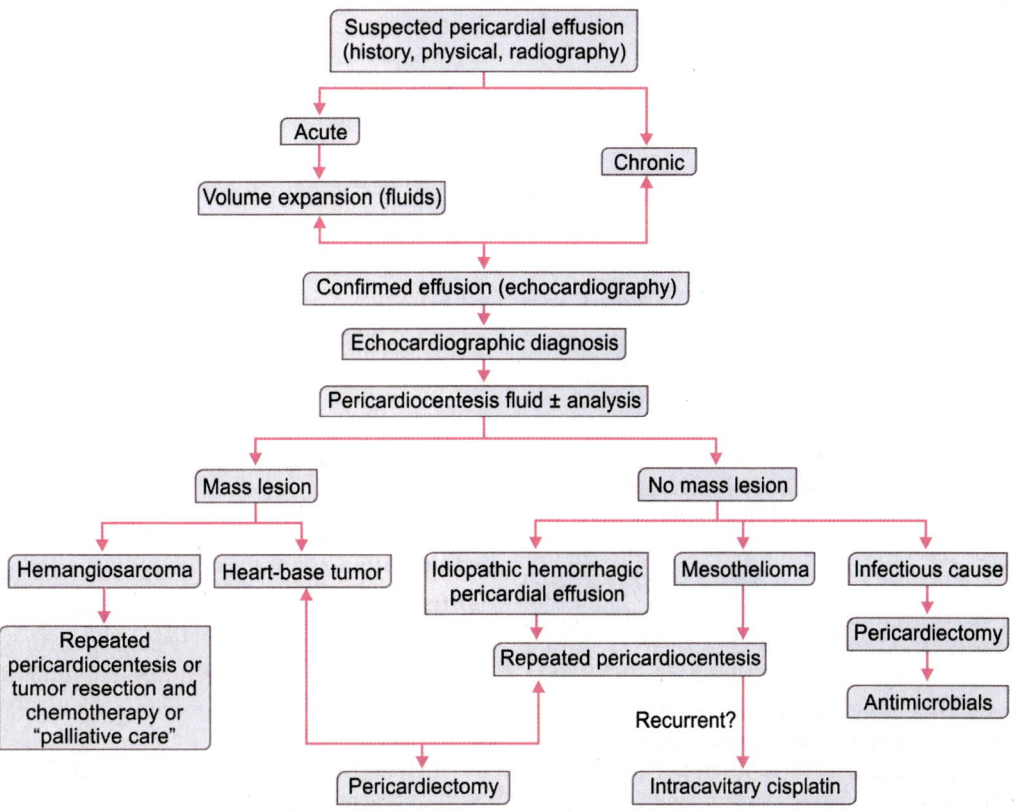

Flowchart 1.4: Diagnostic and therapeutic algorithm

Diagnosis

A. Definite diagnosis of tuberculous pericarditis is based on—demonstration of tubercle bacilli in pericardial fluid or histological section of pericardium

Complete drainage of pericardial fluid should be done, sometimes associated pericardial biopsy in same sitting.

Fluid should be sent for microscopic evaluation and fluid can be inoculated at bedside in double strength Kischner culture medium.

B. Probable diagnosis of tuberculous pericarditis:

i. Evidence of tuberculosis in any other organ in patient having unexplained pericarditis.
ii. If supraclavicular lymph node is palpable—it should be biopsied.
iii. Tuberculin skin testing is of little value in endemic and in non-endemic areas.
iv. Enzyme-linked immunospot test (ELIS POT) detects T cells specific for *Mycobacterium tuberculosis* antigen—more specific for tuberculous pericarditis.

C. Tests for rapid diagnosis of tuberculous pericarditis:

i. *Polymerase chain reaction (PCR),* identifies DNA of *Mycobacterium tuberculosis* rapidly from 1 μl of pericardial fluid (sensitivity 75%, specificity 100%).
ii. *ADA level in fluid*—83% sensitive and 78% specific for tuberculous effusion.
iii. *High interferon γ level*—92% sensitive, 100% specific for pericardial tuberculosis.

Treatment

1. Standard **four-drug antitubercular chemotherapy** for 6 months.
2. **Repeat pericardiocentesis** may be required in 15% patients
3. 10% patients may require **pericardiotomy** during 2 years follow up.
4. Patient may require **steroid therapy.**

RHEUMATIC FEVER

Definition

It is a **systemic autoimmune disorder** related to **prior streptococcal infection**—leading to **acquired heart disease** in adults and children in many parts of the world.

Incidence and Epidemiology

i. In developing world—incidence is 200 per 100000 populations.
ii. In United States—incidence is 1 per 100000 population.

The difference is due to:

i. Improved public health
ii. Living conditions
iii. Development of modern antibiotics
iv. Shifting of endemic strains of group A hemolytic Streptococcus

Rheumatic fever is more common in:

i. Military recruits
ii. Close contacts with school-aged children
iii. Persons of low socioeconomic status

Age incidence: Between the age of 5 of and 18 years, rare before the age of 5.

Sex incidence: It affects both sexes equally, except in Sydenham's chorea—which is more prevalent after puberty

Pathology

This disease occurs 3–4 weeks after throat infection with group A hemolytic streptococci—serotype M (particularly to be 1, 3, 5, 6, 14, 18, 19, 24, 27 and 29).

Pathology is mainly due to antigen mimicry, because antibodies to carbohydrate in the cell wall (anti-M antibodies) of group A Streptococcus cross-react with protein in cardiac valves.

Other tissues are also involved in this disease, e.g.
i. Involvement of connective tissue in joints—arthritis
ii. Involvement of caudate nucleus in brain producing Sydenham's chorea

In case of heart involvement:

i. Pericarditis—commonly occurs.
ii. Myocarditis may produce heart failure and arrhythmia.
iii. Endocarditis involves mitral valve 65–70%, aortic valve 25%, tricuspid valve 10% (but never in isolation)

All the layers of heart develop perivascular foci of eosinophilic collagen surrounded by lymphocytes, plasma cells and macrophages—called **Aschoff bodies.**

Clinical Features

1. **Sore throat**—35–60% patients of rheumatic fever have upper respiratory symptoms in preceding 3–4 weeks ago
2. Patients with rheumatic fever presents with **constitutional symptoms** like:
   a. Fever (101°F–104°F)
   b. Malaise
   c. Weight loss
   d. Pallor
   e. Arthralgia
   f. Epistaxis
3. **Arthritis:**
   i. Occurs in 75% of 1st attack.
   ii. Symmetrically involved large joints—like knee, ankles, elbow and wrists.
   iii. Severe tenosynovitis occurs commonly in adult suggesting diagnosis of gonococcal arthritis.
   iv. Migratory involvement, but overlap can occur. Duration of involvement is 4 weeks for each site.
   v. Resolution is not associated with permanent damage
   vi. Joints are swollen, tender, warm, and red.
   vii. Hands involvement tends to occur in post-strep-tococcal arthritis, a related syndrome without carditis.
   viii. On rare occasions, periarticular fibrosis occurs in rheumatic arthritis—Jaccoud arthritis.
4. **Carditis:**
   i. It occurs in 30–60% of cases, commonly occurs in young children.

ii. Ranges from asymptomatic presentation to progressive congestive heart failure and death, e.g. shortness of breath, dyspnea on exertion, cough, PND, chest pain and/or orthopnea.

iii. *Signs of carditis*—include development of new murmur, cardiac enlargement, CHF, pericardial friction rub and/or pericardial effusion.

iv. *Characteristic murmur:*
   a. High-pitched, blowing holosystolic, apical murmur—**mitral regurgitation**
   b. Low-pitched apical, mid-diastolic flow murmur—**Carey Coombs murmur**—due to relative mitral stenosis.
   c. High-pitched decrescendo, diastolic murmur of **aortic regurgitation.**

5. **Sydenham's chorea:**
   a. It occurs in 25% of patients.
   b. It occurs mainly in children, rare in adult, more common in girls.
   c. It occurs with other symptoms of rheumatic fever or as an isolated finding.
   d. It occurs after **6** months of onset of pharyngitis.
   e. Initial manifestations—difficulty in writing, talking, or walking, handwriting may deteriorate, speech becomes explosive and halting tone.
   f. Symptoms become evident when patient is under stress or awake, but disappears after sleep.
   g. It usually resolves without any residual damage, but may last for 2–3 years.

6. **Erythema marginatum** (Fig. 1.162):
   i. It occurs in 10% of patients.
   ii. This is characterized by non-pruritic, painless, serpiginous, erythematous evanescent macular rash having pale center—tends to disappear within a few days.
   iii. It occurs over the trunk, abdomen, and inner aspect of thigh but not on the face.
   iv. Rash may be induced by heat.
   v. Its presence indicates presence of carditis

7. **Subcutaneous nodules** (Fig. 1.163):
   i. These occur in 20% of RF patients.
   ii. These are usually 0.5–2 cm, firm, painless, freely mobile, nodules, found in clusters.

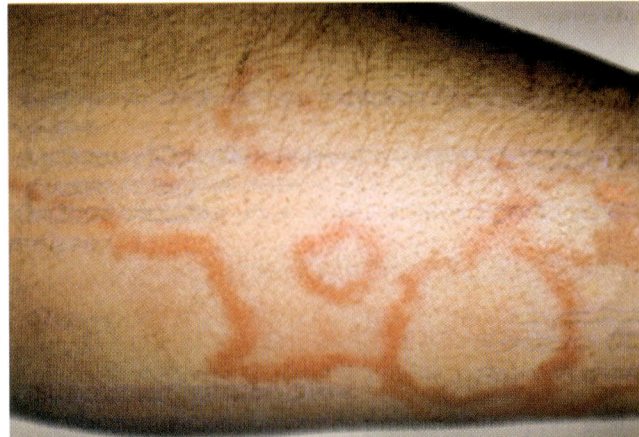

Fig. 1.162: Erythema marginatum

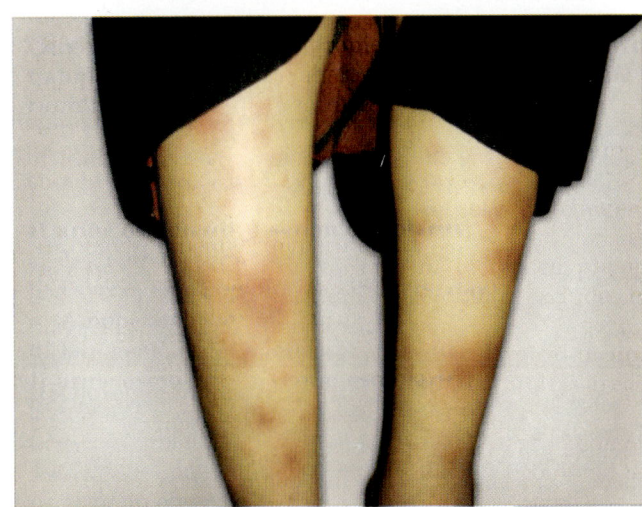

Fig. 1.163: Subcutaneous nodule

iii. They are found over extensor surfaces of joints (knees, elbows and wrists), bony prominences, tendons, dorsum of the foot, occipital regions, and cervical processes.

Flowchart 1.5: Pathogenic pathways, in acute rheumatic fever

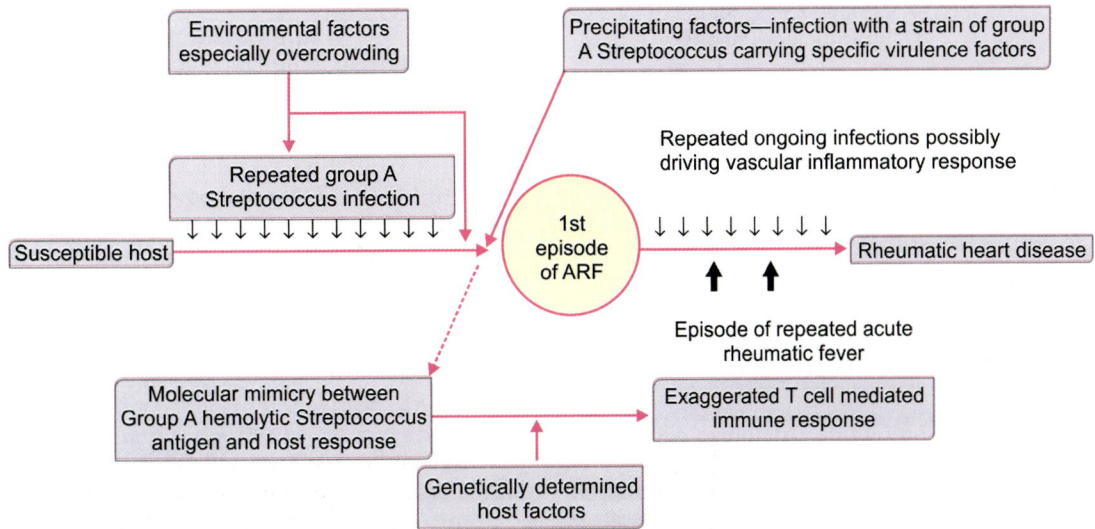

iv. Skin overlying the nodules is freely mobile and shows no sign of discoloration or inflammation.

v. It lasts for few days then disappears.

The **average duration of acute rheumatic fever** is 3 months. Chronic rheumatic fever generally defined as disease persisting longer than 6 months. It occurs in 5% of cases.

8. Fever:

i. It occurs in most case of ARF, although rarely in case of chorea.

ii. Although high-grade fever (≥39°) is the rule.

iii. Low grade temperature may occur.

WHO criteria for diagnosis of rheumatic fever and rheumatic heart disease (based on 1992 revised Jones criteria)

Diagnostic categories	Criteria
Primary episode of rheumatic fever	Two majors or one major and two minor manifestations plus evidence of preceding group A streptococcal infection
Recurrent attack of rheumatic fever in a patient without established rheumatic heart disease	Same as above
Recurrent attack of rheumatic fever in a patient with established rheumatic heart disease.	Two minor manifestations plus evidence of preceding Group A streptococcal infection.
Rheumatic chorea, insidious onset rheumatic carditis Infective endocarditis should be excluded.	Other major manifestations or, evidence of Group A Streptococcus infection not required.
Chronic valve lesions of rheumatic heart disease (patients presenting for the first time with pure mitral stenosis or mixed mitral valve disease and/or aortic valve disease)	Do not require any other criteria to be diagnosed as having rheumatic heart disease
Major manifestations	**Carditis** **Polyarthritis** **Chorea** **Erythema marginatum** **Subcutaneous nodules**
Minor manifestations	**Clinical**—fever, polyarthralgia **Laboratory**—elevated ESR or leukocyte count **Electrocardiogram** **Prolonged PRT interval**
Supporting evidence of preceding streptococcal infection within last 45 days.	Elevated or rising ASO titre. Or other streptococcal antibody. Or positive throat culture. Or rapid antigen test for Group A streptococcus. Or recent scarlet fever.

Recommended tests in case of possible acute rheumatic fever.

Recommended for all cases:

a. White blood cell count

b. Erythrocyte sedimentation rate

c. C-reactive protein

d. Blood culture, if febrile

e. Electrocardiogram (repeat in 2 weeks and 2 months, if prolonged PR interval or other rhythm abnormality)

f. Chest X-ray—if clinical or echocardiographic evidence of carditis

g. Echocardiogram (repeat it after 1 month, if negative).

h. Throat swab culture preferably before administration of antibiotic, for Group-A streptococci.

i. Anti-streptolysin serology—both antistreptolysin and anti-DNase B titre, if available (repeat it 10–14 days later, if 1st is not confirmatory).

Tests for Alternative Diagnoses Depending on Clinical Features

1. Repeat blood culture, if possible endocarditis

2. Joint aspirates (microscopy and culture) for possible septic arthritis

3. Copper, ceruloplasmin and ANA, drug screen for choreiform movement

4. Serology and autoimmune markers for arborival, autoimmune or reactive arthritis.

Radiography

The findings expected:

1. Increased cardiac size.

2. Increased pulmonary vasculature.

3. Pulmonary edema.

Electrocardiogram

1. Sinus tachycardia

2. Prolonged PR interval

3. Low voltage QRS complexes and ST segment changes in acute pericarditis

Echocardiography

1. Evidence of mitral regurgitation

2. Evidence of aortic insufficiency

Biopsy

Aschoff's nodules:

a. A form of granulomatous inflammation, seen in proliferative stage is considered pathognomonic of acute rheumatic carditis.

b. These nodules are found in:

i. Interventricular septum

ii. Wall of left ventricle

iii. Left atrial appendages

Treatment

A. **Treatment of arthritis and arthralgia and fever:**

1. *Aspirin is the drug of choice.* Initial dose—80–100 mg/kg/day in children 4–8 gm/day in adult. In 4–5 divided dose to be given. It may be continued up to 2 weeks.

2. *When acute symptoms subsides*—dose should be reduced to 60–70 mg/kg/day for further 2–4 weeks.

3. *Those who cannot tolerate aspirin:* Naproxen 10–20 mg/kg/day—produces good symptomatic response.

4. *Toxic effects of aspirin*—anorexia, nausea, vomiting and tinnitus

B. Antibiotics:

1. **Penicillin is the drug of choice,** can be given in the following forms
   i. *Phenoxymethyl penicillin* 500 mg orally twice daily in adult and 250 mg for children <27 kg of body weight orally twice daily.
   ii. *Amoxicillin* 50 mg/kg daily (maximum up to 1 gram) for 10 days
   iii. *Benzathine penicillin*—single dose 1.2 million units for adult and 600000 units for children <27 kg weight.

2. *Erythromycin estolate* 20–40 mg/kg/day up to 1 gm/day orally for 10 days.

Secondary Prevention

1. **Benzathine penicillin**—1.2 million units for adults and 600000 units for children <27 kg weight to be given every 4 weeks, but it can be given every 2 or 3 weeks in patient at high risk.
2. **Oral penicillin**—250 mg twice daily, but less effective than benzathine penicillin.
3. **Penicillin allergic patient** can take **erythromycin** 250 mg twice daily.

Duration of secondary prophylaxis depends upon several factors:

1. *Duration since last episode of acute rheumatic fever*. (Recurrence becomes less likely with increasing time)
2. *Age* (recurrence becomes less likely with increasing age)
3. *Severity* of rheumatic heart disease.

Recommended duration of secondary prophylaxis by American Heart Association.

Treatment of Carditis

1. Strenuous physical activity should be avoided
2. Management of congestive cardiac failure
3. In patient with significant cardiac involvement **Corticosteroid is preferred over salicylates.**

Dose: 1 mg/kg/day to start with. It does not affect the course of the disease.

Duration of therapy is guided by:

i. Response to therapy
ii. Severity of the disease

A gradual tapering of dose of steroid is necessary to avoid the relapse.

In case of relapse—salicylates with or without steroid can be given.

Treatment of Chorea

i. Medications do not alter the outcome or duration of chorea.
ii. Milder cases can be managed by providing calm environment.
iii. In severe chorea, carbamazepine or sodium valproate is preferred to haloperidol. Medication should be continued. Sodium valproate—15–20 mg/kg/day for 1–2 weeks.
iv. **In resistant cases**—plasmapheresis, intravenous immunoglobulin have been tried.

Prognosis

1. Untreated ARF lasts for average 12 weeks.
2. With treatment, patients are usually discharged within 1–2 weeks.
3. Inflammatory markers should be monitored every 1–2 weeks—till normalization.
4. Echocardiography should be repeated after 1 month to see any evidence of progression of carditis.

Category of patient	Duration of prophylaxis
1 **Rheumatic fever without**	For 5 years after the last attack or, 21 years of age (whichever is longer)
2 **Rheumatic fever with carditis but no residual valvular disease**	For 10 years after the last attack or 21 years of age (whichever is longer)
3 **Rheumatic fever with persistent valvular disease, evident clinically or on echocardiography**	For 10 years after the last attack or 40 years of age (whichever is longer) sometimes lifelong prophylaxis.

Acid-Base Disorder and Electrolyte Imbalances

ACID-BASE DISORDERS

Acid is a substance—which donates H^+ ions.
Base is a substance—which accepts H^+ ions.

Physiologic balance is maintained through following equations

$$H_2O + CO_2 \rightleftharpoons H_2CO_3 \rightleftharpoons H^+ + HCO_3$$

Acid may be   1. Strong—Hydrochloric acid
                   2. Weak—Carbonic acid

Base may be   1. Strong—sodium hydroxide

$pH = \log (H^+)$

So, pH is inversely related to H^+.

Normally pH = 7.4—which correlates with extracellular H^+—which is 40 nmol/L.

pH—which compatible with life is—6.80 to 7.8—which is equivalent to H^+ in blood 16–160 nmol/L

Acidemia

This can be defined as:
i. Decrease in pH
ii. Increase in H^+ in the blood

Alkalemia

This can be defined as:
i. Increase in pH
ii. Decrease in H^+ in the blood

According to the Genesis of Disorder of Acid and Base Disturbances

A. **Changes in PCO_2**—it is due to respiratory disorder:
  1. Respiratory acidosis:
    i. Decrease in pH
    ii. Increase in PCO_2
  2. Respiratory alkalosis:
    i. Increase in pH
    ii. Decrease in PCO_2

B. **Changes in HCO_3**—due to metabolic disorder:
  1. Metabolic acidosis:
    i. Decrease in pH
    ii. Decrease in HCO_3 in blood

  2. Metabolic alkalosis:
    i. Increase in pH
    ii. Increase in HCO_3 in blood

Buffering

This means an ability of a solution to resist change in pH after administration of strong acid or base. Buffers are of following types:
1. Extracellular buffer—bicarbonate
2. Intracellular buffer—protein, phosphates, hemoglobin
3. Bone—it absorbs significant acid load. But on dissolution, buffer compounds are released. These are:
  i. Calcium carbonate
  ii. Calcium bicarbonate

Ventilatory Response

Respiratory centre and system are able to sense the changes in pH, at the same time control pCO_2 through alveolar ventilation.

In response to acid load
↓
Reduction in PCO_2
↓
Generation of CO_2 and H_2O
↓
Normalization of pH

Normal PCO_2 is 40 mmHg. It is decreased in hyperventilation and increased in alveolar hypoventilation.

Excretion

1. Regeneration and/or reabsorption of HCO_3 to maintain system balance.
2. Through renal elimination of:
  i. Titrable acid (dihydrogen phosphate)
  ii. Nontitrable acids (ammonium)
3. Bicarbonate reabsorption through:
  i. Proximal renal tubular (majority)
  ii. Regulation by plasma HCO_3 levels and effective circulatory volume

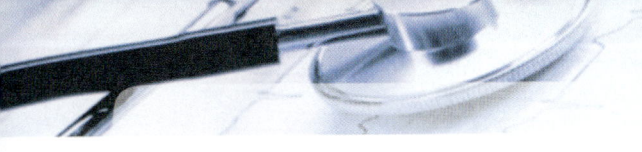

Acidosis occurs due to following factors:

A. *Metabolic insults:*
1. Huge acid load:
   i. Exogenous sources from ingestion of toxin; like ethyl alcohol and other alcohol
   ii. Endogenous sources:
      a. Lactic acidosis
      b. Diabetic ketoacidosis
2. Loss of bicarbonate:
   i. Gastrointestinal loss—diarrhea
   ii. Renal loss—proximal renal tubular acidosis
3. Inability to excrete acid load—distal renal tubular acidosis

B. *Respiratory insult*—by elevation of PCO_2

Alkalosis occurs from the following factors:
Metabolic insult
1. Loss of hydrogen ion rich fluid:
   i. Suction through nasogastric tube
   ii. Increased bicarbonate reabsorption during volume contraction
2. Increased reabsorption of bicarbonate:
   i. Reabsorption of bicarbonate by kidney—stimulated by volume contraction
   ii. Hypochloremia
   iii. Hypokalemia
3. Decrease in PCO_2 due to respiratory hyperventilation

Compensation (Table 2.1)

Alternation of HCO_3 to PCO_2 ratio must be minimized. This can be done by following methods:
A. Metabolic disorders can be compensated by respiratory methods.
B. Respiratory disorders can be compensated by metabolic pathways.

Respiratory Compensation

a. In metabolic acidosis
   i. Decrease in PCO_2
   ii. Alternation in reduction of pH
b. In metabolic alkalosis
   i. Increase in PCO_2,
   ii. Alternation of rise in pH

Metabolic Response

a. In respiratory acidosis—rise in HCO_3 in blood
b. In respiratory alkalosis—decrease in HCO_3
   But all the above compensatory responses take time to generate to show its maximum effect.
   Compensatory response is never complete.

Metabolic Acidosis

Definition

Metabolic acidosis is characterized by:
i. Low pH
ii. Low HCO_3
iii. Respiratory compensation produces low PCO_2 through hyperventilation.

Table 2.1: Effected compensatory responses for acid-base imbalances

Disorder	Primary change	Compensatory response
Metabolic acidosis	Decrease in HCO_3^-	Every 1 mEq/L fall in HCO_3, there is 1–2 mmHg decrease in PCO_2
Metabolic alkalosis	Increase in HCO_3^-	Every 1 mEq/L rise in HCO_3, there is 0.7 mmHg rise in PCO_2
Respiratory acidosis	Increase in PCO_2	Increase in HCO_3
Acute	For every 10 mmHg rise of PCO_2, there is 0.08 decrease in pH	For every 10 mmHg rise in PCO_2, there is 1 mEq/L rise in HCO_3
Chronic	For every 20 mmHg rise in PCO_2, there in 0.03 decrease in pH	For every 10 mmHg rise in PCO_2, there is 3–5 mEq/L rise in HCO_3
Respiratory alkalosis Acute	Decrease in PCO_2 For every 10 mmHg fall in PCO_2, there is 0.08 rise in pH	Decrease in HCO_3 for every 10 mmHg fall in PCO_2, there is 2 mEq/L decrease in HCO_3
Chronic	For every 10 mmHg fall in PCO_2, there is 0.03 rise in pH	For every 10 mmHg fall in PCO_2, there is 4 mEq/L decrease in HCO_3

Etiology

A. Normal anion gap metabolic acidosis:
1. Ureteric diversion
2. Small bowel fistula
3. Ingestion of hydrochloric acid
4. Resolving diabetic ketoacidosis
5. Carbonic anhydrase inhibitor
6. Type 4 renal tubular acidosis
7. Type 1, 2, 3 renal tubular acidosis
8. Pancreatic fistula

B. Increased anion gap metabolic acidosis:
1. Methanol, metformin ingestion
2. Uremia
3. Renal failure due to uric acid nephropathy
4. Diabetic, alcoholic and starvation ketoacidosis
5. Lactic acidosis
6. Salicylates
7. Ethylene glycol
8. Paraldehyde
9. Toluene
10. Isoniazid
11. Carbon monoxide poisoning

C. Low anion gap metabolic acidosis:
1. Increased unmeasured cations
   i. Lithium toxicity
   ii. Hypercalcemia
   iii. Hyperkalemia
   iv. Hypermagnesemia
   v. Multiple myeloma
2. Decreased unmeasured cations (decreased PO_4, albumin):
   i. Hypophosphatemia
   ii. Hypoalbuminemia

3. Chloride overestimation
   i. Iodide toxicity
   ii. Bromide toxicity

Diagnosis

It is very necessary to differentiate various froms of metabolic acidosis.

I. **Step-1:** To differentiate anion gap (AG) from non-anion gap (non-AG), in patient with AG acidosis—acid dissociates into H⁺ ion and "unmeasured" anions.

Simple equation of measurement of anion and cation which is present in extracellular space is

$AG = [Na^+]—[Cl^-] + [HCO_3]$. Normal AG = 10 ± 3 mEq/L

This normal value reflects the presence of unmeasured negative changes from plasma albumin.

So if plasma albumin falls by 1 gm/dl (normal 4 gm/dl), AG decreases by 2.5 mEq/L.

On the other hand, increased AG reflects accumulation of unmeasured anions like lactate, acetate. This increase in AG more or less approximates decrease in HCO_3.

So if there is any disparity between AG and HCO_3 decrease, it indicates superimposed metabolic disorder. These superimposed metabolic disorders are of following types:

1. When $\Delta AG << HCO_3$—there is large disproportionate reduction in HCO_3—it suspects—superimposed non-gap metabolic acidosis.
2. When $\Delta AG >> \Delta HCO_3$—there is attenuation of decrease in HCO_3—it suspects superimposed metabolic alkalosis or chronic respiratory acidosis with increase in serum HCO_3.

To measure the unmeasured anion—following levels are necessary
   i. Lactate levels
   ii. Ketone bodies

II. **Step-2:** To differentiate between non-anion gap (non-AG) and gastrointestinal defect

To differentiate between renal cause and GI cause—urinary anion gap is necessary.

Urine $AG = [Na^+] + [K^+] – [Cl^-]$

1. In normal physiologic state—urine AG is 0–30.
2. **In acidosis,** kidney starts producing large amount of ammonium in response to increased acid load. As a result, this ammonium will be balanced by chloride levels. As a result, large amount of Cl⁻ will be excreted in urine as comparison to Na⁺ and K⁺. As a result, urine AG wll be negative.

In case of renal tabular acidosis—renal ammonium level becomes low, so urine AG will remain positive.

An Ion Gap Metabolic Acidosis

Lactic acidosis—normally human being produces small amount of lactate, product of anaerobic metabolism of pyruvate. Increased production of lactate occurs in following conditions:

   i. Decreased tissue oxygenation, like septic shock
   ii. Excessive energy expenses—seizures, hyperthermia
   iii. Disordered oxidative metabolism—intoxication, malignancy.
   iv. Impaired clearance of lactate—hepatic failure
   v. D-lactic acidosis by D-lactic acid producing organisms

Alcohol or Starvation Ketoacidosis

   i. Here the causes are the combination of poor dietary intake with huge alcohol ingestion.
   ii. Ratio of β-hydroxybutyric acid to acetoacetic acid is 20:1
   iii. Treatment
      a. Volume repletion
      b. Glucose administration
      c. Electrolyte repletion.

Toxic Alcohol (Methanol and Ethylene Glycol) Ingestion

1. Here, the metabolites are:
   a. Formate (in case of methanol)
   b. Glycolate (in case of ethylene glycol)
   These are responsible for high AG.
   Here there is only clue is increased osmolar gap.

   Osmolar gap
   Measured serum osmolarity—calculated osmolarity
   Calculated serum osmolarity = $(2[Na^+] + [glucose]/18) + urea/2.8$

2. If the difference is >15 to 20 mOsm/kg—suggests toxic alcohol ingestion.
   Patient with methanol poisoning—presents with:
   a. Abdominal pain
   b. Vomiting
   c. Headache
   d. Optic neuritis
3. Patients with ethylene glycol poisoning—presents with similar complaints excepts optic neuritis
   Calcium oxalate crystals in urine are suggestive of ethylene glycol poisoning.
4. Most of the morbidities of methanol and ethylene glycol are due to damage produced by their metabolites.
5. Treatment is mainly the blocking the metabolism of toxic alcohol:
   i. Fomepizole—it blocks alcohol dehydrogenase, as a result, metabolism of methanol and ethylene glycol will be retarded.
   ii. Hemodialysis—to enhance toxic metabolic elimination.

Salicylate Overdose

   i. Symptoms:
      a. Nausea
      b. Vomiting
      c. Tinnitus
      d. Alteration in mental status
      e. Coma
      f. Death
   ii. Treatment:
      a. Urine alkalization with HCO_3 infusion—to reduce symptoms
      b. Hemodialysis—indications:
         1. Extremely high levels of toxic metabolites
         2. Severe symptoms
         3. Renal failure
         4. Refractory acidosis

Acetaminophen Ingestion

   i. Symptoms due to accumulation of 5-oxoproline.
   ii. The mechanism is disordered glutathione metabolism
   iii. Cessation of drug improves the symptoms

Characteristics of Renal Tubular Acidosis

Item	Type-I	Type-I	Type-IV
Basic defect	Decreased distal acidification	Diminished absorption of HCO_3 in PCT	Aldosterone resistance or deficiency
Urine pH	>5.3	Variable > 5.3	<5.3
Plasma HCO_3	<10 mEq/L	14–20 mEq/L	>15 mEq/L
Plasma K^+	Usually reduced or normal	Reduced or normal	Elevated
Diagnosis	Response to $NaHCO_3$ or Ammonium chloride	Response to $NaHCO_3$	Aldosterone measurement
Other abnormalities	Nephrocalc-inosis, rickets, renal stones	Osteomalacia	Associated with DM

Treatment of Metabolic Acidosis

1. Treatment of underlying cause.
2. In case of severe acidosis—HCO_3 should be administered for cardiovascular stability.

Initial goal is to raise pH to >7.2. HCO_3 required to correct metabolic acidosis can be calculated by estimating the HCO_3 deficit.

HCO_3 deficit = HCO_3 space (L) × (desired HCO_3—actual HCO_3)

HCO_3 space = 0.5–0.8 × body weight (kg)

HCO_3 space increases with severity of acidosis.

Normally, HCO_3 space is 50% of body weight. But in case of severe acidosis, it may extend up to 80%.

In normal settings, intravenous $NaHCO_3$ (50 mEq in 50 ml)—to be given bolus intravenously followed by continuous intravenous infusion (2–3 ampoules in 5% dextrose).

In chronic metabolic acidosis

i. Oral alkali in the form of sodium bicarbonate tablets.
ii. Sodium or potassium citrate solution.

Dose is—sodium bicarbonate—650 mg—two to three times daily.

HYPERNATREMIA

Definition

Hypernatremia can be defined as serum concentration of sodium more than 145 mEq/L.

Epidemiology

i. Elderly patient usually admits with hypernatremia, whereas, hospital-acquired hypernatremia occurs at any age.
ii. Incidence of hypernatremia is lower than hyponatremia
iii. Incidence of hypernatremia is <2% of all admission, whereas, hospital-acquired hypernatremia is 2 to 5% of all admission.

Cause of Hypernatremia

When water loss will be excess of salt deficit:

i. It may occur with insufficient water intake—if patient does not experience thirst normally.
ii. It may occur less commonly with excess salt.
iii. It may be due to problem in rise in serum osmolarity.

Etiology

A. **Decreased water intake (along with normal fluid loss):**
   i. Abnormally in perception of thirst—normally, increase in 2% osmolarity is associated with increased thirst—hypothalamus.
   ii. Unavailability of environmental water
   iii. Inability to communicate water needs:
   • Coma
   • Cerebrovascular accident
B. **Hypotonic fluid loss (here water loss >salt loss):**
   i. Skin
   a. Sweating
   b. Burns

ii. Gastrointestinal fluid loss
   a. Vomiting
   b. Diarrhea
   c. Fistula
iii. Impaired concentrating ability of kidney:
   a. Diabetes insipidus:
   1. Central cause
   2. Nephrogenic
   3. Drugs:
   • Alcohol
   • Lithium
   • Colchicine
   • Gentamicin
   • Amphotericin B
C. **Osmotic diuresis:**
   i. Mannitol infusion
   ii. Hyperglycemia
   iii. Hypokalemia
D. **Renal disease:**
   i. Nephropathy
   ii. Myeloma
   iii. Tubulointerstitial nephritis
   iv. Polycystic kidney disease
E. **Increased salt:**
   i. Acute salt poisoning
   a. Sea water ingestion
   b. Hypertonic saline
   c. Intravenous bicarbonate
   ii. Increased level of mineralocorticoid
   a. Conn's syndrome (raised blood pressure, low potassium and alkalosis)
   b. Increased glucocorticoid level—Cushing's syndrome
   c. Ectopic ACTH

Pathophysiology

1. Increased sodium concentration in plasma
   ↓
   Increased loss of cellular volume
   ↓
   Rupture of cellular blood vessels
   ↓
   Increased morbidity and mortality

   Patient can tolerate chronic hypernatremia than acute hypernatremia.

2. Cerebrospinal fluid moves into interstitial areas of brain tissue, and
   Increased intracellular electrolytes
   ↓
   Protects the patient from hypernatremia

3. Increased serum osmolarity
   ↓
   Shift of free water from interstitial space to intravascular space
   ↓
   Deceptively normal vital signs
   And
   Cerebral intracellular dehydration
   ↓
   If change in serum sodium concentration is rapid
   ↓
   Rapid shrinkage of brain
   ↓
   Rupture of intracerebral blood vessels

Clinical Signs and Symptoms

Clinical presentation varies according to changes in serum osmolarity:

1. >300 mOsmol/L   Increased thirst
2. >375 mOsmol/L   Irritability, lethargy, weakness
3. >400 mOsmol/L   Tremor, ataxia
4. >420 mOsmol/L   Hyperreflexia, increased spasticity focal neurological defects
5. >430 mOsmol/L   Seizures and coma

Workup of Hypernatremia

1. **Blood tests:**
   i. Renal profile
   ii. Plasma osmolarity
   ii. Serum sodium
   iv. Serum potassium, calcium
   v. Serum lithium level
   vi. Blood sugar
2. **Urine tests:**
   i. Urine osmolarity
   ii. Urine sodium
   iii. Urine potassium
3. **CT scan of brain**

Treatment

Aims of Treatment

i. Ongoing loss should be stopped.
ii. Correction of water deficit.
iii. In case of hypovolemia, correction of sodium deficit.
iv. Treatment of underlying cause.
   1. Hypernatremia should be corrected at a rate of 0.5 mmol/L/h to prevent unwanted complications like brain cellular swelling.
   2. Severe volume depletion with or without hemodynamic instability—should be corrected with normal saline.
   3. If volume depletion is less—it can be treated by 0.2% or 0.45% normal saline.
   4. Once volume status will be restored, 5% dextrose water should be given. Because dextrose will be metabolized in absence of insulin deficiency, and free water will be available.

Complications of Treatment

1. Intracerebral hemorrhage
2. Seizures
3. Cerebral edema
4. Coma

Calculation of Electrolyte Free Water in the Urine from Solute Diuresis

$$CH_2O—\text{urine output/24 hours} \times \{1—(\text{urine sodium} + \text{urine potassium})/\text{serum sodium}\}$$

Calculation of water deficit:

Total body water (TBW) × {(serum sodium – 140)/140}

Current TBW = 40% of total body weight

(Current) Total body sodium = TBW (total body water) × serum sodium

New TBW to get sodium to desired level

Current total body sodium/desired level of sodium

So the difference between current TBW and new TBW along with sensible water loss to be given in 24 hours

HYPONATREMIA

Definition

Hyponatremia can be defined as serum sodium concentration <135 mEq/L and can be defined as severe when serum sodium is below 125 mEq/L.

Acute hyponatremia is defined as fall in serum sodium within 48 hours.

According to severity hyponatremia can be classified into three categories:

1. *Mild hyponatremia*—when serum sodium concentration will be between 130 and 135 mEq/L.
2. *Moderate hyponatremia*—when serum sodium concentration will be between 125 and 129 mEq/L.
3. *Severe hyponatremia*—when serum sodium concentration will be below 125 mEq/L.

Classification according to volume status:

1. *Hypovolemic hyponatremia*—when:
   i. Total body water will be low.
   ii. Total body sodium content will be decreased more.
2. *Euvolemic hyponatremia*:
   i. Increase in total body water content.
   ii. Total body sodium content will be normal.
3. *Hypervolemic hyponatremia*:
   i. Increase in total body sodium content.
   ii. Greater increase in total body water content.

Hyponatremia can be classified according to effective osmolarity:

i. *Isotonic hyponatremia*:
   - It is also called pseudohyponatremia.
   - It occurs due to elevation of plasma lipid and proteins.
   - Here plasma water concentration is 93% of plasma.
   - Plasma lipids and proteins dilute the serum sodium measured by flame photometry.

ii. *Hypertonic hyponatremia*:

Osmolarity of extracellular space in increased
↓
Drawing of water from intracellular space to extracellular space
↓
Increase in aqueous fraction of plasma
↓
Lowering of serum sodium concentration
↓
True hyponatremia

iii. *Hypotonic hyponatremia:* In this condition, extracellular plasma osmolarity will be decreased. It may be due to:
   a. Increased water intake
   b. Impaired water excretion

Etiology

Hypovolemic Hyponatremia

Here Na deficit is excess of water deficit (here urine sodium should be measured):

a. Renal (urinary sodium >20 mmol):
   i. Addison's disease
   ii. Renal failure diuretic stage
   iii. Salt losing nephropathy
   iv. Thiazide and osmotic diuretics
b. Pre-renal loss (urinary sodium <20 mmol):
   i. Gastrointestinal loss—vomiting, diarrhea with continued water intake
   ii. Third space fluid loss—ascites, peritonitis, pancreatitis, burns.
   iii. Excessive sweating
       Associated alkalosis will be present with upper gastrointestinal loss
       Associated acidosis will be present with lower gastrointestinal loss.
c. Cerebral salt-wasting syndrome: It occurs in patients with traumatic brain injury, subarachnoid hemorrhage due to rupture of aneurysm, or intracranial surgery.

Normovolemic Hyponatremia (Measurement of Urinary Osmolarity is Essential)

i. If urine osmolarity < serum osmolarity:
   a. Tea with toast diet
   b. Psychogenic polydipsia (>15 liters/day)
   c. Amphetamine drug
   d. Iatrogenic water overload
ii. If urine osmolarity > serum osmolarity:
   a. CNS:
      1. Encephalitis
      2. Meningitis
      3. Brain absences
      4. Brain tumor
      5. Subarachnoid hemorrhage
   b. Carcinoma from:
      1. Bronchogenic carcinoma
      2. Mesothelioma
      3. Duodenum
      4. Pancreas
      5. Stomach
   c. Pulmonary:
      1. Tuberculosis
      2. Asthma
      3. Abscess
      4. Pneumothorax
   d. Other:
      1. Prolonged exercise
      2. HIV
      3. Idiopathic in elderly
   e. Syndrome of inappropriate secretion of antidiuretic hormone:
   f. Drugs:
      1. MAOI   2. TCA
      3. NSAID   4. Chlorpromazine

Hypervolemic Hyponatremia (Edematous States)

a. Urinary Na <20 mmol/L:
   1. Increased interstitial salt
   2. Secondary hyperaldosteronism

3. Congestive cardiac failure
4. Nephrotic syndrome
5. Hepatorenal syndrome
b. Urinary sodium >20 mmnol/L:
   1. Renal failure
   2. Hypertonic saline, early diuretics
   3. Hypothyroidism

Fictitious Hyponatremia (Pseudohyponatremia)

a. Hyperglycemia (drawing of water to extracellular fluid)
b. Hyperlipidemia
c. Hyperproteinemia
d. Mannitol administration
e. Glycerin washout for TURP

Clinical Manifestations

Severity of symptoms depends upon (Fig. 2.1):
a. Severity of fall
b. Extent of fall:
   1. >125 mmol/L—asymptomatic
   2. 115–125 mmol/L:
      i. Lethargy
      ii. Confusion
      iii. Anorexia
      iv. Nausea
      v. Vomiting
   3. <115 mmol/L:
      i. Muscles cramps   ii. Convulsion   iii. Coma

Physical Findings

1. Neurologic signs:
   i. Level of alertness—from alert to comatose
   ii. Varying levels of cognitive impairment—loss of orientation—time, place, person
   iii. Focal or generalized seizure activity
   iv. In case of severe hyponatremia:
      a. Signs of brainstem herniation
      b. Fixed unilateral dilated pupil
   c. Decorticate posturing
   d. Decerebrate posturing
2. Signs of hypovolemia:
   i. Dry skin, mucous membrane
   ii. Loss of skin turgor
   iii. Tachycardia
   iv. Orthostatic hypotension
3. Signs of hypervolemia:
   i. Pulmonary crepitation
   ii. S3 gallop
   iii. Jugular venous distension
   iv. Peripheral edema
   v. Ascites
4. Non-specific signs:
   i. Muscle weakness
   ii. Cramping
   iii. Rhabdomyolysis

Laboratory Tests (Workup of Hyponatremia)

Preliminary Tests

I. Blood tests:
   i. Renal function tests
   ii. Plasma osmolarity
   iii. Thyroid-stimulating hormone
   iv. Cortisol level
   v. Calculation of osmolar gap:
      a. Calculated plasma osmolarity
         = 2 × [NA]+(BUN/2.8)+(glucose/18)
      b. Osmolar gap =

Measured plasma osmolarity—calculated plasma osmolarity.

II. Urine tests:
   i. Urine osmolarity
   ii. Urine sodium
   iii. Urine potassium
   iv. Urine protein
   v. Urine creatinine

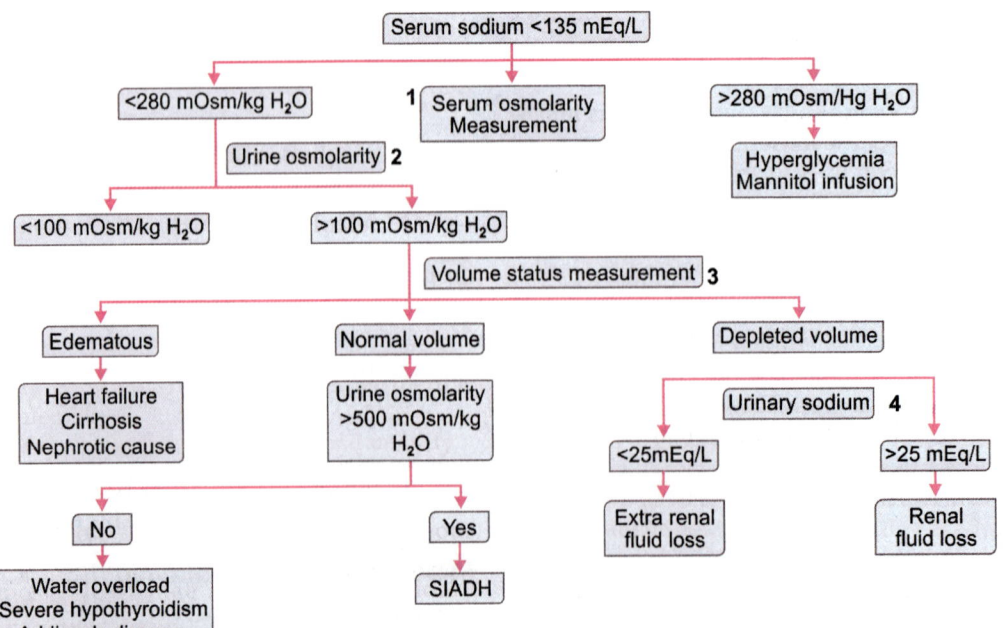

Fig. 2.1: Diagnosis algorithm of hyponatremia

III. Imaging studies:
  i. Computerized tomography of head and brain to evaluate neurological symptoms.
  ii. Chest X-ray—to evaluate pulmonary symptoms.

Urine Osmolarity

Normal value >100 mosmol/kg

Plasma Osmolarity

1. **Isotonic:**
   i. Pseudohyponatremia
   ii. Mannitol (5%)
2. **Hypotonic:** Volume status to be estimated:
   a. Hypovolemic (urine sodium <20 mmol/L and high urine osmolarity >100 mosmol/kg)
   b. Euvolemic:
      • SIDAH (High urinary sodium >40 mmol/L; high urine osmolarity >100 mosm/kg)
      • Primary polydipsia (Low urinary sodium <20 mmol/L; low urine osmolarity <100 mosmol/kg).
   c. Hypervolemic:
      • Congestive cardiac failure (Low urine sodium <20 mmol/L; high urine osmolarity >100 mOsmol/kg).
      • Cirrhosis of liver (low urine sodium <20 mmol/L).
      • Nephrotic syndrome (low urine sodium <20 mmol/L; nephrotic range of proteinuria).
3. **Hypertonic**
   i. Toxin ingestion:
      • Elevated osmolar gap >10 mOsmol/L
      • Elevated anion gap >12 mmol/L
      • Measurement of toxic compound
   ii. Hyperglycemia—normal osmolar gap

Management

Chronic Asymptomatic Hyponatremia

Fluid restriction—it should be guided by measuring urinary electrolyte content

$$\frac{(\text{Urine sodium} + \text{urine potassium})}{\text{Plasma sodium}}$$

1–No free water
0.5 to 1.0–500 ml
≤ 0.5–1000 ml

If the ratio is 1—it means—the patient is not excreting electrolyte free water. Here no free water is given to raise serum sodium, at the same time; insensible water loss will eliminate water (800–1000 ml/day).

If the ratio is 0.4; 60% urine is electrolyte free.

Suppose, the patient is excreting 2000 ml/day so 60% of 2000 ml, i.e. 1200 ml urine is electrolyte free.

So if daily fluid intake is restricted to 1000 ml/day—net result is

1000 – (800 + 1200) = –1000 ml electrolyte free water lost/day.

Treatment of SIDAH—usually does not require pharmacological intervention, unless it is resistant to above intervention.

1. *Lithium:* It induces nephrogenic diabetes insipidus. It has other potential side effects like severe hypernatremia.

2. *Demeclocycline:* It can induce nephrogenic diabetes insipidus and severe hypernatremia without adequate free water intake.
3. *In case of refractory SIADH:* oral urea is safe alternative—dose 30 to 60 gm/d
4. *Vasopressin:* 2 receptors (aquaretics)

Acute or Symptomatic Hyponatremia

1. In case of severe hyponatremia—3% hypertonic saline.
2. In case of moderate hyponatremia—loop diuretics to excrete free water.
3. Sever CNS symptoms usually respond to modest increase in serum sodium.
4. Rate of correction should be 1–2 mmol/L/hour, unless symptoms will be improved.
5. After improvement of symptoms, 8 mmol/L correction of sodium will occur in 1st 24 hours.
6. In next 24 hours, correction should not be more than 10 mmol/L.
7. Serum should be checked at every 1–2 hours to avoid over-correction.
8. Supplementation of potassium can overcorrect the serum sodium.

Dosage of pharmacological agents:

1. Lithium – 900–1200 mg/day — Inhibition of response of kidney to ADA
2. Demeclocycline 300–600 mg/day — -do-
3. V$_2$ receptor antagonist — ADH antagonist
4. Furosemide — Clearance of free water
5. Urea — Osmotic diuresis

Central Pontine Myelinolysis

This is characterized by symptoms of central nervous symptoms due to overcorrection of chronic hyponatremia.

Alcoholic patient, malnourished patients, female, liver transplant are at reisk of developing CPM.

Symptoms of demylination begins 1–3 days after correction of serum sodium level. The symptoms are:
  i. Dysarthria
  ii. Dysphagia
  iii. Seizure
  iv. Altered mental status

So treatment should be gradual correction of sodium level to 120–125 mEq/L. Serum sodium sever should not be allowed to reach normal level or hypernatremic level.

Treatment of Hypervolemic Hyponatremia

  i. Restriction of sodium and water
  ii. Administration of vasopressin receptor antagonist—conivaptan and tolvaptan
  iii. No fluid restriction is necessary.

Calculation of Deficit

No deficit
(Desired sodium—current sodium) × (0.6 × body weight)
In case of asymptomatic hyponatremia: Slow correction at a rate 0.5 mEq/hour (Maximum 12 mEq/24 hours) should be done.

HYPERKALEMIA

Definition

Hyperkalemia is characterized by elevation of serum potassium >5 mEq/L. Normal range is 3.5–5 mEq/L.

Etiopathogenesis

Acute Hyperkalemia

It usually results from transcellular shifting of potassium due to various causes

1. **Very large qualities of oral potassium intake –**
Usually patient can tolerate potassium load up to 135 to 160 mEq/L with no rise of potassium above 3.5 mEq/L.
2. **Intravenous infusion of citrated stored blood –**
It may produce hyperkalemia.
3. **Drugs producing impairment of Na⁺/K⁺ ATPase activity—**digitalis.
4. **Decreased cellular uptake—by**
   i. Insulin deficiency,
   ii. Now selective beta blockade
5. **Release of potassium to extra cellular space due to tissue injury:**
   i. Rhabdomyolysis
   ii. Tumor lysis syndrome
   iii. Burns
   iv. Ischemia
   v. Hemolysis
   vi. Intense physical activity
6. **Metabolic acidosis, but not due to organic acids:**
Diabetic ketoacidosis due to hyperosmolarity from
   a. Hyperglycemia
   b. Insulin deficiency
7. **Pseudohyperkalemia**
   i. Repeated clinching the fist or prolonged tourniquet application during drawing of blood from the limbs.
   ii. Laboratory error
   iii. Leukocytosis, thrombocytosis
8. Hyperkalemic periodic paralysis—Congenital due to mutation of Na⁺ channel in skeletal muscle

Chronic Hyperkalemia

It usually occurs due to decreased renal potassium excretion. Following factors are responsible:

1. **Decreased effect of aldosterone:**
   I. Decreased synthesis of aldosterone: Medical conditions:
      i. Addison's disease
      ii. Acquired immunodeficiency syndrome
      iii. Diabetes mellitus
      iv. Type II pseudohypoaldosteronism (Gordon syndrome).
   II. Medications:
      a. Angiotensin-converting enzyme inhibitors
      b. Angiotensin receptor blockers
      c. Renin inhibitors
      d. Nonsteroidal anti-inflammatory drugs
      e. Low molecular weight heparin
2. **Aldosterone resistance:**
   I. Medications:
      a. Aldosterone antagonists:
         i. Amiloride
         ii. Triamterene
         iii. Spironolactone
         iv. Epleronone
         v. Trimethoprim
      b. Others—cyclosporine
   II. Type I PHA—it occurs due to functional mutation of:
      a. Mineralocorticoid receptor or
      b. Amiloride sensitive epithelial Na⁺ channel
   III. Type II RTA (renal tubular acidosis)
3. **Decreased distal nephron flow:** It occurs in:
   I. Severe hypovolemia
   II. Intense vasoconstriction:
      a. Renal artery stenosis
      b. Congestive heart failure
      c. Cirrhosis

Clinical Manifestations

1. Muscle weakness
2. Lethargy
3. Ascending type fo paralysis
4. Respiratory failure
5. Cardiac arrhythmia

1. **Serum potassium >5.5 mEq/L is associated with abnormalities of repolarization:** Packed T waves (it is the earliest sign).
2. **Serum potassium >6.5 mEq/L is associated with progressive paralysis of the atria:**
   a. P wave widens and flattens
   b. PR segment lengthens
   c. Disappearance of P
3. **Serum potassium >7.0 mEq/L associated with conduction abnormalities and bradycardia:**
   a. Prolonged QRS interval with bizarre morphology of QR.
   b. High-grade AV block with slow junctional and ventricular escape rhythms
   c. Any kind of conduction block, like, bundle branch blocks, fascicular blocks
   d. Sinus bradycardia or slow AF
   e. Development of a sine wave appearance, like preterminal rhythm
4. **Serum potassium level of >9.0 mEq/L causes cardiac arrest due to:**
   a. Asystole
   b. Ventricular fibrillation
   c. PEA with bizarre, wide complex rhythm

Laboratory Workup

1. **Whole blood potassium measurement** to rule out pseudohyperkalemia

2. **TTKG** $= \dfrac{(\text{Urine K}^+ \times \text{serum osmolarity})}{(\text{Serum K}^+ \times \text{urine osmolarity})}$

   i. TTKG <7—decreased effect of aldosterone. But to validate the value of TTKG, following two factors are essential:
      a. Urine osmolarity should be greater than plasma osmolarity

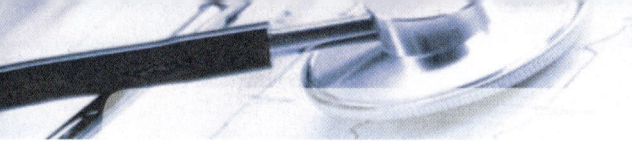

b. Urine sodium is >25 mEq/L.
ii. If TTKG is suggestive of hypoaldosteronism, but clinical presentation is not obvious, then following parameters have to be measured:
   a. Plasma renin activity
   b. Serum aldosterone
   c. Serum cortisol in morning sample after:
      • Either ≥ 3 hours of ambulation
      • Or, after administration of furosemide in the previous evening and in the morning on the date of collection.

Results:
I. Low renin, low aldosterone—hyporeninemic hypo-aldosteronism.
II. High renin, low aldosterone and cortisol—primary adrenal insufficiency.
III. High renin, high aldosterone—drugs—amiloride, triamterene—pseudohypoaldosteronism.

3. **Measurement of anion gap:** Low anion gap—and low urine pH—and decreased aldosterone effect—type IV renal tubular acidosis.
4. **Electrocardiography:** In chronic hyperkalemia—ECG finding may be normal.

Treatment of Hyperkalemia

A. Mode of treatment depends upon:
   i. Presence or absence of neuromuscular symptoms
   ii. Extent of electrocardiographic changes

Correction of the following:
   i. Acidemia
   ii. Hypocalcemia
   iii. Hyponatremia

Intravenous calcium:
   i. Calcium chloride—272 mg of elemental Ca^{++}/gm
   ii. Calcium gluconate—93 mg of elemental Ca^{++}/gm

   So, 1 gm of calcium chloride is sufficient, but, 2 gm of calcium gluconate is usually required.
   Calcium should be given slowly intravenously through central venous line to prevent tissue necrosis.
   Calcium should be given slowly over 5–10 minutes

B. Transcellular shift:
Rapidly acting insulin: Insulin produces intracellular shift of potassium—which lasts for several hours:
   i. 10 units of regular insulin in 25 to 50 gm of dextrose
   ii. Reduction of potassium of 1 to 1.5 mEq/L
   iii. In hyperglycemic patient, insulin can be given alone without adding glucose.
   iv. In normoglycemic patient, he becomes hyperglycemic after giving insulin with 25 gm dextrose.

Beta adrenergic blocking agents—albuterol:
   i. Dose 5–20 mg nebulizer or 0.5 mg intravenous administration.
   ii. Magnitude and duration of effect—similar to insulin.
   iii. Due to risk of rate related ischemia in patient with known IHD, it should be administered with caution.

C. Renal elimination of calcium: This is used in case of mild to moderate hyperkalemia:
   i. Administration of sodium chlorides, sodium bicarbonate and loop diuretics

Mechanism of action—increased load of sodium and anion—will increase potassium excretion.
   ii. In case of severe volume depletion—large volume of fluid should be administered.
   iii. In normovolemic patient—normal saline with loop diuretics should be administered simultaneously.
   iv. In volume overloaded patient, loop diuretic should only the drug of choice.
   v. Patient with type II hypoaldosteronism—thiazide diuretic is the drug of choice.
   vi. Sodium bicarbonate produces intracellular shift of potassium from extracellular space, thus lowers the serum potassium.

Method of administration

> 50 mEq (one ampoule) IV bolus
> ↓
> Followed by slow intravenous infusion

Limitations:
   i. Congestive cardiac failure
   ii. Chronic kidney disease

D. Elimination of potassium through stool: Cation exchange resin (sodium polystyrene sulfonate)—It exchanges sodium for potassium and helps excretion potassium through gastrointestinal tract.
   i. It is usually given orally. Rectal administration should be avoided due to chance of intestinal necrosis.
   ii. Orally – 15 gm or rectally 30–50 gm.
   iii. Each gm of resin exchange 1 mEq of potassium with 1–2 gm of sodium
   iv. Complication—constipation

E. Dialysis—is required when:
   i. There is severe hyperkalemia
   ii. Renal or gastrointestinal is are not feasible.
   iii. It is life saving.

Types of Dialysis

a. Peritoneal dialysis: In patient with serum level 6 mEq/L, 4 rapid exchanges can remove 25–30 mEq of potassium to make the patient out of danger.
b. Hemodialysis: Here dialysate contains 2 mEq/L. In severe hypercalcemia, dialysate may contain 1 mEq/L of potassium.

So correction principles are:
1. Mild hypokalemia (3–6 mEq/L):
   i. Diuretic—furosemide
   ii. Calcium exchange resin—orally 6 hourly
2. Moderate hyperkalemia (6–7 mEq/L):
   i. Glucose insulin (10 units with 50 gm dextrose)—onset—15 minutes, duration—60 minutes.
   ii. Sodium bicarbonate (50 ml 8.4% over 5 minutes) Onset occurs within 5 minutes. Duration—2 hours.
   iii. Albuterol/salbutamol
3. Severe hyperkalemia (>7 mEq/L):
   i. 10% 10 ml calcium chloride over 5 minutes
   ii. 10% 20 ml calcium gluconate over 5 minutes
   iii. Dialysis

HYPOKALEMIA

1. Normal daily potassium intake ~ 80 mEq/day
2. Total body potassium is 50 mEq/kg. Of it:
   i. 98% is intracellular
   ii. 2% is extracellular

Renal Regulation of Potassium

1. Decreased effective circulating blood volume
   or
   Increase in serum potassium
   ↓
   Increased aldosterone production
   ↓
   Increased excretion of potassium through cortical collecting duct
   ↓
   Exchange with sodium producing sodium retention

   Decreased distal flow rate
   ↓
   Reducing potassium excretion
   ↓
   Potassium level will be stable

2. Increased extracellular volume
   ↓
   Decreased aldosterone production
   ↓
   Increased distal flow rate
   ↓
   Maintain potassium homeostasis

Definition

Hypokalemia is characterized by serum level of potassium to <3.5 mEq/L.

Causes of Hypokalemia

I. **Decreased intake:**
   a. Geophagia
   b. Anorexia nervosa
   c. Alcoholism
II. **Increased loss:**
   a. *Gastrointestinal loss:*
      i. Vomiting
      ii. Nesogastric tube
      iii. Diarrhea:
         • Infection
         • Adenoma
         • Enteritis
      iv. Malabsorption
      v. Enteric fistula
   b. *Renal loss:*
      i. Diuretics—Thiazide, loop diuretics
      ii. Licorice ingestion
      iii. Drugs:

   • Sodium penicillin
   • Amphotericin
   c. *Osmotic diuresis:*
      i. Mannitol infusion
      ii. Hyperglycemia
   d. *Aldosterone excess:*
      i. Primary hyperaldosteronism (Conn's syndrome)
      ii. Secondary hyperaldosteronism:
         • Congestive cardiac failure
         • Cirrhosis of liver
         • Hyperproteinemia
   e. *Excess mineralocorticoid:*
      i. Cushing's syndrome
      ii. Chronic use of steroid
      iii. Fanconi's syndrome
   f. *Congenital causes:*
      i. Barter's syndrome
      ii. Liddle's syndrome
      iii. Gitelman's syndrome
   g. *Renal artery stenosis*
III. **Transcellular shifting:**
   a. Metabolic alkalosis
   b. Infusion of dextrose – insulin
   c. Hypomagnesemia
   d. Hypernatremia
IV. **Others:**
   a. Acute myeloid leukemia
   b. Pernicious anemia
V. **Drugs:**
   a. Diuretics:
      i. Thiazide
      ii. Loop diuretics
   b. Antibiotics:
      i. Penicillin
      ii. Amphotericin B
      iii. Gentamicin
   c. Insulin, beta-agonists, salbutamol (Na/K ATPase increased)

Clinical Presentation

1. Potassium level—3–3.5 mEq/L—asymptomatic, but there may be increased mortality in patients on digitalis use.
2. Potassium level—<3 mEq/L —weakness and muscle pain in lower extremities.
3. Potassium level—<2.5 mEq/L:
   i. Paralysis involving muscles of respiration
   ii. Paralytic ileus
   iii. Rhabdomyolysis
4. Nephrogenic diabetes insipidus due to hypokalemia induced non-absorption of water in kidney.
5. Prolonged hypokalemia—may be responsible for:
   i. Irreversible interstitial nephritis
   ii. Renal cyst
   iii. Hypertension
   iv. Glucose intolerance
   v. Hepatic coma—due to increased renal ammonia synthesis in patient with advanced liver disease.

Laboratory Workup

I. **Urine potassium:** 24 hours urinary potassium should be <25 mEq/day—in the background of hypokalemia.

II. **Transtubular K+ gradient:**

$$TTGK = \frac{Urine\ [K^+]\ x\ serum\ osmolarity}{Serum\ [K^+]\ x\ urine\ osmolarity}$$

If TTGK <3—it indicates normal conservation of K+ by kidney

If TTGK >3—the history and physical examination do not suggest any diagnosis, then following investigations should be done:

1. *High renin activity:*
   i. Diuretic use
   ii. Salt loosing nephritis
   iii. GI losses
   iv. Renovascular disease
2. *Low renin/high aldosterone activity:* Primary hyperaldosteronism
3. *Low renin/low aldosterone activity:*
   i. Nonaldosterone mineralocorticoid activity
   ii. Licorice ingestion

III. **Acid-base balance:**
1. *Metabolic alkalosis:*
   i. Diuretics
   ii. Mineralocorticoid excess,
   iii. Vomiting
2. *Metabolic acidosis*—less common:
   a. Type I and II renal tubular acidosis
   b. Diabetic ketoacidosis

IV. **Serum magnesium level:** Hypomagnesemia may be responsible for urinary loss of potassium.

V. **ECG changes:**
1. *Mild to moderate hypokalemia:*
   i. Prominent V waves
   ii. Diminished or inverted T waves
   iii. Depression of ST segment
2. *In severe hypokalemia:*
   i. Prolonged PR
   ii. Wide QRS complex
   iii. Ventricular fibrillation

Treatment

1. **If serum potassium level ~ 3 mEq/L =**
   Total K+ deficit 200–400 mEq

2. **Serum potassium level <3 mEq/L =**
   Total K+ deficit >600 mEq

   This is usually seen in diabetic ketoacidosis. This can be managed by intravenous insulin—which produces transcellular shift of K+ from extracellular space to intracellular space.

Oral Supplement of Potassium

It should be given because of intravenous administration of potassium may produce:
   i. Cardiac arrhythmias
   ii. Venous sclerosis
   iii. Increased cost

   Oral dose of potassium = 40 mEq 4 hourly.

   Potassium salt is important in the form of chloride, because it can correct alkalosis and bicarbonaturia

   Potassium citrate can be given, if associated academia is present.

   Intravenous potassium can be given in the following form:
   i. 40 mEq/L through peripheral line
   ii. 60 mEq/L through central line

   Rate of infusion should not be >10 mEq/hour

   Intravenous infusion of potassium should be given in saline rather than dextrose solution, because release of insulin in response to dextrose will be decreased.

Correction of Metabolic Alkalosis

In case of vomiting, proton pump inhibitor reduces the acidity of gastric secretion and thus prevents loss of acid.

In case of hyperaldosteronism or diuretic therapy (in CCF, HTN), following potassium sparing diuretics can be used:
   i. Spironolactone—it reduces aldosterone synthesis than cures hypokalemia.
   ii. Amiloride and triamterene: These drugs block epical Na+ channel in distal nephron. Side effects of triamterene:
   • Nephrolithiasis
   • Renal insufficiency

Dosage:
   i. In case of mineralocorticoid excess—amiloride 20–40 mg/day orally
   ii. In other cases—amiloride 5–10 mg/day orally.

Amiloride is the drug of choice in:
   i. Liddle's syndrome
   ii. Gillman's syndrome.

METABOLIC ALKALOSIS

Definition

It is a clinical disorder, characterized by elevation of pH due to increase in serum HCO_3.

Causes

1. Gastrointestinal acid loss:
   i. Vomiting
   ii. Nasogastric tube suction
   iii. Ileostomy
   iv. Diarrhea
   v. Dehydration
2. Endocrine:
   i. Hyperaldosteronism
   ii. Cushing's syndrome
   iii. Excess steroid administration
3. Excess acid loss through kidney:
   i. Barter's syndrome
   ii. Gitelman's syndrome,
   iii. Use of diuretics
4. Overdose of base:
   i. Massive Hartmann's transfusion
   ii. Antacids
   iii. Laxative
   iv. Milk alkali syndrome

Diagnostic Testing

1. Chloride responsive:
   i. Vomiting
   ii. Gastric lavage
   iii. Villous adenoma
   iv. Chloride diarrhea
   v. Diuretics
2. Chloride resistant:
   i. Hyperaldosteronism
   ii. Barter's syndrome
   iii. Gitelman's syndrome
   iv. Licorice ingestion
   v. Cushing's syndrome
3. Unidentified:
   i. Alkali administration
   ii. Milk alkali syndrome
   iii. Hypercalcemia
   iv. Massive blood transfusion

Symptoms

Symptoms related to hypocalcemia and hypokalemia: Light headedness, chest tightness, anxiety, dysphasia, laryngospasm.

Diagnostic Tests

In case of chloride sensitive metabolic alkalosis
i. Volume depletion
ii. Low urinary chloride level <25 mEq
   In case of chloride resistant metabolic alkalosis
i. Euvolemia
ii. Elevated urinary chloride level >25 mEq

Treatment

1. If pH is life-threatening (>7.6)—rapid reduction by hemodialysis.
2. In non-urgent cases, treatment depends upon the chloride sensitivity.
   A. In case of chloride responsive metabolic alkalosis:
      i. IV sodium chloride
      ii. Potassium supplements

The result is:
1. Reversion of contraction alkalosis
2. Decrease sodium retention
3. Promotion of HCO_3 excretion

Mode of Administration

50–100 ml/hour in excess of summation of all sensible and insensible water losses should be given.

In edematous states:
a. Diuretics to decrease or prevent pulmonary edema.
b. Acetazolamide 250–275 mg orally twice daily can be given. It is a carbonic anhydrase inhibitor.

Action

1. Decreased absorption of sodium from PCT
2. Increased renal excretion of HCO_3.

Monitoring

Urine pH should increase to >7.0
   i. In case of concurrent hypokalemia—it must be corrected to resolve metabolic alkalosis.
   ii. In case of gastric cause, PPI or H_2 blockers should be used to prevent acid loss.
   iii. In case of diuretic-induced metabolic alkalosis—potassium sparing diuretics should be used to reduce alkalosis.

Chloride Resistant Metabolic Alkalosis

   i. Surgical removal of adrenal adenoma
   ii. Use of potassium sparing diuretics with oral potassium supplement
   iii. NSAIDs, potassium sparing diuretics and potassium supplementation in Barter syndrome.

RESPIRATORY ACIDOSIS AND ALKALOSIS

A. **Acute respiratory acidosis:** It occurs due to acute alveolar hypoventilation, long before buffering defense comes into play.

B. **Chronic respiratory acidosis:** It is characterized by chronic alveolar hypoventilation with renal compensatory mechanisms.

Causes of Acute Respiratory Acidosis

1. **Decreased respiratory drive:**
   a. Central nervous system:
      i. CVA
      ii. Tumor
      iii. Infection
      iv. Hemorrhage
   b. Drugs:
      i. Narcotics
      ii. Sedatives
2. **Diminished movement of chest wall:**
   a. Neurological:
      i. Neuromuscular disorder
      ii. Myasthenia gravis
      iii. Guillain-Barre syndrome
      iv. Tetanus
   b. Toxicity:
      i. Muscle relaxants
      ii. Organophosphorus poisoning
   c. Respiratory (acute):
      i. Trauma
      ii. Surgery
      iii. Chest wall deformity
      iv. Tension pneumothorax
      v. Pleural effusion
      vi. Upper airway obstruction
   d. Equipment—increased deed space
3. Obstructive pulmonary disease
   a. COPD
   b. Asthma
   c. Pneumonia

Clinical Symptoms

   i. Vasodilatation
   ii. Tachycardia
   iii. Mydriasis
   iv. Asterixis
   v. Confusion.

Treatment

   i. Restoration of effective ventilation
   ii. Rise in PCO_2 stimulates respiratory center and increases the minute volume.

Alveolar hypoventilation
↓
Increase in PCO_2
↓
Compensatory increase in HCO_3

Generation of buffering response in acute phase (1st response)

In chronic phase (2nd response), renal compensation will be initiated through increase in NAE.

In third response, there will be restoration of effective ventilation.

RESPIRATORY ALKALOSIS

Causes

A. **Stimulated respiratory drive:**
   I. Central nervous systems:
      a. CVA
      b. ICH
      c. Psychogenic
   II. Hypermetabolic states:
      a. Thyrotoxicosis
      b. Pregnancy
      c. Sepsis.
      d. Anxiety neurosis
      e. Diabetic ketoacidosis
      f. Aspirin
   III. Environmental—hyperthermia
   IV. Drugs:
      a. Aspirin
      b. Progesterone
   V. Liver failure
B. **Hypoxemia induced:**
   I. Lung causes:
      a. Pneumonia
      b. Pulmonary embolism
      c. Asthma
   II. Congenital heart disease
   III. Chronic attitude compensation

Associated Changes

   i. Hypokalemia
   ii. Hypocalcemia
   iii. Hypophosphatemia

Decreased PCO_2
↓
Reduces H+ binding
↓
Increases in negative charge of proteins
↓
Increase binding of calcium to protein
↓
Reduction of ionized calcium in serum
↓
Hypocalcemia
↓
Tetany with carpopedal spasm

Treatment

   i. Treatment of underlying cause
   ii. Rebreathing by mask

Step by Step Diagnosis in Case of Acid-base Disorders

In case of acidosis: The reaction will be shifted to right, so H+ concentration will be higher.

In case of alkalosis: The reaction will be shifted to left, so H+ concentration will be lower.

If carbon dioxide concentration is increased, H+ concentration will be increased, the result is acidosis.

If carbon dioxide concentration is decreased, H+ concentration will be decreased, the result is alkalosis.

If bicarbonate concentration is increased, H+ concentration will be decreased, the result is alkalosis.

If bicarbonate concentration is decreased, H+ concentration will be increased, the result is acidosis.

If PCO_2 is increased, pH will be decreased, the result is respiratory acidosis.

If PCO_2 is decreased, pH will be increased, the result is respiratory alkalosis.

So, if pH is changed due to change in PCO_2—it is termed as change in pH due to respiratory problem.

If pH is decreased due to loss of bicarbonate ions, it is called metabolic acidosis.

If pH is increased due to increase of bicarbonate ions, it is called metabolic alkalosis.

In case of uncompensated respiratory acidosis: PCO_2—increased, pH—decreased, HCO_3—normal.

In case of compensatory respiratory acidosis: PCO_2—increased, pH—normal, HCO_3—increased, because kidney tries to compensate this condition by increasing reabsorption of bicarbonate ion.

In case of uncompensated respiratory alkalosis: PCO_2—decreased, pH—increased, HCO_3—normal.

In case of compensated respiratory alkalosis: Kidney will excrete more HCO_3 ion, as a result PCO_2—decreased pH—normal, HCO_3—decreased.

In case of uncompensated metabolic acidosis: PCO_2—normal, pH—decreased, HCO_3—decreased.

In case of compensated metabolic acidosis: PCO_2—decreased, pH—normal, HCO_3—decreased because respiratory centers will respond by increasing respiration thereby driving off the carbon dioxide.

In case of uncompensated metabolic alkalosis: PCO_2—normal, pH—increased, HCO_3—increased.

In case of compensated metabolic alkalosis: PCO_2—increased, pH—increased, HCO_3—normal, because here lung decrease the respiratory activity, as a result CO_2 will be retained.

Following are the steps in diagnosis of acid-base disorders:
A. First step: Firstly we have to diagnose whether there is acidemia or alkalemia:
   a. If pH <7.4—it indicates acidosis.
   b. If pH >7.4—it indicates alkalosis.
B. Second step: Inspection of serum bicarbonate and carbon dioxide concentration—which change is synchronous with change in pH—it is primary abnormality. But which change is opposite to change in pH—it is secondary abnormality.
C. Third step: We have to determine whether adequate compensation is present or not.

If HCO_3 /CO_2 will move towards same direction—the patient is assumed to have primary disease and expected compensation will be calculated.
- If compensation is adequate—it indicates simple acid-base disorder.
- If compensation is not adequate—it indicates mixed acid-base disorders.

Compensation will be calculated according to the following equations:

In case of metabolic acidosis:
- $PaCO_2 = [1.5 \times HCO_3^-] + 8$, or
- $PaCO_2$ will be decreased by 1.25 mmHg per mmol/L decrease in $[HCO_3^-]$, or
- $PaCO_2 = [HCO_3^-] + 15$.

In case of metabolic alkalosis:
- $PaCO_2$ will be increased by 0.75 mmHg with per mmol/L increase in $[HCO_3^-]$. Or,
- $PaCO_2$ will be increased by 6 mmHg per 10 mmol/L increase in $PaCO_2$ $[HCO_3^-]$. Or,
- $PaCO_2 = [HCO_3^-] + 15$.

In case of acute respiratory alkalosis: $[HCO_3^-]$ will be decreased by 2 mmol/L per 10 mmHg decrease in $PaCO_2$.

In case of chronic respiratory alkalosis: $[HCO_3^-]$ will be decreased by 4 mmol/L per 10 mmHg decrease in $PaCO_2$.

In case of acute respiratory acidosis:
$[HCO_3^-]$ will be increased by 1 mmol/L per 10 mmHg increase in $PaCO_2$.

In case of chronic respiratory acidosis:
$[HCO_3^-]$ will be increased by 2 mmol/L per 10 mmHg increase in $PaCO_2$.

Examples:

First example:
- In 42 years male with hyperventilation: ABG demonstrate: pH—7.55, PCO_2—25 mmHg. PO_2—90 mmHg.
- In this case: pH—indicates alkalosis.
- PCO_2—25 mmHg—it is decreased and it is synchronous with pH increase. So in this case, rise in pH is due to decrease in pCO_2.

So it is case of respiratory alkalosis.

Second example:
- In a patient, ABG shows: PO_2—86 mmHg. PCO_2—55 mmHg. pH—7.1, HCO_3—20 mEq/L
- In this case: pH is low—it indicates acidosis.

Here PCO_2 is increased and HCO_3 is decreased—both indicate respiratory and metabolic acidosis respectively. So it is case of mixed acid-base disorder.

Third example: This patient is showing following ABG:
- pH—7.1, PCO_2—19 mmHg. HCO_3^-—12 mmol/L.

In this case, pH is low—it indicates acidosis.
- PCO_2 is decreased—it indicates respiratory alkalosis.
- HCO_3 is decreased—it indicates metabolic acidosis.
- Now we have to determine whether this compensation is adequate or not.
- Change of HCO_3^-—12 mmol/L.
- Expected change in PCO_2 = 1.25 x 12 mmol = 15.
- But here PCO_2 is decreased more than expected value of 15—it suggests there is associated respiratory alkalosis; hence PCO_2 has been decreased much more.

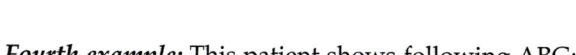

Fourth example: This patient shows following ABG:
- pH—7.1, HCO_3^-—35 mmol/L. PCO_2—62 mmHg
- pH is decreased—it indicates acidosis.
- HCO_3^-—increased (normal value is 24±2)—it indicates metabolic alkalosis.
- PCO_2—increased—it indicates respiratory acidosis
- Since here pH is low, hence this is due to increased PCO_2. Hence it is respiratory acidosis.
- Now we have to determine metabolic alkalosis is adequately compensatory or not.
- Here, PCO_2 is 62, so change is (62 – 40)= 22 mmHg.
- Expected change in HCO_3^- is 2 mmol/L for 20 mmHg change in PCO_2.
- So expected value of HCO_3^- should be 26 mmol/L.
- But the observed value is 35 mmol/L. It suggests a cause other than respiratory acidosis is responsible for this increase in bicarbonate ion.
- So this ABG is an example of mixed respiratory acidosis and metabolic alkalosis.

Mixed Acid-Base Disorder

When more than one primary acid-base disorder coexists independently together it is called mixed acid-base disorder.

It usually occurs in severely ill patients. In the following circumstances, mixed acid-base disorders can be evidenced:
A. Absence of expected compensatory response.
B. When the direction of change of PCO_2 and HCO_3 is just opposite, i.e. one is elevated and the other will be decreased. In simple acid-base disorder, the direction of compensatory response is same as the direction of the initial abnormal change.

C. pH is normal but PCO_2 and HCO_3^- are abnormal.

D. In case of anion gap metabolic acidosis if the change in level of bicarbonate is not proportional to change in anion gap.

E. Delta ratio is greater than 2 or less than 1.

F. In case of simple acid-base disorder, compensatory response will return the pH to normal.

An Ion Gap and Normal Anion Gap Acidosis

Here the delta ratio is less than 1, i.e. bicarbonate reduction is greater than the change in anion gap. So here another process is responsible for buffering of bicarbonate ion. The causes are:
a. Lactic acidosis
b. Diabetic ketoacidosis during treatment
c. Progressive renal failure
d. Type 4 renal tubular acidosis.

Anion Gap Acidosis and Metabolic Acidosis

Here the delta ratio is less than 1, i.e. reduction of bicarbonate ion less than as it should be in relation to change in anion gap. So, here another process is working to increase the bicarbonate without affecting anion gap. The causes are:
a. Lactic acidosis, uremia or DKA patients with active vomiting or on nasogastric suction.
b. DKA patient on bicarbonate therapy.

Normal anion gap acidosis and metabolic alkalosis: This is very difficult to diagnose as both bicarbonate and PCO_2 level move back towards normal value, if metabolic alkalosis will develop.

It occurs in patients with vomiting and diarrhea.

Triple Mixed Acid-base Disorders

A. **Metabolic acidosis with metabolic alkalosis with respiratory alkalosis:** If alcoholic patient vomits—metabolic acidosis + metabolic alkalosis, if patient develop liver disease or gram-negative sepsis, he also develops respiratory alkalosis.
B. **Metabolic acidosis with metabolic alkalosis with respiratory alkalosis:** If patient with chronic obstructive respiratory disease is hypercapnic (respiratory acidosis) and treated with diuretics or develops vomiting, he develops metabolic alkalosis. If this patients develop sepsis, hypotension, he develops metabolic acidosis.

Table 2.2: Acid-base disorders		
Disorders	*Acid-base level*	*Causes*
Metabolic acidosis and respiratory acidosis	pH—low, HCO_3—low, $PaCO_2$—raised	Cardiac arrest Respiratory failure with shock DKA with respiratory disorders.
Metabolic acidosis and respiratory alkalosis	pH—normal, HCO_3—low, $PaCO_2$—low	Salicylate poisoning Gram-negative sepsis Hepatic failure
Metabolic alkalosis with respiratory acidosis	pH—normal, HCO_3—high, $PaCO_2$—high	COPD on diuretics Metabolic alkalosis with severe hypokalemia
Metabolic alkalosis with respiratory alkalosis	pH—increased, HCO_3—increased, PCO_2—decreased	Hepatic failure with vomiting Patient on ventilator with continuous nasogastric suction.
Metabolic acidosis with metabolic alkalosis	pH—normal, HCO_3—normal	DKA with vomiting Vomiting having severe volume depletion producing lactic acidosis
Respiratory acidosis with respiratory alkalosis	Never occur	Never occur

3 Endocrine Disorders

PITUITARY DISORDERS

GROWTH HORMONE AXIS

Growth Hormone – IGF axis

Stimulation	Hypothalamus	Suppression
• Deep sleep • α-adrenergic drugs • Fasting • Acetylcholine • Sex-steroids • Stress • Amine acids • Hypoglycemia • Ghrelin	**+** GHRH SRIF Pituitary	• Obesity • α-adrenergic drugs • Glucocorticoids • High FFA • Hyperglycemia • Hypothyroidism • IGG-I

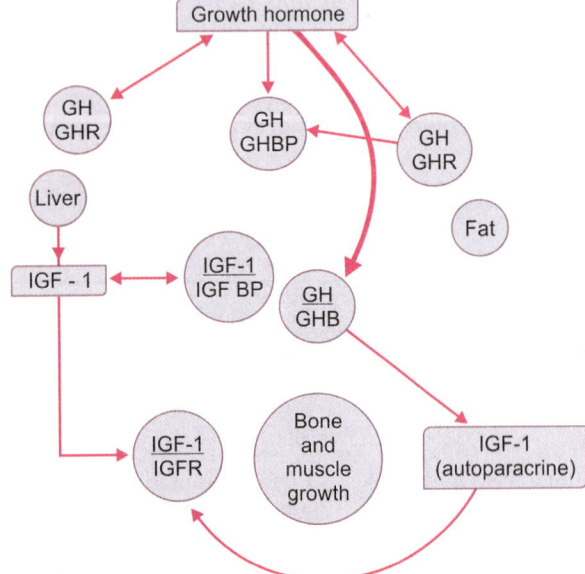

Fig. 3.1: Growth hormone—IGF axis

Somatostatin-releasing inhibitory hormone (SRIF) is produced in medial preoptic areas of hypothalamus and inhibits growth hormone secretion.

IGF-1 is peripheral target for GH, feeds back to inhibit GH.

GROWTH HORMONE

1. Height peak at night; generally correlating with sleep onset.
2. GH release rate decreases with age, so mid-age level is 15% of pubertal levels.

Growth Hormone Measurement

1. **Insulin tolerance test**: Regular insulin IV 0.05–0.15 U/kg
   Blood samples collected:
   i. 30 min before insulin injection
   ii. At the time of insulin injection
   iii. 30, 60, 120 mins after insulin injection

   Glucose and GH have to be estimated.
   Normal response—Glucose <40 mg/dl
   GH >3 mg/L
2. **GHRH test**—1 mg/kg IV
   Blood samples collected at 0, 15, 30, 45, 60, 120 min for GH.
   Value normal of GH >3 mg/L
3. **L-arginine test**—30 gm IV over 30 minutes
   Blood samples collected at 0, 30, 60, 120 minutes for GH.
   Normal value >3 µg/L
4. **L-Dopa test**—500 mg orally
   Blood sample collected at 0, 30, 60, 120 minutes for GH
   Normal value >3 µg/L

Actions

Metabolic Actions

i. It induces protein synthesis and nitrogen retention.
ii. It impairs glucose tolerance by antagonizing action of insulin.
iii. It enhances glucose uptake by cells—insulin like activity.
iv. At whole body levels—it suppresses glucose oxidation, and utilization and enhances hepatic glucose production.
v. It stimulates lipolysis—as a result—increase in FFA levels, reduce in omental fat mass and increase in lean body mass.
vi. It increases sodium, potassium, water in body and elevates serum level of phosphates

196

Bone

1. Linear bone growth

Interactions between IGF-I and GH
↓
Stimulates epiphyseal prechondrocyte differentiation
↓
These precursor cells produce IGF-I locally
↓
Which, in turn, help to proliferate prechondrocyte cells

Skeletal Maturation and Somatic Growth

Growth plate requires following hormonal stimuli:
i. GH
ii. IGF-I
iii. sex-steroids
iv. Thyroid hormones
v. Paracrine growth factors
vi. Cytokines

Growth plate requires following metabolic elements:
i. Calorie energy—10% of normal energy
ii. Amino acids
iii. Vitamin
iv. Trace materials

Linear Growth

i. Mean growth is 6 cm/year in late childhood.
ii. Peak growth rate—during mid-puberty.
a. Bone age is 12 years (girls)
b. Bone age is 13 years (boys)

Bone age is delayed in:
i. All forms of growth hormone deficiency.
ii. Growth hormone receptor defects.

Short stature: It occurs as a result of:
i. Intrinsic growth defect
ii. Extrinsic factors that impair growth.

In short statured person—two types of bone ages are found
1. Delayed bone age: Child with short stature due to:
i. Hormonal disorder
ii. Systemic disorder
2. Normal bone age with short stature:
i. Genetic cartilage dysplasia
ii. Growth plate disorder

ACROMEGALY AND GIGANTISM

Etiology

I. Excess growth hormone secretion:
  A. Pituitary:
   1. Densely granulated growth hormone cell adenoma
   2. Mixed GH and prolactin cell adenoma
   3. Mammosomatrope cell adenoma
   4. Plurihormonal adenoma
   5. GH cell carcinoma
   6. Multiple endocrine neoplasia
   7. McCune-Albright syndrome
   8. Pituitary adenoma
  B. Extra-pituitary tumor:
   1. Pancreatic islet cell tumor   2. Lymphoma
II. Excess growth hormone-releasing hormone secretion:
  A. Central:
   1. Hypothalamic hamartoma
   2. Ganglioneuroma

  B. Peripheral
   1. Bronchial carcinoid
   2. Pancreatic islet cell tumor
   3. Small cell carcinoma of lung
   4. Adrenal adenoma

Clinical Features

1. Acral bony overgrowth results in:
  a. Frontal bossing
  b. Increased hand and foot size
  c. Mandibular enlargement with prognathism
  d. Widened spaces between lower incisor teeth.
2. Growth hormone excess prior to epiphyseal closure of long bones in late puberty leads to long stature, if this process starts in childhood—produces gigantism.

Other Common Features

  i. Excessive perspiration—due to enlarged sweat gland or hypermetabolism.
  ii. Carpal tunnel syndrome—resulting from compression of enlarged or edematous median nerve by fibrocartilagenous tissue of the wrist.
  iii. Joint pain in weight-bearing joints secondary to bony overgrowth and deformity around large weight-bearing joints
  iv. Hypertension due to salt retaining effect of GH
  v. Glucose intolerance—due to anti-insulin effect of GH
  vi. Hypercalciuria and stone formation in kidney.
  vii. Galactorrhea
    a. Due to intrinsic lactogenic properties of GH.
    b. Presence of mixed adenoma—produced by GH and prolactinoma
  viii. Sleep apnea.

Complications

1. Cerebrovascular disease
2. Cardiovascular complications
3. Pulmonary complications

Diagnosis

1. 50–100 gm of glucose orally followed by blood collection at 60–120 minutes—fail to show suppression of GH level <.4 mg/L.
   With newer ultrasensitive GH assay—normal nadir GH level are even lower (0.05 mg/L).
   20% patients show paradoxical rise in GH.
2. 20% patients with acromegaly show raised prolactin level due to development of mixed adenoma in pituitary.
3. TSH, ACTH, LH and FSH levels may be suppressed due to mass effect.
4. Serum IGF level is increased in acromegaly.
5. MRI or CT scan of pituitary fossa.
6. Visual field examination to detect any pressure effect on optic chiasma.

Treatment

Aim

1. To control GH and IGF-I secretion
2. To ablate or arrest tumor growth
3. To alleviate comorbidities
4. To restore mortality rate to normal
5. To preserve pituitary function

Medical Management

Somatostatin analogue

Aim:
a. To produce preoperative shrinkage of large invasive macroadenoma
b. Immediate relief from symptoms
c. Reduction in growth hormone secretion
d. In patient, who:
    i. Is not candidate for surgery
    ii. Avoid or refuse surgery
    iii. Fails to respond to surgery
    iv. Awaiting for the effect of radiotherapy

Mode of actions: It acts through SSTR2 and SSTR5 receptors present on GH secreting tumor.

Drugs: Octreotide

Dose: 50 mg thrice daily subcutaneous injection gradually can be increased up to 1500 mg/day.

Long-acting somatostatin, octreotide and lanreotide.

A. Drugs:
1. *Sandostatin LAR:* Long-acting sustained release formulation incorporated into microspheres
   Intramuscular injection: 20–30 mg monthly injection—suppress GH and IGF suppression to 50%.
2. *Lanreotide autogel:* Slow release depot preparation—suppresses GH and IGF after subcutaneous injection of 60 mg.
   Rapid relief of headache and soft tissue swelling occurs in 75% of patients within days to weeks of somatostatin injection. Improvement of following symptoms will occur:
       i. Headache
       ii. Perspiration
       iii. Obstructive apnea
       iv. Cardiac failure

Side effects

i. Nausea, vomiting, abdominal discomfort, fat malabsorption, diarrhea
ii. Decreased postprandial gallbladder motility
    ↓
Delays gallbladder emptying
    ↓
Accumulation of sludge in gallbladder
    ↓
Gallstones—cholesterol stones
iii. Asymptomatic bradyarrhythmias
iv. Hypoxemia
v. Worsening of glucose in tolerance

B. *Growth hormone receptor antagonists:* Pegvisomant blocks the peripheral growth hormone binding receptors and antagonizes its action—as a consequence IGF-I is suppressed.
    This drug is deprived of 9 essential amino acids, so it binds to the GH receptors but is devoid of action of GH.
    This drugs does not cause any shrinkage of tumor, rather it may increase it theoretically by decreasing the action of native GH to stimulate hypothalamic somatostatin production.

Dose: Subcuteneous injection of 10–20 mg normalizes IGF-I in >90% of patients.

So combined treatment of Pegvisomant and somatostatin analogue has been used effectively in resistant patient.

Dopamine agonist

Mode of action:
1. It lowers the GH and IGF-I level in serum in 10–40% cases.
2. It produces tumor shrinkage in 10% of patient.

Drugs: i. Bromcriptine, ii. Cabergoline

Dose

Bromcriptine: >20 mg/day
Cabergoline: Most useful dopamine agonist—usually begin with 0.25 mg once or twice a week
    ↓
Doses increased to 1–2 mg/week
    ↓
Benefit is gained by increasing the daily dose >3 mg/weeks

Radiation Therapy

External radiation therapy or high energy steriotactic technique.

Effect:
i. GH is suppressed.
ii. Tumor size is reduced.

GH level <5 mg/L—can be achieved by 8 years in 50% patients. Patient should undergo interim medical therapy before full benefit of radiation therapy is achieved.

Disadvantage: Most patients experience hypothalamic–pituitary damage leading to gonadotrophin, ACTH and TSH deficiency. In this case, replacement therapy is needed.

Surgery

Transsphenoidal surgical resection of both microadenoma (cure rate 70%) and macrodenoma (cure rate 50%).

Achievement:
i. Immediate soft tissue swelling improvement.
ii. Growth hormone returns to normal level within 1 hour.
iii. IGF-I level returns to normal within 3–4 weeks.

Disadvantages:
i. Recurrence of acromegaly in 10% patients.
ii. Development of hypopituitarism in 15% patients.

GROWTH HORMONE DEFICIENCY IN CHILDREN

A. GH deficiency:
1. It is autosomal dominant, recessive or X-linked.
2. In 10% cases, GH gone mutations gene deletions.
3. Clinical manifestations:
    i. Short stature
    ii. Micropenis
    iii. Increased fat
    iv. High-pitched voice
    v. Propensity to hypoglycemia
    vi. Fatigue

vii. Low mood, poor concentration
viii. Central obesity
ix. Reduced lean body tissue and bone mineral density.
x. Biochemical abnormalities:
    a. Hyperlipidemia
    b. Glucose intolerance
    c. Microvascular disease—like increased carotid intimal thickness.

B. **GHRH receptor deficiency:** Due to mutation of GHRH receptor gene.

C. **Growth hormone insentivity:** Defect in an receptor structure or signaling pathways. As a result, there is partial or complete GH insentivity and growth failure (Laron syndrome)

Diagnosis is based on:
i. High growth hormone levels
ii. Decreased circulating GHBP level
iii. Decreased IGF-I levels
iv. Defective IGF-I and IGF-II receptor levels

D. **Nutritional short stature:**
i. Calorie deprivation and malnutrition
ii. Chronic renal failure
iii. Uncontrolled diabetes

E. **Psychological short stature:**
i. Emotional, and
ii. Social deprivation

Evaluation of Short Stature

i. Patient's height is >3 standard deviations below the mean for age, or
ii. Growth rate is decelerated.

Skeletal Maturation

Measuring a radiologic bone age—based on:
a. Degree of writs bone growth plate fusion.

Laboratory Evaluation

1. Insulin induced or pharmacologic test or provocative stimuli induced GH level <3 mg/L
2. Serum T_3/T_4, cortisol measurement.

Treatment

Replacement therapy with GH—0.02–0.05 mg/kg/day subcutaneously—resolves growth velocity in GH—deficient children.

POSTERIOR PITUITARY DISORDERS

Neurohypophysis is formed by—axons originating from large cell bodies in the supraoptic and paraventricular nuclei of hypothalamus. It produces two hormones:
i. Arginin vasopressin (AVP)—antidiuretic hormone
ii. Oxytocin

Stimuli of AVP Secretion

I. **Plasma osmolarity:** Main important determinant of AVP secretion.

Change in osmolarity
↓
Stimulate osmoreceptors in supraoptic and paraventricular nuclei of hypothalamus to release antidiuretic hormone

Osmoreceptors contain both inhibitory and stimulatory components—which act as a "set point".
1. Below this set point, plasma AVP is suppressed to permit the development of maximum diuresis.
2. Above this set point, plasma AVP rises steeply in direct proportion to plasma osmolarity to form antidiuresis.

This set point varies from person-to-person, but in average, the set point for AVP release corresponds to plasma osmolarity or sodium concentration which is 280 mosmol/L or 135 mEq/L, respectively.

This set point can be lowered in:
i. Pregnancy
ii. Menstrual cycle,
iii. Estrogen administration.

II. **Arterial underfilling:** It occurs due to bleeding, venous pulling, decreased systemic vascular resistance, third space sequestration.

High pressure mechanoreceptors located in aortic arch and carotid sinus and low pressure receptors located in atria and pulmonary venous system serve as sensors of volume/pressure status.

III. **Other nonosmotic stimuli:**
i. Nausea,
ii. Hypoglycemia
iii. Glucocorticoid deficiency
iv. Smoking
v. Hyperangiotensinemia

Actions

Most important site of action in distal convoluted tubular cells is achieved by increasing the hydro-osmotic permeability of cells.

In absence of AVP: The DCT and collection duct cells are impermeable to water, so little water is absorbed. As a result, large volume of dilute filtrate unless from proximal convoluted tubule and produce maximum diuresis (SpGr-1000, osmolarity 50 mOsmol/L)—this is called water dieresis.

In presence of AVP: The DCT and CD cells become selectively permeable to water, so water will diffuse back down the osmotic gradient produced by hypertonic renal medulla (1000–1200 mOsmol/L).

So urine becomes concentrated and rate of urine flow decreases to about 1 liter.

Antidiuretic effect is mediated via G protein-coupled V_2 receptor.

It increases the concentration of cyclic-AMP → induction of translocation of aquaporin 2 water channel in the apical membrane → which increases the permeability of membrane to water influx into the cells which diffuses water out of the cells through ACP 3 and ACP 4 on the basolateral surface.

Thirst: It is controlled primarily by osmostat, situated in anteromedial hypothalamus and detects little changes in plasma osmolarity and plasma sodium concentration.

Thirst osmostat set point is 5% higher than AVP osmostat.

DIABETES INCIPIDUS

This is a syndrome characterized by production of abnormally large volume of urine as evidenced by:
 i. 24-hour urine volume >50 ml/kg body weight
 ii. Urine osmolarity <300 mOsmol/L

Characteristic symptoms are:
 i. Polyuria
 ii. Nocturia
 iii. Increased frequency
 iv. Daytime fatigue and somnolence

Etiology of Diabetes Incipidus

Pituitary Diabetes Incipidus

A. Primary cause:
  1. Genetic:
      i. Autosomal dominant
      ii. Autosomal recessive
      iii. X-linked recessive
  2. Idiopathic
B. Secondary cause:
  1. Traumatic:
      i. Accidental (head trauma)
      ii. Iatrogenic (surgery)
  2. Tumors:
      i. Craniopharyngioma
      ii. Primary pituitary tumor
      iii. Metastatic tumor
      iv. Acute leukemia
  3. Infection:
      i. Chronic meningitis
      ii. Viral meningitis
      iii. Toxoplasmosis
  4. Inflammatory:
      i. SLE
      ii. Scleroderma
      iii. Wegener's granulomatosis
  5. Granulomatous disease:
      i. Sarcoidosis
      ii. Histiocytosis
      iii. Tuberculosis
  6. Chemical toxins—snake venom:
  7. Vascular:
      i. Sheehan's syndrome
      ii. Aortocoronary bypass
      iii. Hypoxic encephalopathy
  8. Drugs:
      i. Diphenylhydantoin
      ii. Alcohol
  9. Pregnancy

Pathophysiology

When AVP falls below 85% of normal
↓
Urine concentration decreases and rate of urine output rises to symptomatic level, polyuria results in small decrease in body water concentration
↓
Increase in plasma osmolarity and serum sodium concentration
↓
Stimulates thirst osmostat
↓
Results in compensatory increase water intake
↓
As a result hypernatremia and signs and symptoms of dehydration do not occur

But patient has defect in thirst mechanism or fails to drink for some other reasons—signs of dehydration develop gradually.

Clinical presentation:
 i. Polyuria
 ii. Polydipsia—Both occur throughout the day and night.
 iii. More predilections for cold drinks
 iv. Urine volume may be from 1 to 20 liters/day
 v. Serum osmolarity and serum sodium are variable depending upon the activity of thirst mechanism and patient's access to water.

   If thirst mechanism is impaired, patient may develop altered mental status

If diabetes incipidus is due to post-surgical or post-traumatic in the region of hypothalamus—posterior pituitary area, patient may develop triphasic response:
1. In 1st phase—transient DI due to axonal shock—develops within 24 hours of injury and resolve within days.
2. 2nd phase SIADH like phase—ensue within 5–7 days of primary insult. It is secondary to axonal degeneration.
3. 3rd phase—DI may or may not improve or resolve over time.

Diagnosis: Inappropriate dilute urine (pH <1010), low urine osmolarity (50–300 mOsl/kg):
  i. Low AVP concentration
  ii. Raised slightly more than normal plasma osmolarity
  iii. Raised or normal serum sodium concentration
  iv. If fluid is not given overnight, morning urine specific gravity should be at least 1018, if it is lower than the stated range—consider DI
  v. Visual field examination
  vi. Laboratory estimation of all pituitary hormones
  vii. MRI: Enlargement of pituitary stalk above 2–3 mm—due to:
      a. Infiltrative diseases
      b. Malignancy
      c. Infection

Absence of a bright spot in T1-weighted images of the sella—a characteristic finding in central diabetes incipidus.

Nephrogenic Diabetes Incipidus

This is characterized by—hypotonic polyuria resulting from:

i. Renal insensitivity to the action of antidiuretic hormone despite the presence of normal concentration of this hormone in the blood, and

ii. Failure of exogenous ADH to decrease the urine volume significantly or increase in urine osmolarity.

Causes:

I. *Hereditary:*
   1. Familial X-linked recessive (mutation of V_2 receptor)
   2. Autosomal recessive (mutation of aquaporin gene)
   3. Autosomal dominant (mutation of aquaporin gene)

II. *Acquired:*
   A. Drugs
      i. Lithium
      ii. Demedocycline
      iii. Amphotericin B
      iv. Cisplatin
      v. Rifampin
      vi. Foscarnet
   B. Metabolic
      i. Hypocalcemia
      ii. Hypercalciuria
      iii. Hpokalemia
   C. Vascular
      i. Sickle cell disease
      ii. Ischemia
   D. Infiltration amyloidosis
   E. Granulomatous—sarcoidosis
   F. Pregnancy
   G. Idiopathic
   H. Low protein diet

Pathophysiology:

Inability of the collecting duct to increase the water permeability in response to AVP

↓

So inability to conserve water

↓

Increase in plasma osmolarity and sodium concentration

Clinical presentation: In early infancy (in case of familial disease):
   i. Vomiting
   ii. Fever
   iii. Failure to thrive
   iv. Hypotonic polyuria
   v. Electrolyte imbalances
   vi. Hypertonic dehydration

In case of acquired disease—recognition of this disease depends upon:

a. Underlying disease

b. Duration of exposure to medication—may present with moderate polyuria (3–4 liters/min)

Diagnosis:
1. Hypernatremia
2. Elevated plasma osmolarity
3. Normal kidney function
4. Failure to respond to vasopressin after water deprivation test.
5. Serum ADH will be raised.
6. Absent urinary cAMP response after vasopressin administration.
7. Identify carrier mother by measuring urine osmolarity after a 12-hour period of fluid restriction.

Primary Polydipsia

It is of two types:

I. **Dipsogenic diabetes incipidus**: In this case, osmotic threshold for thirst mechanism is lower than that of AVP release—so there is constant hypotonic polyuria in spite of low plasma osmolarity.
   The causes are:
   i. Hypothalamic lesion
   ii. Sarcoidosis

II. **Psychogenic polydipsia**: This is characterized by compulsive water drinking—due to psychogenic disorders. In this case, there is no change in thirst threshold.

Diagnosis of polyuria states:
1. Osmotic causes of polyuria—such as hyperglycemic—should be ruled out by laboratory workup.
2. Presence of psychiatric disease—suggests psychogenic polydipsia.
3. Hypotonic polyuria in the face of increased plasma osmolarity, and serum sodium concentration excludes the diagnosis of primary polydipsia.
4. Sudden development of polyuria after surgical or non-surgical trauma to hypothalamus—pituitary area—suggests central diabetes incipidus.
5. In this situation—provocative test—water deprivation test followed by AVP administration is the most common test used.

Water deprivation test:

A. To minimize discomfort of patient, test should be started in the morning and continued with hourly monitoring of:
   i. Body weight
   ii. Plasma osmolarity
   iii. Plasma sodium concentration
   iv. Urine volume
   v. Urine osmolarity until two end points are reached

   This test should be discontinued, if:
   i. Body weight decreases by 3%.
   ii. Patient has cardiovascular instability
   iii. Urine osmolarity remains stable (3 consecutive urine sample osmolarities vary by <30 mOsml/kg).
   iv. Hypernatremia (>145 mOsol/L).

   Once urine osmolarity has reached a stable value or patient has lost >2% of body weight—samples are obtained for:
   i. Plasma sodium
   ii. Plasma osmolarity
   iii. Vasopressin in plasma

B. Then the patient is given with 0.03 mg/kg of vasopressin subcutaneously or intravenously and repeat urine volume and osmolarity measurement at 30 minutes, 60 minutes, 90 minutes and 120 minutes after the injection.

C. Plasma osmolarity should be measured:
   i. Before commencement of the test
   ii. Before administration of DDAVP and
   iii. After administration of DDAVP

Precaution:
i. Avoid caffeine containing beverages on the day of test.
ii. Alcohol and tobacco should be avoided 24 hours before this test.
iii. During this test, monitoring of the patient is necessary—because nausea, hypotension or vasovagal reactions may occur during and after the test.

Interpretation:
1. *In healthy subject*—water deprivation may lead to maximal stimulus for vasopressin secretion and maximal urine concentration. Hence administration of DDAVP will not lead to increase >10% in osmolarity, because urine is already maximally concentrated.
2. *Primary polydipsia:* Absence of increase in urine osmolarity above the plasma osmolarity—excludes primary polydipsia provided surreptitious drinking is excluded.
3. *Central and nephrogenic DI:*
   1. If urine osmolarity does not >300 mosm/L and urine specific gravity does not >1010, before body weight decreases by >5% or plasma osmolarity/sodium rises above upper limit of normal—patient is suffering from DI of central or nephrogenic origin.
   2. After injection DDAVP, an increase of >50% in urine osmolarity—suggests central DI.
      Absent response suggest nephrogenic DI

Treatment

1. **Maintaining fluid metabolism:** If patient has no intact thirst mechanism—continued monitoring of fluid intake is necessary and balancing with water intake and antidiuretic intervention.
2. **ADH agonist:** It acts through V_2 receptors on collecting duct cells and increases urinary osmolarity.
   The drugs are: Desmopressin—this agent is 2000 times more specific for antidiuresis.
   a. *Intranasal application:* Onset of action 45 min, peak action 1–5 hours
      i. Nasal spray 10–20 mg twice to thrice daily. One dose has an antidiuretic activity of 40 IU.
      ii. Rhinal tube multidose vial—in concentration of 0.1 mg/ml can deliver 5–20 mg into rhinal catheter.
      iii. Stimate nasal spray: Available in concentration of 0.15 mg/ml deliver 0.1 ml (150 mg)—one dose has antidiuretic activity of 600 IU.
   b. *Parenteral administration:* 5–20 times more potent than intranasal application.
      Available as 4 mg/ml solution
      Dose is 1–2 mg subcutaneously or intravenously twice a day.
   c. *Oral administration:* 0.1–0.2 mg tablets. Onset of action is 30–60 minutes. To start with 0.1 mg at bedtimes, it can be increased up to 1.2 mg/day in 2–3 divided doses.

Other agents:
a. *Chlorpropamide:* It enhances the activity of AVP and enhances the release of AVP—decreases polyuria.
   Dose is—100–500 mg orally daily.
b. *Carbamazepine:* It can cause release of ADH. It can be used in partial central diabetes incipidus. Dose—ranges from 20–600 mg/day.
c. *Thiazide diuretics*
d. *Indomethacin*

Treatment of primary polydipsia: Behavior modification

Syndrome of Inappropriate Secretion of Antidiuretic Hormone

Definition

It is a condition of euvolemic hyponatremia secondary to inadequate secretion of antidiuretic hormone which causes:
i. In appropriate urinary concentration
ii. Water retention

Pathophysiology

a. **Hypersecretion of AVP:**
   i. Ectopic inappropriate production and hypersecretion of AVP.
   ii. Inappropriately elevated and non-suppressible basal AVP production.
   iii. Resetting of osmostat triggered by lower than normal osmolarity.
b. **Increased urinary sodium**—due to:
   i. Water retention — pressure-induced natriuresis
   ii. Increased secretion of atrial natriuretic peptide
c. **Hypouricemia** secondary to V_1 receptor stimulated uric acid clearance.
d. **Interleukin 6**—a causative factor in sickness, stress, inflammation.

Etiology

1. Central nervous system disorders:
   i. Vascular
   ii. Infection
   iii. Tumor
   iv. Metabolic
2. Pulmonary conditions:
   i. Pneumonia
   ii. Tuberculosis
3. Neoplasm: Small cell cancer
4. Pharmacologic agents:
   i. Analgesics
   ii. Chlorpropamide
   iii. Barbiturates
5. Others:
   i. Cardiac cause
   ii. Hypothyroidism
   iii. Addison's disease

Symptoms

i. Weakness
ii. Lethargy
iii. Confusion
   If water intoxication occurs:
iv. Vomiting
v. Irritability
vi. Personality changes
vii. Focal neurologic deficits

Diagnosis

i. Hyponatremia
ii. Low serum osmolarity
iii. High urine osmolarity 250 to 1400 mOsm/kg
iv. Normal kidney and adrenal function

v. Urinary Na concentration > 30 mEq/L
vi. Elevated ADH
vii. ↓ Uric acid level
viii. Low urine volume

Acute SIADH—Treatment

Fluid restrictions:

> i. Total fluid intake should be at least 500 ml less than the urinary output per day.
>
> ↓
>
> This increases the serum sodium 1–2% per day and reduces the body water content

ii. If symptoms and signs are more severe: Fluid restriction is to be supplemented with IV infusion of 3% saline (hypertonic saline). This:
a. Corrects sodium deficiency—which is responsible for hyponatremia in SIADH.
b. Produces solute diuresis removing excess water. But rapid correction of hyponatremia produces central pontine myelenosis.

To avoid this complication—rate infusion should be <0.05 ml/kg per minute.

The effect should be monitored continuously by measuring serum sodium 2 hourly.

Infusion should be stopped as soon as the serum sodium increases by 12 mmol/L or 130 mmol/L whichever comes first.

Urine output should be monitored continuously since SIADH may remit spontaneously at any time.

In Chronic SIADH—Treatment

Hyponatremia can be corrected by:
1. Demeclocycline—150–300 mg thrice daily
2. Fludrocortisone—0.65–0.2 mg twice daily
   Effect of demeclocycline manifests in 7–14 days and it is due to production of reversible form of nephrogenic DI.
   Side effects: Photosensitivity, azotemia

Effect of fludrocortisones is:
i. Increased retention of sodium
ii. Inhibition of thirst
iii. Increase urinary potassium excretion—may require oral potassium replacement.

Non-peptide AVP antagonist: It blocks the antidiuretic effect of AVP—it produces: Dose dependent free water excretion, if supplemented by fluid restriction—it reduces body water and corrects—hyponatremia.

The drug is:

1. Combined V2/V1á antagonist (conivaptan)—has been approved for treatment—in congestive cardiac failure and hyponatremia and SIADH.
2. Tolvaptan analogue AVP receptor antagonist with high affinity to AV receptor V_2. It is recommended for hyper/euvolemic hyponatremia. When Na <125 mEq/L. Dose—15–30 mg daily for 3 days ordin continue if Na >140 mEq/L.

THYROID GLAND DISORDERS

THYROID GLAND: ANATOMY AND PHYSIOLOGY

Thyroid gland extracts iodine from circulation in highly efficient manner. Iodine is taken up by a membrane protein presents at basolateral membrane called **sodium-iodide symporter (NIS).** This active process depends upon presence of sodium gradient across the membrane of the cell.

NIS is also present in other iodide concentrating cells, e.g.
i. Salivary gland
ii. Lactating mammary gland
iii. Choroid plexus
iv. Gastric mucosa
v. Cytotrophoblast
vi. Syncytiotrophoblast.

NIS also transport

i. *Pertechnate (TcO₄)* which is used as thyroid scanning tool (radioactive tracer).
ii. *Perchlorate (ClO₄)*—which can block iodide uptake inside the cell.

Transcription of NIS gene and prolongation of half life are increased by TSH.

Low iodine level increases the amount of NIS and increases iodine uptake, whereas **high iodine level** depresses NIS expression.

Another iodine transporter is pendrin—located at the apical surface of the cell—which mediates iodine efflux out of the cell into the lumen.

This transporter is also present in:
i. **Kidney**—plays an important role in acid-base imbalance.
ii. **Inner ear:** Here it is important for generation of endo-cochlear potential.

Mutation of pendrin gene is responsible for development of **Pendred syndrome**—characterized by:
i. Defective organification of iodine.
ii. Goiter.
iii. Sensory neural deafness.

Other protein responsible for iodide efflux is—**chloride channel 5 (ClCN5)**—present at the apical membrane of cells.

In addition to active transport of iodide from extracellular fluid, intracellular iodide is formed by the action of **enzyme iodotyrosine dehalogenase 1 (DEHAL 1)** or **iodotyrosine deiodinase (IYD)**. This iodide is released and immediately reconjugated with thyroglobulin (Tg) into the lumen. This process in interrupted by **thiourea (propylthiouracil)—which is thyroid peroxidase (TPO).**

Organification, Coupling, Storage and Release

At the apical membrane of the thyroid follicular cell, iodide is oxidized by **thyroid peroxidase and hydrogen peroxide—**

iodine atom is added to tyrosyl residue within thyroglobulin molecule (TG) dimeric protein.

The required H_2O_2 is generated by calcium and NADAH dependant DUOX 1 and DUOX 2 oxidase enzymes.

Dual oxidase maturation factor 2 (DUOX A2) a resident ER protein is required for maturation and plasma membrane localization of **DUOX2, for H_2O_2 generation.**

Rate of organic iodination is dependent on degree of stimulation of TSH.

Either T_4 or T_3 can be produced by TPO reaction, depending on number of iodine atoms present in iodotyrosine in TG.

Synthesis of T_4 requires TPO catalyzed fusion of two DIT molecules, and **synthesis of T_3** requires TPO catalyzed fusion of one MIT and one DIT molecules.

In normal iodination state:
i. Three to four T_4 molecules present in each TG molecules.
ii. One in five molecules of TG contains T_3 molecules.

In Graves' disease:
i. Content of T_4 residue remains same.
ii. Number of T_3 residues doubles to an average of 0.4 per molecule.

After coupling, **TG is taken back into the thyroid cells,** where it is processed by lysosomal enzymes to **release T_4 to T_3** which are then deiodenated by enzyme dehalogenase. This iodine will be again reused.

Hormone Release

First step in thyroid hormone release is **endocytosis of colloid** from follicular lumen—which is accomplished by two processes:

i. **Micropinocytosis**—which is predominant in human being.
ii. **Macropinocytosis** by pseudopods formed at apical membrane.

After endocytosis:

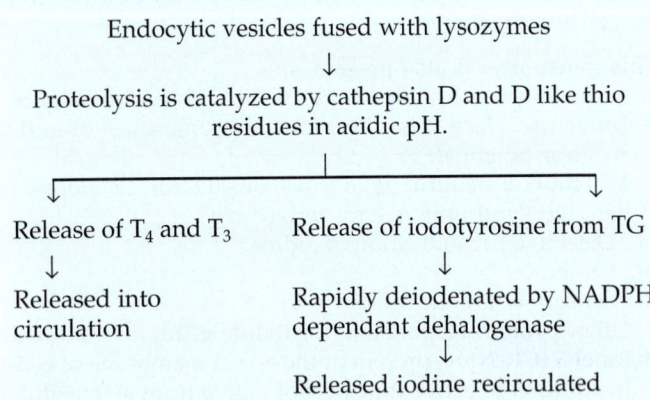

Endocytic vesicles fused with lysozymes
↓
Proteolysis is catalyzed by cathepsin D and D like thio residues in acidic pH.

Release of T_4 and T_3 — Release of iodotyrosine from TG
↓ — ↓
Released into circulation — Rapidly deiodenated by NADPH dependant dehalogenase
↓
Released iodine recirculated

T_4 is accessible to thyroidal type 1 and type 2 deiodinase (D_1 and D_2, respectively). This conversion is usually TSH stimulated.

Normal ratio is T_4 : T_3 = 15:1.

But in Graves' disease, D_1 catalyzes. 5′ deiodination of T_4 in the thyroid contributing to **marked increase in ratio so that T_4 : T_3 become 5 to 10:1.** Propylthiouracil blocks the D_1 catalyzed pathway leading to decreased level of T_3.

In one mediastinal tumor, high expression of D_2 leads to high T_3 and low T_4 level—removal of tumor reverses this condition.

T_4 release from thyroid cells is inhibited by:
1. **Iodide**—Inhibits the:
   i. Secretion of thyroid adenylate cyclase by TSH;
   ii. Stimulatory immunoglobulin in Graves' disease
2. **Lithium**—mechanism of action is not known.
3. **Increased iodination of thyroglobulin molecules.**

Role of TSH

1. **Thyroid-stimulating hormone regulates thyroid gland function through TSH-R,** presents on thyroid cell. TSH-R is G-protein-coupled receptor (G-PCR). TSH has been reported to-couple 7 different G-protein ∝ subunits. When TSH-R combines with a protein ∝ subunits (G∝)
   ↓
   Activates adenylyl cyclase
   ↓
   Increased production of cyclic-AMP
2. **TSH also stimulates phosphatidylinositol turnover** by activating phospholipase C

This phospholipase C and intracellular Ca^{++} pathways stimulate:
   i. Iodide efflux,
   ii. H_2O_2 production
   iii. Thyroglobulin iodination

This cyclic-AMP production regulates:
   i. Iodine uptake
   ii. Transcription of thyroglobulin, thyroid peroxidase (TPD)
   iii. NIS production.

TSH-R also binds to:
   i. TSH-R stimulating antibody
   ii. Thyroid blocking antibodies
   iii. Neutral antibodies
   iv. LH
   v. HCG

HCG binding is responsible of transient hyperthyroidism evidenced in pregnancy.

Plasma transport of thyroid hormones:
1. **Major concentration is T_4**—solely secreted from thyroid gland
2. **T_3:**
   i. 80% derived from enzymatic removal of 5′ iodine peripherally from T_4.
   ii. Small quantity directly from thyroid gland (rT_3)
3. **Trace concentration of other diiodothyronine and mono-iodothyronine** and their conjugates with glucuronic and sulphuric acid.
4. **Deaminated derivatives of T_4 and T_3** bearing acetic acid in side chain.

Binding of Thyroid Hormones

Both T_4 and T_3 are bound to plasma proteins:
a. **Thyroid-binding globulin**—present in very low concentration (1–2 mg/dl) in plasma, but binds 80% of total circulatory hormone with high affinity for T_4 ($T_4 > T_3$).

Low level of thyroid hormone binding globulin seen in:
1. Congenital deficiency TBG.
2. Patient treated with asparaginase.

3. Glycosylation of TBG influences its clearance from plasma seen
   i. In estrogen treated patient
   ii. In patient taking oral contraceptives
   iii. In acute infective hepatitis
4. Post-translational modification in sepsis—(serine proteases released from leukocyte) and cardiopulmonary bypass—in these cases, there is decreased affinity for T_4.

b. **Transthyrectin** (formerly known as prealbumin)—binds 10% of total circulating T_4 and little T_3.

c. **Albumin:** Though it is present in highest concentration in plasma, it binds to 10% of total circulating T_4 and 30% T_3.

Plasma-binding proteins are responsible for:
i. Increase in the pooling of circulating hormones
ii. Daily hormone clearance
iii. Modulation of the hormone delivery to the target tissue

Free Thyroid Hormones in Peripheral Circulation

FT_4 is inversely proportional to the concentration of unoccupied TBG binding sites. It can be estimated by direct or indirect assays.

In normal serum, FT_4 is 1.5 ng/dl.
It is available for:
   i. Intracellular transport
   ii. Feedback regulation
   iii. Induction of metabolic effects
   iv. Deiodination
   v. Degradation

It roughly corresponds to thyroid hormone receptors binding constants for this hormone.

Deiodinase: T_4 is converted into T_3 (more active) by deiodinase system. Three types of deiodinase system are:

1. *Type I deiodinase:*
   i. It is located primarily in thyroid, liver and kidneys
   ii. It has relative low affinity for T_4.

2. *Type II deiodinase:*
   i. It has high affinity for T_4.
   ii. It is formed primarily in pituitary gland, brain, brown fat and thyroid gland.
   iii. It allows concentration of T_3 locally.

It is regulated by thyroid hormone: Hypothyroidism induces enzyme, resulting enhanced $T_4 \rightarrow T_3$ conversion in brain and pituitary.

T_4 to T_3 conversion is decreased in:
   i. Severe sepsis
   ii. Fasting
   iii. Acute trauma
   iv. Oral contrast agents
   v. Medications—propylthiouracil, propranolol, amiodarone, glucocorticoid (high dose)

3. *Type III deiodinase system:*
   i. It inactivates T_4 and T_3
   ii. It is the major source of reverse T_3 (rT_3)
   iii. It occurs in massive hemangioma

Thyroid Hormone Action

Thyroid Hormone Transport

Thyroid hormone enters the cells by:
i. Passive diffusion
ii. Via specific transporters such as monocarboxylate 8 (MCT 8), transporter

So mutations in MCT 8 gene—have been identified in—patients with:
1. X-linked psychomotor retardation and
2. Thyroid function abnormalities (low T_4 and high T_3 and high TSH)

Mechanism of actions: Thyroid hormones bind with high affinity to nuclear thyroid receptors (TR)—μ and b having two gene μ and b—in chromosome number 17 and 3, respectively.

TR has three main functional domains:
   i. One binds to DNA
   ii. One binds to ligand
   iii. Major transcriptional activation domain at C-terminals

Tissue distribution:
1. TR∝—particularly abundant in brain, kidney, gonads, muscles and heart.
2. TRβ—high in pituitary gland and liver

These proteins TR∝ and TRβ are subdivided into:
(i) $TR\propto_1$, (ii) $TR\propto_2$; (iii) $TR\beta_1$; (iv) $TR\beta_2$;

$TR\propto_2$ is thought to be important in hypothalamus and pituitary—where regulation of thyroid hormone occurs.

$TR\beta_2$—is selectively expressed in hypothalamus, pituitary, where it plays a major role in feedback control of thyroid axis.

Thyroid hormone receptor (TR) and retinoid x receptor (R × R) form heterodimers, bind specifically to thyroid hormone responsive elements in the promoter regions of target genes.

1. $\rightarrow T_4$ or T_3 enter the cell through membrane transporter protein.
2. T_3 binding dissociates co-repressors (COR) from TR (thyroid hormone receptors)
3. $\rightarrow T_3$ binding allows recruitment of co-activators (CoA) that enhances transcription.

If TR interacts with co-repressors—activate TR silence gene in absence of hormone binding.

THYROID FUNCTION TESTS

In Vitro Tests

A. **Serum thyroxine (T_4)**—reference range 5–12 mg/dl
   It may be altered in:
   1. Changes in TBG or other binding protein:
      i. Pregnancy
      ii. Oral contraceptives
      iii. Estrogen
   2. Factors altering the concentration of T_4 without changing its metabolism:
      i. Nonthyroidal illness
      ii. Peripheral resistance to thyroid hormone
      iii. Endogenous antibodies to T_4
      iv. Certain drugs

B. **Free thyroxine (FT_4):** Reference range 0.8–2.0 ng/ml
   It is not affected by alteration in serum protein or nonthyroidal illness.

   Calculation: It can be calculated by multiplying the serum T_4 by an indirect assessment of TBG capacity.
   Indirect measurement of TBG may vary. They include:
   a. T_3 uptake test
   b. Thyroid uptake test
   c. Thyroid uptake ratio

Free thyroxine index: This can be estimated by thyroid hormone binding ratio multiplied by total T_4 or T_3 to obtain FT_4I.

C. Serum T_3: Ref range 80–180 ng/dl

D. Serum TSH: Reference range—0.3–3.0 mU/L

Most commercial assays have functional sensitivity of 0.01 mU/L—it can detect mildest term of hyperthyroidism

Causes of elevated TSH:
i. Most common hypothyroidism
ii. TSH secreting pituitary tumor
iii. Thyroid hormone resistance
iv. Assay artifact

Causes of suppressed TSH:
i. Thyrotoxicosis
ii. First trimester of pregnancy
iii. After treatment of hypothyroidism
iv. In response to certain medications—high dose of gluco-corticoid, dopamine.

In vivo Tests

1. **Radioactive iodine uptake:** Administration of ^{123}I and measuring should be done as percent of uptake of radio-iodine dose, 1–24 hours later.

Normal average range of uptake: 8–25%.

Causes of alterations of radioiodine uptake:

A. *High radioiodine uptake:*
   1. Graves' disease
   2. Toxic multinodular goiter
   3. Toxic adenoma
   4. Choriocarcinoma
   5. Hydatidiform mole
   6. TSH producing pituitary tumor
B. *Low RAIU:*
   1. Subacute thyroiditis
   2. Painless thyroiditis
   3. Graves' disease with acute iodine load
   4. Iodine-induced hyperthyroidism
   5. Thyroid hormone therapy
2. **TRH test**
3. **T_3 suppression test**

Other Serological Tests (Figs 3.2 and 3.3)

Antibody Detection Test
i. Antithyroglobulin
ii. Antimicrosomal antibodies
iii. Antibodies to T_4, T_3
iv. Thyroid blocking antibodies

Biochemical Markers of Thyroid Status

Thyrotoxicosis
Increased:
i. Osteocalcin
ii. Atrial natriuretic hormone
iii. Alkaline phosphatase (bone and liver)

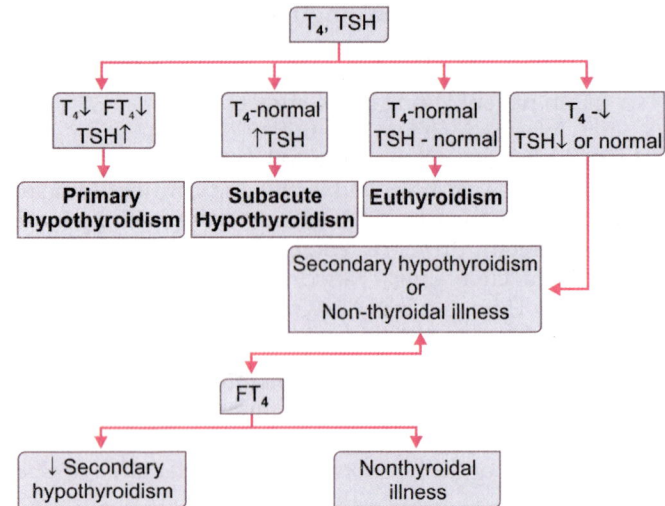

Fig. 3.2: Laboratory evaluation of suspected hypothyroidism

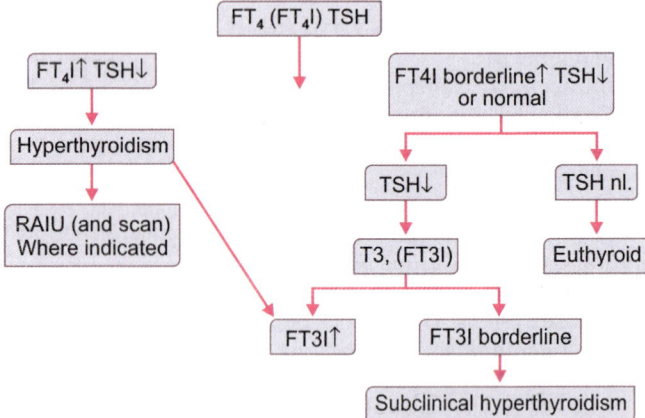

Fig. 3.3: Laboratory evaluation of suspected hyperthyroidism

iv. Von Willibrand factor
v. Ferritin
Decreased—LDL

Hypothyroidism
Increased:
i. CPK (MM forms)
ii. LDL
iii. Plasma norepinephrine
Decreased—vasopressin.

HYPOTHYROIDISM

Definition

It is a clinical condition resulting from lack of the effects of thyroid hormone on body tissues.

Causes of Hypothyroidism

I. **Primary**
   A. *Autoimmune thyroidism:*
      i. Hashimoto's thyroiditis
      ii. Atrophic thyroiditis

B. *Iatrogenic:*
   i. I^{131} treatment
   ii. Subtotal or total thyroidectomy
   iii. External irradiation for lymphoma or cancer
C. *Drugs:*
   i. Iodine excess
   ii. Iodine containing contrast media
   iii. Para-aminosalicylic acid
D. *Congenital hypothyroidism:*
   i. Absent thyroid,
   ii. TSH-R mutation
E. *Iodine deficiency*
F. *Infiltrative disorders:*
   i. Amyloidosis,
   ii. Sarcoidosis
   iii. Hemochromatosis
   iv. Cysteinosis
   v. Riedel's thyroiditis
II. **Transient**
   A. Silent thyroiditis
   B. Subacute thyroiditis
   C. Withdrawal of thyroxine treatment
   D. I^{131} therapy
   E. Subtotal thyroidectomy for Graves' disease.
III. **Secondary**
   A. Hypopituitarism—tumor
   B. Pituitary surgery, irradiation, infiltrative disorders
   C. Isolated TSH deficiency
   D. Bexarotene treatment
   E. Hypothalamic diseases: Tumor, trauma, infiltrative disorder

Congenital Hypothyroidism

Prevalence: One in 4000 population
Causes:
1. *Transient hypothyroidism*—due to:
   i. Mother has TSH-R blocking antibodies
   ii. Mother has received antithyroid drugs
2. *Permanent hypothyroidism:*
   i. Thyroid dysgenesis
   ii. Inborn error of thyroid hormone synthesis

This is more common in girls.

Clinical Manifestations

1. Majority are normal at birth.
2. 10% patients are diagnosed by:
   i. Prolonged jaundice
   ii. Feeding problem
   iii. Hypotonia
   iv. Enlarged tongue
   v. Delayed bone maturation
   vi. Protruding umbilical hernia
   vii. If treatment is delayed, permanent neurological deformity.
3. Typical features of adult hypothyroidism may be present:
   i. Dry coarse skin
   ii. Cold peripheral extremities
   iii. Diffuse alopecia
   iv. Bradycardia
   v. Delayed tendon reflexes
   vi. Carpal tunnel syndrome

Diagnosis:
i. T_4-↓low   ii. TSH↑level

Treatment

> i. T_4—at dose of 10–15 mg/kg/day
> ↓
> Then dose should be adjusted by monitoring TSH level
> T_4 requirement—is high during 1st year of life.
>
> Effect—normalization of IQ level

Autoimmune Hypothyroidism

Classifications

1. It may be associated with goiter—Hashimoto or goitrous thyroiditis.
2. In later stage may be associated with minimal residual thyroid tissue—atrophic thyroiditis.
3. In autoimmune process, there is gradual loss of thyroid function, associated with a phase of compensatory mechanism—when thyroid hormone level is normal with raised level of TSH—in these patients there may be minor symptoms, this state is called subclinical hypothyroidisms.
4. In late stage—T_4, FT_4 level—fall, with further rise in TSH level—(TSH >10 mU/L)—this state is called clinical hypothyroidism.

Clinical Features

A. **In Hashimoto's thyroiditis:**
   i. Onset is insidious
   ii. Present with goiter—it is large, irregular, firm in consistency
   iii. In some cases, only pyramidal lobe can be palpated, normally remnant of thyroglossal duct
   iv. There may be pain over the thyroid gland
B. **In atrophic thyroiditis or in later stage of autoimmune hypothyroidism**
   I. *Skin and appendages:*
      i. Skin is dry, decreased sweating, thinning of epidermis and hyperkeratosis of stratus corneum.
      ii. Increased dermal 'glycosaminoglycans content trap water—called myxomatous tissue—it is characteristically boggy, non-pitting edema (myxedema). These are deposited:
         a. Round the eyes
         b. On the dorsum of the hands and feet
         c. Supraclavicular fossa
         d. It produces enlargement of tongue—producing macroglossia
         e. It produces hoarseness of voice—due to deposition of this tissue
         f. Facies become putty, edematous
         g. Non-pitting pretibial edema
      iii. Skin color is yellowish tinged due to carotene accumulation
      iv. Hair becomes dry, brittle, thin and fall easily
      v. Thinning of outer third of the eyebrows
      vi. Easy bruising due to capillary fragility

II. *Cardiovascular system involvement:*
i. Myocardial contractility, pulse rate is reduced—leading to reduced stroke volume
ii. Bradycardia
iii. Increased peripheral resistance—leads to hypertension—mainly diastolic
iv. Reduction in cutaneous circulation leads to cool-skin and increased sensitivity to cold
v. In extreme hypothyroidism:
a. Enlarged cardiac silhouette
b. Heart sound may be distant or diminished in intensity —all above features are suggestive of pericardial effusion (30% cases) (Fig. 3.4)—fluid rich in protein and glycosaminoglycans
c. Rarely it produces cardiac tamponade

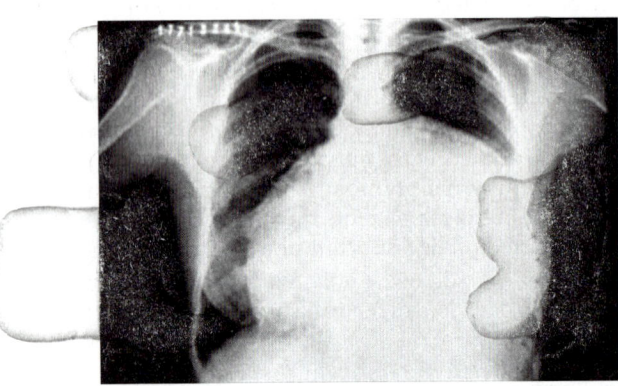

Fig. 3.4: Pericardial effusion

vi. Electrocardiographic changes are:
a. Bradycardia
b. Prolongation of PR internal
c. Low amplitude P wave and QRS complexes
d. Alteration in ST segment
e. Flattened or inverted T waves
f. Low amplitude complexes

III. *Respiratory system:*
i. Ventilatory response to hypoxia and hypercapnea are reduced.
ii. Lung volumes are normal, but maximum breathing capacity and diffusing capacity are reduced.
iii. In severe case, there is carbon dioxide retention—which in turn, can contribute to the development of myxedema coma
iv. Obstructive sleep apnea is common—reversible in euthyroid state

IV. *Alimentary system:*
i. Weight gain—due to retention of fluid containing hydrophilic glycoprotein deposits.
ii. Decreased peristaltic activity together with decreased food intake is responsible for constipation
iii. There may be fecal impaction (myxedema megacolon)
iv. Gaseous distention of abdomen (myxedema ileus) may be associated with colicky abdominal pain and vomiting—mimicking mechanical obstruction
v. Isolated ascites is less common, but in association with pleural effusion, and pericardial effusion, it may be present—fluid contains protein and glycosaminoglycans.
vi. Achlorhydria may be present.
vii. Circulating antibodies against parietal cells may be present in 30% cases—producing pernicious anemia.
viii. In liver function tests—transaminase levels are elevated due to decreased clearance.
ix. Gallbladder may be distended. In female, 3–8-fold increased risk of cholelithiasis.

V. *Renal system:*
i. Reduced excretion of water load—is associated with hyponatremia
ii. Renal blood flow and GFR are reduced, serum creatinine is normal. Delay in water excretion due to—decreased volume of fluid in DCT as a result of diminished renal perfusion—which can be reversed by treatment with thyroid hormone.

VI. *Muscular system:*
i. Arthralgia
ii. Muscle cramps
iii. Stiffness of muscles
iv. Joint effusion
v. Rarely profound increase in muscle mass with slowness of muscular activity may be predominant manifestation (Hoffmann syndrome)
vi. Myoclonus may be present.
vii. EMG shows—exhibit disordered discharge, hyperirritability, and polyphasic action potential.

VIII. *Skeletal system:*
i. Growth failure—is caused by:
a. Impaired general protein synthesis
b. Reduced growth hormone
c. Reduced insulin-like growth factor
ii. Stippled appearance of the epiphyseal center of ossification—epiphyseal dysgenesis.
iii. Impairment of linear growth—in which limbs are disproportionately short in relation to trunk, but cartilage growth is unaffected—dwarfism.
iv. Urinary execution of calcium is decreased, but urinary and fecal excretion of phosphate is variable.
v. Level of PTH is slightly increased, with some degree of resistance to its action. 1, 25 Dihydroxy D_3 level is increased.

IX. *Reproductive system:*
i. Menorrhagia from anovulatory cycle.
ii. Menstruation may become scanty or even cease completely because of deficient secretion of gonadotrophin.
iii. In adolescents—there may be primary amenorrhea
iv. Hyperprolactinemia—due to absence of inhibitory effect of thyroid hormone on prolactin secretion—resulting galactorrhea.
v. Increased incidence of abortion or preterm delivery.
vi. Primary ovarian failure occurs in patient with Hashimoto's thyroiditis—features of polyendocrine syndrome.
vii. In male, loss of libido, oligospermia, erectile dysfunction.
viii. Metabolism of both androgen and estrogen is altered—secretion of androgen is reduced and

metabolism of testosterone is shifted to etiocholanolone.

Metabolism:
  i. Hypothermia—intolerance to cold is common.
 ii. Hypercholesterolemia with increase in serum LDL in blood due to reduced number of LDL receptors.
iii. Hypertriglyceridemia—due to reduced degradation of lipoprotein and reduced lipoprotein lipase activity.

Hypothyroidism in Infants and Children

Severe hyperthyroidism in infancy is called cretinism.

a. Hallmark of cretinism (Fig. 3.5): Retardation of mental development and growth—manifested in late infancy.

As the age advances—mental retardation becomes irreversible even with treatment.

b. During 1st a few months of life:
   i. Feeding problem
  ii. Failure to thrive
 iii. Constipation
  iv. Hoarse cry
   v. Somnolence
  vi. Jaundice

c. As age advances in severe cases:
   i. Protuberant abdomen
  ii. Dry skin
 iii. Poor hair and nail growth
  iv. Delayed eruption of deciduous teeth
   v. Delay in reacting normal, milestone of development
      a. Holding up the head
      b. Sitting
      c. Walking
      d. Talking

d. Mesenchymal involvement: Thyroid hormone receptors are present in osteoclast and osteoblast.

Primary target of thyroid hormone is epiphyseal plates.

As a result:
  i. Impairment of linear growth—result dwarfism, limbs are disproportionately short than trunk.
 ii. Delayed closure of fontanels—leads to larger head in relation to body.
iii. Maldevelopment of femoral epiphyses—results in waddling gait.
 iv. Teeth are malformed and susceptable dental carries.

Characteristic Features

1. Broad flat nose
2. Widely set eyes
3. Periorbital puffiness
4. Large protruding tongue
5. Sparse hair
6. Rough skin
7. Short neck

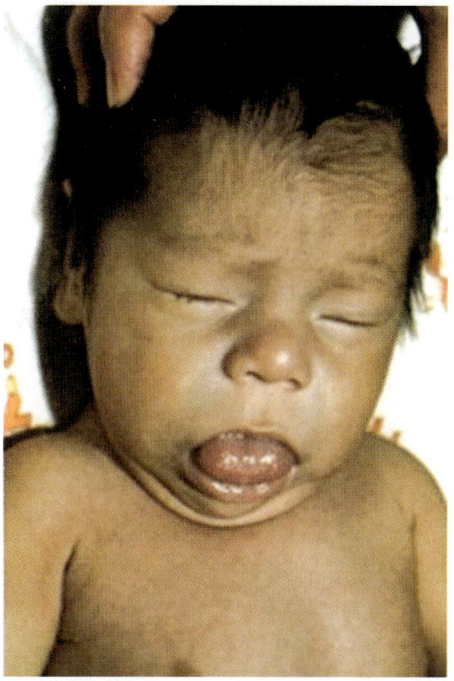

Fig. 3.5: Cretinism

8. Protuberant abdomen with umbilical hernia
9. Mentally retarded.

Radiological Features

1. Skull shows:
   i. Poorly developed bone
  ii. Delayed closure of fontanel
 iii. Widely set orbit
  iv. Short flat nasal bone
   v. Widened pituitary fossa
  vi. Shedding of deciduous teeth and eruption of permanent teeth are delayed

2. Radiological features of epiphyseal dysgenesis—is pathognomonic of hypothyroidism in infancy and childhood
   i. Involve center of endochondral ossification.
  ii. Mainly involve femoral and humeral heads and navicular bone of foot.
 iii. Bone age is retarded in relation to chronological age.
  iv. Multiple small centers are scattered throughout epiphyses.

Laboratory Evaluation (Fig. 3.6)

Serum TSH value:
  i. Normal— 0.4 mU/L
 ii. Subclinical hypothyroidism: TSH value 4–10 mU/L with normal FT_4.
iii. TSH—10–20 mU/L—more severe hypothyroidism.
 iv. >20 mU/L—severe hypothyroidism.

FNAC: If there is any doubt about goiter associated hypothyroidism—FNAC should be done to exclude autoimmune thyroiditis.

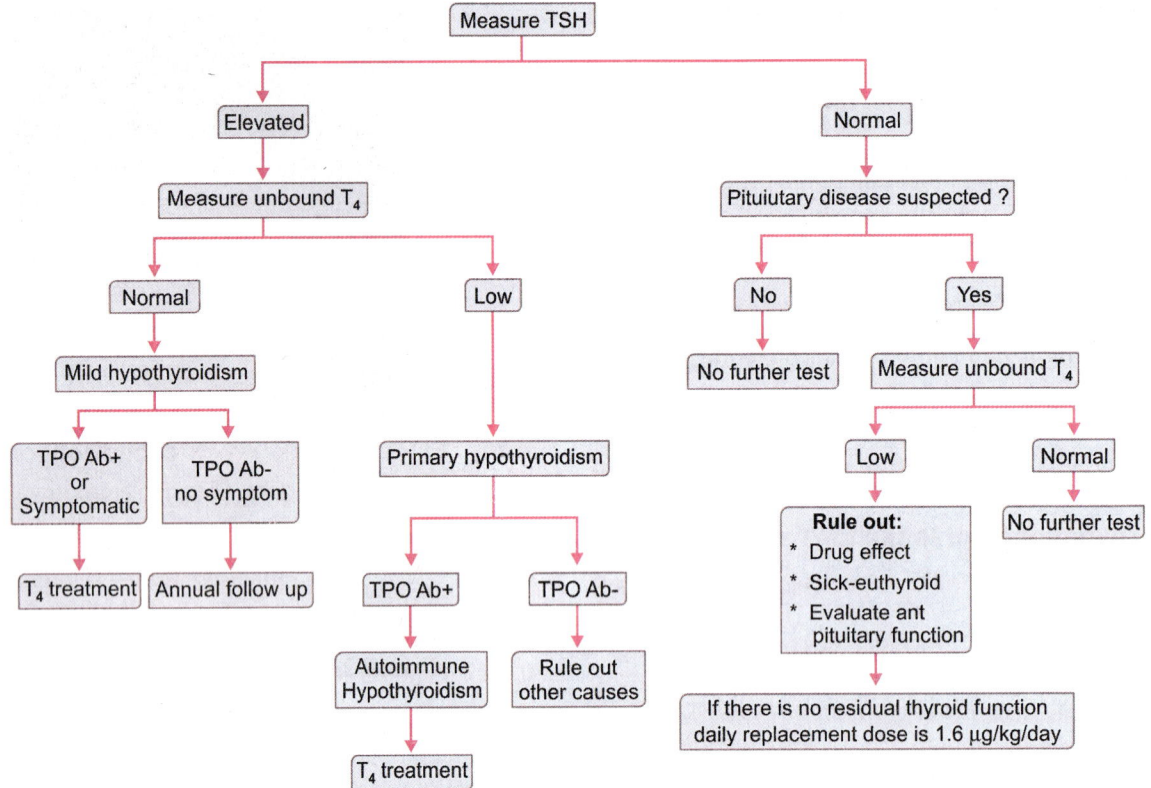

Fig. 3.6: Evaluation of hypothyroidism

Other Causes of Hypothyroidism

I. Iatrogenic hypothyroidism:
  i. It occurs 3–4 months after radioiodine treatment.
  ii. Transient hypothyroidism due to reversible radiation damage.
  iii. Since TSH level is suppressed by hyperthyroidism, FT_4 is the screening for detection of response to treatment.
  iv. Mild subclinical hypothyroidism that develops after subclinical thyroidectomy, may be restored as the gland remnant will be stimulated by TSH.

II. Iodine deficiency:
  i. It is responsible for development of endemic goiter and cretinism but not of adult hypothyroidism, unless there is added factors, example:
    a. Consumption of thiocyanates
    b. Selenium deficiency
  ii. Iodine intake can improve this problem
  iii. Public health measure should be taken to improve iodine deficiency in the community.

III. Paradoxically chronic iodine excess:
i. Individual with autoimmune thyroiditis is mainly susceptible
ii. Patients treated with amiodarone are also at risk

Treatment

A. Levothyroxine:
  i. *If there is no residual thyroid function*—daily dose of levothyroxine—100–150 μg

  ii. *In patients, who develop hypothyroidism after treatment of Graves' disease:* Lower replacement dose 75–125 mg/day
  iii. *In patient under age 60 years:* Treatment may be started with levothyroxine—50–100 mg/day. Dose should be increased with gradual increment 12.5 to 25 mg per shift—it should adjusted by monthly or bimonthly TSH level. Aim isto normalize the TSH level. If TSH level is suppressed, similar decrement in T_4 treatment and regular adjustment with serum TSH level.
B. Desiccated thyroid extract: It is an extract of pig thyroid—T_4: T_3 ratio is 4:1. They are not recommended because the ratio is non-physiologic.
C. The use of levothyroxine combined with liothyronine has been investigated, benefit has not been continued.

Once the full replacement is achieved, and TSH level is stable
↓
Follow up measurement of TSH at annual interval for several years.
↓
If the TSH is stable
↓
Serum TSH level will be measured at 2–3 years interval.

D. In patient with normal body weight, if dose is ≥200 mg/day of levothyroxine, an elevated TSH level is an indication of poor adherence—this is called fluctuating

TSH level despite constant T_4 dosage. These patients have normal or high FT_4 level and elevated TSH level.

Because in these patients, dosage of thyroxine is sufficient to normalize T_4 level but not FT_4 level, this is called **variable adherence**.

In this case one has to consider:
i. A case of missed dose.
ii. Other cases of increased levothyroxine requirement:
   a. Mal absorption syndrome
     1. Celiac disease
     2. Small bowel surgery
   b. Estrogen therapy
   c. Drugs interfering T_3 absorption or clearance:
     i. Cholestyramine
     ii. Ferrous sulphate
     iii. Lovastatin
     iv. Rifampicin
     v. Amiodarone
     vi. Carbamazepine
     vii. Phenytoin.

Subclinical Hypothyroidism

These are not universally accepted recommendation for management of hypothyroidism, but most recent guideline shows:
i. No recommended treatment, if TSH <10 mU/L
ii. Sustained elevation of TSH for more than 3 months is required for initiation of treatment.

But if TSH level is elevated and TPO antibodies are positive, there is every chance of overt hypothyroidism—in this case—start with low dose of levothyroxine at a dose of 25–50 mg/day, regular adjusting with TSH level. Aim is to maintain normal TSH level.

MYXEDEMA COMA

This is most dreadful condition of hypothyroidism.

Precipitating Factors

1. Infections
2. Stroke
3. Sedative drugs from which the patient does not awaken
4. Pneumonia
5. MI
6. CCF
7. GI bleeding
8. Sepsis
9. Exposure to cold

Clinical Features

1. Hypothermia—it can reach as low as 74°F.
2. Bradycardia
3. Alveolar hypoventilation
4. Reduced level of consciousness
5. Seizures

Pathogenesis

Hypoventilation leading to hypoxia and hypercapnea—play a major role in pathogenesis.

Associated risk factors—hypoglycemia, dilutional hyponatremia.

Treatment

1. Levothyroxine IV bolus 500 µg.
       ↓
   Subsequent parenteral dose is—100 µg—T_4 daily IV

2. An alternative is: Intravenously or through nasogastric tube—20–25 µg to be given every 8–12 hour for 1st a few days.
   This is given because T_4 to T_3 conversion is impaired in myxedema coma.

3. Therapy containing both T_4 and T_3 has also been advocated.

   Initial therapy—250 µg T_4 + 25 µg T_3 IV
       ↓
   Followed by 10 µg T_3 every 8 hourly—until the patient responds.

4. Therapy of underlying disease.

Supportive Therapy

1. Correct metabolic disturbances
2. External warming, if temperature <30°C, as it can results in cardiovascular collapse.
3. Special blanket should be used to prevent heat loss.
4. Parenteral hydrocortisone—50 mg every 6 hourly, because of impaired adrenal reserve in hypothyroidism.
5. Precipitating factors and intercurrent illness should be treated by broad-spectrum antibiotics.
6. Ventilatory support with regular blood gas analysis.
7. Hypertonic saline in case of hyponatremia
8. IV glucose in case of hypoglycemia
9. Precipitating drugs must be stopped. Sedative is to be avoided.

THYROTOXICOSIS

Hyperthyroidism is a clinical condition resulting from the effect of excessive amount of thyroid hormone in body tissues.

Causes

I. **Primary hyperthyroidism**
   1. Graves' disease
   2. Toxic multinodular goiters
   3. Toxic adenoma
   4. Functioning thyroid carcinoma
   5. Activating mutation of TSH receptor
   6. Activating mutation of GS∝ (McCune-Albright syndrome)
   7. Struma ovarii
   8. Drugs—iodine excess (Jod-Basedow phenomenon)

II. **Thyrotoxicosis without hyperthyroidism**
   1. Subacute thyroiditis
   2. Silent thyroiditis
   3. Other causes of thyroid dysfunction—amiodarone, radiation, infarction of adenoma)
   4. Ingestion of excess thyroid hormone (thyrotoxicosis factitia)

III. **Secondary hyperthyroidism**
   1. TSH secreting pituitary adenoma
   2. Thyroid hormone resistance syndrome
   3. Chorionic gonadotrophin-secreting tumor.
   4. Gestational thyrotoxicosis.

Pathogenesis

Following factors are responsible for development of Graves disease:

I. **Genetic factors:**
   1. Pleomorphism in HLA-DR, CTLA-4, CD-25, PTPN 22 and TSHR increase the susceptibility for Graves' disease.
   2. Concordance for Graves' disease is: monozygotic twin in 20–30% patients, or dizygotic twin in <5% patients

II. **Environmental factors:**
   1. Stress—presumably through neuroendocrine effects on immune system.
   2. Smoking—minor risk factor for Graves' disease major risk factor for Graves' ophthalmopathy
   3. Sudden increase in iodine excess
   4. In postpartum period—threefold increase
   5. Immune reconstitution phase after highly active anti-retroviral therapy or alemtuzumab therapy.

III. Hyperthyroidism of Graves' disease is caused by TSI, synthesized by thyroid gland, bone marrow and lymph nodes. This antibody can be detected by TBII assay (TSH binding inhibiting immunoglobulin assay).

   This is most important in pregnant mother having thyrotoxicosis; because TSI can cross the placenta and produce neonatal thyrotoxicosis.

IV. TPO-antibodies may occur in 80% patients—which can be readily measured.

V. Sometimes coexisting thyroiditis can also affect thyroid function, hence there is no direct correlation between TSI and Graves' disease.

VI. 15% patients with Graves' disease may develop autoimmune hypothyroidism.

Pathogenesis of Toxic Ophthalmopathy

1. Infiltration of extraocular muscles by activated T cells
   ↓
   Release of cytokines such as IFN-Y, INF, IL-1
   ↓
   Activation of fibroblast and increased synthesis of glycosaminoglycans—that trap water
   ↓
   Characteristic muscle swelling
   ↓
   Later on irreversible fibrosis of the muscles
   Though pathogenesis in thyrotoxic ophthalmopathy is rare, but there is mounting evidence that
   TSH-R may be the shared autoantigen that is expressed in the orbit.
2. Increased fat content
   ↓
   Retrobulbar tissue expansion
   ↓
   Increase in intraorbital pressure
   ↓
   Proptosis, diplopia, optic neuropathy

Clinical Manifestations

Cardiovascular Manifestation

   i. Sinus tachycardia
   ii. Palpitation—occasionally caused by supraventricular tachycardia
   iii. High cardiac output producing:
      a. Bounding pulse, sometimes water hammer pulse
      b. Widened pulse pressure
      c. Aortic systolic murmur
      d. Forceful and diffuse heat beat
   iv. Effort angina
   v. Heart failure in elderly people with pre-existing IHD
   vi. Atrial fibrillation in 50% patients—of these patients, 60% will revert back to sinus rhythm with treatment.
   vii. Loud first heart sound, scratchy systolic sound may be head at left sternal border—resembling pleuro-pericardial friction rub (Means-Lerman scratch).

Protein, Carbohydrate and Lipid Metabolism

a. Due to increased metabolism and heat production, there are:
   1. Increased BMR
   2. Increased appetite
   3. Heat intolerance
b. Since degradation of protein is increased than synthesis, there is net loss of protein leading to:
   1. Weight loss
   2. Muscle wasting
   3. Muscle weakness
   4. Hypoalbuminemia
c. Due to increased lipolysis, there are:
   1. Increased FFA level in serum
   2. Decreased serum cholesterol and triglyceride.

Nervous System

a. Alteration in function of nervous system as manifested by:
   1. Nervousness
   2. Emotional labiality.
   3. Psychiatric manifestations:
      i. MDP
      ii. Paranoid reaction
      iii. Schizophrenia
b. Hyperkinesia can be manifested as:
   1. Shifting the position frequently
   2. Movement will be quick, jerky, and purposeless
c. Fine tremor of hands, tongue or lightly closed eyelids
d. EEG reveals—increased fast wave activity.
e. In patient with convulsive disorder—frequency of seizures is increased.

Muscles

a. Weakness of proximal muscles—as evidenced by:
   1. Difficulty in climbing upstairs
   2. Fatigue from minimal exertion
b. Proximal muscle wasting is out of proportion of overall weight loss (thyrotoxic myopathy)—it affects mainly men.
c. In more severe form of thyrotoxicosis—myopathy involves distal limb muscles, trunk and face muscles.
d. Graves disease occurs 3 to 5% patients with myasthenia gravis and 1% of myasthenia patient develops Graves' disease. This is due to the fact that antibodies develop against TSH and acetylcholine receptors. Here there is female preponderance.
e. Sometimes hypokalemic periodic paralysis may be associated with thyrotoxicosis—which may aggravate the former disorder.

Eyes

a. Retraction of upper or lower or botheyelids—as evidenced by the presence of a rim of sclera present in between lid and limbus—present in all forms of thyrotoxicosis.
b. Lid lag: In which upper lid lags behind the globe when the patient is asked to shift the gaze slowly downward.
c. Globe lag: It is become evident when the globe lags behind the upper eyelid when the patient is asked to look up.
   The ocular manifestations are due to increased adrenergic tone.
d. Thyrotoxic ophthalmopathy: This is characterized by:
   i. Proptosis
   ii. Extraocular muscle swelling and fibrosis causing restriction of ocular mobility and diplopia
e. Exposed eyes become red and tender.
f. Pressure on optic nerve or keratitis can cause blindness. This disorder may be due to autoimmune manifestation and retro-orbital manifestation.
g. Sometimes ophthalmopathy occurs in Hashimoto's thyroiditis and in euthyroid patient without any evidence of thyroid disease.

Eye Sign

Some patients have little clinical evidence of ophthalmopathy but ultrasound or CT scan of orbit may detect enlarged extraocular muscles and other features.

Unilateral signs of ophthalmopathy may be detected in only 10% of patients.

Earliest manifestations of ophthalmopathy are:
i. Sensation of grittiness,
ii. Eye discomfort
iii. Excess tearing

In one-third of patients—proptosis (Fig. 3.7) can be best detected by: Visualization of sclera between lower border or iris and lower eyelid when eye is in primary position.

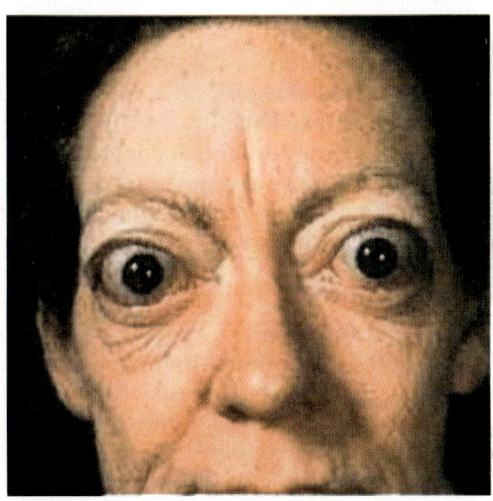

Fig. 3.7: Proptosis

In severe cases—proptosis can produce:
i. Corneal exposure and damages, if eyelid fails to close during sleep
ii. Periorbital edema
iii. Scleral injection
iv. Chemosis

In more severe cases—diplopic occurs when patient looks up and laterally.

Most serious manifestation: Compression of optic nerve at the apex of the orbit leading to:
i. Papilledema
ii. Peripheral field defect
iii. If untreated—permanent loss of vision.

Many scoring systems have been used to gauge the extent and activity of orbital changes. "NO SPECS" scheme derived from following changes:

0 = No sign or symptom
1 = Only sign (lid retraction or lag), no symptom
2 = Soft tissue involvement (periorbital edema)
3 = proptosis (>22 mm)
4 = Extraocular muscles involvement (diplopia)
5 = corneal involvement
6 = sight loss

Following measurements are necessary:
1. Proptosis is usually measured by ophthalmometer
2. Lid tissue width
3. Corneal staining with fluorescein.
4. Evaluation of extraocular muscle function (Hess chart)
5. Intraocular pressure
6. Visual fields
7. Color vision

Skin

a. Warm, moist, velvety, giving youthful appearance
b. Palm is warm and moist
c. Onycholysis—due to retraction of nail from nail bed involving fourth and fifth fingers.
d. Elbow may be smooth and pink, complexion—rosy
e. Palmar erythema—and telangiectasia
f. Vitiligo—an autoimmune disease more common in Graves' disease

Respiratory System

Dyspnea—due to following reason: Vital capacity—reduced due to respiratory muscle weakness.

Gastrointestinal System

1. Decreased food intake—and increased appetite—but there is weight loss.
2. Bowel movements are increased—increased gastric emptying and increased intestinal motility may lead to malabsorption of fat.
3. Celiac and Graves' disease may coexist, pernicious anemia may occur.
4. Hepatic dysfunction may occur in the form of:
   i. Increased SGPT
   ii. Raised bone and liver alkaline phosphatase
   iii. Hepatomegaly with jaundice
5. Splanchnic oxygen consumption is increased but splanchnic blood flow is not proportionately increased—leading to hypoxia and hepatic dysfunction.

Skeletal System, Calcium and Phosphorus Metabolism

a. Increased excretion of calcium and phosphorus in urine and stool.

↓

Leads to demineralization of bone as demonstrated by densitometry

↓

Leads to pathologic fracture in elderly women

Pathology includes: (1) Osteitis fibrosa, (2) Osteoporosis (3) Osteomalacia

b. In postmenopausal women, there may be accelerated reduction in bone density which requires treatment.
c. Serum levels of—total calcium and ionized calcium, heat labile alkaline phosphatase, osteocalcin are elevated.

Hematopoietic System

a. Normal RBC indices but RBC mass is increased.
b. Increased erythropoiesis due to:
    i. Direct effect of thyroid hormone in some marrow
    ii. Increased production of erythropoietin
c. Antibodies
    i. 3% patients have pernicious anemia
    ii. 3% patients have antibodies against intrinsic factor, but normal absorption of vitamin B_{12}.
    iii. Against parietal cell.
d. White blood cell:
    i. Total WBC count is low due to decreased number of neutrophils.
    ii. Lymphocyte, eosinophil and monocyte count may be increased.
e. There may organomegaly:
    i. Splenomegaly
    ii. Enlargement of thymus
    iii. Enlargement of lymph nodes.
f. Platelet level and clotting system:
    i. Factor-VIII is often increased—returning to normal after treatment of thyrotoxicosis.
    ii. There may be enhanced sensitivity to warfarin—because of accelerated clearance of vitamin-K dependent clotting factors.

Reproductive System

a. Impaired fertility in women, oligomenorrhea
b. In male—azoospermia, importance
c. Gynecomastia be in male due to increased peripheral conversion of androgen to estrogen despite high testosterone level.
d. Increased in thyroid binding globulin level, thus raised total testosterone and estradiol level.
e. Serum LH and FSA levels are normal or increased.

Pituitary and Adrenocortical Function

1. Hepatic inactivation of cortisol is accelerated with increased level of 5∝/5β reductase

↓

Disposal of cortisol will be accelerated but its rate of secretion is also increased

↓

So serum cortisol level is unchanged and normal.

Thyroid Gland

Enlarged in size. Its size and consistency depends upon underlying pathology. Hyperfunctioning of the gland may be evidenced by bruit over the thyroid gland.

Skin manifestation:
a. Thyroid dermopathy occurs in <5% of patients, almost always is associated with moderate to severe ophthalmopathy.
b. Typical lesion is:
    i. Non-inflamed, indurated plaque with deep pink or purple color looking like "orange, skin" appearance— pretibial myxedema (Fig. 3.8).
    ii. Nodular lesion can occur.

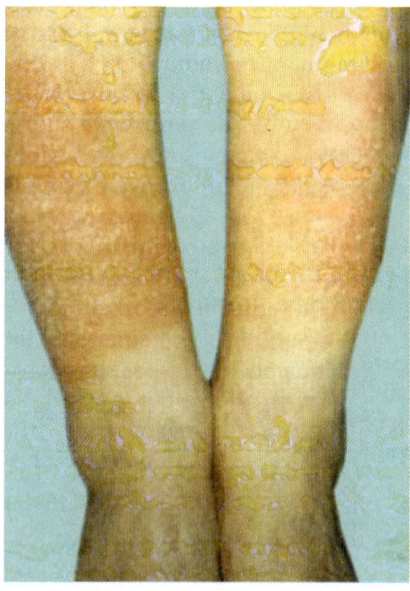

Fig. 3.8: Thyroid dermopathy (pretibial myxedema)

Site:
    i. Anterior and lateral aspect of the lower leg (hence— called pretibial myxedema).
    ii. This lesion may rarely extends and involves whole lower leg and foot—mimicking elephantiasis.
c. Thyroid acropachy: It is a form of clubbing found in <1% of patient with Graves' disease.

Laboratory Investigation

I. **Test for thyroid function:**
    i. Serum free thyroxine or free thyroxine index increased.
    ii. Serum FT_3, FT_3 index—increased.
        But in T_3 thyrotoxicosis, FT_3—raised but FT_4—normal.
    iii. Serum TSH—undetectable
        If serum TSH—is raised in hyperthyroid patient— indicates TSH induced hyperthyroidism
    iv. Radioactive iodine intake at 4, 6, or 24 hours is increased in patients with increased production of thyroid hormone and decreased when gland is lacking thyroid hormone.

II. **Test for etiology:**
    a. Thyroid stimulating immunoglobulin (TSI)—if positive—it indicates—hyperthyroidism is the result of Graves disease.

b. TSH receptor antibody measurement—the binding of patient's IgG to a TSH receptor. It is positive in 90% patient with active Graves' disease.
c. Antiperoxidase antibody: Positive in:
   i. Graves' disease
   ii. Hashimoto's thyroiditis
d. Thyroid scan is useful in patients with modular goiter with hyperthyroidism to determine:
   i. Whether there is autonomous hyperfunctioning nodule that concentrates all the radio-iodine and suppresses all the glandular tissue.
   ii. Whether multiple nodules concentrate radio-iodine
   iii. Whether the nodules are cold and hyperfunctioning tissue is between the palpable nodules.

Therapy

Hyperthyroidism of Graves' disease can be treated with following aims:
1. Reducing thyroid hormone synthesis by antithyroid drugs.
2. Reducing the amount of thyroid tissue—with radio-iodine or by thyroidectomy.

Antithyroid drugs are predominant therapy in many centers of Europe and Japan.

Radioiodine is 1st line of treatment in North America.

Functions of Antithyroid Drugs

i. Inhibit the function of TPO
ii. Reduce oxidation and organification of iodide
iii. Reduce thyroid antibody levels
iv. Enhance the rate of remission
v. Propylthiouracil inhibits deiodination of T_4 to T_3—it is most important in severe thyrotoxicosis.

Drugs are: Thionamides:
i. Propylthiouracil   ii. Carbimazole
iii. Active metabolites of carbimazole—methimazole

Treatment Regimen

1. Carbimazole or methimazole—10–20 mg—every 8–12 hourly
$$\downarrow$$
After euthyroidism once daily dosing
2. Propylthiouracil 100–200 mg 6–8 hourly—throughout the course. The dose should be reduced as the thyrotoxicosis improves.
3. High dose of antithyroid drugs with levothyroxine to be given to avoid drug-induced hypothyroidism (Block—replace regimen)

Monitoring of Treatment

Thyroid hormone assay should be started 3–4 weeks after starting the treatment. TSH measurement is not sensitive marker.
$$\downarrow$$
Euthyroidism should be achieved after 6–8 weeks of treatment.

Maintenance dose: Carbimazole or methimazole 2.5–10 mg/day or propylthiouracil—50–100 mg/day.
   In block—replace regimen
i. Antithyroid drug should be constant.
ii. Levothyroxine should be adjusted to maintain normal T_4.

Maximum remission rate are achieved by 18–24 months by titration regimen and by 6 months by block—replace regimen.

Relapse

1. Close follow up for relapse during 1st year after treatment
2. Patient with severe hyperthyroidism and large goiter are most likely to relapse after treatment.

Common side effects:
i. Rash
ii. Urticaria
iii. Fever
iv. Arthralgia—these may resolve spontaneously or after substitution or treatment.

Rare side effect (major):
i. Hepatitis
ii. SLE like syndrome
iii. Agranulocytosis
   In these cases—all antithyroid drugs must be stopped and not to be started further.
   Agranulocytosis is of major concern (sore throat, fever, mouth ulcer)—It is idiosyncratic and abrupt.

Propranolol

Mechanism of action:
i. Block excessive adrenergic activity
ii. Modest reduction in serum T_3 concentration by blocking conversion of T_4 to T_3.

Propranolol 20–40 mg every 4–6 hourly. The dose should be adjusted to maintain heart rate 70–80 beats/min.

Drug should be tapered as hyperthyroidism is controlled, and should be discontinued as euthyroid is achieved.

Effective β blockade—eliminates:
i. Tachycardia
ii. Tremor
iii. Asterexis
iv. Nervousness.
v. Sweating

Atenolol—is long acting and less likely to cause depression.

β-adrenergic blockade is indicated in rate related heart failure.

Contraindication: (i) Asthma, (ii) COPD, (iii) Diabetes

Radioiodine Treatment

Indications:
i. Destroy thyroid cells
ii. Initial treatment or for relapse after trial of antithyroid drugs.

Risk is thyroid crisis—after radio-iodine treatment.

This can be minimized by pretreatment with antithyroid drugs for at least 1 month to deplete the iodine store from thyroid gland mainly in elderly persons.

The antithyroid drugs should be stopped before the initiation of radio-iodine treatment:
i. Methimazole or carbimazole should be stopped 2 days before radio-iodine administration.
ii. Propylthiouracil—because of prolonged effect, it should be stopped 2 weeks prior to radio-iodine treatment.

Dose: A practical strategy is to give fixed dose based on clinical features such as:

i. Severity of thyrotoxicosis
ii. Size of goiter
iii. Level of radioiodine uptake

Usual dose is: 5–15 mCi.

To deliver 80–120 mCi/gm of thyroid tissue, estimated dose should be 5000–15000 rad to the thyroid gland. There will be gradual restoration of euthyroid state in most patients over a period of 6 months.

Early relapse occurs mostly in males and in patients <40 years of age.

Most patients ultimately progress to hypothyroidism over 5–10 years.

Certain safety precautions are required in 1st a few days after radioiodine treatment:

1. Patient needs to avoid close and prolonged contact with children and pregnant women for several days, because of possible transmission of residual isotope and exposure to radiation from thyroid gland.
2. Mild pain due to radiation thyroiditis—within 1–2 weeks of commencement of treatment. Hyperthyroidism can persist up to 2–3 months before radioiodine takes its full effect.
3. β-adrenergic drugs to be given to block the peripheral effect of thyroid drug.
4. Persistant hyperthyroidism can be treated by 2nd dose of radio-iodine; usually 6 months after 1st dose.
5. Pregnancy and breastfeeding are absolute contraindication to radioiodine treatment.
6. Presence of severe ophthalmopathy requires caution:
   Prednisolone—40 mg/day at the time of radioiodine treatment tapered over 2–3 months to prevent exacerbation of ophthalmopathy.
7. Radioiodine can be safely administered in older children.

Thyroidectomy

Indications:
i. Relapse with antithyroid drugs
ii. Patient who prefers treatment with surgery than radio-iodine treatment
iii. When goiter is large.

Complications of treatment:
i. Bleeding:
ii. Laryngeal edema
iii. Hypothyroidism
iv. Damage to recurrent laryngeal nerve
   All above complications can be prevented by skilled surgeon.
v. Chance of thyrotoxicosis—which can be prevented by administration of antithyroid drugs followed by potassium iodide (3 drops SSKI orally thrice daily) prior to surgery.

Treatment of Drugs during Pregnancy

1. During pregnancy, titrating regimen should be used rather than blocking, which can produce fetal hypothyroidism.

2. Propylthiouracil—should be given at lowest possible dose because it has:
   i. Very low transplacental transfer.
   ii. Ability to block T$_4$ to T$_3$ conversion will be low.
3. Carbimazole and methimazole produce:
   i. Fetal aplasia cutis
   ii. Chonal atresia
4. It is better to stop the drugs at third trimester of pregnancy.
5. There is every chance of transplacental transfer of antibodies producing fetal thyrotoxicosis as evidenced by:
   i. Poor intrauterine growth
   ii. Fetal heart rate >160 beats/min (because high level of maternal antibodies present in last trimester of pregnancy).
   Hence, fetus of hyperthyroid mother should be treated for 1–3 months after delivery until maternal antibodies disappear from the blood.
6. Hyperthyroidism will relapse in postpartum period; hence, she should be treated with low dose of antithyroid drugs.

Treatment of Graves' Ophthalmopathy

1. Mild to moderate ophthalmopathy does not require any treatment because of spontaneous improvement.
2. Meticulous control of thyroid hormone, cessation of smoking.
3. Discomfort can be relieved by:
   i. Artificial fears (1% methylcellulose)
   ii. Eye ointment
   iii. Use of dark glasses with side frames
4. Periorbital edema may respond to:
   i. Upright sleeping position.
   ii. Diuretics.
5. Corneal exposure during sleep can be avoided by— patches or taping the eyes shut.
6. Minor degree of diplopia can be improved with prism fitted with spectacles.
7. Severe degree of ophthalmopathy can be treated by:
   i. Prednisolone 40–80 mg daily sometimes combined with cyclosporine
      Glucocorticoid dose can be tapered by 5 mg every 2 weeks.
   ii. Pulse therapy with IV methylprednisolone 500–1000 mg in 200 ml of saline infused over 2 hours daily for 1 week followed by oral therapy.
8. If glucocorticoid is refractory—orbital decompression through transsphenoidal route—thereby displacing fat and swollen extraocular muscles.
   Proptosis recedes at average of 5 mm per week.
9. Once eye disease becomes stabilized—surgery may be indicated for (i) relief of diplopia, (ii) correction of appearance.
10. External beam radiotherapy.

Treatment of Thyroid Dermopathy

i. Usually does not require any treatment.
ii. Topical or high potency glucocorticoid.

EVALUATION OF THYROTOXICOSIS

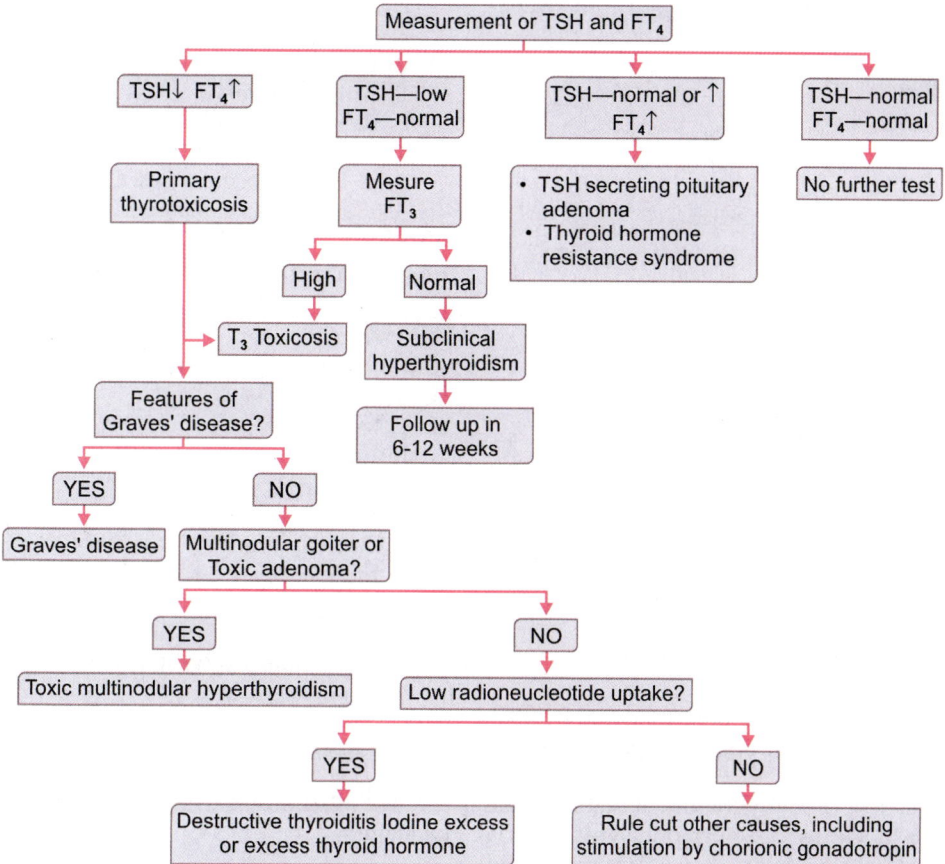

Fig. 3.9: Patient with symptoms and signs suggesting thyrotoxicosis, no amiodarone, serum TSH <0.2 mU/L, free T_4 and T_3—raised

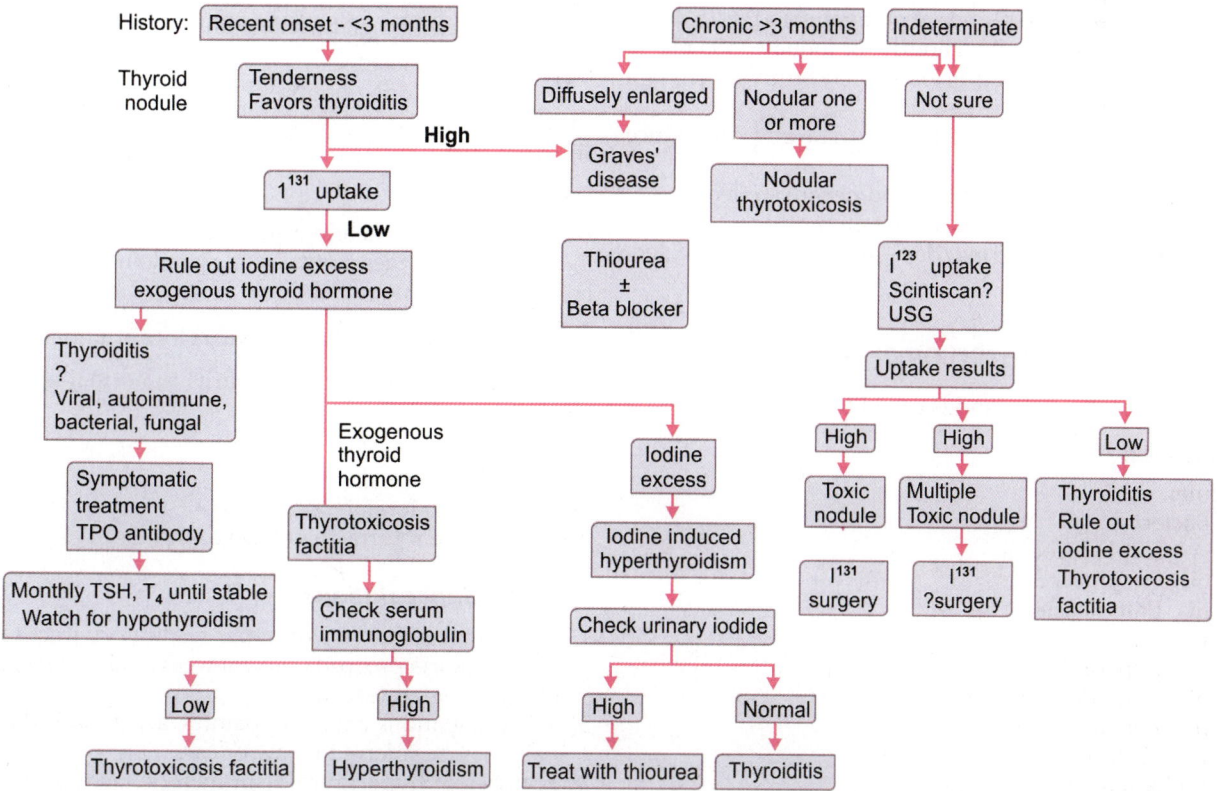

Fig. 3.10: Algorithm of management of hyperthyroidism

THYROTOXIC CRISIS

This is a dangerous condition of decompensated thyrotoxicosis.

Clinical Presentation

i. Tachycardia
ii. Fever
iii. Agitation
iv. Restlessness,
v. Psychosis
vi. Nausea
vii. Vomiting
viii. Diarrhea
ix. Jaundice

It results from—long-term neglected hyperthyroidism, the additive risk factors—intercurrent illness:
a. Gastroenteritis
b. Pneumonia
c. Emergency surgery
d. Stroke
e. Trauma
f. DKA

Mortality

i. Cardiac failure
ii. Arrhythmia
iii. Hyperthermia

Management

1. Intensive supportive cure with bedside continuous monitoring.
2. Identification of cause and their specific treatment
3. Antithyroid treatment:
   i. Propylthiouracil 600 mg loading dose followed by 200–300 mg 6 hourly—orally or through nasogastric tube or per rectum.
   ii. One hour after 1st dose of propylthiouracil, stable iodide is to be given to block thyroid hormone synthesis via Wolff-Chaikoff effect (the delay allows the antithyroid drug to prevent excess iodine from being incorporated into new hormone).
4. **Iodide salt:** Saturated solution of potassium iodide (5 drops SSKI) may be given orally 6 hourly, or ipodate (500 mg 12 hours) may be given. Sodium iodide may be given 0.25 IV 6 hourly fort 2 weeks:
   a. Propranolol (2 mg every 2 hourly) to be given to reduce peripheral manifestation.
   b. Caution must be needed to avoid negative effect
   c. Control of high rate circulatory failures
   d. Dexamethasone—4–8 mg/day—unless contraindicated, in severe infection.

THYROIDITIS

Inflammation of thyroid gland is called thyroiditis.

Classification

I. Acute:
  1. Bacterial:
     i. Staphylococcal
     ii. Streptococcal
     iii. Enterobacter
  2. Fungal:
     i. Aspergillus
     ii. Candida
     iii. Pneumocystis
     iv. Histoplasma
  3. Radiation
  4. Amiodarone

II. Subacute:
  1. Viral
  2. Silent
  3. Mycobacterial
III. Chronic:
  1. Autoimmunity
  2. Riedel's thyroiditis
  3. Parasitic thyroiditis:
     i. Echinococcus   ii. Cysticercosis

Subacute Thyroiditis

It is also called De Quervain thyroiditis.

Etiology

Most likely viral origin. The viruses responsible are:
  i. Mumps,
  ii. Coxsackie
  iii. Influenza
  iv. Adenovirus
  v. Echoviruses
     Clinical prodrome—viral like prodrome—myalgia, arthralgia, fever.

Epidemiology

i. Peak incidence at 30–50 years
ii. Women: Men—3:1

Pathophysiology

There are three stages in this disease:

1st stage

Histology shows:
  i. Patchy inflammatory infiltrate
  ii. Disruption of thyroid follicles
  iii. Multinucleated giant cells within some follicles

Blood level of hormones
  i. Release of thyroglobulin
  ii. $\uparrow T_4$ and T_3
  iii. Low TSH

2nd stage

Destructive phase: Histology shows:
i. Follicular changes progress to granuloma
ii. Fibrosis of some follicles

  Blood level: Radioiodine uptake is low or undetectable.

  3rd stage: Thyroid gland returns to normal after several weeks to months.

Blood level shown:
  i. Low T_3, T_4
  ii. $\uparrow$ TSH (moderately increased)
  iii. I^{131} uptake returns to normal or increased

Clinical Manifestations

1. Prodromal symptoms of upper respiratory tract infection, fever, malaria proceeds several weeks before emergence of thyroid related features.
2. Thyroid gland is enlarged, painful, accompanied by fever. Pain may be referred to jaw or ear.
3. Features of hyperthyroidism include tachycardia, palpitation, weight loss, nervousness, and diaphoresis.

4. As the disease progresses—pain often migrates to contralateral side.
5. On physical examination:
   i. Tender, hard ill-defined mass, usually unilateral, sometimes tenderness may be present on opposite side.
   ii. Tachycardia
   iii. Warm and moist skin
   iv. Fine tremor of hands
6. There may be permanent features of hypothyroidism, if there is associated development of autoimmunity
7. Disease course is prolonged over many months with one or two relapses.

Laboratory Evaluation

I. **Thyroid function tests evolve through three different stages:**
   1. *Thyrotoxic phase:*
      i. T_4 and T_4 levels are increased—reflecting discharge from thyroid follicle.
      ii. TSH level is suppressed.
      iii. T_4/T_3 ratio is greater than in Graves' disease
   2. *Hypothyroid phase:*
      i. T_3 and T_4 level depressed.
      ii. TSH level will be raised.
      Diagnosis is confirmed by raised ESR and raised while blood cell count.
   3. *Normothyroid phase (recovery phase)*
II. **Thyroid antibodies:** Antimicrosomal (TPC) and anti-thyroglobulin—mildly elevated for several weeks after onset of symptoms and returns to normal after several months.
   Transient antibody elevation is probably a response to the release of thyroglobulin into circulation.
III. **Thyroid radioactive iodine uptake:** Suppressed during acute phase, usually <2% at 24 hours—it is due to disruption of iodine trapping mechanisms as result of inflammation and cell destruction.

Clinical Course and Treatment

I. **In the initial phase**—the symptoms are pain, features of hyperthyroidism and suppressed RAIU.
   Pain may be relieved by prednisolone—40–60 mg/day. Pain usually abates within a few hours after 1st dose. If it is not relieved, then the diagnosis of SAT is in doubt.
   Indicators of response:
   i. Improvement of symptoms
   ii. Lowering of ESR.
   After symptomatic improvement, dose of the steroid is gradually tapered as 5 mg every 2–3 days.
   In these patients, radioactive iodine uptake tests have to be done when it will be normalized, then the treatment can be gradually stopped.
   If there is evidence of relapse after tapering the dose of steroid, again the dose of steroid will be increased followed by gradual tapering.
   Symptoms of hyperthyroidism are to be treated by beta adrenergic drugs. Antithyroid drugs are not indicated.
II. **In second phase**—thyroid gland is depleted of all hormones and emerges as a state of hypothyroidism. It lasts for 2–3 months. During this phase—hormone replacement should be done in the form of:

   i. Levothyroxine 50–100 µg/day.
   After several months of treatment, levothyroxine treatment should be discontinued and TSH level should be checked after 6–8 weeks after the cessation of levothyroxine.
III. **During recovery phase:** Plasma thyroid hormone is normal. But RAIU is temporary elevated because of avoidance of iodine trapping by thyroid gland. But this test should not be done during this phase—except to confirm the diagnosis.
   Though uncommon, in a few cases—frank hypothyroidism may occur.

Painless Thyroiditis

This disorder is characterized by:
   i. Symptoms of thyrotoxicosis
   ii. Elevated T_3, T_4 level
   iii. Suppressed TSH level
   iv. Painless non-tender goiter

Etiology

It is autoimmune disease, variant of Hashimoto's thyroiditis. Women are mostly affected
   Genetic predisposition: $HLADRW_3$ and HLA DRW_5

Clinical Features

1. Features of hyperthyroidism—varying mild to moderate in severity depending upon severity of disease process.
2. Mildly enlarged, non-tender goiter. 50% patients have no palpable goiter.

Differentiation from Graves' Disease

Clinical features	Painless thyroiditis	Graves disease
1. Onset	Abrupt	Gradual
2. Severity	Mild to moderate	Moderate to severe
3. Duration of symptoms	<3 months	>3 months
4. Goiter	Firms, diffuse mildly enlarged	Mild to moderate firm, diffuse
5. Thyroid bruit	Absent	Present
6. Exophthalmos	Absent	May be present
7. T_4/T_3 ratio	<20:1	>20:1
8. RAIU	Suppressed	Elevated

Laboratory Studies

T_3 is less elevated in comparison to T_4—it is opposite in Graves disease—because of preferential secretion of T_3 by thyroid stimulating immunoglobulin.

Clinical Course and Treatment

1. In initial phase: Lasts for 6 weeks to 4 months.
   Treatment—relief of hyperthyroid symptoms with beta blocker.
   Anti-thyroid drugs should be avoided.
2. Euthyroid phase—3–6 weeks: During this phase, thyroid gland is depleted of hormones.
3. This is followed by in 25 to 40% patients—hypothyroid period—last no longer than 2–3 months.

During this phase, supplemental thyroxine is required.
4. Following this hypothyroid phase, clinical euthyroid state is achieved. During this phase, relapse may occur. Postpartum thyroiditis—occurs in 25% patients with type 1 diabetes mellitus.

Hashimoto's Thyroiditis

This is an autoimmune disorder—most common inflammatory thyroid disease.

Etiology

Genetic predisposition: HLA DR-5, HLA-B8 occurrence in this disease. It occurs in middle aged woman.

Pathology

Due to abnormal suppression of suppressor T lymphocytes
↓
Helper T lymphocytes interact with specific antigen of thyroid cell.
↓
Inflammation of thyroid gland

Clinical Presentation

This disease has a wide-spectrum of presentation.
1. Most common presentation is middle aged female with a symptomatic goiter.
2. Occasionally, patient may present with mild anterior neck discomfort—due to gradually enlarging thyroid gland.
3. Symptoms of hypothyroidism may be present depending on degree of hypothyroidism.
4. Physical examination: Symmetrically enlarged, very firm goiter, pebbly or knobby in consistency, occasionally patient may present with single nodule.
5. A small subsets of patients (2 to 4%) present with hyperthyroidism known as "hashitoxicosis". In these patients—TSI is detected in serum.

Laboratory Tests

i. 80% patients with HT have—normal T_4 and TSH.
ii. >90% patients have antimicrosomal antibodies.
iii. Thyroid ultrasound reveals a heterogenous micronodular pattern, often with increased blood flow.

Treatment

1. Levothyroxine (L-T_4)—treatment of choice in HT with hypothyroidism. It should be continued indefinitely in hypothyroid patient with Hashimoto's thyroiditis.
2. Patient with mild thyroid failure (normal T_4 and elevated TSH) may become overt hypothyroid.
3. Glucocorticoid is usually administered in HT patient with rapidly enlarging thyroid having pressure symptoms.
4. Surgery is indicated with enlarge thyroid producing pressure symptoms.

RIEDEL THYROIDITIS

i. It is extremely rare, fibroid variant of Hashimoto's to thyroiditis. Female: Male = 3:1, age between 30 and 60 years.
ii. These patients present with pressure symptoms. On examination, an extremely hard, woody, immobile thyroid gland palpated.
iii. Associated sclerosing symptoms:
   a. Retroperitoneal fibrosis
   b. Mediastinal fibrosis
   c. Ascending cholangitis
iv. Thyroid function test shows—hypothyroidism in 30% patients
v. Thyroid antibody test –ve
vi. Ultrasound of thyroid reveals invasive type picture with obliteration of normal thyroid margin.
vii. Surgical treatment in patient presenting with compression symptoms.
viii. Tamoxifen—may be helpful in some patients because of its inhibitory effect on growth factor.

PARATHYROID GLAND DISORDERS

PARATHYROID GLAND

Osteoblast synthesizes and secretes organic matrix. Osteoblast is derived from mesenchymal osteoblast progenitor.

Mesenchymal osteoblast progenitor cell
  ←Bone morphogenic protein (regulatory protein)
↓
Osteoblast
  ←PTH, vitamin D, IGF, BMP
↓
Active osteoblast
↓
Secretes organic matrix
↓
This becomes mineralized to form bone

Actions of Parathyroid Hormone

I. **On kidney:**
   a. Almost all the calcium of initial filtrate is absorbed—from renal tubule:
      • 65–70% in proximal convulated tubules
      • 10%—in ascending, limb of loop of Henle
      • 10%—in distal convulated tubule—in this part parathormone helps in absorption by a transcellular active transport mechanism.
   b. Phosphate absorption in PCT and DCT is strongly inhibited by PTH.
   c. PTH stimulates the 25α hydroxylase to form 1, 25(OH)$_2$ D$_3$ (calcitriol) from I(OH) D$_3$ by inducing transcription of 25 (DH) D 1-hydroxylase gene.

II. **Effect on bone:** PTH has some direct and indirect effects on bone.
   a. Chronic effect of PTH is to:
      i. Increase in number of bone cells—both osteoblast and osteoclast,

ii. Increase remodeling of bone, this effect becomes apparent within a few hours of PTH administration.

b. Continuous administration of PTH leads to increased osteoclastic resorption of bone.

c. Intermittent administration of PTH—leads to net effect of bone formation rather than bone resorption—involved bones are mainly hip and spine.

Osteoblast has PTH receptors but osteoclast has no PTH receptors.

So, stimulation of osteoclast is indirect through release of cytokines from osteoblast to activate osteoclast.

III. **Effect on metabolism of vitamin D and calcium**

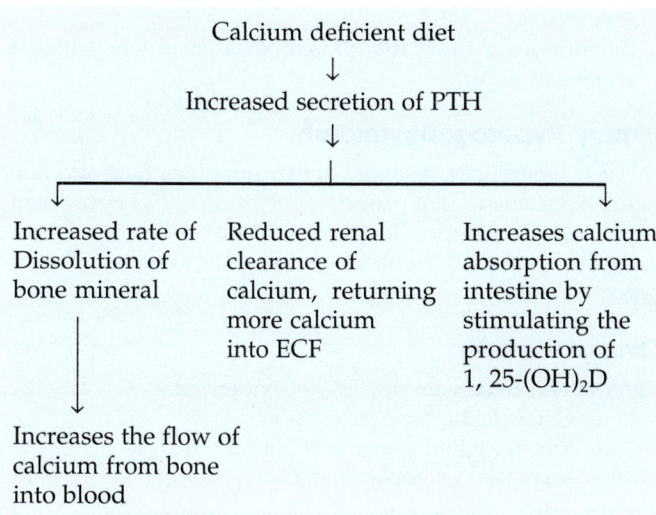

Structure of PTH

PTH is 84-amino acid containing single chain peptide.
1. Aminoterminal portion PTH (1–34) is highly conserved and critical for biologic actions of the molecule.
2. Aminoterminal fragment PTH (1–11) is sufficient to activate the PTH receptors (PTH/PTHrP)
3. Carboxy terminal end of full length PTH binds to separate binding protein (cPTH-R)

Calcitonin

It is 32-amino acid peptide—secreted by parafollicular C cells in thyroid gland.

These cells are stimulated by rise in extracellular calcium and are inhibited by fall in extracellular calcium.

A. **Functions:**
1. It reduces the bone resorption by inhibiting osteoclastic activity.
2. At the kidney level—it increases renal clearance of calcium and phosphate by reducing tubular absorption.
3. Homeostatic function of calcitonin is to buffer calcium absorbed through intestine.

The net effect is lowering the level of calcium and phosphorus.

B. **Calcitonin gene-related peptide:** It is 37-amino acid residue containing peptide produced by alternative expression of calcitonin gene from neuroendocrine cells of hypothalamus. It acts as:
  i. Neurotransmitters
 ii. Vasodilator
iii. Exerts effect directly on the cells.

PTH and PTHrP Hormone Actions

1. Both PTH and PTHrP bind to PTH/PTHrP receptors (known as PTH-1 receptor) and produce common physiologic functions.
2. PTH-2 receptor is primarily expressed in brain, pancreas and testes—it responds efficiently to PTH but not to PTHrP.
3. PTH-3 receptor has been identified for carboxy-terminal PTH.

Action

PTHrP is important in maintaining growth regulation in fetal and adult tissues—these are local actions:

PTHrP has been demonstrated in following tissues
  i. Cardiovascular musculature
 ii. Breast
iii. Epidermis
 iv. Hair follicle
  v. Cartilage
vii. Skeletal tissue
viii. CNS tissues
 ix. Placenta
  x. Prostate

It functions in utero to modulate mineral homeostasis.

Fibroblast growth factor: It is a systemic factor—is an important regulator of serum phosphate concentration and responsible for pathogenesis of both hypophosphatemic and hyperphosphatemic disorders.

FGF 23 binds to several FGF receptors.

Elevation of serum FGF 23 lowers serum phosphate concentration and serum $1, 25 (OH)_2 D_2$.

Calcium Phosphate Homeostasis

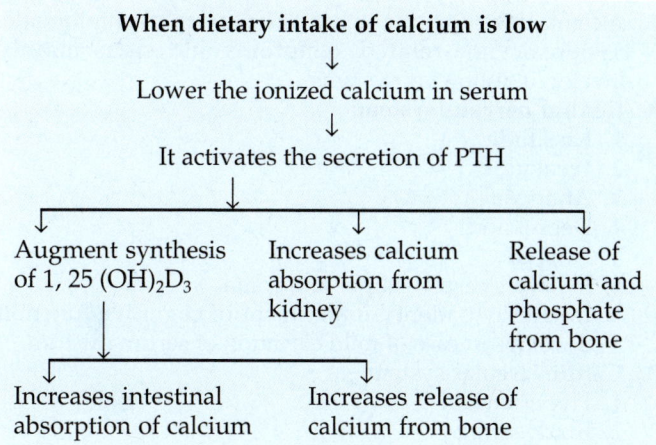

HYPERCALCEMIA

Classifications

I. **Parathyroid related:**
  a. Primary hyperparathyroidism:
    1. Adenoma
    2. Carcinoma
    3. Multiple endocrine neoplasia
  b. Lithium therapy
  c. Familial hypocalciuric hypercalcemia

II. Non-parathyroid related:
a. *Malignancy related:*
1. Solid tumor with metastasis
2. Solid tumor with humoral mediators of hypercalcemia
3. Hematologic malignancies

b. *Vitamin D related:*
1. Vitamin D intoxication
2. Increased 1, 25 (OH)₂D
3. Sarcoidosis

c. *Associated with high bone turnover:*
1. Hyperthyroidism
2. Immobilization
3. Thiazide
4. Vitamin A intoxication

d. *Associated with renal failure:*
1. Severe secondary hyperparathyroidism
2. Aluminum intoxication
3. Milk–alkali syndrome.

Clinical Features

A spectrum of presentations starting from asymptomatic hypercalcemia, detected only during routine investigation to severe life-threatening presentation, culminating death. Symptoms and signs of hypercalcemia depend upon:
1. Age of patient:
   a. Elderly patient is frequently sensitive to serum calcium alteration.
   b. Young individual can tolerate severe hypercalcemia.
2. Underlying primary disease process
3. Concurrent medical disorders
4. Degree, duration and rate of development of hypercalcemia. Slowly developing severe hypercalcemia may not produce any symptom; again mild to moderate hypercalcemia developing acutely may be severely symptomatic. Hypercalcemia-related symptoms and signs mainly develop in following systems:

A. **Central nervous system:**
1. Lassitude
2. Weakness
3. Anorexia
4. Depression
5. Fatigue
6. In severe cases—stupor and coma
7. In elderly patient—impairment of cognitive function develops in case of mild elevation of serum calcium.

B. **Cardiovascular system:**
1. Hypertension
2. Bradycardia
3. Short QT interval
4. Increased sensitivity to digitalis glycosides

C. **Renal manifestation:**
1. Impaired urinary concentrating ability
2. Polyuria
3. Reduced GFR
4. Nephrocalcinosis
5. Nephrolithiasis
   Nephrolithiasis and nephrocalcinosis occur in case of chronic hypercalcemia

D. **Gastrointestinal manifestation:**
1. Nausea
2. Vomiting
3. Anorexia
4. Gastroesophageal reflux
5. Peptic ulcer
6. Constipation
7. Uncommon but serious presentation—acute pancreatitis.

Relation of Calcium Levels with Clinical Presentation

1. At calcium level 11.5–12 mg/dl—symptoms are common.
2. At calcium level 13 mg/dl—ectopic calcification occurs in kidney, skin, vessels, lungs, heart and stomach and renal insufficiency may develop—if the serum phosphate is severe.
3. Calcium level 15–18 mg/dl is medical emergency, cardiac arrest can occur.

Primary Hyperparathyroidism

This is a generalized disorder of calcium phosphate and bone metabolism due to inappropriate secretion of PTH producing hypercalcemia, hypophosphatemia, phosphaturia, loss of cortical bone, and various chronic sequelae of chronic hypercalcemia.

Clinical Features

I. **Skeletal involvement:** This is evidenced by:
   i. Osteoclastic bone resorption
   ii. Fibrovascular marrow replacement
   iii. Increased osteoblastic activity

The following are the radiographic appearences:
   i. Generalized demineralization of bone, with coarsening of trabecular pattern (due to osteoclastic resorption of smaller trabeculae)
   ii. Subperiosteal bone resorption is phalanges of hands—giving rise to irregular serrated appearance of outer subperiosteal cortex—progressing to extensive cortical resorption.
   iii. Bone cyst is multiple, containing brownish serous or mucoid fluid, occurs in central medullary portion of shaft of metacarpals, ribs and pelvis.
   iv. Brown tumor composed of—numerous multinucleated osteoclasts (giant cells), mixed with stromal cells and matrix—found in trabecular portion of jaw, long bones, ribs.
   v. Pathological fractures.
   vi. Skull X-ray shown—finely mottled salt and paper like radiographic appearance, loss of delineation of outer and inner cortices.
   vii. Dental radiography shows—loss of lamina dura due to subperiosteal bone resorption, with extension to adjacent mandibular bone.
   viii. As a result of bone resorption, following bones may be disappeared:
      a. Tuft of distal phalanges of hands
      b. Inferolateral cortex of distal third of clavicles
      c. Distal ulna
      d. Interior margin of femoral neck and pubis
      e. Medial aspect of proximal tibia
   As a result, following skeletal deformity may occur:
      a. Bowing of shoulders
      b. Kyphosis
      c. Loss of height

d. Collapse of lateral ribs and pelvis
e. Pigeon breast
f. Triradiate deformities

II. Renal manifestation:
i. Recurrent nephrolithiasis
ii. Nephrocalcinosis
iii. Renal calcium abnormalities
iv. Impaired concentrating ability
v. End stage renal failure.

Patient may present with flank pain, polyuria, polydipsia. Stone may be composed of:
i. Calcium
ii. Oxalate
iii. Calcium and oxalate

III. Gastrointestinal manifestation:
i. Vague abdominal discomfort
ii. Nausea
iii. Vomiting
iv. Constipation
v. Peptic ulcer disease
vi. Features of acute or chronic pancreatitis

IV. Eye manifestations:
i. Conjunctival calcification
ii. Band keratopathy

V. Cardiovascular manifestations:
i. Left ventricular hypertrophy
ii. Cardiac function defect
iii. Endothelial dysfunction.

VI. Neuropsychiatric manifestations:
i. Symmetrical muscle weakness
ii. Gait disturbances
iii. Muscle atrophy
iv. Characteristic electromyographic abnormalities
v. Generalized hyperreflexia
vi. Tongue fasciculation

Causes of Hyperparathyroidism

A. Parathyroid
i. Solitary adenoma
ii. Rarely parathyroid carcinoma
iii. May be all the parathyroid glands are hyperfunctioning.

Chief cell parathyroid hyperplasia—it may be associated with other endocrine abnormalities.

B. Hereditary syndrome and multiple parathyroid tumors
1. *Multiple* endocrine neoplasia (Werner's syndrome): It consists of:
   i. Hyperparathyroidism
   ii. Pancreatic tumor—associated with gastric hypersecretion and peptic ulcer disease (Zollinger-Ellison syndrome)

   Other hormones—glucagon, VIP, pancreatic polypeptide may be secreted from this tumor.
   iii. Pituitary tumor—commonly prolactinoma, but ACTH and growth hormones may be hypersecreted.

   This disease occurs due to expression of inactivating mutation of a tumor suppressor gene (Menin/MEN1 gene) located in chromosome 11q13.

2. *Multiple endocrine neoplastic type 2a (Sipple syndrome):* This disease consists of:
   i. Medullary carcinoma of thyroid
   ii. Pheochromocytoma
   iii. Parathyroid hyperplasia

   This disease is caused by activating mutation of RET proto-oncogene on chromosome 10.

3. *Hyperparathyroidism—Jaw tumor syndrome:* Autosomal dominant disease characterized by:
   i. Recurrent adenoma of parathyroid gland
   ii. Bone lesion punched out cystic lesion in mandible and maxilla.

4. *Familial isolated hyperparathyroidism.*

Diagnosis

1. **Hypercalcemia:** Majority of patients may present with intermittently elevated hypercalcemia or marginally elevated hypercalcemia—in that case ionized calcium measurement is most essential.

   But in case of vitamin D deficiency—serum calcium is low, in that case—administration of vitamin D (vitamin D challenge test) may unmask hypercalcemia.

2. **Parathyroid hormone level:** Level of immumoreactive PTH—can be measured by different types of assay:
   i. First generation assay
   ii. Double antibody or immunometric assays—this is second generation assay.
   iii. Third generation assay—it can defect large PTH fragments devoid of extreme amino terminal portion of PTH molecule.

   Second and third generation assays are useful for detecting:
   i. Primary hyperparathyroidism
   ii. High turnover bone disease in chronic kidney disease

3. **Measurement of urinary excretion of total or nephrogenous cyclic adenosine monophosphate**—it can assess the PTH action on kidney.

4. **Urinary calcium excretion:** This measurement depends upon:
   i. Serum calcium level.
   ii. Filtered load of calcium by kidney.
   iii. Intestinal absorption of calcium
   iv. Dietary intake.
   v. Level of parathormone level.

   Normal urinary calcium excretion in presence of hypercalcemia is of greater diagnostic value than increased urinary calcium (it occurs in elevated level of 1, 25 $(OH)_2D$).

5. **Hypophosphatemia:** It is observed in 50% of cases where renal threshold for phosphorus reabsorption is low.

6. **Chloride: phosphorus ratio:**
   i. Normal value is >32
   ii. It will be elevated in 60 to 70% of primary hyperparathyroidism.

7. **Biochemical markers of bone remodeling:**
   a. Formation biomarker:
   i. Osteocalcin
   ii. Alkaline phosphatase
   b. Resorption biomarkers:
   i. Hydroxyproline
   ii. Deoxypyridinoline
   iii. Collagen-C telopeptide

Preoperative and intraoperative parathyroid localization procedure:

1. *Ultrasound of parathyroid gland:* It is diagnosed in 80% of cases. It can be used intraoperatively to detect successful operation of parathyroid gland.
2. *Magnetic resonance imaging:* Detect parathyroid abnormalities.
3. ^{99m}Tc—*sestamibi scintigraphy:* Widely used as sensitive localization procedure for parathyroid adenoma.
4. *Parathyroid angiography:* This angiography combined with selective venous sampling is used:
   i. To identify a gradient in PTH levels
   ii. To localize hyperplastic glands or adenoma in most cases
5. *Intraoperative parathyroid localization:* By hand-held gamma-radiation detector (gamma probe) can rapidly locate an abnormal gland.

Treatment

1. **Removal of parathyroid adenoma or removal of all four glands:** Preoperative radioactive scan of parathyroid adenoma and intraoperative sampling of PTH just before and after operation at 5 minutes interval commonly down to normal postoperatively—suggests successful removal of adenoma.
2. **If hypercalcemia is severe**—it may be parathyroid carcinoma; in such cases neck exploration with wide excision of tissues should be done. But care should be taken to prevent rupture of capsule so that local seedling of malignant cells can be avoided.
3. **In case of parathyroid hyperplasia**—two methods can be undertaken:
   i. Removal of 3 glands and partial excision of fourth gland is of choice; but care should be taken to preserve good blood supply to remaining glands.
   ii. Total removal of all four glands with implantation of a portion of removed parathyroid gland into the muscles of forearm.
4. **In a few cases, no abnormality is found in neck parathyroid gland.** In such cases, adenoma can be found in mediastinum.

Status of Calcium Level in Blood

Decline in serum calcium occurs within 24 hours after successful surgery and it comes to normal level in 3–5 days. Acute postoperative hypocalcemia occurs, if:
i. Severe bony mineral deficit is present
ii. Injury to all parathyroid glands occurs during surgery.

The complication in single parathyroid adenoma is less in following situations:
i. Who do not have symptomatic bone disease.
ii. Who do not have large deficit in bony mineral.
iii. Who have sufficient vitamin D and magnesium in serum.
iv. Who have good renal and gastrointestinal functional reserve.

Symptomatic hypocalcemia occurs when:
i. If all glands are biopsied—hypocalcemia is transiently symptomatic but prolonged.
ii. After second parathyroid operation—hypocalcemia is symptomatic—mainly when normal parathyroid tissue is removed in 1st operation and when remaining glands are manipulated and/or biopsied.

Signs and symptoms of hypocalcemia—are evidenced by
a. Muscle twitching
b. Anxiety
c. Positive Chvostek's sign
d. Trousseau's sign coupled with—Serum calcium <8 mg/dl

Parenteral calcium therapy should be instituted—rate and duration of therapy are determined by severity of signs and symptoms of hypocalcemia.

> Infusion of 0.5–2 mg/kg of body weight—is sufficient to relieve symptoms.
> ↓
> If symptoms worsen
> ↓
> Addition of oral calcium (2–4 gm/dl)
> and
> Vitamin analogue (calcitriol 0.51 mg/day)

Rise in serum calcium after several months of vitamin D replacement—may indicate restoration of parathyroid gland to normal.

Since concomitant magnesium deficiency may impair the secretion of PTH, hypomagnesemia must be corrected, when defected by:
i. Orally $MgCl_2$ or $Mg(OH)_2$
   Or
ii. 0.5–1 mmol/kg of body weight—in severe hypomagnesemia
   But total dose 20–40 mmol is sufficient.

Guideline for surgery in asymptomatic primary hyperparathyroidism

Parameter	Guideline
1. Serum calcium (above normal)	Along the upper limit of normal
2. 24 hour—urinary calcium	More than 400 mg/day
3. Creatinine clearance	If <60 ml/mm
4. Bone density	T score < –2.5 at any of 3 sites (spine, hip, distal radius)
5. Age	<50 years

Medical therapy: In patients with poor surgical risk:
1. *Administration of orthophosphate salts:* 1–3 gm/day of phosphorus can control:
   i. Hypercalcemia
   ii. Nephrolithiasis
   This treatment should not be given in patient with:
   i. Serum calcium >12 mg/dl
   ii. Renal insufficiency
   iii. Habitual poor hydration
   Side effect:
   i. It can induce calcium phosphate stone formation
   ii. It increases the level of PTH
2. *Estrogen* can antagonize the PTH-induced bone resorption.
3. *Bisphosphonate:* Alendronate—it preserves the bone density in these patients.

4. *New class of drugs: Calcimimetics (cinacalcet)*—acts as calcium sensor receptor antagonist. It reduces serum calcium and parathhormone level for up to 5 years.

But US FDA accepts this drug in patient with:
  i. Dialysis
  ii. Parathyroid carcinoma

Investigation of Hypercalcemia (Figs 3.11, 3.12)

Calcium Hemostasis

1. 98% body calcium is found in skeleton—extracellular calcium.

2. Intracellular calcium is less than extracellular calcium by a factor of 100,000.

ICF calcium—control following intracellular processes
  i. Activity of many enzymes
  ii. Cell division
  iii. Exocytosis

In plasma, calcium exists in three different forms:
  i. 50% as ionized or the biologically active form
  ii. 45% bound to plasma proteins (mainly albumin)
  iii. 5% complexed with phosphate and citrate

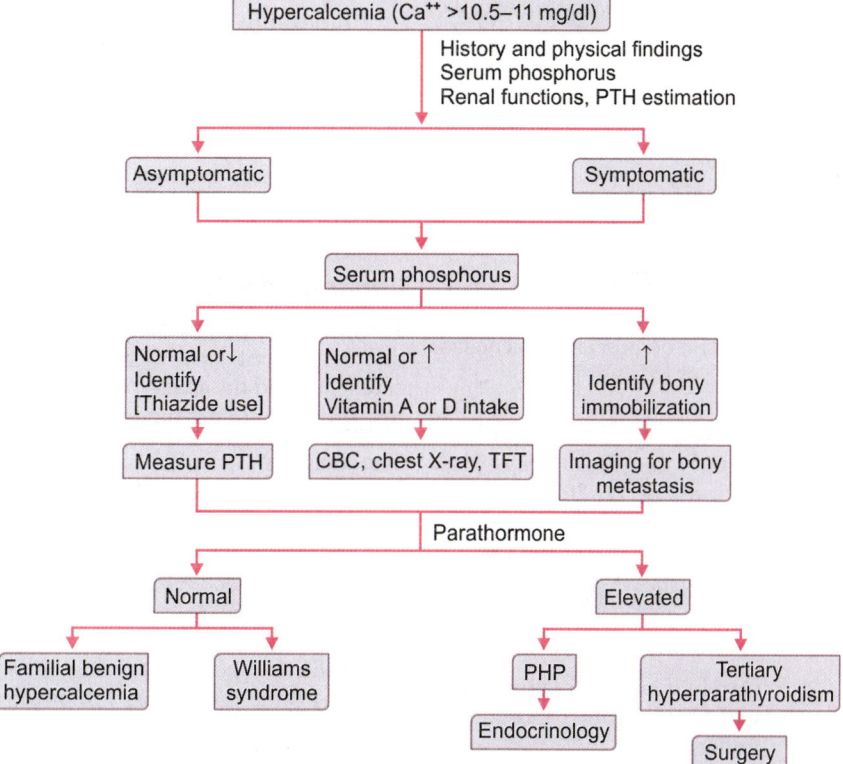

Fig. 3.11: Investigations for hypercalcemia

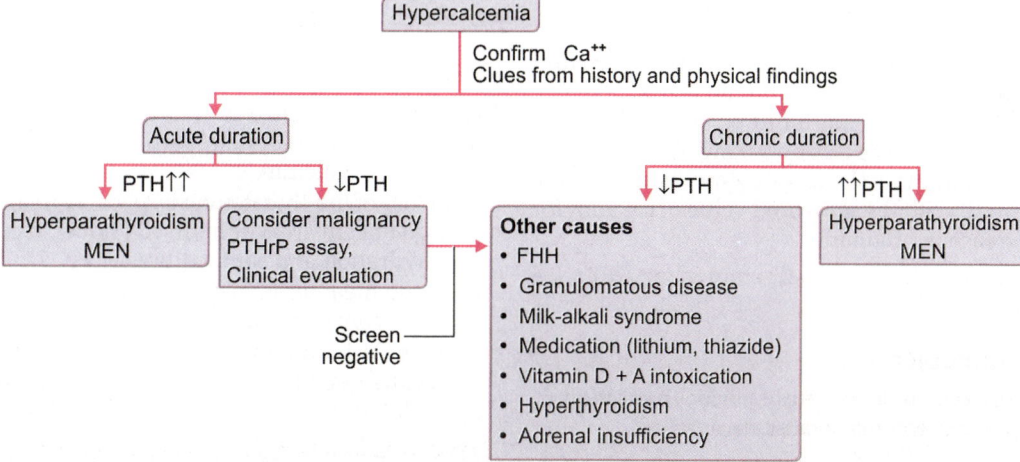

Fig. 3.12: Evaluation of hypercalcemia according to severity

In absence of acidosis and alkalosis, albumin is the major factor determining the amount of calcium that is bound.

Decrease in extracellular calcium concentration

↓

Stimulates parathyroid gland to increase secretion of PTH

↓

PTH increases distal renal tubular absorption of calcium within minutes
Stimulates osteoclastic activity

↓

Release of calcium from skeleton within 1–2 hours
More prolonged PTH stimulation

↓

Stimulates 1α hydroxylase activity in proximal tubular cells

↓

Increased production of 1, 25 $(OH)_2D$

↓

Increased absorption of calcium from intestine

All above mechanisms help to maintain serum calcium within limits.

Level of Calcium in Different Conditions

A. Normal serum calcium—8–10 mg/dl
B. Hypercalcemia >10.5 mg/dl—it can be subclassified based on total serum calcium and ionized calcium levels:

a. Mild	i. Total calcium	10.5–11.9 mg/dl
	ii. Ionized calcium	5.6–8 mg/dl
b. Moderate	i. Total calcium	12–13.9 mg/dl
	ii. Ionized calcium	8–10 mg/dl
c. Severe	i. Total calcium	14–16 mg/dl
	ii. Ionized calcium	10–12 mg/dl

Exchangeable form of calcium is 1–2% of total body calcium

↓

| One-half in active ionized form | One-half bound to albumin, globulin and other inorganic molecules |

In metabolic acidosis:

1. Reduced protein binding leads to increased ionized calcium.
2. Increased protein binding leads to decreased ionized calcium.

Unbound ionized term is biologically active; serum calcium level must be adjusted for abnormal albumin levels.

Every 1 gm/dl drop in serum albumin below 4 gm/dl measured serum calcium decreases by 0.8 mg/dl.

So, to correct for an albumin level below 4 gm/dl, one should add 0.8 gm/dl with the measured value of calcium for each 1 gm/dl decrease in albumin.

So, corrected calcium {(4-plasma albumin in gm/dl) × 0.8 + serum calcium}

Treatment of Hypercalcemia

Firstline of treatment: Aim is to restore normal hydration. Hypercalcemia patients are dehydrated because of:
  i. Vomiting
  ii. Inanination

iii. Hypercalcemia-induced defect in urinary concentrating ability
iv. Decrease in renal tubular sodium and calcium clearance.
  I. *Intravenous saline:*
    i. Restores normal ECF volume
    ii. Increase urinary calcium excretion by 100–300 mg/day
    iii. Increase in sodium excretion (400–500 mmol/day) further increases the calcium excretion.
  II. *Forced diuresis with diuretics:* Diuretics can be given twice daily—prevents calcium absorption from renal tubule. This modality of treatment can increase calcium excretion to 500 mg/day and decrease the serum calcium 1–3 mg/dl within 24 hours.
    Caution: Depletion of potassium and magnesium is inevitable accompaniments, if not treated properly, pulmonary edema develops.
    Potential complications can be reduced by:
    i. Proper monitoring of central venous pressure
    ii. Plasma and urinary electrolytes measurement
    iii. Urinary bladder catheterization
  III. *If renal function is compromised*—hemodialysis is the treatment.

Bisphosphonates

They have a high affinity in the areas of increased bone turn over—concentrated in these areas. They are taken up by osteoclast and the action of osteoclast will be inhibited, so bone resorption will be inhibited.

The drugs:
1. *Pamidronate:* 30 to 90 mg single dose 1% over few hours—returns serum calcium to normal in 24–48 hours and persists for few a weeks.
2. *Zolendronate:* 4–8 mg/5 minute infusion. Duration of action >3 weeks
3. *Alendronate*
   All the above bisphosphonates have high favorable ratio of blocking bone resorption: inhibiting bone formation.

Complications
  i. Fever
  ii. Hypophosphatemia
  iii. Hypocalcemia
  iv. Hypomagnesemia
  v. Rarely jaw necrosis

Calcitonin

Mechanism of action: It blocks through receptors on osteoclast to block bone resorption and reduce the tubular absorption of calcium.
  i. In case of life-threatening hypercalcemia, calcitonin can be used effectively within first 24 hours in combination with rehydration and saline diuresis.
  ii. In the meantime, bisphosphonate will be administered and it comes into action.
  iii. After 24 hours, the action of calcitonin will be reduced because of tachyphylaxis. This phenomenon can be inhibited by glucocorticoid administration.

Dose: 2–8 units/kg of body weight. IV, SC or IM every 6–12 hours.

Calcitonin, because of its low toxicity, is usually used though it produces modest reduction in serum calcium level.

After single daily dose of 15–25 mg/kg, calcium lowering effect can occur within 12–24 hours. Sustained lowering of calcium can last for 1–3 weeks. So it can be used in case of hypercalcemia with malignancy.

Plicamycin

It inhibits bone resorption. But it is now seldom used because of its toxicities (bone marrow depression, renal and hepatic dysfunction) and effectiveness of bisphosphonates.

Gallium Nitrate

i. It inhibits bone resorption
ii. It alters the structure of bone crystals.

It inhibits bone resorption by adsorbing and reducing solubility of hydroxyproline in bone matrix.

Administration: Continuous administration for 5–10 days for severe hypercalcemia—usual dose is 100 mg/m^2

Duration of action is 24–48 hours.
Duration of normocalcemia will be 6–10 days.

Important side effect is nephrotoxicity; so this drug should be used with caution when serum creatinine level >2.5 mg/dl

Glucocorticoid

Mode of action:
I. In general:
  i. It increases urinary calcium excretion
  ii. It decreases intestinal calcium absorption when steroid is given in pharmacologic dose.
II. In normal person and in patient with primary hyperparathyroidism—glucocorticoid neither decrease nor increase serum calcium concentration.
III. In glucocorticoid responsive malignancies (multiple myeloma, leukemia, Hodgkin's disease, other lymphoma, carcinoma of breast)—steroid reduces hypercalcemia.
IV. In certain osteolytic malignancies
V. Hypercalcemia due to vitamin D intoxication, sarcoidosis
VI. In certain autoimmune disorders

Dose: 40–100 mg in divided doses

Phosphate Therapy

By correction of hyperphosphatemia, It inhibits calcium absorption and promotes calcium phosphate deposition.

Dose: Oral dose—1000–1500 mg elemental phosphate in divided doses, not exceeding 3000 mg/day.

Parenteral administration is 1000 mg/24 hours infusion over 4–6 hours period.

Ectopic soft tissue calcification occurs when calcium phosphorus product >40—so for the reason, phosphate treatment should not be given when serum calcium level >12–13 mg/dl.

Milk-Alkali Syndrome

Triad of hypercalcemia, metabolic alkalosis and renal failure—it may produce metastatic calcification

Cause: Ingestion of calcium and absorbable alkali.

Pathogenesis: It involves a vicious cycle—in which alkalosis decreases renal calcium clearance and leads to hypercalcemia = which in turn maintains metabolic alkalosis.

Clinical presentation:
i. Nausea, vomiting
ii. Nephrocalcinosis
iii. Nephrogenic diabetes incipidus
iv. Renal failure

Diagnosis: PTH level is invariably low in hypercalcemic patient.

Treatment:
i. Clearance of calcium by hydration
ii. Dialysis

As a result of treatment of renal failure, patient returns to normal unless this disorder has been severe and long standing.

Williams' Syndrome

This is characterized by:
1. Supravalvular aortic stenosis
2. Elfin facies
3. Mental retardation
4. Hypercalcemia occurs transiently in first 4 years of life.

Pathophysiology: Increased absorption of calcium from intestine and associated elevation of calcitriol, that fails to normal as blood calcium level normalizes.

Levels of 25 (OH)D is normal.

Treatment:
i. Dietary manipulation
ii. Bisphosphonates

Familial Hypocalciuric Hypercalcemia

In this case, major clue to the diagnosis is family history of hypercalcemia.

It is autosomal dominant disease—expressed very early in life.
i. There is inactivating mutation of CSR (calcium sensing receptor).
ii. There is other mutation in long arm of chromosome 3
iii. There is also mutation involving long and short arm of chromosome 19.
  a. So there is higher threshold of serum calcium to suppress PTH hormone secretion—hence there is mild to moderate hypercalcemia.
  b. Mutated CSR in kidney produces variable reduction in urinary calcium to produce hypocalciuria.

Biochemical features are:
i. Variable degree of hypocalciuria.
ii. Hypercalcemia
iii. Hypermagnesemia
iv. Hypomagnesuria
v. Ratio of calcium clearance to creatinine clearance (Cca/Ccr)—it is more sensitive index of renal calcium excretion—than total calcium excretion.
  In familial hypocalciuric hypocalcemia—ratio is <0.1
vi. Parathhormone is normal or slightly elevated.

Response to parathyroid surgery is very poor in FHH. But the development of acute pancreatitis in FHH may necessitate total parathyroidectomy.

Agents those Reduce Intestinal Absorption of Calcium

Enteric absorption calcium is mainly responsible for maintenance of hypercalcemia.

a. In disorder of vitamin D excess: Treatment with glucocorticoid is highly effective in reducing calcium absorption.
b. Reduction of dietary intake of calcium may be useful maneuver in:
   i. Vitamin D—excess state
   ii. Milk–alkali syndrome
c. Cellulose phosphate which complexes with calcium in intestine, prevents intestinal absorption of calcium.
d. Ketoconazole—reduces plasma level of 1,25 $(OH)_2$ D.

Hypocalcemia Disorders

Causes

A. Parathyroid-related disorder:
1. Surgical hypoparathyroidism—surgical removal of parathyroid tissue.
2. Idiopathic hypoparathyroidism
3. Congenital:
   i. Digeorge's syndrome
   ii. X-linked or autosomal inherited hyperparathyroidism
   iii. Autoimmune polyglandular syndrome
4. Infiltrative disorder:
   i. Sarcoidosis
   ii. Hemochromatosis
   iii. Wilson's disease
   iv. Metastases
5. Impaired secretion of PTH:
   i. Hypomagnesemia
   ii. Respiratory alkalosis
6. Target organ resistance:
   i. Hypomagnesemia
   ii. Pseudohypoparathyroidism—type 1 and 2

B. Vitamin D-related disorder:
1. Vitamin D deficiency:
   i. Poor dietary intake
   ii. Malabsorption
2. Accelerated loss:
   i. Impaired enterohepatic circulation.
   ii. Anticonvulsant medication
3. Impaired 25, hydroxylation:
   i. Liver disease
   ii. Isoniazid
4. Impaired 1α hydroxylation: Renal failure
5. Vitamin D dependant rickets type 1.
6. Osteogenic osteomalacia
7. Target organ resistance:
   i. Vitamin D dependant rickets type 2
   ii. Phenytoin

C. Other causes:
1. Excessive deposition into skeleton:
   i. Osteoblastic malignancy
   ii. Hungry bone syndrome
2. Chelation:
   i. Foscarnet
   ii. Phosphate infusion
   iii. Fluoride
   iv. Infusion of citrated blood products
3. Neonatal hypocalcemia:
   i. Asphyxia   ii. Hyperparathyroid mother

4. HIV infection
5. Critical illness

Clinical Signs and Symptoms

The signs and symptoms of hypocalcemia are the function of:
1. Level of serum calcium
2. Serum level of magnesium
3. Serum level of potassium
4. Disturbance of acid base balance
5. Age of onset and duration of symptoms
A. Increased neuromuscular irritability resulting in muscle cramping (tetany), classic sign of tetany is:
   1. Carpopedal spasm—Trousseau sign
   2. Chvostek's sign: Increased irritability of fifth cranial nerve
   3. Other neuromuscular sign:
      i. Paresthesia
      ii. Laryngospasm
      iii. Bronchospasm
      iv. Abdominal cramping
      v. Generalized hyperreflexia
      vi. CNS disturbances include:
         a. Seizure (hypocalcemic seizures).
         b. Grand mal and petit mal seizures.
         c. Syncope
         d. Impaired memory
         e. Psychosis
         f. Disturbances in extrapyramidal system function—such as parkinsonism, choreoathetosis.
         g. EEG—are non-specific—mainly increases in burst of high voltage, slow wave activity
B. Most ocular manifestation of chronic hypocalcemia:
      i. Cataracts—calcium deposits in subcapsular, anterior, posterior zonular location.
      ii. Papilledema
      iii. Pseudomotor cerebri
C. Cardiovascular disturbances:
      i. ECG disturbances include
         a. Prolongation of QT interval
         b. Non-specific T wave changes
      ii. Refractory congestive heart failure resistant to digitals therapy
      iii. Hypotension resistant to conventional does of pressor agents.
D. Soft tissue calcification—and exostoses:
   1. Periarticular calcification—chondrocalcinosis, pseudogout.
   2 Basal ganglia calcification
E. Macrocytic megaloblastic anemia—due to deficient binding of vitamin B_{12} to intrinsic factor in presence of hypocalcemia.
   Chronic hypocalcemia produces following dermatological manifestations:
   1. Coarse hair
   2. Brittle nails
   3. Psoriasis
   4. Dry skin
   5. Chronic pruritus
   6. Poor dentition
   7. Cataracts

Physical Examination

Neural hyperexitibility due to acute hypocalcemia—produces:
a. Smooth muscle contraction
b. Skeletal muscle contraction
c. Dementia.
d. Psychosis

On head and neck examination:
a. hair is coarse
b. Alopecia
c. Signs of surgery of the neck (scar over thyroid region)
d. Perioral anesthesia
e. In adult with chronic hypocalcemia—increased risk of dental caries and enamel hypoplasia
f. Subcapsular cataracts
g. Papilledema

On respiratory examination:
a. Inspiratory or expiratory wheezes
b. Smooth muscle contraction—produces
    i. Laryngospasm
    ii. Bronchospasm
    iii. Dysphagia

On cardiac examination:
a. Bradycardia
b. Tachycardia
c. Third heart sound
d. Signs of heart failure

Dermatological examination:
a. Dry skin
b. Psoriasis
c. Eczema
d. Excoriation

Tests for Chvostek's sign (10% of patient): Tapping the skin over facial nerve—about 2 cm anterior to external auditory meatus:
- Ipsilateral contraction of facial muscles → positive sign
- Depending on calcium level, graded response will occur
- Twitching first at angle of the mouth → nose → eye → facial muscles.

Test for Trousseau sign: Place blood pressure cuff on the patient's arm—inflate it to 20 mmHg above systolic blood pressure for 3–5 minutes.

Results:
i. This increases irritability of nerves.
ii. Flexion of the wrist and metacarpophalangeal joints.
iii. Extension of interphalangeal joints.
iv. Abduction of thumb.
    This test is more specific.

Movement abnormalities:
a. Choreoathetosis
b. Dystonic spasm
c. Parkinsonism
d. Hemiballism.

Peripheral nervous system findings include:
a. Tetany
b. Focal numbness
c. Muscle spasms

Smooth muscle involvement:
a. Biliary colic
b. Intestinal colic
c. Dysphagia

Pseudohypoparathyroidism

This is a group of disorders with:
    i. Biochemical and clinical features of hypoparathyroidism
    ii. Target organ resistance to parathyroid hormone
    iii. Elevated level of parathyroid hormone
       Two types of pseudohypoparathyroidism

Type I Pseudohypoparathyroidism

This is characterized by:
a. Biochemical features of hypoparathyroidism
b. Characteristic developmental and somatic features
    i. Short stature
    ii. Round facies
    iii. Obesity
    iv. Brachydactyly
    v. Pseudoclubbing of the neck
    vi. Subcutaneous calcification
    vii. Ossifications
    viii. Forshortened fourth and other metacarpals
c. Mental retardation: The above somatic features are called Albright hereditary osteodystrophy.

The etiology: Diminished activity of $G_s\alpha$—α subunit of stimulatory G protein—though different types of mutation—missense mutation, chain terminating mutations.

Associated other hormone resistance syndrome may be associated with type 1A pseudohypoparathyroidism of
    i. TSH resistance syndrome (hypothyroidism)
    ii. Glucagon resistance syndrome (no clinical disorder)
    iii. Gonadotrophin resistance syndrome (amenorrhea)

Diagnosis:
1. Presence of features of Albright hereditary osteodystrophy
2. Reduced $G_s\alpha$ protein activity (reduced by 50% in RBC membrane)
3. Evidence of end organ resistance to PTH
        i. Hypocalcemia
        ii. Hyperphosphatemia
        iii. Elevated level of PTH
   or iii. Blunted rise in excretion of nephrogenous cyclic AMP
        iv. Absence of PTH stimulation of renal production of 1, 25 $(OH)_2$ D.
        v. Low calcitriol level
        vi. Blunted calcemic response (skeletal resistance)
In some patients, hypocalcemia is intermitted, but PTH is persistently elevated as a result urinary calcium excretion is low due to action of PTH on DCT of kidney—producing normocalcemia.

Pseudohypoparathyroidism type IA—characterized by:
1. Somatic features of Albright hereditary osteodystrophy
2. Patients are normocalcemic, but lack in evidence of PTH resistance
3. Inheritance of same abnormal $G_s\alpha$ gene:
    i. If patient inherits mutant gene from father side, he develops pseudopseudohypoparathyroidism.

ii. If patient inherits mutant gene from mother side—he develops only pseudohypoparathyroidism
4. Subcutaneous calcifications, mainly progressive osseous heteroplasia almost exclusively seen.

Pseudohypoparathyroidism type IB: This is characterized by:
1. Isolated PTH resistance
2. Normal $G_s\alpha$ protein activity
3. Absence of features of Albright hereditary osteodystrophy
4. Expression of PTH resistance is similar to type 1:
   i. Absent rise in urinary cyclic-AMP
   ii. Absent phosphaturic response to exogenous PTH.

Pseudohypoparathyroidism type IC: This is characterized by:
   i. Feature of AHO syndrome
   ii. Multiple forms of hormone resistance syndrome to similar to that of type 1A.
   iii. Defect in Gsα protein activity—which cannot be demonstrated with current assay.

Type II Pseudohypoparathyroidism

PTH raises the cAMP normally, but fails to increase the level of serum calcium or urinary phosphate excretion—it occurs due to defect is located downstream of generation of cyclic-AMP.

Signs are:
   i. Hypocalcemia.
   ii. Hypophosphatemia.
   iii. Elevated immumoreactive PTH level.

This finding can occur with vitamin D deficiency—which can be differentiated by administration of vitamin D.

Hypomagnesemia

This hypomagnesemia can lead to hypocalcemia which is resistant to administration of calcium and vitamin D.

Causes of Hypomagnesemia

I. Loss via—kidney:
   i. Osmotic diuresis
   ii. Drugs
II. Gastrointestinal tract:
   i. Chronic diarrhea
   ii. Severe pancreatitis
   iii. Resection of small bowel.
III. The mechanism of hypocalcemia includes:
   i. Resistance to parathormone to kidneys and bones
   ii. Decrease in parathormone secretion—due to decreased release of PTH from parathyroid gland

Administration of magnesium increases the release of PTH.

Hepatic Disease

The causes of hypocalcemia in liver disease are:
1. Impaired 25 hydroxylation of vitamin D
2. Decreased bile salts with malabsorption of vitamin D
3. Decreased synthesis of vitamin D-binding protein
4. Other factors interfere with vitamin D function
5. Decreased sun exposure

Hungry Bone Syndrome

1. As a consequence of surgical correction of primary or secondary hyperparathyroidism—rapid increase in bony remodeling—this exceeds the osteoclast medicated bone resorption.
2. Correction of thyrotoxicosis
3. After institution of vitamin D for osteomalacia
4. Tumors associated with bone formation (prostate, breast, leukemia)

Hypocalcemia in Emergency Department

1. Rhabdomyolysis: Increased phosphate from creatinine phosphokinase and other anions (lactate and bicarbonate) chelates calcium
2. Toxic shock syndrome—can cause hypocalcemia
3. High calcitonin level
4. Malignancy:
   i. Osteoblastic metastases (breast and prostate cancer)
   ii. Tumor lysis syndrome
5. Infiltrative disease:
   i. Sarcoidosis
   ii. Tuberculosis
   iii. Hemochromatosis—infiltrating parathyroids
6. Toxicologic cause—hydrofluoric acid burn
7. Trauma patients with massive transfusion

In severe sepsis: The causes are:
   i. Hypomagnesemia
   ii. Acute renal failure
   iii. Transfusion
   iv. Gram-negative sepsis—due to:
      a. Elevated levels of cytokines (interleukin level 6, interleukin 1, TNF-alfa)
      b. Hypoparathyroidism
      c. Vitamin D deficiency or remittance.

Hypocalcemia workup:
1. Liver function test
2. Renal parameter
3. Coagulation parameter
4. Serum calcium level
5. Serum parathormone level
   To measure hypocalcemia, measurement of serum albumin is essential to distinguish true hypocalcemia—which involves—reduction in ionized serum calcium from factitious hypocalcemia.
   To correct for hypoalbuminemia—substract 0.8 mg/dl from the total serum calcium for each 1.0 gm/dl decrease in albumin below 4.0 gm/dl.
   Serum ionized calcium: Serum calcium <8 mg/dl or ionized calcium <1 mmol/L—is considered as hypocalcemia.
   Blood should be unheparinized.

Falsely Elevated Calcium Level

1. Heparin
2. Oxalate
3. Citrate
4. Hyperbilirubinemia

Serum Electrolytes

1. Combination of hypocalcemia and elevated phosphorus level—suggests hypoparathyroidism or pseudohypoparathyroidism.
2. Hypocalcemia, hyperphosphatemia and raised PTH level—renal failure.

3. Hypocalcemia, hypophosphatemia—vitamin D deficiency
4. Serum magnesium—low due to low dietary intake

Parathyroid Hormone

1. PTH level will be raised—in PTH resistance pseudohypoparathyroidism
2. Low or normal PTH:
   a. Hereditary or acquired hypoparathyroidism
   b. Severe hypomagnesemia

Vitamin D Metabolites

1. Measurement of 25 (DH)D—low in vitamin D deficiency—due to:
   a. Poor dietary intake
   b. Lack of sunlight
   c. Malabsorption
2. **Low 1, 2 (OH)$_2$D**—with high PTH—suggests ineffective PTH from lack of vitamin D—occur in:
   i. CRF
   ii. Vitamin D deficiency rickets
   iii. Pseudohypothyroidism
3. **Urinary cyclic-AMP:** If differentiates hypoparathyroidism (where it is elevated) from type 1 and 2 pseudohypoparathyroidism.

Electrocardiogram

Acute hypocalcemia—produces QT interval—which leads to ventricular dysrhythmia—ventricular tachycardia.

Treatment of Hypocalcemia

It depends upon:
   i. Cause
   ii. Severity
   iii. Presence of symptoms
   iv. Rapidity of development.

Since hypocalcemia is a symptom of a definite cause—so the etiology must be treated early to recover hypocalcemia.

Mild Hypocalcemia

The goal is to correct symptomatic hypocalcemia without inducing the development of hypercalcemia.

Therapeutic end point is to maintain:
i. Serum calcium levels in the range of 8.5 to 9.5 mg/dl
ii. Urinary calcium level below 400 mg/day

Oral supplement: If there is no malabsorption, in case of moderately severe hypocalcemia—3 to 7 gm of elemental calcium per day in divided doses.

This form of treatment is effective in short-term basis.

Drugs	Calcium content
1. Calcium carbonate	400 mg/1 gm
2. Calcium gluconate	9 mg/1 gm

Severe Hypocalcemia

1. Supportive treatment
   i. IV fluid replacement
   ii. Oxygen
2. IV calcium replacement: Dose 100–300 mg of elemental calcium (10 ml of calcium gluconate contains 90 mg of elemental calcium, 10 ml of calcium chloride contains 272 mg of elemental calcium) in 50–100 ml of 5% dextrose water to be given over 5–10 minutes. Calcium chloride 10% solution delivers higher amount of calcium—where rapid correction is needed—but it should be given via central venous access.
3. Calcium infusion—0.5 mg/kg/hr increased up to 2 mg/kg/hr—with an arterial line placed for frequent measurement of ionized calcium—to maintain calcium level 8–9 mg/dl.
4. In patient with cardiac arrhythmia, or patient is on digoxin therapy—continuous ECG monitoring during IV calcium replacement—because calcium potentiates digitalis toxicity.
5. Patient with hyperparathyroidism, oral calcium with vitamin D for 1–2 days prior to parathyroid surgery can prevent severe postoperative hypocalcemia.

Chronic Hypocalcemia

Treatment here depends upon the etiology:
1. Patient with hypoparathyroidism and pseudohypoparathyroidism:
   i. Oral calcium supplements
   ii. Thiazide diuretic
2. In patient with severe hypoparathyroidism:
   i. Since PTH is necessary for conversion of Vitamin D to calcitriol, hence 0.5–2 µg of calcitriol or 1α hydroxyl D$_3$ should be given.
   ii. Those that have undergone parathyroidectomy—there is a considerable difficulty in maintaining serum calcium level
      a. So oral calcium should be given in between meals.
      b. Active vitamin D (calcitriol)—enhances the absorption of calcium.
3. In patient with severe nutritional vitamin D deficiency—from lack of sunlight or reduced oral intake of vitamin D$_3$:
   i. Oral calcium 1–2 gm elemental calcium 1 day
   ii. Calcitriol

Vitamin D 1000 units/day (2–3 mg/day)

Calcitriol—0.25–1 mg/day can be given to prevent rickets in normal individual.

40000–120000 V of vitamin D$_3$—is required in hypoparathyroidism.

In low 25 (OH) vitamin D state—60000 unit of vitamin D (cholecalciferol) is given weekly for 8 weeks.

PANCREAS

DIABETES MELLITUS

Insulin synthesis occurs in the beta cells at the tail end of pancreas—these are one million in number.

Biosynthesis of insulin occurs in two stages:
- Human insulin gene is located in the region P_{13} of the short arm of chromosome number 11.
- Insulin gene expression and biosynthesis occurs on the beta cell at the tail end of pancreas.

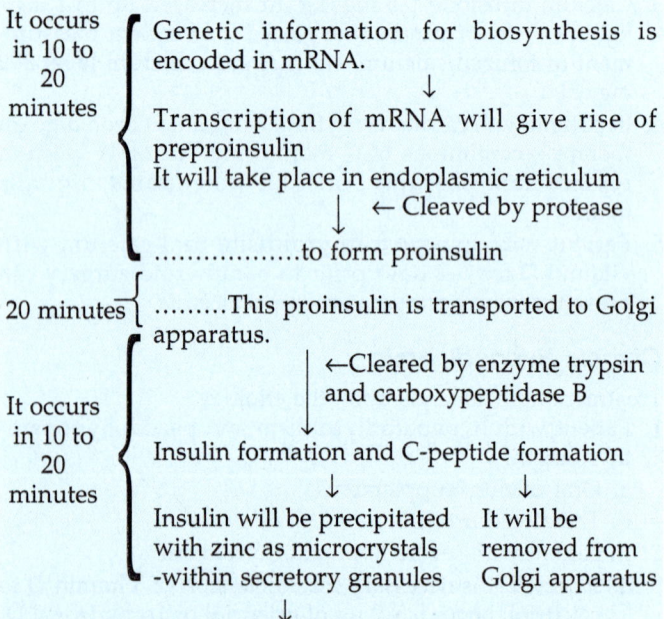

It occurs in 10 to 20 minutes {
Genetic information for biosynthesis is encoded in mRNA.
↓
Transcription of mRNA will give rise of preproinsulin
It will take place in endoplasmic reticulum
↓ ← Cleaved by protease
..................to form proinsulin

20 minutes { ....This proinsulin is transported to Golgi apparatus.

It occurs in 10 to 20 minutes {
←Cleared by enzyme trypsin and carboxypeptidase B
↓
Insulin formation and C-peptide formation
↓   ↓
Insulin will be precipitated with zinc as microcrystals -within secretory granules | It will be removed from Golgi apparatus
↓

It will be stored as granules for hours to days (total quantity of insulin stores is about 200 units).

Function of C-peptide is to facilitate the correct folding of á and β chains and alignment of their disulphide bridges, before their eventual cleavages.

Insulin and C-peptide are stored in the granules as equimolar amounts.

Structures

Insulin has molecular weight of 6000 Daltons.

Two subunits:
1. α chain—21 amino acid residues
2. β chain—30 amino acid residues

Two chains are linked by disulfide bridges.

C-peptide—has 35-amino acid. It is released in equimolar concentration—hence plasma level of C-peptide is a good index of insulin secretion.

Biological actions of C-peptide:
1. It stimulates glucose transport in skeletal muscles
2. Restores Na–K-ATPase action
3. Induces vascular smooth muscle dilatation
4. Relieves autonomic neuropathy.

Insulin Secretion

Stored granules containing insulin move along the network of microtubules and microfilaments pathway from Golgi apparatus to the plasma membrane. Mechanical structures within the microtubules are action and myosin. These play an active role in this secretory process. This whole process is called exocytosis (emiocytosis).

There are two pathways of biosynthesis and processing of insulin:
1. Regulated pathway
2. Cosecutive pathway

In type 2 diabetes mellitus and insulinoma, cosecutive pathway will be in action, as a result, proinsulin and its split products are released before conversion to insulin.

Regulator of Insulin Secretion

Nutrient

Glucose Main source is carbohydrate—glucose.

Glucose is first transported into beta cells by glucose transporter (GLUT 2 isoform): Glucose stimulated insulin release is biphasic.

| Acute insulin response, it lasts for 5–10 minutes (1st phase) | Prolonged second phase of insulin response—which persists till the stimulus will be present |

1. Beta cells are sensitive to changes in blood glucose as low as 2 mg%.
2. Blood sugar level of <90 mg%—will not affect the insulin release.
3. Blood sugar level between 99 and 300 mg%—insulin secretion occurs.

Role of acute insulin response:
1. It maintains normal glucose tolerance.
2. It suppresses the endogenous glucose production.
3. Early insulin secretion primes insulin sensitive tissues.
4. It prevents postprandial hyperglycemia.
   I. *In β cells* — at basal state K^+ dependent channel is open and voltage dependent Ca^{++} channel will be closed.
      But as glucose enters in the cells—K^+ channels will be closed and Ca^{++} channel will open, as a result, Ca^{++} influx releases stored insulin into the cytosol by emiocytosis.

Released insulin enters in portal circulation in seconds
↓
It reaches the liver
↓
Half of the insulin will be cleared by liver in first pass.

Early entry of insulin prevents or suppresses hepatic glucose output.
   i. In fasting state, normal blood glucose will be maintained by hepatic glucose output.
   ii. In fed state—as plasma glucose rises, it will give signal to liver to suppress hepatic glucose output.

In absence of acute insulin response, hepatic glucose output results rise in postprandial blood glucose level.
   II. *Primary stimulus*—then can provoke insulin release.
   These are—glucose, other carbohydrate sources like:
   a. Arginine
   b. Lysine

c. Ketone bodies
d. Free fatty acids
e. Drugs (sulphonureas).
III. *Potentiators:* These are inactive by themselves but they promote insulin release in response to stimulators. The potentiators are:
   a. cyclic-AMP
   b. Neurotransmitter (acetylcholine)
   c. Gut peptides—glucagon, GLP-17–36 amide, GIP, secretin

Hormones

Gut hormones:
i. They mediate "incretin" effect, and enhance insulin release in response to oral glucose rather than intravenous glucose; this is **"enteroinsular" axis.**
   These hormones are:
   • Gastric inhibitory polypeptide
   • Glucagon-like peptide 1 (GLP 17–36 amide)
ii. They increase the intracellular cyclic-AMP level; as a result, enhance the nutrient-mediated insulin secretion.
iii. Neural: This is mediated by hypothalmoenteroinsular axis—this is under control of vagus nerve.

This is cephalic phase of insulin secretion in response to smell, sight and expectation of food.

This phase prevents early rise in postprandial glucose.

Beta cell functions in normal persons: Total insulin secretion in 24 hours is 30–40 units.

50% of it is secreted in based conditions.

50% of it is secreted in response to meals.

This pulsatile insulin secretion occurs at every .5–2 hours. It will be amplified postprandially.

This pulsatile fashion is called "ultradian pulse". On this pulse, rapid oscillations in beta cell activity will be superimposed—it occurs every 8–16 minutes. This rapid oscillation has some important biologic functions.

Advantages of pulsatile insulin release:
1. Receptor numbers will be maintained.
2. It potentiates hormone action.
3. It maximizes insulin responsiveness.
4. It effectively inhibits hepatic glucose output.

In type-1 diabetes mellitus: There is total destruction of beta cells, so no insulin will be released. So here replacement of insulin is the treatment of choice.

In type-2 diabetes mellitus:
i. Abnormality in oscillatory activity in stimulation of beta cells is the earliest manifestation of beta cells dysfunction.
ii. Absent first phase secretory response to intravenous glucose.

Insulin Action on Target Tissues

Substrate phosphorylation

1. Insulin release	1. Glucose uptake
2. Adipolysis	2. Glucose oxidation
3. Fatty acid synthesis	3. Glycogen synthesis
4. Ion transport	4. Protein synthesis
5. Amino acid uptake	5. Antiapoptosis
6. DNA synthesis	6. Gene expression

Receptor Events *(Fig. 3.13)*

Gene for insulin receptor lies on chromosome no 19.

Insulin receptor on target cell has four extracellular subunits:
i. Two α subunits
ii. Two β subunits.

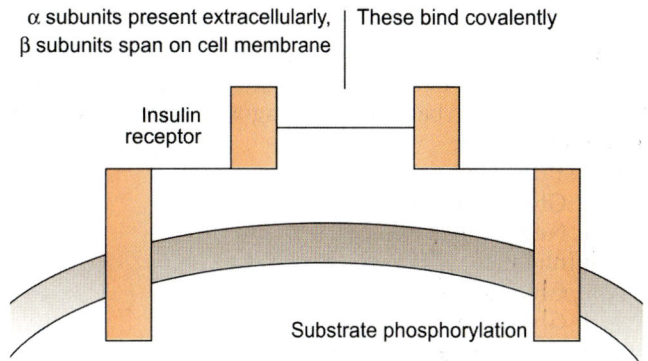

α subunits present extracellularly, β subunits span on cell membrane | These bind covalently

Insulin receptor

Substrate phosphorylation

Fig. 3.13: Receptor-insulin interaction

Post-Receptor Events

Insulin lowers the cAMP concentration by activating one or more membrane associated phosphodiesterase
↓
This is responsible for following postreceptor actions
Inhibition of   i. Gluconeogenesis in liver
                ii. Glycogenolysis in liver
               iii. Lipolysis in adipose tissue

The postulated mechanisms of insulin action:
1. Tyrosine kinase activity cascade
2. Cyclic-GMP activity
3. Glycosylated inositol phosphate activity.

Insulin action on peripheral tissues:
1. Increased glucose uptake by muscles and fat.
2. Recruits more and more glucose transporters (GLUT-1 toll) which catalyses glucose influx into the cells.
3. It modifies intrinsic activity of these glucose transporters.
4. It activates several intracellular enzymes in the pathway of fatty acid and triglyceride metabolism—leading to lipogenesis.

Insulinopathies

Definition

In this condition, mutation of insulin gene leads to abnormal synthesis and secretion of insulin.

Inheritance

It is inherited as heterozygous state for normal and mutant allels. They have additional abnormalities:
i. In insulin secretion process
ii. At insulin receptor site

Features

i. Hyperinsulinemia
ii. Varying degrees of glucose intolerance
iii. Normal response to exogenous insulin.

Glucagon

It is a major catabolic hormone—produced by α cell of pancreas.

At rest:
i. Arterial plasma glucose requires 56 mg/ml to deliver glucose in brain.
ii. Brain utilizes glucose at rate of 6 gm/hour
iii. Other tissue utilizes glucose at a rate of 4 gm/hour
iv. Whole body utilizes glucose at a rate of 10 gm/hour

So it is very much necessary for constant supply of glucose for the body—it can be done by glucagon, even in fasting state.

Action: In the liver:
1. It stimulates:
   i. Glycogenolysis
   ii. Neoglucogenesis
2. It inhibits:
   i. Glycogenesis
   ii. Glycolysis

Inhibitors of ghlucagon secretion:
i. Glucose
ii. Fatty acid
iii. Ketones
iv. Gastrointestinal polypeptide
v. Gastrin
vi. Secretin in portal vein

Stimulators of glucagon secretion:
i. Amino acids
ii. Hypoglycemia
iii. Stress
iv. Exercise

Somatostatin

It is a 14-amino acid residue containing polypeptide. It is synthesized by:
i. D cells of ilet cells of Langerhans
ii. Gut
iii. In specific neurons

Actions: It inhibits the secretion of:
i. Growth hormone
ii. Insulin
iii. Glucagon
iv. Gut peptides

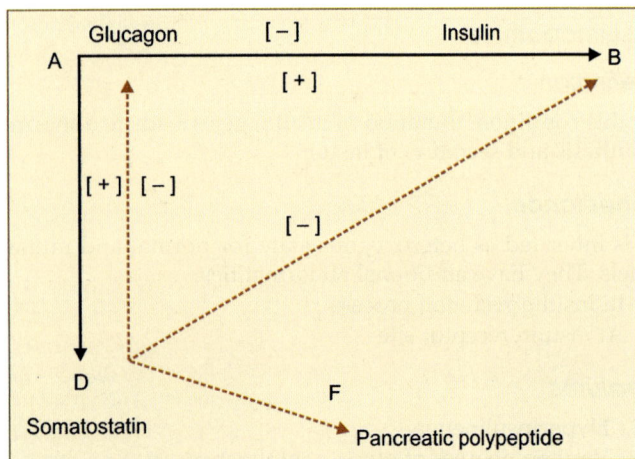

Fig. 3.14: Interrelationship of different norms to maintain euglycemia

Stimulators of somatostatin:
i. Glucose
ii. Amino acids
iii. Insulin deficiency.

Amylin

It takes part in glucose regulation. It is secreted from pancreatic beta cells.

Actions:
i. It controls the gastric emptying; thereby it shows intestinal absorption of glucose and makes a correlation with the uptake in peripheral tissues.
ii. It suppresses the hepatic glucose output by inhibiting glucagon secretion after meal ingestion.
iii. It induces postprandial satiety.
   a. In type-1 diabetes: There is absolute amylin deficiency.
   b. In type-2 diabetes: There is progressive decline in amylin levels in proportion to decline in insulin secretion.

Etiologic Classifications of Diabetes Mellitus

I. **Type 1 diabetes mellitus** (beta cell destruction—leading to absolute insulin deficiency):
   1. Immune mediated
   2. Idiopathic
II. **Type 2 diabetes mellitus:** It ranges from predominantly insulin resistance with relative insulin deficiency to predominantly insulin secretory defect with insulin resistance.
III. **Other specific types of diabetes:**
   A. Genetic defects in beta cell function—due to mutation in different genes.
   B. Genetic defects in insulin action.
   C. Disease of exocrine pancreas.
   D. Endocrinopathies: Acromegaly, Cushing's syndrome, pheochromocytoma, glucagonoma, hyperthyroidism, somatostatinoma.
   E. Drug-induced: Glucocorticoids, dizoxide, thiazide, hydantoin, α-interferon, epinephrine.
   F. Infections: Congenital rubella, cytomegalovirus, coxsackie virus.
   G. Uncommon forms of immune-mediated diabetes: Stiff-person syndrome, anti-insulin receptor antibodies.
   H. Other genetic syndrome associated with diabetes:
      • Down's syndrome
      • Klinfelter's syndrome
      • Turner's syndrome
      • Huntington's chorea
      • Laurence-Moon-Biedl syndrome
   I. Gestational diabetes mellitus

Risk Factors of Type 2 Diabetes Mellitus

1. Family history of diabetes (parent or sibling with type 2 diabetes mellitus)
2. Obesity (BMI ≥29 kg/m^2)
3. Physical inactivity
4. Race/ethnicity—African, American, native American
5. Previously identified with IFG, IGT, A1c–5.7–6.4%
6. History of GDM

Table 3.1: Spectrum of glucose homeostasis and diabetes mellitus					
Type of diabetes	Normal	Impaired GT (prediabetes)	Diabetes		
			Not insulin requiring	Insulin required for control	Insulin requires for survival
Type-1					
Type-2					
Others					
GDM					
FPG	<100 mg/dl	100–125 mg/dl	>126 mg/dl		
2 hours PG	<140 mg/dl	140–199 mg/dl	>200 mg/dl		
HbA1c	<5–6%	5.7–6.4%	>6.5%		

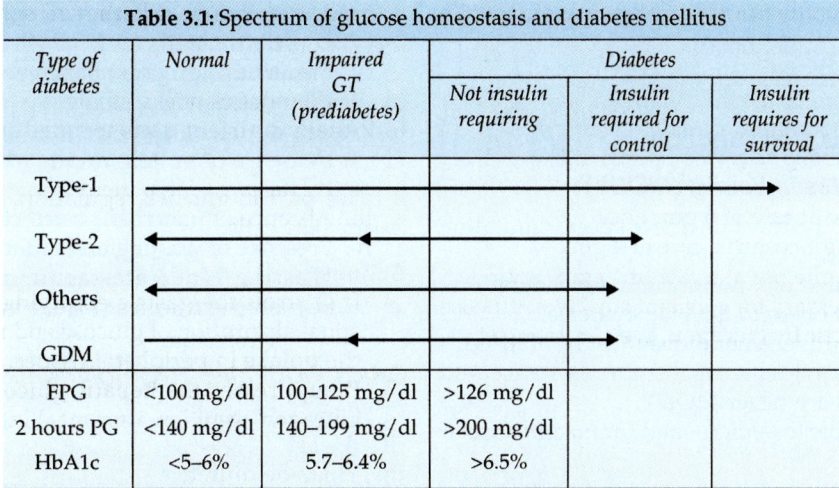

Table 3.2: Criteria for diagnosis of diabetes mellitus				
Test	Normo-glycemia	Impaired fasting glucose	IGT	High risk	Diabetes
Fasting plasma glucose (mg/dl)	<100	100–125	—	—	≥126
2 hour post-prandial glucose (mg/dl)	<140	—	140–199	—	≥200
Hemoglobin A1c	—	—	—	—	≥6.5
Random plasma glucose	—	—	—	—	≥200 mg/dl + Symptoms of diabetes

7. Hypertension (Blood pressure ≥ 140–90 mm Hg)
8. HDL cholesterol <35 mg/dl, triglyceride level <250 mg/dl
9. Polycystic ovary syndrome or acanthosis nigricans.
10. History of cardiovascular disease.

FPG and HbA1c is used as screening for T2DM because:
1. Large number of patients meet the current criteria for DM but are asymptomatic.
2. Epidemiologic studies show—Type 2 DM may be present up to a decade before diagnosis.
3. Some individuals have one or more diabetic complications at the time of diagnosis.
4. Treatment of type 2 DM favorably alters the natural history of DM.

So screening is required for:
i. Individuals >45 years—every 3 years
ii. If patient is obese (BMI >25 kg/m²)—at earlier age and have additional risk factor.

Type-1 Diabetes Mellitus

1. Onset—mostly in childhood, adolescence, but may occur at any age.

2. Strong positive genetic association with HLA-B8-DR3 and/or DR4.
3. Their survival depends upon insulin.
4. On withdrawal of insulin—they develop hyperglycemia, diabetic ketoacidosis, and coma.
5. Onset—is abrupt, or may be protracted in course:
   i. Slow onset type 1 diabetes mellitus
   ii. Late onset autoimmune diabetes of adult (LADA)
6. The following factors are responsible:
   i. Genetic factors
   ii. Autoimmune factors
   iii. Environmental factor.
7. It can be subclassified into two types:
   i. Type-1A—antibodies to islet cells, GAD (glutamic acid decarboxylase), 1A-2 -2B, insulin autoantibodies.
   ii. Type 1B—no evidence of autoimmunity—idiopathic
8. Associated autoimmune disorders:
   i. Graves' diseases
   ii. Thyroiditis
   iii. Autoimmune Addison's disease
   iv. Ovarian failure
   v. Vitiligo
   vi. Pernicious anemia
   vii. Celiac disease
9. Absence or very low level of glucagon stimulated "C" peptide—are the diagnostic of type-1 diabetes mellitus.

Type-2 Diabetes Mellitus

1. It occurs mostly in middle age or after 40 years, but may occur in third decade of life.
2. The causative factors are:
   i. Impaired beta cell function
   ii. Marked increase in peripheral insulin resistance at:
      a. Receptor level
      b. Post-receptor level.
3. Circulating level of insulin and C-peptide varies from very high level to normal level, but never low level.
4. This type-2 diabetes mellitus can be subclassified into:
   a. Obese type
   b. Non-obese type
5. Coma is rare phenomenon—but it can develop from:
   a. Hyperglycemia
   b. Hyperosmolarity.

6. Ketoacidosis can occur only from—acute increase in insulin requirement.
7. Lactic acidosis is rare.

Genetic Defect in Beta Cell Function

Maturity Onset Diabetes in Young (MODY)

1. It results from beta cell dysfunction due to specific mutation in MODY related gene.
2. It is autosomal dominant and non-insulin dependent.
3. These patients are not obese to develop diabetes.
4. Three or more consecutive generations must be affected.
5. Young diabetes with evidence of insulin resistance and acanthosis nigricans—are never MODY.
6. They are less susceptible to—micro- and/or macrovascular complications.
7. In type MODY—mutation of 6 genes are demonstrated.
    i. Hepatocyte nuclear factor—4a (type 1 MODY)
    ii. Glucokinase—(MODY type 2)
    iii. Hepatocyte nuclear factor 1a (MODY type 3)
    iv. Insulin promoter factor 1 (MODY type 4)
    v. Hepatocyte nuclear factor 1B (MODY type 5)
    vi. Neurogenic differentiation factor 1 (MODY type 6)

Genetic Defect in Insulin Action—Type A Insulin Resistance

Insulin resistance means hyperinsulinemia with hyperglycemia. It is associated with following congenital or acquired syndromes:
    i. Leprechaunism   ii. Lipoatrophy
    iii. Acanthosis nigricans.

Insulin resistance associated acanthosis nigricans can be subdivided into two types:
    i. Type-A—hereditary—defects in insulin receptor number and function. It affects young women.
    ii. Type-B autoimmune—due to development of antibodies against insulin receptor. It affects women having other evidence of autoimmune diseases.

Malnutrition Related Diabetes Mellitus (MRDM)

It is restricted to tropical countries. The diagnostic criteria are the following:
    i. Age of onset <30 years
    ii. Body mass index <19
    iii. Patient living in tropic—with history of malnutrition in childhood.
    iv. Stigmata of present or past malnutrition
    v. Variable exocrine pancreatic deficiency
    vi. High dose of insulin requirement
    vii. Not prone to ketosis in absence of stress.

Classification

MRDM will be Classified into two subgroups:
a. **Fibrocalculous pancreatic diabetes (FCPD):**
    i. Less than 1% diabetes in India
    ii. Etiological factors:
        1. Malnutrition   2. Dietary toxin
        3. Genetic susceptibility
    iii. Classical triad are:
        1. Diabetes
        2. Recurrent abdominal pain since childhood.
        3. Pancreatic calculi—calculi are often large, lying within the duct.
    iv. Presence of exocrine pancreatic efficiency.
    v. Presence of sticky stools.
b. **Protein deficient diabetes mellitus:**
    i. Evidence of protein calorie malnutrition
    ii. It affects young patients
    iii. Absence of pancreatic calcification
    iv. Presence of wasting and stunting
        Wasting—indicates acute nutritional deprivation
        Stunting—indicates chronic nutritional deprivation.

Drugs Producing Hyperglycemia

    i. Glucocorticoid
    ii. ACTH
    iii. Thiazide diuretics
    iv. Phenytoin
    v. Pentamidine
    vi. Vacor (rodenticide)

Endocrinopathies

1. In acromegaly, overt diabetes can occur—improves with treatment.
2. In case of growth hormone deficiency, which is being treated with insulin—can produce severe hypoglycemia.
3. In patient having autoimmune disorders—involving adrenal and thyroid gland—producing Addison's disease or hypothyroidism may coexist with diabetes.
4. Excess production of cortisol (Cushing syndrome), catecholamine (pheochromocytoma), and growth hormone (gigantism or acromegaly) from tumor of endocrine gland may produce diabetic state also; since the above hormones are counter-regulatory hormones.
5. Schmidt's syndrome—polyglandular autoimmune states—it is autosomal recessive state—it is characterized by autoimmune thyroiditis, adrenal failure and type 1 diabetes mellitus.

Genetic Syndrome

    i. Down's syndrome—Type 1 diabetes mellitus
    ii. 2/3rd of Turner syndrome.   ⎱ Diabetic glucose
    iii. 1/4th of Klinefelters syndrome ⎰ tolerance curve

    iv. Alstorm syndrome   ⎱ Mild diabetes with
    v. Lawrence-Moon-Biedal syndrome ⎰ inherited insulin
    vi. Prader willi syndrome   resistance (Group I)

    vii. Dystrophia myotonica   ⎱ Severe diabetes
    viii. Leprechaunism   ⎰ with inherited
    ix. Rabson-Mendenhall syndrome   Group II insulin
    x. Lipodystrophic syndrome   resistance

Gestational Diabetes Mellitus (GDM)

GDM can be defined as impaired glucose tolerance, developed or recognized during pregnancy.

Fate of GDM: In postpartum phase:
1. It may revert back to normal.
2. It may continue as impaired glucose tolerance.
3. It may progress to frank diabetes after few years.

Monitoring

Oral glucose tolerance test with 75 gm glucose:
  i. Six weeks after delivery
  ii. Repeated after 6 months
        ↓
  iii. Then once a year

Risk

There is risk of development of diabetes in future.

Impaired glucose tolerance: It can be defined as glucose tolerance which is above the conventional normal range but below the range, which is being considered as diabetes.

2-hour postprandial glucose 140–190 mg/dl

It is a transient stage—present in between normal glucose tolerance and type 2 diabetes mellitus.

Impaired fasting glucose: It can be labeled as: Fasting glucose concentration of 100–125 mg/dl, but postprandial glucose <140 mg/dl.

Criteria for GDM:

- Fasting blood sugar >92 mg/dl
- Postprandial blood glucose level 75 mg/dl
- One value is sufficient.

Pathogenesis of IGT and IFG:

i. Phase 1 insulin secretion is impaired.
ii. Phase 2 insulin secretion and insulin sensitivity is normal.

In IGT:

i. Basal insulin secretion is normal.
ii. Glucose stimulated 1st and 2nd phase insulin secretion and peripheral insulin sensitivity will be reduced.

Combined glucose intolerance (CGI): These patients have both impaired glucose tolerance and impaired fasting plasma glucose. Here pathogenesis will be:
i. Insulin resistance
ii. Impaired insulin secretion of IGT and IFG.

Blood Biochemical Parameter Characteristic

1. **In case of both IGT and IFG:** Plasma concentration of glucose will be raised for 60 minutes.
2. **Then, in case of IGT:** Plasma glucose concentration will be rising after 60 minutes and it may be elevated at 120 minutes.
3. **In case of IFG:** In 30–60 min—plasma glucose can be elevated little more than normal level—due to hepatic insulin resistance.

   But by 120 minutes, plasmas glucose concentration returns to normal.

Table 3.3: Difference between IFG and IGT

Impaired fasting glucose	Impaired glucose tolerance
1. Increased hepatic insulin resistance	1. Increased peripheral resistance to insulin
2. Stationary beta cell dysfunction and/or chronic low beta cell mass	2. Progressive loss of beat cell function
3. Normal peripheral sensitivity to insulin	3. Near normal hepatic sensitivity to insulin
4. Altered GLP-1 secretion	4. Reduced secretion of GLP-1
5. Inappropriately elevated glucagon secretion	5 Inappropriately elevated glucagon secretion

Importance

1. IFG is risk factor and risk marker for diabetes.
2. IGT is a risk marker for cardiovascular disease.

Treatment

1. IFG, since there is hepatic resistance to insulin, is more likely to get benefit from oral hypoglycemic, metformin.
2. IGT—since there is impaired insulin secretion as well as skeletal muscle resistance to insulin, these patient can be benefited from such drug which improves skeletal muscle resistance to insulin. So treatment—peroxisome proliferator-activated receptor δ against (PPAR-δ).

        +

    Insulin secretagogue—GLP-1 analog—glimeperide or glinides.

From pathophysiological stand point, T2DM demonstrates three cardinal abnormalities:

1. Resistance to the action of insulin in peripheral tissues, particularly muscles, fat, and also liver.
2. Defective insulin secretion, in response to glucose stimulus
3. Increased glucose production.

Clinical Presentation of Type 2 DM in Children

1. Unrecognized hypoglycemia
2. Polyuria
3. Hispanic
4. Black
5. Caucasians
6. Mean age 14.3 years
7. Acanthosis nigricans
8. Type-2 family histories
9. Hypertension
10. Mean glucose 397 mg/dl
11. HbA1c 9.3%
12. Average insulin level 76.8 mIU/L
13. C-peptide 5.5 ng/dl
14. Elevated total cholesterol, LDL
15. Weight >120% of total ideal body weight or BMI—85th percentile for age and sex
16. DKA

Diagnosis of Diabetes Mellitus

Diagnostic values for oral glucose tolerance test for diabetes mellitus and other types of hyperglycemia

Types	Venous glucose
1. **Diabetes mellitus:**	
i. Fasting value	≥ 126 mg/dl
ii. 2 hours after 75 gm of glucose load	≥ 200 mg/dl
2. **Impaired glucose tolerance (IGT)**	
2 hours after 75 gm of glucose load	140–199 mg/dl
3. **Impaired fasting glucose (IFG)**	
i. Fasting value	>100–125 mg/dl
ii. 2 hours after 75 gm of glucose load	<140 mg/dl.

Diagnostic Criteria

1. Glucose tolerance is normal when fasting and the 2 hours postprandial value are <100 mg/dl and <140 mg/dl respectively.

2. The patient will be diagnosed as diabetic, if:
   Fasting plasma glucose value—≥126 mg/dl
              Or
   2 hours postprandial plasma glucose value ≥200 mg
3. Impaired glucose tolerance, if 2 hours value 140–199 mg/dl.
4. Impaired fasting glucose—if fasting level ≥100 mg/dl and two hours postprandial value in ≤140 mg%.

ETIOPATHOGENESIS

Type 1 Diabetes Mellitus

Epidemiology

i. More occur in population of Sweden, Finland, but rare in Japan.
ii. Mostly it occurs in people under 21 years age, but may occur at any age.
iii. Season—It occurs in autumn and spring.
iv. Sex—Female suffer most than males.

Etiology

a. Genetic factors:
   i. 10% type 1 DM has history of diabetes in his or her family (siblings or parents)
   ii. Concordance rate in twin is 30–50%.
   iii. Histocompatibility antigen
Three classes of MHC genes present on short arm of chromosome 6:
1. Class 1 molecules (HLA—A, E, C and B)—expressed on the surface of most nucleated cells.
2. Class 2 molecules (HLA-DR, DQ and DP)—expressed on macrophages, B lymphocytes.
3. Class 3 molecules (complement C_4, C_2, properidien Bf gene, 21-hydroxylase gene)

Function: The function of HLA is to present the processed antigens to cell receptor.

Association with HLA gene:
   i. DM with HLA-B8 genes—DR3-DQ2 and DR4-DQ8—high risk of diabetes in Caucasians.
   ii. In Caucasian population, there is association with HLA-B15. But In Indian population, there is no association.
   iii. Aspartane at 57 position of DQ beta and non-Arg at position 52 of DQ alpha—give protection against diabetes—it is seen in Caucasian, but not in Japanese.
   iv. Non-HLA association: Hypervariable region near insulin gene in chromosome 11 with pleomorphism of T cell receptor in β chain.

Risk of type 1 diabetes:
   i. In general population   - 0.4%
   ii. In off spring of diabetic father   - 6.1%
   iii. In offspring of diabetic mother   - 2%
   iv. In offspring of diabetic parents   - 3.6%

b. Immunologic factors: Both humoral and cell-mediated autoimmune mechanism are responsible for insulitis and beta cell destruction.
Progressive decline in serum insulin level varies with amount of beta cell destruction.
   i. Islet cell antibodies (ICA)—IgG class—detected by conventional direct immunofluorescence; antibodies are directed against cytoplasm of these cells.

To start with, titer of this antibody will be very high, but over years, in 80% cases, antibody disappears.
These antibodies react with cytoplasm of:
1. α cells containing glucagon.
2. Delta cells containing somatostatin.
3. Beta cells containing insulin
   ii. Islet cell surface antibodies (ICSA): This antibody has separate specificity to α, β and delta cells.
   iii. Autoantigen—glutamic acid decarboxylase (GAD 65)—it facilitates biosynthesis of inhibitory neurotransmitter—GABA. The antibody against this antigen is present in >80% of newly diagnosed diabetic patients. This is beta cell specific.
   iv. Insulin autoantibodies have been demonstrated recently in newly diagnosed type I DM.

c. Viruses/toxin:
   i. There is correlation of Coxsackie B4 virus with type I DM.
   ii. Other virus involved is congenital rubella infection.

Mechanism of action:

1. Virus invades beta cells
      ↓
   It interferes with metabolic and secretory functions.
2. Virus triggers immunological response—producing beta cell death.

d. *Dietary factors:* Consumption of cow's milk during early life.

Mechanism of action:

Bovine serum albumin (BSA)—acts as antigen
      ↓
Enters in intact form through gut of neonates
      ↓
Stimulates immune response against beta cells

Sequence of Events in the Development of Type 1 DM

Genetic susceptibility
↓
Environmental triggering (virus/toxins)
↓
Immunological activation (autoimmunity)
↓
Progressive beta cell destruction
↓
Type 1 diabetes mellitus

Honeymoon Phase

a. At the onset of type 1 diabetes:
   i. Insulin secretion in response to secretagogue is low
   ii. Requirement of exogenous insulin is high.
b. After correction of hyperglycemia:
   i. There is recovery of endogenous insulin secretory capacity.
   ii. Requirement of exogenous insulin will be low.

This is called honeymoon phase.

Follow-up of this honeymoon phase:

1. This period lasts for few months to years.
2. After a variable period,
   With the total destruction of beta cells
   ↓
   Absolute insulin deficiency occurs.

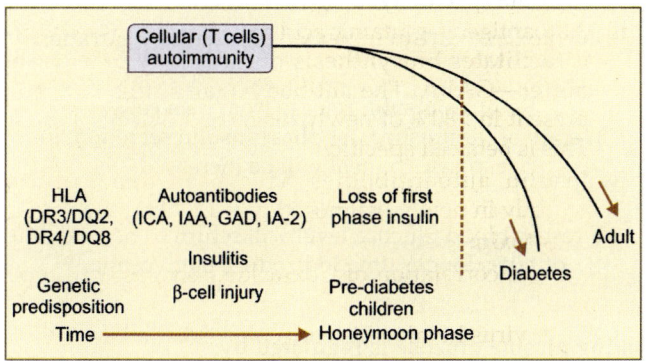

Fig. 3.15: Natural history of type 1 diabetes mellitus

Etiopathogenesis of Type 2 Diabetes Mellitus

Epidemiology

1. 100% concordance in case of identical twins.
2. Diabetic genotype is influenced by:
   i. Central obesity—it produces diabetes in susceptible individual
   ii. Dietary habits—independent of obesity—reduce intake of fibre
   iii. Physical indolence
   iv. Stress of life
   v. Urbanization

Type 2 diabetes mellitus—may be due to following type of abnormalities.

A. **Impaired pancreatic insulin secretion**—Here beta cell dysfunction is of two types:
   i. Loss of pulsatile insulin delivery even in presence of normal glucose tolerance.
   ii. Loss of compensatory mechanisms:
      a. Increased beta cell mass
      b. Insulin output
      c. Maximum secretory capacity

Insulin secretion in T2DM:
- Normal level is 5 to 15 mU/ml
- In case of high sensitivity to insulin, it may be <5 mU/ml.
- In case of decreased sensitivity to insulin, it may be >15 mU/ml.

Two types of insulin delivery occur:
i. Pulsatile delivery of insulin every 90–120 minutes in response to meals or secretagogues—it is also called ultradian oscillations.
ii. Rapid oscillation of insulin delivery—every 8–16 minutes—it inhibits hepatic glucose output.

Response of insulin secretion to glucose load:
1. *First phase:* Within 1st 4–5 minutes of glucose load, there is acute insulin response (AIR)—released from stored granules. This response abates within 10 minutes.

2. *Second phase:* In response to ambient rise of blood glucose, insulin promotes glucose utilization in peripheral tissues (muscle, and adipose tissue).

   In type 2 diabetes mellitus—ultradian oscillation of insulin delivery will be lost.

B. **Beta cell dysfunction:**
   i. There is deposition of islet amyloid polypeptide get accumulated extracellularly in close contact with beta cells and form fibrils—there by reduces insulin secretion.
   ii. Amylin lowers the basal and insulin stimulated glycogen synthetase in the muscles.
   iii. Amylin reduces glucose-stimulated insulin secretion. But non-glucose (arginine, neurotransmitters and hormones) stimulated insulin secretion will be present.

Insulin Secretory Abnormalities in Type 2 Diabetes Mellitus

1. Sensing of glucose is impaired.
2. Failure of ability to respond for elevation or reduction of blood glucose level during glucose infusion.
3. Reduction or absence of first phase insulin secretion during intravenous glucose administration.
4. Reduction or absence of early insulin secretory response to oral glucose.
5. Alteration in rapid oscillation of insulin secretion.
6. Impaired ability of gastrointestinal hormones to potentiate glucose-mediated insulin secretion.
7. No correlation between insulin secretion and magnitude of hyperglycemia.

Insulin Resistance

Definition

It is a state where normal amount of insulin produces a subnormal amount of insulin response or, large amount insulin produces normal response.

Types

Insulin resistance falls in two categories:
1. Decreased sensitivity—here large amount of insulin produces normal effective response.
2. Decreased response: Here not even supramaximal insulin level can produce normal response. These patients present with:
   i. Diabetes
   ii. Impaired glucose tolerance, and euglycemic, because they compensate the defect with large amount of insulin.

At molecular level, insulin resistance can occur at following levels:
   i. At insulin—receptor interaction sites
   ii. After insulin receptor binding and kinase function
   iii. Post-receptor signal pathway

Causes of Insulin Resistances

A. **Genetics of insulin resistance:** Type A syndrome and its variants:
   i. Leprechaunism
   ii. Lipoatrophic diabetes

B. **Immune disorders:** Type B syndrome:
   i. Anti-insulin antibodies
   ii. Anti-insulin receptor antibodies
C. **Endocrine and metabolic disorders:**
   i. Obesity
   ii. Type-2 diabetes mellitus
   iii. Type-1 diabetes mellitus on insulin therapy
   iv. Cushing syndrome
   v. Acromegaly
D. **Physiologic conditions:**
   i. Pregnancy   ii. Puberty   iii. Aging

In liver:

> After glucose ingestion
> ↓
> Insulin is released into portal vein
> ↓
> Insulin is carried to liver
> ↓
> Insulin binds to specific receptors on hepatocytes
> ↓
> Suppression of glucose output

In insulin resistance, liver fails to perceive this signal → increase in hepatic glucose output.

In muscles: The defects in actions are:
   i. Diminished insulin receptor tyrokinase activity
   ii. Diminished glucose transporters
   iii. Diminished glycogen synthetase and pyruvate kinase

As a result of above defects, disturbances in major intracellular pathways of glucose disposal like synthesis of glycogen, oxidation of glucose.

Post-receptor defects are:
   i. Impaired generation of insulin's second messenger
   ii. Diminished transport of glucose into cells
   iii. Post-glucose transport abnormalities

In type 2 diabetes mellitus—post-receptor defect in insulin action is responsible for insulin resistance.

Insulin resistances occur in three stages:
A. First phase: Due to hyperinsulinemia, plasma glucose remains normal in spite of insulin resistance.
B. Second phase: As insulin resistance progresses, there is postprandial hyperglycemia despite of hyperinsulinemia.
C. Third phase: Ultimately insulin level will decline, but insulin resistance will not change, as a result there will be fasting hyperglycemia.

> The presence of fasting and postprandial hyperglycemia stimulates the beta cell further.
> ↓
> The resultant effect is hyperinsulinemia
> ↓
> Downregulation of receptor number and post-receptor events.

Insulin secretory defect—a primary event:

> Earliest abnormality in T2 DM is loss of ultradian oscillation of insulin secretion.
> ↓
> Excessive and prolonged increase in plasma glucose concentration.
> ↓
> Glucotoxicity due to increased glucose concentration
> ↓
> Reduces insulin release from beta cells
> In spite of diminished 1st phase insulin secretion, in response to meal will be increased.
> ↓
> As a result, blood glucose level will return to normal, but of takes longer time to produce euglycemia.

Fasting plasma glucose is regulated by:
   i. Fasting plasma insulin
   ii. Hepatic sensitivity to insulin
   iii. Fasting substrate availability

In type 2 diabetes:
   i. Basal insulin secretion impaired
   ii. Decreased hepatic sensitivity to insulin impaired

Postprandial glucose is regulated by:
   i. Fasting plasma insulin
   ii. Hepatic sensitivity to insulin
   iii. Fasting substrate availability

In type 2 diabetes:
   i. Impaired secretion of 1st phase insulin
   ii. Increased in resistance of liver and muscles to insulin
   iii. Lack of suppression of glucagon

So pathogenesis in type 2 diabetes mellitus (Fig. 3.16):
1. Pancreas   Defect in insulin secretion
2. Liver   Excess glucagon production
3. Muscle   Reduced glucose uptake
4. Adipose tissue   Increased lipolysis

Stages of progression to frank type 2 diabetes mellitus
1. Stage-1   Impaired glucose tolerance
2. Stage-2   Postprandial hyperglycemia
3. Stage-3   Phase 1 type 2 diabetes mellitus
4. Stage-4   Phase 2 type 2 diabetes mellitus
5. Stage-5   Phase 3 type 2 diabetes mellitus

Lipotoxicity: Adipose tissue—is the site for (Fig. 3.18):
1. Energy storage
2. Adipokine production

The adipokines are:
1. TNFα   2. Angiotensin II
3. Resistin   4. IL-6
5. Leptin   6. CRP
7. Free fatty acid

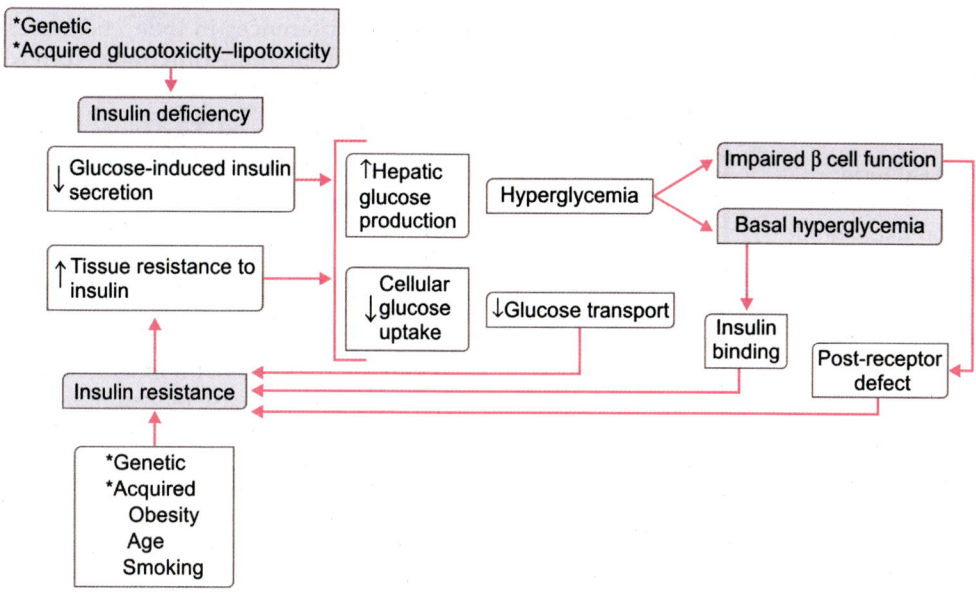

Fig. 3.16: Pathogenic sequences of the events in type-2 diabetes mellitus

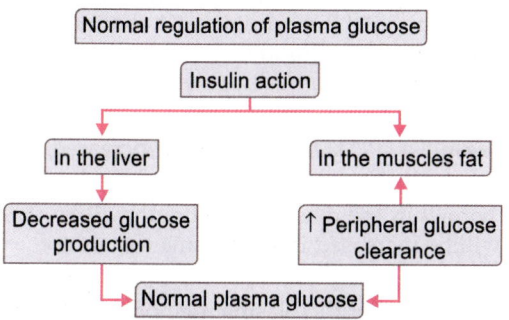

Fig 3.17: Natural history of type 2 diabetes mellitus

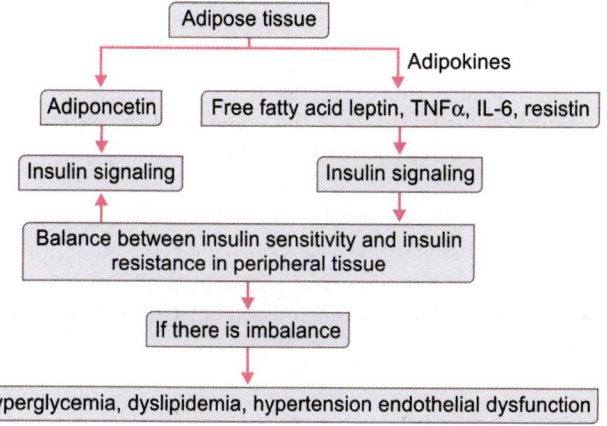

Fig 3.18: Function of adipose tissue

1. **Tumor necrosis factor α (TNFα):** Its production increases with the increasing adipocyte mass.

   TNFα downregulates the insulin sensitive glucose transporters (GLUT 4 in adipocyte).

2. *Leptin:*
   i. Its concentration varies with percentage of body fat and serum insulin concentration.
   ii. It inhibits food intake, reduces body fat and stimulates energy expenditure

3. *Resistin:*
   i. It has inhibitory action on hepatic glucose output.
   ii. It has a putative role in mediating insulin resistance in obesity.

4. *Adiponcetin:* It is an adipocyte product: It ameliorates insulin resistance both in muscle and liver. So its low level correlates with obesity and increased insulin resistance.

MANAGEMENT OF DIABETES MELLITUS

Weight Reduction and Exercise

1. **Normalize:**
   i. Blood sugar
   ii. HbA1c
   iii. Control hypertension
   iv. Control hyperlipidemia

2. **Lifestyle changes:**
   i. Aerobic and resistance exercise
   ii. Increase muscle mass
   iii. Reduce body fat—visceral fat
   iv. Reduce level of triglyceride and free fatty acids
   v. Food rich in antioxidants to be taken
   vi. Increase physical activity
   vii. Reduce mental and physical stress
   viii. Increase intake of dietary fiber
   ix. Decrease consumption of saturated fat and trans-fat
   x. Decrease consumption of high refined foods.
   xi. To take a healthy breakfasts every day
   xii. Adequate sleep

Oral Antidiabetic Drugs

Drugs:	*Mode of action*
A. 1. Suphonylureas 2. Glimeperide 3. Meglitinide-repaglinide 4. D-phenylalanine-nateglinide 5. GLP-1 (glucagon like peptide-1) 6. Amylin antagonists	Insulin secretogogues
B. 1. Metformin: 2. Thiozolidinediones (rosiglitazone pioglitazone) 3. Antiobesity drugs	Insulin sensitizers
C. 1. á-glucosidase inhibitors: (acarbose, meglitol, voglibose 2. Amylin analogue (pramlintide)	Inhibitors of gastrointestinal glucose absorption
D. 1. Antilipolitic and antihyper-lipidemic agents, fatty acid oxidation inhibitors	Inhibitors of intermediary metabolism
E. 1. Insulin analogue 2. Insulin-like growth factor-1 3. Vanadium salts	Insulin mimetic drugs
F. 1. Sitagliptins 2. Vildagliptin	Gliptin
G. 1. Canagliflozin 2. Empagliflozin 3. Dopagliflozin	$SGLT_2$ inhibitor

Sulphonylureas

Three generations of drugs are:
1. **First generation:**
   a. Tolbutamide (short actions)—250–3000 mg/day in divided does
   b. Chlorpropamide (long acting)—50–5000 mg/day
2. **Second generation** (started with "G")
   a. Glibenclamide   1.25–20 mg/day
   b. Glipizide   2.5–40 mg/day
   c. Gliclazide   80–240 mg/day
3. **Third generation:**
   a. Glimeperide   1–8 mg/day

Pharmacokinetics (Table 3.4):
i. It is orally taken, absorbed through gastrointestinal tract, metabolized to varying extent in the liver.
ii. Since genetic factors may be responsible for its pharmacokinetics in different patients, hence these drugs may not produce same effects in all individuals.

iii. Slight differences in their chemical structures are responsible for their functional differences, duration of action and potency of action.

Mechanism of actions: Two types of actions:
a. In short-term administration—there is enhancement of insulin release while paradoxically insulin biosynthesis will be inhibited. So they prime the beta cells to the hyperglycemia—producing beta-cytotrophic effect).

   Thus they correct the blood glucose level to normal physiological range.
b. In chronic administration—they increase the number of receptors on different peripheral organs as well as augment post-receptor increase in insulin sensitivity.

   As a result, subsequent euglycemia will be maintained throughextra pancreatic effect of the drugs without augmentation of insulin release—so they:
   i. Decrease in hepatic glucose output.
   ii. Promote utilization of glucose in muscles, adipose tissues
Sulphonylureas increase insulin level by—reducing hepatic clearance of the hormones:

Mechanism of insulin secretion and risk of sulphonylurea:

1. In normal person, plasma membrane is polarized by keeping open ATP modulated K^+ channel and at the same time keeping closed Ca^{++} channel.
2. Glucose metabolism produces large numbers of ATP.
↓
As a result ATP/ADP ratio will be increased.
↓
K^+ channel in the plasma membrane will be closed; K^+ ion will be increased in the plasma membrane
↓
Depolarization of the plasma membrane will occur
↓
There is opening of voltage dependent Ca^{++} channel
↓
Large number of Ca^{++} ion will enter into the cell
↓
Increased cytosolic Ca^{++} stimulates secretion of insulin
↓
Sulphonylurea binds to the receptor at the extracellular site of ATP dependent K^+ channel.
↓
As a result, K^+ channel will be closed.
↓
Due to depolarization of plasma membrane, Ca^{++} ion enters the cell and large amount of insulin released from the cell.

Table 3.4: Pharmacokinetics of sulphonylurea					
Compound	Duration of action (hr)	Daily dosage	Metabolite activity	Hypoglycemia	Excretion
Glibenclamide	20–24	2.5–20	-/+	-/+	Kidney—50%; Bile—50%
Glipizide	12–24	2.5–20	—	—	Kidney—80%; Bile—20%
Gliclazide	10–15	40–320	—	—	Kidney—70%; Bile—30%

Therapeutic applications:

Glibenclamide: It used to be widely used agent in obese type 2 diabetes mellitus not controlled by diet alone.

The adverse effect is hypoglycemia due to its sustained effect of this drug. It inhibits ischemic preconditioning, therefore is no longer a preferred agent.

Glipizide: It has short duration of action, requiring multiple doses and maintains better control of glucose.

Satisfactory control of sugar can be achieved in type 2 diabetic patient by combining glipizide with insulin therapy. It can be used on diabetics with renal impairment.

Gliclazide: It has following effects:
1. Favorable influence over platelet aggregation and fibrinolysis.
2. It has insulinotropic effect in pancreas.
3. It has extra pancreatic effect.
4. It has protective effect in preventing vascular complications.
5. Patients on gliclazide will not gain weight as the drug restores normal physiologic secretion of insulin.

Choice of sulphonylurea drug: Following factors detect the sulphonylurea drugs:
1. Intrinsic antidiabetic drugs
2. Rapid of onset of action
3. Duration of action
4. Mode of metabolism and excretion
5. Side effects of the drugs.
   a. Second generation sulphonylurea drugs are more potent than first generation drugs.
   b. Therapeutic dose should be in milligram/day than gm/day

Drug failure: There are two types of failure

A. *Primary failure:* This can be diagnosed when—patient is strictly on prescribed diet, patient has no overt or occult infection, patient is on maximum allowable dosage of the sulphonylurea, but fail to get full glycemic control within one month of initiation of the above drug.

B. *Secondary failure:* This can be diagnosed when in initial phase, there is good glycemic response to the sulphonylurea drug, but ultimately, it will be ineffective in future.

Common causes of secondary failure:
A. Patient-related factors:
   i. Over eating and weight gain
   ii. Poor patient compliance
   iii. Stress
   iv. Intercurrent illness
B. Disease-related factors:
   i. Decreased beta cell function
   ii. Increased insulin resistance
C. Drug-related factors:
   i. Inadequate dosage of drugs
   ii. Impairment of absorption of drug due to hyperglycema.
   iii. Concomitant therapy with diabetogenic drugs

Contraindication to sulphonylurea therapy:
   i. Insulin dependent diabetes mellitus
   ii. Pregnancy (except glibenclamide)
   iii. Severe infections
   iv. Allergy to drugs
   v. Severe liver and kidney diseases
   vi. Surgery

Glimeperide

   i. It binds to the receptors (65 kDa) which are different from receptors (140 kDa) to which sulphonylurea binds.
   ii. It is 3 times faster in binding to receptor and 9-fold faster in dissociation from receptors than sulphonylureas.
   iii. Its onset of action is very rapid, and duration of action is long.
   iv. It has highest total blood glucose lowering activity but lowest insulin releasing activity.
   v. It has inhibitory effect on platelet aggregation
   vi. It has no cardiovascular side effect.
   vii. It is being excreted equally through liver and kidney; hence, it is safer in mild renal failure.
   viii. It enhances the glucose transport to peripheral tissues by enhancing GLUT-4 translocation from intracellular pool to cell membrane.
   ix. It stimulates insulin secretion stimulated by postprandial glucose, but fasting insulin and C-peptides being normal.

Dosages: 1–4 mg/day—to maximum 8 mg/day.

Repaglinide

   i. It stimulates postprandial glucose-stimulated insulin secretion by regulating ATP sensitive K+ channels at different binding sites than by sulphonylurea and glimeperide.
   ii. Recommended dosage—0.5 to 6 mg/day to maximum 16 mg/day
   iii. Due should be increased at least at weekly interval
   iv. It should be taken just before meals.
      a. To provide immediate hypoglycemic activity
      b. To decrease the risk of hypoglycemia between meals

Nateglinide

   i. It has shorter and faster duration of action in controlling postprandial glucose control.
   ii. It is rapidly absorbed after its oral administration just prior to meal.
   iii. Dose is 60 mg twice to thrice daily, maximum being 360 mg/day.

Indication:
   i. It acts as monotherapy in type 2 DM, who fails to meal plan and physical exercise.
   ii. It can be given in patients having erratic food habits just prior to meal.
   iii. It can be given in combination with metformin who fails to respond to metformin only.

Insulin Sensitizers

Biguanides—Metformin:

Mechanism of action: It has effect both on carbohydrate and lipid metabolism. It has action on whole body and at cellular level.

On whole body:
i. Reduction of excessive HGP
ii. It induces insulin-mediated glucose uptake in liver and muscles.
iii. It inhibits lipolysis and reduces free fatty acid availability.

On cellular level:
i. Its affinity for binding with insulin is high.
ii. It stimulates insulin receptor tyrosine kinase activity.
iii. It enhances glucose transport (GLUT-4).
iv. It increases glycogen synthetase.

The effect on carbohydrate metabolism:
i. It has anorexogenic effect.
ii. It inhibits absorption of glucose from the intestine.
iii. It prevents hepatic neoglucogenesis.
iv. It increases the number of receptors.
v. It increases GLUT-4 glucose transporters in insulin sensitive cells.

The cumulative effect of above actions:
i. It reduces plasma glucose by 25% both fasting and postprandial glucose.
ii. It is more effective in patients with insulin resistance than patients with insulin deficiency.
iii. It does not reduce basal plasma glucose below physiological level in diabetic or nondiabetic patients.

The effect on lipid metabolism:
i. It decreases hepatic triglyceride synthesis and lowers the serum triglyceride level.
ii. It converts atherogenous LDL to non-atherogenous lipid through its actions on carrier lipoproteins.

Other actions: It has favorable effect on fibrinolysis and platelet aggregation.

Therapeutic indications:
1. Type II diabetes, refractory to treatment by diet.
2. In type II brittle diabetes.
3. Patient whose blood sugar is refractory to sulphonylurea.
4. In case of true insulin resistance, to reduce insulin requirement
5. Non-alcoholic steatohepatitis.
6. Polycystic ovarian disease

Indications for transient discontinuation:
i. Major surgery
ii. Radiographic procedure involving intravenous contrast
iii. Hospital admission with serious medical disorder.

Relative or absolute contraindications:
i. Impaired renal function (serum creatinine 1.5 mg/dl in male and ≥ 1.4 mg/dl in women, GFR <70 ml/mm)
ii. Symptomatic CCF requiring pharmacological treatment
iii. Chronic liver disease with liver transaminase ≥3-folds above upper limit of normal.
iv. Elderly (≥80 years) patients, if creatinine clearance ≤70 ml/mm
v. Pregnancy

vi. Lactation
vii. Type 1 diabetes
viii. History of excess alcohol intake.

Side effects:
1. Major side effects are gastrointestinal:
   i. Anorexia
   ii. Nausea
   iii. Vomiting
   iv. Diarrhea
   v. Abdominal discomfort
   vi. Metallic taste
2. Potential side effect
   i. If metformin does is >2000 mg, there is chance of vitamin B_{12} malabsorption, but clinically there is no anemia.
   ii. Lactic acidosis—it may result from:
      a. Over production of lactic acid from tissue hypoxia, in case of septicemic shock, myocardial infarction or congestive cardial failure
      b. Decreased removal in case of hepatic failure.
      c. Failure of conversion to pyruvate, as in alcohol ingestion, it inhibits lactate dehydrogenase.

Advantages:
1. Absence of weight gain.
2. Lowering of LDL cholesterol.
3. Increase in HDL cholesterol.
4. Decrease in plasminogen activator inhibitor-1

Thiazolidinediones: The drugs are:
i. Ciglitazone
ii. Pioglitazone
iii. Englitazone
iv. Rosiglitazone
v. Troglitazone

Troglitazone: It has insulin sparing action, restores pancreatic response to external stimuli.

It exerts its action through the activation of the peroxisome proliferator activated receptors (PPAR).

These drugs have effects in following different tissues:
A. *Adipose tissue:*
   i. Increased glucose uptake
   ii. Increased fatty acid uptake
   iii. Lipogenesis
B. *Muscles:*
   i. Increased glucose uptake
   ii. Glycolysis
   iii. Increased glucose oxidation
   iv. Glycogenesis
C. *In liver:*
   i. Glycogenolysis
   ii. Neoglucogenesis
   iii. Lipogenesis
   iv. Increased glucose uptake

Side effects:
1. Weight gain—it is due to increase in subcutaneous fat but not the visceral fat—on the contrary hepatic, myocellular fats are reduced—it reduces the cardiovascular risk.
2. Ankle edema
3. Fluid retention
4. Bone fracture

5. Congestive cardiac failure: In patients, who prone to develop fluid retention, glitazone should be avoided.

6. In patient with moderate to severe hepatocellular disease, with SGPT level >2.5 upper limits of normal. Hence serum SGPT level should be monitored before the initiation of therapy and then every 2 months for the first year and intermittently their after.

Rosiglitazone has been banned because of increased incidence of congestive cardiac failure and myocardial infarction.

Dosages:

Pioglitazone: To start with 7.5 mg/day—it may be increased intermittently to 30 mg/day.

This drug has been withdrawn from European countries because of increased reported incidence of bladder cancer.

So this drug should be 2nd or 3rd line of drug.

The drugs under trial are:
  i. Muraglitazar
 ii. Tesaglitazar
iii. Ragaglitazar.

Alpha-Glucosidase Inhibitor

It is a nitrogen containing pseudotetrasaccharide. The drugs are:

Acarbose:

a. It is reversible competitive inhibitor of brush border alpha-glucosidase and alpha-amylase inhibitors—which are present in juxtaluminal epithelium of jejunum. As a result:
  i. Digestion of starch, maltose and sucrose
 ii. It delays digestion of carbohydrates—thereby absorption of glucose, disaccharides, oligosaccharides and polysaccharides are inhibited.
    But digestion of glucose and monosaccharides is normal. The carbohydrates, which are not absorbed, will be metabolized by colonic bacteria into short chain fatty acids and absorbed.
b. It decreases meal-stimulated secretion of gastric inhibitory polypeptide and other gastrointestinal hormones.
c. It decreases synthesis of VLDL, thus reduces the serum triglycerides in patients with hypertriglyceridemia.
d. It produces dose-related decrease in postprandial hyperglycemia, but it never produces hypoglycemia, when it will be used alone.

Primary elements necessary for effective glycemic control:
  i. High carbohydrate diet
 ii. This drug to be started a low dose
iii. Slow and gradual titration of dose with the diet
 iv. Maximal glycemic improvement, measured by hemoglobin A can be achieved by long-term therapy with lowest dose.

Dosage: It should be taken with the first bite of food.

It has to be started as 25 mg with the first bite of food. The dose may be increased up to 200 mg/day in divided doses.

Effects:
  i. Mean decrease in postprandial glucose is 50 gm/dl.
 ii. HbA1c fall will be in the range of 0.6–1.4%
iii. Fall in fasting plasma glucose is 21.8 mg%

In case of type 1 diabetes mellitus:
  i. Addition of acarbose in patient with insulin improves glycemic control.
 ii. It decreases nocturnal hypoglycemia

Contraindication:
  i. Hypersensitivity
 ii. Diabetic ketoacidosis
iii. Cirrhosis
 iv. Inflammatory bowel disease
  v. Colonic ulceration

Caution: If patient on acarbose with sulphonylurea and become hypoglycemic, oral glucose tolerance test should be done with dextrose rather than sucrose.

Side effects:
1. Gastrointestinal side effects—flatulence, diarrhea, abdominal discomfort—which will be alleviated within few months of continued therapy.
2. Regular check up of liver function tests—if it shows any abnormality, it will be revert back to normal after withdrawal of drug.

Interference with other drug:
  i. Concomitant use of bile acid resin or digestive enzyme preparations, antacids interfere with effectiveness of acarbose.
 ii. Acarbose does not interfere with absorption of sulphonylurea, ACE inhibitors, β-adrenergic blockers, warfarin.

Miglitol 25 mg and 50 mg tablets

Voglibose:
  i. It prevents postprandial increase in plasma glucose in type 2 diabetes—delays absorption of glucose.
 ii. It is a competitive inhibitor of a glucosidase in the intestinal mucosa and thus prevent the absorption of dietary starch and glucose.

Dose: 0.2 to 0.3 mg to be taken after 1 bite of food.

Side effects:
  i. Mild to moderate gastrointestinal discomfort
 ii. Flatulence

Sulphonylurea and insulin combination:

Insulin	i. Suppresses the hepatic glucose output
	ii. Acts on receptor level
Sulphonylurea	i. Acts on beta cells
	ii. Acts on receptor level
	iii. Acts on post-receptor level

By the above combination, ultimate insulin requirement will be reduced.

Combination of metformin with insulin:

Insulin—suppresses hepatic glucose production
Metformin—acts as insulin sensitizer

The result of combination therapy:
  i. Reduction of blood glucose
 ii. Reduction of insulin requirement by 25% of required dose.

Combination of sulphonylurea, metformin and insulin:

Insulin—suppresses glucose production
Metformin—acts as insulin sensitizer
Insulin—reduces hepatic glucose production

The result of the above combination:
 i. Reduction of quantity of insulin
 ii. Reduction of oral antidiabetic dose
 iii. Minimizes the side effects of oral antidiabetic drugs

Rationale of bedtime insulin and daytime sulphonylurea:
Normal glucose homeostasis depends upon the balance between dynamic interactions between:
 i. Insulin
 ii. Insulin sensitivity
 iii. Insulin secretion.

Metabolic benefits of insulin therapy:
1. Reduces fasting and postprandial glucose levels
2. Suppresses hepatic glucose production
3. Stimulates peripheral glucose utilization
4. Increases glucose oxidation/storage in skeletal muscles
5. Improves abnormal lipoprotein composition .
6. Reduces glucotoxicity
7. Improves endogenous secretory ability
8. Reduces glycosylated end products.

Table 3.5: Types of insulin

Insulin preparation	Onset of action (hr.)	Peak of activity (hr.)	Total duration of action (hr.)
Short acting			
Regular	0.5–1	2–4	4–6
Semilente	1–2	3–6	8–12
Intermediate acting			
NPH	3–4	10–16	20–24
Lente	3–4	10–16	20–24
Long acting			
PZI	6–8	14–20	32
Ultralente	6–8	14–20	32
Biphasic			
Premixed (NPH + Reg)	0.5	2–10	12–18

Analogous
Short acting

Lipro (humalog)	Within a few minutes
Aspart (novorapid)	
Gulisine (apidra)	

Long acting

Glargine (lantus)	←— Peak less actions for 24 hours
Detemir (lev emir)	
Degludec (tresiba)	

Premixed
Novomix (30/70 and + 50/50)
Humalog mix (25: 75 and 50: 50)

Factors affecting Disposal of Injected Insulin

Injection Site

a. Anatomic site: Absorption varies depending on the site of absorption:
 i. It is fastest in abdomen.
 ii. Followed by upper limb.
 iii. Then to thigh and gluteal region.
b. Rate of absorption: It is enhanced by exercise of the limbs within 30 minutes of injection.

c. Local insulin degradation at injection sites by protease
d. Depth
e. Insulin concentration
f. Mixing insulin preparation
g. Intra-subject coefficient variation

Plasma:
a. Insulin antibodies in the circulation
b. Physical state of modified insulin in serum

Insulin receptors: Disposal of insulin by liver, kidney.

Dosage of insulin: Initial dose:
1. 0.5 units/kg of body weight—for type 1 DM
2. 0.2 units/kg of body weight—for type 2 DM

a. If the patient is not symptomatic (polyuria, polydipsia, polyphagia and severe weight loss)
 50% of calculated dose should be the starting dose
 ↓
 It should be gradually increased by 4 units every 4th day.
b. If the patient is symptomatic, calculated dose should be given in divided doses in morning and evening.

Monitoring (Figs 3.19, 3.20)

a. The best time to monitor the effectiveness of morning dose is to measure fasting blood glucose in next morning.
 If the fasting blood sugar is high—in addition to morning dose of insulin, 50% of morning dose of intermediate-acting insulin may be given at dinner time.
b. If the prelunch blood sugar is high, regular insulin is usually necessary in the morning to control post-breakfast hyperglycemia, because of long period to work by intermediate-acting insulin.

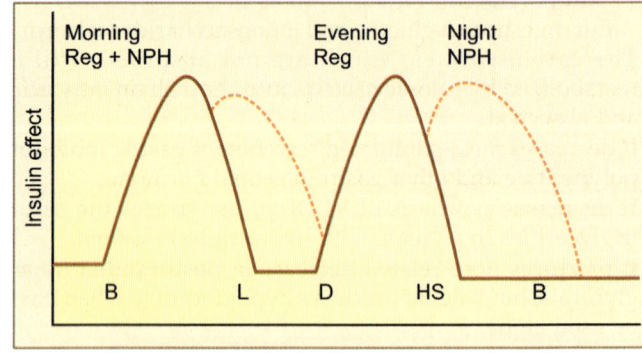

Fig. 3.19: Type A—split and mixed insulin regimen

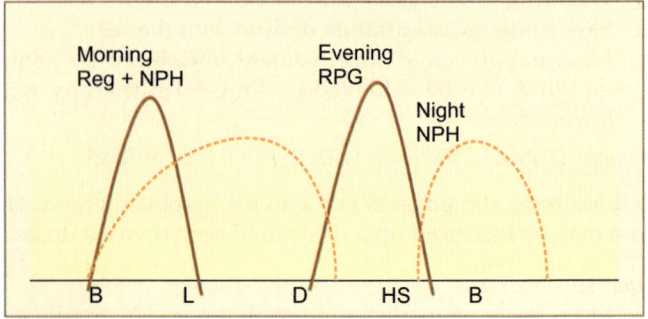

Fig. 3.20: Type-B—lente or NPH shifted towards bedtime to cover pre-breakfast hyperglycemia

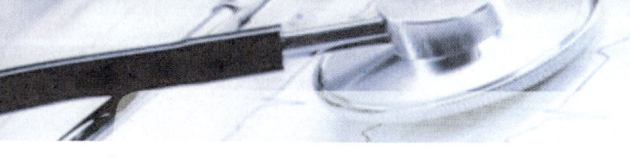

c. If post-dinner blood sugar is high, combination of regular and intermediate-acting insulin is necessary.

The combination of short- and intermediate-acting insulin in the morning and evening is known as "mixed and split" dose of insulin regimen. Here 2/3rd of total dose should be given in the morning and 1/3rd given in the evening.

Again of this combination, 1/3rd should be regular insulin and 2/3rd should be intermediate-acting insulin.

If patient develops prebreakfast hyperglycemia; intermediate-acting insulin should be given at bedtime.

Incretin Based Therapy

Definition of Incretin Effect

It implies that ingestion of carbohydrate (glucose) causes release of substances from the intestinal mucosa—which enhances the release of insulin beyond the release of insulin caused by absorbed glucose itself. The incretin hormones are:
i. Glucose dependent insulinotropic polypeptide (GIP)
ii. Glucagon like polypeptide-1 (GLP-1)

The differences between above hormones are:

GLP-1	GIP
1. It is released from I cells	1. It is released from K cells in duodenum
2. It stimulates insulin response from beta cells in glucose-dependent manner	2. It releases insulin from beta in glucose-dependent cells manner
3. It inhibits gastric emptying	3. It has no effect on gastric emptying
4. It inhibits glucagon secretion from ∝ cells in glucose dependent manner	4. It has no effect on body weight
	5. It reduces food intake and body weight
	6. It will not inhibit glucagon secretion from ∝ cells
	7. Little risk of hypoglycemia

When GLP-1 is administered subcutaneously—it will be susceptible to degradation by dipeptidyl peptidase 4 inhibitor. So there is GLP-1 analogue which is resistant to this enzyme.

Exenatide (Byetta)

It is GLP-1 receptor against:
i. Isolated from the venom of Gila monster,
ii. It is resistant to degradation by dipeptidyl peptidase

The actions of exenatide are:
i. Glucose dependent enhancement of insulin secretion.
ii. Restoration of 1st phase of insulin response.
iii. Suppression of inappropriately high glucagon secretion.
iv. Slows gastric emptying.
v. Reduction of food intake.

In presence of elevated blood glucose concentration, exenatide acutely stimulates beta cells to release insulin. This drug is also apparently cleared from kidney only by glomerular filtration.

Dose: It should be administered subcutaneously at 5 µg twice daily, within one hour period before the morning and evening meals, or between two meals at least 6 hours apart

Precaution: It must be avoided in:
i. Type 1 diabetes
ii. Diabetic ketoacidosis
iii. Renal failure
iv. Hepatic insufficiency
v. Severe gastrointestinal disease
vi. Pediatric patients

Liraglutide (Victoza)

1. It is a long-acting GIP-1 analogue—provides 24 hours glycemic control.
2. It is usually administered subcutaneously—absorbed very slowly to reach its maximum concentration.
3. The actions of liraglutide:
   i. Glucose dependent enhancement of insulin secretion
   ii. Suppression of glucagon secretion
   iii. Slowing of gastric emptying
   iv. Promotion of increased β cell mass in type 2 diabetes mellitus.
   v. Reduction of body weight
4. Risk of hypoglycemia is very low.
5. Dosage: Starting dose 0.6 µg daily subcutaneously—the dose may be increased to 1.2 µg. Maximum dose 1.6 µg per day.

Once weekly GLP1 analogue is Dulaglutide.

DPP 4 Inhibitors

These drugs protect endogenous GPI inhibitors from degradation DPP 4 inhibitor. Functions:
i. Improvement of beta cell function
ii. Increase in peripheral tissue sensitivity.

As a result: There is reduction of fasting and postprandial glucose concentration and thus HbA1c. But there is no elevation of insulin level during DPP4 inhibitor treatment.
iii. DPP-4 inhibitor has little effect on gastric emptying
iv. There is no change in body weight.

The effect of DPP 4 inhibitors is mainly mediated by GLP-1.

The DPP 4 inhibitors are:
i. Sitagliptin
ii. Vildagliptin
iii. Saxagliptin
iv. Linagliptin
v. Alogliptin

Dosage:

1. Sitagliptin   100 mg/once daily
2. Saxagliptin   2.5, 5 or 10 mg once daily
3. Alogliptin   12.5–25 mg/daily
4. Vildagliptin   50 mg twice daily
5. Linagliptin   5 mg daily

Elimination: All the drugs excreted through:
1. Kidney—sitagliptin, alogliptin
2. Liver and kidney—saxagliptin, vildagliptin

Dose adjustment: In case of sitagliptin, saxagliptin, alogliptin.

Newer Antidiabetic Drugs *(Fig. 3.21)*

Sodium Glucose Co-transporter-2 (SGLT-2) Inhibitors

All the glucose filtered through glomerulus are subsequently reabsorbed by two active transport mechanisms
a. Sodium glucose linked transporters (SGLT)
B. Facilitative glucose transporters (GLUTs)

SGLT are of two types:
i. SGLT-1
ii. SGLT-2

SGLT-2 transporters are present in proximal convulated tubule, which reabsorbs almost all the glucose till the blood glucose level reaches its threshold value of renal excretion.

So inhibition of SGLT-2 inhibits glucose reabsorption from proximal table and responsible for normal glycemic control.

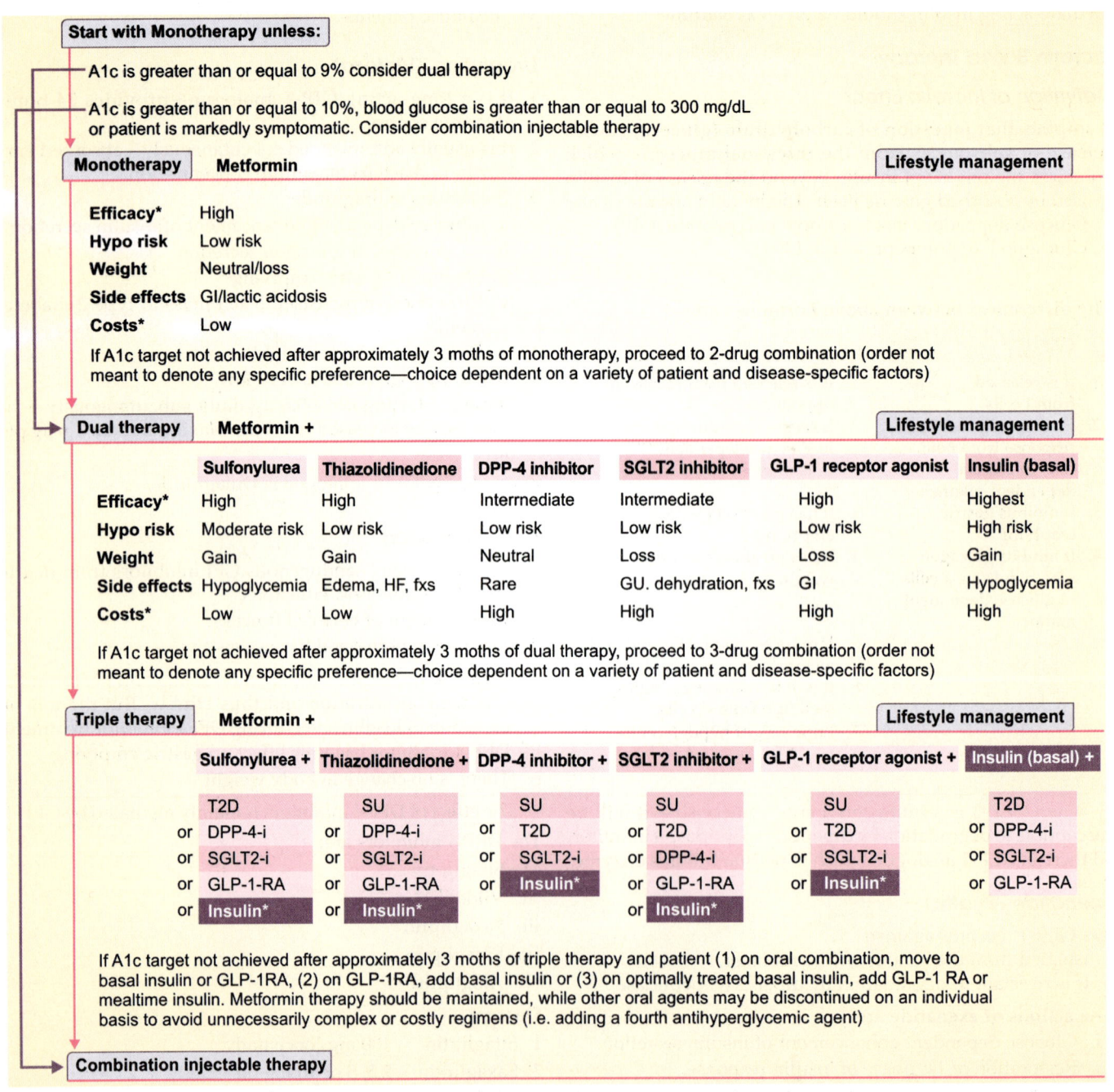

Fig. 3.21: Antihyperglycemic therapy in type 2 diabetes: general recommendations. The order in the chart was determined by historical availability and the route of administration, with injectable to the right; it is not meant to denote any specific preference. Potential sequences of antihyperglycemic therapy for patients with type 2 diabetes are displayed, with the usual transition moving vertically from top to bottom (although horizontal movement within therapy stages is also possible, depending on the circumstances). DPP-4-i, DPP-4 inhibitor; fxs, fractures; GI, gastrointestinal; GLP-1 RA, GLP-1 receptor agonist; GU, genitourinary; HF, heart failure; Hypo, hypoglycemia; SGLT2-i, SGLT2 inhibitor; SU, sulfonylurea; T2D, thiazolidinedione. "See ref 21 for description of efficacy and cost categorization. Usually a basal insulin (NPH, glargine, detemir, degludec). Adapted with permission from inzucchi, et al. (21)"

SGLT-2 inhibitors are:

1. Dapagliflozin
2. Canagliflozin
3. Empagliflozin

Amylin (Pramlintide)

i. It is a soluble analogue—it does not aggregate and accumulate in islet tissue
ii. It improves glycemic control in type 1 and type 2 diabetes mellitus.
iii. **Physiologic actions:**
  1. It inhibits food intake (through central mechanism)
  2. It slows gastric motility
  3. It inhibits postprandial glucose secretion
  4. It suppresses postprandial hepatic glucose production
  5. It suppresses arginine—stimulated glucagon secretion
  6. It inhibits insulin secretion in response to secretagogues
  7. It inhibits gastric acid secretion

DIABETIC KETOACIDOSIS

Clinical Manifestations

Symptoms

1. Patient with uncontrolled DM may present with non-specific illness.
2. If the disease progresses an indolent course—patient may present with profound cachexia, prostration.
3. If the patient is under physical or emotional stress, metabolic decompensation may occur—over few hours to days.

  Patient may present with:
  i. Nausea
  ii. Vomiting
  iii. Abdominal pain—acute in nature, may be associated with distension
  iv. Deep and slow breathing (Kussmaul's breathing)
  v. Fruity odor from mouth—acetone
  vi. Thirst
  vii. Polyuria

Signs

1. Tachycardia
2. Dehydration
3. Hypotension
4. Tachypnoea—Kussmaul's respiration
5. Distended abdomen with paralytic ileus
6. Lethargy, obtundation, cerebral edema
7. Coma

Precipitating Events

1. Inadequate insulin administration
2. Infections (pneumonia, urinary tract infection, gastroenteritis sepsis)
3. Infarction (cerebral, coronary, mesenteric, peripheral)
4. Drugs (cocaine)
5. Pregnancy.

Pathophysiology

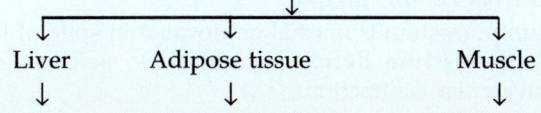

1. Relative or absolute insulin deficiency
and
Counter-regulatory hormone excess (glucagon, catecholamine, Cortisol and growth hormone)
↓
Ratio of insulin: glucagon will be decreased
↓

Liver	Adipose tissue	Muscle
↓	↓	↓
Promotes -	mobilized free fatty acid to liver	mobilize amino acid to liver

  i. Gluconeogenesis
  ii. Glycogenolysis
  iii. Ketone body formation

2. Markers of inflammation (cytokines, CRP) are elevated in DKA.
3. Insulin deficiency and hyperglycemia

  i. Reduce hepatic level of fructose 2, 6-bishosphate
  ↓
  This alters the activity of
  a. phosphofructokinase
  b. Fructose 1, 6-bisphosphatase

  ii. Increase the activity of phosphoenolpyruvate carboxykinase
  Glucagon excess—decreases activity of pyruvate kinase.
  The above changes shift the handling of pyruvate:
  a. Towards glucose synthesis.
  b. Away from glycolysis.
4. Insulin deficiency reduces

  I. the level of GLUT4 glucose transporter
  ↓
  As a result impairment of glucose uptake into
  i. Muscles
  ii. Fat

  II. Intracellular glucose metabolism
5. Reduced insulin level with combination of catecholamine and GH increases lipolysis → releases free fatty acids.

  In DKA, carnitine palmitoyl transferase transports the free fatty acids into mitochondria.
  ↓
  Beta oxidation and conversion to ketone bodies

  Normally, FFA is converted to triglyceride or VLDL in liver.
6. At physiologic pH—ketone bodies exist as ketoacid which is neutralized by bicarbonate.
  As bicarbonates are depleted, ketoacids start accumulation—ensuing metabolic acidosis.
7. Due to decreased activity of insulin sensitive lipoprotein lipase—in case of insulin deficiency, VLDL excretion is reduced in the face of increased triglyceride and VLDL production from muscles and fat.

As a result, hypertriglyceridemia ensues—this may result acute pancreatitis.

Laboratory Investigations (Fig. 3.22)

1. Serum glucose—250–600 mg/dl. It may be minimally elevated
2. Serum bicarbonate <15 mEq/L
3. Arterial pH 6.8–7.3
4. Serum Na 125–135 mEq/L
5. Serum potassium is normal or elevated in spite of total body potassium deficit secondary to acidosis and intravascular contraction.
6. Serum chloride, phosphorus and magnesium are reduced
7. Raised serum BUN and creatinine—due to prerenal cause as a result of intravascular volume depletion.

   Serum sodium is reduced as a consequence of hyperglycemia—1.6 mmol/L reduction of serum sodium for each 100 mg/dl rise in serum glucose.
8. Serum osmolarity = 300–360 mmol/ml
   Calculated serum osmolarity =

$$\frac{\{2 \times (Na^+ K^+) + Plasma\ glucose\ (mg) + BUN/2.8\}}{18}$$

9. Three principal ketone bodies are:
   i. β-hydroxybutyrate
   ii. Acetoacetate
   iii. Acetone

   If measured, total ketone concentration is usually >3 mmol/L
   - to as high as 30 mmol/L (normal value are up to 0.15 mmol/L)
   a. Serum acetone concentration (nonenzymatic decarboxylation of acetoacetate) is 3–4 times higher than the concentration of acetoacetate—it does not contribute to acidosis.
   b. Ratio of β-hydroxybutyric acid: acetoacetate
      i. In normal individual—1:1
      ii. In mild DKA—3:1
      iii. In severe DKA—15:1

   Standard nitroprusside reagents—react with acetoacetate but not with β-hydroxybutyrate
   Hence small ketone does not exclude ketoacidosis.
   Again with treatment β-hydroxybutyric acid will be converted to acetoacetate—giving stronger reaction with nitroprusside reagents—it does not indicate worsening of DKA.
10. Anion gap = (Na – {Cl + HCO₃})—Normal 14 mEq/L
    In most DKA patient, it is ≥20 mEq/L, in some patient >40 mEq/L.

    Acidosis is due to:
    i. Accumulation of β-hydroxybutyric acid and acetoacetate in serum
    ii. Some degree of acidosis
    iii. Hyperchloremic acidosis especially after intravenous therapy during recovery.
11. Leukocytosis—ranges from 15,000 to 20,000/L, occurs frequently in DKA.

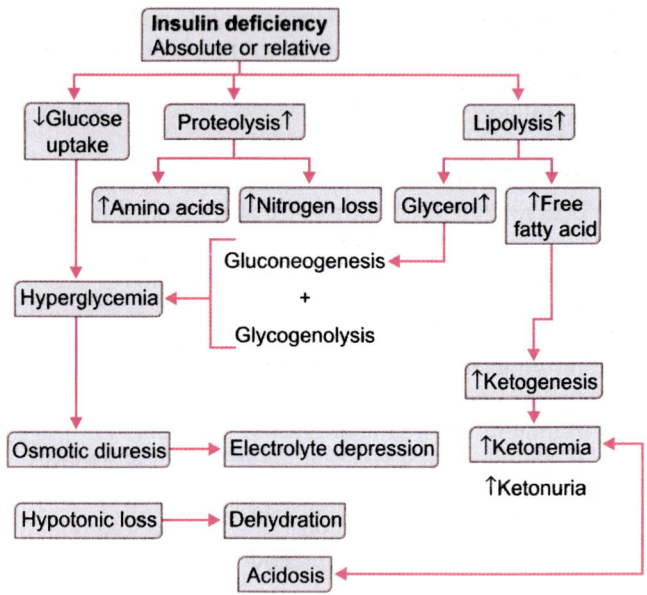

Fig. 3.22: Algorithm of pathophysiology of diabetic ketoacidosis

12. Serum amylase is raised—may be of pancreatic or salivary gland origin.

Management of Diabetic Ketoacidosis

I. **Confirmation of diagnosis:**
   i. Plasma glucose—increased.
   ii. Serum ketone—increased.
   ii. Metabolic acidosis.

II. **Assess:**
   i. Serum electrolytes (Na⁺, K⁺, Mg⁺⁺, Cl⁻, bicarbonate, phosphate)
   ii. Acid base status (pH, HCO₃, PCO₂, beta hydroxybutyrate)
   iii. Renal function (urea, creatinine)

III. **Replacement of fluid:**

   2–3 liters of 0.9% saline over 1–3 hour
   (15–20 ml/kg/hour)
   ↓
   Depending upon serum sodium concentration
   <0.45% saline 250–500 ml/hour.
   ↓   Measure plasma glucose hourly
   When plasma glucose <200 mg/dl
   ↓
   5% glucose in 0.45% saline at 150–250 ml/hour to allow continued insulin administration until ketonemia is controlled to avoid hypoglycemia.

IV. **Insulin administration**

   0.1 unit/kg body weight as intravenous bolus as short acting insulin
   ↓
   0.1 unit/kg per hour as continuous infusion
   (Goal is: rate of reduction of serum glucose 50–75 mg/hour)

(Contd.)

(Contd.)

↓ Measure plasma glucose and K⁺ per hour
When plasma glucose <200 mg/ml
↓
Changes fluid to 5% dextrose 0.45% NS
And
Reduce the insulin 0.05 unit/kg/hour
↓
Thereafter adjust insulin infusion to maintain glucose level to between 150 and 200 mg/dl until pH is >7.3

If serum K⁺ level <3.3 mEq/L	If serum K⁺ >5.2 mEq/L
↓	↓
First potassium correction followed by IV insulin administration	No potassium administration till serum K⁺ will be corrected

V. Potassium supplementation

i. If potassium >5 mEq/L—no supplementation is required.
ii. If serum potassium 4 to 5 mEq/L, 20 mEq/L to each litre of replacement fluid after adequate renal function is established (normal urine flow and normal creatinine is documented)
iii. If serum potassium is 3 to 4 mEq/L, 40 mEq/L has to be added in each litre of replacement fluid
iv. If serum potassium <3 mEq/L

Stop insulin
↓
Start 10–20 mEq per hour
↓
Measure K⁺ hourly
↓
If K⁺ >3.3 mEq/L
↓
Add 40 mEq/L of potassium in each litre of replacement fluid.

VI. Bicarbonate

i. If arterial pH <7.0 or bicarbonate <5 mEq/L
↓
50 mEq in 200 mg of H_2O and to be infused over 1 hour until pH will be >7.0
ii. If arterial pH > 7.0, no infusion of bicarbonate
iii. If pH <5.9, 100 mEq of bicarbonate + 20 mEq of potassium chloride in 400 ml of water and to be infused over 2 hours until pH >7.0

VII. Phosphate

If phosphate level <1 mEq/L

↓

20–30 mmol potassium phosphate over 24 hours
Serum calcium level has to be measured.

Assessment of patient:

i. Presence or absence of infection
ii. Trauma
iii. Myocardial infarction

Monitoring:

i. Blood pressure
ii. Pulse
iii. Respiration
iv. Mental status
v. Fluid intake and urine output per 24 hours.
Continue all the above till:
a. Blood glucose <150–250 mg/dl
b. Acidosis is resolved, pH >7.30
c. Bicarbonate >18 mEq/L

Transition to Subcutaneous Insulin

To prevent recurrence of DKA during transition period of conversion of subcutaneous insulin—intravenous insulin has to be continued for at least 2–3 hours.

Administer long-acting insulin as soon as patient is eating.

Complications in Diabetic Ketoacidosis

1. With proper therapy mortality in <1%
2. Related to precipitating factors:
   i. Infections
   ii. Myocardial infarction
3. Complications, those may occur in DKA:
   i. Venous thromboembolism
   ii. ARDS
   iii. Acute gastrointestinal bleeding
   iv. Cerebral edema—it usually occurs during therapy specially in children

Monitoring Glycemic Control

Presently following methods are used:
1. Testing urine for presence of glucose
2. Occasional blood glucose test to be done in laboratory
3. Estimation of glycosylated hemoglobin and serum fructosamine levels
4. Self-monitoring of blood glucose level

Methods of Estimating Blood Glucose Level

Blood glucose levels must be estimated using latest acceptable methods such as the:
- Glucose oxidase or hexokinase technique
- Folin Wu method
- Somogyl-Nelson method
- Ferricyanide technique
- Orthotoludine technique

Some drugs or medications which will not allow a correct evaluation of glucose levels:
i. Benzodiazepine
ii. Chlorfibrate
iii. Corticoids
iv. Diazoxide
v. Furosemide
vi. Lithium
vii. MAO inhibitors
viii. OCP
ix. Phenothiazines
x. Thiazide diuretics

Elapses time between collection of blood sample and its estimation also affects the result, e.g.:

i. Blood glucose levels will decrease at a rate of about 7–10 mg/dl per hour of room temperature unless the red cells are removed or their enzyme systems inhibited. For this purpose, fluoride will be used.

So, greater the interval between the time of collection and the estimation of sample, the lower will be the results.

ii. Rough handing—produces RBC breakdown

iii. Contamination of blood sample

iv. Inadequate refrigeration

COMPLICATIONS OF DIABETES MELLITUS

I. **Acute complications**
   a. Diabetic ketoacidosis
   b. Hyperglycemic hyperosmolar coma
II. **Chronic complications:**
   a. *Microvascular*
      1. *Eye disease:*
         i. Retinopathy —— Non-proliferative / Proliferative
         ii. Macular edema
      2. *Neuropathy:*
         i. Sensory and motor (mono- and polyneuropathy)
         ii. Autonomic neuropathy
      3. *Nephropathy*
   b. *Macrovascular:*
      1. Coronary artery disease
      2. Peripheral artery disease
      3. Cerebrovascular disease
   c. *Others:*
      1. Gastrointestinal
         i. Gastroparesis
         ii. Diarrhea
      2. Genitourinary
         i. Uropathy
         ii. Sexual dysfunction
      3. Dermatologic
      4. Infections
      5. Glaucoma
      6. Cataracts
      7. Periodontal disease
      8. Hearing loss.

DIABETIC NEUROPATHY

Somatic Neuropathy

Gradual Onset

Distal symmetrical polyneuropathy:

i. Chronic symmetric symptoms—affecting peripheral nerve

ii. Longest nerve involves first

iii. Though sensory and motor functions affected, but sensory will be predominant

iv. Associated often with autonomic dysfunction

v. Symptoms:
   a. Tingling and numbness bilaterally symmetrically involve
      Feet—then spreading proximally as in stocking like fashion
   b. Later on, upper extremity is involved in similar fashion in gloves like manner.
   c. Loss of balance in eye closed position
   d. Painless injuries due to loss of sensation

Acute Onset

1. **Painful symmetric polyneuropathy:** Finding is similar to above, but is usually acute onset, associated with burning, stabbing, crushing, aching sensations, increases severity at night.

2. **Mononeuropathy and mononeuropathy multiplex:** Individual nerve is usually affected:
   i. Median nerve in wrist
   ii. Ulnar nerve at elbow

   Symptoms—usually comprises of pain, tingling, numbness wasting and weakness.

   It may involve in the form of solitary nerve involvement or in combination.

3. **Cranial mononeuropathy:**
   i. Cranial III, IV and VI nerves involvement can manifest as:
      a. Acute headache or eye pain followed by diplopia developing over few hours.
      b. Muscle weakness in the distribution of single nerve
      c. Pupillary light reflexes are spared.
   ii. Facial neuropathy—manifests as acute or subacute facial muscle weakness—can be recurrent or bilateral.

4. **Diabetic radiculoplexopathy** (also known as proximal neuropathy):
   i. Sudden severe unilateral pain in low back, hip, high, it may occur in shoulder or back.
   ii. Weakness or atrophy—develops over brief time
   iii. Reflexes—depressed
   iv. Numbness and paresthesia
   v. Depression, anorexia, weight loss
   vi. Seen in older people

5. **Diabetic radiculopathy:**
   i. Burning, stabbing, boring, belt-like or deep acting pain, in the territory of nerve root
   ii. It begins unilaterally, and becomes bilateral
   iii. Numbness is most prominent in distal distribution of nerve root
   iv. Skin hypersensitivity
   v. Weakness presents in the distribution of affected nerve root
   vi. Co-existing diabetic distal symmetric polyneuropathy may be present
   vii. Single or multiple roots may be involved

6. **Diabetic neuropathy cachexia:** Presents with:
   i. Severe weight loss in older subject
   ii. This is followed by severe pain, signs and symptoms of autonomic neuropathy.

Autonomic Neuropathy

Clinical Manifestations

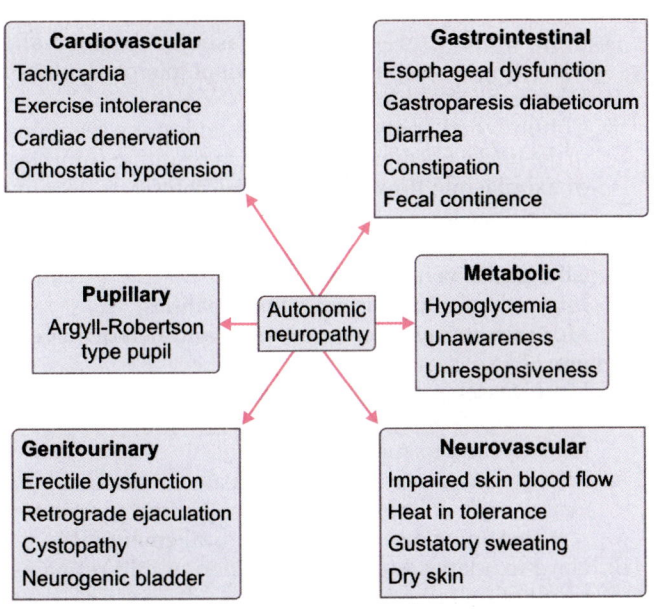

Fig. 3.23: Manifestations in autonomic neuropathy

Diagnosis *(Table 3.6)*

A. Careful history taking:
   i. Sensory (tingling, numbness, anesthesia, paresthesia, incoordination)
   ii. Motor (wasting, washing, nocturnal muscle cramps)
   iii. Autonomic (gastrointestinal, bladder symptoms, sexual dysfunction, postural light headedness)

B. Tests for peripheral sensation:
   i. Touch (cotton)
   ii. Pain (pin prick)
   iii. Vibration (calibrated timing fork)
   iv. Monofilament test: This is a very simple but clinically important study of sensation of feet.

C. Motor involvement—muscle wasting and power

D. Reflexes

E. Detection of autonomic neuropathy.

Management

A. Aggressive diabetic control—to improve nerve conduction velocity.
B. Risk factors for neuropathy hypertriglyceridemia, hypertension should be treated
C. Avoidance of risk factors—smoking, alcohol intake.
D. Supplementation of vitamin B_{12} and folic acid
E. Avoidance of trauma to feet where there is devoid of sense because of risk of ulceration.
F. Pain test neuropathy can respond to:
   1. Antidepressant (tricyclic antidepressant—amitryptyline, desipramine, nortryptyline, imipramine)
   2. Selective serotonin norepinephrine reuptake inhibitors (duloxeline)
   3. Anticonvulsants (gabapentin, pregabalin, carbamazepine, lamotrigine)
   Since the pain is of acute nature—it may resolve overtime.
G. Therapy of orthostatic hypotension—secondary to autonomic neuropathy—by a variety of agents with limited success
   Fludrocortisone, midodrine clonidine, octreotide, yohmbine.
H. Non-pharmacologic maneuvers:
   i. Adequate salt intake
   ii. Avoidance of dehydration
   iii. Avoidance of diuretics
   iv. Lower extremity support
I. Gastroparesis diabeticorum—treated by
   i. Metoclopramide
   ii. Domperidon
   iii. Levosulpride
J. Diabetic diarrhea
   i. Clonidine
   ii. Cholestyramine
   iii. Loperamide
   iv. Metachlopramide
K. Cystopathy can be treated by:
   i. Bethanecol   ii. Doxazosin
L. Erectile dysfunction can be treated by:
   i. Sildenafil
   ii. Tadlafil
   iii. Vardenafil
   iv. GMP—type-5 phosphodiesterase inhibitor

DIABETIC RETINOPATHY

Eye disease is a serious complication of diabetes mellitus, can often presents without any visual symptoms.

Factors Affecting the Onset and/or Progression of Retinopathy

   i. Duration of diabetes
   ii. Uncontrolled hyperglycemia
   iii. Proteinuria
   iv. High blood pressure
   v. Dyslipidemias
   vi. Pregnancy and puberty
   vii. One undefined factor—that modulate and development of complications, e.g.
       a. In a few patients with long-standing diabetes—they never develop nephropathy or retinopathy

Table 3.6: Tests in autonomic neuropathy			
Test for autonomic neuropathy		*Normal response*	*Abnormal response*
Resting heart rate			>100/mm
Heart rate response to standing	Measure R-R interval at beat 15 and 30 second after patient stands	A	30:15 ratio of less than 1.03 is abnormal
Systolic blood pressure changes on standing	Measure SBP in lying down then standing position	Decrease <10 mmHg	Decrease >30 mmHg
Heart rate response to deep breathing	Measure heart rate response to deep breathing	Increase rate >15 beats/min	Increase <10 beats/minute

b. In a few patients in spite of rigid control of glycemia, they can develop complications.

This factor is genetic susceptibility.

Pathophysiology (Fig. 3.24)

Stages of Diabetic Retinopathy

Stage-1: Mild non-proliferative retinopathy—characterized by increased capillary permeability

Stage-2: Moderate to severe non-proliferative retinopathy—characterized by vascular closure.

Stage-3: Proliferative diabetic retinopathy—characterized by—growth of new blood vessels on the retina and posterior surface of vitreous.

Macular edema, characterized by retinal thickening from leaking blood vessels—can develop in all stages of retinopathy.

Symptoms

i. Blurring of vision
ii. Difficulty in reading and writing
iii. Double vision
iv. Eyes get red and stay that way
v. Feeling of pressure in eyes
vi. Seeing of spots or floaters
vii. Straight lines do not like straight.

Clinical Signs—Ophthalomoscopic Findings

Non-proliferative Retinopathy

1. **Mild:**
   i. Microaneurysm—an easy vascular abnormality consisting of outpouching of retinal microvasculature.
   ii. Hemorrhages—blot shaped
   iii. Cotton wood spots—gray or white lesions seen along in the nerve fiber layer of the retina resulting from stasis of axoplasmic flow caused by microinfarcts of retinal nerve fiber layer.

2. **Moderate:**
   i. Changes in venous vessel caliber
   ii. Intraretinal microvascular abnormalities
   iii. More numerous microaneurysms and hemorrhages

3. **Severe:**
   i. More vessels are blocked; parts or retina is deprived of blood supply and set the stage of new blood vessels are to be formed to supply these parts.
   ii. *Macular edema*—fluid and lipid leak from retinal blood vessels may collect in macula—called macular edema. It should be considered as medical emergency.
   iii. Hard exudates: Lipid accumulation within retina as a result of increased permeability.

Proliferative Retinopathy

i. Newly formed blood vessels appear near optic nerve and/or macula

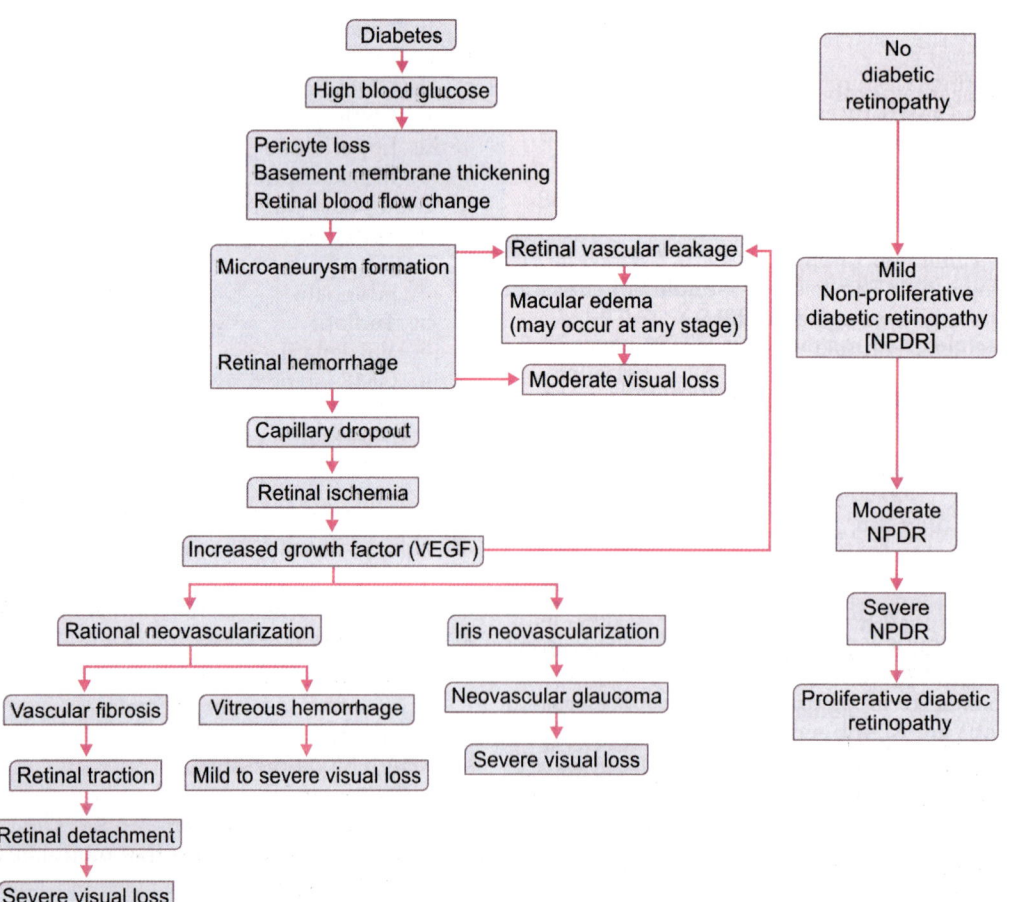

Fig. 3.24: Pathophysiology of diabetic retinopathy

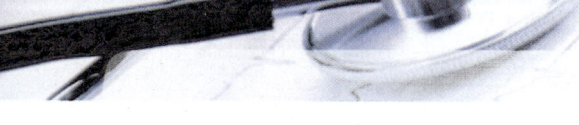

ii. Rupture of these blood vessels
iii. Vitreous hemorrhage
iv. Scar in retina—producing retinal detachment

Amsler's chart is very useful for early detection of macular problem and thus very important as this may be the early sign of macular problems leads to loss of central visions.

Therapy

Most important therapy of retinopathy is prevention.

The following are preventive measures:
1. *Lifestyle:*
   i. 30–60 minutes exercise in a day
   ii. Moderate alcohol consumption only
   iii. Control of obesity—if possible, balanced diet containing 5 portions of vegetable or fruits a day
   iv. Very low salt.
2. *Blood pressure:*
   i. In non-proteinuric patient   130/80 mm Hg
   ii. In proteinuric patient   125/75 mm Hg
3. *HbA1c:*
   i. 6.5% or less is preferable
   ii. ACE-I unless young/pregnant/very low blood pressure/poorly tolerated
4. *Cholesterol:* <4.66 mmol/L, statin is recommended
5. *Smoking:*
   Smoking 20/day—triples retinopathy
   Passive smoking from roommates increases at least 20%.

Specific Therapy

1. **Laser photocoagulation**—is very effective in preventing:
   i. Proliferative retinopathy (postretinal laser photocoagulation)
   ii. Macular edema by—focal laser photocoagulation
2. **Vitrectomy**—In: i. Vitreous hemorrhage
                        ii. Retinal detachment
3. Anti-VEGF drugs:
   i. Bevacizumab
   ii. Ranibizumab
   iii. Lapatinib
   iv. Sorafenib

GLYCOSYLATED HEMOGLOBIN

An estimation of glycosylated hemoglobin level allows the glycemic control to be judged over a span of time.

Hemoglobin, an oxygen transporter, is located inside the RBC.

Lifespan of RBC is 120 days. So lifespan of hemoglobin is related to the lifespan of RBC in which it resides.

During the span of 120 days, hemoglobin is exposed to glucose, as a result, hemoglobin is glycated with glucose—this glycosylated hemoglobin is usually measured.

The conditions which reduce the lifespan of RBC also affect the value of HbA1c—it is falsely low HbA1c.
1. Hereditary spherocytosis
2. Hemolysis
3. Sickle cell anemia
4. Thalassemia
5. Acute and chronic blood loss

The conditions which lengthen the lifespan of RBC, increase falsely HbA1c:
1. Vitamin B_{12} deficiency
2. Folate deficiency
3. Iron deficiency
   a. HbA1c of 6%—represents mean glucose—130 mg/dl
   b. Each 1% increase in HbA1c glucose increases approximately 30 mg/dl

HbA1c Interpretation

HbA1c	5.5% represents mean glucose	100 mg/dl
HbA1c	7.0% represents mean glucose	150 mg/dl
HbA1c	8.0% represents mean glucose	180 mg/dl
HbA1c	9.0% represents mean glucose	220 mg/dl
HbA1c	10% represents mean glucose	250 mg/dl

Following patients should monitor their blood glucose levels:
1. All patients on insulin therapy, especially those on multiple dose regimens.
2. Patients with widely fluctuating blood glucose level
3. Patients prone to severe ketosis or recurrent hypoglycemia
4. Those manifesting hypoglycemia "unawareness".
5. Patient in whom "tight" control is essential
6. In preoperative period
7. Those with abnormal renal thresholds

HYPERGLYCEMIC HYPEROSMOLAR STATE

It occurs commonly in type-2 diabetes mellitus patients.

Symptoms

Symptoms present: Several weeks of history of polyuria, weight loss, diminished weight loss—followed by:
   i. Mental confusion
   ii. Lethargy
   iii. Stupor
   iv. Coma

The symptoms which are absent:
   i. Nausea
   ii. Vomiting
   iii. Abdominal pain
   iv. Kussmaul's respiration

Physical Signs

   i. Profound dehydration
   ii. Hyperosmolarity
   iii. Profound hypotension
   iv. Tachycardia
   v. Altered mental status

Precipitating Factors

   i. Stroke
   ii. Sepsis
   iii. Pneumonia
   iv. Myocardial infarction
   v. Other intercurrent infections
   vi. Social situation compromising water intake

Pathophysiology

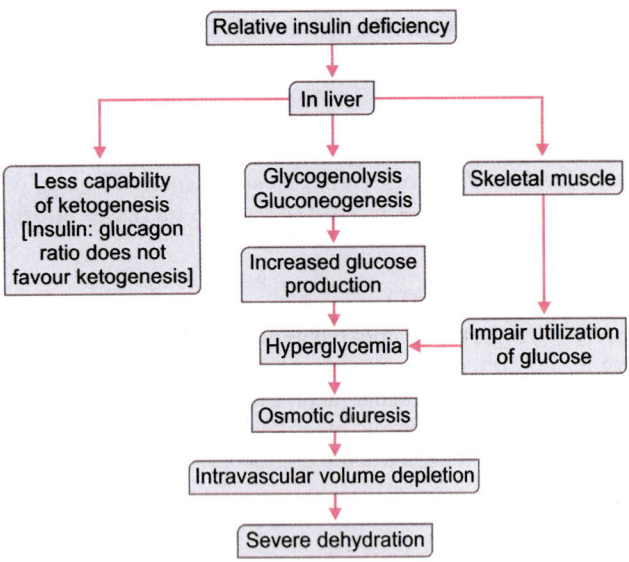

Fig. 3.25: Effect of insulin deficiency in liver

Laboratory Abnormalities

1. Glucose — 600–1200 mg/dL
2. Sodium — 135–145 mEq/dL
3. Potassium — Normal
4. Magnesium — Normal
5. Chloride — Normal
6. Phosphate — Normal
7. Creatinine — moderately raised
8. Plasma osmolarity — 330–380 mosm/mL
9. Plasma ketone — +/-
10. Serum bicarbonate — Normal to slightly ↓
11. Arterial pH — >7.3
12. Anion gap — Normal or slightly ↑

Treatment

Prominent features are: Volume depletion and hyperglycemia.

So urgent requirements are:
1. Fluid replacement
2. Insulin therapy

Fluid Replacement

1. 1–3 liters 0.9% normal saline has to be given over 1st 2–3 hours.

    Fluid deficit occurs over periods of days to weeks in HHS—hence rapid reversal of fluid balance may produce cerebral edema.

2. If serum sodium >150 mmol/L or >150 mEq/L, 0.45% saline should be started.

3. After hemodynamic stability has been achieved, rapid reversal of free water deficit can be corrected by

    0.45% saline initially
    ↓
    5% dextrose water

4. Calculated free water deficit (9–10 liters) should be corrected over next 1–2 days (infusion rate 200–300 mL/hour of hypotonic fluid)

    Electrolyte replacement

5. Potassium should be corrected with regular check up of serum potassium.

6. If patient is using diuretic—severe potassium deficiency is usually with magnesium deficiency.

7. Phosphate level will be lower during therapy and can be corrected by:
    i. Potassium phosphate infusion
    ii. Starting nutrition

Insulin Therapy

0.1 unit/kg IV bolus followed by constant infusion of 0.1 units/kg/hour
↓
If blood glucose level does not fall
↓
Double the infusion rate of insulin (0.2 units/kg/hour)
↓
When plasma glucose falls to 250–300 mg/dl
↓
Dose of infusion will be reduced to 0.05 unit/kg/hour
↓
When the patient starts taxing food orally change the IV insulin to subcutaneous insulin with few hours of combination of IV and SC insulin to prevent recurrent hyperglycemia
↓
Patient can be discharged by either
    i. SC insulin
Or ii. OHA

HYPOGLYCEMIA

Hypoglycemia is really a mismatch between "Insulin-food-activity".

Definition of hypoglycemia: According to American Diabetic Association/Endocrine Society

A. All the episodes of abnormally low plasma glucose concentration that expose the diabetic patients to potential harm (so a single threshold value of plasma glucose cannot define hypoglycemia).

B. Shift of glycemic threshold for development of symptoms towards:
    a. Lower side in case recent antecedent hypoglycemia
    b. Higher side in case of poorly controlled diabetic patients and infrequent hypoglycemia

C. Alert value of plasma glucose in a diabetic patient treated with either insulin or sulfonylurea or glinide at risk of hypoglycemia is <70 mg/dl.

D. In case of neonates, plasma glucose value of <45 mg/dL during first 24 hours of life.

Glucose homeostasis:

A. Plasma glucose will be lowered by insulin.

B. Plasma glucose will be increased by counter-regulatory hormones, like, catecholamine, glucagon, cortisol and growth hormone through following mechanisms:
   a. Glycogenolysis, i.e. mobilizing glycogen from the liver.
   b. Gluconeogenesis, i.e. glucose synthesis from non-glucose sources.

So, in case of hypoglycemia, there will be surge of counter-regulatory hormones mainly catecholamine and glucagon mobilize the endogenous sources of glucose as well as appearances of adrenergic symptoms. So, if this safety mechanism fails the patient will show the signs of hypoglycemia.

Pathophysiology of Hypoglycemia

A. Human brain physiologically consumes 5 gm of glucose per hour.
B. Again blood flow to brain is 1 liter per minute.
C. Thousand millions of brain cells require glucose concentration of 100 mg/dL
D. Brain can store up to 1.5 gm of glycogen as reserve. It can be mobilized to glucose during brief period of emergency to maintain brain function.
E. If blood glucose falls below 45 mg/dL the hypothalamic center acts in the three following places:
   a. Hunger center will be stimulated and it creates the need for sugar.
   b. In bulbar reticular system, activation of sympathetic and parasympathetic systems leading to release of counter-regulatory hormones.
   c. In the pituitary gland, release of growth hormone and ACTH.

Causes of Hypoglycemia

Reactive Hypoglycemia

a. Early stage of maturity onset diabetes.
b. Post-gastrectomy
c. Idiopathic postprandial syndrome
d. Inborn error of metabolism:
   • Galactosemia
   • Hereditary fructose intolerance

Fasting Hypoglycemia

A. Decrease glucose production in case of normal insulin level:
   a. Liver dysfunction:
     • Glycogen storage disease
     • Hepatoma
   b. Dysfunction of endocrine glands:
     • Addison's disease
     • Glucagon deficiency
     • Hypopituitarism
   c. Sepsis: In case of endotoxemia, different cytokines increase insulin release.
B. Over-utilization of glucose in case of elevated insulin level:
   a. Hyperinsulinemia:
     • Insulinoma
     • Autoantibody against insulin or insulin receptors
     • Nesidioblastosis
   b. Inappropriate insulin level:
     • Extra-pancreatic tumor
     • Cachexia with depletion of fat
     • Systemic carnitine deficiency

C. Deficiency of substrate:
   a. Chronic starvation
   b. Chronic renal failure
   c. Ketotic hypoglycemia in infancy
D. Compromised glucose counter-regulation:
   a. Fixed syndrome:
     • Defective glucose counter-regulation.
     • Hypoglycemic unawareness.
   b. Dynamic syndrome: High blood glucose threshold resulting from:
   • Effective intensive insulin therapy
   • Recent antecedent hypoglycemia
   • Adrenergic antagonist therapy
   c. Drug-induced hypoglycemia:
     • Sulfonylurea   • Exogenous insulin
     • Propranolol   • Salicylates
     • Pentamide   • Quinine

According to ADA/Endocrine Society Classification of Hypoglycemia

A. **Severe hypoglycemia:** Event requiring assistance of another to take corrective action, like, active administration of carbohydrate, glucagon or others.
B. **Documented symptomatic hypoglycemia:** Here typical symptoms of hypoglycemia with blood glucose of ≤70 mg/dL.
C. **Asymptomatic hypoglycemia:** Here blood glucose of ≤70 mg/dL but without any typical symptom.
D. **Probable symptomatic hypoglycemia:** Here symptoms typical of hypoglycemia not accompanied by blood glucose that was presumably caused by a value of ≤70 mg/dl.
E. **Pseudo-hypoglycemia:** Here the person with diabetes reports any of the typical symptom of hypoglycemia with blood glucose concentration >70 mg/dL, but is approaching to that level. Here rapid fall of blood sugar from 400 to 140 mg/dL may produce hypoglycemic symptoms but the blood glucose level is well above the classical hypoglycemic range.

Risk Factors of Hypoglycemia

A. Advanced age
B. Frailty
C. Low health literacy
D. Polypharmacy
E. Comorbidity:
   a. CRF
   b. CHF
   c. Cognitive impairment
F. African American race
G. Irregular eating patterns
H. Intense glycemic control
I. History of prior hypoglycemia

Clinical Features

Symptoms and signs are due to following causes:
A. Due to adrenergic activation:
   a. Pallor   b. Tremor
   c. Palpitation   d. Hypothermia
   e. Vomiting   f. Tachycardia
   g. Systemic hypotension   h. Raised temperature

B. Due to parasympathetic activation:
   a. Eructation   b. Cold sweating
   c. Hypotension   d. Mitigation of expected tachycardia
C. Signs and symptoms of neuroglycopenia:
   a. Frequent yawning
   b. Perioral numbness
   c. Headache: Early morning headache indicates nocturnal hypoglycemia.
   d. Dizziness
   e. Fatigue
   f. Irritability
   g. Disturbed vision and/or diplopia
   h. Paresthesias
   i. Motor dysfunction
   j. Cognitive impairment
   k. Mental confusion
   l. Transient hemiparesis or focal neurological defects
   m. Convulsions
   n. Semi-coma
   o. Coma

Neuroglycopenia is usually developed as a result of insufficient glucose entry into the cells due to:
A. Decreased concentration of glucose in the blood
B. Block of further metabolism after entry of glucose into the cells.

Predisposing factors:
A. In case of constant dose of insulin, regular timely meal and accustomed exertion, increased insulin absorption from the site of injection or release of insulin from insulin-insulin-antibody complexes
B. In case of chronic renal failure, decreased clearance of insulin through the kidney.
C. In case of gastroparesis, delayed absorption of nutrients.
D. Increased alcohol consumption
E. Depletion of glycogen storage in the liver.

Difference between insulin-induced and oral anti-diabetic drug (OAD) induced hypoglycemia: In case if insulin-induced hypoglycemia, hypoglycemia is predictable and it depends on the sourec, site of injection and strength of insulin.

In case of OAD, hypoglycemia is prolonged and relapsing and occurs at unexpected time.

Biguanide never produces hypoglycemia as its mechanism of action is extra-pancreatic.

In case quinine administration, hypoglycemia occurs due to:
A. Increased insulin secretion
B. Consumption of glucose by malarial parasite.

In some cases, following drugs can potentiate the primary action of sulfonylurea:
A. Phenylbutazone
B. Sulfa antibiotics
C. Beta adrenergic antagonists (propranolol)

In case of type 1 diabetes mellitus, hypoglycemia occurs due to following reasons:
A. Compromisation of physiological defenses against hypoglycemia which in turn leads to defective glucose counter-regulation.
B. In long-standing diabetes:
   a. Selective deficient secretion of glucagon in early cases.
   b. Deficient secretion of epinephrine in late cases.

Hypoglycemic unawareness: It can be defined as the failure of an individual to develop autonomic symptoms, like, tremor, sweating, hunger, which are usually present when the blood glucose will be level nearly 60 mg/dL but before the development of neuroglycopenic symptoms. Neuroglycopenic symptoms usually occur when the blood glucose level is 50 mg/dL.

Features of reactive hypoglycemia:
A. It is more common in obese or overweight insulin resistant patients.
B. It may be a frequent precursor to type 2 diabetes mellitus.
C. Possible high-risk patients with family history of type 2 diabetes mellitus.

In case of gestational hypoglycemia, following features are present:
A. It is more frequent in women of 25 years old.
B. It is more frequent in women with pre-existing medical condition.
C. It is less frequent in women with prepregnancy body mass index $\leq 30 \text{ kg/m}^2$.

Diagnosis

Diagnosis is based on Whipple's triad:
A. Low plasma glucose
B. Symptoms of hypoglycemia
C. Correction of glucose and normalization blood glucose.

Following factors are responsible for:
A. Overuse of basal insulin.
B. Long period between meals.
C. Inconsistent insulin absorption from the injection sites.
D. Delayed effect of exercise from the prior day.
E. Overcorrection of bedtime dosing
F. Overnight insulin sensitivity
G. Poor epinephrine counter-regulation with sleep
H. Impaired hypoglycemia awareness at night.

Difference between hypoglycemic sweating and sweating due to autonomic neuropathy: In case of diabetic autonomic neuropathy, there is anhidrosis of lower half of the body and compensatory hyperhydrosis of the trunk and face. In case of hypoglycemia, sweating occurs all over the body.

Management of Hypoglycemia

A. **In case of conscious patient,** sweetened drink or fruit juice should be given.
B. **In case of unconscious patient:**
   a. 25% glucose intravenously over a few minutes
   b. 1 mg glucagon intramuscularly or, 0.5 cc adrenaline subcutaneously. It will immediately mobilize the glucose from the liver.
      The patient will recover his consciousness within 5–10 minutes after intravenous glucose.
   c. If the patient cannot recover his consciousness, intravenous hydrocortisone 100 mg as bolus intravenous doses at the time the administration of intravenous glucose. This cortisol helps entering of glucose into neural cells and aggravating the recovery from hypoglycemia.
   d. If the above measures fail, 40 grams mannitol intravenously over 20 minutes along with 8 mg dexamethasone intravenously every 6 hours.

e. After recovery from hypoglycemia, following questions should be enquired:
- Excessive dose of insulin
- Unusual exertion
- Missed meal
- Delayed meal
- Use of wrong syringe for type and strength of insulin
- In patient taking sulfonylurea whether the patient takes phenylbutazone, sulfa, salicylate or anticoagulant, because these drugs will potentiate the action of antidiabetic drug by competitive binding with protein.

C. In case of fasting hypoglycemia:
a. If dietary therapy is inadequate, intravenous glucose can be infused.
b. Intravenous octreotide can be given intravenously to prevent endogenous insulin secretion.

c. Avoidance of exercise as exercise will burn carbohydrate and increases the sensitivity to insulin.
d. Definitive treatment is surgical resection of tumor. Success rate in case of benign islet cell adenoma is good. But in case of malignant islet cell, tumor is nearly 50%.

D. In case of reactive hypoglycemia:
a. Refined carbohydrate should be restricted.
b. One should avoid simple sugar
c. One should increase the frequency of meals but reduce the size of meals.
d. Protein and fiber are increased in the diet.
e. Alfa glucosidase inhibitor can be administered because it can cause reversible inhibition of pancreatic alfa amylase as well as membrane bound intestinal alfa glucoside hydrolase enzymes. As a results glucose absorption will be delayed, this leads to inhibition of postprandial hyperglycemia and thus reactive hypoglycemia will be prevented.

ADRENAL DISORDERS

ADRENAL CORTEX

Regulation of Control of Steroidogenesis

Production of glucocorticoids and adrenal androgens is under control of hypothalamic–pituitary–adrenal (HPA) axis.

Production of mineralocorticoids is under control of renin–angiotension–aldosterone (RAA) axis.

ACTH is the principal hormone stimulating glucocorticoid biosynthesis.

ACTH is produced by following pathway:

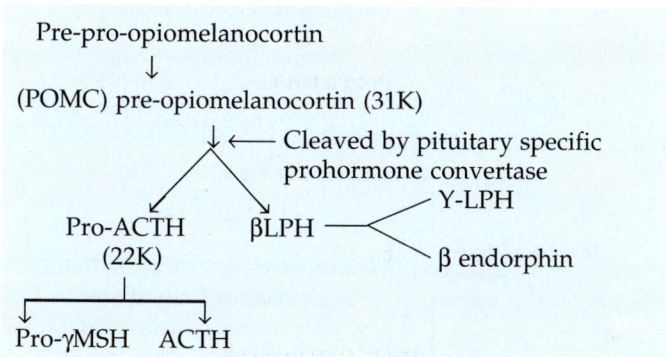

Excess control can suppress ACTH and CRH by inhibiting anterior pituitary and hypothalamus, respectively (Fig. 3.26).

Aldosterone synthesis is under control of three principal factors: (1) Angiotensin-II, (2) Potassium, (3) to some extent, ACTH.

The factors those directly inhibit aldosterone syntheses are: (1) Somatostatin, (2) heparin, (3) atrial natriuretic factor, (4) dopamine:
A. Renin secreted by juxtaglomerular cells in the kidney is dependant on renal arterial blood pressure.
B. Renin converts angiotensinogen to angiotensin-I.

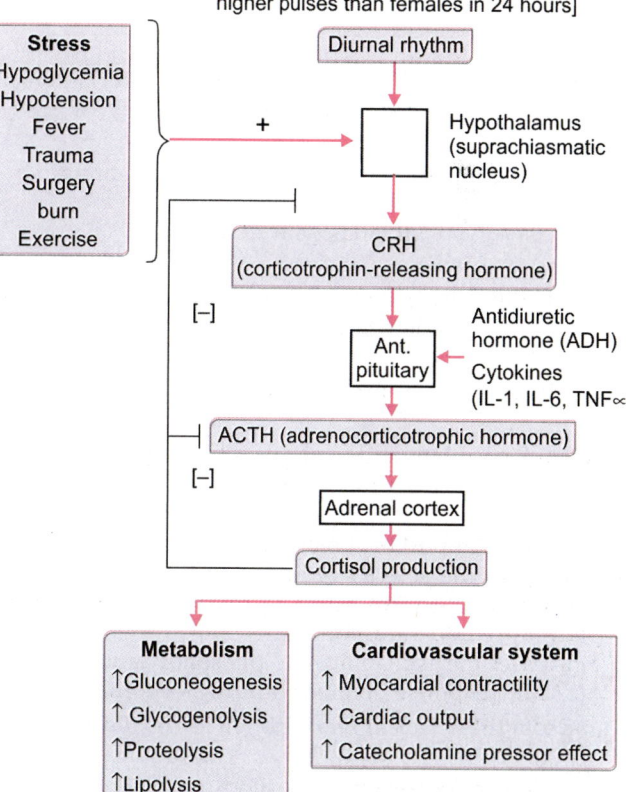

Fig. 3.26: Regulation of cortisol secretion

C. Angiotensin-I is converted in the lungs by angiotensin converting enzyme to angiotensin-II.
D. Angiotensin-II stimulates adrenal aldosterone synthesis.
E. Extracellular fraction of potassium has an important direct inhibitory influence on aldosterone secretion.

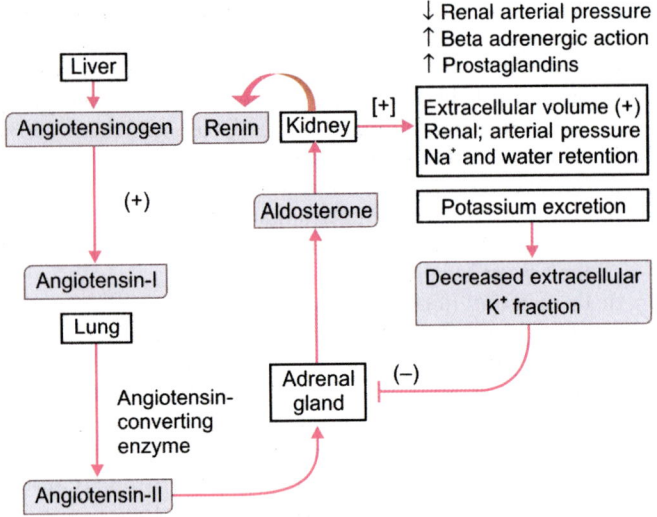

Fig. 3.27: Control of mineralocorticoid hormone secretion

Synthesis of Steroids (Fig. 3.28)

Cholesterol is the precursor of steroid synthesis. This is provided from following:
1. Low density lipoprotein cholesterol
2. It can be generated endogenously within adrenal cortex from acetyl co-enzyme A.
3. Uptake of high density lipoprotein through putative HDL receptor.

ACTH receptor MC2R (melanocortin 2 receptor) interacts with MRAD.
↓
This complex is transported to cell membrane
↓
It binds with ACTH
↓
ACTH stimulates generation of cyclic-AMP by increasing adenylate cyclase activity
↓
cAMP upregulates protein kinase signaling pathways.
↓
Protein kinase activation impacts steroidogenesis in three distinct ways:

i. Increased import of cholesterol esters.
ii. Increases the activity of hormone sensitive lipase—it cleaves cholesterol esters to release cholesterol and introduce into mitochondria.
iii. increases the availability and phosphorylation of CREB (cAMP response element binding)—it enhances the transcription of CYP11A1 and other enzymes required for glucocorticoid synthesis.

Zona glomerulosa—synthesize aldosterone
Zona fasciculata—synthesize glucocorticoid
Zona reticularis—synthesize androgens

Star protein (steroidogenic acute regulatory protein)
↓
Helps the cholesterol to cross from outer to inner mitochondrial membrane

Majority of steroidogenic enzymes are cytochrome 450 (CYP) enzymes which are either located:
i. In mitochondrion (side chain cleavage enzyme, 11 β hydroxylase, aldosterone synthetase, or
ii. In endoplasmic reticulum membrane – 17 ∝ hydroxylase, 21 hydroxylase, aromatase)

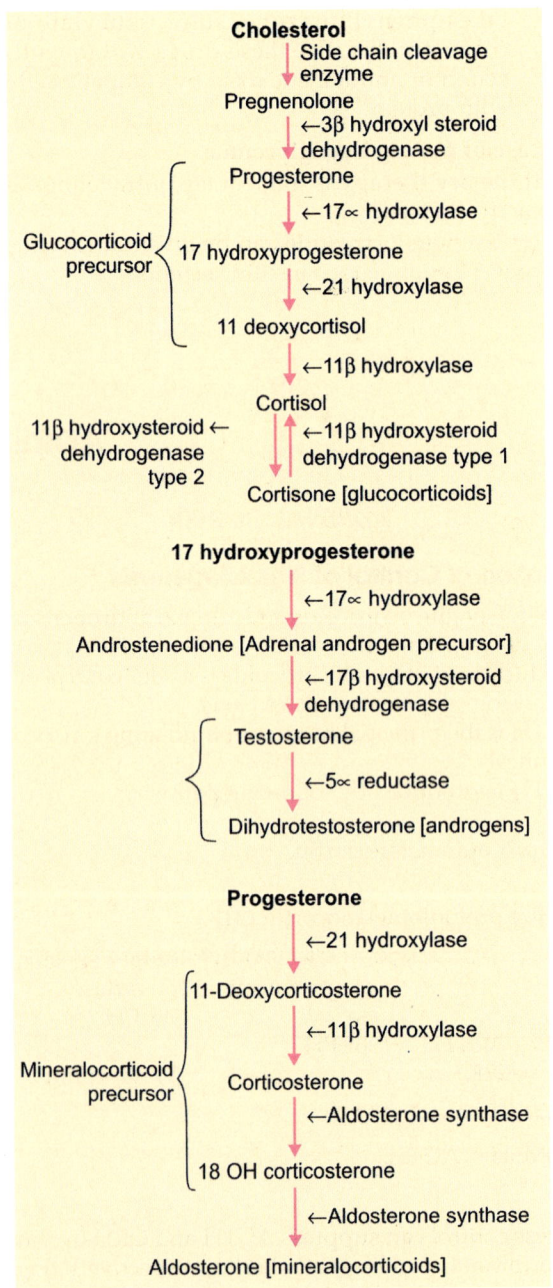

Fig. 3.28: Synthesis of steroid hormone

CUSHING SYNDROME

Three distinct pathogenic disorders of Cushing syndrome are:
1. **Pituitary Cushing syndrome:** Small pituitary micro-adenoma produces excess amounts of adrenocorticotropic hormone (ACTH).
   - This is called Cushing disease

2. **Adrenal Cushing syndrome:** This occurs from autonomous cortisol production from adrenal tumor (adenoma or carcinoma) or adrenal hyperplasia—which may be micronodular or macronodular.
3. **Ectopic Cushing syndrome:** It results from ACTH producing extra pituitary malignancy—producing markedly elevated ACTH.

Causes of Cushing's Syndrome

A. **ACTH-dependent Cushing's syndrome:**
  1. Cushing's disease (ACTH-producing pituitary adenoma)
  2. Ectopic ACTH-producing hormone:
      i. Bronchial carcinoma
      ii. Pancreatic carcinoma
      iii. Carcinoid tumor
      iv. Small cell carcinoma of lung
      v. Medullary carcinoma of thyroid
      vi. Pheochromocytoma
  3. Macronodular adrenal hyperplasia
  4. Iatrogenic treatment with ACTH
B. **ACTH independent Cushing's syndrome:**
  1. Adrenocortical adenoma
  2. Adrenocortical carcinoma
  3. Primary pigmented nodular adrenal hyperplasia
  4. Carney's syndrome
  5. McCune-Albright syndrome
  6. Aberrant receptor expression (gastric inhibitory polypeptide)
  7. Iatrogenic—pharmacologic dose of prednisolone, dexamethasone
C. **Pseudo-Cushing's syndrome:**
  1. Depression
  2. Obesity

Clinical Pictures

A. **Body fat:**
  i. Obesity centripetal in nature
  ii. In pediatric patient there may be generalized obesity
  iii. Development of fat depots over
      1. Thoracocervical spine (buffalo hump)
      2. In the supraclavicular region
      3. Over the cheeks and temporal region (rounded moon like face)
  iv. Abnormal fat accumulation in epidural space—lead to neurologic deficit
B. **Skin:**
  i. Thinning of skin and separation with exposure of subcuteneous vascular tissue.
  ii. Wrinkling of the skin on the dorsum of the hand.
  iii. Facial plethora—secondary to thinning of skin
  iv. Easy bruising
  v. Loss of facial subcutaneous tissue fat
  vi. Red purple livid striae greater than 1 cm width most frequently found on the abdomen, upper thigh, breast and arms—common in younger patient, less common in patient more than 50 years
  vii. Skin pigmentation is rare in Cushing's disease, but common in ectopic ACTH syndrome results from over stimulation of melanocyte receptors.
  viii. Acne
  ix. Hirsutism.

C. **Reproductive organs:**
  i. Menstrual irregularity in female
  ii. Loss of libido in both sexes.
  iii. Hirsutism—vellus hypertrichosis on the face: This should be differentiated from darker terminal hirsutism—occurring due to ACTH-mediated androgen excess.
  iv. Hypogonadotrophic hypogonadism—occurs due to direct inhibitory effect of cortisol on growth hormone releasing hormone and LH/FSH.
D. **Psychiatric features and CNS features:**
  i. Agitated depression and lethargy are most common
  ii. Insomnia
  iii. Memory and cognitive dysfunction

Lowering of cortisol by pharmacological or surgical treatment results rapid improvement of psychiatric problem.

E. **Bone:**
  i. Loss of linear growth in children
  ii. Loss of height due to osteoporotic vertebral collapse
      (It can be assessed by patient's sitting height or comparing the height with arm span.)
      In normal subject, both arm span and height should be equal.
  iii. After minor trauma—there will be pathological fracture, painless rib fracture.
      Radiological appearance is typical, like, exuberant callus formation at the site of healing of fracture.
  iv. Osteonecrosis of femoral or humeral heads
  v. Hypercalciuria—may lead to renal calculi, but there is no hypercalcemia.
F. **Muscles:**
  i. Myopathy
  ii. Bruising—these two are most distinct features of Cushing's syndrome
      Myopathy of proximal muscles of lower limb and shoulder girdle—as a result, patient is:
      a. Unable to climb upstairs.
      b. Unable to get up from deep chair.
G. **Cardiovascular:**
  i. Hypertension—it is much more common in Cushing's syndrome than in patient with simple obesity.
  ii. Atherosclerosis—due to metabolic effect—diabetes, hyperlipidemia.
  iii. Thromboembolic events are much more common.
H. **Infection:**
  i. It is much more common because depression of normal inflammatory response.
  ii. Fungal infections of skin (Tinea versicolor) and nail.
  iii. Wound infection is much more common
I. **Hematopoietic system:**
  i. Increased white blood cell count
  ii. Eosinopenia
  iii. Hypercoagulability—increased risk of DVT and pulmonary embolism.
J. **Metabolic and endocrine effect:**
  i. Glucose intolerance—leads to diabetes mellitus
  ii. Hepatic lipoprotein synthesis stimulated—leading to hypercholesterolemia and hypertriglyceridemia
  iii. Hypokalemic alkalosis—due to raised control—it is more common in ectopic ACTH-producing tumor

because of higher cortical production rates, than with Cushing's syndrome.

iv. Direct suppression effect of cortisol on pituitary gland suppressing TSH and gonadotropin.

K. Eye:

i. Raised intraocular pressure

ii. Exophthalmos—due to accumulation of retro-orbital fat

iii. Cataract—well-recognized complication of corticosteroid therapy—is uncommon now.

Investigation

1. **Plasma cortisol level:**

   a. Normally—highest value in the early morning and reaches nadir at mid-night (<50 nmol/L)

   b. In patient with Cushing's syndrome: Normal at 9 AM but nocturnal level is raised, mid-night control value >200 nmol/L or >7.5 mg/dL indicates Cushing's syndrome, value: 5.0 mg/dL—unlikely, <2 mg—exclude Cushing's syndrome.

   False +ve:

   i. Intercurrent illness

   ii. Stress

   iii. Admission in hospital

   (Midnight sleeping serum cortisol ≥1.8 mg/dL—suggests 100% sensitive for Cushing syndrome)

2. **Urinary free cortisl:** This is a direct measurement of cortisol not bound to plasma protein—it is most reliable and useful test for assessing cortisol secretion. Upper range of normal is 220–330 nmol/24 hour or 90–100 mg/24 hours.

   HPLC-based measurement—upper level is 50 mg/24 hours. It is elevated—3 times than normal in Cushing syndrome. It can be elevated in:

   i. High water intake

   ii. Drugs: carbamazepine

   It can be decreased in:

   i. Low urine output

   ii. Incomplete urine collection

   iii. Renal failure (false –ve)

3. **Dexamethasone overnight suppression test:** It is a screening test for hypercortisolism as outpatient basis.

   Procedure:

   1. Dexamethasone 1 mg orally—at 11 to 12 pm.

   2. Sample collection for plasma cortisol—at 8 AM in the morning.

      a. Normal response—plasma cortisol level <5 mg/dl

      b. Level between 2 and 7 mg/dL—may be difficult to interpret. This level is commonly seen in subject with:

         i. Mental retardation

         ii. Alcohol or stress-induced (pseudo-Cushing's disorder)

      c. Accelerated metabolism of dexamethasone by alcohol, drugs (nefidepine, rifampin, hydantoin, carbamazepine, phenobarbitone, tamoxifen), induction of enzyme CYP3A4 produces false negative test.

d. Suppression of cortical level is incomplete in:

   i. Chronic renal failure—because of decrease clearance

   ii. High estrogen states—because of increased cortisol binding globulin.

e. Serum cortisol level >50 μg/L—suggest Cushing syndrome.

4. **Salivary cortisol level:** Value >2 μg/dl (5.5 nmol/L) is 100% sensitive and 96% specific for diagnosis of Cushing syndrome.

5. **48 hours low dose dexamethasone suppression test:**

   Procedure:

   a. Plasma cortical to be measured at 9 AM on day 0.

   b. 0.5 mg dexamethasone orally 6 hourly as started from 9 AM for 48 hours.

   c. Collect plasma after 48 hours for plasma cortisol measurement.

   Interpretation:

   a. In normal person, <2 mg/dl plasma cortisol

   b. In patient with Cushing syndrome, plasma cortisol >50 nmol/L.

6. **Standard two-day 2 mg test:**

   Procedure:

   a. Baseline—collection of 24-hour urine sample for urinary free cortisol and 17-hydroxy corticosteroid

   b. Day-1:

      i. Administration of dexamethasone 0.5 mg orally 6 hourly as of 9 AM.

      ii. Collect the urine sample for 24 hours for UFC and 17 OHCS

   c. Day-2:

      i. Administration of dexamethasone 0.5 mg orally 6 hourly with last dose administered at 6 AM on the day-3 morning.

      ii. Collect 24 hours urine sample for UFC and 17 OHCS

   d. Day-3: Collect blood sample for serum cortisol at 8 AM.

   Interpretation: In normal subject—suppression of 24 hours urinary free cortisol excretion <10 mg/24 hours and 17 OHCS <2.5 mg/day

7. **Serum ACTH with serum control:** Sample should be collected.

   a. 8 AM under basal conditions.

   Concomitant serum cortisol measurement along with ACTH—establish—whether hypercortisolism is due to ACTH over production or not.

      i. ACTH value >10 pg/mL with high plasma control suggests hypercortisolemia is due to pituitary tumor or ectopic ACTH production.

      ii. ACTH value <5 pg/dL with raised plasma cortisol level suggests—adrenal adenoma

8. **High dose dexamethasone suppression test:** Collection of 24 hours urine samples for UFC and 17 OHCS after administration of large doe (8 mg/day for 2 days) of dexamethasone—shows:

   i. Suppression of >50% of baseline urinary UFC and 17 OHCS on day 2 indicates—pituitary Cushing's disease.

   ii. Failure of suppression:

      a. Adrenal adenoma or adrenal carcinoma

      b. Ectopic Cushing syndrome

iii. Lack of suppression of cortisol and or its metabolites in subjects having large pituitary macrodenoma.

9. **Metyrapone test:**

Metyrapone blocks the conversion of 11-deoxycortisol to cortisol and dexycorticosterone to corticosterone
↓
These lower the serum level of cortisol and corticosterone
↓
This via—negative feedback increases the ACTH level in blood by stimulating pituitary gland
↓
This in turn increases the secretion of adrenal steroids proximal to block.
750 mg metyrapone 6 hourly orally
↓
This raises plasma ACTH
↓
Which in turn stimulates adrenal cortex to release 11 deoxycortisol >1000 nmol/L.

In patient with ectopic ACTH syndrome—little or no response and level of 11 deoxycortisol is similar to that of Cushing's disease

10. **Corticotropin-releasing hormone test:**

CRH from hypothalamus
↓
Stimulates pituitary to release ACTH
↓
Stimulates adrenal gland to release cortisol
Procedure
1 mg/kg IV. Human CRH or fixed dose of 100 mg IV
↓
Increases ACTH and cortisol level up to 90% in patient with Cushing syndrome due to pituitary cause.

But in case of ectopic ACTH-secreting tumor or adrenal tumor—there is no release of ACTH or cortisol in response to CRH.

So it can distinguish ACTH dependent Cushing syndrome from ACTH independent Cushing's syndrome.

Localization Procedure

1. **MRI of pituitary fossa**—detect 2 mm size tumor with or without gadolinium administration.
2. **CT scan of adrenal gland**—is the initial test of choice because it can detect most of the tumor, because surrounding tissue will be atrophied and suppressed.
3. **MRI of adrenal gland**—may compensate the CT scan of adrenal gland
4. **Ectopic Cushing syndrome:** Full lung CT scan of MRI scan: It can detect bronchial carcinoid, small cell carcinoma of lung hence the procedure of choice. It can also detect:
   i. Thyroid medullary carcinoma producing ACTH
   ii. Ectopic CRH stimulating tumor
5. **Octreotide scintigraphy:** Some ACTH secretory neuroendocrine tumors express somatostatin receptor type-2 and

5—hence can be detected by radiolabeled somatostatin analogs.

Inferior Petrosal Sinus Sampling

Than can distinguish pituitary from non-pituitary ACTH secretion.
i. Samples for ACTH are obtained simultaneously from each inferior petrosal sinus before as well as 2 to 3 and 5–6 minutes after CRH administration.
ii. Inferior petrosal sinus to peripheral ACTH ratio >2.0–3.0—confirms the presence of pituitary ACTH-secreting tumor.
   If ratio is ≤ 1.8—suggests ectopic ACTH-producing tumor.

Treatment (Fig. 3.29)

A. **In ACTH independent Cushing's syndrome:** Removal of adrenal tumor is the treatment of choice.
B. **In Cushing's disease**

Transphenoidal removal of pituitary corticotropic tumor.
↓
After initial remission following surgery followed by late relapse in significant number of patients.

In this case following methods of therapy can be done:
   i. Second surgery
   ii. Radiotherapy
   iii. Steriotactic radiosurgery
   iv. Bilateral adrenalectomy
C. **In severe overt Cushing syndrome:** Where there is difficult to control hypokalemic hypertension or acute psychosis—drugs to control cortisol excess prior to surgery.
D. **Patients with metastasized glucocorticoid producing carcinoma:** Long-term antiglucocorticoid drugs administration.
E. **In case of ectopic ACTH-producing tumor, where tumor cannot be located:** Bilateral adrenalectomy—facilitates immediate cure following by lifelong corticosteroid treatment.

Oral Agents

1. **Metyrapone**—inhibits 11β hydroxylase and thus cortisol synthesis.
   Dose: 500 mg thrice daily—maximum dose—6 gram to start with.
2. **Ketokonazole**—it inhibits early steps in steroidogenesis
   Dose: 200 mg thrice daily.
3. **Mitotane**—an adrenolytic drug—because of its side effect profile—it is most commonly used in adrenocortical carcinoma.
   But low dose treatment (500–1000 mg/day) is used in the treatment of benign Cushing's.
4. **In severe case:** Etomidate can be used to lower cortisol.

Postsurgical Removal of Tumor—Oral Replacement Therapy

Hydrocortisone replacement needs to be started at the time of surgery and slowly tapered following recovery.

This allows physiologic adaptation to normal cortisol levels.

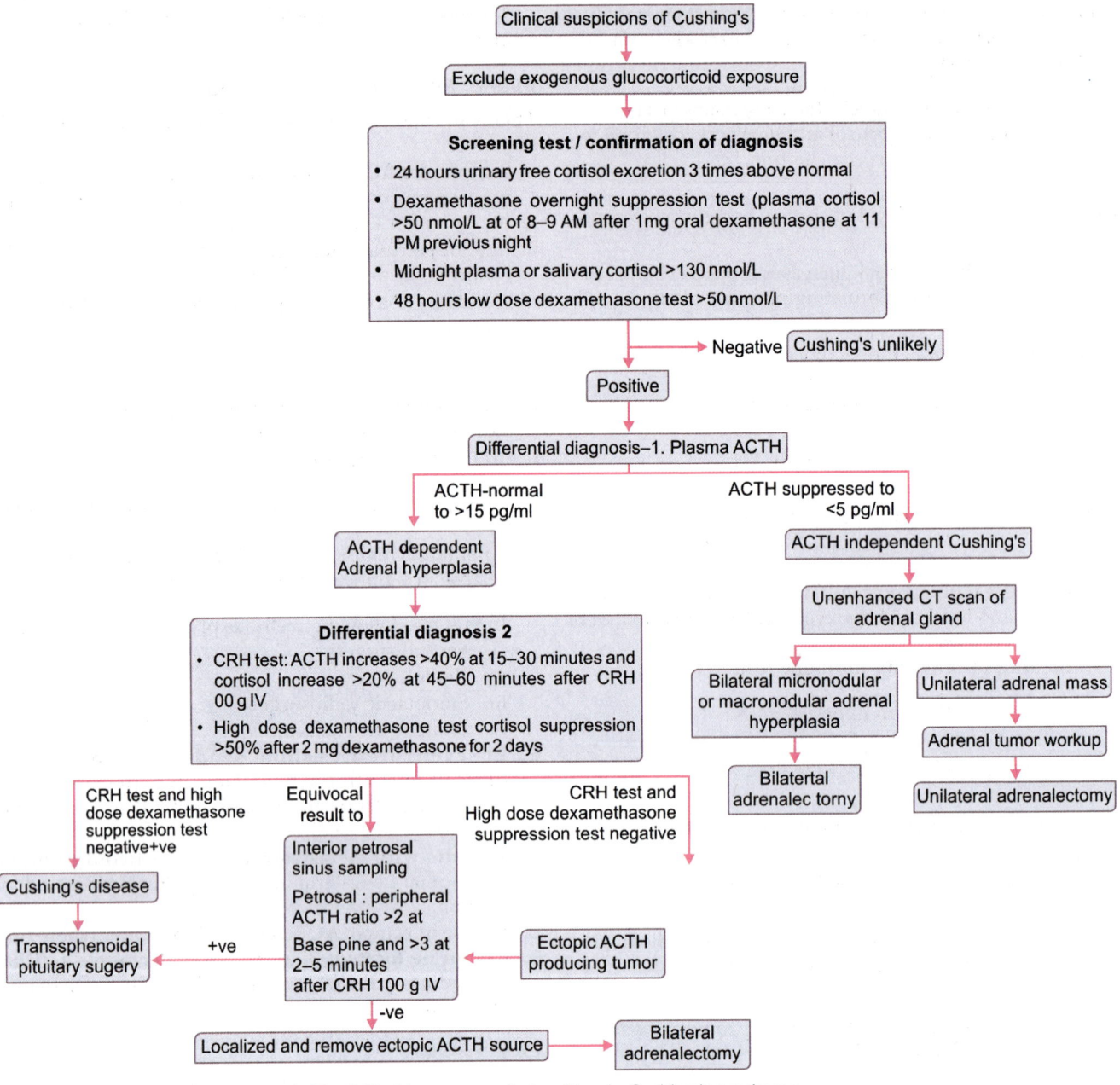

Fig. 3.29: Management algorithm in Cushing's syndrome

ADRENAL INSUFFICIENCY

Causes

I. Primary:
  a. Idiopathic adrenal atrophy
  b. Granulomatous disease
    1. Tuberculosis
    2. Histoplasmosis
    3. Sarcoidosis
  c. Neoplastic infiltration
  d. Hemochromatosis
  e. Amyloidosis
  f. Following bilateral adrenalectomy
  g. ACTH resistance syndrome

II. Secondary:
  a. Tumor

    i. Craniopharyngioma
    ii. Pituitary tumor
    iii. Tumor of third ventricle
  b. Pituitary infarction or hemorrhage.
  c. Postpartum necrosis (Sheehan syndrome).
  d. Hemorrhage in tumor.
  e. Granulomatous disease—Sarcoidosis.
  f. Following hypophysectomy.
  g. Steroid withdrawal.

Clinical Presentation

A. Symptoms and signs caused by glucocorticoid deficiency
  1. Fatigue, lack of energy
  2. Weight loss, anorexia
  3. Malaise
  4. Joint pain

5. Gastrointestinal discomfort ranging from mild diffuse tenderness to chronic or acute abdominal pain, vomiting, diarrhea.

   Gastrointestinal symptoms are more dominant in primary than secondary hypoadrenalism.
6. Hematological—anemia, lymphocytosis eosinophilia.
7. Hypoglycemia—more common in children
8. Low blood pressure, postural hypotension
9. Hyponatremia—due to loss of feedback inhibition of AVP release.

B. Signs and symptoms caused by mineralocorticoid deficiency:
1. Dizziness, postural hypotension
2. Abdominal pain, nausea, vomiting
3. Salt craving
4. Low blood pressure, postural hypotension.
5. Increased serum creatinine (due to volume depletion).
6. Hyponatremia.
7. Hyperkalemia.

C. Signs and symptoms caused by adrenal androgen deficiency:
1. Lack of energy
2. Dry itchy skin (in women)
3. Loss of libido (in women)
4. Loss of axillary and public hair (in women)

D. Other signs and symptoms:
1. In primary adrenal insufficiency due to compensatory increase in ACTH leading to mucocutaneous hyperpigmentation—as ACTH binds to melanocyte receptor-1, which is responsible for pigmentation. Hyperpigmentation can be diffuse, but may be spotty.

   Site of pigmentation:
   i. Lips
   ii. Inner buccal mucous membrane
   iii. Exposed pressure areas, e.g.
       a. Knuckles
       b. Knees
       c. Feet
       d. Elbows
       e. Belt and brassiere lines
2. Multiple freckles and generalized tan—seen along with areas of vitiligo in autoimmune adrenalitis.
3. Alabaster-colored pale skin—in secondary adrenal insufficiency.

Acute Adrenal Insufficiency

Triggering factors:
1. Intercurrent illness
2. Surgical or other stress
3. Increased glucocorticoid inactivation

It occurs after prolonged period of non-specific complaint and observed in patient with primary adrenal insufficiency.

Clinical presentation:
i. Postural hypotension leading to hypovolemic shock
ii. Features of acute abdomen with abdominal tenderness nausea, vomiting, fever

iii. Neurological symptoms—decreased responsiveness, stupor and coma.

Diagnosis of Adrenal Insufficiency

I. Routine biochemical tests:
1. Hyponatremia
2. Hyperkalemia—present in primary adrenal insufficiency, absent in secondary adrenal insufficiency.
3. Increased vasopressin—resulting in increased free water retention.
4. Hyponatremia—depletional in primary but dilutional in secondary with normal blood urea.
5. Hypercalcemia—particularly marked in patient with coexisting thyrotoxicosis.
6. FT_4—is normal but TSH is elevated.

II. Mineralocorticoid status: In primary hypoaldosteronism:
i. Elevated PRA
ii. ↓ Aldosterone

III. Assessment adequacy of function of the HPA axis:
1. *Serum cortisol* > 14.5 mg/dL—indicative of intact HPA axis.

   <3 mg/dl—hypoaldosteronism

2. *ACTH stimulation test (rapid ACTH stimulation test):* IV or IM administration of 250 mg tetracosactin—followed by measurement of plasma cortisol at 0 and 30 minutes:
   i. Normal response >20 mg/dL plasma cortisol—normal value rules out primary adrenal insufficiency
   ii. In secondary adrenal insufficiency—blunted response

3. *ACTH level in serum:*
   i. In primary insufficiency—50–100 pg/mL
   ii. In secondary insufficiency—low or normal 10 pg/mL.

4. *Insulin tolerance test:* It should be carried out under direct supervision of specialist. Induction of hypoglycemia is contraindicated in:
   i. Diabetes patient
   ii. Cardiovascular disease
   iii. History of seizures
   iv. Severe hypopituitarism

   Adequate hypoglycemia (blood glucose (2.2 mmol/L) with signs of neuroglycopenia—sweating, tachycardia

   In normal subject, peak cortisol in plasma is >18 mg/dL.

5. *Low dose (1 μg) ACTH test:* This test is more sensitive and accurate than sensitive that of 250 μg ACTH test. It can detect partial adrenal insufficiency especially in patient with secondary adrenal insufficiency due to:
   i. Chronic glucocorticoid treatment.
   ii. Pituitary tumor

6. *Single dose metyrapone test:* It activates HPA axis by blocking cortisol production at 11 hydroxylase step and lowering control levels.

This test is done to confirm diagnosis of secondary adrenal insufficiency:

i. In normal response—level of 11 deoxycortisol is >7 mg/dl.

ii. In primary or secondary insufficiency level of 11 deoxycortisol will be <5 mg/dl.

An abnormal metyrapone test in patient with near normal ACTH stimulation tests suggests secondary adrenal insufficiency.

Diagnosis of Etiology

1. CT scan: Enlarged or calcified adrenals, suggestive of infective, hemorrhagic or malignancy
2. Chest X-ray
3. Tuberculin test
4. Early morning urine test for—culture of *Mycobacterium tuberculosis*
5. CT-guided adrenal biopsy:
   i. Malignancy
   ii. Tuberculosis
   iii. Sarcoidosis
6. Measurement of circulating level of VLCFA Adrenoleukodystrophy.
7. Pituitary MRI

Treatment (Fig. 3.30)

Acute Adrenal Insufficiency

1. Immediate initiation of rehydration by saline infusion at 1 litre/hour with continuous cardiac monitoring.
2. Glucocorticoid replacement: Bolus injection of 100 mg hydrocortisone will be followed by 100–200 mg over 24 hours, by continuous infusion.
3. Mineralocorticoid replacement—can be initiated when dose of hydrocortisone has been reduced to 50 mg because higher dose of hydrocortisone provides sufficient stimulation of mineralocorticoid receptors.

Chronic Adrenal Insufficiency

1. **Glucocorticoid replacement:** A dose that replaces the physiologic daily cortisol production, e.g.
   i. 15–30 mg hydrocortisone in 2–3 divided doses
   ii. In 3rd trimester of pregnancy increasing dose is required.
   ½ of total dose is to be given in the morning.

   Long-acting glucocorticoid—prednisolone is not preferred because of increased glucocorticoid exposure due to extended glucocorticoid receptor activation.

   Dose equivalency:
   - 1 mg hydrocortisone = 1.6 mg cortisone acetate = 0.25 mg prednisone
   - 30 mg of hydrocortisone or more will affect bone metabolism—hence at regular interval bone mineral density should be measured.
   - In case of fever with intercurrent illness, doubling of daily dose of hydrocortisone is required
   - In case of prolonged vomiting, surgery and trauma—daily 100 mg hydrocortisone injection is required.

2. **Mineralocorticoid replacement:** 100–200 mg fludrocortisones should be initiated.

   Adequacy of treatment can be evaluated by:
   i. Measuring blood pressure—sitting and standing to detect postural hypotension.
   ii. Serum sodium potassium, plasma renin should be measured regularly.

   Change in glucorticoid dose may have also impact on mineralocorticoid replacement because cortisol binds to mineralocorticoid receptors.

   40 mg hydrocortisone is equivalent to 100 mg fludrocortisone.

   The dose of fludrocortisones should be increased during summer.

3. **Adrenal androgen replacement:** This can be achieved by administration of 25–50 mg DHEA. Treatment should be monitored by—measurement of:
   i. DHEA
   ii. Androsterodione
   iii. Testosterone
   iv. SHBG 24 hours after the last dose of DHEA.

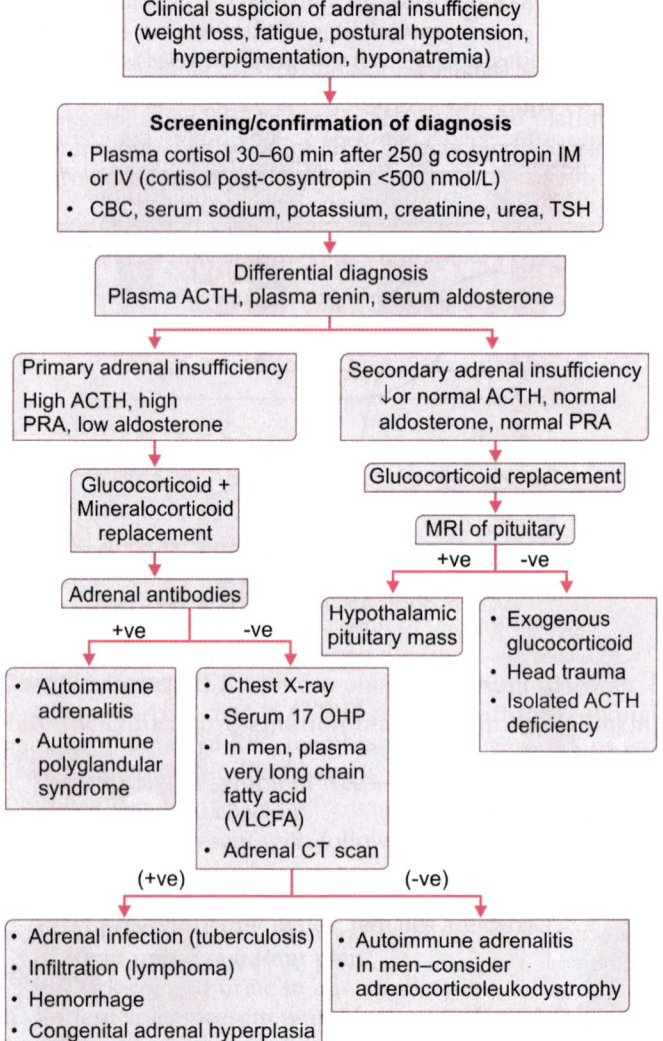

Fig. 3.30: Algorithm for management of patient with suspected adrenal insufficiency

CONGENITAL ADRENAL HYPERPLASIA

21 Hydroxylase deficiency

Disrupts glucorticoid synthesis and mineralocorticoid
synthesis
↓
Negative feedback on HPA axis
↓
Increased secretion of ACTH
↓
Increased synthesis of androgen precursor
↓
Excess androgen production

Diagnostic Marker

i. Glucocorticoid and mineralocorticoid deficiency
ii. Excess androgen production
iii. Excess ACTH production

Diagnostic Marker Steroid in Serum

1. 17 Hydroxyprogesterone
2. 21 deoxycortisol (pregnantriol, 17 hydroxypregnanolone)

Features of Virilizations

1. Virilization of external genitalia in neonatal girl.
2. Hirsutism and oligomenorrhea in young women
   Patient may die in 1st a few weeks of life due to adrenal
crisis (salt wasting crisis)

MINERALOCORTICOID AND GLUCOCORTICOID SYNTHESIS

MINERALOCORTICOID EXCESS

Zona glomerulosa of adrenal cortex secretes aldosterone.
Dexycorticosterone (DOC) is nonaldosterone steroid
having most potent mineralocorticoid efficacy.
Under physiologic conditions—renin–angiotensin system
is the main regulator of aldosterone secretion

A. This renin–angiotensin system responds variably to
volume status of the body.
1. Volume depletion
↓
Induces renin secretion
↓
Angiotensin I
↓
Angiotensin II
↓
Stimulates adrenal cortex (zona glomerulosa)
↓
Aldosterone secretion
↓
Retention of sodium and water
↓
Restoration of blood volume
2. Volume expansion
↓
Reduction of renin, angiotensin I and II and
aldosterone secretion
↓
Facilitation of sodium and water excretion

(Contd.)

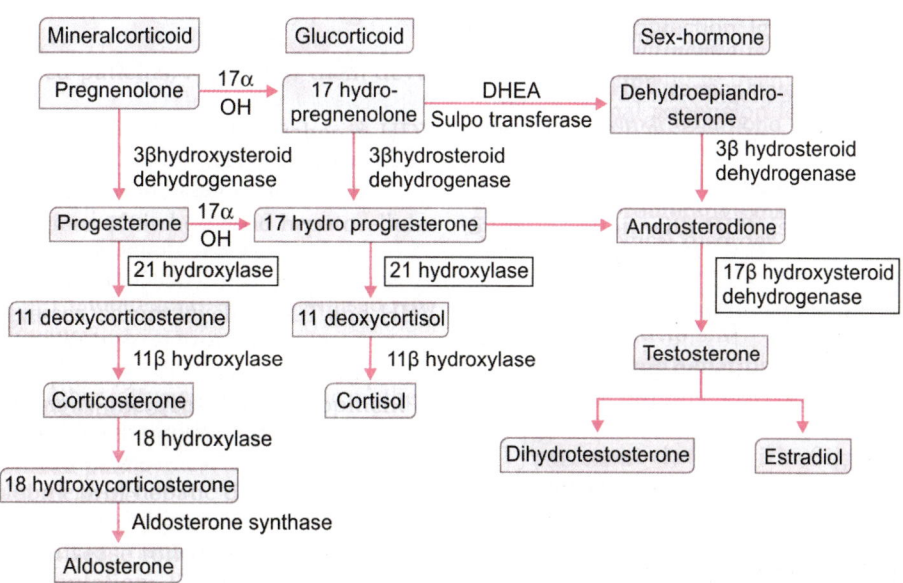

1. 21 hydroxylase deficiency
2. 11β hydroxylase deficiency
3. 17 hydroxylase deficiency

Fig. 3.31: Synthesis of mineralocorticoid and glucocorticoid

(Contd.)

B. Potassium and ACTH stimulates aldosterone secretion directly independent of volume changes.
   1. Increase in serum potassium
      ↓
      Significant stimulation of aldosterone secretion
      ↓
      In turn facilitation of potassium excretion in urine
   2. Low potassium in serum
      ↓
      Decreases in aldosterone level in serum
      ↓
      Diminishes excretion of potassium in urine.

Etiology

Primary aldosteronism implies autonomous hypersecretion of aldosterone. There are five distinct forms:
1. Adrenal aldosterone producing adenoma
2. Idiopathic hyperaldosteronism with bilateral micronodular hyperplasia of adrenal gland
3. Unilateral micronodular adrenal hyperplasia
4. Glucocorticoid—remediable hyperaldosteronism—characterized by bilateral adrenal hyperplasia with reversal of clinical and biochemical abnormalities following glucocorticoid administration.
5. Aldosterone producing adrenal carcinoma.

Clinical Manifestations

Most of the pathophysiological abnormalities in primary hyperaldosteronism can be explained by—effect of excessive aldosterone on sodium and potassium transport so the following features develops gradually:
i. Increased renal tubular resorption of sodium and water leading to volume expansion and hypertension.
ii. Renal excretion of potassium and hydrogen leading to hypokalemia and metabolic alkalosis.

So the clinical features are:
1. Hypertension—most prominent and universal findings.
2. Hypokalemia: If it is <3.5 mEq/L—patient may present with:
   i. Features of volume depletion
   ii. Muscle weakness
   iii. Fatigue
   iv. Cramping
   v. In severe cases—muscle paralysis
   vi. Concentrating defect—leading to polyuria, polydipsia—these are resistant to vasopressin.
       Chronic hypokalemia—may lead to electrographic abnormalities
       a. Widened QT interval   b. U waves
3. Swelling of legs—due to accumulation of extracellular fluid
4. Mild metabolic alkalosis—due to direct aldosterone effect or due to hypokalemia
5. Hypomagnesemia—due to decreased tubular absorption of magnesium

Physical Examination

1. Peripheral edema
2. Bradycardia
3. Postural hypotension
4. Blunted peripheral reflexes.

Diagnosis

Classic triad of biochemical criteria for diagnosis of primary hyperaldosteronism:
1. Hypokalemia with inappropriate kaliuresis
2. Suppressed plasma renin activity
3. Elevated aldosterone level that does not fall appropriately in response to volume expansion or sodium load.

Screening Tests

1. **Plasma aldosterone/renin ratio** (Spironolactone, eplerenone and high dose amiloride must be discontinued for at least 6 weeks prior to testing. In case of mild hypertension, drug withdrawal must be 2–4 weeks prior to testing) If ARR >750 pmol/L:ng/ml/hr—suggests primary aldosteronism.
2. **Plasma renin activity:** Plasma renin activity is suppressed in primary hyperaldosteronism—it occurs in 60 to 80% patient because:
   i. Hypertensive patients are initially treated with diuretics and vasodilators—that stimulate plasma renin activity
   ii. Low PRA is found in elderly.
3. **Aldosterone measurement**: >450 pmol/L
4. **Confirmation tests:** Aldosterone suppression tests—salt loading test: This test is not recommended in:
   i. Severe hypertension   ii. Renal failure
   iii. Congestive heart failure   iv. Cardiac arrhythmia.

Procedure

A. *Saline infusion test:*
   1. Patient should be on regular diet.
   2. Obtain serum K^+, if the level ≥4 mmol/L—this test can be done.
   3. Baseline aldosterone level should be measured.
   4. Infusion of 0.9% sodium chloride at a rate of 500 ml/hour for 4 hours—total 2 litres.
   5. Repeat blood samples for K^+ and aldosterone
      Following infusion, plasma aldosterone will normally drops to 50% for below 5 ng/dl.
      But in case of primary hyperaldosteronism, aldosterone level will be more than 10 ng/dl.

B. *Oral salt loading test:*
   1. Increase sodium intake to >200 mmol/L.
   2. Add slow release potassium chloride tablet to keep potassium level in normal level.
   3. 24-hour urine will be collected to verify that intended intake has been attained.
   4. 24 hours urine collection—to be started on the morning of 3rd day for measuring urinary aldosterone
      Urinary aldosterone excretion >12 to 14 µg/24 hours—suggests primary aldosteronism.
      <10 mg/24 hours excludes the diagnosis of PA.

D. *Test to differentiate adrenal adenoma from benign adrenal hyperplasia:*
   1. Adrenal CT scan and MRI
   2. Adrenal vein sampling for aldosterone concentration
      Episodic secretion of aldosterone should be avoided by:
      i. Simultaneous sampling from both adrenal glands
      ii. If samples are collected following injection of ACTH.
   3. Adrenal radioisotope scanning with iodocholesterol or NP-59 is often helpful in differential diagnosis of primary hyperaldosteronism:

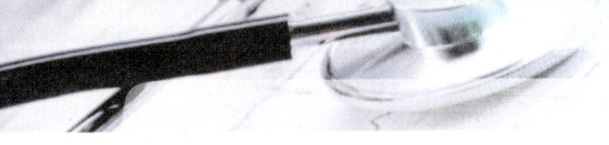

i. Unilateral and asymmetrical uptake indicates adrenal adenoma.
ii. Bilateral diffuse uptake—suggests adrenal hyperplasia.

Ancillary tests in equivocal cases—Posture test: Aldosterone producing adenoma—responsive to ACTH but not to angiotensin II.

But benign adrenal neoplasia is responsive to angiotensin.

Procedure:
1. Blood samples for PRA and plasma aldosterone are obtained between 8 to 9 AM after patient becomes in supine position for 30 minutes.
2. Patient becomes upright position and ambulates moderately for 4 hours—during this times blood samples are collected again.

Interpretation:
i. In normal person: In upright posture—PRA—aldosterone
ii. In case of aldosterone secreting adenoma: ↓PRA, ↓↓ Aldosterone

iii. In benign adrenal hyperplasia: ↑PRA, ↑aldosterone in upright posture—indicates—partially intact renin response and enhanced sensitivity to adrenal gland.

Plasma 18 hydroxycorticosterone:
i. >100 ng/dL—suggests APA
ii. <50 ng/dL—suggests BAH

Treatment (Fig. 3.32)

1. **Aldosterone producing tumor:**
   i. Surgical removal of gland is the treatment of choice.
   ii. Potassium repletion by oral potassium supplementation.
   iii. Preoperative treatment with mineralocorticoid antagonist.

2. **Benign adrenal hyperplasia:** This patient should be treated medically:
   i. *Spironolactone* (12.5 to 200 mg daily) is the drug of choice, but long term treatment is associated with:
      a. Impotence
      b. Gynecomastia, c. menstrual disorder.

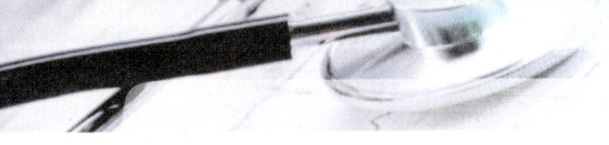

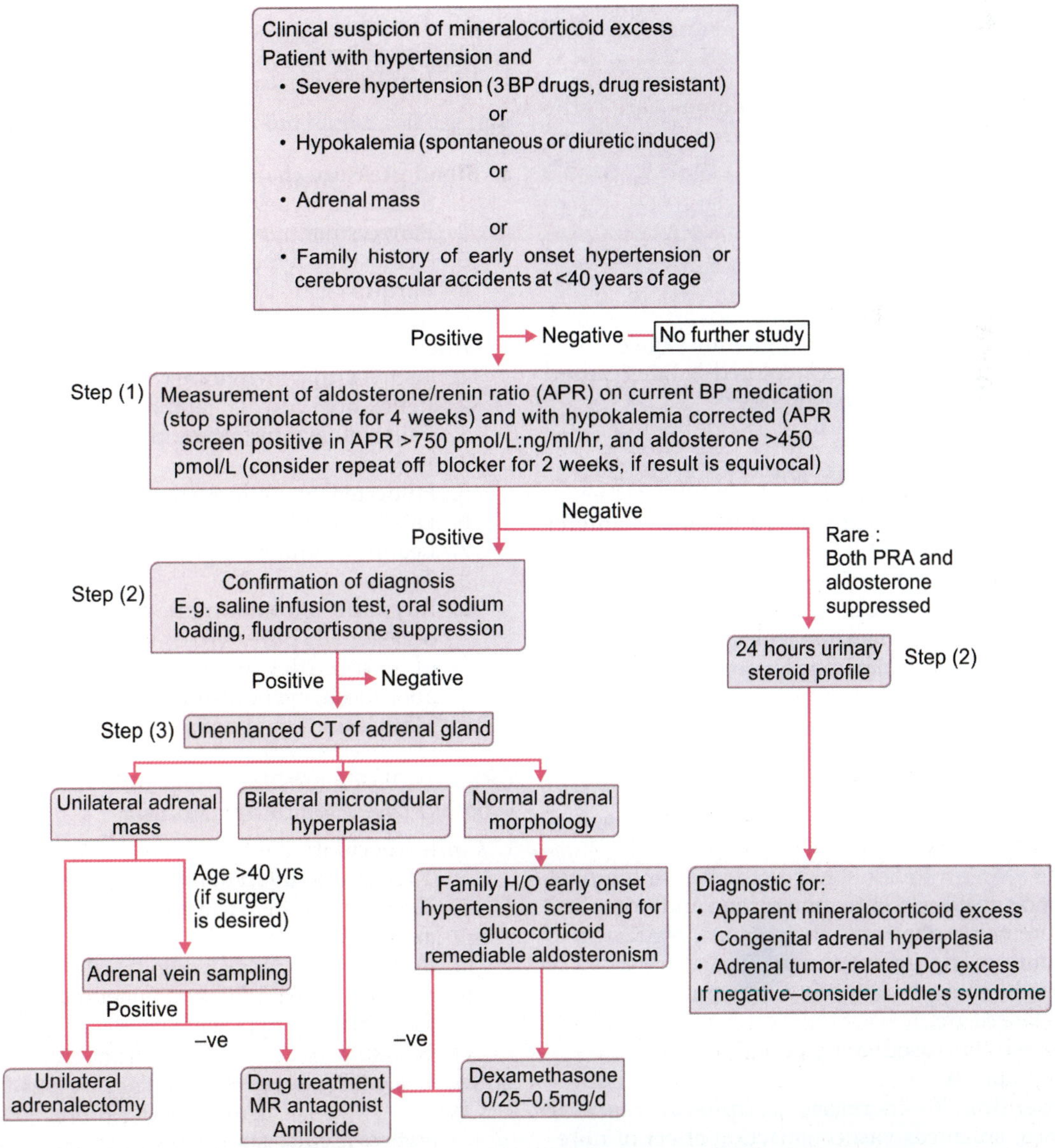

Fig. 3.32: Algorithm for management of patient with mineralocorticoid excess

ii. *Eplerenone*: Alternative mineralocorticoid receptor antagonist—if does not interact with androgen or progesterone receptor—it is not available now.

iii. *Amiloride:* 40 mg/day—acts on renal tubular cells independent of aldosterone activity.

It is successful therapeutic agent in the treatment of primary aldosterotism.

Liddle Syndrome

i. Familial disorder.

ii. Hypertension and hypokalemic alkalosis

iii. Absence of excessive secretion of any of known mineralocorticoids

iv. Defect is increased reabsorption of sodium and chloride and enhanced secretion of potassium in distal convulated tubule.

v. Hypertension and hypokalemia are relieved by either amiloride (10 to 40 mg daily) or triamterene (100 mg 4 times daily in divided doses)

vi. ↓PRA and ↓aldosterone

PHEOCHROMOCYTOMA

Definition

Pheochromocytoma and paraganglioma are the catecholamine producing tumor derived from sympathetic and parasympathetic nervous system.

Etiopathogenesis

Pheochromocytoma and paraganglioma are well vascularized tumor—arising from:

1. Adrenal medulla—sympathetic
2. Parasympathetic—carotid body and glomus vagale.

Pheochromocytoma—reflects black-colored staining caused by chromaffin oxidation of catecholamines.

Anatomy

Pheochromocytoma presents as:

i. Benign, vascularized, encapsulated lesions, diameter 5 cm, weight <70 gm.

ii. 10% becomes malignant.

iii. Adrenal pheochromocytoma—more frequent in adult.

iv. Extra-adrenal pheochromocytoma—locations:
   a. Superior and inferior para-aortic areas—80% cases
   b. Thorax
   c. Bladder
   d. Head
   e. Neck
   f. Pelvis

Biochemistry

i. Pheochromocytoma secretes epinephrine and norepinephrine, more norepinephrine

ii. It can produce only norepinephrine

iii. It rarely produces epinephrine and dopamine

iv. Other substances are:
   a. Adrenomedulin (vasodilating peptide)
   b. Chromogranin A,
   c. Neuropeptide Y—increases peripheral vascular resistance, enhances vasoconstricting effect of norepinephrine.

Clinical Manifestations

Symptoms

a. Common:
1. Headache
2. Sweating
3. Palpitations with or without tachycardia
4. Nervousness
5. Weight loss
6. Chest and abdominal pain
7. Nausea with or without vomiting
8. Weakness or fatigue

b. Less common:
1. Visual disturbances
2. Constipation
3. Warmth
4. Dyspnea
5. Paresthesia
6. Flushing
7. Polyuria
8. Polydipsia
9. Tightness by throat
10. Tinnitus
11. Dysarthria
12. Painless hematuria

Signs

a. Blood pressure changes:
1. Sustained hypertension
2. Paroxysmal hypertension
3. Orthostatic hypotension
4. Paradoxical blood pressure response to some antiarrhythmic drugs

b. Other signs:
1. Tachycardia, arrhythmia
2. Reflex bradycardia, fetal heart beat
3. Pallor of face and upper part of body
4. Anxious, frightened
5. Hypertensive retinopathy
6. Dilated pupils
7. Leanness, underweight
8. Tremor
9. Raynaud's phenomenon or livedo reticularis—occasionally puffy, red cyanotic hands in children, skin of extremities is wet, cold, clammy, and pale, gooseflesh, cyanotic nail beds
10. Mass lesions in abdomen or neck

Manifestations Related to Complications of Co-existing Diseases or Syndromes

1. Cardiovascular:
   i. Myocardial infarction
   ii. Congestive heart failure with or without cardiomyopathy
   iii. Arrhythmias
   iv. Cardiac arrest following general anesthesia
   v. Unexplained hypotension
   vi. Shock
   vii. Dissecting aneurysm

2. CNS:
   i. Cerebrovascular accident
   ii. Hypertensive encephalopathy

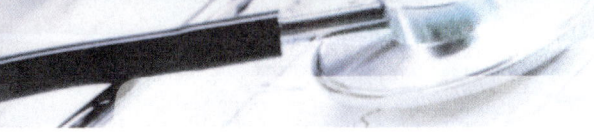

3. Gastrointestinal:
  i. Ischemic enterocolitis
  ii. Cholelithiasis
4. Renal: Azotemia
5. Pregnancy related: Severe pre-eclampsia during pregnancy, fever, shock, sudden death.

Urine should be assayed for:
1. Fractionated metanephrines (normetanephrine and metanephrine)
2. Free catecholamines (epinephrine and norepinephrine)
3. Vanilmandelic acid

  Serum level: Catecholamine >2000 pg/mL.
  Measurement of plasma metanephrine is most sensitive and is less susceptible to false positive elevation from stress including venipuncture.

Drugs those may increase measured level of fractionated catecholamines:
  i. TCA
  ii. Levodopa
  iii. Drugs containing adrenergic receptor agonists (decongestants)
  iv. Amphetamines
  v. Prochlorperazine
  vi. Reserpine
  vii. Withdrawal of clonidine
  viii. Illicit drugs (cocaine, heroin)
  ix. Ethanol

Treatment (Fig. 3.33)

Main aim is removal of tumor.

Preoperative Preparation

1. α-adrenergic blocker (phenoxybenzamine)—initiated with 5–10 mg three times per day, gradually increasing the dose up to 20–30 mg three times daily.
2. Paroxysms can be controlled by: Oral prazosin or intravenous phentolamine
     Before surgery blood pressure should be consistently <160/90 mmHg.
3. Beta-blockers – 10 mg propranolol orally three to four times daily to control tachycardia.
4. Calcium channel blocker or angiotensin-converting enzyme inhibitor.

Medications during and Postoperatively

1. Nitroprusside infusion is useful for intraoperative crises
2. Hypotension can be lived by volume infusion

Methods of Surgery

1. Endoscopic surgery—transperitoneal or retroperitoneal approach
2. Open surgery.

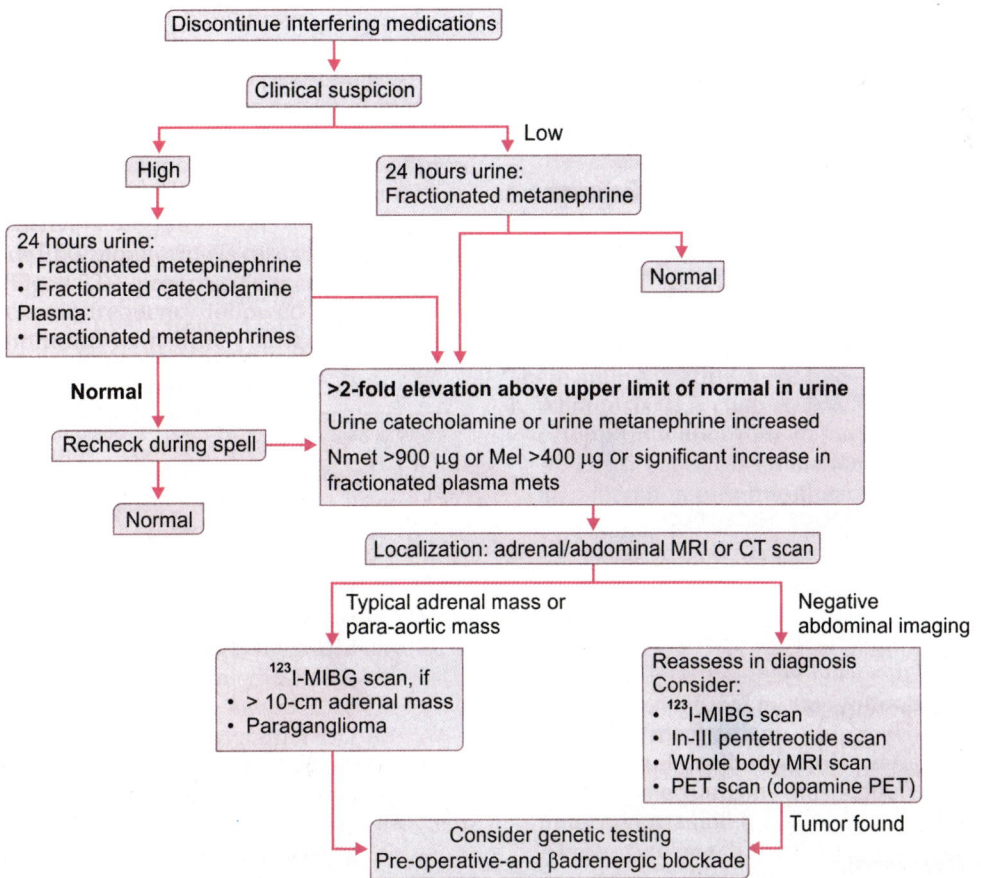

Fig. 3.33: Algorithm for management of pheochromocytoma

* I-MIBG—Metaiodobenzyl guanidine using radioiodine—diagnostic value 78% specificity; III I—somatostatin analogues

4

Gastrointestinal Disorders

LUMINAL GASTROENTEROLOGY

ESOPHAGUS

ESOPHAGEAL MOTOR DISORDERS

Dysphagia

This is characterized by impediment in the movement of food from mouth to stomach.

Swallowing involves three phases:

1. In 1st phase: This is called preparatory phase. During this stage, there is evidence of chewing, mixing with saliva, shaping and positioning of food bolus with the help of teeth, tongue or oral cavity.
2. In 2nd phase: The bolus is being propelled from the oral cavity into the pharyx, during which airway will be protected.
3. In the 3rd phase: The bolus will be transported thoughout the esophageal cavity.

Odynophagia: This is pain during swallowing.

Globus hystericus: There is no difficulty in swallowing, but there is sensation of lump or fullness in the throat.

Aphagia: This is characterized by impaction of food bolus in the esophageal cavity, so that no food (solid or liquid) will pass beyond the site of impaction.

Commonest Causes of Globus Sensation

i. Anxiety disorders
ii. Gastroesophageal reflux disease
iii. Goiter
iv. Early case of hypopharyngeal cancer

Classifications of Dysphagia

Two types of dysphagia are (Table 4.1):
1. Oropharyngeal dysphagia
2. Esophageal dysphagia

Oropharyngeal Dysphagia

This dysphagia usually involves 1st and 2nd phases of swallowing during which the food will be prepared as blus

Table 4.1: Differences between oropharyngeal and esophageal dysphagia

Esophageal dysphagia	Oropharyngeal dysphagia
1. Organ specific—esophageal cancer, esophageal motor disorders	1. Systemic—Parkinson's disease, myasthenia gravis
2. Expandable organ—one function only	2. Non-expandable organ—functions like, speech swallowing, respiratoion
3. Treatable—operation or dilatation	3. Non-treatable usually
4. Associated symptoms—chest pain, water brush, regurgitation	4. Associated symptoms—weekness, ptosis, cough

and transferring the prepared bolus from oral cavity to esophageal cavity. The causes of oropharyngeal dysphagia are:

I. **Propulsive disorders:**
  A. *Neurological causes:*
    a. Cerebrovascular accident
    b. Parkinson's disease
    c. Amyotrophic lateral sclerosis
    d. Multiple sclerosis
  B. *Degenerative diseases:*
    a. Cerebral palsy
    b. Recurrent laryngeal nerve palsy
    c. Alzheimer disease
    d. Friedreich ataxia
  C. *Muscular causes:*
    a. Muscular dystrophy
    b. Eaton-Lambert syndrome
    c. Myasthenia gravis
    d. Dermatomyositis
  D. *Metabolic causes:*
    a. Hypothyroidism
    b. Hyperthyroidism
    c. Myxedema
  E. *Inflammatory causes:*
    a. Systemic lupus erythematosus
    b. Amyloidosis

F. *Infectious causes:*
   a. AIDS
   b. Syphilis
   c. Meningitis
   d. Diphtheria
II. **Structural causes:**
   A. *Benign causes:*
      a. Cricopharyngeal web
      b. Hypopharyngeal diverticulum
      c. Cervical spondylosis
   B. *Neoplasm*
   C. *Dental causes:*
      a. Dental abnormality
      b. Toothache
      c. Gingivitis
   D. *Infections:*
      a. Pharyngeal ulceration
      b. Pharyngeal abscess
      c. Pharyngitis
   E. *Autoimmune disorders:*
      a. Crohn's disease
      b. Behcet disease
   F. *Extrinsic compression:*
      a. Goiter
      b. Cervical lymphadenopathy
III. **Iatrogenic causes:**
   A. Radiation induced:
      a. Xerostomic
      b. Myopathy
   B. Drug induced:
      a. Steroid-induced myopathy
      b. Tardive dyskinesia
      c. Chemotherapy induced mucositis.
   C. Surgery
   D. Prosthetic
      a. Ill-fitted denture

Clinical presentation of oropharyngeal dysphagia:
a. Inability to initiate swallowing process
b. Coughing
c. Choking sensation
d. Nasopharyngeal regurgitation
e. Drooling of saliva during deglutination
f. Ptosis
g. Photophobia, visual changes
h. Progressive weakness of oropharyngeal muscles during swallowing at the end of the day.

In case of brainstem stroke: Swallowing centers present bilaterally in reticular substance below the tractus solitarius nucleus. From here, efferent fibers go to motor nucleus of ambiguous controlling musculature of swallowing. So in brainstem stroke:
i. Difficulty in initiating swallow
ii. Absence of swallow response

But most of the stroke-related dysphagia will be recovered within 2 weeks. If symptomatic and no improvement occur in 2 weeks, then swallowing function should be evaluated.

In case of myasthenia gravis: There is progressive destruction of acetylcholine receptors striated muscles in esophagus. Hence during repeatitive swallowing process, there is progressive worsening of dysphagia due to weakness of striated muscles in esophagus.

But after taking some rest, patient can start swallowing due to improvement of the swallowing controlling muscles, because, there will be reaccumulation of acetylcholine near the acetylecholine receptor.

Esophageal Diverticula

According to location, this can be subdivided into three types:
1. **Epiphrenic diverticula:** This is associated with achalasia or distal esophageal stricture
2. **Mid-esophageal diverticula:** It is caused by traction from adjacent inflammation as in case of traction by tuberculosis lymph nodes.

   It involves all the layers of esophageal wall. It may be associated with esophageal motor disorder pulsion diverticulum.

   Symptoms: Usually they are assymptomic, but when they enlarge sufficiently, they produce:
   i. Dysphagia due to pressure on esophageal wall due to retention of food
   ii. Regurgitation of the accumulated food

   Treatment: It can be removed surgically in conjunction with myotomy.

   Small epiphrenic diverticula should not be resected since it is usually associated with motility disorder, manometry should be performed and it will dictate the operative procedure—which may include long myotomy of lower esophageal sphincter.

   There may be recurrence after myotomy.
3. **Zenker's diverticulum (hypopharyngeal diverticulum)**
   Causes: Increased intraluminal pressure with distal obstruction. Here obstruction is at the cricopharyngeal muscle (upper esophageal sphincter)

   The herniation is at hypopharynx in the area of natural weakness (Killan's triangle).

Presentation:
i. Small diverticulum is usually asymptomatic
ii. In case of large Zenker's diverticulum:
   a. Dysphagia
   b. Halitosis
   c. Food aspiration

Treatment:
i. Surgical diverticulectomy and cricopharyngeal myotomy
ii. Marsupialization—endoscopic staping device

   Complications following endoscopic therapy for Zenker's diverticulum:
   i. Aspriation
   ii. Sedation
   iii. Perforation
   iv. Bleeding

Esophageal Ring and Web

Lower Esophageal Mucosal Ring (B Ring)

   i. It is a thin membranous ring.
   ii. It is present at squamocolumnar junction.
   iii. It occurs in 15% of people

Clinical presentation:
a. It is usually asymptomatic.
b. When its diameter is <13 mm, it is called Schatzki ring.

These patients present with:
1. Episodic solid food dysphagia
2. These patients are [3] 40 years of old.
3. These rings are usually acquired.
4. These may be responsible for intermittent food impaction—which is also called "steakhouse syndreome".

Treatment: Dilatation of ring by large diameter bougie repeatedly.

Upper Esophageal Ring or Web (A Ring)

Site: It usually originates along the anterior aspect of upper esophagus.

Origin: It may be congenital or acquired inflammatory.

Clinical presentation:
1. It occurs in 10% of people.
2. It is usually asymptomatic.
3. If it is circumferential, it may produce intermittent dysphgtia.

Treatment: Dilatation of the ring

Association: If this upper esophageal web is associated with iron deficiency anemia in middle aged women, it is called Plummer-Vinson syndrome.

Dysphagia Lusoria

Lusoria mean "a trick of nature". So it is characterized by impringement of aberrant vasculature on proximal esophagus.

This involves abnormal subclavian artery arising from left side of aortic arch compresses esophagus.

Diagnosis:
1. Barium swallow with marshmallow or barium pill
2. Manometry
3. Magnetic resonance imaging

Hiatus Hernia

This is characterized by herniation of stomach into the mediastenum through esophageal hiatus or diaphragm.

Hiatus hernia is of four types:
1. **Type-I:** It is commonest, 95% of total hiatus hernia.
   Anatomical pathology: Here gastroesophageal junction and gastric cardia ascend upwards due to weekening of phrenoesophageal ligament, which attaches gastroesophageal junction to the diaphragm at the hiatus. The causes of sliding type hiatus hernia are:
   a. Increased abdominal pressure:
      i. Obesity
      ii. Pregnancy
      iii. Heredietary cause
   b. Swallowing
   c. Respiration
   Clinical presentation: The patient is usually presents with symptoms of GERD.
2. **Type-II:** It is a paraesophageal hernia, where gastric fundus herniates along with other structure into the mediastinum. In this type, sometimes stomach will be up side down.
3. **Type-III:** It is a paraesophageal hernia, when gastric fundus along with gastroesophageal junction herniates into the mediastinum. In case of large paraesophageal hernia, stomach may be up side down producing volvulus.

So surgical repair is required in case of large para-esophageal hernia.
4. **Type-IV:** In this type of paraesophageal hernia, abnormal structures other than the stomach herniates into the mediastinum.

In case of type I esophageal hernia, head end of the bed should be elevated to prevent the ascent of food into esophagus.

Achalasia Cardia

Achalasia cardia is characterized by following cardinal features:
i. Failure of lower esophageal sphincter to relax.
ii. Aperistalsis or severe hypoperistalsis of body of the esophagus. Age incidence is 25 to 60 years.
   Prevalence is 8 cases per 1000 population.
   Sex incidence—it is equal in both sexes.

Pathophysiology: There are two types of neurons present in esophageal wall:
i. Excitatory ganglionic neuron (cholinergic)—it is variably affected.
ii. Inhibitory ganglionic neuron (nitric oxide)—it is mostly affected.

Inhibitory neuron—is:
i. Responsible for relaxation of LES.
ii. Responsible for propagative peristalsis of the body of the esophagus.

So absence of inhibitory neuronal function is responsible for:
i. Inability of LES relaxation
ii. Aperistalsis of esophagus

Here at the site of involvement, there is accumulation of inflammatory infiltrate involving mainly mononuclear cells, in myenteric plexus.

Vigorous Achalasia

This is characterized by prominent contraction in the body of the esophagus—which can be diagnosed by manometry or radiography. Here the contraction is simultaneous and fulfil the definition of aperistalsis which is required for the diagnosis of achalasia.

This should be separated from isoberic waves which can be evidenced in patient with achalasia. This wave is being generated by bolus of food—this is bolus-induced passive fluctuations in pressure within common cavity of dilated esophagus.

Etiology

Though etiology is not known specifically, but following may be the possibilities:
1. **Viral etiology:** Herpes virus or measles virus may be responsible, because in some myotomy specimen, there is presence of herpes virus.
2. **Autoimmune etiology:** Because of the following evidences—it has been speculated to be an autoimmune disease:
   i. Immunohistochemical evidence of T cell infiltrates in the myenteric plexus.
   ii. This disease may be associated with certain class II human leukocyte antigens like DQB1, DQA1, DQW1.

Causes of Achalasia

1. It is mostly acquired disease occurs in both sexes, rare below the age of 20 years.

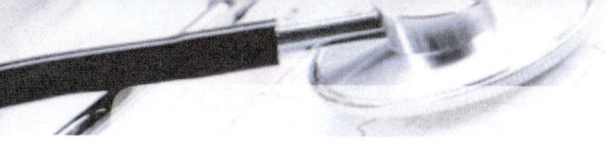

2. There may be evidences of familial cases:
   i. Triple A syndrome—achalasia, alacrima and resistance to adrenocorticotropic hormone are the characteristics of this disease.
   ii. Alport syndrome

Clinical Presentation

1. **Dysphagia:**
   i. Dysphagia though may occur due to ingestion of solid and liquids, but solid food dysphagia is the characteristics than liquid food.
   ii. Some patient may present with dysphagia in the region of LES.
2. Regurgitation of food:
   i. It may be active
   ii. It may be induced by recumbent position or bending
   iii. Sometimes, in the morning after wakening, the patient may find the remnants of previous night food in the mouth
3. Weight loss
4. Pulmonary symptoms
   i. Aspiration pneumonia
   ii. Lung abscess
5. Chest pain—two types of chest pain:
   i. Obstructive type—this is due to swallowing of food bolus—which will be relieved after passage of food through LES to stomach cavity.
   ii. Second type—it is unrelated to eating—it is present in vigorous achalasia—the cause may be due to abnormalities in sensory pathways. Pain may be radiated to neck, arm, jaw and back.
6. Heart burn—it may be due to:
   i. Lactic acid production due to bacterial breakdown of retained food.
   ii. Reflux of true acid from stomach cavity.

Associated Involvement

Stomach and pylorus may also be involved due to absence of inhibitory nerve in those places.

Investigations

1. Barium meal of esophagus—shows:
   i. In early case, normal size esophagus and prominent non-peristaltic contraction.
   ii. Sigmoid esophagus—this is evidenced by elongated dilated esophagus—it is seen in long-standing disease
   iii. Smoothly narrowed gastroesophageal junction—giving rise to bird's beak appearance.
   iv. Only small amount of barium will pass through LES into stomach cavity.
2. Endoscopic findings:
   a. Normal in early cases
   b. In obvious cases:
      i. Esophageal dilatation
      ii. Varying amount of esophageal secretions or food material seen in esophageal cavity
      iii. Lack of contractions or vigorous contractions in esophageal body.
3. Esophageal muscosa shows:
   i. Erythema
   ii. Erosion or
   iii. Ulcerations

It may be due to:
   i. Candida infection, or
   ii. Retained food material
4. Tight but elastic feeling at gastroesophageal junction during passage of endoscope through GE junction.
   But in ability of passage of endoscope through GE junction inspite of giving moderate amount of pressure—is mainly due to:
   i. Inflammatory
   ii. Neoplastic structure

Secondary achalasia: The causes are:
   i. Cancer
   ii. Chagas disease
   iii. Amyloidosis
   iv. Other infiltrative disorders
   v. Mixed connective tissue disorder
   vi. Endocrine disorders

Manometric feature: Two cardinal features are:
   i. Lack of peristalsis of the body of the stomach
   ii. Abnormal relaxation of LES in response to swallowing—which is >90% relaxation.

Chance of malignancy in achalasia cardia:
   i. Achalasia is premalignant.
   ii. It occurs in mid-stomach.
   iii. It is squamous cell carcinoma.
   iv. Symptoms occur until late stage.
   v. Prevalence of carcinoma in achalasia is 3%.

Causes of malignancy in achalasia:
   i. Long-standing stasis of food in esophageal cavity
   ii. Secondary changes in esophageal epithelium

Treatment of Achalasia Cardia

Treatment is palliative.
A. Pharmacological treatments:
   i. Calcium channel blocker
   ii. Nitrates
      The above drugs produce smooth muscle relaxation
   iii. Botulinum toxin injection at LES: This drug—blocks exitatory neural input in LES by inhibiting release of ACh
B. Mechanical treatment: Balloon dilatation— it produces partial tear at LES.
C. Surgical treatment: Surgical myotomy—it is straight forward therapy

Dosage of drugs:
a. Isosorbide dinitrate 5–10 mg sublingually. Action starts within 15 minutes and it lasts for 90 minutes.
b. Nifedipine—it is more effective than verapamil. Action starts within 45 minutes and lasta >1 hour

Dosage of botulinum toxin: Botulinum toxin A has to be diluted in a normal saline to produce a solution 20U/ml

In LES region, it will be injected 1 cm above z line.

Diffuse Esophageal Spasm

Definition: This is characterized by episodes of dysphagia along with chest pain, which may be due to abnormal contraction of esophagus

Pathophysiology: It is ill defined.

Clinical Presentation

Chest pain—it is episodic, non-exertional, prolonged pain. It is aggravated by meals, it interrupts sleep. It is relieved by antacids.

Associated symptoms:

i. Heart burn
ii. Dysphagia
iii. Regurgitation

Radiologically: Presence of tertiary contractions; known as "cork screw esophagus", "rosary bead esophagus" pseudo-diverticula.

Manometric studies: The following are the spectrum of findings:

i. Incoordinate activities of distal esophagus
ii. Spontaneous and repetitive contracts of wall of esophagus
iii. Contraction of high amplitude and prolonged character

High resolution manometric studies show:

i. In diffuse esophageal spasm—there is evidence of propagated contraction at the onset of contraction, but later on it becomes non-propagated.
ii. In nutcracker exphagus extraordinary vigorus and repetitive contractions—this is propagating.

Treatment

1. **Medical therapy:** Followings drugs can be given but with less benefit.
   a. Nitrates,
   b. Calcium channel blocker
   c. Vasodilator hydralazine
   d. Botulinum toxin
   e. Anxiolytics
2. **Surgical therapy (rare):**
   a. Long myotomy
   Or b. Esophagectomy

BARRETT'S ESOPHAGUS

This is defined as metaplastic changes at the lower end of esophagus, where squamous epithelium of esophageal mucosa will be changed to intestinal epithelium, a pre-malignant epithelium.

Diagnosis of Barrett's Esophagus

Mainly two techniques are necessary:

1. Endoscopy—it can recognize abnormal esophageal epithelium.
2. Biopsy—it can detect intestinal metaplasia.
   Newer technically advanced methods have been discovered. These are:
   i. Confocal microendoscopy
   ii. Spectroscopy
   iii. Fluorescence imaging
   iv. Optical coherence tomography
   v. High resolution endoscopy.

Extent of Barrett's Esophagus

i. Tongue-shaped intestinal metaplasia in distal esophagus
ii. Circumferential intestinal metaplasia in entire length.

Following people should be screened for Barrett's esophagus
1. Old white men
2. Reflux symptoms for long duration

3. Smokers
4. Obesity

Treatment

Aims of Treatment

1. Control of reflux symptoms
2. Healing of erosive esophagitis
3. Prevention of adenocarcinoma

Treatment Option

Medical treatment: Proton pump inhibitor
Surgical treatment: Laparoscopic fundoplication

Indications of Surgery

1. For younger patients:
   i. Who are non-complaint.
   ii. Who are not willing to take daily medication.
2. For all patients—who are not adequately controlled with medications.

Future Advances

1. Newer endoscopic technique should be searched to remove dysplastic and metaplastic epithelium.
2. Searching for biomarkers which will be helpful for detection of subgroup of patients who are at risk of development of Barrett's esophagus.

ESOPHAGITIS

Eosinophilic Esophagitis

This is characterized by combination of:

i. Typical esophageal symptoms
ii. Histological demonstration of eosinophilic infiltration of squamous epithelium of esophageal mucosa

Age incidence: It occurs in both children and adults.

Etiology

A. primary—idiopathic
B. Secondary:
   i. GERD
   ii. Drug-induced hypersensitivity
   iii. Connective tissue disorders
   iv. Infections
   v. Hypereosinophilic syndrome
   vi. Allergen:
      1. Dietary
      2. Aeroallergens

Clinical Presentation

i. Dysphagia with food impaction—EOE should be considered first in children and adult in absence of organic cause
ii. A typical chest pain
iii. Heart burn refractory to therapy with proton pump inhibitor
iv. History of allergy, eczema, asthma and allergic rhinitis

Laboratory Working

1. Serum level of the following will be elevated:
   i. Cytokines—IL-5, exotoxin
   ii. Thymus-related chemokines

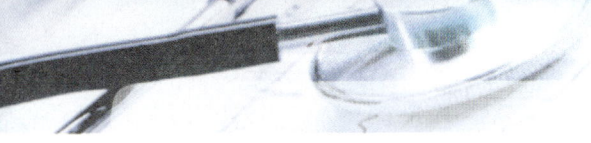

2. Endoscopic finding:
   i. Multiple esophageal rings
   ii. Linear furrows
   iii. Punctate exudates
   iv. Narrowed esophagus
   v. Esophageal stricture
3. Histologically:
   i. Demonstration of increased eosinophils in esophageal squamous epithelium—it is ≥15 eosinophils/HPF
   ii. Evidence of fibrosis.

Complications

i. Food impaction
ii. Esophageal perforation

Treatment

1. Dietary restriction—especially allergic food should be avoided

2. Proton pump inhibition + dietary restriction
   ↓
   If the symptoms persist even after PPI
   ↓
   Topical glucocorticoids (fluticasone propionate or budesonide
   +
   Dietary restriction
   ↓
   If symptoms persist
   ↓
   Systemic glucorticoids

3. Surgical treatment
   Esophageal dilatation

Infectious Esophagitis

Commonest causes are:
A. In normal person:
   i. Candida albicans
   ii. Herpes simplex
B. In immunocompromised individual:
   i. Cytomegalovirus
      When CD4 count >200—it is rare
      When CD4 count <100—it is common
   ii. Self-limited IRIS syndrome

Candida Esophagitis

It is present in:
i. Normal individual
ii. Association with motor disorder
iii. Association with diverticula

Clinical Presentation

A. Most common symptoms:
   i. Odynophagia
   ii. Dysphagia
B. Less common symptoms:
   i. Heart burn
   ii. Chest pain
   iii. Nausea
   iv. Dysgeusia
   v. Bleeding

Signs: Oral thrush may be present.

Endoscopic findings: Discrete adherent creamy friable white plaque with or without exudates.

Microscopic examination:
i. Mucosal invasion by budding yeast
ii. Presence of mycelial forms

Barium swallow of esophagus: It is very much less sensitive. The following findings may be seen:
i. Multiple nodules
ii. Diffuse mucosal ulcerations

Risk Factors for Production of Candida Esophagitis

   i. HIV infection
   ii. Hematologic malignancies
   iii. Non-hematologic malignancies
   iv. Diabetes mellitus
   v. Adrenal dysfunction
   vi. Alcoholism
   vii. Advanced age
   viii. Radiation therapy for thoracic malignancies
   ix. Immunosuppressive treatment in case of transplant individual.

Treatment

1. Orally fluconazole 200 mg—1st day
   ↓
   100 mg daily × 7–12 days
   ↓
   Refractory to fluconazole
   ↓
   Itraconazole—200 mg/day × 7–14 days.

2. Refractory to oral drugs or poorly responsive
   i. Intravenous echinocandin (capsufungin) 50 mg daily × 7–21 days
   ii. Intravenous amphotericin B = 10–15 mg infusion for 6 hours daily up to total dose of 300–500 mg

Herpetic Esophagitis

Etiology

i. Herpes simplex type 1 and 2
ii. Varicella zoster virus in children with chickenpox and in case of adult with zoster

Lesions

Endoscopic findings:
i. Small discrete vesicles in esophagus
ii. Punched out ulcers
   All the lesions are limited to squamous epithelium

Histological examination of biopsy taken from the margin of the ulcers:
i. Ground glass nuclei
ii. Eosinophilic Cowdry's type A inclusion bodies
iii. Giant cells.

Culture or PCR can identify acyclovir resistant strain.

Treatment

A. Usually, this patient may not require treatment. But if the treatment will be started in early course of infection, duration of symptom can be reduced. The treatment will be:

Acyclovir 250 mg/m² —8 hourly intravenously till the patient can swallow.

↓

Valcyclovir 100 mg 3 trimes daily orally × 7–10 days

B. In case of immunocompromised patient or acyclovis resistant cases: Foscarnet 40 mg/kg thrice daily × 2 weeks

Cytomegalovirus Esophagitis

CMV esophagitis may occur in following patients:

i. Immunocompromised patients—in transplanted individual
ii. Transfusion of blood or blood products.

Endoscopic findings:

i. Serpiginous ulcer in normal mucosal epithelium of distal esophagus.
ii. Differences in endoscopic findings between CMV and herpes esophagitis.

In HSV esophagitis:

i. Small vesicles in middle or distal esophagus
ii. Vesicles coalesce to form circumscribed ulcers having raised yellow edges—volcano ulcer.
iii. These may be diffuse ulcerations, devoid of squamous epithelium.

In CMV esophigitis:

i. Presence of linear serpiginous ulcers in mid and distal esophageal mucosa.
ii. These ulcers may coalesce to form giant ulcers
iii. These ulcers produce stricture of esophageal lumen.

Histology shows: Large nuclear or cytoplasmic inclusion bodies are pathognomonic.

Immunohistology shows: Monoclonal antibodies to CMV in situ hybridization test.

Treatment

1. Gancyclovir—5 mg/kg—12 hourly intravenously × 3–6 weeks
   It is the treatment of choice.
   Valgancyclovir—900 mg twice daily orally
   Or
2. Foscarnet 90 mg/kg intravenously 12 hourly × 3–6 weeks.

ESOPHAGEAL CARCINOMA

Introduction

1. Two types of esophageal carcinoma are:
   i. Squamous cell carcinoma
   ii. Adenocarcinoma

2. Barrett's esophagus is a premalignant condition where squamous cell epithelium will be replaced by intestinal epithelial cells.
3. The incidence of squamous cell carcinoma is gradually decreasing, whereas incidence of adenocarcinoma is gradually increasing in white men.
4. This disease is rare in women for unknown reason.

Causes

1. Exposure to carcinogenic materials—location of malignancy is proximal and distal esophagus. Incidence increases with age.
2. As a consequence of generic mutation of normal squamous epithelial at gastroesophageal junction mainly in patient with GERD. Because in GERD, continuous reflux of gastric acid bathes the gastroesophageal junction and contributes to generic mutation of the epithelium.
3. Barrett's esophagus:
   Squamous epithelium → intestinal metaplasia → low grade dysplasia → adenocarcinoma

Risk Factors

A. In case of squamous cell carcinoma—risk factors are:
   i. Chronic tobacco smoking
   ii. Chronic alcohol intake
   iii. Breast irradiation
   iv. Ingestion of hot liquids
   v. Mediastinal irradiation
   vi. Human papilloma virus 16 or 18.
   vii. Achalasia
   Heavy alcohol intake and tobacco smoking increase the incidence of cancer to 100-fold.
B. For adenocarcinoma of esophagus, the risk factors are:
   i. Barrett's esophagus
   ii. GERD
   iii. Obesity
   iv. Scleroderma
   v. History of colonic cancer
   vi. Medications
      a. Chronic theophylline
      b. Beta agonists
   Protective factor is *Helicobacter pylori* infection.
C. In patient with long-standing GERD, there is chance of developing Barrett's esophagus, which is premalignant.

Clinical Presentation

History of:
   i. Dysphagia
   ii. Weight loss
Past history of:
   i. Tobacco use
   ii. Chronic alcohol intake
   iii. GERD
Clinically:
   i. Patient becomes thin and emaciated
   ii. Pallor
   iii. Cervical lymphadenopathy

Screening for Carcinoma

In patient with long-standing GERD to detect Barrett's esophagus in elderly (>50 years old).

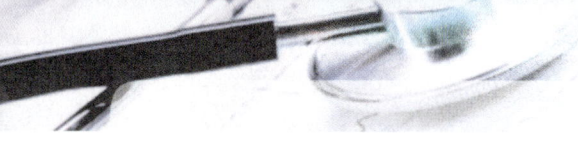

Surveillance for Endoscopy

In patient having Barrett's esophagus—endoscopic surveillance depends upon grades of dysplasia.

i. If no dysplasia—endoscopy should be repeated yearly interval.

↓

If no dysplasia is found in two consecutive specimen of annual screening

↓

Endoscopy should be done 2–3 years interval

ii. In case of low grade dysplasia—endoscopy should be done at every 6 months interval

↓

If high grade dysplasia is found

↓

Endoscopy should be done at every 3 months

In case of high grade dysplasia and endoscopic mucosal abnormalities, endoscopic mucosal resection and ablation should be of choice.

Stages of Esophageal Carcinoma (Table 4.2)

This stage should include:
1. Clinical examination
2. Blood counts
3. Endoscopic findings
4. CT scan of chest and abdomen

Endoscopic ultrasound should be done to assess:
i. Depth of invasion of tumor tissue
ii. Lymph node involvements

Position emission tomography is helpful to detect distant metastasis.

Table 4.2: Stages of esophageal carcinoma	
Stage	*Findings*
A. Primary tumor	
Tx	Primary tumor cannot be assessed
To	No evidence of primary tumor
Tis	Carcinoma in situ
Ty	Tumor invades lamina propria or submucosa
T2	Invasion of muscularis propria
T3	Tumor invasion of adventitia
T4	Tumor invasion of adjacent structures
B. Regional lymph nodes	
Nx	Regional nodes cannot be assessed
No	No distant metastasis
N1	Metastatis to regional lymph node
C. Distant metastasis	
Mx	Cannot be assessed
Mo	No distant metastasis
M1	Distant metastasis
Stages are	
O	Tis N0M0
I	T1 N0M0
IIA	T2N0M0; T3 N0M0
IIB	T1 N1M0; T2N1M0
III	T3N1M0; T4NM0
IVA	Any T any NM1a
IVB	Any T any NM1b

Prognosis

In stage I and IIA—5 years survival is 34 to 60%.
In stage IIB and III—5 years survival is 15 to 25%.

Prognosis is bad in case of squamous cell carcinoma than adenocarcinoma of esophagus for following reasons:
i. Location of tumor
ii. Propensity for lymphatic spread
iii. Comorbidities of the patients.

Laboratory Workup

1. Barium swallow:
   i. Mass in esophageal lumen
   ii. Evidence of compression from adjacent structure
2. Endoscopy shows: Ulcerated polypoidal lesion—which may or may not prevent the endoscope to pass beyond the lesion.

Biopsy should be done from that lesion—to prove it as carcinoma—which is the gold standard.

After its diagnosis—it has to estimate its resectibility by following methods:
i. Endoscopic ultrasound
ii. CT scan of chest
iii. CT scan of abdomen
iv. Positron emission tomography

These are usually done to detect:
i. Depth of invasion
ii. Regional metastasis
iii. Distant metastasis

Treatment

For stage I disease—curative surgery is the treatment of choice in case of localized squamous cell carcinoma or adenocarcinoma and if submucosa or muscularis mucosa will be involved.

Endoscopic mucosal resection of adenocarcinoma presents on superficial layers of esophagus in the treatment of choice.

The procedures of choice are:
i. Suction cap fitted with a snare
ii. Electrocautery
iii. Argon plasma coagulation
iv. Photodynamic therapy

Surgical Therapy

i. Resection of tumor with anastomosis of cervical esophagus with stomach.
ii. Interposition of colon to maintain gastrointestinal continuity.

For stage IIA—III:
- If the patient is willing to go for surgery: Chemotherapy + Radiotherapy + Surgery
- If the patient is not willing to go for surgery: Chemotherapy + Radiotherapy

For stage IV: In case of distant metastasis, cancer is not at all curable: Radiotherapy + Chemotherapy

STOMACH

GASTRITIS

This is characterized by—histologically documented inflammation in the gastric mucosa.

Classification with Etiology of Gastritis

A. Acute gastritis:
    a. *Helicobacter pylori* infection
    b. Other infective gastritides:
        i. Bacterial
        ii. *H. heilmannii*
        iii. Phlegmonous
        iv. Mycobacterial
        v. Syphilitic
        vi. Viral
        vii. Parasitic
        viii. Fungal
B. Chronic gastritis (atrophic type):
    a. Type A gastritis autoimmune involving mainly body
    b. Type B gastritis—*Helicobacter pylori* related, mainly involving antrum
C. Uncommon form:
    a. Lymphocytic
    b. Eosinophilic
    c. Crohn's disease
    d. Sarcoidosis
    e. Granulomatous

Acute Gastritis

A. *H. pylori* infected acute gastritis—is characterized by:
    i. Acute abdominal pain
    ii. Nausea
    iii. Vomiting
    iv. Histology showed—marked neutrophilic infiltrate, edema and hyperemia.
    v. If untreated, it may turn into chronic gastritis
    vi. Hypochlorhydria
B. Bacterial or phlegmonous gastritis is characterized by:
    i. Acute inflammatory infiltrate involving entire gastric wall may be associated necrosis.
    ii. High-risk people are:
        a. Elderly
        b. Alcoholic
        c. AIDS affected patients
        d. Patients undergone gastric polypectomy
        e. Mucosal injection with India ink
        f. Treatment—supportive measures or gastrectomy

Chronic Gastritis

This is characterized by the following features:
    i. Histologically—mucosa is infiltrated with lymphocytes, plasma cells and scanty neutrophils
    ii. Distribution—patchy
    iii. Involved areas—superficial mucosa, glandular portion.
    iv. Progression—Glandular destruction → mucosal atrophy → Intestinal metaplasia
    v. Classification
        a. Superficial gastritis
        b. Gastric atrophy

Three stages of chronic gastritis are:
Stage-1: Superficial gastritis—here the inflammation is limited to lamina propria of surface mucosa.
Stage-2: Atrophic gastritis—here, the inflammation extends to deeper layer of the mucosa with distortion and destruction of glands.
Stage-3: Gastric atrophy—here, inflammatory infiltrate will be less as well as glandular structures.

Endoscopic View Description

Mucosa will be thinned through which background blood vessels can be visualized.

At the end of stage 3, there will be intestinal metaplasia which denotes conversion of gastric glands to intestinal phenotype. This is a predisposing factor for gastric cancer.

Classification of Chronic Gastritis

I. Type A—body predominant form (mainly autoimmune):
This is characterized by the following:
1. Fundus and body are involved with sparing of antrum
2. This is also called autoimmune gastritis
3. Antibody to parietal cells present in
    i. 50% patients with this type gastritis
    ii. 90% patients with pernicious anemia
    iii. This parietal cell antibody is directed against—H^+K^+ ATPase
    iv. 20% patients with Vitiligo and Addison's disease
    v. 20% patients over 60 years of age.
4. Antibody to intrinsic factor is more specific for type A gastritis
5. Higher incidence in specific familial histocompatibility haplotypes—HLA B8, HLA DR-3.

The result is:
    i. Achlorhydria
    ii. Vitamin B_{12} deficiency
    iii. Due to sparing of antrum and G cells in antral mucosa, there is evidence of hypergastrinemia (>500 pg/cm)
    iv. Enterochromaffin cell hyperplasia due to tropic effect of gastrin

II. Type B antral predominant gastritis (*H. pylori* related):
The characteristics are:
1. Though it is antral predominant, it may extend to body and fundus—it is called pangastritis—it requires 15–20 years to develop.
2. At ≥70 years age, 100% patients develop gastritis.
3. During antral predominant condition
    i. Quantity of *H. pylori* is highest.
    ii. Dense chronic inflammatory infiltrate in lamina propria.
    iii. Epithelial cell infiltration with PMNS.

The stages of type B gastritis are:

Multiple atrophic gastritis

Gastric atrophy

Intestinal metaplasia
↓
Gastric adenocarcinoma

H. pylori has been regarded as isolated risk factor for adenocarcinoma. Because, *H. pylori* seropositivity will be increased to 3–6 folds in case of gastric cancer.

Chronic T cell stimulation caused by *H. pylori* infection
↓
Production of cytokines
↓
Promotion of B cell tumor

Development of gastric MALT lymphoma

Eradication of *H. pylori* with treatment is responsible for regression of tumor—it takes more than a year to regress.

This can be diagnosed serially by CT scan and EUS in every 2–3 months.

In few cases, in spite of *H. pylori* treatment, low grade lymphoma may progress to high grade lymphoma.

PEPTIC ULCER DISEASE

This is characterized by denudation of the stomach or duodenal mucosa extending up to muscularis propria, exposed to gastric acids:

- If the size is >5 mm, it is ulcer.
- If the size is <5 mm, it is erosions.

Gastric Physiology

Anatomy of Gastric Glands

Gastric epithelial lining consists of rugae, it contains microscopic gastric pits.

Each pit will branch into 4 to 5 gastric glands which is made up of highly specialized different types of cells that vary according to the areas of stomach.

A. In the fundus, <5% of gastric gland area contains:
   i. Mucous cells
   ii. Endocrine cells
B. In the oxyntic mucosa, >75% of gastric gland area contains following cells:
   i. Mucous neck cells
   ii. Parietal cells
   iii. Endocrine cells
   iv. Enterochromaffin cells
   v. Enterochromaffin like-cells.
C. In the pyloric gland area—the gland contains:
   i. Mucous cells
   ii. Endocrine cells—contain gastrin cells

Parietal cell is also known as oxyntic cells. Unstimulated oxyntic cells contain:
i. Tubulovesicles containing $H^+K^+ATPase$ on its membrane
ii. Intracellular canaliculi with prominent microvilli along the apical surface.

In stimulated oxyntic cells: Tubulovesicular membrane along with its apical membrane will be converted into dense network of canaliculi.

In this apical canalicular process, high energy requiring acid secretion process occurs, where numerous mitochondria are involved.

Mucosal Defense in Stomach and Duodenum

Gastric and duodenal mucosa is exposed to variety of injurious agents:
a. Endogenous noxious factors:
   i. Hydrochloric acids
   ii. Pepsinogens or pepsin
   iii. Bile salts
b. Exogenous noxious factors:
   i. Medications
   ii. Alcohol
   iii. Bacteria

So, there is defense mechanisms will come into play to protect against the above agents. This mucosal defense consists of:
a. Pre-epithelial layer
b. Epithelial layer
c. Subepithelial elements

Pre-epithelial layer is mucus–bicarbonate phospholipid layer.

Mucus is being secreted by gastroduodenal mucosal epithelial cells—it consists of:
   i. Water (95%)
   ii. Phospholipid
   iii. Glycoprotein.

This mucus layer acts as unstirred water layer and prevents the diffusion of ions and molecules like pepsin.

Bicarbonate is also secreted by gastroduodenal epithelial layer—into mucus. As a result, pH of mucus will be:
   i. 1–2 on the gastric luminal surface
   ii. 6–7 on the epithelial surface

Epithelial cell layer provides defense through following mechanisms:
1. Mucus production
2. Epithelial cell ionic transporters
3. Maintenance of intracellular pH
4. Bicarbonate production
5. Maintaining intracellular tight junctions
6. Heat shock protein productions—it:
   i. Prevents protein denaturation
   ii. Protect cells from certain factors:
      a. Temperature
      b. Oxidative agents
      c. Cytotoxic agent
7. Generation of trefoil factor family peptides and cathelicidins—they:
   i. Provide cell protection
   ii. Cell regeneration

In case of any small breach in pre-epithelial layer, epithelial cells of stomach migrate, border to restore the site of injury—it is called restitution. Restitution process requires:
   i. Uninterrupted blood flow
   ii. Alkaline pH in surrounding area
   iii. Modulation by following growth factors:
      a. Epidermal growth factor
      b. Basic fibroblast growth factor
      c. Transforming growth factor

In case of large breach—epithelial cells require regeneration to repair the breech. This is regulated by:
   i. Prostaglandin
   ii. Epidermal growth factor
   iii. Transforming growth factor-α

During the regeneration of epithelial cells, regeneration as well as multiplication of blood vessels occurs—which is aided by:
i. Vascular endothelial growth factor
ii. Fibroblast growth factor

Subepithelial Defense (Fig. 4.1)

Microvascular system of subepithelial layer:
i. Provides—HCO_3^-—it neutralizes acid generated by parietal cells.
ii. Provides micronutrients and oxygen—these remove all toxic products.

Prostaglandins play a central role in epithelial defense/repair by performing following:
i. Regulation and release of mucosal bicarbonate and mucus
ii. Inhibition of parietal cell secretion
iii. Maintenance of mucosal blood flow
iv. Epithelial cell restitution.

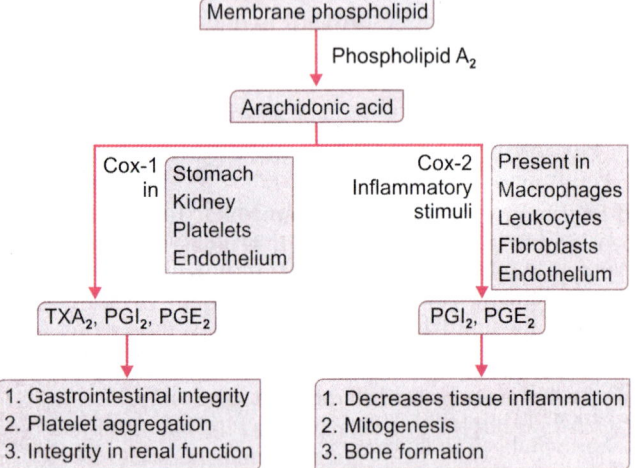

Fig. 4.1: Fate of membrane phospholipid

NSAID:
1. Inhibits cox-2—reduces inflammation
2. Inhibits cox-1—GI mucosal ulcerations, renal dysfunction.
So selective cox-2 inhibitors are responsible for:
i. Reduction of inflammation
ii. Reduction of GI side effects
iii. Adverse effect on cardiovascular system—increased risk of myocardial infarction.

Nitric oxide: Nitric oxide produced by nitric oxide synthatase present on mucosa is responsible for cytoprotection through following mechanisms:
1. Gastric mucus production
2. Increase in mucosal blood flow
3. Maintenance of epithelial cell barrier function.

Central nervous system: It is responsible for regulating mucosal defense by following factors:
i. Corticotropin-releasing factor
ii. Thyrotropin-releasing factor
iii. Melanocortin.

Hormones: It plays an important role in regulation of gastric mucosal defense by following factors:
i. Gastrin
ii. Cholecystokinin
iii. Ghrelin

iv. Growth factors
v. Cytokines
vi. Adrenal corticoids

Pathophysiology of Gastric Secretion

Hydrochloric acid: It is usually secreted in two conditions:
a. Basal acid production occurs in circadian rhythm:
   i. Highest level occurs at night
   ii. Lowest level occurs in the morning.
   Two principal enhancing inputs are responsible for basal acid productions:
   i. Cholinergic input—via vagus nerve
   ii. Histaminergic input from local gastric sources.
b. Stimulated acid production—occurs in three phases:
   i. *Cephalic phase:* In this phase, sight, smell and taste of the food stimulate vagus nerve to secrete gastric acid secretion.
   ii. *Gastric phase:* In this phase:

   a. As the food enters the stomach
   Amino acids and amine
   ↓
   Directly stimulate G cells
   ↓
   Release of gastrin
   ↓
   Activation of parietal cells (direct and indirect mechanism)
   b. Distension of stomach
   ↓
   Release of gastrin
   ↓
   Stimulation of parietal cells
   ↓
   Release of acid from cells

   iii. *Intestinal phase:* In this phase, as the food enters intestine, luminal distension and nutrient assimilation simultaneously gastric acid secretion.

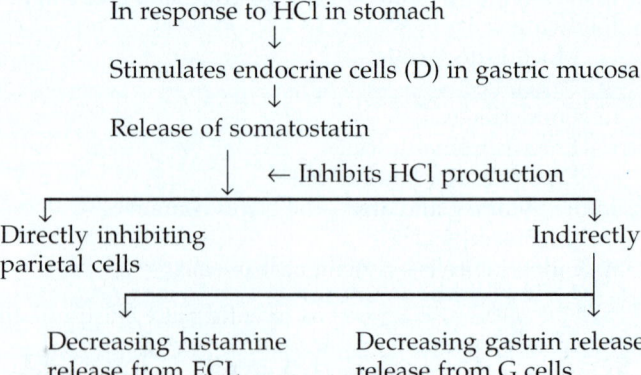

Other Inhibitors of Acid Secretion

A. Neural:
   i. Central
   ii. Peripheral
B. Humoral:
   i. Amylin
   ii. Atrial natriuretic peptide

iii. Cholecystokinin
iv. Ghrelin
v. Obestatin
vi. Secretin
vii. Serotonin

Ghrelin, appetite—regulating hormone may stimulate acid secretion through vagus nerve stimulation.

Parietal cells in oxyntic gland—functions:
i. Acid secretion
ii. Secretion of intrinsic factor
iii. Receptors for:
  1. Histamine (H_2)
  2. Gastrin (cholecystokinin B)
  3. Acetylcholine (muscarinic—M_3)

Histamine binds to H_2 receptors
↓
Activation of adenylate cyclase
↓
Increased concentration of cyclic-AMP
↓
Release of HCl
Gastrin receptors and acetylcholine receptors
↓
Activation of protein kinase C/phosphoinositol signaling pathway
↓
Release of HCl

Activates H_2 receptors on D cells
↓
Inhibition of somatostatin release

When three signaling pathways are combined, there will be potentiation of acid secretion.

Hence administration of H_2 blocker which inhibits acid secretion by blocking H_2 receptors also inhibits acid secretion by inhibiting other pathways (gastrin and acetylcholine) H^+K^+ ATPase— it is responsible for generation of HCl.

H^+K^+ ATPase is a membrane e bound protein.
↓
Two subunits

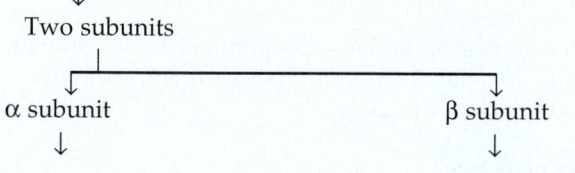

α subunit | β subunit
↓ | ↓
In it, active catalytic site is found | Activity unclear

H^+K^+ ATPase (found in secretory canaliculi and in non-secretory tubulovesicles)
←— With the help of ATP

Transfer H^+ ion from parietal cell cytoplasm to secretory canaliculi in exchange of K^+.

H^+K^+ ATPase pump is inactive in tubulovesicles due to impermeability to K^+.

So according to activity of parietal cells, the H^+K^+ ATPase distribution varies.

Chief cells in fundus
↓
Synthesize and secretes pepsinogens in the stomach
↓
In acid environment
↓
Pepsinogens will be cleaved into pepsin

Activity of pepsin:
i. Highest pepsin activity in pH ≤2.
ii. Significantly diminished activity of pepsin at pH 4
iii. Irreversible inactivated pepsin—≥ 7 pH.

Pathophysiology of Peptic Ulcer Disease

Epidemiology

Duodenal ulcers: Incidence of duodenal ulcers declines gradually in Western population. As a result, death rates, incidence of surgery has been reduced.

It may be due to reduction of frequency of *Helicobacter pylori* infection.

Gastric ulcer:
i. It usually occurs in later life than duodenal ulcer
ii. Peak incidence is at 6th decade of life.
iii. It is more common in males.
iv. According to autopsy, incidence of both GU and DU is similar.

Pathology

A. Duodenal ulcer:
  i. 95% cases, it occurs in 1st part of duodenum, amongst them 90% occurs within 3 cm from pylorus.
  ii. Diameter is usually ≤1 cm, but in case of giant ulcer it is 3–6 cm in diameter.
  iii. Margin—sharply demarcated
  iv. Depth—it may reach the muscularis mucosae.
  v. Base—it may be clear or may contain zone of eosinophilic necrosis with surrounding fibrosis.
  vi. Malignant ulcer is very rare.

B. Gastric ulcer:
  i. Malignant ulcer is most common than benign ulcer, hence the entire ulcer in stomach must be biopsied.
  ii. Benign ulcer is usually present in the area distal to antrum and proximal to acid secretory mucosa
  iii. Benign gastric ulcer is rare in fundus.
  iv. If gastric ulcer is *H. pylori* associated, it should be associated with antral gastritis.
  v. In case of NSAID-induced gastric ulcer, there will be no evidence of chronic gastritis.
  vi. In case of NSAID-induced chemical gastropathy, there may be:
    a. Foveolar hyperplasia
    b. Edematous lamina propria
    c. Epithelial regeneration
    d. Absence of *H. pylori* infections.

Pathophysiology

A. Duodenal ulcer:
  i. Majority of duodenal ulcer is due to:
    a. *H. pylori*   b. NSAID

ii. Average basal and nocturnal gastric acid secretion will be increased, but there may be overlap between control and duodenal ulcer patients.

iii. Altered acid secretory status may be due to:
   a. *Helicobacter pylori* infection
   b. Significantly decreased bicarbonate secretion in duodenal ulcer.

B. Gastric ulcer:
   i. *Helicobacter pylori* and NSAID are mainly involved in gastric mucosal damage.
   ii. In case of prepyloric ulcer or ulcers in gastric body associated with duodenal ulcer scar or active duodenal ulcer, the pathogenesis is similar to that of duodenal ulcer.
   iii. Basal and stimulated acid output will be normal or decreased in case of gastric ulcer.
   iv. In case of gastric ulcer with minimal acid level, the pathology may be the damage of mucosal defense.
   v. Classifications of gastric ulcer:
      a. Type-I   Ulcer in gastric body + low gastric acid secretion
      b. Type-II   Ulcer in gastric antrum + gastric acid may vary from low to normal.
      c. Type-III Ulcer within 3 cm of pylorus + normal or high gastric acid + associated duodenal ulcer may be present.
      d. Type-IV   Ulcer in gastric fundus + low gastric acid
   vi. Delayed gastric emptying may be responsible for development of gastric ulcer.
   vii. Abnormalities of basal and stimulated pyloric sphincter pressure may be responsible for duodeno-gastric bile reflux in gastric ulcer patient, where, bile acid, pancreatic enzymes, lisolecithin may damage gastric mucosal defense.

Helicobacter pylori and Peptic Disorders

H. pylori is responsible for:
   i. Peptic ulcer disease;
   ii. Mucosa-associated lymphoid tissue lymphoma
   iii. Gastric adenocarcinoma

The cause is not clear that *H. pylori* resides in gastric mucosa but is responsible for duodenal ulcers.

Description of Bacteria

Helicobacter pylori:
   i. Spiral shaped, Gram-negative organism
   ii. Multiple sheathed with unipolar flagella—it is responsible for movement in the mucus layer of stomach.
   iii. Its potent urease activity is essential for colonization and survival.

Residence

   i. It resides in deeper portion of gastric mucus gel in gastric mucosa.
   ii. It may also reside between the mucus layer of gastric epithelium.
   iii. It usually resides in antrum but it may migrate into the proximal segments of the stomach.

The organism is capable of transforming to coccoid from—which is in dormant state.

Genetic of *H. pylori*

Genome of *H. pylori* encodes 1500 proteins—amongst which the following proteins are responsible for colonization and pathogenesis:
   i. Outer membrane protein
   ii. Urease proteins
   iii. Vacuolating cytotoxin

Genomic fragments of *H. pylori* encode cag-pathogenicity islands (cag-PAI).

Genes that encodes cag-PAI; help cag-PAI to translocate into host cell.

In the cell, Cag-PAI activates series of cellular events and is responsible for:
   i. Cell cytokines production and release
   ii. Cellular growth

Two points are essential for pathogensis of duodenal ulcer due to *H. pylori*:
   i. Bacterial motility
   ii. Urease production

Urease enzyme produces ammonia from urea which is responsible for alkalizing the surrounding pH. Other bacterial factors are:
   i. Catalase
   ii. Lipase
   iii. Adhesins
   iv. Platelet activation factors
   v. Pic B—it induces cytokines.

Epidemiology

The risk-factors of infections:
1. Socioeconomic status
2. Less educations
3. Birth or residence in developing countries
4. Domestic crowding
5. Poor sanitation
6. Unclean food or water.
7. Exposure of gastric content of an infected individual

Routes of Transmission

   i. Oral to oral transmission
   ii. Few oral transmissions

Nowadays, rate of infection is gradually declining in developing countries.

In developing countries—80% population are infected by the age of 20 years. In United States, organisms are rare in childhood.

Pathophysiology

Particular end results of *H. pylori* infection are:
   i. Gastritis
   ii. Peptic ulcer diseases
   iii. Gastric MALT lymphoma
   iv. Gastric cancer

This is determined by following factors.

Bacterial factors: *H. pylori*—avoid host defense, facilitates gastric residence, they induce mucosal injury.

Different strains induce different virulent factors:
   i. Cag-PAI (pathogenicity islands) encodes following virulence factors:

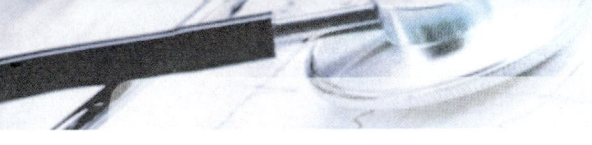

a. Cag-A
b. Pic-B
ii. Vac A is also responsible for pathogenicity—but it is not encoded in the island.

Bacterial virulence factors + other bacterial constituents
↓
Disturb the functions of immune cells
↓
Produces mucosal damage

a. Vac A targets following cells:
　i. Inhibits proliferation of human CD4+ T cells
　ii. Disrupts normal function of B cells
　iii. Disrupts normal function of CD8+ cells
　iv. Disrupts normal function of macrophages
　v. Disrupts normal function of mast cells
b. *H. pylori* positivity is associated with high risk of
　1. Peptic ulcer disease
　2. Malignant gastric carcinoma

Urease positive *H. pylori*
↓
c. Urease allows the bacteria to reside in acidic environment in stomach
↓
Generation of NH_3
↓
Damage of gastric epithelial cells
d. Bacteria produce surface factors which are chemotactic for—neutrophils and monocytes
↓
Responsible for epithelial injury
e. *H. pylori* produces proteases and phospholipases
↓
Breakdown glycoprotein lipid complex of mucus gel
↓
Reduce the efficacy of mucus gel.
↓
Produces mucosal injury
f. H. *Pylori* expresses adhesins (OMPs, BabA)
↓
Aggravation of attachment of bacteria to gastric epithelial cells

g. *H. pylori* secretes lipopolysaccharide
　i. It is responsible for infection
　ii. It has low immunologic activity
h. *H. pylori* is responsible for smouldering chronic inflammation.

Host factors:
a. There is genetic predisposition to acquire *H. pylori* infection in human being.
b. There is increased production of inflammatory cells like, neutrophils, plasma cells, macrophages, T and B lymphocytes.

c.
Pathogen
↓
Binds to class II MHC on gastric epithelial cells
↓
Cell death (apoptosis)

d. Cag-PAI positive *H. pylori* strain
↓
Introduce CagA into the cells → increased production of cytokines
↓
Aggravation of cell injury　(It is found in gastric epithelium of *H. pylori* infected individual)
↓
The cytokines are
　i. Interleukin　　1α/β
　ii. Interleukin　　2
　iii. Interleukin　　6
　iv. Interleukin　　8
　v. Interferon
　vi. Tumor necrosis factor-α

e. *H. pylori*-induced systemic and humoral response—it is responsible for compound epithelial injury.
f. Other factors responsible for *H. pylori*-induced epithelial cell injury:
　1. Activated neutrophils mediated production of reactive oxygen or nitrogen species
　2. Apoptosis related to interaction with T cells and IFN-γ

Following are the possible reasons for development of *H. pylori*-induced duodenal ulcers.

This is more virulent than *H. pylori*-induced gastric ulcers:
　i. Duodenal ulcer promoting gene A (dupa A) is responsible for promoting duodenal ulcer.
　ii. Gastric metaplasia in duodenal mucosa is aggravating the promotion of gastric ulcer in case of high exposure to *H. pylori*.
　iii. Increased acid production and increased exposure of duodenal mucosa to acid and thus production of mucosal injury.
　iv. Basal, meal and gastrin releasing peptide induced gastrin recreation will be increased in *H. pylori*-infected individual.
　v. Number of somatostatin secreting D cells will be decreased.
　vi. Direct and indirect interactions of *H. pylori* and pro-inflammatory cytokines on G, D and parietal cells.
Following are the possible factors in case of *H. pylori* induced gastric ulcers (Fig. 4.2).
　i. Evidence of pangastritis with normal or low gastric acid secretion.
　ii. Decreased duodenal mucosal bicarbonate production.

NSAID-Induced PUD

NSAID-induced PUD has a wide spectrum of presentation which ranges from nausea and dyspepsia at one end to severe gastrointestinal bleeding or perforation at other end.
* 4–5% patients develop symptomatic ulcer in 1 year.
* 80% patients with serious NSAID-related complication have not preceding history of dyspepsia.

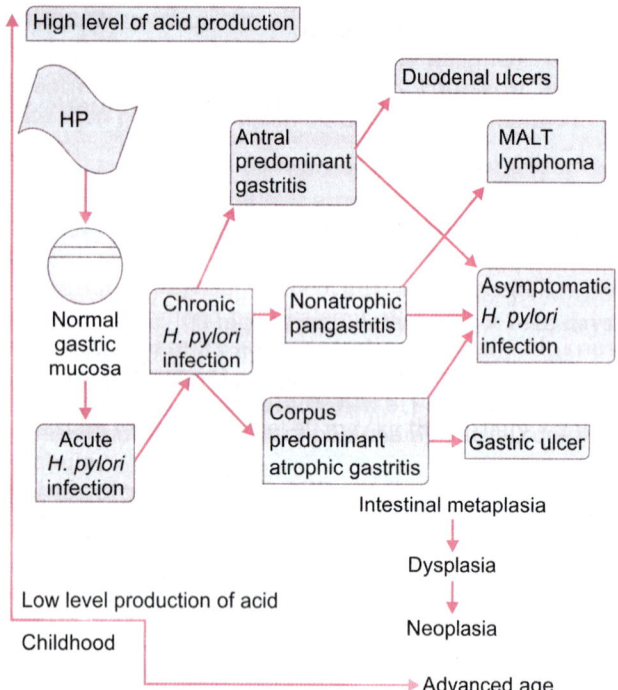

Fig. 4.2: Effect of *H. pyloxi* on gastric mucona

There is no dose relation of NSAID with PUD-related morbidity and mortality.

There are following risk factors in case of NSAID-induced PUD:

i. Advanced age
ii. History of ulcer
iii. Concomitant use of glucorticoids
iv. High dose of NSAID
v. Multiple NSAIDs
vi. Concomitant use of anticoagulants
vii. Clopidogrel
viii. Serious or multisystem diseases
ix. Concomitant infection with *H. pylori*
x. Cigarette smoking
xi. Consumption of alcohol

Pathophysiology

Role of prostaglandin

NSAID
↓
Interruption of prostaglandin synthesis
↓
Impairment of mucosal defense and repair
↓
Facilitation of mucosal injury

1. Aspirin and NSAIDs
↓
It is present in nonionized lipophilic form in acid environment in stomach
↓
It migrates across the lipid membrane into the cytoplasm
↓
This is trapped intracellularly in ionized form
↓
Responsible for cellular injury

2. Topical NSAID
↓
Alteration of surface mucous layer
↓
Back diffusion of H⁺ ion and pepsin
↓
Result is severe mucosal injury

H. pylori and NSAID are the isolated risk factors for PUD. Again combinations of *H. pylori* and NSAID synergistically are responsible for gastrointestinal bleeding.

Pathogenesis of other risk factors in case of duodenal ulcers: Cigarette smoking is responsible for gastric or duodenal ulcers by following mechanisms:

1. Decreased healing rates.
2. Impaired response to therapy.
3. Increasing incidence of ulcer-related complications, like perforations.

Factors responsible for generation of peptic ulcers in smokers:

i. Decreased gastric emptying
ii. Decreased proximal duodenal bicarbonate secretion
iii. Increased risk of *H. pylori* infection
iv. Generation of toxic, noxious mucosal free radicals.

Other factors related to development of peptic ulcers:

1. Genetic factors—1st degree relatives are three times more prone to develop peptic ulcers.
2. Blood group O
3. Non-secretory status
4. Psychological factors
5. Dietary factors—certain foods and beverages may be responsible for dyspepsia, but association with ulcer has not yet proven.

Following chronic diseases are associated with peptic ulcer disease:

a. **Strong association:**
   1. Cirrhosis
   2. Chronic renal failure
   3. Chronic pulmonary
   4. Systemic mastocytosis
   5. Nephrolithiesis
   6. Systemic mastocytosis
   7. α-1 antitrypsin deficiency.

b. **Possible associations:**
   1. Coronary artery disease
   2. Hyperthyroidism
   3. Chronic pancreatitis
   4. Polycythemia vera

Drugs responsible for peptic ulcer disease:

1. Glucocorticoid when combined with NSAID
2. Bisphosphonate
3. Clopidogrel
4. Chemotherapeutic agent
5. Mycophenolate mofetil
6. Potassium chloride

Systemic diseases responsible for PUD:
1. Crohn's disease
2. Radiation therapy
3. Infiltrating disease
4. Basophilia in myeloproliferative disease
5. Sarcoidosis

Clinical Pictures

A. 10% patients on NSAID may present with complications of PUD, like, perforation, bleeding without any previous presenting symptoms.
B. Abdominal pain:
   a. It is epigastric in origin.
   b. Character—burning or growing, or acting or hunger pain
   c. Timing:
      i. In case of duodenal ulcer, it usually occurs 90 minutes to 3 hours after taking food.
      ii. Sometimes it may awake the patient from sleep (midnight to 3 AM). This may occur also in patient with non-ulcer dyspepsia.
   d. In case of gastric ulcer, it will be aggravated by food, in case of DU, aggravation factor is empty stomach.
   e. Nausea with or without vomiting—may occur in gastric ulcer patient.

Mechanism of occurrence of abdominal pain in ulcer patient:
   i. Acid-induced activation of chemoreceptors in duodenum
   ii. Enhanced duodenal sensitivity to bile acid and pepsin.
   iii. Altered gastroduodenal motility

Site of Ulcers

A. **In case of duodenal ulcer:**
   i. Age of onset—young age
   ii. May occur in 30–55 years of age.
   iii. Site of ulcer—at duodenal bulb and pyloric channel.
   In this site, the mechanism of ulcer formation:
   i. Decreased bicarbonate secretion
   ii. Increased parietal cell mass and acid secretion
   As a result:

Small islands of gastric metaplasia in duodenal bulb
↓
Colonization of those areas with *H. pylori*
↓
Development of duodenitis
↓
Duodenal ulcer

B. **In case of gastric ulcer**
   i. Age incidence is 35–70 years—peak incidence sixth decade.
   ii. Sites of ulcer are:
      a. Antral mucosa
      b. Lesser curvature at the junction of gastric body and antrum.
C. **In case of combined gastric and duodenal ulcers:** Sites of gastric ulcers are in pyloric antrum or pyloric channel.

Following symptoms or change of previous symptoms indicate complications of PUD:

1. Constant dyspepsia, pain radiating to back, not relieved by antacids and foods—it indicates penetrating ulcer to pancreas.
2. Sudden severe right abdominal pain with severe sweating and card-board rigidity on examination and rebound tenderness indicate perforation.
3. Postprandial nausea and vomiting of undigested food suggest—gastric cutlet obstruction.
4. Coffee ground vomiting and/or black tarry stool—suggest bleeding from ulcers.

Examinations

A. In uncomplicated cases, epigastric tenderness is the only finding. In 20% cases, it may be present at right of midline.
B. In complicated cases:
   1. Tachycardia, orthostatic hypotension, indicates vomiting or upper gastrointestinal bleeding.
   2. Severe tender board-like abdomen—indicates perforation.
   3. Succussion splash—suggests fluid in the stomach—gastric outlet obstructions.

Complications of Peptic Ulcer Disease

A. **Gastrointestinal bleeding (common complication):**
   1. It occurs in >60 years age.
   2. It occurs in 15% of elderly individual.
   3. Mortality is 5–10%.
   4. It occurs mostly in NSAID user.
   5. 20% patient may bleed without any preceding warning symptoms.
B. **Perforation:**
   1. It is 2nd most common complication.
   2. It occurs in 6–7% of PUD patients.
   3. Incidence in elderly is progressively increasing due to increased use of NSAID.
C. **Penetrating ulcers:**
   Ulcer may penetrate to adjacent organ
   1. Duodenal ulcer may penetrate posteriorly to pancreas.
   2. Gastric ulcer may penetrate to left hepatic lobe.
   3. Gastric ulcer may penetrate to colon producing gastrocolic fistula.
D. **Gastric outlet obstruction:**
   a. Relative obstruction: It may occur in ulcer in prepyloric region producing sever inflammatory edema. But during ulcer healing, this edema as well as obstruction will be resolved.
   b. Fixed obstruction: It occurs due to severe fibrosis and scar formation in peripyloric region producing fixed narrowing or deformity.

Following diseases may produce ulcer-like symptoms:
1. Gastroesophageal reflux disease
2. Essential dyspepsia
3. Vascular disease
4. Biliary colic—due to presence of gallstones
5. Chronic pancreatitis
6. Crohn's disease involving stomach and duodenum

Diagnostic Workup

Barium Studies

In case of single contrast barium meal study—diagnosis of DU is >80%.

In case of double contrast barium meal study—diagnosis of DU is >90%.

Sensitivity is decreased in following conditions:
   i. Small ulcers
   ii. Presence of previous scarring
   iii. In case of postoperative patients.

In case of duodenal ulcer:
   i. Ulcer in the bulb
   ii. Presence of discrete crater

In case of benign gastric ulcer:
   i. Presence of discrete crater
   ii. Origination of radiating mucosal fold from the ulcer

In case of malignant ulcer:
   i. Ulcer size >3 cm
   ii. Presence of associated mass

Endoscopy

This is the most specific and sensitive method for diagnosing ulcer in gastrointestinal tract.

In case of gastric ulcer (since 5% of gastric ulcer is malignant)—biopsy sample should be taken from the margin in newly diagnosed ulcer or follow-up case of ulcer after 12 weeks treatment with acid suppressing medications and to be sent for histopathological examination.

Proper evaluation of Zollinger-Ellison syndrome should be considered in following conditions:
   i. Multiple ulcers
   ii. Refractory ulcers
   iii. Ulcers at unusual sites—like jejunum or post-bulbar area of duodenum
   iv. History of diarrhea and weight loss.

Diagnostic Tests for Helicobacter pylori

Tables 4.3 and 4.4 describe the diagnostic tests for *H. pylori*.

Treatment

Medical Management

Aim:
   i. Healing of ulcer
   ii. Prevention of ulcer recurrence
   iii. Prevention of future complications
   iv. All ulcers should be treated with anti *H. pylori* regimen, even there is presence of clear history of intake of NSAID.

Effects of intravenous proton pump inhibitor:
   i. It decreases transfusion requirement.
   ii. If decreases the need for surgery.
   iii. It decreases the duration of hospitalization.
   iv. It decreases the need for homeostasis therapy.

Antacids: These are rarely used for symptomatic relief. The drugs are:
1. Combination of aluminum hydroxide and magnesium hydroxide
2. Calcium carbonate
3. Sodium bicarbonate

Dose: 100–140 mEq/L—1 and 3 hours after meals and at night.

Complications:
a. Aluminum hydroxide:
   i. Constipation
   ii. Phosphate depletion

Table 4.3: Invasive test

Methods	Sensitivity	Specificity	Comments
1. Rapid urease test	93–97%	95–100%	False negative in i. Recent case of PPI ii. Antibiotic use or bismuth iii. Gastrointestinal bleeding
2. Culture	70–80%	100%	i. Time consuming ii. Skilled personnel required iii. Expensive iv. Determination of antibiotic susceptibility
3. Histology	80-90%	95%	i. Good staining and processing is required ii. Histological information can be obtained.

Table 4.4: Non-invasive tests

Test	Sensitivity	Specificity	Comment
1. Serology (ELISA)	85%	79%	i. Inexpensive ii. Convenient iii. Should not be used for early follow up
2. Urea breath test	95%	>90%	i. Simple ii. Rapid iii. Used for early follow up
3. *H. pylori* antigen in stool	91–97%	94–98%	i. It confirms successful cure ii. It is used for initial diagnosis iii. It is inexpensive iv. Convenient

b. Magnesium hydroxide—loose stool
c. Calcium carbonate—it will be converted into calcium chloride in stomach and responsible for milk alkali syndrome which is characterized by:
   i. Hypercalcemia
   ii. Hyperphosphatemia
   iii. Renal calcinosis
   iv. Renal insufficiency
d. Sodium bicarbonate—systemic alkalosis

In chronic renal failure:
i. Magnesium-containing antacid—hypermagnesemia
ii. Aluminum-containing antacids—chronic neurotoxicity

H₂ receptors, antagonists: The drugs are:
A. Cimetidine:
   1. Dose—400 mg twice daily before meals or 800 mg at bedtime
   2. Side effects: Week antiandrogenic effects:
      i. Reversible gynecomastia
      ii. Impotence

iii. Confusion (rare)

iv. Raised blood level of aminotransferase, creatinine prolactin

   3. Drug interaction—cimetidine inhibits cytochrome P-450, hence monitoring of the following drugs should be required:
      i. Warfarin
      ii. Theophylline
      iii. Phenytoin

B. *Ranitidine*—300 mg at bedtime

C. *Famotidine*—40 mg at bedtime

D. *Nizatidine*—300 mg at bedtime

   Other rare reversible complications of H_2 blocker:
   i. Pancytopenia
   ii. Neutropenia
   iii. Anemia
   iv. Thrombocytopenia

Proton pump inhibitors: The drugs are:

A. Omeprazole

B. Esomeprazole

C. Lansoprazole

D. Rabeprazole

E. Pantoprazole

   These are benzimidozole derivatives. They bind and irreversibly inhibit H^+K^+ ATPase.

   Omeprazole and lansoprazole are acid labile, hence they are enteric-coated granules—they will be dissolved in the intestine at pH 6.

   Lansoprazole tablet can be used in patient having significant dyspepsia.

   Omeprazole and sodium bicarbonate combination can be used because here the effects of sodium bicarbonate are:
   i. Protect omeprazole from acid degradation
   ii. Promote rapid gastric alkalization
   iii. Help in activation of PPI—thus facilitates its action

Pantoprazole and rabeprazole:
   i. They are enteric coated tablets.
   ii. These are lipophilic compounds. After entering parietal cell they are potonated and trapped in acid environment.
   iii. Onset of action—2–6 hours after administration.
   iv. Duration of action—72–96 hours.
   v. Half life—18 hours.

Side effects:
1. Mild to moderate hypergastrinemia—it will be reversibly reduced within 1–2 weeks after drugs cessation.
2. Rebound gastric hyperacidity—it may last up to 2 months after discontinuation of PPI (in case *H. pylori* negative patient).

   Mechanisms: Hyperplasia and hypertrophy of histamine containing enterochromaffin like cells.

   Clinical importance in case of gastroesophageal reflux disease or dyspepsia.

   Prevention: This can be prevented by gradual tapering the dose and switching over to H_2 blockers.

   In case of *H. pylori* positive patient, this acid rebound will not occur due to *H. pylori*-induced inflammation followed by suppression of acid production.

3. Intrinsic factor will not be produced—but vitamin B_{12} deficiency anemia is uncommon.
4. Long-term suppression of acid may be responsible for:
   i. Community-acquired pneumonia
   ii. Hospital-acquired *Clostridium difficile* infection.
5. Competitive inhibition of clopidogrel. Hence this drug should be used at 12 hours in interval from rabeprazole or pantoprazole. Because, both PPI and clopidogrel have affinities for cytochrome P450 (CYP2C19).
6. Other drug, interaction—monitoring of the following drugs must be done who are on omeprazole or lansoprazole:
   i. Warfarin
   ii. Theophylline
   iii. Diazepam
   iv. Phenytoin
7. PPI interfere with the absorption of following drugs
   i. Ketoconazole
   ii. Ampicillin
   iii. Iron
   iv. Digoxin

Two newer PPIs are:

1. *Tenatoprazole:*
   i. Contains imidazopyridine ring
   ii. Irreversible proton pump inhibition
   iii. Longer half-life than other PPIs
   iv. It significantly reduces nocturnal acid secretion.

2. *Potassium* — competitive acid pump antagonists (P-CABs) These drugs inhibit gastric acid secretion through potassium competitive binding of H^+K^+ ATPase.

Dosages:
1. Omeprazole—20 mg/day
2. Lansoprazole—30 mg/day
3. Rabeprazole—20 mg/day
4. Pantoprazole—40 mg/day
5. Esomeprazole—20 mg/day

Cytoprotective agents:

A. *Sucralfate:* It is a complex sucrose salt. In it, hydroxyl group will be replaced by aluminum hydroxide and sulfate.

   It produces a viscous paste in the ulcer bed in stomach and duodenum and responsible for following actions:
   i. It acts as physic-chemical barrier
   ii. It binds with growth factor (EGF) and promotes tropic action
   iii. It enhances prostaglandin synthesis.
   iv. It stimulates mucus and bicarbonate secretion
   v. It enhances mucosal defense and repair.

Complication:
   i. Constipation
   ii. Hyperphosphatemia (rare)
   iii. Bezour formation.
   iv. In case of renal insufficiency—aluminum related toxicity

   Dose: 1 gm—4 times daily 15 minutes before meals.

B. *Bismuth containing compounds:* The drugs are:
   i. Colloidal bismuth subcitrate
   ii. Colloidal bismuth subsalicylate

Mechanism of action—unclear
Adverse effect:
   a. Short-term use:
      i.   Black stool
      ii. Constipation
      iii. Darkening of tongue
   b. Long-term use—neurotoxicity
C. *Prostaglandin analogue:*
   Mechanism of action:
      i. It enhances mucosal defense and
      ii. Repair of mucosal integrity
   Toxicity:
      i.   Diarrhea
      ii. Uterine bleeding
      iii. Uterine contraction
   Misoprostal is contraindicated in:
      i. Pregnant women
      ii. Women of child bearing age
   Dose: 200 mg four times daily.

H. pylori Positive PUD

Triple therapy

Proton pump inhibitor	twice daily	
+		
Clarithromycin (500 mg)	twice daily	× 7–14 days
Or		
Metronidazole (400 mg)	twice daily	
+		
Amoxycillin (1 gm)	twice daily	
Or, proton pump inhibitor	twice daily	
+		
Clarithromycin (500 mg)	twice daily	× 7–14 days
+		
Metronidazole (400 mg)	twice daily	

Quadruple therapy

Bismuth subsalicylate (525 mg)	4 times daily before meals	
+		
Metronidazole (200 mg)	4 times daily	× 10–14 daily
+		
Tetracycline (500 mg)	4 times daily	
+		
Proton pump inhibitor	twice daily	

Levofloxacin based triple therapy

Proton pump inhibitor	twice daily	
+		
Levofloxacin (250–500 mg)	twice daily	× 10 days
+		
Amoxycillin (1 gm)	twice daily	

Sequential therapy

Proton pump inhibitor	twice daily	× 10 days
+		
Amoxicillin (1 gm)	twice daily	× 5 days
+		
Clarithromycin (500 mg)	twice daily	
and		x next
Tinidazole (500 mg)	twice daily	5 days

Eradication rate:
1. Triple therapy   73–85%
2. Quadruple therapy   75–90%
3. Levofloxacin based therapy   60–80%
4. Sequential therapy   83–98%

Recommendation:
1. Triple therapy should be the 1st line of therapy.
2. In penicillin allergic patient—2nd triple therapies should be given.
3. Quadruple therapy should be given to those patients who fail to respond to triple therapy.
4. Levofloxacin based triple therapy should be second line of rescue therapy.
5. Sequential therapy:
      i.   May be initial therapy
      ii. 2nd line therapy
      iii. Rescue therapy

The above therapy should be given to following patients:
   i.   First degree relatives of gastric adenocarcinoma
   ii. Atrophic gastritis
   iii. Intestinal metaplasia.
   iv. *H. pylori* infected patient with unexplained iron deficiency.

After successful eradication treatment for *H. pylori*, reinfection is rare. If recurrence occurs within 6 months after discontinuation of treatment, it is due to recrudescence of infection.

Treatment for NSAID-Induced PUD

I. In case of active ulcer:
   A. First step: Discontinuation of NIAIDs
   B. Second step: H$_2$ receptor antagonist or proton pump inhibitor:
      a. Continuation of NSAIDs—at lowest effective dose
      b. Proton pump inhibitor

II. Prophylactic therapy:
   1. Lowest effective dosage of nonselective NSAID having lower GI toxicity:
      i.   Diclofenac
      ii. Aceclofenac
      iii. Ibuprofen
   2. Mesoprostol—200 mg 4 times daily or proton pump inhibitor.
   3. Highly selective cox-2 inhibitors:
      i. Celecoxib
      ii. Rofecoxib

These are 100 times more potent than standard NSAID, but due to their increased cardiovascular event and thrombotic events they are withdrawn from the market. Because cox-2 inhibitors produce following functions to produce cardiovascular events:
   i.   Irreversible platelet aggravation
   ii. Vasoconstriction
   iii. Smooth muscle proliferation

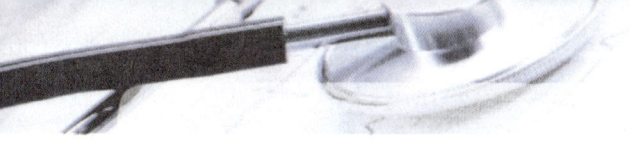

Use of NSAIDs as per guideline of American College of Physicians		
	No/low NSAID risk	*NSAID risk*
No cardiovascular risks		
No aspirin	Traditional NSAID	Coxib Traditional NSAID + PPI, or misoprostol Consider—non-NSAID therapy
Cardiovascular risk (consideration) of aspirin)	Traditional NSAID + PPI, or Misoprostol If gastrointestinal risk requires gastro-protection.	Gastroprotective drugs must be added in case of traditional NSAID
	Consider non-NSAID therapy	Consider non-NSAID therapy

Operations for Duodenal Ulcers

The procedures involved:
1. Vagotomy with drainage:
   a. Pyloroplasty
   b. Gastroduodenostomy (Billroth I)
   c. Gastrojejunostomy (Billroth II)
2. Highly selective vagotomy—it does not require drainage
3. Vagotomy with antrectomy

The choice of procedures depends upon the following:
1. Elective or emergency
2. Degree and extent of duodenal ulceration
3. Expertise of surgeon.

Specific operative procedures for gastric ulcers: Presence of associated ulcer usually dictates the operation for gastric ulcer:
1. In case of antral ulcer—antrectomy with Billroth I anastomosis
2. If duodenal ulcer is present—vagotomy is performed.
3. If ulcer is present in esophagogastric junction—subtotal gastrectomy with Roux-en-Y esophagogastrojejunostomy (Csende's procedure)
4. In patient with high duodenal ulcer—antrectomy, intraoperative biopsy from ulcer and vagotomy (Kelling-Madlener procedure). Chance of ulcer recurrence is 30%.

Complications of surgery:
I. *Ulcer recurrence:* Causes are:
  i. Incomplete vagotomy—this can be diagnosed by analysis of gastric acid output in response to sham feeding and chewing of food.
    a. Increase in gastric acid output in response to sham feeding—vagus nerve is intact.
    b. Rise in serum pancreatic polypeptide >50% within 30 minutes of sham feeding—intact vagus nerve.
  ii. Retained antrum—Fasting serum gastrin level will be elevated and Zollinger-Ellison syndrome must be excluded.

  iii. Inadequate drainage
  iv. Persistent or recurrent *H. pylori* infection

II. *Afferent loop syndrome:* This usually occurs after partial gastrectomy with Billroth II anastomosis. Two types of syndrome are:
1. *Type-I syndrome:* Bacterial over growth is more common, symptoms are:
  i. Abdominal pain—postprandial
  ii. Abdominal bloating
  iii. Diarrhea
  iv. Malabsorption of fat and vitamin B_{12}.
    This type is refractory to antibiotic. It requires surgical revision of the affected loop.
2. *Type-II afferent loop syndrome:* Symptoms are:
  i. Abdominal pain
  ii. Bloating
  iii. Postprandial vomiting—this gives relief to abdominal pain and bloating. Vomitus contains bile salts and pancreatic secretion.

    This syndrome is refractory to dietary measures. It usually requires surgical revision.

III. *Dumping syndrome:* This syndrome is characterized by—constipation of vasomotor and gastrointestinal signs and symptoms in patients having vagotomy with Billroth type drainage procedure. Two types of dumping syndrome are:
1. *Early dumping syndrome:*
  i. It occurs 15–30 minutes after intake of meals
  ii. Symptoms and signs are:
    a. Cramping abdominal pain
    b. Light headedness
    c. Nausea
    d. Vomiting
    e. Diarrhea
    f. Belching
    g. Tachycardia
    h. Diaphoresis
  iii. Pathophysiology

Rapid entry of hyperosmolar gastric content into intestinal lumen
↓
Rapid shift of fluid from blood vessels into intestinal lumen
↓
Rapid contraction of plasma volume

Acute distention of intestinal content
  * Release of vasoactive gastrointestinal hormones.
2. *Late dumping syndrome:*
  i. It occurs 90 minutes to 3 hours after meals
  ii. *Clinical features:*
    a. Light headedness
    b. Diaphoresis
    c. Palpitations
    d. Tachycardia
    e. Syncope
  iii. *Pathophysiology:*
    a. Secondary to hypoglycemia
    b. Excessive insulin release

Factors responsible for dumping syndrome:
   a. Ingestion of simple carbohydrate (sucrose) and high osmolarity
   b. Ingestion of large amount of fluid.

  vi. *Treatment:*
    A. Dietary modification:
      1. Dietary modification is the main stay of treatment:
        a. Small, multiple meals, devoid of carbo-hydrates
        b. Elimination of liquids during meals.
      2. Use of anti-diarrheal and anticholinergic agents
      3. Use of Guar and pectin to increase the viscosity of the intraluminal content.
      4. Use of acarbose (α-glucosidase inhibitor)—because it delays the digestion of ingested carbohydrates—useful in late phase of dumping syndrome.
    B. Diet refractory cases:
      1. Subcutaneous administration of octreotide—50 µg thrice daily
      2. Long-acting depot octreotide

IV. *Post-vagotomy diarrhea:*
  i. In case of truncal vagotomy—intermittent diarrhea occurs 1–2 hours after meals.
  ii. This occurs due to:
    a. Interruption of vagal fibers—which supply the gut wall.
    b. Decreased absorption of ingested nutrients
    c. Increased excretion of bile acids
    d. Release of luminal factors that promoter secretion.
  iii. Treatment:
    a. Diphenoxylate or loperamide—can symptomatically control the symptoms.
    b. Cholestyramine
    c. Surgical reversal of 10 cm segment of jejunum

V. *Bile reflux gastropathy:*
  1. Symptoms:
    i. Abdominal pain
    ii. Early satiety
    iii. Nausea vomiting
  2. Endoscopic finding—mucosal erythema of gastric remnant
  3. Histological examinations: Minimal inflammation, with epithelial cell injury.
  4. Treatment: Prokinetic agents—cholestyramine and sucralfate

MENETRIER'S DISEASE

This is rare disease, characterized by the following:
  i. Large tortuous gastric mucosal folds—more prominent in body and fundus
  ii. Histologically foveolar hyperplasia—which replaces chief and parietal cells and produces prominent folds.
  iii. Pits of gastric gland elongate and extremely tortuous
  iv. Lamina propria contains chronic inflammatory infiltrate.

Clinical Features

  a. Epigastric pain
  b. Nausea
  c. Vomiting
  d. Anorexia
  e. Weight loss
  f. Occult bleeding, overt bleeding is rare but may occur due to superficial erosions
  g. Hypoproteinemia and edema due to—protein loosing gastropathy
  h. Gastric acid secretion will be reduced.
    i. Endoscopy—large gastric folds can be detectable.

Treatment

  i. Anticholinergic agents
  ii. Prostaglandin
  iii. PPI
  iv. Prednisolone
  v. H$_2$ receptor antagonists
  vi. High protein diet—it is given to replace protein and hypoalbuminemia
  vii. Subtotal gastrectomy—in some cases, it may be associated with high morbidity and mortality.

STRESS ULCERS

This ulcer is characterized by—acute erosive gastric mucosal changes with or without frank ulceration.

Causes

1. Shock
2. Sepsis
3. Burns
4. Severe trauma
5. Head injury
6. Respiratory failure requiring mechanical ventilation
7. Underlying coagulopathy

Symptoms

Gastrointestinal bleeding—it may be minimal or life-threatening.

Laboratory Workup

Elevated gastric acids are usually found in case of:
  i. Head trauma (Cushing's ulcer)
  ii. Severe burns (Curling ulcer)

Histology

  i. Mucosal ischemia
  ii. Breakdown of normal protective barrier of stomch

Management

1. Improved general management in intensive care unit—it reduces the incidence of bleeding from 20% to <5%.
2. Use of preventive measures (medical therapy)—in following high-risk patients:
    a. Mechanically ventilated patients
    b. Severe burns
    c. Multiorgan failure
    d. Coagulopathy
    The aim is to maintain gastric pH >3.5 by continuous infusion of PPI or H$_2$ blockers.
    Sucralfate can be given in the dose of 1 gm every 4–6 hours.

Risk:
  i. Constipation
  ii. Aluminum toxicity

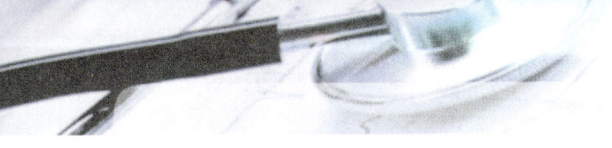

iii. In case of endotracheal intubated patient—chance of aspiration pneumonia

If bleeding will be continued inspite of giving PPI
↓
Intra-arterial vasopressin
↓ If fails
Intra-arterial embolization
↓← If fails
Surgery
↓

Vagotomy   Total gastrectomy
+
Antrectomy

ZOLLINGER-ELLISON SYNDROME

This syndrome is characterized by evidence of severe peptic ulcer due to unregulated released gastrin-induced hyper-secretion of gastric acid. This gastrin is being released by non-β-cell endocrine tumor (gastrinoma).

Epidemiology

1. Sex—males are more commonly affected than females.
2. Age—it is common between 30 and 50 years of age.
3. Sporadic tumor is more common.
4. Some tumors are associated with type 1 multiple endocrine neoplasia.

Pathophysiology

Increased gastrin secretion from autonomous neoplasm
↓

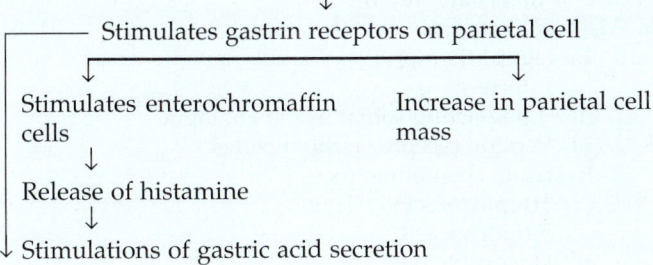

Tropic action on gastric epithelial cells
Ultimate results are:
 i. Development of peptic ulcer
 ii. Erosive esophagitis
iii. Diarrhea

Sites of Tumor

1. Pancreatic site
2. Extrapancreatic sites:
   i. Hypothetical gastrinoma triangle
      a. Confluence of cystic and common bile duct—superiorly
      b. Inferiorly—junction of 2nd and third part of duodenum
      c. Medially junction of neck and body of pancreas.
   ii. Duodenal tumor—smaller and slow growing
   iii. Stomach

iv. Bone
 v. Liver
vi. Lymph node
vii. Heart
viii. Ovaries

Histology

Gastrin producing cells:
 i. Well differentiated
ii. Expression of markers of endocrine neoplasm—chromogranin neuron specific enolase

Clinical Features

A. **Peptic ulcers:**
   i. Sites:
      a. Usually in duodenal bulb
      b. Unusual location—2nd or beyond 2nd part of duodenum
   ii. This is refractory to medical therapy.
   iii. Recurrence after ulcer surgery
   iv. Presence of frank complications
      a. Perforation
      b. Bleeding
      c. Obstruction
   v. It may be present in absence of *H. pylori* or NSAID ingestion.
B. **Esophageal involvement:**
   i. Mild esophagitis
   ii. Esophageal ulcerations
   iii. Esophageal stricture
   iv. Barrett's mucosa.
C. **Diarrhea:** It is present in 50% patients. It may be present with peptic ulcers or isolatedly. The causes of diarrhea are:
   i. Marked volume overload to small bowel.
   ii. Pancreatic enzyme inactivation by acid
   iii. Intestinal epithelial cell damage by acid
   Results of intestinal epithelial cell damage are:
      a. Maldigestion
      b. Malabsorption
   iv. Direct stimulatory effect of gastrin or enterocytes
   v. Co-secretion of additional hormones like VIP from tumor.
D. **Association with MEN-1 syndrome:** It is autosomal dominant. The organs involved in this syndrome are:
   i. Parathyroid glands
   ii. Pancreas
   iii. Pituitary gland

   Here the defect lies in long arm of chromosome 11.

   Hyperparathyroidism produces hypercalcemia—it produces direct effect on parietal cells.

   High incidence of gastric carcinoid tumor in type 1 MEN.

Diagnosis

Fasting serum gastrin level: Normal <150 pg/mL

Following are the causes of hypergastrinemia:
1. Gastric hypochlorhydria or achlorhydria with or without pernicious anemia
2. Retained gastric antrum
3. G-cell hyperplasia

4. Gastric outlet obstruction
5. Renal insufficiency
6. Massive small bowel obstruction.
7. Systemic diseases:
   a. Rheumatoid arthritis
   b. Diabetes mellitus
   c. Vitiligo
   d. Pheochromocytoma
   8. Use of antisecretory agent
9. *H. pylori* infection

Before estimation of serum gastrin level, PPI should be stopped for at least 1 week before testing and H_2 blocker should be stopped for 2 days before testing.

Serum gastrin concentration of >1000 pg/ml with pH of stomach <2.0—is the diagnostic of ZE syndrome.

But it occurs in 5–9% of ZES.

40% patients show serum gastrin level <500 pg/ml.

Special Tests

A. Secretin stimulation test: It is a provocative test of high sensitivity method.

Baseline serum gastrin level to be measured

↓

2 units/kg of body weight secretin to be injected intravenously over 1 minute.

↓

Serial estimations of serum gastrin at 2, 5, 10, 15 and 20 minutes to be done

↓

Absolute increase in serum gastrin by ≥ 200 pg/ml

↓

Suggest ZES
Sensitivity and specificity >83%)

B. Ratio or basal acid output to pentagastrin stimulated maximum acid output:
   • >0.6—suggestive of ZES
   • <0.6—exclude the diagnosis.
C. Basal acid output:
   • >15 mEq/hour
      Or
   • >5 mEq/hour in patient with prior vagotomy or partial gastrectomy are suggestive of ZES.
D. Basal gastric pH ≥ 3—exclude the ZES
E. Calcium infusion test is less sensitive and difficult to perform

Imaging

CT scan shows:
1. 80% of gastrinoma—is present in gastrinoma triangle area.
2. 80% of duodenal gastrinoma—is present in 1st and 2nd portion of duodenum—it is smll and multiple.
3. Pancreatic gastrinoma is >1cm.
   Somatostatin receptors bind to octreotide—based in this, two followed methods are used:
   i. Somatostatin receptor scintigraphy with [111]Indium pentaoctreotide—it is more sensitive.
   ii. Single photon emission computerized tomography—sensitivity of CT scan is 54–56%.

Endoscopic ultrasonography: It is useful for:
 i. Preoperative tumor localization
ii. Staging of ZES—specially in head and body of pancreas

Special examinations:
1. Portal venous sampling
2. Intra-arterial injection of secretin combined with venous sampling.
   The above tests are useful for regionalization of the tumor—it is useful to find duodenal gastrinoma.
3. Endoscopic transillumination of the duodenal wall
4. Intraoperative ultrasonography

The above two methods are useful for detection of small duodenl tumor.

Treatment

Aims are:
 i. Control of gastric acid hypersecretion—it reduces symptoms and their complications.
ii. Surgical resection to—control tumor growth.

Medical Treatment

a. Proton pump inhibitors—60 mg/day in divided doses. The aim is
   i. To reduce BAO <10 mEq/hour in surgery negative patients
   ii. To reduce BAO <5 mEq/hour in patient with previous history of surgery.
b. Somatostatin analogue—has inhibitory effect on gastrin release—it can be given as an adjunct.

Surgical Therapy

Surgical removal of tumor.

In case of metastatic tumor:
A. *Medical therapies:*
   1. Biological therapies
       i. Interferon-α
      ii. Long-acting somatostatin analogue
      iii. Peptide receptor radionuclides
   2. Systemic chemotherapy
       i. Streptozotocin
      ii. 5-fluorouracil
      iii. Doxorubicin
   3. [111] Indium pentetreotide
B. *Several other surgical therapies:*
    i. Radiofrequency ablation
   ii. Cryoablation of liver lesions
   iii. Agents that block vascular endothelial growth receptor pathway (sunitinib, bevacizumab)
   iv. Debulking surgery, liver transplantation.

SMALL INTESTINE

ACUTE INFECTIVE DIARRHEA

Definition

On western diet, if stool volume is >200 gm/day, it is called diarrhea.

This should be differentiated from the following types of motions:

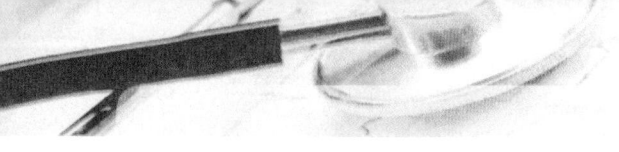

i. **Pseudodiarrhea:** It is characterized by frequent passage of small volume of stool, associated with rectal tenesmus. It is usually accompanied by irritable bowel syndrome or proctitis.

ii. **Fecal incontinence:** This is characterized by involuntary discharge of rectal contents. It is usually caused by:
   a. Neuromuscular disorders.
   b. Anorectal structural abnormalities.

Diarrhea is subdivided into three types:
   i. Acute diarrhea—if it persists less than 2 weeks.
   ii. Persistant diarrhea—if it persists for 2–4 weeks.
   iii. Chronic diarrhea—it persists more than 4 weeks.

The organisms responsible are:
1. *Toxin-producing organisms:*
   a. Preformed toxin:
      i. *Bacillus cereus*
      ii. *Staphylococcus aureus*
      iii. *Clostridium perfringens.*
   b. Enterotoxin:
      i. *Vibrio cholerae*
      ii. *Enterotoxigenic E. coli*
      iii. *Klebsiella pneumoniae*
2. *Enteroadherent organisms:*
   a. Enteropathogenic and enteroadherent:
      i. *E. coli*
      ii. *Giardia*
      iii. *Cryptococcus*
      iv. *Helminths*
   b. Cytotoxin producers:
      i. *Clostridium difficile*
      ii. Hemorrhagic *E. coli.*
3. *Invasive organisms:*
   a. Minimal inflammation:
      i. Rotavirus
      ii. Norovirus
   b. Variable inflammation
      i. *Salmonella*
      ii. *Campylobacter*
      iii. *Vibrio parahemolyticus*
      iv. *Yersinia*
   c. Severe inflammation:
      i. Enteroinvasive *E. coli*
      ii. *Shigella* species
      iii. *Entamoeba histolytica*

There are five risk groups recognized:
1. *Travellers:*
   a. Latin American, African and Asian travelers develop diarrhea due to enterotoxigenic or enteroinvasive *E. coli, Campylobacter, Shigella, Aeromonas,* norovirus, coronavirus and *Salmonella.*
   b. Visitors to Russia develop *Giardia* associated diarrhea.
   c. Visitors to Nepal—risk of *Cyclospora*
   d. Cruise strips may be affected by noroviral diarrhea.
2. *Certain food consumers:*
   a. Chicken—*Salmonella, Campylobacter, Shigella.*
   b. Undercooked hamburger—enterohemorrhagic *E. coli.*
   c. Fried rice—*Bacillus cereus*
   d. Mayonnaise or cream—*Staphylococcus* aureus.
   e. Eggs — *Salmonella*
   f. Uncooked food or soft cheeses—*Listeria.*
   g. Seafood—*Salmonella, Vibrio* species, hepatitis A virus

3. *Immunodeficient persons:* The patient may be:
   a. Primary immunodeficient (hypogammaglobulinemia IgA deficiency).
   b. Secondary immunodeficiency—AIDS, pharmacologic suppression.
      i. The agents may transmit through rectum
         * *Neisseria gonorrhoeae*
         * *Treponema pallidum*
         * *Chlamydia*
      ii. Patients with hemochromatosis are prone to develop fatal infection with *Vibrio* species.
4. *Day care attendance and their family members:* These persons are prone to develop with:
   i. *Shigella*
   ii. *Giardia*
   iii. *Cryptosporidium*
   iv. Rotavirus
5. *Institutionalized persons:* In many hospitals, the patients may suffer from variety of microorganisms, specially *Clostridium difficile.*

Pathologic Mechanism

There are a number of factors on which the infectivity and severity of the disease depend. These are:
1. **Size of inoculums:** This varies from organism to organisms.
   a. In case of *Shigella*, enterohemorrhagic *E. coli, Entamoeba, Giardia lamblia*—10 to 100 bacteria or cysts
   b. In case of *Vibrio cholerae*—10^5 to 10^8 organisms.
   c. In case of *Salmonella* and other organisms—doses vary according to species, host and food vehicle—like:
      i. *Shigella*, enterohemorrhagic *E. coli, Entamoeba* and *Giardia* spread from person to person.
      ii. *Salmonella* has to grow for several hours to reach infecting dose.
2. **Adherence:** The virulent organisms compete with normal bowel flora to colonize and adherent to the gastrointestinal mucosa by specific cell surface proteins
   a. *Vibrio cholerae* adheres to enterocytes via specific surface adhesins including toxin-coregulated pilus.
   b. Enterotoxigenic *E. coli* by adherence protein called colonization factor antigen adheres to upper small intestine.
   c. Enterohemorrhagic and enteropathogenic *E. coli* attach to the efface of brush border epithelium to produce virulence determinants.
3. **Toxin production:** Production of several enterotoxins is important in producing diarrhea by several organisms:
   a. Enterotoxin acting directly on the secretory mechanisms in the intestinal mucosa.
   b. Cytotoxin: Destruction of mucosal cells is responsible for inflammatory diarrhea.
   c. Neurotoxin: It affects directly on central or peripheral nervous system.

The enterotoxins are:
   i. Cholera toxin—composed of one A and five B subunits. A subunit contains enzymatic activity. B subunits bind holotoxins to the enterocytes surface receptor ganglioside G_{M1}.
   ii. Enterotoxigenic *E. coli*—produces heat-labile enterotoxin, similar to cholera toxin—produces secretory diarrhea.

iii. Some enterotoxigenic *E. coli*—produces heat-stable enterotoxin.

The cytotoxin producing organisms are

i. *Shigella dysenteriae* type 1
ii. *Vibrio parahemolyticus*
iii. *Clostridium difficile*

The neurotoxins: It is produced by bacteria outside the host—The toxins are:

i. Staphylococcal toxin
ii. *Bacillus cereus toxin*

These toxins act on CNS to produce vomiting.

4. **Invasion:** Usually dysentery results from:
   i. Cytotoxin production
   ii. Bacterial invasion of intestinal mucosal cells
   iii. Destruction of intestinal mucosal cells.

In case of *Shigella* and enteroinvasive *E. coli:*
   i. Invasion of mucosal epithelial cells
   ii. Intraepithelial multiplication
   iii. Subsequent spread to adjacent cells

In case of *Salmonella typhi*—inflammatory diarrhea occurs due to:
   i. Invasion of the bowel mucosa.
   ii. Multiply intracellularly in Payer's patches and intestinal lymph nodes.
   iii. Spread through bloodstream

Host Defenses

Normal hosts have some interest protective facts to combat with the pathologic factors of organizations

1. **Normal bowel flora:** These organisms are mainly anaerobic. They produce—acidic pH and volatile fatty acids. These are responsible for preventing colonization by potential enteric pathogens.
2. **Gastric acid:** Gastric acidic pH is mainly responsible to act as a barrier against pathogenic organisms like, *Salmonella*, *Giardia lamblia* and some helminths.
   Hence, the following factors increase the risk of entry of the above organisms:
   i. Gastric surgery
   ii. Use of proton pump inhibitors
   iii. Use of antacids.
3. **Intestinal motility:** Intestinal normal peristalsis prevents colonization of bacteria in proximal small intestine. So, impaired intestinal motility is responsible for colonization of organisms. The factors are:
   i. Treatment with opiates or other antimotility agents
   ii. Anatomic abnormalities
   iii. Hypomotility states.
4. **Immunity:** The immunities responsible for protection against invasive organisms are:
   i. Cellular immunity
   ii. Humoral immunity including IgM, IgA and IgG.

The process of developing immunity is bacterial antigen binds with M cells on luminal surface in distal small intestine.

↓

Presentation of antigen to subepithelial lymphoid tissue

↓

Lymphocyte sensitization

↓

Proliferation of lymphocytes

↓

These lymphocytes circulate and populate in mucosal tissue of the body as IgA secreting plasma cells.

5. **Genetics of hosts:** Genetic variations are responsible for susceptibility of some hosts to a particular type of organism.
   i. Patients with blood group-O—increased susceptibility to variety of organisms—like *Vibrio cholerae*, *Shigella*, *E. coli* (0157), norovirus.
   ii. Genetic polymorphism: It is responsible for outcome of different infections like, enterotoxigenic *E. coli*, *Salmonella*, *Clostridium difficile*, *Vibrio cholerae*.

Epidemiology

A. 20–50% of travelers from temperate climate to tropical climates may develop diarrhea 3 days to 2 weeks after leaving resource-heavy areas. The disease is self-limiting. The organisms are:
   a. Bacteria:
      i. Enterotoxigenic *E. coli*
      ii. Enteroinvasive *E. coli*
      iii. *Campylobacter jejuni*
      iv. *Shigella*
      v. *Salmonella*
   b. Virus:
      i. Norovirus (as in case of ship cruise)
      ii. Rotavirus.
   c. Parasites:
      i. *Giardia lamblia*
      ii. *Cryptosporidium*
      iii. *Entamoeba histolytica.*
   d. Other:
      i. Acute food poisoning
      ii. Unidentified pathogen
B. **Locations**
   a. *Day care centers:*
      i. Rotavirus—in young children <2 years old
      ii. *Giardia lamblia*—in older children
      The characteristic features are high attack rate of associated family members.
   b. *Hospital sites:*
      i. Nosocomial route: *Clostridium difficile*—in adult.
      ii. *Klebsiella oxytoca*—antibiotic associated hemorrhagic colitis.
      iii. Rotavirus—in pediatric wards
      iv. Cytotoxin producing *Clostridium. difficile*—in chronic care center.
   C. **Age:** Globally, mortality is highest in children <5 years of age.
      Breastfed infants get some protection by maternal antibodies.
      In infants—rotaviral diarrhea is common.
      In older children and adults—norovirus, enterotoxigenic, enteroinvasive *E. coli*, *G. lamblia*, *V. cholerae*, *shigella*, *C. jejuni*.
   D. **Host immune status:**
      a. In impaired cell-mediated immunity:
         i. Salmonellosis
         ii. Shigellosis

Clinical Features

	Pathogens period	Incubation period	Vomiting	Abdominal pain	Fever	Diarrhea
I.	Toxin producing					
	a. Preformed toxin					
	i. *B. cereus, Staph. aureus*	½ to 8 hrs	+++	++	-/+	Watery ++++
	ii. *C. perfringens*	8–24 hrs	++++	++	-/+	Watery [++++]
	b. Enterotoxin	8–72 hrs	+++/++++	++	+	-do-
II.	Enteroadherent	1–8 days	+	+++	+/++	++ watery/mushy
III.	Cytotoxin producing					
	i. *C. difficile*	1–3 days	+/-	+++	+/++	++ watery/bloody
	ii. Hemorrhagic *E. coli*	1/2 to 3 days	+/-	+++	++	++/+++ watery/bloody
IV.	Invasive					
	i. Minimal	1–3 days	+/++	++	+++	watery
	ii. Moderate	1–11 days	-/++	+++	+++	Watery/bloody
	iii. Severe	1–8 days	-/+	++/+++	+++/+++	bloody

    iii. Listeriosis
    iv. Cryptosporidiosis
  b. In case of hypogammaglobulinemia
    i. *Clostridium difficile*
    ii. *Giardia lamblia*
  c. Patients on cancer chemotherapy: *Clostridium difficile*

The immune uncompromised patients are liable to develop bacteremia and metastatic seeding of infections.

Signs of Dehydration

i. **Mild dehydration**: Thirst, dry mouth, decreased axillary sweat, decreased urine output, weight loss.
ii. **Moderate dehydration**: Hypotension, orthostatic hypotension, loss of skin turger, sunken eyes, depressed fontanelle.
iii. **Severe dehydration:** Obtundation, lethargy, rapid and thready pulse, severe hypotension, shock.

Laboratory Investigations

I. Stool microscopy:
  i. In non-inflammatory diarrhea
    a. No fecal leukocytosis
    b. Mild or no increase in fecal lactoferin
  ii. In case of inflammatory diarrhea
    a. Fecal polymorphonuclear leukocytes
    b. Increase in fecal lactoferin
  iii. In case of invasive diarrhea, severe fecal polymorphonuclear leukocytosis
  iv. Cyst, trophozoites—*G. lamblia, E. histolytica*
II. Stool culture:
  i. Cholera—thiosulfate—citrate—bile salts—sucrose or tellurite—taurocholate—gelatin agar
  ii. *Salmonella, shigella*, in MacConkey agar as non-lactose fermenting colonies—which can be grown in *Salmonella–Shigella* agar or selenite enrichment broth—which inhibit other organisms.

  iii. *Campylobacter*
  iv. *C. jejuni*—incubation of fresh stool in selective growth medium at 42°C in microaerophilic atmosphere.
  v. Enterohemorrhagic *E. coli*—as lactose fermenting, Indole positive colonies on sorbitol MacConkey plates.

III. Rapid detection in stool:
  i. Latex agglutination test—for rotavirus
  ii. Reverse-transcriptase PCR and specific antigen enzyme immunoassay—for norovirus in stool.
  iii. Immunofluorescence based rapid assay—*Giardia lamblia* (less sensitive), *Cryptosporidium*
  iv. Rapid enzyme immune assay and latex agglutination tests—detect toxin A and B of *Clostridium difficile*.

Treatment of Acute Diarrhea

Mainstay of treatment is replenishment of water and electrolytes in the body. This can be done is two ways:
A. Oral rehydration by ORS: The compositions in:
- Sodium chloride   3.5 gm
- Sodium bicarbonate   2.5 gm
- Potassium chloride   1.5 gm
- Glucose   20 gm
  Or
- Sucrose   4.0 gm

It may cause secretory diarrhea, but with less electrolyte loss than in cholera.

The other solution is: Reduced osmolarity/reduced salt—it is better tolerated and more effective. The composition is:
- Sodium chloride   2.6 gm
- Trisodium citrate   2.9 gm
- Potassium chloride   1.5 gm
- Glucose   13.5 gm
  Or
- Sucrose   27 gm.

The composition above is per liter of water.

But rice or cereals-based solutions are more effective than glucose-based solution.

In case of severe dehydration—intravenous solutions ringer lactate.

Specific Treatment

1. Most secretory form of traveler's diarrhea can be treated by:
   i. Rehydration
   ii. Antimotility agents
   iii. Antimicrobial agents to reduce the duration of illness
   iv. Probiotics
2. Bloody diarrhea or dysentery should be treated by:
   i. Antimicrobial drugs
   ii. Rehydration
   iii. Antispasmodics
   iv. Probiotics
3. Campylobacter diarrhea can be effectively treated by—Macrolide group of antibiotics—erythromycin, azithromycin, due to resistance against fluoroquinolone.
4. In case of salmonellosis, antimicrobial agents may interfere with intestinal colonization with *Salmonella*, hence, these drugs should be administered in following types of patients:
   i. Young children
   ii. Elderly individual
   iii. Patients having prosthetic devices
   iv. Immunocompromised patients.

Antibiotics

Travel to high-risk countries other than Thailand.

Adult:

a. *Fluoroquinolones:*
   i. Ciprofloxacin 750 mg single dose or 500 mg twice daily × 3 days.
   ii. Levofloxacin 500 mg as single dose or 500 mg 4 times daily × 3 days.
   iii. Norfloxacin—800 mg as single dose or 400 mg twice daily × 3 days.
b. *Macrolide group:* Azithromycin—1000 mg as single dose or 500 mg 4 times daily × 3 days
c. **Rifaximin**—200 mg thrice daily or 400 mg twice daily × 3 days. It is not used in dysentery.

Pediatrics:
- Azithromycin or fluoroquinolone
- Travel to Thailand (fluoroquinolone resistant): Azithromycin as above dosage.

Post-Diarrheal Complications

A. Chronic diarrhea:
   i. Lactase deficiency
   ii. Malabsorption syndrome
   iii. Small bowel bacterial overgrowth.
B. Irritable bowel syndrome (10% of traveler's diarrhea)
C. Acute exacerbation of inflammatory bowel disease
D. Reactive arthritis—in case of *Shigella, Salmonella, Campylobacter* and Yersinia *enterocolitica* infection
E. Hemolytic uremic syndrome—in case of shiga-1 toxin producing bacteria and enterohemorrhagic *E. coli* infection.
F. Guillain-Barre syndrome—in case of *Campylobacter* infection.

Prophylaxis

Prevention of possible feco-oral transmission of infection
Traveler:
   i. Takes hot, fresh cooled food
   ii. Avoid raw vegetables, ice, salads, unpeeled fruits
   iii. Takes boiled or treated water
   iv. Prophylactic drugs—Bismuth subsalicylate (525 mg)—to be taken 4 times daily for up to 3 weeks.

   Possible complications:
   a. Darkening of tongue
   b. Tinnitus
   v. Antibiotics, should be avoided except in the following conditions
   a. Immunocompromised patient
   b. Comorbid illness
      But non-absorbable antibiotics, like, rifaximin can be given in Latin America to prevent infection with non-invasive *E. coli*, because rifaximin is not effective against invasive organisms.
   vi. Vaccine against rotavirus is nowadays available—but protection is short lived and incomplete.

EOSINOPHILIC GASTROENTERITIS

Definition

This is characterized by mature eosinophils in the stomach, small intestine and colonic mucosa with pronounced peripheral eosinophilia in 50% of cases.

Pathology

Chemokines (Eotaxin 1 and Eotaxin 2)
↓
Recruitment of eosinophils to the gut
↓
Activation of eosinophils to release proinflammatory mediators. Mediators are major basic protein, eosinophilic peroxydase, eosinophilic cationic protein and leukotrienes
↓
Initiates inflammation

Clinical Features

Three major patterns of clinical symptoms and signs are present

First type: This is associated with eosinophilic infiltration of mucosa and submucosa:
1. Diarrhea
2. Steatorrhea
3. Abdominal pain
4. Nausea
5. Vomiting.

Associated signs:
i. Iron deficiency anemia
ii. Hypoalbuminemia

Imaging studies show:
i. Small bowel wall thickening
ii. Mucosal nodularity

Second type: This pattern is associated with eosinophilic infiltration of visceral mucosa and muscle.

Features are like obstructive symptoms
 i. Nausea
 ii. Vomiting
 ii. Abdominal pain
 iv. Weight loss
 v. May be diarrhea

Imaging studies show evidence of mass lesion in visceral wall mimicking malignancy.

Third type: Here the symptoms are due to eosinophilic infiltration in serosa and subserosa. The clinical features are:
 i. Abdominal discomfort
 ii. Diarrhea
 iii. Nausea

Diagnosis

Diagnosis stands on following findings:
 i. Presence of gastrointestinal symptoms
 ii. Eosinophilic infiltration of visceral wall
 iii. Eosinophilic ascites
 iv. Exclusion of other causes producing eosinophilia and gastrointestinal symptoms:
   a. Parasitic disease
   b. Food allergies
   c. Drug allergies
   d. Mastocytosis
   e. Polyarteritis nodosa
   f. Churg-Strauss syndrome
   g. Lymphoma
   h. IBD
   i. Hypereosinophilic syndrome

Treatment

Oral prednisolone—20–40 mg/day for 2–4 weeks
↓
Followed by gradual tapering of the steroid

Follow-up

a. Most of the patients show sustained remission
b. Only a few patients show relapses—requiring second course of corticosteroids
c. A few patients require continuous steroid therapy.
d. A few patients become resistance to corticosteroid.

Diet: Diet should be eliminated based on skin sensitivity to foods.

INTESTINAL MALABSORPTION

Typical western diet contains
 • Fat   100 gm
 • Carbohydrate   400 gm
 • Protein   100 gm
 • Fluid   2 liters
 • Electrolytes—sodium, potassium, calcium, chloride, vitamin—adequate.

During digestion, following secretions are added:
 i. Salivary
 ii. Gastric
 iii. Intestinal
 iv. Hepatic
 v. Pancreatic
Amount 7–8 liters.

During passage through small and large intestines—the total amount of fluid will be reduced to 200 ml. This contains:
 • Fat   <8 gm
 • Nitrogen   1–2 gm
 • Electrolytes <20 mEq (Na$^+$, K$^+$, Cl$^-$, HCO$^-_3$, Ca^{++}, Mg^{++})

Now, if there is deficient absorption in any or all steps—malabsorption may occur. It may be:
 i. Selective malabsorption—like, lactose deficiency
 ii. Generalized malabsorption

Classifications of Malabsorption

1. Diseases associated with impaired intraluminal digestion:
   i. Pancreatic diseases
   ii. Liver and biliary diseases
   iii. Postoperative post-gastrectomy malabsorption
2. Diseases which are responsible for impaired digestion, uptake and transport of nutrients:
   i. Celiac disease
   ii. Tropical sprue
   iii. Eosinophilic gastroenteritis
   iv. Radiation enteritis
   v. Whipple disease
   vi. Systemic mastocytosis
   vii. Crohn's disease
   viii. Abetalipoproteinemia
3. Diseases which are responsible for defect in intraluminal digestion and mucosal function:
   i. Short bowel syndrome
   ii. Intestinal bacterial overgrowth
   iii. Zollinger-Ellison syndrome
4. Diseases which are responsible for defect in post-mucosal transport.

Lymphangiectasia
— Primary
— Secondary

Clinical Features

 I. Gastrointestinal symptoms:
   1. *Diarrhea*—it may be >10 times/day to ~1 voluminous loose stool/day—volume is >200 gm/day.
   Causes are:
     i. Malabsorption of nutrients
     ii. Secretions of small intestines
     iii. Unabsorbed fatty acids will be converted to hydroxyl fatty acids by colonic flora, thus impairs absorption and increases the secretion of electrolytes and water by colon.
     iv. Unabsorbed bile acids—impairs absorption
   2. *Weight loss*—causes are:
     i. Impaired absorption from intestinal mucosa
     ii. Decreased oral intake of nutrients
   3. *Excessive flatus and abdominal bloating:*
     i. It occurs due to excessive gas production—due to fermentation of unabsorbed carbohydrate which

may occur in primary or secondary disaccharidase deficiency.

ii. Malabsorption of dietary nutrients and intestinal fluid secretion due to inflammation of small intestinal mucosa.

iii. Evidence of vitamin deficiency—like, glossitis, cheliosis, stomatitis

4. *Abdominal pain*—it may be due to:
   i. Abdominal muscle spasm
   ii. Stretching pain of bowel wall as a result of distention of bowel. Example:
      a. Chronic pancreatitis
      b. Pancreatic cancer
      c. Crohn's disease

II. Hematopoietic system:

1. Anemia—It may be of macrocytic:
   i. Vitamin B_{12} deficiency
   ii. Pyridoxine deficiency
2. Bleeding—it may be:
   a. Petechiae
   b. Purpura
   c. Subconjunctival hemorrhage—it may be due to hypoprothrombinemia, due to vitamin K deficiency.

III. Musculoskeletal system:

1. Calcium deficiency due to vitamin D malabsorption producing—osteomalacia, rickets
2. Calcium, magnesium and vitamin D deficiency—producing carpopedal spasm—tetany

IV. Endocrinological changes:

1. Secondary hyperparathyroidism due to protracted calcium, and vitamin D deficiency.
2. Amenorrhea, infertility, impotence—occur due to:
   i. Poor dietary intake
   ii. Malabsorption of nutrients

V. Skin:

1. Edema or/and ascites—due to:
   i. Protein loosing enteropathy due to:
      a. Severe mucosal inflammation
      b. Lymphatic obstruction
   ii. Poor dietary absorption of protein.
2. Hyperpigmentation—it may be due to:
   i. Adrenal insufficiency
   ii. Secondary hypopituitarism
3. Purpura—It may be due to vitamin K deficiency
4. Dermatitis herpetiformis

VI. Nervous system:

1. Vitamin A deficiency:
   i. Night blindness
   ii. Xerophthalmia
   iii. Corneal xerosis
   iv. Complete blindness
2. Peripheral neuropathy:
   i. Vitamin B_{12} deficiency
   ii. Vitamin A deficiency
   iii. Malabsorption of essential fatty acids.

Laboratory Investigations

A. Stool studies:

i. *Macroscopic appearances:* Stool is pale, greasy, bulky, often frothy with rancid odor.

ii. *Stool fat estimation:*
   a. Diet containing 80–100 gm fat for a day or two, unabsorbed fat like, mineral oil, olestra and fat based suppositories should be avoided.
   b. Stool should be kept in refrigerator to prevent bacterial degradation of long chain fatty acid
   c. Excretion of >7–8% of fat intake—denotes steatorrhea.
   d. Excretion of >9.5% of stool fat—suggests intra-luminal maldigestion
   e. Excretion of <9.5% of stool fat—suggests mucosal disease

iii. *Stool elastase:*
   a. Low, moderate and severe pancreatic in sufficiency
   b. In mucosal disease—may be low due to dilution.

iv. *Stool for ova and parasite:*
   a. Positive in parasitic biliary cholangiography
   b. In mucosal disease—it may diagnose:
      1. Giardia   4. Microsporidia
      2. Isospora   5. Tapeworm
      3. Cryptosporidia

B. Serum biochemistry:

i. Serum carotene—decreased
ii. Serum cholesterol—decreased
iii. Serum calcium:
   a. Decreased—in:
      1. Mucosal disease of intestine
      2. Lymphatic obstruction
   b. Normal in pancreatic disease
iv. Serum albumin—decreased in
      1. Mucosal disease
      2. Lymphatic obstruction
      3. Bacterial overgrowth in the intestine
v. Serum 25 OH vitamin D—decreased
vi. Serum iron:
   a. Decreased—in mucosal disease of intestine
   b. Normal in maldigestion, lymphatic obstruction.
vii. Serum folate:
   a. Normal in maldigestion in intestine
   b. Low in malabsorption
viii. Prothrombin time—prolonged in liver disease

C. Serology:

IgA—anti-tissue transglutaminase antibody
         And
IgA—anti-endomycelial antibody
   The above are present in celiac disease.

D. Complete blood count:

i. Anemia
   a. Microcytic anemia
   b. Macrocytic anemia
   c. Dimorphic anemia
   In Whipple's disease—interferes with iron and folate absorption
ii. Intestinal bacterial overgrowth and severe pancreatic exocrine deficiency—interferes with vitamin B_{12} absorption—producing macrocytic anemia
iii. Normocytic or microcytic anemia—may occur in:
   a. Crohn's disease
   b. Intestinal lymphoma
   c. Whipple's disease

iv. Peripheral eosinophilia:
   a. Eosinophilic enteritis
   b. Some parasitic diseases.
v. Profound lymphopenia—intestinal lymphangiectesia
vi. Thrombocytosis—reflects hyposplenism.

Specific Absorption Tests

i. D-xylose test:

It is a pentose sugar—absorbed by facilitated diffusion
25 gm of D-xylose is administered orally

| |
5 gm of xylose will be   Blood level will be 25 mg/dl
excreted in urine in 5 hours

If this level is low in urine as well as in blood—suggests mucosal malabsorption—celiac disease

Limitations of this test:
1. Delayed gastric emptying—it produces very low level in blood as well as in urine.
2. Impaired renal excretion—It produces normal blood level but low urinary level.
3. Ascites and edema—responsible for sequestration of absorbed xylose—produces false positive results.
4. In bacterial overgrowth, in proximal small intestine, as some bacteria metabolize glucose—this test will be positive.

ii. Breath hydrogen test

Orally administration of lactose and sucrose
↓
In case of lactase deficiency
↓
Lactose is not absorbed
↓
It travels to distal intestine
↓
Here bacterial flora metabolize sugar
↓
Release of hydrogen
↓
It is excreted through lung
↓
It can be measured in the breath

Test dose is 2 gm/kg—maximum 25 gm
Result <10 part per million—normal
>20 parts per million—suggest lactase deficiency

Limitations of this test:
a. Following factors are responsible for false negative results
   1. Delayed gastric emptying
   2. Chronic pulmonary disease
   3. Recent antibiotic use
   4. Absence of hydrogen producing bacteria
b. Following factor is responsible for false positive results

   1. Intestinal bacterial overgrowth
   ↓
Hydrogen will be released before absorption of sugar.

iii. Direct measurement of disaccharidase enzyme: All the above tests cannot discriminate between primary and secondary lactase deficiency.

iv. ^{14}C-xylose test:

Orally administration ^{14}C-xylose (xylose is absorbed in proximal intestine)
↓
Rapid metabolism of it by bacteria in proximal small intestine
↓
Release of $^{14}CO_2$
↓
Released through lung
↓
Measurement of $^{14}CO_2$
This test is positive in small intestinal bacterial overgrowth in proximal small intestines.

v. Schilling test

Imaging Studies

The following tests are used for diagnosis
1. Endoscopic retrograde cholangiopancreatography (ERCP)
2. Magnetic resonance cholangiopancreatography (MRCP)
3. Computerized scan of abdomen
4. Abdominal magnetic resonance imaging
5. Abdominal ultrasonography
6. Barium contrast studies—these are the following:
   i. Barium follow through small intestine
   ii. Double contrast enteroclysis—this is performed by instilling—both barium and carboxymethy lcellulose into duodenal lumen.

   ↓

   Transit of contrast material through small intestine (This can be seen by fluoroscopically)
   iii. Computed tomographic enterography (CTE) for evaluation of:
      a. Crohn's disease
      b. Assessment of remaining length of small intestine after major intestinal resection
      c. Detection of focal abnormalities in intestine—like:
         1. Intestinal stricture
         2. Neoplasm
         3. Lymphoma
   iv. MRA enterography

Small Intestinal Biopsy

Indications
i. In patient with suspected steatorrhea or chronic diarrhea
ii. Diffuse or focal abnormalities of small intestine

Types of Biopsy
Three types of biopsies are usually seen:
A. Diffuse and specific lesions:
   1. *Whipple's disease:* Macrophages containing PAS +ve material seen lamina propria of small intestinal mucosa.
   2. *Abetalipoproteinemia:* Fat containing vacuoles seen in epithelial cells postprandially
   3. *Agammaglobulinemia:* Absence of plasma cells in lamina propria, normal or flat architecture of villi.
B. Patchy and specific lesions:
   1. Intestinal lymphangiectasia:
      i. Normal mucosal architecture
      ii. Dilated lymphatics in lamina propria

2. Intestinal lymphoma:
   i. Infiltration of epithelium, submucosa, lamina propria with malignant lymphoma cells
   ii. Widened, shortened villi
3. Eosinophilic enteritis:
   i. Normal or flat mucosal architecture
   ii. Aggregates of eosinophils infiltration in lamina propria in patch.
4. Mastocytosis:
   i. Normal or flat mucosal architecture
   ii. Mast cell infiltration of lamina propria
5. Amyloidosis:
   i. Normal mucosal architecture
   ii. Amyloid deposits in lamina propria seen.
6. Giardiasis:
   i. Normal or flat mucosal architecture
   ii. Trophozoites are found in:
      a. Lumen
      b. Surface of absorptive cells.
7. Crohn's disease: Non-caseating granuloma and inflammation in lamina propria.

C. Diffuse but nonspecific:
1. Celiac disease:
   i. Short or absent villi
   ii. Mononuclear cell infiltration in lamina propria
   iii. Cryptic hyperplasia
   iv. Damage of absorptive cells.
2. Tropical sprue:
   i. Normal or flat mucosa
   ii. Mononuclear cell infiltration of lamina propria
   iii. Damage of absorptive cells
3. Bacterial overgrowth:
   i. Patchy mucosal damage
   ii. Lymphocytic infiltration of mucosa
4. Folate, vitamin B_{12} and radiation enteritis:
   i. Shortened villi
   ii. Megalocytosis
   iii. Decreased mitosis in crypts
5. Zollinger-Ellison syndrome: Ulceration of mucosa

CELIAC DISEASE

Other names of this disease:
 i. Non-tropical sprue
 ii. Gluten sensitive enteropathy
 iii. Adult celiac disease
 iv. Celiac sprue

Hallmark of Celiac Disease

 i. Presence of abnormal small intestinal biopsy.
 ii. Response of symptoms and histological changes to the gluten-free diet.

Symptoms

Wide-spectrum of presentations are seen in this disease:
1. Symptoms may start in infant with the introduction of gluten in diet—which may remit spontaneously during 2nd week of life. This is usually followed by:
   i. Either spontaneous and permanent remission, or
   ii. Reappearance of symptoms in adult life and persists throughout the adult hood.

2. In many patients, there may be evidence of spontaneous exacerbation and remissions of symptoms and signs.
Following symptoms are usually present:
   i. Diarrhea
   ii. Steatorrhea
   iii. Weight loss
   iv. Symptoms of deficiency of different nutrients—anemia of metabolic bone disease
   v. Absence of gastrointestinal symptoms.
3. In case of asymptomatic relatives of celiac disease:
   i. Small intestinal biopsy suggestive of celiac disease
   ii. Positive serologies—like:
      a. Antitissue transglutaminase antibody
      b. Antiendomysial antibodies.

Etiology

The etiology is unknown. But following factors may be considered as etiological targets for the development of celiac disease.

A. Environmental factors: Glidin, component of gluten present in wheat, barley, rye, triggers the disease.

In patient with celiac disease, instillation of glidin in rectum and distal ileum produces morphological and histological changes within few hours.

Again restriction of gluten in the diet reverts the abnormal morphological and histological changes in intestine in patient with celiac disease.

B. Immunological factors: This involves both adaptive and innate immune response. These are three antibodies present in these patients although the link between these antibodies and development of the disease is unknown. The antibodies are:
 i. IgA antiglidin antibody
 ii. IgA antiendomysial antibody—90–95% specific and sensitive
 iii. IgA antitissue transglutaminase antibody.

tTG recognizes antiendomysial antibody, tTG deaminates glidin—it is presented to HLA-DQ2 and HLA-DQ8. Prednisolone treatment induces remission as well as converts abnormal mucosal histology in intestine to normal inspite of continued intake of gluten in diet.

C. Genetic factors:
1. This disease is present in different populations
   i. High in whites
   ii. Low in black and Asians
   iii. 10% in first degree relatives
2. All patients express following allele
   i. HLA-DQ2
   ii. HLA-DQ8

Absence of above allele excludes the diagnosis of celiac disease

Diagnosis

A high index of suspicion is required for diagnosis of this disease. Following investigations should be done in suspected case of celiac disease.

A. Serology:
 i. IgA antiendomysial antibody
 ii. IgA anti-tissue transglutaminase antibody

These are 90–95% sensitive and specific.

Celiac disease diagnosis requires:
  i. Presence of suggestive signs and symptoms
 ii. Characteristic histological changes in intestinal mucosa.
iii. Signs and symptoms of positive improvement and histological changes with gluten-free diet.
    Serological test may be negative in case of IgA deficiency. In that case, IgG anti-tTG antibody and IgG antiendomysial antibody can be detected.

Recently, it has been demonstrated that IgA and IgG anti-deamidated glidin antibodies are available—they are highly specific and sensitive than IgG anti-tTG—and it is the test of choice in IgA deficient individual.

B. Intestinal biopsy: Following are the features of celiac disease:
  i. Increased intraepithelial lymphocytes
 ii. Flattened villi architecture
iii. Cryptic hyperplasia
 iv. Loss of villus structure followed by villus atrophy
  v. Cells are cuboidal in appearance and presence of nuclei at the base of the cells
 vi. Increased infiltration of lymphocytes and plasma cells in the lamina propria
vii. Reversion of the above clinical and histological picture in response of gluten-free diet.

Failure to Respond to Gluten-Free Diet

90% patients respond to gluten-free diet, rest 10% patients will not respond to this diet. These patients are called refractory sprue. These patients have following characteristics:
1. They will respond to other dietary protein, e.g. soy protein
2. They will respond to corticosteroids.
3. These clinical pictures are temporary because they will disappear after few months or years.
4. They will fail to respond to above treatment, and they will turn into T cell lymphoma.

Pathophysiology of Diarrhea

Following are the pathologic mechanisms of diarrhea:
  i. Steatorrhea—due to changes in jejunal mucosa
 ii. Changes in jejunal brush border enzyme function producing secondary lactase deficiency.
iii. As a result of bile salt malabsorption, there will be bile salt induced water secretion in colon—producing diarrhea.
 iv. As a result of cryptic hyperplasia, there will be endogenous fluid secretion.

Associated Diseases

1. Dermatitis herpetiformis—There is characteristic papulo-vesicular lesion—responding to dapsone.
2. Type 1 diabetes mellitus
3. IgA deficiency
4. Down syndrome
5. Turner's syndrome

Complications

1. Gastrointestinal and non-gastrointestinal cancer—when the patient with celiac disease responding well to gluten-free diet suddenly do not respond to gluten-free diet—it may be an indication of development of gastrointestinal cancer.

2. Intestinal ulcerations independent of lymphoma
3. Refractory sprue
4. Collagenous sprue—here a layer of collagen-like material will be present in basement membrane.
    These patients will never respond to gluten-free diet. They have poor prognosis.

Treatment of Celiac Disease

Initial Treatment

1. Barley, wheat, rye, oat gluten must be avoided.
2. Safe diets are—rice, millet, corn, potato, buck wheat, soya beans.
3. Avoid the milk, until disappearance of diarrhea
4. Micronutrients like iron, folate deficiencies should be replaced.
5. If there is evidence of osteopenia, calcium and vitamin D should be prescribed.
6. If there is presence of hyposplenism, pneumococcal vaccine should be administered.

Follow-up
  i. Every 6–12 months, dietary compliance should be monitored.
 ii. Serological tests should be repeated 6–12 months after commencement of gluten-free diet.
iii. Annually, following should be checked
    a. Hematocrit
    b. Hemoglobin
    c. Stool for occult blood
    d. Monitoring of bony density.

Refractory Sprue

This disease is similar to classical celiac disease from clinical and histological point of view; but gluten withdrawal from diet will not improve symptoms and histology. Few patients again are refractory to gluten withdrawal from the very outset. These patients are also serologically negative.

Before the conclusion as refractory sprue, one must exclude following diseases:
  i. Eosinophilic enteritis
 ii. Tropical sprue
iii. Lymphocytic colitis
 iv. Intraluminal bacterial overgrowth.

There are two types of refractory sprue:
1. *In type 1 patient:* The increased as well as expanded population of intraepithelial lymphocytes (IEL)—consists of phenotypically normal polyclonal T cells.
These patients should be treated with:
  i. Corticosteroids
 ii. Immunosuppressive agents (azathioprine)
iii. Gluten withdrawal

Oral budesonide
↓
If not responded
↓
Systemic corticosteroids
↓ If no response
Immunosuppressive agents

2. *In type 2 patients:* Here there is evidence of clonal expansion of phenotypically aberrant intraepithelial

lymphocytes due to over-expression of epithelial cell interleukin-15. This abnormal T cells express CD3 in the cytoplasm, but do not express surface CD3, CD8 on T cell receptors for β chain.

Type 1 may progress to Type 2 occasionally.

Progression of type 2 refractory sprue:

i. Intractable nutritional deficiencies

ii. T cell lymphoma

Following immunosuppressive agents fail to treat type 2 patients:

i. Infliximab

ii. Cladribine

iii. Autologous stem cell transplantation.

TROPICAL SPRUE

This disease is characterized by the following:

1. Chronic diarrhea
2. Steatorrhea
3. Weight loss
4. Nutritional deficiency—like folate , vitamin B_{12} deficiency.
   Other infectious agents responsible for chronic diarrhea in tropical environment are:
   i. *Giardia lamblia*
   ii. *Yersinia enterocolitica*
   iii. *C. difficile*
   iv. *Cryptosporidium parvum*
   v. *Cyclospora cayetanesis.*

Etiology

The etiology and pathogenesis is uncertain because of the following:

1. It is found mainly in India, Philippines, and several Caribbean islands rather than in all tropical areas.
2. Few individual will develop symptoms long after leaving the endemic areas. Hence the celiac disease was referred as non-tropical sprue.
3. Microorganisms found in jejunal aspirate were implicated as an etiological factor in some cases, whereas bacterial toxins were found as etiological factors.
4. Due to improvement in sanitations in tropical areas, incidence of tropical sprue will be increased.

Clinical Pattern

The pattern of clinical picture varies in different countries.

i. In India, it may present with acute enteritis before the appearance of steatorrhea.

ii. In Puerto Rico, it is usually insidious and responds to antibiotics.

Diagnosis

Small intestinal biopsy:

i. Normal or flattened villus throughout small intestine

ii. Mononuclear cell infiltration in lamina propria

It can be distinguished from celiac disease by following features

i. Recent history of exposure to endemic region

ii. Absence of anti-tTG antibody and anti-endomysial antibodies

iii. Presence of vitamin B_{12} deficiency

iv. Absence of response to gluten-free diet

v. Response to folic acid and antibiotics.

Treatment of Tropical Sprue

1. **Antibiotics:** Tetracycline—500 mg twice daily for 6 months. Signs of improvement will be evidenced within 1–2 weeks.
2. **Folic acid:** It will improve:
   a. Appetite
   b. Weight gain
   c. Morphological changes in biopsy.
3. Nutritional deficiency relating to vitamin B_{12}, vitamin D_3, calcium should be corrected.

Prognosis

i. Response to treatment with antibiotics and folic and is excellent and prompt.

ii. Relapse may occur several months to years after treatment.

WHIPPLE'S DISEASE

Definition

This is a multisystem disease involving:

i. Gastrointestinal system

ii. Central nervous system

iii. Cardiovascular system

iv. Joint

Causative Organism

Tropheryma whipplei—it is an actinobacterium, it is less virulent but highly infective.

Clinical Presentation

1. Gastrointestinal manifestations:
   a. Diarrhea   b. Steatorrhea
   c. Weight loss   d. Abdominal pain
2. Joint symptoms
   a. Arthralgia
   b. Arthritis involving multiple joints
3. Systemic symptoms—fever
4. Central nervous system:
   a. Cognitive deterioration
   b. Ophthalmoplegia
   c. Hypothalamic dysfunction
   d. Oculomasticatory or oculofacial myorhythmia
   e. Ataxia
5. Cardiac involvement:
   a. Pericarditis
   b. Culture negative endocarditis
   c. Pleuropulmonary involvement
      i. Pleural effusion
      ii. Sarcoid-like pulmonary infiltrate
      iii. Cough

Physical Findings

1. Skin hyperpigmentation
2. Peripheral lymphadenopathy
3. Cardiac murmurs
4. Arthritis—signs
5. Anemia

Lab Diagnosis

1. Hematological—anemia
2. Biochemical

a. Albumin level ↓↓
b. Hypocalcemia
3. Histology:
   a. Light microscopy—intestinal mucosa shows:
      i. Demonstration of *T. whipplei*
      ii. Infiltration of lamina propria with PAS positive macrophages.
      iii. Distortion of mucosal architecture by macrophages
      iv. Dilatation of mucosal and submucosal lymphatics
   b. Electron microscopy of small intestinal mucosa.
      Demonstration of *T. whipplei* bacterium in mucosa of proximal small intestine.

   Here care must be taken to exclude *Mycobacterium avium* especially in immunocompromised patients.
4. Polymerase chain reaction amplification of the small intestinal mucosa is used for diagnosis.

Treatment

1. Due to chance of development of CNS manifestation, following antibiotics can be given:

Ceftriaxone—1–2 gm per day for 2 weeks
↓
Trimethoprim—160 mg
+
Sulfamethoxazole—800 mg
The above treatment must be continued for 1–3 years

2. Correction of nutritional difficulties

Prognosis

i. In absence of CNS manifestation, prognosis is excellent.
ii. Patient should be monitored to identify the early signs of relapse. CNS signs are the first sign of relapse:

MESENTERIC VASCULAR ISCHEMIA

This is an uncommon vascular disease—which can be classified according to etiology.
 i. Arteriooclusive mesenteric ischemia (AOMI)
 ii. Nonocclusive mesenteric ischemia (NOMI)
 iii. Mesenteric venous thrombosis (MVT)

   Mesenteric venous thrombosis—occurs in case of hypercoagulable state which is responsible for chronic ischemia, like:
a. Antithrombin III deficiency
b. Protein S deficiency
c. Protein C deficiency
d. Polycythemia vera
e. Carcinoma

Risk Factors of Acute Arterial Ischemia

a. Atrial fibrillation
b. Valvular heart disease
c. Recent myocardial infarction
d. Recent cardiac catheterization.

   Ischemic colitis is the most common form of acute ischemia which is a common complication of cardiovascular surgery.

Arterial Anatomy and Pathophysiology

Blood supply of intestines

Involved circulation	Mesenteric artery	Adjoining artery	Collateral artery
Systemic	Celiac	Descending aorta	Phrenic artery
Systemic	**IMA	Hypogastric	Middle hemorrhoidal
Mesenteric	Celiac	*SMA	Superior/inferior pancreaticoduodenal
Mesenteric	*SMA	**IMA	Arch of Riolan
Mesenteric	*SMA	Celiac/**IMA	Intramesenteric
Mesenteric	*SMA	**IMA	Marginal

* SMA—Superior mesenteric artery
** IMA—Inferior mesenteric artery

   There are extensive collateral circulation between major mesenteric trunk and mesenteric arcades.

   In case of small bowel, the collateral circulations are numerous and present in:
i. Duodenum and
ii. At the bed of pancreas.
   In case of large bowel, collaterals in colon are present at:
i. Splenic flexure—Griffith's point
ii. Descending/sigmoid colon—Sudeck's point
   The above two areas are at risk of ischemia.
   Protective responses to prevent ischemia are:
 i. Abundant collateralization
 ii. Autoregulation of blood flow
 iii. Increased oxygen extraction from the blood.

Two types of ischemia are:
A. *Occlusive ischemia:*
   i. Embolus—more than 75% from cardiac origin. It obstructs distal to the origin of middle colic artery from superior mesenteric artery.
   ii. Progressive thrombosis—involving at least two major vessels supplying intestines.
B. *Non occlusive ischemia:* Severe vasoconstriction in response to:
   i. Dehydration
   ii. Shock.

Presentation

Acute ischemia from arterial embolus or thrombosis:
 i. Severe non-remitting abdominal pain which is out of proportion of physical finding.
 ii. Nausea
 iii. Vomiting
 iv. Transient diarrhea
 v. Bloody stool

Physical findings are:
 i. Hypoactive bowel sounds
 ii. Minimal abdominal distension

Late findings:
 i. Peritonitis
 ii. Cardiovascular collapse

Laboratory Workup

1. Complete blood count
2. Serum biochemistry
    i. Liver functions
    ii. Amylase
    iii. Lipase
    iv. Lactic acid
    v. Cardiac enzymes
    vi. Blood gas analysis
3. Coagulation profile

Other Investigations

1. Electrocardiogram: Arrhythmia—suggests the embolic cause.
2. Plain radiography of abdomen:
    a. Evidence of free intraperitoneal air—suggests perforation of viscus.
    b. Bowel wall edema "thumb printing" like appearance
    c. Air in the wall of bowel (pneumatosis intestinalis)
    d. Air within portal venous system
    e. Calcification in the aorta indicates atherosclerotic heart disease.
3. Dynamic CT scans of abdomen with oral or intravenous contrast—with three-dimensional reconstruction—very sensitive for acute mesenteric ischemia.
4. Intraoperative mesenteric angiography
5. Mesenteric duplex scan—shows high peak velocity of flow in superior mesenteric artery.
    Negative duplex scan excludes mesenteric ischemia.
6. Visible light spectroscopy—it can diagnose chronic ischemia

Treatment

i. Gold standard for management of acute ischemia is laparotomy followed by selection of the affected intestine.
ii. Restoration of blood supply—by intraoperative and preoperative arteriography followed by intra-arterial heparinization.
    Small and large bowel should be checked starting from ligament of Treitz.
iii. When superior mesenteric artery proximal to origin of middle colic artery is occluded, proximal jejunum may be spared, but remain small bowel up to transverse colon will be affected.
iv. Mesenteric thrombosis can be treated by angioplasty with or without endovascular stent placement.

Nonocclusive Intestinal Ischemia

Clinical Presentation

1. Hematological—leucocytosis
2. Biochemical
    i. Metabolic acidosis
    ii. Raised amylase
    iii. Raised CPK
    iv. Lactic acidosis.

All the above parameters are indicative of advanced intestinal ischemia.

Investigational markers of intestinal ischemia:
    i. D-dimer
    ii. Glutathione

iii. S-transferase
iv. Platelet activating factor
v. Mucosal pH monitoring.

Management

These patients should be admitted in intensive care unit. Following measurement should be undertaken:
i. Aggressive fluid resuscitation
ii. Proper oxygen delivery through nasal prongs.
iii. Blood transfusion should given to combat anemia
iv. Broad-spectrum antibiotic—for coverage of:
    a. Enteric pathogens
    b. Gram-negative organisms
    c. Anaerobic organism
v. Monitoring of:
    a. Blood pressure
    b. Urine output
    c. Blood gases.

CHRONIC INTESTINAL ISCHEMIA

Symptoms

1. Postprandial abdominal cramping pain
2. Weight loss
3. Chronic diarrhea

Signs

1. Abdominal bruit
2. Other manifestations of atherosclerosis.

Investigations

1. Duplex ultrasound for evaluation of mesenteric vessels.
    In absence of obesity and increased bowel gas—following findings may be found:
    a. Flow disturbances with the vessels
    b. Lack of vasodilatation in response to feeding.
2. Mesenteric arteriography—this is the gold standard method for diagnosing the mesenteric vascular occlusion. Following evaluations are carried out: Identification and intervention for the treatment of thrombus.

Limitations

i. Renal failure
ii. Contrast allergy

In case of above limitations—magnetic resonance angiography can be done.

Management

a. Management of atherosclerosis by:
    i. Administration lipid lowering agents
    ii. Exercise
    iii. Cessation of smoking
b. Cardiac evaluation
c. Endovascular procedure—endovascular stenting following angiography and if required, angioplasty.
d. Entire length of small and large bowel should be checked.

PROTEIN-LOSING ENTEROPATHY

Definition

It is characterized by a group of disorders (gastrointestinal or non-gastrointestinal) with evidence of hypoproteinemia with or without edema, but in absence of proteinuria or defective protein synthesis, like, chronic liver disease.

Normally, only 10% of total protein is catabolized through gastrointestinal tract. But more than 65 different conditions produce excess protein loss through gastrointestinal tract. This can be classified into three groups:

1. Excessive protein loss through ulcerated mucosa of intestine. Example—ulcerative colitis, peptic ulcer, carcinoma of gastrointestinal tract.
2. Excessive protein loss through non-ulcerated mucosa due to altered permeability across the epithelium. Example—celiac disease, Menetrier's disease of intestine.
3. Lymphatic disease of intestine:
   i. Primary lymphangiectesia
   ii. Secondary lymphatic obstruction—due to:
      a. Cardiac disease
      b. Enlarged lymph nodes

Clinical Features

Hypoproteinemia with or without edema in absence of renal or hepatic disease may occur. In this disease:

i. There may be selective albumin loss with normal serum globulin—suggests the absence of hepatic or renal disease.
ii. In presence of reduced serum albumin, but reduced serum globulin—suggests decreased globulin synthesis, rather than increased globulin excretion into intestine.

Investigation

1. Increased excretion of administered radiolabeled protein loss and measurement of protein in stool during 24–48 hours, it suggests protein loosing enteropathy.
2. α1 antitrypsin protein estimation in stool—since it is resistant to proteolysis, it can be assessed in stool.

   It cannot be used to assess gastric protein loss, because it will be degraded in acid milleu of stomach.

   So, α1 antitrypsin clearance is measured by—estimating:
   i. Stool volume
   ii. Estimation of α1 antitrypsin in plasma as well as stool.
3. In case if lymphatic obstruction—lymphocytes may be lost via lymphatics. So, presence of lymphopenia in presence of increased protein loss in gastrointestinal tract—suggests protein losing enteropathy, due to lymphatic obstruction.

In these patients, there is presence of steatorrhea due to lipid-containing chylomicron excretion through intestinal epithelial cells, from intestinal lymphatics.

In intestinal lymphangiectasia: There is intestinal lymphatic dysfunction in absence of mechanical or anatomic lymphatic obstruction and absence of lymphatic dysfunction in peripheral extremities.

In Milroy's disease: There is intrinsic peripheral lymphatic disease in association with intestinal lymphangiectasia and hypoproteinemia.

Other Causes

a. Cardiac disease:
   i. Chronic pericarditis
   ii. Right-sided valvular heart disease
b. Menetrier's disease

Treatment

1. Treatment of underlying causes rather than treating hypoproteinemia
   a. Celiac disease should be treated by gluten-free diet.
   b. Ulcerative colitis should be treated by mesalamine.
2. In case of lymphatic obstruction, nature of obstruction should be measured—imaging should be done to diagnose lymphoma or mesenteric obstruction.
3. Cardiac disease should be diagnosed by:
   i. Echocardiography
   ii. Right-sided cardiac catheterization
4. Hypoproteinemia can be treated by:
   i. Low fat diet
   ii. Administration of medium chain triglyceride.

SHORT BOWEL SYNDROME

50% of small bowel resection can maintain the function of bowel, if:

1. Duodenum is not resected or absent of any disease
2. Proximal jejunum is not resected or free of disease
3. 100 cm distal ileum is not resected or free of disease.

   Following factors are responsible for type and degree of symptoms:
   i. Specific segment (jejunum vs. ileum)
   ii. Total length of resection
   iii. Patency and integrity of ileocecal valve
   iv. Associated large intestine whether is removed or not.
   v. Pressure of any disease in remaining parts of large or small intestine (Crohn's disease)
   vi. Speed and degree of adaptation of remaining small intestine.

   This syndrome occurs at any age, from neonates to elderly.

Causes of resection of intestines are mainly the following:
1. Mesenteric vascular diseases:
   a. Vasculitis
   b. Thrombosis
   c. Embolic
   d. Atherosclerosis
2. Disease of mucosa—Crohn's disease
3. Trauma

   After resection of small bowel, adequate intake of dietary nutrients and calories is required to stimulate adaptation of both structural and functional integrity of the small intestine by following methods:
   i. Direct contact of food with intestinal mucosa
   ii. Release of one or more pancreatic hormones
   iii. Release of intestinal hormones
   iv. Biliary secretion

   This adaptation requires 6–12 months for regaining its full functions. Hence in early postoperative period enteral nutrition must be maintained even in presence of extensive resection.

   In absence of small intestinal mucosa, many factors are responsible for diarrhea and steatorrhea.

i. Removal of ileum with ileocecal valve—produces severe diarrhea.
ii. In absence of whole ileum, excessive bite salt stimulated colonic secretion of fluid and electrolyte produces diarrhea.
iii. Absence of ileocecal valve—responsible for:
    a. Decrease in intestinal transit time
    b. Bacterial overgrowth from colon.
iv. Presence of colon is responsible for fewer diarrheas and less likelihood of intestinal failure—due to fermentation of non-absorbed carbohydrate to SCFAs—it is absorbed from colon and stimulates absorption of sodium and water—thus reduces intensity of diarrhea.
v. Gastric acid hypersecretion is responsible for diarrhea.
vi. Removal of lactase enzyme in brush border of intestinal mucosa is responsible for lactase intolerance.

There may be presence of extraintestinal symptoms in case of short bowel syndromes:

1. Increased incidence of calcium oxalate calculi—due to increased absorption of oxalate from intact large intestine—this is followed by hyperoxaluria (enteric hyperoxaluria). The mechanisms of increased oxalate absorption are following:
    i. Increased permeability of colonic mucosa to oxalate due to presence of excess bile acids and fatty acids

    ii. Increased fatty acids bind to calcium
    ↓
    Results increased soluble oxalate
    ↓
    Absorbed through colonic mucosa

    So cholestyramine (an ion binding resin) and calcium can prevent hyperoxaluria.
2. Increased incidence of gallstones—due to decreased bile acid pool size—which, in turn produces cholesterol super-saturation in bile.
3. Gastric acid hypersecretion occurs due to:
    i. Increased serum gastrin due to reduced small intestinal catabolism of gastrin.
    ii. Reduced hormonal inhibition of acid secretion.
4. Reduced pH in duodenal cavity produces steatorrhea by following mechanisms
    i. Inactivation of lipase
    ii. Precipitation of bile acids
    iii. Inhibition of gastric acid secretion.

SMALL INTESTINAL BACTERIAL OVERGROWTH

Proximal intestine normally contains $<10^5$ bacteria/ml of intestinal content. These are usually derived from oro-pharyngeal flora. The excessive accumulation of bacteria in the proximal small intestine can be inhibited by:
    i. Normal intestinal motor function
    ii. Normal gastric acid secretion
    iii. Secretion of immunoglobulin into the lumen of the gut.

Causes of bacterial overgrowth in proximal intestine:
1. Motility disorders:
    i. Scleroderma
    ii. Diabetic autonomic neuropathy
    iii. Pseudo-obstruction

    iv. Irritable bowel syndrome
    v. Amyloidosis
2. Structural abnormalities:
    i. Diverticular disease
    ii. Strictures
        a. Crohn's disease
        b. Radiation enteritis
    iii. Afferent loop syndrome in Billroth II gastrectomy
    iv. Fistulas:
        a. Gastrocolic
        b. Jejunocolic
        c. Jejunoileal
3. Hypochlorhydria:
    i. Atrophic gastritis
    ii. Vagotomy with gastric resection
    iii. Long-term use of PPI
4. Hypergammaglobulinemia

Pathophysiology for Malabsorption

Normally: Bile salts secreted by liver into small intestine
↓
Conjugated to glycine and taurine derivatives
↓
Absorbed by active transport from distal ileum

In Small Bowel Bacterial Overgrowth

1. Bacterial enzymes deconjugates bile salts in small intestine
    ↓
    These are absorbed in proximal intestine by passive nonionic diffusion
    ↓
    Decreased availability in the lumen of intestine

2. Deconjugated bile salts are:
    i. Less effective detergents
    ii. Poorly soluble at intraluminal pH
    The results are less effective dispersion of intraluminal dietary lipids for absorption.
3. Bacteria produce—following intraluminal:
    i. Proteases
    ii. Glycosidases
    iii. Toxins
    These damage brush border epithelium and enzyme like hydrolase—which interfere with last phase of carbohydrate and protein digestion.
4. Interaction of bacteria with intestinal mucosa produces mucosal inflammation—thus impairs with dietary absorption.
5. In the gut lumen: Bacteria bind with B_{12} vitamin thus metabolize the vitamin. As a result, absorption of vitamin B_{12} will be hampered in distal ileum.

Clinical Presentations

Following symptoms are usually present:
1. Diarrhea
2. Steatorrhea
3. Flatulence
4. Abdominal distension
5. Weight loss

In elderly people, SIBO may be undetected due to their mild presentation. These patients may present with features of vitamin B_{12} deficiency, like pernicious anemia.

Investigations

1. Quantitative culture of duodenal fluid—it is the diagnostic test.
   Limitations:
   i. Costly
   ii. Invasive
   iii. Requirement of fastidious growth media
2. Breath tests utilizing lactose, xylose, and glucose: In absence of ileal disease, two-stage vitamin B_{12} absorption test is helpful.
   Bacteria impair absorption of free vitamin B_{12} and intrinsic factor bound vitamin B_{12}, so urinary exctaction will be low.
3. Biopsy from small intestinal mucosa:
   i. Blunting of villus architecture
   ii. Cryptic hyperplasia
   iii. Damaged absorptive cells
   iv. Submucosal inflammation

Treatment

i. In case of surgically correctable lesions (structure in small intestine or gastrocolic fistula)—reconstruction surgery is of choice.
ii. Antibiotics are the choice of treatment in case of following abnormalities:
   a. Chronic motor abnormalities
   b. Multiple jejunal diverticula.
   c. Non-correctable anatomic abnormalities

The antibiotics are:

i. Amoxicillin—clavulanate alone
ii. Amoxicillin—clavulanate along with metronidazole
iii. Rifaximin poorly absorbable antibiotics

Duration of Treatment

1. 3 weeks course of therapy—may produce prolonged remission.
2. Frequent intermittent courses of antibiotics during symptomatic period.
3. Sometimes, continuous treatment is of benefit.
4. Antibiotic—1 week per month may be more effective even in absence of symptoms.

Other Treatment

i. Administration of vitamin B_{12} in case vitamin B_{12} deficiency
ii. Folic acid replacement
iii. Mineral replacement:
   a. Calcium
   b. Magnesium
   c. Zinc
   d. Iron
iv. Home parenteral replacement—can be maintained for many years.
v. Administration of trophic hormones—like glucagon-like peptide (GLP-2) may improve absorptive functions.
vi. Administration of opiates—reduces stool output

Dietary Treatment

1. To minimize diarrhea due to fatty acid-induced colonic fluid secretion—low fat, low carbohydrate diet.
2. Low lactose diet
3. Various soluble fiber containing diet.
4. In case of diarrhea due to gastric acid hypersecretion—protein pump inhibitor should be of choice.

INFLAMMATORY BOWEL DISEASE

Epidemiology

Items	Ulcerative colitis	Crohn's disease
Incidence	2.2–14.3/19999 population	3.1–14.6/1000 population
Age incidence	15–30 years 60–80 years	15–30 years 60–80 years
Ethnicity	Jewish is more common than non-Jewish. 2-fold to 4-fold increased frequency in Jewish. Frequency decreases progressively in non-Jewish while African, American Hispanic and Asian population	
Male: Female ratio	1:1	1:1—1.8:1
Smoking	It may prevent disease	2-fold increase in CD
Oral contraceptives	No evidence of increased risk	Odds ratio is 1.4
Appendicectomy	It is protective against VC	Increased risk
Monozygotic twins	6% concordance rate	58% concordance rate
Dizygotic twins	0% concordance	4% concordance

Following genetic syndromes are associated with inflammatory bowel disease:

1. Turner syndrome (loss of part or all of X chromosome)—ulcerative colitis and colonic Crohn's disease.
2. Hermansky-Pudlak syndrome (autosomal recessive)—granulomatous colitis
3. Wiskott-Aldrich syndrome (X-linked recessive disorder). Loss of WAS protein function:
   i. Severe immunodeficiency
   ii. Dysfunctional platelet
   iii. Thrombocytopenia
   iv. Colitis
4. Glycogen storage disease (glucose-6-phosphate transport protein deficiency):
   i. Granulomatous colitis
   ii. Neutropenia
   iii. Hepatomegaly
5. Immune dysregulation polyendocrinopathy: Loss of Fox P3 transcription factor, loss of T-regulatory cell function:

i. Ulcerative colitis-like features
ii. Endocrinopathy

Etiopathogenesis

Etiopathogenesis of IBD is depicted in Fig. 4.3.

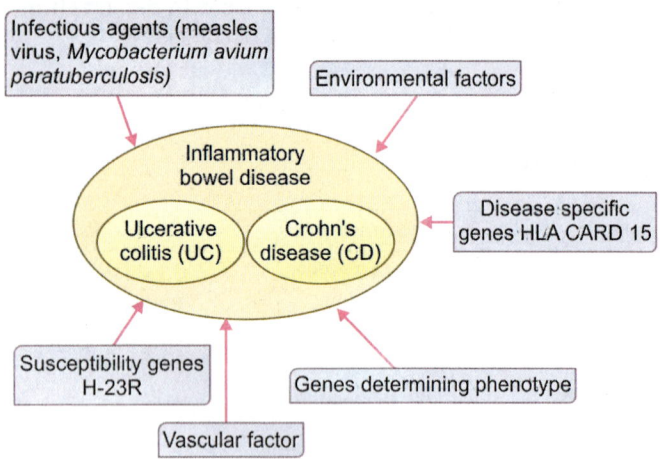

Fig. 4.3: Etiopathogenesis of IBD

Genetic Factors (Fig. 4.4)

Approximately 100 diseases associated loci are present on different chromosomes. One-third of genetic risk factors are commonly centered by both UC and CD.

The disease and genetic risk factors that are shared by IBD are the following:

1. Rheumatoid arthritis—TNFAIP3
2. Psoriasis (IL23R, IL 12B)
3. Ankylosing spondylitis (IL23R)
4. Type 1 diabetes mellitus (IL-10, PTRN2)
5. Asthma (ORMDL 3)
6. Systemic lupus erythematosus (TNFAIP3, IL-10)

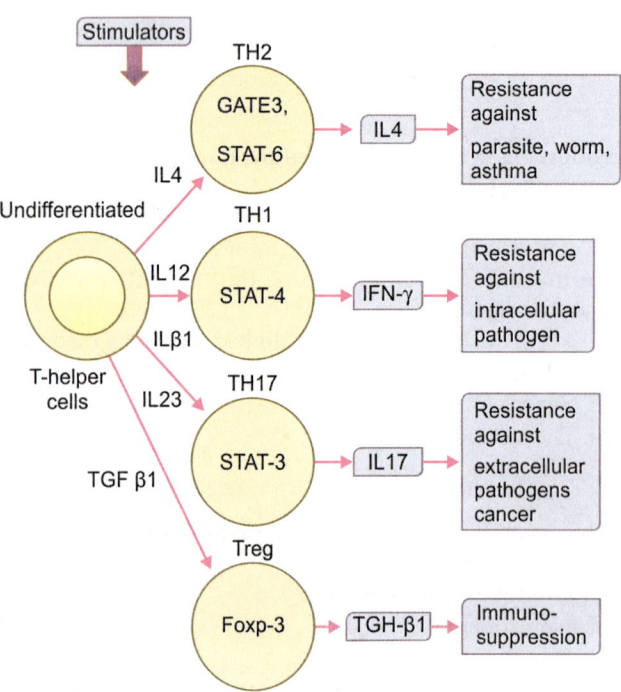

Fig. 4.4: Genetic factors in IBD

Examples of Genetic Associations with Inflammatory Bowel Disease

Gene	Chromosome	Associations with UC/CD	Biological functions
CARD 15	16	Crohn's disease, ileal involvement	Innate immunity Involvement of intracellular receptors for muramy dipeptide
ATG16L1	2	Crohn's disease	Destruction of cellular contents by autophagy
IL23R	1	Crohn's disease Inflammatory bowel disease	It helps in differentiation of T cell to TH^{17} cells
IBD 5	5	Crohn's disease	?
IBD 3	6	Crohn's disease ulcerative colitis	It is involved in antigen recognition

Normally

Figure 4.5 depicts normal function of T cells.

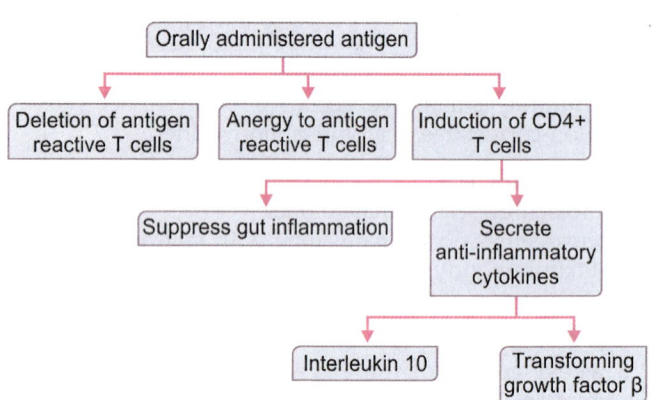

Fig. 4.5: Normal function of T cell

But in IBD—this suppression will be altered, which leads to uncontrolled inflammation (Fig. 4.6).

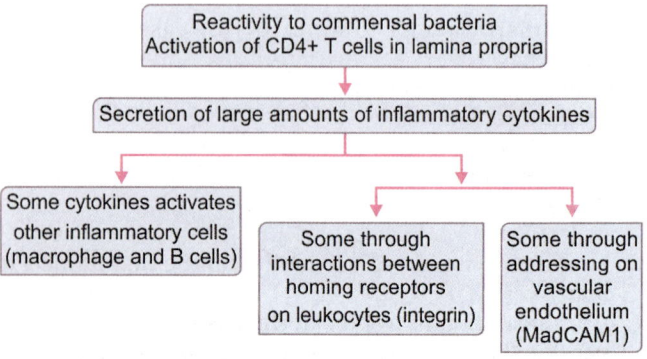

Fig. 4.6: Functions of T cells in IBD

Three types of CD4+ T helper cells promoting inflammations:
1. TH^1: It secretes interferon.
2. TH^2: It secretes IL4, IL-5, and IL-13.
3. TH^{17}: It secretes IL-17, IL-21.

TH^1—induces transmural granulomatory inflammation like Crohn's disease.

IL-13 induces superficial mucosal inflammation like UC.

TH^{17} is responsible for neutrophil recruitment.

Activated macrophage secretes tumor necrosis factor (TNF and IL-6) 30.

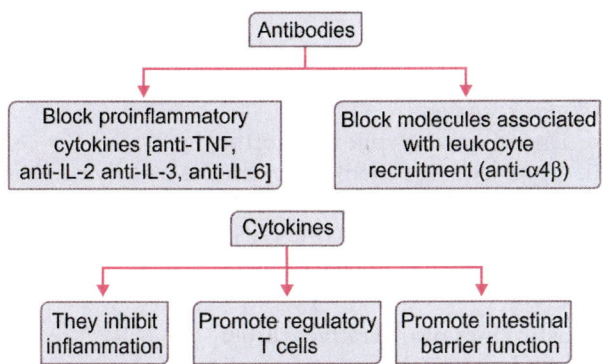

Fig. 4.7: Functions of antibodies in IBD

Inflammatory Cascade in IBD

Abnormal innate immune sensing of bacteria by parenchymal cells (intestinal epithelial cells) and hematopoietic cells (dendritic cells)

↓

Abnormal T cell activation

↓

Release of inflammatory cytokines—IL-1, IL-6, TNG

Functions

i. Promotion of fibrogenesis
ii. Promotion of production of collagen
iii. Activation of tissue metalloproteinase
iv. Production of other inflammatory mediators
v. Activation of co-agulation cascade in local blood vessels

In Case of Infection

Released cytokines normally produce limited tissue damage.

But in IBD—the activity of released cytokines is dysregulated—which results in imbalance between proinflammatory and anti-inflammatory mediators.

Exogenous Factors

In inflammatory bowel disease

1. Multiple pathogens (*Salmonella, Shigella, Campylobacter, Clostridium difficile*)

↓

Trigger uncontrollable inflammatory response

2. Commensal intestinal microbial composition will be altered in ulcerative colitis and Crohn's disease
3. Anaerobic organisms—Bacteroides, Clostridia species are responsible for induction of inflammation.

4. Dietary products or drugs (metronidazole, ciprofloxacin) alter the intestinal flora and produce improvement in CD.
5. Probiotics inhibit inflammation in intestine.

Psychological Factors

Following factors may increase the incidence of IBD:
  i. Illness
 ii. Death in the family
iii. Divorce
iv. Separation
 v. Interpersonal conflict.

Acute daily stress many increase the symptoms of IBD

Other Theories Regarding the Etiology of IBD

1. *Vascular inflammation:* Small vessels of mesentery may lead to inflammation and infarction.
2. *Microparticles:* Some particles in toothpaste may produce foreign body reaction with granulomatous inflammation.
3. *MMR vaccine:* It has combined effect on over all immune system.

Pathology of Inflammatory Bowel Disease

Following are the differential diagnoses of ulcerative colitis:
1. Indeterminate colitis
2. Acute self-limiting colitis
3. Drug-induced colitis
4. Ischemic colitis
5. Diverticular disease
6. Eosinophilic colitis

Differential diagnosis of Crohn's disease:
1. Ulcerative colitis
2. Acute self-limiting colitis
3. Drug-induced colitis
4. Ischemic colitis
5. Diverticular disease
6. Intestinal tuberculosis
7. Microscopic colitis

Commonest of above differential diagnoses are:
1. Acute self-limiting colitis:
   i. Absence of cryptic distortion
   ii. Absence of basal plasmacytosis
   iii. Neutrophilic infiltration of lamina propria and surface epithelium
2. *Drug-induced colitis:*
   i. Increased surface epithelial apoptosis
   ii. Large number of eosinophils and pigmented macrophages in superficial lamina propria
3. *Diverticular disease:*
   i. Inflammation of cryptic epithelium
   ii. Presence of granulomas
   iii. Distortion of villus architecture
   iv. Loss of plasma cells
4. *Microscopic colitis:*
   i. Lymphocytic colitis—it is characterized by >20–100 intraepithelial lymphocytes.
   ii. Collagenous colitis—it is characterized by increased thickness of subepidermal collagen plates which will be >10 μm.

Pathology of Crohn's Disease

The key features for diagnosis:
1. Focal inflammation
2. Transmural inflammation
3. Presence of granulomas

Macroscopic appearances:
   i. Presence of stricture
   ii. Granular appearance of serous coat
   iii. Wrapping of fat around affected intestine
   iv. Presence of skip lesions
   v. Mucosa looks like cobble stoning appearance
   vi. Ulcer becomes skipped with intervening normal mucosa, shape of ulcer become serpiginous.
   vii. Right-sided colonic involvement mainly occurs. Rectum will be spared.

Microscopic appearances:
   i. Presence of deep penetrating ulcer extending up to bowel wall
   ii. Presence of transmural inflammation with lymphocyte aggregates
   iii. Presence of granulomas near the vessels
   iv. Inflammation of crypts with or without abscess formation
   v. Presence of skip lesions with preservation of normal cryptic architecture in normal mucosa
   vi. Metaplasia of pyloric gland and paneth cells
   vii. Presence of goblet cells
   viii. Presence of submucosa edema
   ix. Fibrosis of intestinal wall
   x. Neuronal hyperplasia
   xi. Inflammation of serosa may be present

Following are the diagnostic features of Crohn's disease:
   i. Presence of granuloma
   ii. Involvement of small bowel
   iii. Transmural lymphoid aggregates

Pathology of Ulcerative Colitis

Ulcerative colitis usually involves whole mucosa of large bowel starting from rectum up to cecum, but it may extends up to 1–2 cm of ileum beyond ileocecal valve producing "backwash" ileitis.

Macroscopic appearance:
   i. Diffuse involvement of colonic mucosa—it is confined to large bowel only.
   ii. Mainly it involves left side of the colon.
   iii. Usually no evidence of fissuring, fistula, sinus.
   iv. No evidence of stricture
   v. No evidence of thickening of bowel wall
   vi. No evidence of involvement of serosa
   vii. Presence of friable ulcerated granular mucosa—in early cases.
   viii. In late cases—pseudopolyps, linear ulcerations

In some cases of ulcerative colitis, following features of Crohn's disease may be present:
   i. Presence of ileal involvement—backwash ileitis
   ii. Patchy involvement or discontinuous involvement
   iii. Appearance of extracolonic inflammation

   iv. Presence of aphthous ulceration
   v. Granulomatous involvement in the areas of ruptured crypts.
   vi. Transmural inflammation.

Microscopic appearance of ulcerative colitis: There are two types of changes:

A. *Active changes:*
   i. It is mostly involved distally.
   ii. Presence of cryptitis or cryptic abscess
   iii. Ulceration
   iv. Mucin depletion
   v. Basal plasmacytosis with loss of inflammatory cell gradient in lamina propria

B. *Chronic changes:*
   i. Distortion of cryptic architecture
   ii. Metaplasia of paneth cells which is usually present on right side of the colon
   iii. Hyperplasia of endocrine cells
   iv. Regenerative epithelial changes
   v. Presence of pseudopolyps

Diagnostic clues of ulcerative colitis:
   i. Continuous involvement of mucosa of colon
   ii. Presence of pseudopolyps
   iii. Absence of granuloma
   iv. Absence of fissuring and sinuses.
   v. Rectal involvement is must.

In long-standing ulcerative colitis—there may be evidence of dysplasia—which may be seen in either in flat mucosa or as a mass lesion—which is called dysplasia associated lesion.

This must be distinguished from sporadic adenoma by following features:
   i. Polyps are usually present outside the active disease.
   ii. Histological features of sporadic adenoma
   iii. Uneventful course following polypectomy

Dysplasia in IBD

   i. It can be detected by surveillance colonoscopy with biopsy
   ii. Four to six quadrant biopsy should be taken
   iii. It can precede cancer in almost all cases
   iv. It is rare in case of retained rectal segment after operative anastomosis

Microscopic appearance of dysplasia: These are three grades of dysplasia:

A. *Low-grade dysplasia:*
   i. Nuclei are oriented at base
   ii. Mild nuclear enlargement
   iii. Crowding of nuclei
   iv. Hyperchromatic nuclei

B. *High-grade dysplasia:*
   i. More hyperchromatic nuclei
   ii. Pleomorphic nuclei
   iii. Prominent nuclear stratification
   iv. Severe architectural distortion
   v. Villus or nodular growth pattern.

C. *Indefinite dysplasia:*
   i. Acute and active inflammation and regeneration
   ii. Epithelial changes

Clinical Features

Both ulcerative colitis and Crohn's disease frequently relapse and remit, produce flares of variable duration and severity.

Ulcerative colitis (UC) usually involves different parts of colon as a whole or in parts.

Crohn's disease involves the mucosa from anus to stomodium either in continuity or in segmental manner producing constellation of symptoms.

Different classifications were done to classify the disease and their severity.

Recently Montreal classification has aimed to classify the disease.

Crohn's Disease

Luminal symptoms:

I. *Small bowel involvement:* Symptoms are mainly due to:
   i. Inflammation of intestinal mucosa
   ii. Indirectly due to varying degree of functional loss.

   Symptoms:
   1. Diarrhea:
      a. It is the cardinal feature: It usually persists at night producing disturbances in sleep.
      b. In case of involvement of terminal ileum—there may be varying degree of fat and bite salt malabsorption producing steatorrhea—in the form of pale stool—which is difficult to flush.

      The causes of diarrhea may be:
      i. Bacterial overgrowth, in proximal stenotic segments
      ii. Reduced capacity of inflamed mucosa to absorb water.
   2. Abdominal pain—it occurs due to:
      i. Bowel wall edema
      ii. Bowel wall stricture—it occurs usually 1–2 hours after taking food mainly high fiber diet.
   3. Nausea with or without vomiting—it occurs in case of stricture.
   4. Weight loss—it may be due to:
      i. Catabolic state of inflammatory response
      ii. Malabsorption
      iii. Avoidance of food to avoid post prandial abdominal pain

II. *Large bowel involvement:*
   1. Diarrhea: It usually occurs due to:
      i. Reduced capacity of inflamed mucosa to absorb water.
      ii. Alteration in transit times.
   2. Rectal bleeding: It occurs due to extensive inflammation of colonic mucosa. It is more pronounced in case of distal colon involvement.
   3. Urgency and incontinence—due to reduced capacity of inflamed rectum.
   4. With distal involvement of the mucosa—stool becomes mucoid.
   5. Abdominal pain—it is cramping like, will be relieved by defecation.

Fistulae formation: It occurs in one-third of Crohn's disease. It may present in following forms:
   1. Between segments of bowel, producing:
      i. High output diarrhea
      ii. Abdominal pain
      iii. Electrolyte depletion
   2. Between small intestine and urinary bladder:
      i. Urinary tract infection
      ii. Pneumaturia
      iii. Faecaturia
   3. Between small intestine and female reproductive organ—abnormal vaginal discharge

III. *Perianal involvement:* This involvement depends upon the distribution of luminal involvement:
   i. >90% in cases of Crohn's colitis
   ii. <12% in case of small bowel involvement

   The following are the common findings:
   i. Skin tags
   ii. Hemorrhoids
   iii. Anal fissures—it is painless.
   iv. Perianal abscess
   v. Perianal fistula
   vi. Anal canal stenosis
   vii. Cancer

IV. *Esophagus—stomach:* In case of involvement of esophagus:
   i. Odynophagia
   ii. Dysphagia

   In case of involvement of stomach:
   i. Epigastric pain
   ii. Nausea
   iii. Vomiting.

Luminal symptoms in case of ulcerative colitis (UC):

I. *Proctitis:*
   1. Passage of blood with mucus, or fresh blood or mixed with stool or streak of blood in stool.
   2. Tenesmus
   3. Urgency
   4. Fecal incontinence
   5. Constipation rarely occurs.

II. *Left-sided extensive disease:* When the disease extends beyond the rectosigmoid junction—the presentation will be:
   i. Variable amount of bloody diarrhea
   ii. Stool containing pus
   iii. Nocturnal episodes of diarrhea, which may produce sleep disturbance.
   iv. Abdominal pain—it may be:
      a. Lower abdominal discomfort
      b. Cramping abdominal pain

Extraintestinal Manifestations

These occur in 25–30% of UC and CD patients. In this UC or CD, following systems are involved:

I. **Cutaneous manifestation:** It occurs in 10% patients with IBD.
   A. **Erythema nodosum:** This is characterized by:
      i. Sudden onset painful bilateral nodules.
      ii. Size—around 2 cm.

iii. These commonly occur in shins but may occur in calves, face trunk.

iv. It is in most common in ulcerative colitis.

B. *Pyoderma gangrinosum:* This is characterized by:

   i. Pain precedes the development of pustules.

   ii. Rapid formation of necrotic ulcer having bluish borders.

   iii. It usually appears in lower legs.

C. *Oral manifestations:*

   i. Aphthous ulcerations—it occurs in 10% of patients

   ii. Pyostomatitis vegetans—it is looking like painful mucosal cobble stoning.

II. **Musculoskeletal manifestations:**

A. *Central arthropathies:*

   a. Asymptomatic sacroilitis—it can be diagnosed radiologically. It occurs in UC and CD.

   b. Ankylosing spondylitis—it is characterized by following:

      i. It occurs in 5% of patients.

      ii. Inflammatory low back pain—mainly occurs at night or at rest and relieved with movement.

      iii. It usually radiates to buttock.

      iv. History of morning stiffness occurs more than 30 minutes.

      v. It is relieved by nonsteroidal anti-inflammatory drugs.

      vi. Course is continuous, progressive, producing permanent skeletal damage and deformity.

B. *Peripheral arthropathies:* It occurs in 5–20% of patients with IBD. This is divided into the following subgroups:

   a. *Type-1:* This is characterized by the following:

      i. Pauciarticular—<5 joints are involved.

      ii. Joint involvement is asymmetrical.

      iii. There is evidence of swelling and effusion of the joints.

   b. *Type 2:* This is characterized by the following:

      i. Polyarticular—>5 joints are involved.

      ii. Joints are asymmetrically involved.

      iii. There is evidence of swelling and effusion occurs in involved joints.

Type-1 arthritis-like condition may occur in post-enteric infection—it is called reactive arthritis.

Hence, in patient with asymmetrical large joint arthritis with evidence of gastrointestinal symptoms, rectal biopsy is necessary to see the signs of IBD.

Ocular Manifestations

It occurs in 10% of IBD patients.

1. Episcleritis: It is the commonest ocular complication in IBD. It usually occurs during flare up of IBD.

2. Scleritis

3. Uveitis

These patients complain of:

   i. Unilateral or bilateral redness in eyes

   ii. Burning sensation of the eye

   iii. Irritations

If there are added symptoms, like:

   i. Photophobia

   ii. Reduction of visual acuity

   Patient will develop scleritis or uveitis.

Hepatobiliary Diseases

Primary sclerosing cholangitis—it occurs in 3% of cases in this case, patient will present with

   i. Jaundice

   ii. Pruritus

   iii. Biliary sepsis

Symptoms related to malabsorption of following nutrients:

Elements	Symptoms related to deficiency
1. Albumin	i. Dependent edema, ii. Cardiac failure
2. Calcium	a. Neuromuscular i. Perioral tingling, ii. Carpopedal spasm b. Neurological i. Depression, ii. Seizures, iii. Changes in behavior c. Cardiac—i. Congestive cardiac failure ii. Shortness of breath d. Cuteneous—i. Brittle nails, ii. Psoriasis iii. Dry skin
3. Magnesium	i. Weakness, ii. Muscle wasting
4. Niacin	Pellagra
5. Vitamin B_{12}	i. Megaloblastic anemia ii. Peripheral neuropathy

Symptoms related to excess of elements: Oxalates—i. Renal colic, ii. Painful hematuria

Thromboembolic events:

1. Venous thromboembolism, as evidenced by: Swelling of legs

2. Pulmonary embolism—as evidenced by:

   i. Pleuritic chest pain

   ii. Shortness of breath

3. Cerebral venous sinus thromboses

4. Axillary/subclavian thromboses

Montreal classifications of ulcerative colitis—to see evidence of extent

Extent of the disease	Anatomical sites involved
E-1: Ulcerative proctitis	Disease limited to rectum, it does not exceed rectosigmoid junction
E-2: Left-sided ulcerative colitis	Disease limited to portion colon distal to splenic flexure
E-3: Extensive ulcerative colitis	Disease extends proximal to splenic flexure

Montreal classification of ulcerative colitis to see evidence of disease severity

Severity grade	Anatomical sites involved
1. S0—clinical remission	Asymptomatic
2. S1—mild ulcerative colitis	i. Number of motions 1–4/day ii. Stool contains blood or absence of blood iii. No systemic illness iv. Normal inflammatory markers

(Contd.)

(Contd.)

Severity grade	Anatomical sites involved
3. S2—moderate ulcerative colitis	i. Motions >4 times/day ii. Minimal sign of systemic toxicity

4. S3—severe ulcerative colitis	i. Motions—6 times/day
	ii. Systemic toxicity
	   a. Pulse—90/minutes
	   b. Temperature—37.5%
	   c. Hemoglobin—10.5 gm/100 ml
	   d. ESR—≥30 mm/1st hour

Laboratory Investigations

A. **Full blood count:**
1. Low hemoglobin—from:
   i. Iron loss
   ii. Decreased folate absorption
   iii. Decreased vitamin B_{12}—it indicates terminal ileum is involved.
2. Raised platelet count—in acute inflammation
3. Raised white blood cell count—in acute inflammation
But raised WBC with neutrophilia—suggests acute infection or abscess formation.

B. **Blood biochemistry:**
1. In case of chronic diarrhea—serum potassium and magnesium will be low.
2. In case of extensive CD, malabsorption:
   i. Serum calcium level will be low.
   ii. Serum albumin level will be low.
3. In case of IBD with liver involvement in the from of primary sclerosing cholangitis: Raised alkaline phosphatase.

C. **Inflammatory markers**—following are raised:
   i. C-reactive protein
   ii. Erythrocyte sedimentation rate
But in some cases of UC or CD, the above markers are normal.

D. **Stool microscopy, culture and sensitivity**—if it is negative, it excluders infective causes of diarrhea.
   But three consecutive samples should be taken to exclude the causes.

E. **Clostridium difficile**—*Clostridium difficile* toxin (CDT) should be tested in the following patients:
   i. In case of chronic diarrhea
   ii. In patient with coexistent IBD
   iii. In patient present with diarrhea in outpatient department
   In a few patients with *Clostridium difficile*-associated diarrhea, CDT test is negative; in that case, preceding history of antibiotic therapy should be taken and as endoscopic biopsy should be considered.

F. **Stool test:**
1. Stool for ova, parasite and cyst to be examined
2. Fecal lactoferrin—it is highly sensitive and specific for detecting intestinal inflammation.
3. Fecal calprotectin—calprotectin, a protein, is released by neutrophils. Its level correlates with:
   i. Histologic inflammation
   ii. Prediction of relapse
   iii. Detection of pouchitis
   It can distinguish functional bowel disorders.

G. **Sigmoidoscopy:**
   a. *Rigid sigmoidoscopy:*
      Advantages:
      i. It can be performed without any bowel preparation
      ii. In case of rectal involvement, it is diagnosed quickly.
      iii. In case of established ulcerative colitis—it is used to monitor disease activity.
      Disadvantages:
      i. It will not allow to estimate the disease activities, if the lesion extends beyond rectum.
      ii. If the CD spares rectum, rigid sigmoidoscopy is less effective.
   b. *Flexible sigmoidoscopy:*
      i. It can be performed in unprepared bowel.
      ii. It usually does not require any sedation.
      iii. It can be performed quickly.
      iv. It can be used to monitor left-sided colitis.
      v. Biopsies should be taken to exclude superimposed infection like *Clostridium difficile* and cytomegalovirus.

Ileoscopy

   i. It can visualize entire colon up to terminal ileum.
   ii. It can differentiate UC from CD both by endoscopic and histologic appearances.
   iii. Bowel should be prepared properly to visualize mucosa.
   iv. It can determine the extent and activity of the disease both by endoscopic and histologic appearances.
   v. It can be used for surveillance for colorectal cancer in case of IBD.
   vi. In case of chemo-endoscopy, indigo carmine can be sprayed to detect mucosal irregularities—from where mucosa can be taken for histological examination.

Appearance in Endoscopic Examination

In case of UC:
   i. Loss of vascular pattern
   ii. Edema
   iii. Mucosal granularity
   iv. Mucosal ulceration
   v. Friable mucosa—which bleeds on touch

   In case of long-standing UC: Appearance of pseudopolyps—these are not adenomatous or neoplastic.

In case of CD:
   i. Focal asymmetric inflammation in colonic mucosa with or without ulceration in terminal ileum
   ii. Ulcer may be apthoid or deep serpiginous
   iii. Mucosal cobble stoning of the mucosa

In case of UC: Gradation can be done in following ways:
1. *In mild cases:*
   i. Erythematous mucosa
   ii. Decreased vascular pattern
   iii. Mucosal friability
2. *In moderate cases:*
   i. Marked erythematous mucosa
   ii. Absent vascular pattern
   iii. Mucosal friability
   iv. Mucosal erosions

3. *In severe cases:* Spontaneous bleeding from ulcerations.

Capsule endoscopy:

i. It can diagnose CD in case of occult gastrointestinal bleeding.
ii. It can assess small bowel disease
iii. It is more sensitive than contrast studies

Complications:

i. Non-retrieval of capsule
ii. Intestinal obstruction
iii. Perforation

Radiology

In case of UC

A. Plain X-ray of abdomen:

i. Colonic edema—giving rise to thumb printing appearance
ii. It can assess the disease extent.
iii. It can identify proximal constipation in patients with left-sided colitis.
iv. It can detect toxic megacolon:
   a. A long segment .6 cm in diameter—containing air with dilatation.
   b. Follow up radiograph after 24 hours—it can monitor course of dilatation—whether it needs emergency colectomy.

B. Double contrast barium enema:

i. It is inferior to colonoscopy because biopsy cannot be taken by this method.
ii. It can detect loss of colonic haustrations and destruction of colonic mucosa.
iii. It is contraindicated in case of moderate to severe colitis—because of risk of:
   a. Perforation
   b. Formation of toxic megacolon.

C. Small bowel imaging: In CD:

i. Segmental narrowing with loss of normal mucosal pattern.
ii. Fistula formation
iii. String sign—it is characterized by narrow flow of barium through inflamed or scarred area. It is seen in terminal ileum.
iv. "Rose thorn" ulcers seen in inflamed loops of bowel.

CT Scanning

It is helpful in following circumstances:

i. If colonic or small intestinal perforation is suspected.
ii. It can estimate the extent of the disease.
iii. It can delineate the anatomy of complexes inflammatory masses in Crohn's disease.
iv. It can detect adherent multiple loops.
v. It can detect multiple strictures.
vi. It can detect mural thickening (>1.5 cm) in homogenous wall density.
vii. Presence of perirectal and presacral fat
viii. Presence of adenopathy

While cell scanning: This method is safe and non-invasive. This process is useful in following conditions:

i. In investigation of atypical symptom
ii. To detect any localization of white cells to the bowel

Magnetic Resonance Imaging (MRI)

It is a non-invasive and nonionization radiation technique.

Indications:

i. It can localize the disease precisely.
ii. It can identify the site of fistulae in CD, mainly in pelvis and perineum.
iii. It is used to assess the response to therapy.

Serological Markers

Due to presence of different immune response to different microorganisms, following biomarkers are evident:

1. Antibodies to *Escherichia coli* outer membrane protein C (Omp C)—55% of CD.
2. Antibodies to I_2, homologue of bacterial transcription factor families from *Pseudomonas* fluorescence associated sequence—50–54% CD.
3. Antibody to saccharomyces cerevisia (ASCA)
4. Antibody to perinuclear antineutrophil antibody (PANCA)
5. Antiflagellin antibody (anti-Cbir1)—it is associated with small bowel disease, fibrostenosing disease and internal penetrating disease.

These serological markers are marginally helpful for diagnosis of UC or CD.

- PANCA is positive in 60–70% of UC and 5–10% of CD.
- ASCA in positive in 10–15% of UC and 60–70% of CD.

PANCA/ASCA serology is 64% sensitive and inspecific.

If CD patient will show all biomarkers to be positive—they are more aggressive, takes shorter time to progress to internal perforating and/or stricturing disease.

Complications

In Case of Crohn's Disease

Since it is a transmural process—it produces:

i. Fistula
ii. Reduced incidence of perforation—1–2% of patients. Sites are:
   a. Ileum
   b. Jejunum
   c. As a complication of toxic megacolon
   d. Colonic perforation is usually fatal produces peritonitis.
iii. Abscesses:
   a. Intra-abdominal abscess
   b. Pelvic abscess
iv. Intestinal obstruction—40% of cases
v. Massive hemorrhage in the intestine
vi. Malabsorption
vii. Serve perineal disease

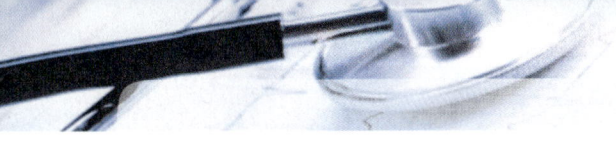

In Case of Ulcerative Colitis

i. Massive hemorrhage—in this case, if a patient requires 6–8 units of blood within 24–48 hours—colectomy is indicated.
ii. Toxic megacolon:
    a. Site—right colon or transverse colon
    b. Pathology:
       1. Diameter— 6 cm
       2. Loss of haustrations
    c. Triggering factors:
       1. Narcotics
       2. Electrolyte abnormalities
    d. 50% will be resolved with medical therapy, but colectomy may be required.
iii. Perforation—it occurs mainly in patients receiving glucocorticoids. In patient with toxic megacolon, rate of perforation is 15%.
iv. Stricture—in 5–10% patients
v. Malignancy—if the strictured area cannot be negotiated by colonoscope in patient with UC—chance of malignancy is very high.
vi. Anal fissure
vii. Perianal abscess
viii. Hemorrhoids.

Management of Inflammatory Bowel Disease

Principles of Management

1. Establishment of the diagnosis—excludes:
    i. Infection
    ii. Bile salt malabsorption
    iii. Functional dyspepsia
2. Induction of remissions
    a. Acute severe form of disease—this patient requires in-patient management or surgery.
    b. Active disease—this patient can be treated as out patient.
3. Alleviation of symptoms—treatment with analgesics
4. Maintenance of remission

Choice of therapy depends upon following factors:
1. Extent of the disease:
    i. Topical therapy for distal UC
    ii. Budesonide for ileal CD
2. Severity of the disease—severe patient may require steroid
3. Patient adherence
4. Drug regimen

Drugs

5-ASA agents: Sulfasalazine is the mainstay of treatment.

Indications:
i. It is indicated in mild to moderate UC.
ii. It has limited role in remission of CD but no clear role in maintenance of CD

Actions: This drug is combination of
    sulfapyridine (antibacterial activity)
       +
    5-ASA (anti-inflammatory)
This drug will pass through small intestine after oral intake
    ↓

It is broken down in the colon by bacterial azo-reductase
    ↓
It clears azo bond between two molecules
    ↓
Sulfapyridine shows its effectiveness in colon

Side effects: Following are due to sulfapyridine moiety:
1. Allergic reactions
2. Intolerable side effects:
    i. Headache
    ii. Nausea
    iii. Vomiting

Following are independent of sulfapyridine moiety.

Hypersensitivity reactions:
a. Rash
b. Fever
c. Hepatitis
d. Agranulocytosis
e. Hypersensitive pneumonitis
f. Pancreatitis
g. Worsening of colitis
h. Reversible abnormalities in sperm

Following are due to sulfasalazine: Impairment of folate absorption—Newer sulfa-free aminosalicylate preparations deliver increased amount of 5-ASA at the site of action. Here, Peroxisome proliferator-activated receptor-γ (PPAR-γ) mediates the action of 5-ASA by decreasing nuclear localization of NF-KB.

The sulfa-free formulation includes:
1. Alternative azo-bond carrier
2. 5-ASA dimmers
3. pH dependent tablets
4. Delayed release preparation
5. Controlled release preparation.

Olsalazine: Here two 5-ASA radicals are linked by an azo-bond. In the colon, bacterial azo reductase breaks the azo-bond of the drugs to release two AGS molecules.

Action is similarly effective as sulfasalazine.

Side effect: 17% patients may produce non-bloody diarrhea.

Balsalazide: Here, Azo-bond binds mesalamine with the carrier molecule 4-aminobenzoyl-β-alanine

This drug is effective in colon.

Asacol: it is an enteric coated formulation of 5-ASA which is released into active form in the intestine from small intestine up to splenic form at pH >7.

Pentasa: It is an ethyl cellulose coated tablet of mesalamine. It will be disintegrated in the stomach by absorption of water. Mesalamine will be released as microspheres. They then disperse throughout the colon and small intestine in both fasted and fed conditions.

Once a day formulation of mesalamine: It is prepared in Multi Matrix System technology. This technology incorporates mesalamine into lipophilic matrix within hydrophilic matrix. This drug is then encapsulated in polymer resistant to low pH (<7).

Apriso is an encapsulated granule. It delivers mesalamine to terminal ileum and colon.

Uncapsulated variation of mesalamine has been used in Europe for induction and maintenance of remission.

Table 4.5: Drugs in ulcerative colitis

Drugs	Formulation	Dosage/day	Site of action
A. Azo-bond Sulfasalazine (500 mg)	Sulfapyridine + 5-ASA	3–6 gm (in acute case) 2–4 gm (Maintenance)	Colon
Olsalazine (250 mg)	ASA + 5-ASA	1–3 gm	Colon
Balsalazide (750 mg)	Aminobenzoyl alanine	6.75–9 gm	Colon
B. Delayed release drugs Mesalamine (400–800 mg)	Eudragit	2.4–4.8 gm (acute case) 1.6–4.8 gm (Maintenance)	Small intestine + colon
Mesalamine (1–2 gm)	MMX technology	2.4–4.8 gm	Ileum, colon
C. Controlled release Mesalamine (250, 500, 1000 gm)	Ethyl cellulose microgranules	2–4 gm (acute case) 1.5–4 gm (maintenance)	From stomach to color
D. Delayed and extended release Mesalamine [. 375 gm]	Apriso	1.5 gm (Maintenance)	Ileum to colon

Topical mesalamine: This is used in case of mild to moderate ulcerative colitis distal to splenic flexure.

Combination therapy: Oral and enema mesalamine is effectively used in case of mild to moderate distal or extensive ulcerative colitis.

Mesalamine suppositories: This is used in case of ulcerative proctitis.

Glucocorticoids:

A. Oral glucocorticoids—prednisolone—it can be started as 40–60 mg/day in case of active ulcerative colitis unresponsive to 5-ASA therapy.
B. Parenteral glucocorticoids:
   1. Hydrocortisone—300 mg/day
   2. Methylprednisolone—40–60 mg/day
   This can be used in extensive colitis.
C. Topical corticosteroids—it can be used in:
   i. Distal colitis
   ii. Rectal involvement associated with more proximal disease.

The following forms are:

Hydrocortisone enema and foam: This form of drug is extensively absorbed from rectum, which can lead to adrenal suppression in case of prolonged therapy.

So, topical 5-ASA is more effective than topical steroid from side effects point of view.

In case of Crohn's disease: Moderate to severe disease can be treated with a remission rate of 60 to 70%.

To avoid systemic side effect, newer steroid is being used.

Budesonide—It is less well absorbed and has increased first pass metabolism.

Dose: In case of ileocolic Crohn's disease—9 mg/day for 2–3 months, then it can be tapered.

6 mg/day—this dose can reduce the relapse at 3–6 months but not at 12 months.

Methods of tapering the dose of steroid:
i. Glucorticoids can be tapered at a rate of 5 mg/week.
ii. This can be tapered to 20 mg/day within 3–4 weeks.
   It can be discontinued within several months to avoid side effects.

The side effects are:
   i. Fluid retention
   ii. Redistribution of fat
   iii. Abdominal striae
   iv. Osteoporosis
   v. Hyperglycemia
   vi. Subcapsular cataract
   vii. Osteonecrosis
   viii. Myopathy
   ix. Emotional disturbances
   x. Withdrawal symptoms

All the above side effects except osteonecrosis can develop from:
1. Dose of steroid
2. Duration of steroids

Antibiotics:

A. In case of UC, the indications of use of antibiotics are:
   1. IPAA
   2. Pouchitis after colectomy
B. In case of CD, the indications are:
   1. Active inflammatory conditions
   2. Fistulous CD
   3. Perianal CD
   4. Prevention of recurrence after ileal resection.

The antibiotics are:
1. *Metronidazole*—15–20 mg/kg/day in three divided doses—it can be continued for several months.
   Side effects are:
      i. Nausea
      ii. Metallic taste
      iii. Disulfiram-like reaction
      iv. Peripheral neuropathy—it may be permanent on rare occasion despite discontinuation of therapy
2. *Ciprofloxacin:* Dose is 500 mg twice daily.

   Side effects: Tendo-Achilles tendinitis and rupture.

Immunosuppressive: The drugs are: Azathioprine and 6-mercaptopurine.

Indicatioins:
   i. As steroid sparing agents
   ii. As maintenance therapy in UC or CD
   iii. Active perianal disease in CD

iv. Active fistulas in CD

Azathioprine is rapidly absorbed

↓

Converted to 6 mercaptopurine

↓

It is then metabolized to active end products—thioino-sinic acid

i. It is inhibitor of purine ribonucleotide synthesis
ii. It inhibits cell proliferation
iii. It inhibits immune response

Efficacy: It is usually seen within 3–4 weeks and it is taken up fully within 3–6 months.

Dosage:
- Azathioprine—2–3 mg/kg/day
- 6 mercaptopurine—1–1.5 mg/kg/day

Drug adherence can be checked by monitoring the level of the following:
i. 6-thioguanine
ii. 6-methyl mercaptopurine

Side effects:
1. Pancreatitis—it can be seen within a few weeks of therapy—it is completely reversible after stoppage of drug
2. Nausea
3. Fever
4. Rash
5. Hepatitis
6. Bone marrow suppression—mainly leucopenia which is dose-related and delayed. Hence regular monitoring of complete blood count is absolutely necessary.
7. Congenital deficiency of thiopurine methyltransferase produces increased accumulation of thioguanine metabolites which may lead to entrancement of toxicity.
8. Lymphoma—there is fourfold risk of developing lymphoma in these patients which may be due to:
   i. Medication
   ii. Underlying disease
   iii. Both

Methotrexate

Actions:
i. It inhibits dihydrofolate reductase inhibitor—as a result DNA synthesis is being impaired.
ii. It has anti-inflammatory properties—due to decreased IL-1 production.

Dose:
i. 25 mg/week—intramuscular or subcutaneous
   - Induction of remission
   - Reduces the dose of glucocorticoids
ii. 15 mg/week—it is helpful for maintaining remissions in Crohn's disease.

Toxicities:
i. Leucopenia
ii. Hepatic fibrosis—hence regular complete blood count and liver function test is absolutely necessary.
iii. Hypersensitivity pneumonitis—rare but serious complications.

Cyclosporine: It is a lipophilic peptide.

Mechanism of actions: It mainly inhibits humoral and cellular immune system.
i. It blocks production of IL-2 by T lymphocytes.
ii. It binds to cyclophilin

   ↓

   It inhibits calcunurin, a cytoplasmic phosphatase enzyme

   ↓

   Inhibits the T cell activation
iii. It blocks the T helper cells

   ↓

   Inhibits B cell function

Indications:
i. In severe ulcerative colitis refractory to intravenous glucocorticoids
ii. It is alternative to colectomy.

   Dose: 2–4 mg/kg/day intravenously.

Toxicities:
i. Hypertension
ii. Gingival hyperplasia
iii. Hypertrichosis
iv. Paresthesia
v. Tremor
vi. Headache
vii. Electrolyte imbalance
viii. Seizures—it may occur, if there is presence of hypomagnesemia
ix. Opportunistic infection—*Pneumocystis jirovecii* pneumonia—when combined immunosuppressive therapy will be instituted.
x. Nephrotoxicity—it is major side effect—it requires dose adjustment.

Tacrolimus: It is a macrolide antibiotic. It has immunomodulatory activity.

Indications:
i. In children with refractory IBD
ii. In adult with extensive involvement of small bowel
iii. In adult with steroid-dependent UC and CD
iv. In adult with refractory UC or CD
v. In case of refractory fistulizing CD

It is not dependent on bile or mucosal integrity for its absorption.

Biologic Therapies

First biologic is infliximab—it is chimeric IgG$_1$ antibody to INF-α.

Indication:
i. Moderately severe ulcerative colitis.
ii. CD with refractory perianal and enterocutaneous fistula
iii. CD—refractory to glucocorticoid, 6-MP, 5-ASA
iv. Refractory UC

Dose: Intravenous dose—5 mg/kg—1/3rd cases will enter into remission.

Side effects:
a. Development of antibodies to infliximab (ATI). As a result, there will be:
   i. Increased infusion reaction
   ii. Decreased response to treatment
   In this case, efficacy of the drug can be restored by following methods
   i. Decreasing dose interval
   ii. Increasing the dose to 10 mg/kg
b. Increased risk of lymphoma—both Hodgkin's disease and non-Hodgkin's disease:
c. Hepatosplenic T cell lymphoma—universal fatal lymphoma—it mainly occurs in Crohn's disease.
d. Acute infusion reaction
e. Severe serum sickness
f. Increased risk of infections
   1. Reactivation of pulmonary tuberculosis
   2. Opportunistic fungal infections
      -Disseminated histoplasmosis
      -Coccidiomycosis
g. Optic neuritis
h. Seizures
i. New onset or acute exacerbations of clinical symptom and radiological features of demyelinating disorders like multiple sclerosis.

Adalimumab: It is recombinant human monoclonal IgG_1 antibody. It contains human peptide sequences. It is injected subcutaneously.

Actions: It binds to TNF
$$\downarrow$$
Blocks the interactions between TNF and cell surface receptors
$$\downarrow$$
Neutralization of its function

It is less immunogenic than infliximab.

Indication: It is approved for treatment of moderate to severe Crohn's disease

Certolizumab Pegol:
   i. It is a pegylated form of anti-TNF antibody.
   ii. It is administered subcutaneously once in months
   iii. It is useful in active inflammatory CD.

Natalizumab: Integrins are expressed on the surface of leukocytes. It serves as a mediator of: Leukocyte adhesion to vascular endothelium. The integrins are:
 i. Alpha 4
 ii. Beta 1 or beta 7 subunits
   Interactions between α4 and β7 are important in lymphocyte tracking to gut mucosa.
   Natalizumab is a human recombinant immunoglobulin G4 against α4 integrin. It is effective in induction of remission and maintenance of CD.

Indications: In patient with refractory or intolerant to TNF therapy for Crohn's disease

Side effect: Annual risk of promyelocytic leukemia is 1 in 1000 population.

Newer Therapies
1. Monoclonal antibodies against IL-12, and IL-23:
   • IL-12 is derived from intestinal antigen presenting cells, it initiates Th1-mediated inflammation.
   • It-23 is a cytokine. It is composed of P19 subunit together with P40 subunit of IL-12. It promotes Th17 cells and inhibits T regulatory cells.
   So, newer antibodies inhibit IL-12 and IL-23 by neutralizing IL-12 P40.
2. Monoclonal antibodies directed against IL-6.

Nutritional Therapy
In Crohn's disease; since dietary antigen stimulates immune response in intestinal mucosa, hence, the treatment in active CD is:
  i. Bowel rest
  ii. Total parenteral nutrition—all the above methods are useful for induction of remission on which is as effective as glucocorticoids.
  iii. Enteral diet, in the form of elemental or peptide-based diet:
      a. It is as effective as TPN and glucocorticoids.
      b. It is very vital for cell growth.
      c. It has no complications of TPN.

In case of ulcerative colitis: Dietary intervention does not reduce the inflammation in UC.

Surgery in Case of Inflammatory Bowel Disease
Indications in case of ulcerative colitis:
1. Intractable disease
2. Fulminant colitis
3. Toxic megacolon
4. Colonic perforation
5. Severe hemorrhagic colitis
6. Long continued ulcerative colitis
7. Colonic obstruction
8. Extracolonic disease

Indications in case of Crohn's disease:
A. *Small intestine:*
   1. Small intestinal stricture with obstruction
   2. Formation of fistula
   3. Hemorrhage massive
   4. Refractory to medical therapy
B. *Colon:*
   1. Intractable colitis
   2. Fulminant colitis
   3. Refractory fistula
   4. Colonic obstruction
   5. Cancer prophylaxis
   6. Perianal disease which is refractory to medical therapy

In case of ulcerative colitis: Choice of surgery is IPPA

Side effects: 6–10 bowel movements per day

Complication: Most frequent complication is pouchitis—it is characterized by the following:
  i. Fever
  ii. Arthralgia

iii. Increased stool frequency

iv. Watery stools

v. Cramping pain

vi. Urgency

vii. Nocturnal leakage of stools

viii. Malaise

Histology confirms pouchitis.

Treatment (Fig. 4.8):

a. Responds to antibiotics

b. In 3–5% cases, patients may respond to:

    i. Glucocorticoids

    ii. Immunomodulators

    iii. Anti TNF therapy

    iv. Pouch removal

Prevention of recurrent pouchitis can be done by—probiotics preparations to be taken daily. This preparation contains—4 strains:

a. Lactobacillus—4 strains

b. Three strains of *Bifidobacterium*

c. One strain of *Streptococcus salivarius*

In case of Crohn's disease (Fig. 4.9): Needs of surgery are related to:

i. Duration of disease

ii. Site of involvement

In case of small intestinal—80% chance of surgery

In case of large intestinal involvement—50% chance of surgery.

In case of small intestine: Choice of treatment will be:

i. Resection of diseased small bowel

ii. Stricturoplasty—when, already large segment of bowel will be resected, stricture is short and intervening mucosa is normal.

Risk factor for recurrence of CD in postoperative cases:

i. Cigarette smoking

ii. Penetrating disease

    a. Internal fistula

    b. Abscess

iii. Multiple surgeries

iv. First surgery at younger age

Treatment of postoperative recurrences:

i. Azathioprine

ii. 6-MP

iii. TNF therapy

iv. Infliximab

In case colonic disease: Choice of surgery:

i. Temporary loop ileostomy

ii. Resection of the disease segment of colon

iii. Segmental colon resection with primary anastomosis

iv. Diverting colostomy to heal severe perianal disease or rectovaginal fistula

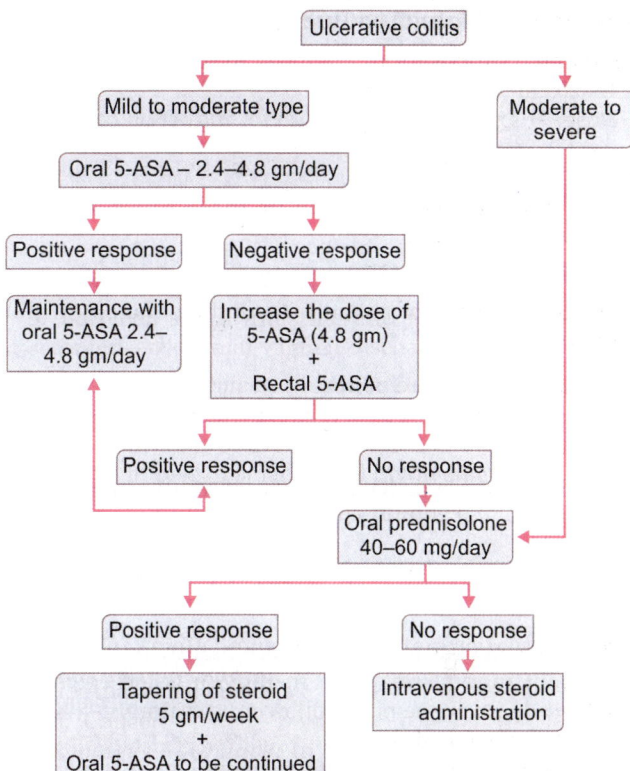

Fig. 4.8: Management of ulcerative colitis

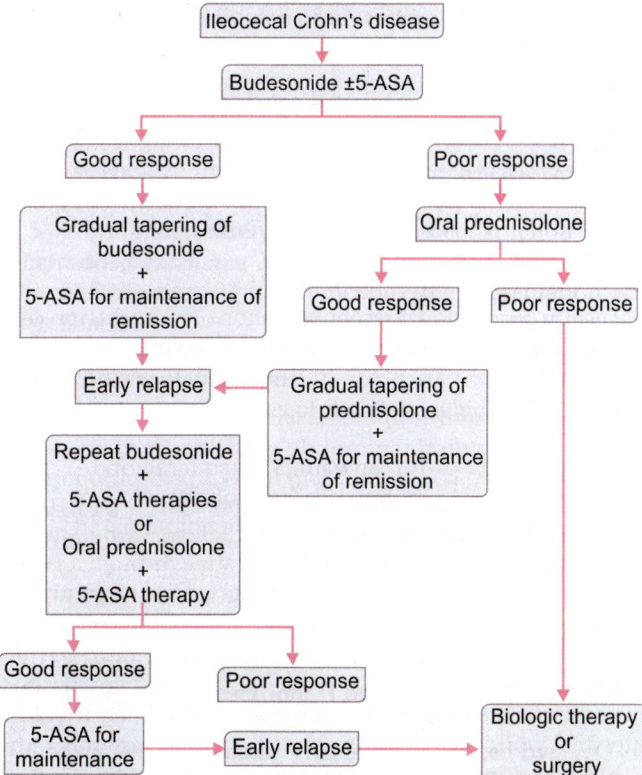

Fig. 4.9: Management of ileocecal Crohn's disease

Treatment of Ulcerative Proctitis

Mesalamine suppositories (Pentasa, Asacol)
i. 15–20 cm above anal verge
ii. Dose—1 gm. Daily for 1 month for induction of remission

> 1 gm every third day or three times weekly to maintain remission

↓

Small percentage of patients discontinue therapy without relapse

In case of left-sided colitis
Pentasa enema or Asacol foam enema (every night)

↓

Reach up to splenic flexure or distal transverse colon

Improvement occurs with 2–4 weeks (induction of remission)

↓

Rectal enema has to be given once nightly or once weekly to maintain remission. Oral therapy or liquid enema may substitute foam enema in following conditions
 i. If foam enema is irritant.
 ii. If patient is unable to retain enema

↓

If no response occurs in 2–4 weeks

↓

Corticosteroid can be administered rectally along with foam enema—one foam enema in the morning and other foam enema in the evening.

↓

If no response occurs after giving above two topical therapies.

↓

Oral 5-ASA along with rectal 5-ASA preparation can be added.

LARGE BOWEL DISEASE

DIVERTICULAR DISEASE OF COLON

In western population, half of population of more than 60 years of age suffer from diverticular disease of colon.

Again 20% of patients with diverticular disease become symptomatic.

Anatomy and Pathophysiology

There are two types of diverticula of intestine:
A. True diverticulum: This is characterized by sac-like herniation of entire wall of the intestine through a gap.
B. Pseudo-diverticulum: This is characterized by protrusion of mucosa through muscularis propria of the colon.

The protrusion usually occurs at a point through which nutrient artery, i.e. vasa recta, penetrates muscularis mucosae—since here there is a breach in the integrity of the intestinal wall.

Site: It usually occurs in sigmoid colon but in 5% of case it occurs throughout the colon.

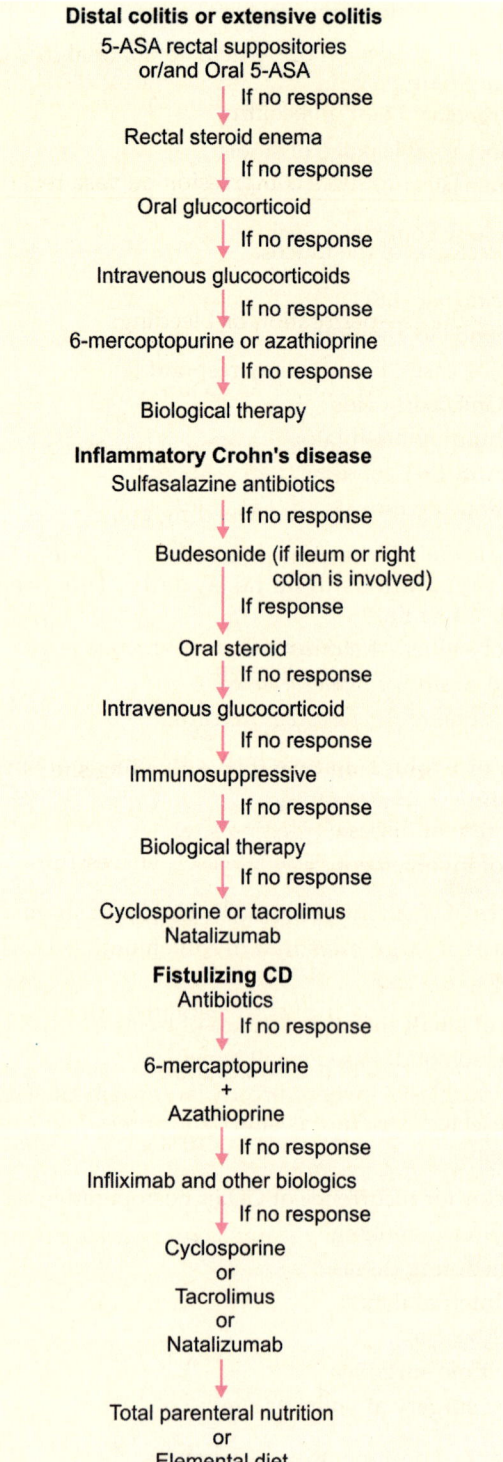

Fig. 4.10: Stepwise therapeutic approach in IBD

Cause of Development

High amplitude contraction in a patient with chronic constipation
 +
High fat content of the diet within sigmoid colonic lumen results in formation of colonic diverticula.
Diverticulitis is nothing but inflammation of diverticula.

(Contd.)

(Contd.)

$$\left\{ \begin{array}{l} \textbf{Cause} \quad \text{Retention of particulate material in the sac} \\ \qquad\qquad + \\ \qquad\quad \text{Formation of fecolith} \end{array} \right\}$$

↓

This produces compression on vasa recta

↓

Erosions of the mucosa

↓

Produces—perforation or bleeding.

Presentation

Commonest presentation is bleeding. It is most common cause of hematochezia in patient >60 years old.

Risk factors for diverticular bleeding are:
  i. Hypertension
 ii. Atherosclerosis
iii. Use of NSAIDs

Fate: Most of the bleeding stops spontaneously with bowel rest. Risk of rebleeding will be 25%.

Investigations and Management

1. **Colonoscopy:** It can localize the bleeding site.
2. **Mesenteric angiography:**
     i. It can localize the bleeding site.
    ii. It occludes the bleeding vessels successfully in 81% of cases.
   Follow-up should be done by colonoscopy.
3. **Segmental resection of colon:** It eliminates the risk of further bleeding.
   Advantages: It is useful in patient with chronic blood thinners.
4. **Highly selective coil embolization**
   Advantages:
   a. Rate of colonic ischemia is <10%.
   b. Risk of acute bleeding is <25%.
   c. The result will be long term.
5. **Selective infusion of vasopressin: It can stop hemorrhage.**
   Complication:
     i. Myocardial ischemia or myocardial infarction
    ii. Intimal ischemia
6. If patient with bleeding from diverticular disease is unstable and has lost 6 units of blood within 24 hours—the choice of operation is total colectomy.

Diverticulitis

Presentation

  i. Fever
 ii. Left lower quadrant pain
iii. Anorexia
iv. Obstipations
 v. In <25% of cases, evidence of generalized peritonitis due to perforation of diverticula.
vi. In case of localized abscess in pericolonic area—patient may present with localized abdominal distention and tenderness.

Diagnosis

1. Leukocytosis
2. In plain abdominal film—presence of air fluid level in left lower quadrants—suggests giant diverticulum in sigmoid colon—this can be managed by resection before impending rupture.
3. CT scan findings in case of diverticulitis
     i. Sigmoid diverticula
    ii. Wall of the colon thickened by >4 mm
   iii. Inflammation within pericolic fat
   iv. Presence or absence of collection of contrast material or fluid.
    v. In 16% cases, presence of pericolic abscess.

Mimicking with irritable bowel syndrome—since symptoms may suggest IBS, hence, absence of leukocytosis, absence of CT scan diagnostic criteria, absence of fever will virtually exclude the diagnosis of diverticulitis.

Barium enema and colonoscopy should not be performed in acute setting, because air insufflations during colonoscopy or pressure insertion during barium enema may produce perforation of diverticulum. Hence colonoscopy should be performed 6 weeks after attack of diverticular disease.

Complicated Diverticular Disease

This can be defined as diverticular disease associated with following features:
  i. Abscess
 ii. Perforation
iii. Stricture
iv. Fistula formation
   a. Cutaneous
   b. Vesicle
   c. Vaginal

Colovaginal fistula—occurs in women who has undergone hysterectomy.

Stages of Performation

Stage-I: Perforated diverticulitis confined to paracolic abscess.
Stage-II: Perforated diverticulitis—which is closed spontaneously along with distant abscess formation.
Stage-III: Non-communicating perforated diverticulitis with focal peritonitis.
Stage-IV: Perforation and free communication with the peritoneum—producing peritonitis.

Medical Management of Diverticular Disease

Dietary modifications:
  i. Fibers enriched diet—30 gm per day
 ii. Supplementary fiber to be added are—metamucil, fibercon, citrucel.
iii. Avoidance of smoking—because smoking may increase the complication related to diverticular disease.
iv. In case of diverticular disease with infection—
   broad-spectrum antibiotics

   Co-trimoxazole

   Or

   Ciprofloxacin
   +
   Metronidazole

Target bacteria are aerobic gram-negative rods or anaerobic bacteria.

In case of non-responders: Ampicillin can be added

Alternative antibiotics are

Intravenous piperacillin

Or

Oral penicillin/clavulanic acid

Total duration of administration is 7–10 days.

For long-term management in diverticular disease:

i. Rifaximin—poorly absorbable antibiotics can be given.
ii. Use of prebiotics:
  • It decreases the incidence of recurrent attacks.
  • It decreases the presence of *Clostridium* species and increase in *Lactobacillus* and *Bifidobacterium* species.

Surgical Management

Preoperative risk factors which are responsible for postoperative mortality follow American Society of Anesthesiologists Physical status classification system—it includes:

P_1 — Normal healthy patients
P_2 — Presence of mild systemic disease
P_3 — Presence of severe systemic disease.
P_4 — Presence of severe systemic disease—which is a constant threat to life
P_5 — Morbid patient who is not expected to survive without operation
P_6 — A declared brain dead patient whose organs are being removed for donation

The goal of surgical treatment in diverticular disease:

1. Control of sepsis
2. Removal of complication
3. Removal of diseased colonic segment
4. Restoration of intestinal continuity
5. Minimization of morbidity rate
6. Decrease in length of hospitalization
7. Improvement of quality of life.

Methods of operation: Removal of diseased sigmoid up to rectosigmoid junction is the method of choice.

Current recommendation is open or laparoscopic sigmoid resection.

Benefits of laparoscopic resection include:
  i. Early discharge of the patient
 ii. Less narcotic use
iii. Less postoperative complications

Methods of management of complicated diverticular disease:

1. Proximal diversion of fecal matter through ileostomy or colostomy
2. Closure of distal bowel with formation of Hartmann's pouch
3. Coloproctostomy
4. Resection with anastomosis and diversion (coloproctostomy with loop ileostomy)

Recurrence of Diverticular Disease

A retained segment of diseased rectrosigmoid colon is the common cause of recurrence of diverticular disease. Choice of operation according to complicated diverticular disease:

Hinchey state	Operative procedure
1.	Resection with primary anastomosis without diverting stoma
2.	Resection with primary anastomosis with or without diversion
3.	Hartmann's procedure vs. diverting colostomy with omental pedal graft.
4.	Hartmann's procedure vs. diverting colostomy and omental pedal graft.

ISCHEMIC COLITIS

Here colonoscopy is needed to observe:
i. Integrity of colonic mucosa
ii. Integrity of rectosigmoid junction

It occurs in:
i. Nonocclusive ischemia
ii. Occlusive ischemia—in case of aortic surgery

These are three grades of colonic ischemia

  i. In mild type—minimal erythema of mucosa
 ii. In moderate type:
      a. Pale mucosa with ulceration
      b. Lesion extends to muscular layer of bowel wall.
iii. In severe type: Extensive severe ulceration results in black or brown discoloration.

Predictors of degree of reversibility mucosal findings:

1. Mild erythema—100% reversible
2. Moderate erythema—50% reversible
3. Severe and frank necrosis—dead intestine.

Indications of laparotomy in case of non-occlusive ischemia:

1. Appearance of peritonitis
2. Gradual worsening of endoscopic findings
3. Non-improvement of medical conditions in spite of aggressive resuscitation.

Ischemia due to Mesenteric Venous Thrombosis

Symptoms

1. Vague abdominal pain
2. Nausea
3. Vomiting

Signs

1. Abdominal distention
2. Abdominal tenderness
3. Signs of dehydration

Diagnosis

Abdominal spiral CT scan with oral and intravenous contrast
Findings are:
a. Bowel wall thickening
b. Ascites
c. Delayed arterial phase with clot in superior mesenteric vein.

Management

1. Massive intravenous fluid resuscitation for
   a. Optimizing hemodynamics
   b. Correction of electrolyte abnormalities
2. Intravenous broad-spectrum antibiotics
3. Anticoagulation
4. In case of laparotomy:
   i. Heparin anticoagulation
   ii. Resection of compromised bowel

Prognosis

Intestinal ischemia due to mesenteric vascular insufficiency has best prognosis.

IRRITABLE BOWEL SYNDROME

Introduction

Irritable bowel syndrome is the most common functional bowel disorder, which usually affects women (>70% of total IBS patients are women)—it may be due to the following facts:
1. Women more easily complain of abdominal bloating and pain and altered bowel habit.
2. It may be due to hormonal difference between men and women that may affect the function of the gut and altered perception of pain related to abdominal distention.
   Age of occurrence: IBS predominantly affects the people in the prime of their lives, mostly between the ages of 20–40 years having average duration of symptoms of 11 years. But in one-third of patients, it may be much longer.

It was reported that women with IBS have history of 71% abdominal surgeries than women without IBS (34%), and rate of cholecystectomies, hysterectomies and appendectomies were twice more common than patients without IBS.

One study demonstrated that patients with IBS were absent from their work or school for average of 13 days per year as compared to patients without IBS.

Only 25% of IBS patients actually consult primary care physician for their symptoms and a few patients visit gastroenterologists—again, of these patients, 60% have psychological disturbances and rest 30% have history of sexual abuse.

Pathogenesis

The following factors are responsible for development of IBS:

Disturbences in the Intestinal Motility

Disturbences in motility is diurnally variable, and it can be anticipated only by long-term motility studies. The type of disturbances are:
1. Frequency and duration of discrete cluster of contractions (DCC) will be increased.
2. Frequency of migratory motor complex (MMC) will be increased.

3. Jejunal and duodenal retrograde contractions will be more.
4. Exaggerated response to meal ingestion, ileal distention,
5. Colonic distention dose not decrease duodenal motility—it suggests impaired intestine—intestinal inhibitory complex.
6. Colonic motility to meal ingestion will be exaggerated—it is the most consistent abnormality.
7. Reduced rectal compliance and increased rectal lesion will be detected.

Visceral Hypersensitivity

Abdominal pain is mostly responsible for considerable morbidity in IBS patients—this is due to visceral hypersensitivity, as a result of involvement of both central and peripheral nervous systems.

↓

Following episodes of gut inflammation in acute gastroenteritis

↓

Release of immune and inflammatory mediators, such as, prostaglandins, leukotrienes, serotonin, histamine, neurotrophic factors and reactive metabolites

↓

Intracellular signaling pathways activation

↓

This in turn, upgrades their sensitivity and excitability. (This phenomenon is known as peripheral sensitization)

↓

This is responsible for primary hyperalgesia (increased sensitivity to painful stimuli) as well as allodynia (increased sensitivity to non-painful stimuli, like colonic or rectal distention)

↓

This phenomenon is followed by secondary hyperalgesia, which means increased area of hypersensitivity in the surrounding uninvolved tissue due to recruitment and amplification of both non-nociceptive and nociceptive inputs.

There is evidence of central sensitization, an important mechanism for the development of visceral hypersensitivity as suggested from following important observations:
The patients with IBS:
1. Have greater radiation of pain to other somatic structures.
2. May develop fibromyalgia.
3. May demonstrate proximal area of gut hypersensitivity.

Altered brain processing signals from following areas of brain may responsible for visceral hypersensitivity:
   a. Anterior cingulate gyrus   b. Thalamus
   c. Insula   d. Prefrontal cortices

Post-Infection IBS

11.9% patients suffering from acute gastroenteritis develop IBS in near future, if the following risk factors persist:
1. Severe acute illness of recurrent nature
2. Bacterial toxigenicity
3. Female sex

4. Range of adverse psychological factors, including:
   a. Neuroticism
   b. Hypochondriac condition
   c. Anxiety
   d. Depression
   e. Adverse event in the patient's life.

IBS is usually reported after gastroenteritis due to infection by following organisms:

   1. Shigella   2. Salmonella   3. Campylobacter

Histological studies in colon in post-infection IBS demonstrate increased lymphocytes in lamina propria.

Histological studies in terminal ileum demonstrate increased mast cell infiltration.

Histological studies in throughout large and small intestine show enterochromaffin cells hyperplasia, which in turn release large amount of 5-HT, it is shown in post-infection IBS and diarrhea-related IBS.

Stress Response

The interplay between the autoimmune nervous system and hypothalamic-pituitary-adrenal axis (HPA axis) is regulating gut mucosal immunology and it is mostly responsible for post-infectious IBS when following stress factors may be active:

   1. Prior life stress   2. History of childhood abuse
   3. Anxiety   4. Hypochondriasis
   5. Depression

Symptoms

A. **Altered bowel habit:** It has following characteristics:
   1. Constipation resulting from complaints of hard stool having narrow caliber, painful or infrequent defecation and intractability to laxatives.
   2. Diarrhea which means small volumes loose stools, evacuation preceded by urgency and frequency.
   3. Post-prandial urgency for defecation.
   4. Characteristically, one feature predominates in one patient, but significant variability in bowel habits exist among patients.

B. **Abdominal pain:** It may have following important characteristics:
   1. Non-radiating pain is frequently diffuse.
   2. Common site of pain is left lower quadrant region
   3. Acute episodes of sharp pain may be superimposed on more constant dull aching sensation.
   4. Meal may be precipitating factor of pain.
   5. Defecation may improve pain but never relieve it.
   6. Pain produces presumed gas pockets in splenic flexure—it may mimic anterior chest pain or left upper quadrant abdominal pain.

C. **Abdominal distention**

D. **Clear or white mucorrhea of non-inflammatory etiology**

E. **Heart burn**

F. **Nausea and/or vomiting**

G. **Dyspepsia**

H. **Non-gastrointestinal symptoms:**
   1. Sexual dysfunction including dyspareunia and poor libido
   2. Worsening of symptoms in premenstrual period
   3. Comorbid fibromyalgia
   4. Backache
   5. Headache
   6. Stress-related symptoms

Symptoms inconsistent with IBS which may alert the clinician to exclude any organic cause (flag sign):

   1. Onset in middle age or older.
   2. Progressive symptoms
   3. Nocturnal symptoms
   4. Acute symptoms
   5. Anorexia and weight loss
   6. Steatorrhea
   7. Lactose intolerance
   8. Gluten intolerance
   9. Fever
   10. Rectal bleeding
   11. Painless diarrhea
   12. Recent change in symptoms
   13. Family history of colonic and ovarian cancer

Subtyping of IBS

A. Symptom-based diagnostic criteria are not at all unique in the field of gastroenterology. But this type of criteria has become increasingly sophisticated. Thus "Manning criteria" has been developed in 1978, and it has been proven to be reasonable tool for diagnosis of IBS.

   These criteria: (Presence of any four of the six symptoms)
   i. Abdominal pain that is relieved with a bowel movement.
   ii. Pain associated with more frequent stools.
   iii. Loose stools at the onset of pain.
   iv. Sensation of incomplete evacuation.
   v. Passage of mucus per rectum.
   vi. Abdominal distension.

B. Rome criteria have been evolving from the first set of criteria and presented in 1989 through Rome Classification system for functional GI disorders in 1990. There are three Rome criteria:
   i. Rome criteria I for IBS (1992)
   ii. Rome criteria II for IBS (1999)
   iii. Rome criteria III for IBS (2006)

   Rome criteria III: Recurrent abdominal pain or discomfort at least 3 days per month in last 3 months associated with 2 or more of the following:
   1. Improved with defecation.
   2. Onset is associated with a change in frequency of stool (straining, urgency, or feeling of incomplete evacuation).
   3. Onset is associated with a change in the form of the stool (lumpy/hard or loose/watery stool).

C. **To differentiate the different subtypes more efficiently, the Bristol Stool form scale has been very helpful clinically in defining the spectrum of constipation to diarrhea:**
   1. Type 1: Separate hard lumps like nuts (difficult to pass).
   2. Type 2: Sausage shaped but lumpy.
   3. Type 3: Lake sausage, but with cracks on its surface.
   4. Type 4: Like sausage or snake, smooth and soft.
   5. Type 5: Soft blobs with clear cut edges (Passed easily).
   6. Type 6: Fluffy pieces with ragged edges, a mushy stool.
   7. Type 7: Watery, no solid pieces, entirely liquid.

D. **Subtyping of IBS by predominant stool pattern:**
   1. IBS—C (Constipation predominant): Description of stool: Hard lumpy stool passed >25% of the time and loose stool passed <25% times of bowel movements.

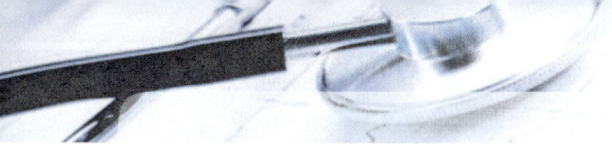

2. IBS—D (Diarrhea predominant): Description of stool: Loose stool passed >25% of the time and hard lumpy stool passed <25% of bowel movements.
3. Mixed IBS: Stool description: Hard lumpy stool >25% of the time and loose stool >5% times of bowel movements.
4. Unsubtyped IBS Insufficient abnormality in the stool consistency to meet the criteria for IBS—C, IBS—D and mixed subtype.

To elicit psychological factors as an important cause of IBS, doctor has to ask following questions:
1. Do you feel down or have you lost interest in things you normally enjoy.
2. Have you had sudden attacks of fear or anxiety?
3. Do you feel worry or anxious most o the time?

Differential Diagnoses

1. Celiac disease
2. Lactose intolerance
3. Bile salt malabsorption.
4. Thyroid disease—hyperthyroidism, hypothyroidism
5. Microscopic colitis
6. Inflammatory bowel disease
7. HIV enteropathy
8. Giardiasis

To exclude the organic diseases, we have to ask a few questions:
1. Bleeding per rectum.
2. Blood and mucus with stool.
3. History of intolerance to lactose, wheat, flour, etc.
4. History of exposure.

Physical Examination

1. Edema
2. Tachycardia
3. Thyroid function test abnormalities
4. Lymphadenopathy
5. Any abdominal masses
6. Rectal examination to exclude:
   a. Anal fissure   b. Anal fistula
   c. Skin tags   d. Any mass in rectum
   e. Any blood in anus.
7. To exclude abdominal wall pain—carnett test.

Method: Ask the patient to fold their arms across the chest and raise their head of from the pillow, while the clinician palpates the abdomen.

Results with interpretations:
i. If local tenderness improves or disappears, the etiology is likely to be visceral origin.
ii. If tenderness worsens with this maneuver, the etiology is of abdominal wall origin—muscles, trapped nerve or hernia.
iii. Resolution of pain after trigger point injection with 1% xylocaine with or without 20–40 mg triamcinolone—confirm the origin as abdominal wall.

Investigations

Investigations required to exclude organic causes:
A. Hematology:
  1. Complete blood count—increased in infection, IBD, microscopic colitis.
  2. Raised ESR: It indicates activity of organic disease.
  3. Anti-tissue transglutaminase antibody, antiendomycelial antibody, IgA antiglidin antibody—its absence excludes celiac disease.
  4. Thyroid test (FT4, TSH)—to exclude thyroid disease mainly hypothyroidism.
  5. Comprehensive metabolic panel—to exclude metabolic disorders, to rule out dehydration, electrolyte abnormality.
  6. Serum calcium—Normal or low level exclude hyperparathyroidism.
  7. P-ANCA, C-ANCA—to exclude inflammatory bowel disease (IBD).

B. Stool:
  1. Stool for occult blood: to exclude perianal disease, IBD, carcinoma.
  2. Stool—for parasite—to exclude giardiasis.

C. Endoscopy:
  1. Long colonoscopy—it can diagnose IBD, colonic and rectal carcinoma, perianal disease.
  2. Upper GI endoscopy with culture of duodenal aspirate—to exclude bacterial overgrowth.
  3. Hydrogen breath test—to exclude bacterial overgrowth.

D. Dietary studies:
  1. Direct lactose free diet for 1 week in conjunction with lactose supplementation—if it demonstrate improvement it indicates lactose intolerance.
  2. Direct 48 hours fasting—persistent diarrhea—it suggest secretary pathology.
  3. Fructose free diet followed by rechallanged with gradual addition of fructose—improvement followed by gradual deterioration—suggests Fructose intolerance.
  4. Excess secretion of artificial bile salts (selenium homocholic acid taurine (SeHCAT).

E. History specific imaging studies:
  1. Upper gastrointestinal studies with small bowel follow through to screen tumor, inflammation, obstruction and Crohn's disease. We can take biopsy to detect mucosal abnormality in the duodenal wall.
  2. Double contrast barium enema—to screen colorectal neoplasm and inflammation.
  3. Upper abdominal ultrasonography—to exclude gall bladder.
  4. Abdominal CT scan—it excludes tumor, obstruction, pancreatic disease and abdominal lymphoma.

F. Histological studies:
  1. Biopsy of small bowel shows shortened or blunted villi with elongated crypts with increased inflammatory cells in lamina propria—its absence exclude tropical sprue.
  2. Biopsy of the colon shows increased sub epithelial collagen and intra epithelial lymphocytes—its absence exclude microscopic colitis.

G. Manometry: Anal Manometry reveals specific response to rectal distention.

Complications

1. Increased morbidity
2. Time off from work and school
3. Multiple physician visits
4. Personal expenses and medications
5. Psychological problems:

Treatment

To treat the patient, firstly the clinician should establish why the patient is seeking for cure from this chronic ailment.
1. What is the patient's belief regarding the cause of the symptom.
2. Is there any fear of cancer suffering from?
3. Is there any psychological factor responsible?

Initial General Treatment of IBS

1. Proper education improves clinical outcome by giving the patient knowledge and skills to manage IBS.
2. Life style modification:
   a. Keeping the daily record of diet to identify the factors that trigger symptoms—certain foods like, cabbage, beans, broccoli, and cauliflower may produce abdominal bloating, pain.
   b. If bloating is the main problem—carbonated beverages, gum, artificial sweetener containing sucrose—should be avoided.

Medical Treatment

Medical treatment should be tailored to the predominant symptoms of such individual.
A. **Treatment with fibres:**
   1. Increased fibers in the diet or fiber supplements—it improves stool consistency and regulate bowel movement.
   2. It is commonly used for—mixed variety. In can be used in IBS—C, but with antispasmodics because increased fibers distends the colon and thus producing stretching pain.
   3. But there is no high quality evidence based study supporting the benefits of fiber in treating IBS in IBS- D because it increases diarrhea in these patients.
B. **Regarding antidiarrheal agents:**
   1. Loperamide and Diphenoxylate hydrochloride decrease number of motion as well as amount of stool in diarrhea.
   2. Cholestyramine binds bile salt and slows down the diarrheal activity.
      But all the above have no effect on abdominal pain and bloating, hence antispasmodics can be provided as pre-needed therapy in IBS –D.
C. **Regarding laxatives:**
   1. Stimulant laxatives (senna, bisacodyl, cascara):
      a. They may produce permanent damage to myenteric plexus by constant stimulation of these nerve endings—but studies are conflicting.
      b. They may produce abdominal cramps and bloating in chronic cases.
   2. Osmotic laxatives: a. Non gas forming laxatives: Polyethylene glycol—it is of choice in IBS—C. But these laxatives increase the bulk of the stool and thus produce stretching pain arising from the intestinal wall and produce abdominal bloating and cramps, so these drugs can be given in conjunction with antispasmodics.
D. **Antispasmodics:**
   1. Minimal evidenced based studies show antispasmodics can treat pain component of IBS.
   2. The drugs responsible are:
      a. Dicyclomine hydrochloride
      b. Hyoscyamine sulfate
      c. Scopolamine   d. Phenobarbital

3. They are prescribed before meals to:
   a. Inhibit abdominal pain and bloating.
   b. Inhibit and uncontrolled bowel movement.
E. **Tricyclic antidepressant:**
   1. It is prescribed to:
      i. Reduce abdominal cramping
      ii. Reduce gut motility in IBS—D due to its anticholinergic properties.
   2. Side effects: Dry eyes, dry mouth, urinary retention, constipation, fatigue, weight gain.
   3. The approach will be—to start with low dose (10 mg daily), followed by gradual increase of the dose by 10 mg. every 2–3 weeks as tolerated or according to symptomatic response.
F. **Regarding selective serotonin reuptake inhibition:** Same serotonin is a key neurotransmitter in the central processing of visceral afferent information—serotonin has a positive effect on gut motility.
   So, its reuptake inhibitors alleviate abdominal pain associated with constipation by reducing motility. The drugs are:
   a. *Citalopram:* It:
      i. Improves symptomatic abdominal pain and cramps and bloating.
      ii. Improves quality of life.
      iii. Improves over all wellbeing.
   b. *Fluoxetine hydrochloride:*
      i. It decreases abdominal discomfort and bloating.
      ii. It increases bowel movements.
G. **$5-HT_3$ antagonists:** Alosertan—it is approved for severe IBS—D on women who have failed with conventional therapy.
   Mode of actions:
   i. It decreases colonic transit.
   ii. It decreases rectal urgency.
   iii. It decreases abdominal pain.
   Complications:
   i. Severe constipation   ii. Ischemic colitis
This drug was launched in February 2000, and was temporarily withdrawn from the market for its severe complications. Again it reentered in the market but with following modifications:
   1. Dose—1 mg twice daily.
   2. It is restricted to women with chronic IBS—D refractory to other therapies.
   3. Patients taking alosertan must sign patient–physician agreement indicating that they have been informed of and undersigned the associated risk.
H. **Tegaserod:**
   1. It is $5-HT_4$ receptor agonist.
   2. Its actions: It:
      i. Stimulates peristalsis.
      ii. Increases velocity of propulsions through the colon.
      iii. Reduces firing rate of rectal afferent nerves.
      iv. Alters the chloride secretion in the intestine.
      v. Reduces visceral sensitivity.
   3. Effects:
      i. Bowel function will become normal.
      ii. Patient gets relief from abdominal pain.
   4. Indications:
      i. IBS–C in women.
      ii. Chronic constipation of men and women.

5. Side effects: Cardiovascular ischemic events. In patients with pre-existing cardiovascular abnormalities.

So, this drug should be prescribed in women with:
1. Younger than 55 years of age.
2. Do not have cardiovascular risk factors.
3. Chronic constipation.
4. IBS–C.   5. Does not respond to other treatments.

I. Lubiprostone:
1. Mechanism of actions: Chloride channel—2 activator:
   i. It increases fluid secretion into the lumen
   ii. It increases the bowel movements and stool will be softened.
2. Recommended dose:
   i. In IBS—C, 8 mcg. Twice daily.

   ii. In chronic constipation—24 mcg twice daily.
3. Side effects: It prodces
   i. Nausea   ii. Diarrhea

J. Rifaximin:
1. It is a nonsystemic, semisynthetic antibiotic.
2. Its spectrum of activity is over gm-positive, gm-negative, both aerobic and anaerobic organisms.
3. Dose: 400 mg thrice daily for 10 days.

K. Probiotics:
Bifidobacterium infantis alleviates:
1. Abdominal pain and bloating.
2. Slow down the stool.
3. Reduces the bowel movements.

HEPATOLOGY

LIVER FUNCTION TESTS

To evaluate the patients with liver disorders, one has to classify the patients into following categories:

A. Test to detect the capacity of the liver to transport the organic anions and metabolize drugs.
   i. Serum bilirubin
   ii. Sulfobromophthalein sodium
   iii. Serum indocyanine, green
   iv. Serum bite acids
   v. Serum caffeine
   vi. Serum lidocaine metabolites
   vii. Breath tests
   The above tests measure the ability of the liver to clear the exogenous and endogenous metabolites from the circulation.
B. Tests to detect the injury to the hepatocytes:
   i. Alanine aminotransferase
   ii. Aspartate aminotransferase
   iii. Alkaline phosphatase
C. Tests to detect the synthetic capacity of the liver:
   i. Serum albumin
   ii. Serum ceruloplasmin
   iii. Serum ferritin
   iv. α_1-antitrypsin
   v. Serum lipoproteins
   vi. Blood clotting factors.
   The above substances are produced in the liver and consequently released into circulation.
D. Tests to estimate the fibrosis of liver:
   i. Serum type IV collagen   ii. Serum hyaluronate
   iii. Procollagen III   iv. Laminin
   v. Fibro-test—it is multiparametetric tests.
E. Tests to detect chronic inflammation and immune dysregulation:
   i. Specific serum antibodies
   ii. Serum immunoglobulins.

Bilirubin

Bilirubin is produced from:
   i. Breakdown of hemoglobin in senescent red blood cells.
   ii. Premature destruction of erythroid cells in bone marrow.
   iii. Turnover of hem proteins in tissues throughout the body.

First Step

In reticuloendothelial cells of liver and spleen
↓
With the help of microsomal enzyme heme-oxygenase clearage of the alfa-methane bridge of porphyrin group, opens heme ring.
↓
Production of equimolar amount of biliverdin and carbon monoxide

Second Step

With the help of cytosolic enzyme biliverdin reduction, biliverdin will be converted to bilirubin.
↓
This bilirubin is lipid soluble and water insoluble.
↓
Bilirubin will bind with album in blood and is carried to liver
↓
Here bilirubin will be taken up by the hepatocytes by carrier-mediated membrane transport mechanism.
↓
In hepatocyte, bilirubin will be coupled to glutathione-s-transferases (ligandin)
↓
The bilirubin will be conjugated with glucuronic acid to from bilirubin monoglucuronide and bilirubin diglucuronide—these salts are water-soluble and are called direct-acting bilirubin.
This reaction is catalyzed by enzymes of endoplasmic reticulum in hepatocyte.
↓
This conjugated bilirubin then transported to biliary canaliculi by ATP dependent transport process—this is a rate limiting step in hepatic bilirubin excretion. This process is mediated by a protein in bile canaliculi membrane—multi-drug resistance associated protein
↓
This conjugated bilirubin will be transported into duodenal cavity.
↓

(Contd.)

(Contd.)

This will be carried distally to ileum and colon.

↓

In distal ileum and colon, conjugated bilirubin will be hydrolyzed to unconjugated form by bacterial β-glucuronidases.

↓

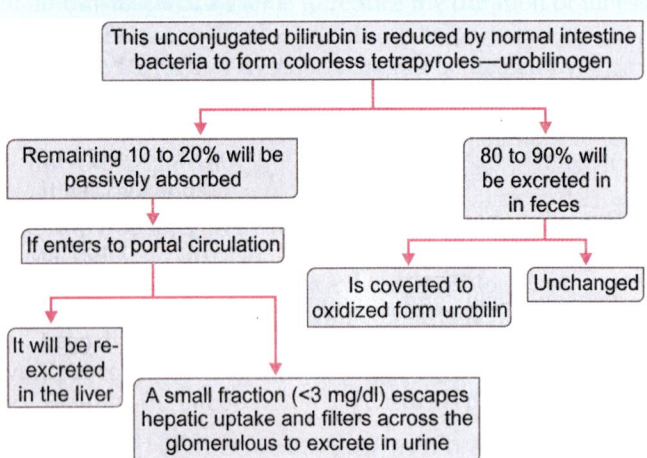

Appearance of urobilinogen in urine depends upon following factors:

i. Urine pH   ii. Rate of urine flow

Normal level of bilirubin is 0.2 to 0.9 mg/dl.

Abnormal Rise in Bilirubin

Rise in unconjugated bilirubin occurs in:

i. Over production from hemolysis
ii. Familial
iii. Impaired uptake or conjugation

Rise in conjugated bilirubin occurs in:

i. Leakage of conjugated bilirubin as a result of damage of hepatocytes
ii. Decreased excretion of conjugated bilirubin.

Rise in total bilirubin is not a sensitive indicator of hepatic dysfunction, because:

i. Hyperbilirubinemia may not be associated with elevation of enzyme levels.
ii. Hyperbilirubinemia may not be present in moderate to severe hepatic parenchymal damage or partially obstructed common bite duct.

Capacity of human liver to remove bilirubin from circulation is twofold greater than the daily pigment load, before hyperbilirubinemia occurs.

Serum albumin level controls the serum bilirubin level, because

i. Serum substance like salicylates, sulphonamide or free fatty acids displaces the bilirubin from attachment with serum albumin and transfers it into tissues.
ii. Increase in serum albumin temporarily shifts the bilirubin from tissues into circulation.

Unconjugated hyperbilirubinemia can be detected when serum level of indirectly acting bilirubin is >1.2 mg/dl and directly reacting fraction will be less than 20% of total serum bilirubin.

Increase in direct fraction to more than 0.3 mg/dl—usually indicates mild liver injury.

Methods of Detection of Serum Bilirubin and its Fractionation

  i. Vandenberg diazo reaction
 ii. Alkaline methanolysis with chloroform extraction
iii. High performance gas liquid chromatography
 iv. Thin layer chromatography
  v. Spectrophotometric determination.

Urine Bilirubin

1. In case of unconjugated bilirubinemia, no bilirubin will appear in urine due to its water insolubility.
2. In case of conjugated bilirubinemia, in spite of normal serum bilirubin, conjugated bilirubin appears in the urines, as many laboratory methods can detect urinary bilirubin at as low as 0.05 mg/dl of urine.

Serum Enzyme Tests

These tests indicate—whether the liver damage is:

  i. Hepatocellular
 ii. Cholestatic
iii. Infiltrative

But the following enzymes cannot differentiate intra-hepatic from extra-hepatic cholestasis. The enzymes are:

 i. Alanine aminotransferase (ALT)
ii. Aspartate aminotransferase (AST)

The above enzymes catalyze the transfer of an amino-group of alanine and aspartic acid to a keto group of keto glutaric acid to form pyruvic acid and oxaloacetic and respectively (Fig. 4.11).

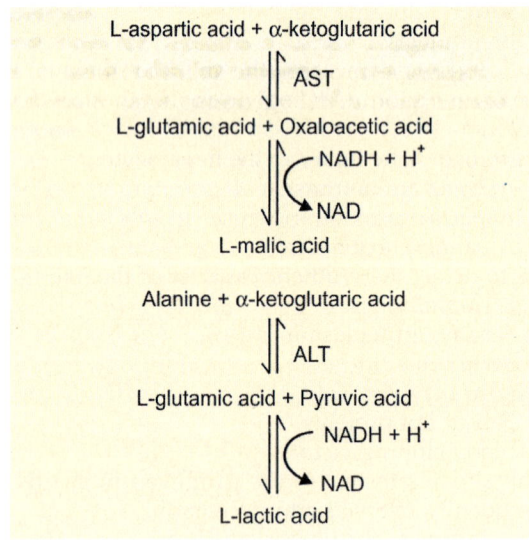

Fig. 4.11: Mechanism of action of AST and ALT

As NADH absorbs light at 340 nm, this reaction allows spectrophotometric analysis of these enzymes.

Aspartate Aminotransferase (AST)

1. It is present in following tissues from highest concentration to lowest concentration:
  a. Liver
  b. Heart
  c. Skeletal muscles
  d. Kidneys

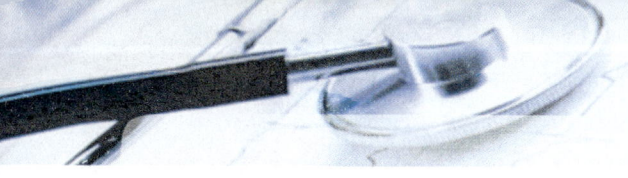

e. Brain
f. Pancreas
g. Lung
h. Leukocytes
i. Erythrocytes
2. It is usually present in cytoplasm and mitochondria of the above tissues.
3. Macro-AST—it is rare benign condition—characterized by isolated AST elevation due to binding of AST within immunoglobulins—which cannot be cleared by blood or kidneys.
4. Low level of AST can be found in:
   i. Chronic hemodialysis
   ii. Pyruvate kinase deficiency.
5. There is no correlation between rise in transaminase level and degree of hepatocyte necrosis.
   Causes of raised aminotransferase level:
   I. Unexpected rise in aminotransferase level
      i. Non-alcoholic fatty liver disease
      ii. Alcohol abuse
      iii. Hemochromatosis
   II. Less common causes of rise:
      i. Autoimmune hepatitis
      ii. α_1 antitrypsin deficiency
      iii. Wilson's disease
      iv. Drug-induced liver disease
      v. Non-hepatic disorder
         a. Addison's disease
         b. Anorexia nervosa
         c. Celiac disease
   III. Markedly elevated transaminase:
      i. Viral hepatitis
      ii. Paracetamol-induced hepatotoxicity
      iii. Ischemic hepatitis
      iv. Autoimmune hepatitis
   IV. Very high level of enzymes:
      i. ALD coexisting with paracetamol toxicity
      ii. ALD coexisting with viral hepatitis
6. Ratio of AST to ALT:
   i. Greater than 2—alcoholic liver disease. This occurs due to:
      a. Damage of mitochondria which release large amount of AST.
      b. ALT is more sensitive to pyridoxal 5-phosphate deficiency—leading to lowering of ALT.
   ii. Raised in advanced hepatic fibrosis or cirrhosis

Alkaline Phosphatase (ALP)

It is a group of enzymes that catalyses the hydrolysis of phosphate esters at neutral pH. The important co-factors are magnesium and zinc.
   ALP is present in differ organs in gradual decreasing quantity:
   i. Placenta
   ii. Ileal mucosa
   iii. Kidney
   iv. Bone
   v. Liver
   80% of ALP is present in liver, bone and kidney and 20% of ALP is secreted from intestine with blood group O and B.
   Blood level of alkaline phosphatase will be increased after fatty meal.

Bone, liver, kidney ALPs:
i. Coded by some genes.
ii. Share common protein structure, but differ in carbohydrate content.

The common causes of increased synthesis of ALP are (Fig. 4.12):
i. Increased hepatobiliary synthesis
ii. Increased canalicular leakage

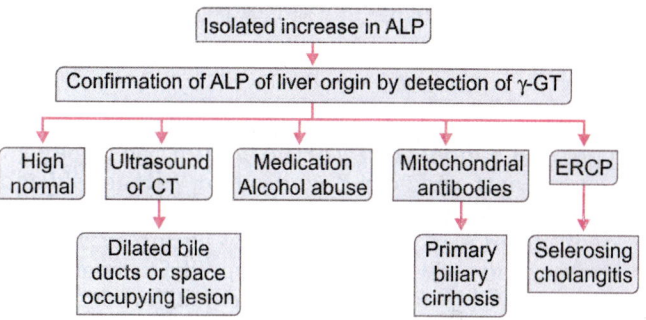

Fig. 4.12: Causes of increased ALP

Hepatic ALP can be differentiated from bone ALP by:
i. Isoenzyme fractionation
ii. Rise in gamma glutamyltransferase in hepatic involvement.

Rise in ALP are observed in (without jaundice):
i. Primary and secondary hepatic tumors
ii. Infiltrative diseases in liver
   a. Amyloidosis
   b. Abscess
   c. Lymphoma
   d. Granuloma

Nonspecific mild elevation of ALP in case of non-hepatobiliary involvement (Stauffer's syndrome):
i. Hodgkin's disease
ii. Heart failure
iii. Hyperthyroidism
iv. 15% cases of renal cell carcinoma

Low ALPs are seen in:
i. Hypothyroidism
ii. Wilson's disease
iii. Hemolysis
iv. Congenital hypophosphatasia
v. Pernicious, anemia
vi. Zinc deficiency
vii. Severe hepatic insufficiency
viii. Children recovering from severe enteritis.

In individual:
i. In 15 to 50 years old age group—level is higher in men than women.
ii. In older than 60 years—level in women is normal or exceeds than men.
iii. In children, alkaline phosphatase level is considerably elevated.
iv. In healthy adolescent male—level is three times higher than in healthy adult.

If raised alkaline phosphatase is only abnormal finding, then the source of it must be identified by following means:

i. By observing the different mobilities in electrophoresis
ii. Difference in susceptibility to inactivation by heat or 2 mol. urea—placental ALP is heat stable, but bone, liver and intestinal ALP will be partially inactivated.
iii. Estimation of level GGT and 5' neucleotidase are measured to substantiate the diagnosis—because these enzymes will be elevated only in liver disease.

5' neucleotidase: It catalyses the hydrolysis of nucleotides, like, adenosine 5' phosphate, and inosine 5'-phosphate. Presence of alkaline phosphatase in serum complicates the assay of 5' neucleotidase. So correlation for ALP activity can be made in two ways:
i. Incubation of serum in proper concentration of ethylenediaminetetraacetic acid selectively inactives ALP.
ii. The assay in presence and absence of nickel—because it specifically inactivates 5' neucleotidase.

Normal level: 0.3 to 3.2 Bodansky units. Its level is not clearly influenced by sex or race.

Importance:
i. Its level is increased in hepatobiliary disease along with rise in ALP.
ii. It can differentiates the raise in ALP—whether it is of bone or liver origin.

It is found in
i. Liver
ii. Intestine
iii. Brain
iv. Heart
v. Blood vessels;
vi. Endocrine pancreas.

γ-glutamyl Transpeptidase

This enzyme catalyses the transfer of γ-glutamyl group from γ-glutamyl peptides or other peptides or other peptides to L-amino acids.

It is present in cell membranes of kidneys, pancreas, liver, spleen, heart, brain and seminal vesicles.

Value: i. Normal value is 0–30 IU/L
ii. Children more than 4 years have normal value of adults.

Importance:
i. Main importance is to confirm the raised ALP is of hepatobiliary origin or not.
ii. It is also raised in alcohol abuse in absence of liver disease.
iii. It may be raised non-specifically in the following diseases:
   a. Hepatobiliary disease
   b. Alcoholism
   c. Chronic obstructive lung disease
   d. Diabetes mellitus
   e. Hyperthyroidism
   f. Rheumatoid arthritis
   g. Severe medications like, barbiturates, cimetidine, carbamazepine, furosemide oral contraceptives
iv. It has high predictive value for screening of biliary tract disease, like, intrahepatic cholestasis. But there are following exceptions:
   a. Progressive familial intrahepatic cholestasis (type 1 or Byler's disease, and type 2)
   b. Benign recurrent intrahepatic cholestasis type 1 (Summerskill's syndrome)

Lactic Dehydrogenase

This enzyme is present in cytoplasm of different tissues in the body.

There are five isoenzymes present in the body—these can be separated by various electrophoretic techniques. Raised level is found in:
i. Neoplasm
ii. Ischemic hepatitis
iii. Hepatic involvement in neoplasm.

ALT: LDH ratio:
1. >1.5 → acute viral hepatitis
2. <1.5 → ischemic hepatitis, paracetamol overdose.

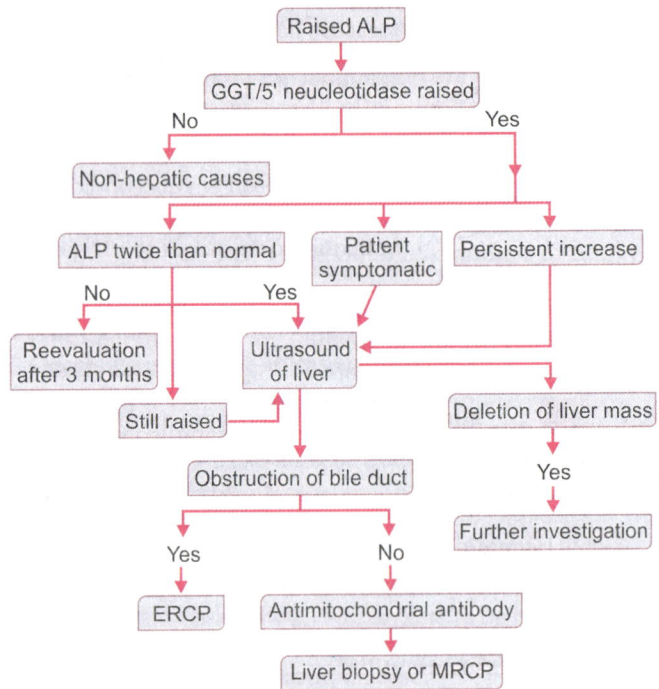

Fig 4.13: Algorithm of raised alkaline phosphatase

Tests for Liver Biosynthetic Capacity

Liver produces a large number of plasma proteins—these are synthesized on polyribosemes bound to rough endoplasmic reticulum—then they are secreted into serum.

The proteins are:
i. Albumin
ii. Fibrinogen
iii. α_2-antitrypsin
iv. Haptoglobin
v. Ceruloplasmin
vi. Transferrin
vii. Severe coagulation factors.

The following proteins are acute phase reactants; because, these are raised in tissue injury like, inflammation:
i. Fibrinogen
ii. Haptoglobin
iii. α_2-antitrypsin
iv. C3 component of ferritin
v. Ceruloplasmin.

The factors responsible for raised acute phase reactant

Cytokines (IL-1, IL-6, TNF-α)
↓
Binds to cell surface receptors
↓
Send messages from hepatocyte membrane to the hepatocyte nucleus
↓
Induction of specific nuclear factors
↓
They interacts with promoter elements at the 5' end of several acute phase reactants genes
↓
Increased synthesis of acute phase reactants

Cytokine also inhibits synthesis of:
a. Albumin
b. Transferrin
c. Other non-acute phase reactant proteins.

Immunoglobulins

These are synthesized by B cells of lymphoid system. Their levels are increased in all cirrhotic as non-specific response to bacteremia.

Haptoglobin

i. It is a glycoprotein, composed of α and β polypeptide attached by disulphide bonds.
ii. It is synthesized by hepatocytes
iii. Significance:
   a. Hereditary deficiencies in American black people
   b. Low values are seen in:
      1. Heaptocellular disease
      2. Megaloblastic anemia
      3. Hemolytic crisis

Ceruloplasmin

It is a glycoprotein, containing 6 copper atoms per molecule. It is a major copper binding protein.

   Low concentration found in:
   i. 95% of homozygous for Wilson's disease
   ii. 10% heterozygous for Wilson's disease
   iii. Decompensated cirrhosis not due to Wilson's disease

   High values are found in:
   i. Pregnancy
   ii. Patient is on estrogen therapy
   iii. Large bile duct obstruction

   Values normal to high is found in—patients with Wilson's disease, who have liver transplant.
   Ceruloplasmin level should be measured in all patients with chronic hepatitis.

Transferrin

i. It is an iron transport protein. It is synthesized by many cells, but hepatocytes are the major source.
ii. There is inverse relationship between iron level and transferrin synthesis, i.e. in iron deficiency, transferrin synthesis will be increased and reduced during iron overload.

iii. Two important functions of transferrin
   1. Transportation of iron into ferric state
   2. Delivery of iron to cell surface transferrin receptors
iv. In untreated idiopathic hemochromatosis, 90% of transferrin is saturated with iron.
v. Low values are found in—cirrhosis.

C$_3$ Component of Complement

1. Low value is seen:
   i. Alcoholic fatty liver
   ii. Alcoholic cirrhosis with or without hepatitis—it is due to reduced hepatitis synthesis.
2. It is increased in chronic hepatitis
3. It is increased in compensated primary biliary cirrhosis.
4. Transient reduction of this complement is seen in—immune complex stage of acute hepatitis B.

α-Fetoprotein

It is normal component of plasma protein in fetus of more than 6 weeks of gestation.
↓
It reaches maximum between 12 and 16 weeks of fetal life
↓
But after birth, it will disappear.

Its level is increased in:
   i. Primary liver cancer
   ii. Secondaries in liver
   iii. Chronic viral hepatitis
   iv. Embryonic tumors of ovary and testis
   v. Embryonic hepatoblastoma
   vi. Gastro intestinal tract carcinoma
   vii. Ataxia telangiectesia.

   Value: More than 400 ng/ml—is diagnostic of primary liver cancer, but normal value cannot exclude it.

Albumin

It is most important plasma protein, exclusively synthesized by liver.
   Normal value is 3.5 to 4.5 gm/dl. It is synthesized 15 gm/day.
   Its half-life is 20 days.

Albumin synthesis is regulated by:
   i. Nutritional status
   ii. Osmotic pressure
   iii. Systemic inflammation
   iv. Hormonal levels
   v. Amino acids like tryptophan, phenylalanine, glutamic acid, and lysine.
   vi. Amino acids (ornithine and arginine)—that increase urea synthesis.
   vii. Corticosteroid and thyroid hormones—by increasing the mRNA and transfer RNA concentration.

Factors decreasing albumin synthesis:
   i. Alcohol inhibiting the formation of polysomes.
   ii. Inflammation through inhibitory effects of interleukin-1 and tumor necrosis factor.

Serum albumin level is normal in:
   i. Acute viral hepatitis,
   ii. Drug-related hepatotoxicity
   iii. Obstructive jaundice.

Serum albumin level is low in:
i. Chronic hepatitis
ii. Cirrhosis
iii. Chronic malnutrition:
  a. Protein loosing enteropathy
  b. Chronic infection
  c. Nephritic syndrome.

In ascites—hypolbuminemia is due to increased volume distribution in spite of normal or increased albumin synthesis.

Prothrombin Time

Usually clotting involved—13 clotting factors, of which 11 factors are synthesized by liver. These factors are:

Factor-I — Fibrinogen
Factor-II — Prothrombin
Factor-V — Proaccelerin, labile factor
Factor-VII — Stable factor
Factor-IX — Christmas factor
Factor-X — Stuart factor
Factor-XII and XIII—preallikrein

Liver is involved in clearing some clotting factors from serum.

The abnormalities in liver function—can be assessed by prothrombin time—it can measure the rate and by which prothrombin is converted to thrombin. In presence of tissue extracts, calcium ions, a series of coagulation factors will be activated followed by polymerization of fibrinogen to fibrin. The result is expressed in seconds:
i. Normal range is 9–11 seconds.
ii. Prolongation of 2 seconds or more—is considered as abnormal.
iii. Prolongation of more than 4 seconds—is at risk of uncontrolled bleeding.

INR (international normalized ratio)
i. It is used to express the degree of anticoagulation in patients receiving sodium.
ii. It standardizes prothrombin time measurement, according to the characteristics of thromboplastin reagent used in our laboratory.

Factors II, VII, IX and X require carboxylation at glutamic acid residues—which can be possible in presence of vitamin K.

Absence of vitamin K allows the release of des-γ-carboxy prothrombin (abnormal prothrombin)—which can be detected by radioimmunoassay.

Presence of prothrombin in serum is more sensitive indicator of vitamin K deficiency than measurement of prothrombin time, because, abnormal prothrombin is present in high concentration despite normal prothrombin time.

Prolonged prothrombin time is seen in following conditions
A. Hematological disorders:
  i. Congenital deficiency of coagulation factors
  ii. Consumption of coagutation factors.
  iii. Ingestion of drugs affecting prothrombin time.
B. Hypovitaminosis
  i. Prolonged obstructive jaundice
  ii. Steatorrhea
  iii. Dietary deficiency
  iv. Intake of antibiotics affection intestinal flora
  v. Poor utilization of vitamin K.

After single perenteral injection of vitamin K:
i. Prothrombin time will be normal:
  a. Hypovitaminosis K
  b. Obstructive jaundice.
ii. Slight improvement—hepatitis.

In case of severe cirrhosis, prothrombin time may be normal or slightly prolonged.

It has high prognostic value mainly in hepatocellular disease.

Prolongation of prothrombin time >5–6 seconds—indicates:
1. Acute fulminent hepatic necrosis, in case of acute hepatitis
2. Alcoholic steatonecrosis.

Such rise in prothrombin time—that does not respond to perenteral administration of vitamin K—indicates:
1. Extensive parenchymal damage
2. Acetaminophen overdose

Tests to Detect Fibrosis of Liver

The following tests are useful:
i. Hyaluronan level   ii. Type IV collagen
iii. Procollagen III   iv. Laminin

Multiparameter tests:
i. AST to platelet ratio index
ii. Fibro test biomarker

Hyaluronan

It is glucosaminoglycan synthesized in mesenchymal cells and widely distributed in extracellular space.

It is degraded by hepatic sinusoidal cells in a specific receptor mediated process.

It is found to be elevated in cirrhosis.

If the level is:
>100 mg/dl   78% specificity, 83% sensitivity
>300 mg/dl   96% sensitivity
It is an indicator of advanced fibrosis in:
i. Alcoholic liver disease
ii. Hepatitis C
iii. Hepatitis B

Lipid and Lipoprotein Metabolism

Lipid Metabolism

Cholesterol:

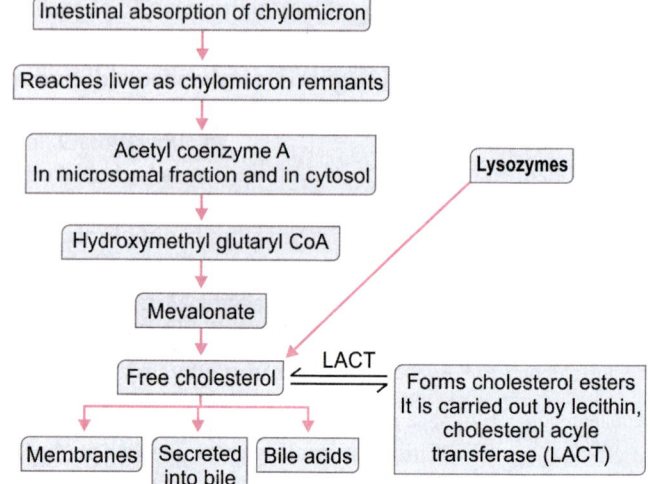

Synthesis is increased in:
i. Biliary duct obstruction
ii. Terminal ileal resection
iii. Biliary or intestinal lymph fistula
iv. Medications—cholestyramine, corticosteroids, thyroid hormones

Cholesterol synthesis is inhibited by:
i. Bile acids
ii. Cholesterol feeding
iii. Fasting
iv. Medications—clofibrate, nicotinic acid, statins

Phospholipids: It is an important constituent of cell membrane and participates in many reactions.

Phosphatidylcholine (lecithin) is 60% of total phospholipids and is most abundant in plasma and most cellular membranes. It is secreted in greater quantity than cholesterol in bile.

This secretion of phospholipids into the biliary canaliculi is prompted by bile salts. Here the canalicular bile acid transporter is responsible for transport.
↓
There is vesiculation of outer canalicular membrane
↓
There is increased supply of phospholipids to inner cytoplasmic membrane—here transporter protein phosphotidylcholine transfer protein
↓
To biliary canaliculi

Lipoprotein

Two metabolic cycles for lipoproteins:
1. First one is fat absorbed from small intestine.
2. Second one is responsible for handling of endogenous lipid.

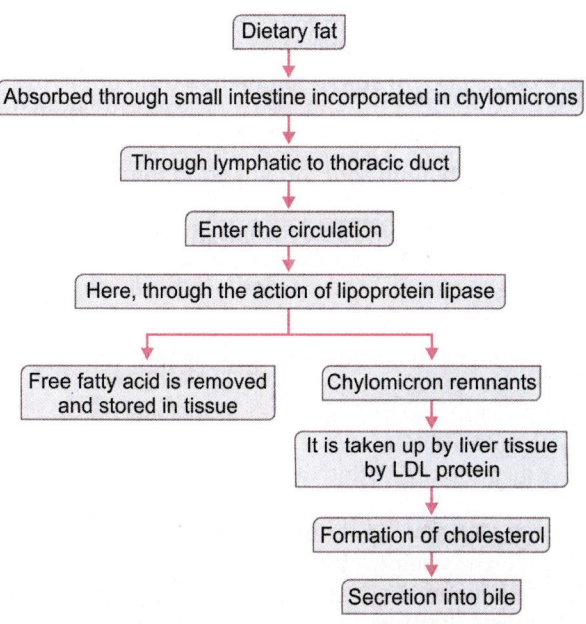

Fig 4.14: Algorithm of effect of dietary fat

In endogenous pathway:

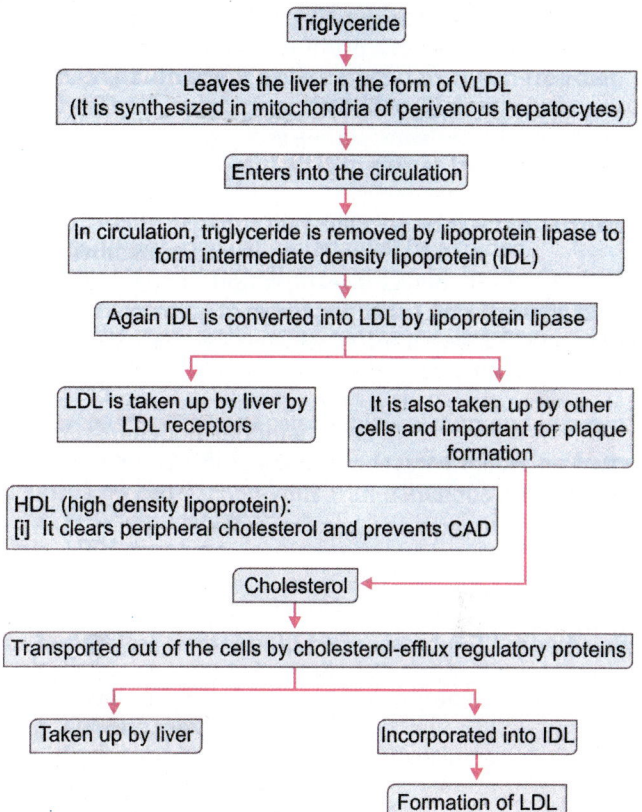

Fig 4.15: Endogenous pathway of metabolism of triglycerides

Changes in Liver Disease

Cholestatic Liver Disease

Total and free cholesterol is erased in circulation due to following factors:
i. Regurgitation of biliary cholesterol into circulation
ii. Increased hepatic synthesis of cholesterol
iii. Reduced plasma LCAT activity.
iv. Regurgitation of biliary lecithin.

Causes are:
i. 1.5–2 times normal in acute cholestasis
ii. ≥ 2 times normal in chronic cholestasis
   a. Postoperative stricture
   b. Cholestatic liver disease
   c. Primary biliary cirrhosis

Significance: Values more than 5 times than normal—associated with cutaneous xanthoma

Lowering level of cholesterol seen in:
i. Malnutrition
ii. Carcinoma of biliary tract—associated with anorexia
iii. Congenital LCAT deficiency

Red cell changes in cholestasis are related to—abnormalities in cholesterol and lipoprotein.

Parenchymal Liver Inquiry

1. In cirrhosis, total cholesterol level is normal. If the level is low—it indicates:
   i. Malnutrition
   ii. Decompensation

2. In fatty liver disease, due to alcohol—triglyceride and VLDL levels are increased.

   Microsomal triglyceride transfer protein (MTTP) is necessary for incorporation of triglyceride into VLDL—but the activity of this protein is inhibited by:
   i. Alcohol
   ii. HIV
   iii. Rarely genetic defect
   The net result is hepatic steatosis.
3. The drug usually affects apolipoprotein synthesis, as a result, there is defect in exportation of triglyceride into VLDL—the result is hepatic steatosis.
4. The Apolipoprotein B-100, which is associated with VLDL may be absent in
   i. Due to genetic reasons
   ii. Deficiencies in amino acids like, threonine or
   iii. Due to generalized malnutrition (kwashiorkor)
5. Low level of Apolipoprotein A-1—occurs in Tangier's disease—this disease is characterized by:
   i. Low level of HLD
   ii. Accelerated atherosclerosis

Bile Acids

1. It is mainly produced by liver.
2. 250–500 mg is produced as well as lost every day.
3. It is stored in gallbladder, in case of cholecystectomy; it is usually accumulated in proximal duodenum.
4. Bile acid synthesis is under negative feedback control.
5. Primary bile acids are:
   i. Cholic acid
   ii. Chenodeoxy cholic acid
6. Main substrate is cholesterol—which produces bile acids in two different pathways:
   i. Classical pathways
   ii. Alternate pathways

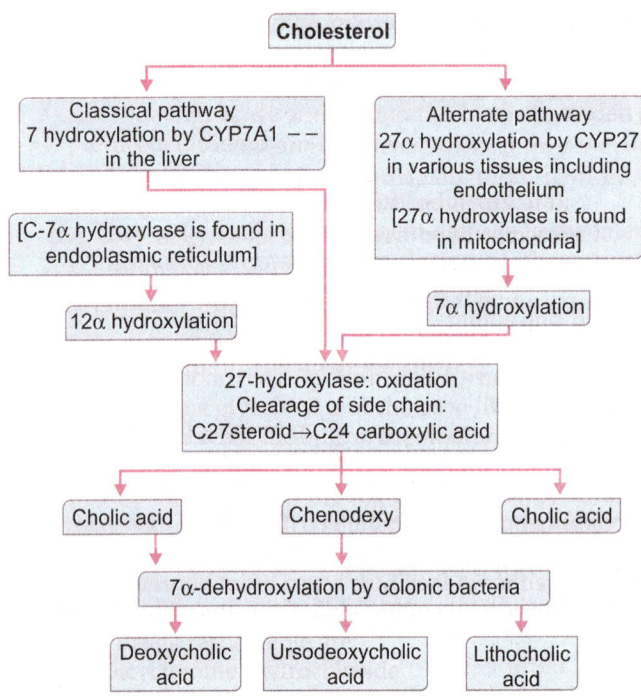

Fig 4.16: Metabolism of cholesterol

In Human Bile

Amount of cholic acid ≃ chenodeoxycholic acid
+
Deoxycholic acid

In the liver—bile acids conjugate with amino acids, glycine and taurine at ratio of 3:1 to form glycocholale and taurocholate salts.

Functions of Bile Acids

i. Bile acids achieve a high concentration in the intestinal lumen to facilitate fat digestion and absorption.
ii. Conjugation prevents precipitation at physiological pH. In cirrhosis and cholestasis, sulphation and glucoronidation will be increased.

In colon, colonic bacteria deconjugate the bile salts to bile acids and amino acid, taurine and glycine.

Bile salt's excretion into bile canaliculi against enormous concentration gradient between liver and bile depends upon three factors:
i. Negative potential approximately—35 mV which is responsible for facilitated diffusion.
ii. ATP-stimulated transporters.
iii. Extent of conjugation:
   1. In the upper small intestine—bile salt micelles are large and hydrophilic—so it cannot be absorbed.
      Bile salts are responsible for digestion and absorption of lipids.
   2. In terminal ileum and proximal colon, 95% of bile acids are absorbed by active transport process—through apical sodium-dependent bile acid transporters.
   3. Through out the intestine, non-ionic, passive diffusion of unconjugated dihydroxy bile acid occurs.

The above bile salt absorption can be inhibited by orally administered ursodeoxycholic acid.

After absorption, bile salts enter the portal circulation
↓
Liver
↓

Enter hepatocyte through basolateral membrane by sodium taurocholate co-transport system—which use sodium ion as gradient force across the sinusoidal membrane, chloride ion is also involved. (90% trihydroxy bile acids and 80% dihydroxy bile acids are absorbed
↓

Hydrophobic bile acids (unconjugated mono- and dihydroxybile acids) enter hepatocyte by simple diffusion through lipid membrane.

In hepatocyte, bile acids are reconjugated and reexcreted into bile.

But lithocholic acid is not reexcreted but non-toxic and become sulphated in liver.

Enterohepatic circulation of bile salts occurs 2–15 times per day.

Bile salts, phospholipids, and cholesterol combine to form micelles which is helpful for:
i. Emulsification of fat
ii. Pancreatic lipolysis
iii. Release of gastrointestinal hormones
iv. Mucosal phase of absorption

Normal serum bile salt concentration depends upon:
i. Normal hepatic blood flow
ii. Hepatic uptake and secretion
iii. Intestinal motility
Disorder of any of the above leads to altered serum bile acid levels.

Diminished bile salt excretion leads to:
i. Defect in biliary micelle formation—which is responsible for formation of gallstones.
ii. Steatorrhea
iii. Cholestasis

In case of bacterial overgrowth
↓
Bile acids are deconjugated
↓
Generation of free bile acids
↓
It is absorbed through intestine
↓
Micelle formation and absorption of fat are impaired
↓
Steatorrhea

In case of terminal ileal resection
↓
Interruption of enterohepatic circulation of bile

Large amounts of bile acids reach colon

Here they are dehydroxylated by colonic bacteria
↓
Reduction of bile salt pool in the body

Altered bile salts produce secretory diarrhea
↓
Large amount of electrolytes and water are lost
Lithocholic acids are mostly excreted in feces

In case of cessation of bile acid synthesis, following incidences may occur:
i. Inability to excrete cholesterol
ii. Stoppage of bile acid dependent bile flow
iii. Malabsorption of fat-soluble vitamins
iv. Irreversible fecal loss.

Estimation of bile acids:
1. Enzymatic assays based on use of bacterial 3-hydroxy steroid dehydrogenase
2. Bioluminescence assay
3. Radioimmunoassay

Amino Acid Metabolism

1. Amino acids derived from diet and tissue breakdown
↓
They reach liver via portal vein
↓
They enter hepatocytes through Na^+ independent and Na^+ dependent systems across sinusoidal membrane
↓
Some are transaminated or deaminated to ketoacids
↓
They then are metabolized by tricarboxylic acid cycle.

2.
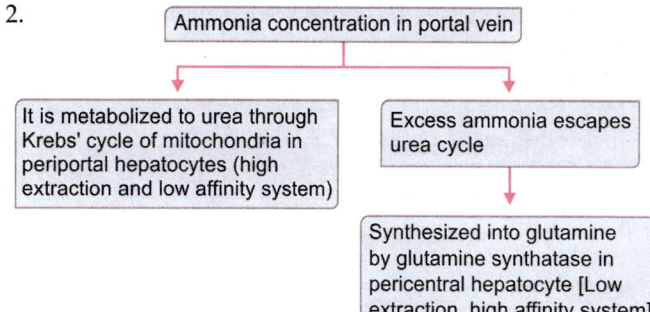

In acute liver failure: Hyperammonemia is due to:
1. Elevated arterial ammonia due to dysfunction of Krebs'
2. Low blood urea level cycle

In decompensated cirrhosis: Hyperammonemia is due to:
i. Dysfunction of glutamine synthesis
ii. Portal systemic shunting from small and large intestine.

Significance

1. In severe liver disease:
   i. Increase in one or both aromatic amino acids like, tyrosine and phenylalanine with methionine
   ii. Reduction in branched chain amino acid—like, valine, leusine, isoleusine
   The above changes are due to:
   i. Impaired hepatic function
   ii. Portal systemic shunting of blood
   iii. Hyperinsulinemia
   iv. Hyperglucagonemia
2. Patient with minimal liver disease demonstrates:
   i. Reduction in plasma protein—indicating increased collagen production.
   ii. No change in ratio between branched chain amino acid and aromatic amino acid, even in presence of hepatic encephalopathy.
3. In acute liver failure—generalized aminoaciduria—involving cysteine, and tyrosine.

HEPATITIS

HEPATITIS A VIRUS

This virus is responsible for hepatitis in developing countries of Africa, Asia and Latin America—here seroprevalance rate is 100%.

But in Industrial countries—due to improvement of socio-economic conditions, there will be shift of age, so adults and elderly people are mostly affected.

Method of Transmission

a. Feco-oral route—by:
   i. Ingestion of contaminated food
   ii. Ingestion of contaminated water
   iii. Person to person contact
b. Parenteral transmission due to use of contaminated products—rare.
c. Vertical transmission—uncommon

Risk groups are:
 i. Travelers from endemic areas
 ii. Military personal
 iii. Day-care workers
 iv. Institutionalized patients
 v. Homosexuals
 vi. Multiple sexual partners
 vii. Intravenous drug users

Hepatitis Virus A

 i. It is an RNA virus, member of Picornaviridae family.
 ii. HAV genome is linear, positive sense, single-stranded RNA.
   It has two ends:
   a. At 5'NCR end VPg protein is attached with covalent bond.
   b. At 3' NCR end, poly A tail is attached.
 iii. This genome codes a single protein—polyprotein—it has been divided into three functional domains—P_1, P_2 and P_3.
 iv. P_1 encodes viral capsid protein—VP_1, VP_2, VP_3 and VP_4.
 v. P_2 and P_3 encode non-structural proteins—which includes:
   a. RNA helicase
   b. Protease
   c. RNA polymerase

Natural History

1. Age incidence:
   i. In child—it is usually asymptomatic
   ii. With advancing of age—patient becomes symptomatic
   iii. 90% of adolescents may develop jaundice
2. Fate of infection:
   i. Usually HAV infection is followed by lifelong immunity.
   ii. 1% adult patient having pre-existing chronic liver disease, if develops acute HAV infection, may enter into the stage of acute fulminant hepatic failure.
   iii. Uncommon clinical features include:
   a. Cholestatic hepatitis
   b. Relapsing hepatitis (less commonly)

Immunopathogenesis

This cytopathic virus along with immune response of the patient against HAV is responsible for necroinflammatory lesions of liver.

These inflammatory sites may demonstrate increased number of CD4 and CD8+ T cell receptors:
 i. In acute phase or early phase of illness—dominant IgM and IgG response against VP_1 develop
 ii. In late phase of illness—dominant IgM and IgG response to VP_3 and VP_0 develop.
 iii. Non-secretory IgG antibody to HAV usually persists lifelong.

Treatment

 i. Usually no specific therapy except bed rest
 ii. Maintenance of strict hygiene
 iii. Vaccination programme—Available vaccine usually induces long-lasting (>20 years) immunity

iv. Routine vaccination is recommended for following patients:
   a. Young children in endemic areas
   b. Travelers to endemic areas
   c. Homosexual men
   d. Intravenous drug users
   e. Patients having chronic liver disease

HBV VIRAL HEPATITIS

HBV is hepatotropic containing deoxyribonucleic acid, virus of Hepadnaviridae family.

HBV virion is called Dane particle—42 nm in diameter—it has outer lipoprotein layer—it encodes viral envelop protein, HBsAg antigen and surrounds nucleocapsid core, HBcAg.

Nucleocapsid core contains:
 i. Viral genome
 ii. Viral polymerase

HBV infected serum also contains two subviral particles—which are spherical or filamentous in shape. These consist of:
 i. Envelope glycoprotein
 ii. Host-derived lipid

The exact biologic significance of the overproduction of envelop particles is not known.

Double-stranded DNA of HBV encodes partially relaxed four open reading frames:
 i. Surface gene   ii. Core gene
 iii. Polymerase   iv. X-gene

52 end of minus strand is covalently attached with a polymerase protein.

5' end of plus strand is attached with a capped oligoneucleotide.

S gene codes for hepatitis B surface antigen.

Core (c) gene codes for hepatitis c core antigen.

Polymerase gene codes for DNA polymerase/reverse transcriptase.

X-gene encodes for HBX protein—this protein is responsible for transcriptional transactivating function—which is, in future, responsible for hepatocellular carcinoma.

S gene is preceded by pre-S_1 and pre-S_2 regions—that code large, middle and small surface protein.

Core (C) gene has pre-c region—it encodes hepatitis c antigen (HBcAg) and hepatitis e antigen (HBeAg).

The terminal 5' ends of both plus and minus strands maps the direct repeat regions in viral DNA, known as DR_1 and DR_2.

Process of Viral Replication

1. **Entry and uncoating**
   Virus is attached to the cell membrane of hepatocyte with the help of pre-S_1 domain in L-envelope region
   ↓
   Membrane fusion occurs
   ↓
   Envelope of B virus will be stripped off
   ↓
   Nucleocapsid will be released into cytoplasm
   ↓
   Nucleocapsid helps the viral DNA to enter into nucleus
   ↓
   In the nucleus, with the help of DNA polymerase, double-stranded DNA will be converted into covalently closed circular DNA (cccDNA)—by following processes:

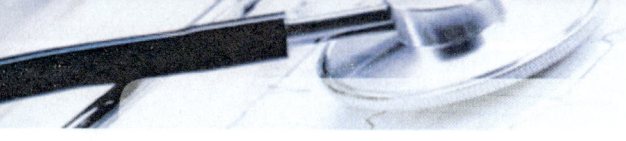

i. Repair of single stranded gap region.

ii. Removal of its terminal RNA and P protein.

iii. Covalent ligation of DNA termini.

Transcription

cccDNA acts as template for transcription by host RNA polymerase II.

In chronic hepatitis, persistence of virus in infecting cells depends upon generation and maintenance of pool size of cccDNA in the cell.

Two types of transcripts are synthesized from cccDNA:

i. Subgenomic transcripts act as mRNA for translation of envelope proteins (L, M and S proteins) and HBX proteins.

ii. Genomic transcripts act as mRNA for translation of precore, core and polymerase protein.

Genomic mRNA is encapsulated inside immature core particles
↓
Firstly, minus (-) strand of HBV DNA will be synthesized by reverse transcriptase of genomic RNA.
↓
Secondly—plus (+) strand HBV DNA will be produced as a result of replication of minus (-) strand of HBV DNA
↓
Subsequently, secretion of incomplete partially double-stranded DNA particle occurs into endoplasmic reticulum.

S protein, L protein and M protein will be synthesized by rough endoplasmic reticulum by subgenomic mRNA transcript
↓ ↓
Surface protein, L and M protein will be implicated in HBV DNA during development.
↓
Finally fully synthesized HBV DNA will be transferred to Golgi apparatus
Then it will be secreted into liver cells.

Importance of cccDNA

Cellular pool of cccDNA is maintained by:

i. Superinfection of hepatocytes by additional virions

ii. Import of nucleocapsid from hepatocyte cytoplasm

Nucleoside analogue for treatment of hepatitis B infection has very little or no inhibitory effects on cccDNA.

The causes are:

i. Inhibition of reverse transcription of genomic RNA.

ii. Longer life of infected hepatocytes—this is responsible for psot-treatment viral relapse.

Serotypes and Genotypes of HBV

HBV are serotyped based on antigenic determinants present of "S" protein.

i. The common determinant is "a"

ii. The other determinants are "y" versus "d" and "w" versus "r"

So four major serotypes are: ayw, ayr, adw, adr.

HBV are classified into eight genotypes A, B, C, D, E, F, G and H. These genotypes are determined based on nucleoside sequences distributed variable in different geographic regions.

Importance of HBV Genotype

i. It determines the activity of the disease.

ii. It determines the progression of liver disease.

iii. It determines the response to antiviral therapy.

HBV Variants

Reverse transcriptions of HBV progenomic RNA is responsible for HBV replication. But reverse transcriptase is deficient in proofreading ability. So there is large number of errors occur during viral replication. As a result, there is development of HBV quasispecies, which is a mixture of viral strains with variation of viral sequences)

It occurs mainly in chronically infected patient.

Predominant strain will be selected by following factors:

A. Endogenous factors:

i. Host immune response

ii. Replication fitness of the variant

iii. Replication space

B. Exogenous factors:

i. Antiviral neucleoside analogue

ii. Immune based therapies

a. Vaccine

b. Immunoglobulin (HBIG)

Mutation occurs mainly in pre-core, core and core promoter regions.

i. Precore and core regions are responsible for synthesis of precore protein—which is processed into small soluble HBe antigen.

ii. Core promoter region is present in the upstream of precore and core regions. It overlaps with "x" gene.

This region:

Regulates the transcription of pregenomic RNA and precore RNA
↓
Thus regulates HBV replication and HBeAg production

Mutations in Precore Region

1. Point mutation of nucleoside 1896 of HBV genome:

Result of this mutation is development of premature stop codon. It prevents production of HBeAg. It is found in:

a. Mostly in genotype D

b. Genotype B, C, E to a lesser extent

c. Genotype A, F and H rarely

This mutant is found in:

i. Fulminant hepatitis.

ii. Severe forms of chronic liver disease.

iii. Inactive carrier state.

2. Common core promoter variant—it includes:
   - Dual mutation—at A1762T and G1764A
   - Result is downregulation of HBeAg production.

   It is found in all the genotypes—but most commonly found in C.

Mechanism of Hepatocyte Injury

HBV related liver injury is not directly cytopathic, so here liver injury is related to host immune response against infection. In HBV related liver injury, total loss of HB$_S$Ag from serum will never occur. So:

1. Quiescent phase or inactive phase—host immune response to virus will suppress the viremia.
2. In chronic active infection in liver—there is strong imbalance between HBV replication and host immune response.
3. In case of resolving acute infection—strong polygonal T cell response (CD8+ cells)
4. In chronic infection—T cell response is weak and poorly functional.

Epidemiology

Rate of chronic HBV infection in different parts of the world
   i. In low prevalence areas (USA, Australia, New Zealand)—0.1–2%
   ii. In intermediate prevalence areas (Mediterranean countries, India, Singapore) 3.5%
   iii. In high prevalence areas (South-East Asia, Sub-Saharar Africa) 10–20%

Mode of Spreads According to Prevalence Areas

   i. High prevalent areas: Perinatal transmission—is major mode of spread:
      1. At the time of birth
      2. Close contact during first 2 years of life
   ii. Intermediate prevalence areas: During child hood, close contact with tooth brushes, cuts, abrasions, sharing of razors, contaminated needles
   iii. In low prevalence areas: Infections occur during adult life:
      1. Unprotected sex
      2. Injection drug use

Mode of Transmissions

HBV spreads more easily than HCV or HIV infections due to:
   i. Much higher level of viremia (12 log 10^{10}/ml)
   ii. Its ability to survive in human body for up to 7 days
      Blood transfusion is nowadays a rare source because blood is screened for:
   i. HBsAg
   ii. Anti-HBc
   iii. Anti-HBV—DNA

A transmission occurs through:
a. Patient to patient
b. Patient to health care personnel

   The methods are:
   1. Contaminated surgical instruments
   2. Accidental needle stick
c. Surgeons to patients
   Methods—cut in gloves
d. Maternal–infant transmission—perinatal transmission—at the time of birth and within 2 years of life

In uterus, infection is very uncommon but may occur.
e. Sexual transmissions—it is the major mode of spread in developed countries. It is increased in:
   i. Multiple sexual partners
   ii. Sexually transmitted disease
   iii. High risk behavior
f. Renal failure patient on hemodialysis
g. During transplantation of extrahepatic organs, such as kidney from HBsAg the donors.

Clinical Manifestations

In acute phase—manifestations vary from:
   i. Subclinical hepatitis
   ii. Anicteric hepatitis
   iii. Icteric hepatitis
   iv. Fulminant hepatitis

In chronic phase:
   i. Chronic hepatitis
   ii. Cirrhosis
   iii. Liver failure
   iv. Hepatocellular carcinoma

In perinatal or childhood infection:
   i. Little or no symptoms
   ii. High level of chronicity

In adult infections:
   i. Presence of symptoms
   ii. Long level of chronicity

Acute HBV Infection

10% patients have subclinical or anicteric hepatitis
Incubation period—1–4 months
   Prodromal period serum sickness like syndrome: Symptoms are:
   i. Malaise
   ii. Anorexia
   iii. Nausea
   iv. Vomiting
   v. Right upper abdominal discomfort
   vi. Jaundice
   vii. Temperature

Follow-up symptoms:
   i. Symptoms and jaundice will disappear within 1–3 months.
   ii. Some patients develop persistent fatigue in spite of normal ALT levels.

Signs:
   i. Jaundice
   ii. Low grade temperature
   iii. Spider nevi may be present
   iv. Soft tender hepatomegaly
   v. Rarely splenomegaly

Laboratory Tests

   i. Elevation of liver enzyme (ALT and AST)— ≥ 1000–2000 IUIL—hallmark of diagnosis in acute phase—it may precede the symptoms.
   ii. ALT level is higher than AST level.
   iii. In patient with icteric hepatitis—raised bilirubin level lag behind raised ALT levels. Peaked ALT levels—

reflect hepatocellular injury, but there is no correlation between raised ALT levels and the prognosis.

iv. Prothrombin time will be abnormal—it reflects decreased synthesis of factors II, VII, IX, X.
    Since, half life of clotting factor VII is 6 hours, hence PT reflects instantaneous function of liver.

v. Serum albumin—its half life is 21 days. Hence it is not a good marker of acute hepatitis.

vi. Mild leucopenia with relative lymphocytosis

vii. Red cell survival is shortened—but hemoglobin and hematocrit level is within normal limit.

viii. In patients with resolving infection
    a. ALT level will return to normal within 1–4 months followed by normalization of serum bilirubin.
    b. Persistently raised ALT for more than 6 months—indicates chronic liver injury.

Serological tests:

	HBsAg	HBeAg	IgM anti-HBC	IgG anti-HBc	Anti-HBs	Anti-HBe	HBV DNA	
Acute HBV infection	=	=	=		–	–	+++	Early phase
	–	–	+		–	+	+	Window phase
	–	–	–	+	+	+	±	Recovery phase
	+	+	–	+	–	–	+++	HBeAg chronic hepatitis

Interpretation of HBV serological markers:

1. Hepatitis B surface antigen (HBsAg) — Acute or chronic HBV infection
2. Hepatitis B e antigen (HBeAg) — High levels of HBV replication and infectivity
3. Anti-HBe antibody — Low level HBV replication and infectivity.
4. Anti-HBc IgM — Recent HBV infection
5. Anti-HBc IgG — Recovered or chronic HBV infection
6. Anti-HB$_s$ antibody — HBV infection immunity
7. Anti-HBc (IgG) + Anti-HBs antibody — Past HBV infection
8. Anti-HBC (IgG) + HBsAg — Chronic HBV infection

Following patients should be screened for hepatitis B virus:

A. Individuals from high and intermediate prevalent areas for HBV including immigrants and whose 1st generation is HBsAg positive:
    i. All countries of Asia, Africa, South East pacific islands
    ii. European Mediterranean: Malta and Spain
    iii. Arctic countries (Alaska, Canada, Greenland)
    iv. South America, Ecuador, Guyana, Suriname, Venezuela, Haiti, Amazon region of Bolivia, Brazil, Colombia and Peru.
    v. All countries of Eastern Europe except Hungary.

vi. Carrabian—Antigua, Barbuda, Dominica, Haiti, Jamaica, St. Kitts and Nevis. St. Lucia and Turks, Caicos
vii. Central America, Guatemala, Honduras

B. Others groups for screening:
    i. Non-vaccinated infant in US of parents born in highly endemic areas
    ii. Household and sexual contact with HBsAg +ve persons.
    iii. Intravenous drug user
    iv. Male homosexuals
    v. Persons having multiple sexual partners
    vi. Persons having history of sexually transmitted diseases
    vii. Person with chronically raised SGPT or SGOT
    viii. HCV or HIV infected persons
    ix. Patient on maintenance hemodialysis
    x. All pregnant women
    xi. Persons on immunosuppressive therapy

Status of HBsAg and anti-HBsAb:

1. HBsAg can be detected 1–10 weeks of exposure
2. HBsAg can be detected 2–6 weeks prior to onset of symptoms or elevation of SGPT
3. If the patent recovers
    a. The HBsAg will disappear after 4–6 months
    b. There is a definite window period of several weeks to months—when HBsAg and anti-HBsAb cannot be detected.
    c. Anti-HBsAb—ultimately appears and may persist for lifelong.
    d. In case of carrier—anti-HBsAb may be detectable—it may be due to development of antibody against subtype determinants and not against 'a' determinants.

HBcAg and anti-HBcAg antibody: HBcAg cannot be detected in serum only anti-HB$_C$Ab can be detected. Two types of anti-HBcAb are:

1. Anti-HBcAb IgM—this antibody appears early—it can be detected along with HBsAg or anti-HBs antibody.
    Sometimes during window period, when neither HBsAg nor anti-HBs can be detected, it is the only representer of HBsAg infection.
2. Anti-HBc IgG—this antibody appears late and present for longtime in the blood. It can be detected with anti-HBs antibody representing past HBV infection.
    Again this antibody along with HBsAg in serum represents chronic HBV infection.
    HBV DNA is usually present in liver. So when liver from patient with positive anti-HBc antibody will be transplanted into seronegative patient, risk is higher.

HBeAg and anti-HBc:

1. HBeAg is usually derived from processing of precore protein of HBV.
2. It is a marker of active viral replication and infectivity.
3. Seroconversion from HBeAg to anti-HBe antibody is associated with decrease in HBV DNA level associated with remission in liver disease.
4. It, in presence of anti-HBc antibody, high HBV DNA level indicates the presence of precore and core promoter HBV variants—these prevent or decrease the production of HBeAg.

HBV DNA:
1. Presence of HBV DNA—in serum indicates viremia and infectivity hence:
   i. It can be detected 2–3 weeks before the appearance of HBsAg in serum in acutely infective patient.
   ii. Its level fluctuates during chronic viral infection.
2. Its level can be detected even after HBsAg seroconversion. So serial monitoring of HBV DNA is necessary to determine the phase of infection in any infected patient.
3. In real time PCR assays—detection limit is less than 10 IU/ml with highest range up to 10^8 IU/ml.

Liver biopsy: This can assess:
   i. Degree of necroinflammation in the liver
   ii. Extent of fibrosis
   iii. Rule out the other causes of liver disease
   iv. Assess the efficacy of antiviral treatment—by immune histochemical staining for:
      a. HBsAg
      b. HBcAg
      c. PCR for HBV DNA
   v. Liver stiffness by elastography—liver stiffness can be influenced by:
      a. Fibrosis
      b. Inflammation
      c. Edema

Chronic HBV Infection

Symptoms

   i. No symptom
   ii. Mildly symptomatic—like fatigue, anorexia, nausea, jaundice
   iii. Rarely features of hepatic decompensation

Physical Examination

   i. Normal
   ii. Stigmata of chronic liver disease, like, spider nevi
   iii. Mild hepatomegaly
   iv. In patient with persistent chronic liver disease:
      a. Splenomegaly
      b. Pedal edema
      c. Ascites
      d. Jaundice
      e. Hepatic encephalopathy

Laboratory Tests

   i. In case of compensated cirrhosis—normal
   ii. May be mild to moderate elevation of ALT and AST
   iii. During exacerbations:
      a. ALT level >1000 U/L or may be 5-fold higher than normal
      b. Evidence of marked impaired hepatic dysfunction
         1. Prolonged prothrombin time
         2. Decreased albumin
         3. Increased bilirubin
      c. α-fetoprotein level may be as high as 5000 ng/ml
      d. AST: ALT—greater than 1

Histological Changes in Liver Biopsy

A. In case of acute HBV hepatitis:
   1. Lobular disarray
   2. Acidophilic hepatocyte degeneration
   3. Focal lobular necrosis
   4. Bile canaliculi disruption with cholestasis
   5. Inflammatory cell infiltration in portal and parenchymal area
      a. Predominantly lymphocytes
      b. Macrophages
      c. Eosinophils
      d. Neutrophils
      e. Rarely plasma cells
      f. Hypertrophy and hyperplastic of Kuffer cells and macrophages
B. Resolution phase is characterized by:
   1. Reduction in amount of inflammatory cell infiltration.
   2. Regeneration of parenchymal cells.
C. In case of severe form of hepatitis—bridging necrosis in adjacent lobules.

In Chronic HBV Infection

Histological changes in chronic hepatitis can be divided into following categories
A. Chronic persistent hepatitis:
   1. Periportal necrosis—if severe may disrupt limiting plate—piecemeal necrosis or interface hepatitis
   2. Inflammatory cells like, mononuclear cell infiltration in portal zone.
B. Chronic active hepatitis: Fibrous tissue initially within portal tract, which may extend to centrilobular areas and adjacent portal areas producing bridging necrosis.
C. Chronic lobular hepatitis:
   1. Spotty necrosis
   2. Lobular inflammation
   3. Minimal portal tract inflammation

In HBV chronic infection: Ground glass hepatic cells—stain positive for HBsAg.

According to international panel, histological diagnosis include:
   i. Etiology of hepatitis
   ii. Grade of necroinflammatory activity;
   iii. Stage of liver disease

Immunohistochemical staining of liver tissue demonstrates:
1. Presence of HBV in chronic HBV infection—it may be:
   a. Cytoplasmic or
   b. Membranous
2. Presence of HBcAg in nucleus of hepatocyte. But it may be distributed in cytoplasm in acute exacerbation of disease.

Extrahepatic Manifestation

A. **Serum sickness-like syndrome:** Sometimes, HBV hepatitis may be preceded by:
   i. Fever
   ii. Rash
   iii. Arthralgia
   iv. Arthritis

The skin and joint manifestation may subside with the appearance of jaundice.

B. **Polyarteritis nodosa:**
  i. 10–30% of PAN patients develop HBsAg positive hepatitis.
  ii. HBV-related PAN gradually decreases with gradual decline in incidence of HBV related hepatitis.
  iii. Deposition of immune complexes containing HBV antigen and antibodies in large, medium and small vessels—producing immune-mediated injury—vasculitis.
  iv. It involves cardiovascular, gastrointestinal, musculoskeletal, neurological and dermatological systems.
  v. Symptoms related to systems:
    a. Pericarditis, hypertension, cardiac failure (CVS)
    b. Hematuria, proteinuria (renal)
    c. Abdominal pain, mesenteric vasculitis (gastrointestinal)
    d. Arthralgia, arthritis (musculoskeletal)
    e. Mononeuritis, central nervous system involvement (neurological)
    f. Rashes (dermatological)
    Most severe manifestations are:
    i. Gastrointestinal bleeding
    ii. Intestinal perforation

C. **Glomerulonephritis:** Following types of glomerulonephritis can be run:
  i. Membranous—most common
  ii. Membrane—proliferative
  iii. Mesangio-capillary
  iv. Focal proliferative
  v. Minimal change disease
  vi. IgA nephropathy
  Pathology demonstrates—deposition of immune complexes containing HBsAg, core antigen and associated antibodies with complement components—in glomerular basement membrane and mesangium.
  Follow-up:
  i. Children with membranous glomerulonephritis may recover spontaneously.
  ii. Some adults may undergo renal failure, and some patients may require maintenance hemodialysis.
  Treatment:
  i. Corticosteroid is usually effective, it may aggravate HBV replication.
  ii. Interferon can induce remission in Asian adults
  iii. Lamivudine can produce remission.

D. **Essential mixed cryoglobulinemia:**
  i. It is small vessel disease
  ii. It may present with glomerulonephritis, arthritis and purpura.
  iii. Cryoprecipitate contains:
    a. HBsAg
    b. Anti-HBs
    c. HBV-like particle.

E. **Papular acrodermatitis (Gianotti-Crosti syndrome):**
  i. It is usually associated with HBsAg antigenemia in children under 4 years of age.
  ii. Circulating immune complexes are—HBsAg and anti-HBs
  iii. This patient presents with:

a. Symmetric erythematous maculopapular non-itchy eruptions seen over:
  1. Buttock
  2. Limbs
  3. Trunk
  These rashes persist for 15 to 20 days.
b. Mucous membrane is not involved.
c. Associated axillary, inguinal lymph nodes are enlarged.
d. Acute hepatitis may coincide with acute dermatitis.

F. **Aplastic anemia:**
  i. It can occur in early phase of hepatitis.
  ii. But according to recent published data, aplastic anemia associated with hepatitis is not related to B virus, rather than related to immunopathologic mechanisms.

Course of the Disease

Course of the HBV hepatitis depends upon following factors:
  i. Virus related
    a. HBV replication
    b. HBV genotype
    c. Viral variants
  ii. Host related
    a. Age
    b. Sex
    c. Race
    d. Genetic makeup
    e. Immunity
  iii. Environment related
    a. Alcohol
    b. Obesity
    c. Infections with other viruses, like CD, HIV
    d. Carcinogen—aflatoxin

In Case of Acute HBV Infection

Recovery from infections depends upon:
i. Age of the patient at the time of infection
ii. Immune status of the patient—which can be amplified in the following findings:
  a. Absence of HBsAg from the serum
  b. Detection of anti-HBs antibody

HBV DNA can be found in very low titer in the serum or in liver for long time after recovery from infection; hence this disease can be reactivated in any time in life when his immune response declines from any cause.

In Case of Chronic HBV Infection

Chronic HBV infection passes through four phases. Though the entire patients will not go through all the phases, but, childhood or adult acquired HBV infection may never progress to reactivation phase (Fig. 4.17).

Four following phases are:
1. **Immune tolerant phase**: In this phase:
  a. Viral markers:
    i. Presence of HBeAg
    ii. High levels of HBV DNA
  b. Conditions of liver—minimal liver injury
  c. Liver enzyme—normal ALT
  d. Prognosis—favorable in short-term follow-up—in patient under age 40 years and spontaneous HBeAg seroconversion.

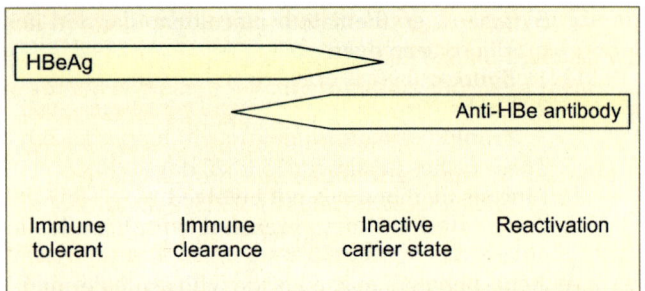

Fig. 4.17: Different phases of chronic HBV infection, alanine amino transferase (ALT)

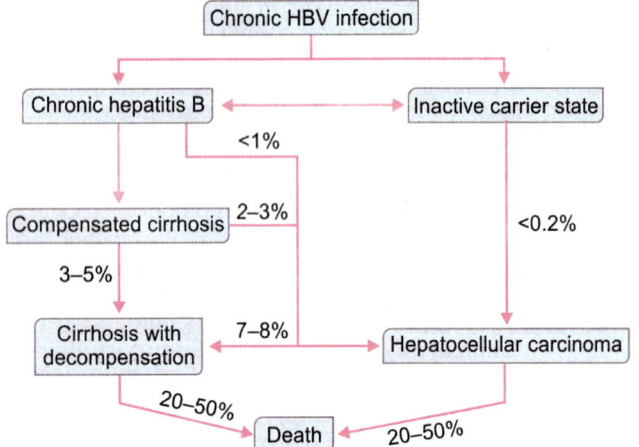

Fig. 4.18: Serological profile of acute HBV infection, ALT

e. Patient involved—young Asians perinatally acquired HBV infections.
f. Duration of this phase is 10–30 years.

2. **Immune clearance phase (HBeAg positive chronic hepatitis):** In this phase:
   a. Fate of viral markers:
      i. Presence of HBeAg in serum
      ii. High titer of HBV DNA
      iii. Persistent or intermittent ALT flare due to immune mediated hepatocyte lysis.
      iv. Liver biopsy showed hepatocyte inflammation
   b. Effect of ALT flare:
      i. Patient may be asymptomatic
      ii. Features of acute hepatitis
      iii. High jaundice
      iv. Occasionally liver failure
      v. ALT flare is associated with lowering HBV DNA in serum but HBeAg remain positive.
      vi. It occurs more frequently in men than women—which accounts for high rate of cirrhosis and hepatocellular carcinoma in men.
   c. Outcome of this phase:
      i. HBeAg seroconversion
      ii. Factors responsible for HBeAg seroconversion
         a. Older age
         b. Higher ALT
         c. Other ethnic people other than Asian.

3. **Inactive chronic HBV hepatitis:** In this phase, there is:
   i. Absence of HBeAg
   ii. Normal ALT
   iii. Presence of anti-HBe
   iv. Low or undetectable HBV DNA

   In case of minimal liver injury in preceding immune clearance phase, the patient in this phase has favorable prognosis.

   These patients will develop HBeAg negative chronic hepatitis having normal ALT level and inflammation with fibrosis in liver histology.

   This occurs in patient with high serum level of HBV DNA with abnormal ALT level.

4. **Reaction phase (HBeAg negative chronic hepatitis):** In this phase—there are:
   i. Absence of HBeAg
   ii. Presence of anti-HBeAg
   iii. High level of HBV DNA
   iv. Intermittent or persistently elevated ALT
   v. Necrotic hepatic inflammation.

In this phase:
i. Some patients enter into HBeAg negative chronic hepatitis.
ii. Older patients may develop advance chronic liver disease.

In these patients, core or precore mutants prevent or decrease production of HBeAg.

Spontaneous HBsAg Clearance

There is spontaneous clearance of HBsAg at a rate of 1% per year—but it does not occur at linear rate. This is associated with:
i. Undetectable HBV DNA.
ii. Normalization of ALT.
iii. Normal liver histology.

Prognosis depends upon the patient age at which HBsAg is cleared. As for example:
i. Prognosis is excellent, if patient's age is less than 50 years.
ii. If patient's age is more than 50 years—patient may develop:
   a. Cirrhosis   b. Hepatocellular carcinoma

Occult HBV Infections

This is characterized by:
   i. HBV DNA—in most cases it is detected in liver, but undetectable or present in low concentration in serum.
   ii. Absence of HBsAg in serum
   iii. Vast majority of patients have positive anti-HBc—it indicates prior HBV infection.
   iv. It is present in higher number of patients with hepatitis infection associated with HCC.
   v. Presence of HCC—indicates prior HBV infection.

Clinical outcomes: The outcome includes:
   i. Progression to cirrhosis
   ii. Liver failure
   iii. Hepatocellular carcinoma
The following factors responsible for clinical outcome
   i. Host factor
   ii. Environmental factor
   iii. Viral factor

Co-infection with following viruses responsible for HCC in HBV infected patient:

i. HIV
ii. HCV
iii. HDV

Viral factors and clinical outcomes:

A. Different studies showed that high HBV DNA level, late conversion of HBeAg and HBV reactivation are associated with increased risks of:
   i. Cirrhosis
   ii. Hepatocellular carcinoma
   iii. Mortality related to liver failure
B. Different studies showed—HBV genotype B and genotype C are associated with:
   i. Rapid progression to cirrhosis
   ii. Rapid progression to hepatocellular failure
C. HBV genotype C is associated with:
   i. Delayed seroconversion of HBeAg
   ii. Core promoter mutations
D. Dual mutation of A1762T and G1764A in core promoter region is associated with:
   i. Severe active hepatitis or fulminant hepatitis
   ii. Increased risk of hepatocellular carcinoma

Treatment of Chronic HBV Hepatitis

The Goal of Treatment

Prevention of:

a. Cirrhosis
b. Hepatocellular carcinoma
c. Hepatic failure

Parameters used to Assess the Response of Treatment

i. Decrease in HBV DNA.
ii. Loss of HBsAg with or without seroconversion to anti-HBsAg antibody.
iii. Loss of HBeAg with or without seroconversion to anti-HBeAb.
iv. Normalization of ALT
v. Hepatic histology improvement.

The treatment should be started in:

i. Life-threatening liver disease
ii. High risk of cirrhosis or hepatocellular carcinoma in next 10 years.

Indications for Hepatitis B Treatment

1. Acute liver failure
2. Decompensated cirrhosis with detectable HBV DNA level
3. Compensated cirrhosis and serum HBV DNA >2000 IV/ml.
4. Acute exacerbation of chronic hepatitis B.
5. HBsAg positive patients receiving cancer chemotherapy or immunosuppressive therapy for nonrelated medical or oncological condition.

   This prevents reactivation of HBV replication.

If there is HBV DNA replication—it manifests as:

i. Progressive rise in HBV DNA
ii. Asymptomatic increase in ALT level

iii. Symptomatic hepatitis
iv. Acute liver failure
v. Death
vi. Frequent disruption of chemotherapy regimen with increased risk of cancer death.

Treatment should be given in following patients:

1. HBeAg positive chronic hepatitis with:
   i. Elevation of ALT >2 times upper limit of normal
   ii. HBV DNA level >20000 IV/ml
2. HBeAg negative chronic hepatitis with
   i. Elevation of ALT >1 times the upper limit of normal
   ii. HBV DNA level >20000 IV/ml
3. HBeAg positive chronic hepatitis with:
   i. ALT level is 1–2 time the upper limit of normal
   ii. Age is more than 40 years.
4. HBeAg negative chronic hepatitis with:
   i. ALT level 1–2 times the upper limit of normal
   ii. HBV DNA level 2001–20000 IV/ml.

Treatment should be deferred in following patients:

1. In young patient in immune tolerant phase when HBeAg will be positive.
2. Some patients may undergo spontaneous HBeAg seroconversion and they enter into inactive carrier stage as they never require antiviral therapy in future.
3. Other group may not undergo spontaneous HBeAg seroconversion as they enter into immune clearance phase (HBeAg positive chronic hepatitis).
4. Patients in true inactive carrier state. In these patients, serum ALT and HBV DNA level should be done thrice a year to observe any evidence of—any recrudescence of hepatitis in future, because these selected patients may require antiviral therapy.

In case of pregnant patient:

1. If the patient is in 1st trimester of pregnancy—lamivudine and tenofovir may produce birth defect in fetus.
2. In third trimester of pregnancy, if there is high incidence of viremia, there is high risk of maternal–infant transmission of virus—the antiviral drugs may be given, but safety of ART is limited.

Drugs

1. Two types of interferon
   i. Conventional interferon
   ii. Pegylated interferon
2. Five nucleoside analogues:
   i. Lamivudine
   ii. Adefovir dipivoxil
   iii. Entecavir
   iv. Telbivudine
   v. Tenofovir disoproxil fumerate

Interferon

i. Conventional interferon—can be administered daily or three times per week.
ii. Pegylated interferon—can be used weekly.

Predictor of response to interferon: In case of HBeAg positive hepatitis, following are the predictors of seroconversion.

i. Elevated pretreatment ALT level.
ii. High liver histology index
iii. Low serum HBV DNA level
iv. Genotype A and B than genotype C and D

Predictor of long-term response: Decline in HBeAg and HBsAg titers in first 12 to 24 weeks of commencement of treatment is associated with long-term prognosis.

Side effects:
1. Flu-like syndrome
2. Fatigue
3. Anorexia
4. Weight loss
5. Mild increase in hair loss
6. Emotional lability
    i. Anxiety
    ii. Irritability
   iii. Depression
7. Bone marrow suppression
8. Exacerbation of autoimmune diseases

Contraindications:
1. In patient with decompensated cirrhosis, because of risk of:
    i. Sepsis
    ii. Liver failure
2. HBV related acute liver failure
3. Severe exacerbation of chronic hepatitis B
4. In patient on immunosuppressive therapy or cancer chemotherapy, but may require HBV prophylaxis.

Nucleos(t)ide Analogues

They are divided into three groups:
A. L-nucleosides:
    i. Lamivudine
    ii. Telbivudine
B. A cyclic nucleoside phosphonates:
    i. Adefovir dipivoxil
    ii. Tenofovir disoproxil fumerate.
C. Deoxyguanosine analogues—Entecavir

Site of action: These drugs inhibit reverse transcription of pregenomic RNA to HBV DNA.

After withdrawal of treatment, viral relapse is very common, which is due to following reason.

These drugs have no direct inhibitory effect on cccDNA—since it is a template of viral replication, virus replicates after withdrawal of treatment.

From the point of potency: Entecavir, tenofovir and telbivudine are more potent followed by lamivudine, lastly adefovir.

Resistance to Antiviral Drugs

The effect of long-term use of antiviral drug is the development of antiviral drug resistance in the form of virological break-through.

Virological break through means:
i. Increase in serum HBV DNA level more than 1 log from nadir, or
ii. Redetection of HBV DNA in serum whose blood level previously showed absence of HBV DNA in serum.

Initially, drug resistant mutants fail to show replication fitness but in late, compensatory mutation help these mutants to develop or to restore replication capability, so that they can multiply enormously.

This virological break through may be associated with or precede the biochemical break through, the results are:
i. Hepatic flares
ii. Hepatic decompensation

The causes of virological break through:
i. Long-term use of antiviral drugs
ii. Non-adherence to drugs

Monitoring of HBV DNA:
i. In case of adherence to drug—every 3–6 months
ii. In case of non-adherence to drug
    a. Counseling regarding drug intake
    b. Retesting of HBV DNA after 1–3 months before instituting rescue therapy unless patient develop decompensated liver disease

Mutations responsible for virological break through occur in reverse transcriptase region of HBV polymerase gene.

Drugs responsible for resistance	Mutations in the area of reverse transcriptase
1. Lamivudine	Substitution of methionine for valine or isolucine in tyrosine—methionine-aspartate—aspartate motif
2. Adefovir	Substitution of alanine for threonine or valine
3. Tenofovir	Substitution of alanine for threonine

Predictors of response:
1. High pretreatment of ALT is strongest predictor of response in HBeAg positive patients.
2. In case of HBe negative patient, there is no predictor.

Table 4.6: Dosage of drugs	
Drugs	Dosage
1. Lamivudine	100 mg daily
2. Adefovir dipivoxil	10 mg daily
3. Entecavir	0.5 mg daily Or in case of lamivudine resistance 1 mg daily
4. Telbivudine	600 mg daily
5. Tenofovir disoproxil fumerate	300 mg daily

Side effects
1. Mitochondrial toxicity and myopathy—telbivudine
2. Lactic acidosis—Entecavir in patient with liver failure
3. Nephrotoxicity with rise in serum creatinine ⎞ Adefovir
   Renal tubular acidosis—Fanconi syndrome ⎠ Tenofovir

4. Myopathy and peripheral neuropathy—Telbivudine
5. peripheral neuropathy—combination of telbivudine and pegylated interferon

Advantages of interferon therapy:
1. Definite duration of treatment
2. Higher rate of HBsAg in patients infected with genotype A
3. Antiviral resistance—not identified.

Disadvantages of interferon therapy:
1. Parenteral administration
2. Frequent and severe side effects
3. Modest antiviral activity.

Advantages of nucleoside therapies:
1. Oral administration
2. Well tolerated
3. Very potent antiviral activity
4. Negligible side effects

Disadvantages of nucleoside therapies:
a. High chance of antiviral resistance
b. Long duration of treatment

Indications for use of nucleos(t)ide drugs:
1. Patient with decompensated liver disease
2. In case of contraindication to interferon therapy
3. If the patient who prefers oral long-term therapy.

Choice of oral antiviral drugs:
1. Entecavir and tenofovir—best profile regarding efficacy, safety drug resistance.
2. Entecavir is preferred in patient with renal insufficiency.
3. Tenofovir is preferred in:
   i. Young female contemplating pregnancy
   ii. Patient exposed to lamivudine in past.
4. Lamivudine and telbivudine should not be used as 1st line of therapy because of high chance of drug resistance.
5. Adefovir is less used because it has weak antiviral activity.

Choice of interferon therapy:
Interferon is recommended in following conditions:
1. Patient having compensated cirrhosis having
   i. Normal synthetic function
   ii. No evidence of portal hypertension
2. Young patient, who is unwilling for continuation of long-term treatment.
3. HBeAg positive patient with genotype A, because in this case, high rate of HBeAg seroconversion and HBsAg loss.

Interferon is not recommended in following conditions:
1. Decompensated liver disease
2. Medical contraindication
3. Psychiatric contraindication
4. On immunosuppressive therapy

Combination Therapy

Advantage of lamivudine with pegylated interferon over monotherapy:
i. Synergistic viral activity
ii. Prevention of antiviral drug resistance against lamivudine

But this viral suppression is not sustained, because, after stoppage of treatment, virus activation may start.

Again, entecavir and tenofovir have low rate of viral resistance when used alone.

Hence, nowadays, entecavir or tenofovir is used as monotherapy.

Time of Termination of Treatment

A. In case of pegylated interferon—there is definite duration of treatment, which is usually 48 weeks for both HBeAg positive and HBeAg negative patients.
B. In case of nucleos(t)ide analogue:
   a. In case of decompensated cirrhosis, lifelong treatment is usually required to prevent acute flares
   b. In case of compensated cirrhosis:
      i. Lifelong treatment is usually required.
   Or ii. Treatment may be stopped, if:
      1. There is reversal of cirrhosis
      2. Loss of HBsAg
      3. HBeAg seroconversion will occur
   In the above cases, close monitoring should be done to see any evidence of biochemical changes or clinical relapse.
C. In case of HBeAg positive precirrhotic liver disease—it should be completed when:
   i. HBeAg seroconversion occurs (HBeAg negative, anti-HBe positive and absent HBV DNA)
   ii. Treatment should be continued at least 12 months of consolidation therapy.
   But a few percentage of patients remain HBV DNA positive in spite of HBeAg seroconversion months for months or years.
D. In case of HBeAg negative precirrhotic liver disease, duration of treatment is unclear.

Treatment Failure

This treatment failure is tailored to:
i. Type of treatment failure
ii. Type of treatment that the patient is receiving
iii. History of prior treatment
iv. Characteristics of pretreatment

In these cases, following change in therapy can be done:
i. Switch to another mode of therapy
ii. Addition of another drug in the persistent therapy.

Lack of initial response may occur in case of lamivudine, adefovir or telmivudine therapy. This lack of initial response can be characterized by slow decline in serum HBV DNA level during first 12–24 weeks of nucleotide treatments.

These patients develop antiviral drug resistance during continued therapy.

This type of viral resistance may not be seen with the treatment entecavir and tenofovir.

Virological Break Through

This virological break through may occur due to:
i. Antiviral resistance
ii. Non-adherent to medicine

Here HBV DNA must be retested after 1–3 months. In case of virological break through—rescue therapy should be started immediately in case of:
i. Decompensated liver disease
ii. Severe hepatitis flares.

The choice of rescue therapy depends upon (Table 4.7):
i. Current or any prior treatment given to the patient
ii. Pattern of resistance mutation, if any
iii. Susceptibility of these mutations to other nucleos(t)ide analogues.

Table 4.7: Antiviral drugs		
Type of resistance of drugs	*Preferred treatment to be given*	*Alternative treatment*
1. Lamivudine or telbivudine	Tenofovir can be added or switch to tenofovir	Addition of adenovir. Lamivudore or telbivudine should be stopped and switch to truvada
2. Adefovir	Entecavir can be added or switch to entecavir	Addition of lamivudine or telbivudine Adefovir should be stopped and switch to truvada
3. Entecavir	Tenofovir can be added or switch to tenofovir	Entecavir should be stopped and switch to truvada.
4. Tenofovir	Entecavir can be added or switch to entecavir	Tenofovir should be stopped and switch to truvada

Truvada is the combination of emtricitabin and tenofovir—it is not approved for HBV till now.

HEPATITIS C

Hepatitis C virus disease is a burning public health problem. It is one of the 10 leading causes of infectious disease death worldwide. Again HIV and HBV coinfection will add burden to this disease.

Highest prevalence is seen in Africa (Egypt), Asia.

Lower prevalence is seen in industrialized countries of West.

Transmission

Hepatitis C virus can be transmitted through three routes:
1. Parenterally:
   i. Intravenous drug users—80% cases of acute HCV infections.
   ii. Introduction of blood products
2. Permucosally (sexually)—due to high-risk traumatic sexual practice.
3. Vertical transmission: In case of HIV-infected individual, super added acute HCV infections differ from HCV monoinfection in following categories:
   i. Epidemiology
   ii. Natural history
   iii. Immunology
   iv. Virology

Virology

Hepatitis C virus is small enveloped RNA virus, being member of family Flaviviridae.

RNA genome contains positive sense RNA containing 9400 nucleotides. It comprises of one long open reading frame encoding polyprotein of 3010 to 3033 amino acids.

At the 5′ end of the genome, nucleocapsid and envelope structural protein are being encoded.

At the 3′ end of the genome, non-structural proteins are present.

Nucleocapsid is formed by—non-glycosylated capsid protein C complexed with genomic RNA.

Two glycoprotein products are present in viral envelope. These are:
i. E1 or gp35
ii. E2 or gp70.

These sites are:
a. Highly antigenic
b. Their variability is very important for persistence of infection and immunopathogenesis.

Carboxyterminal end of E2 will be cleaved into small protein p7.

Non-structural region of HCV genome will be divided into NS2 to NS5 regions.

NS3 has two functional domains:
i. Protease—it is involved in the cleavage of remainder non-structural regions. NS4A acts as a cofactor.
ii. Helicase—it is involved in RNA replication.

HCV NS5 is cleared to form:
i. NS5a
ii. NS5b—it is viral RNA dependent RNA polymerase.

HCV has six genotypes and more than hundred subtypes.

Pathology and Pathogenesis

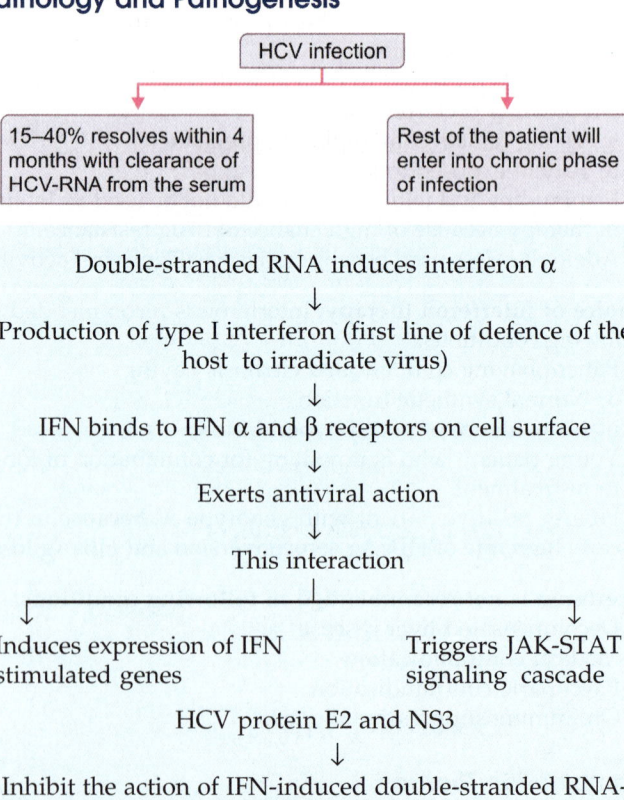

The abrogated innate antiviral immune responses within the infected hepatocytes are:
i. Retinoic acid—inducible gene 1
ii. IFN regulatory factor 3 pathway

Following pathologic immune mechanisms are nvolved in acute viral hepatitis C:
i. HCV specific HLA class I restricted cytotoxic T cell lymphocytes—it recognizes epitopes in variable region or envelope or non-structural proteins.
ii. CD4+ cell T lymphocyte response to recombinant viral antigens.
There is positive correlation between CD4+ T cell response to HCV core and benign course of infection in minimal hepatitis.
iii. HCV specific CD8+ cytotoxic T cells are responsible for elimination of HCV during incubation phase.

So, viral mutation against T cell recognition may be responsible for immune escape phenomenon which ultimately produces chronicity.

Again, downregulated cytotoxic activity of NK cells against HCV virus—may also produce chronicity.

Different genotypes of HCV are mainly responsible for:
i. Difficulty in immunological control
ii. Development of prophylactic vaccines
iii. Development of therapeutic vaccines

In case of chronic infection:
i. HCV-related cytotoxic T cells weakly detectable.
ii. HCV is resistant to the effect to antiviral cytokines.
iii. There is exhaustion of T cells

Development of Fibrosis

Inflammatory process
↓
Induces cytokines and other signaling molecules
↓
Deposition of extracellular matrix proteins
↓
Fibrosis begins around portal tract
↓
Gradual extension of fibrosis into lobules
↓
To around central vein
↓
Extensive fibrosis

Following factors are responsible for acceleration of fibrosis:
i. Older age
ii. Male gender
iii. Heavy alcohol intake
iv. Coinfection with HIV and HBV
v. Steatosis

Diagnostic Tests for HCV

Since detection of viral antigen is very difficult, hence antibody to HCV by ELISA is prime importance in confirmation of acute recent or past infection.

The antibody level usually declines over time after resolution of infection.

In case of acute infection:
i. Anti-HCV is undetectable at presentation.
ii. But at the peak level of ALT, this antibody can be detected.
Again IgM antibody to HCV detection is not available in our country. So IgG antibody to HCV will be of choice.
Third generation immunoassay will include:
i. Antigen from nucleocapsid (C22)
ii. Other non-structural regions of the genome.
Routine testing of anti-HCV in blood donors reduce the risk of spread of infection to the community.

In low-risk population, the following method is used to detect HCV infection.

Recombinant immunoblot assay (RIBA): In this method, antibodies to recombinant HCV protein are sought.
i. If antibodies to two or more protein are found—sample is confined as positive.
ii. It antibodies to single HCV protein is found, sample is confirmed as in determinate.

Detection HCV RNA: It can:
i. Confirm the viremia
ii. Quantify the viremia.
If the patient is HCV RNA negative, but anti-HCV antibody positive—it signifies past and resolved infection.

It the patient presents with unexplained raised alkaline phosphatage, Anti-HCV antibody test must be done.

HCV RNA

1. This can be detected in blood and other tissues by real-time PCR.
2. Limit of detection of HCV RNA in plasma is 10–15 IU/ml.
3. It can be detected within 1–2 weeks of transfusion of blood products and will be present for decades in untreated patients.
   Hence, it is not justified to estimate the level of HCV RNA repeatedly in untreated patient.
4. It should be tested prior and after antiviral therapy to detect the efficacy of treatment.

Genotyping

There are six major genotypes and 100 subtypes of HCV RNA. This can be differentiated by:
i. Restriction fragment length polymorphism
ii. PCR reactions
iii. Hybridization with type specific probes

But the definite method for viral genotype is sequencing.

Following are the viral genotypes with areas of distribution:
1. Genotype 1a and 1b—Europe and United States
2. Genotype 1b—Southern Europe
3. Genotype 3a and 1a—young individual with H/O intravenous drug user.
4. Genotype 1b—More than 50 years of age
5. Genotype 4—In Egypt, many areas of Middle East, Africa
6. Genotype 5—In South Africa, France, Spain.

Acute Hepatitis C

Incubation period (time of exposure to onset of symptoms) is on 2–12 weeks (average 7 weeks).

In case of large inocula (administration of factor VIII concentrate)—incubation period will be shorter.

Symptoms:
1. The disease may be mild and unrecognized.
2. The other patients may present with nonspecific symptoms, like:
   a. Fatigue
   b. Anorexia
   c. Lethargy
   d. Right upper quadrant pain
   e. Jaundice in 25% of patients.

Indicators of chance of clearance of virus:
1. Icteric patient
2. Severally affected female with jaundice
   HIV coinfected patient has less chance of clearing the virus.
   Chance of fulminant hepatitis is rare in HCV infection except during:
   i. Following chemotherapy, or
   ii. Withdrawal of chemotherapy.

Blood Biochemistry

1. 25% patients show mildy elevated bilirubin.
2. Elevation of ALT is less than with hepatitis A or B virus.
3. HCV RNA is intermittently negative during acute phase.

Fate of Acute Hepatitis C

i. Higher rate of spontaneous recovery occur in most cases.
   a. It occurs in those patients with single nuclear polymorphism which lie in or near IL28B gene on chromosome 19, encoding IFN-γ3.
   b. Spontaneous resolution also occurs in c/c genotype at rs 12979860 in European and African peoples.
ii. Chronic hepatitis C—it is major complication of hepatitis C.

Pathology

Liver biopsy shows:
1. Parenchymal cell necrosis
2. Histiocytic periportal inflammation
3. Preservation of reticulin framework
4. Multifocal centrilobular massive or submassive necrosis
5. Hepatocytes are swollen, also shown ballooning, sometimes shrinks—giving rise to acidophilic bodies.
6. Infiltration of mononuclear cells in portal zones
7. Proliferation of bile ductules, Kupffer cells and endothelial cell
8. Cholestasis in early phase in viral hepatitis due to plugging of bile thrombi in bile canaliculi

Management

Since this disease is usually silent, and 70% patients present with non-specific symptoms, hence treatment should be started as:
1. Conventional supportive management
2. Antiviral therapy

HCV RNA testing should be repeated to differentiate transient and permanent viral clearance.
Early antiviral treatment should be:
 i. Interferon
ii. Pegylated interferon and ribavirin

The patients who will not be under convalescent phase even after 2–4 months should be under antiviral treatment, because, these patients may enter into chronic phase and chronic HCV infection is less responsive to treatment.

In acute infection, interferon monotherapy usually produces sustained virological response in 6 months.

Treatment should be given in following conditions:
1. If serum alanine aminotransferase level will be elevated
2. HCV RNA remains detected 2–4 months after first detection
3. Patient will not be in convalescent phase ever after 2–4 months after initiation of infection.

Chronic Hepatitis C Infection

Chronic hepatitis C infection may be defined as persistence of HCV RNA in serum for more than 6 months.

The progression of acute to chronic phase is silent and insidious and may be unnoticed (Fig. 4.19).

Epidemiological Risk Factors

 i. Blood transfusion
ii. Intravenous drug users
iii. Sexual risk

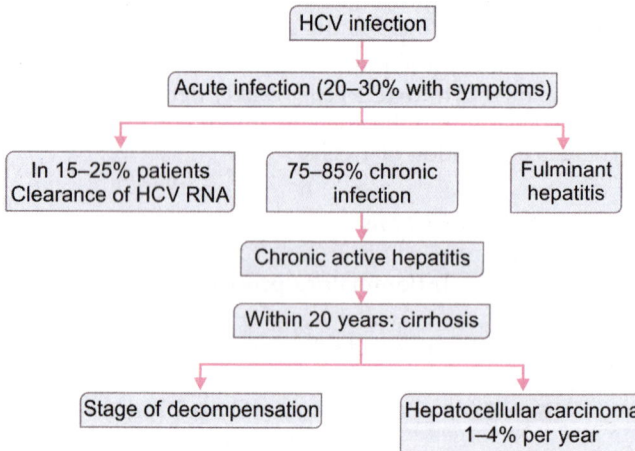

Fig. 4.19: Progression of chronic hepatitis C

Following factors are responsible for morbidity of disease:
1. Age of acquisition
2. Concomitant alcohol abuse
3. Male gender
4. Co-existence with other viral infections like HBV and HIV infection
5. Host immune response.

Effectiveness of the treatment can be judged by following:
1. HCV genotype
2. HCV RNA viral load

In case of progressive chronic hepatitis C disease, following laboratory values are abnormal:
1. AST level is greater than ALT.
2. Low serum albumin.
3. Prolonged prothrombin time.
4. Low platelet count.
5. Low level of autoantibodies.
6. Positive for LKM1 antibody.

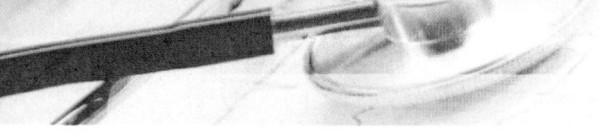

7. Anti-HCV antibody persists—for decades.
8. HCV RNA is usually detectable in patient with raised ALT and AST level and persistent HCV antibodies.

Variations in chronic hepatitis: There may be presence of low grade hepatitis as well as hepatic fibrosis in chronic hepatitis C infection, but it is less rapid in females than males with low or normal ALT.

Extrahepatic manifestations: The extrahepatic manifestations are:
1. Autoimmune hepatitis
2. Cryoglobulinemia
3. Vasculitis
4. Lichen planus
5. Porphyria cutanea tarda
6. Lymphocytic sialoadenitis
7. Membranous glomerulonephritis

Association of other Diseases with Hepatitis C

1. Non-Hodgkin's lymphoma
2. Insulin resistance and type 2 diabetes mellitus due to:
   i. Inhibition of insulin signaling pathway
   ii. Increased reactive oxygen species production
3. Direct genotypic association with metabolic effect, i.e. association of genotype 3 with steatosis in liver

Followings are factors for poor prognosis:
1. Insulin resistance
2. Obesity
3. Overt diabetes

Following factors are responsible for increased hepatic fibrosis:
1. Steatosis
2. Inflammatory process
3. Insulin resistance
4. Impaired response to interferon

Pathology in Chronic Hepatitis C

There is positive correlation of HCV RNA with hepatic involvement
i. Presence of HCV RNA with some degree of hepatitis
ii. Disappearance of HCV RNA after treatment is associated with histological improvement in liver.

Following histological findings are present:
1. Inflammation of portal tract with lymphoid aggregates
2. Mild periportal piecemeal necrosis
3. Parenchymal steatosis, apoptosis
4. In late stage, portal fibrosis, portal central fibrosis
5. HCV antigen can be detected in scattered hepatocytes
6. Large number of CD4 lymphocytes found in periportal areas.
7. Some degree of hepatic steatosis may be present.
8. There is evidence of positive correlation between serum hepcidin and both hepatic neuro-inflammation and fibrosis.

In chronic hepatitis, the level of hepcidin will be low, leading to iron accumulation in liver.

Minor histological abnormalities are found in:
i. HCV RNA negative person
ii. Patient with anti-HCV antibody positivity
iii. Normal alanine aminotransferase

Management

Prior to initiate the therapy in chronic hepatitis, following investigations should be required:
1. Quantification of HCV RNA
2. Liver function test to detect—hepatic involvement
   i. ALT
   ii. Bilirubin
   iii. Alkaline phosphatase
3. Genotype of HCV—should be determined
4. In coinfection with viruses:
   i. HBsAg, for HBV
   ii. HIV
5. To exclude associated autoimmune hepatitis
   i. Anti-smooth muscle cell antibodies
   ii. Anti-liver, kidney microsomal antibodies
According to recent guidelines, the entire patient with chronic hepatitis C must get antiviral therapy, liver biopsy is not at all mandatory for all patients.

Nowadays, following non-invasive methods are used to estimate the stage of the disease:
1. Aspartate aminotransferase to platelet ratio index (APRI)

$$\frac{\text{Aspartate aminotransferase (U/L) upper limit of normal}}{\text{Platelet count } (10^9 \times L)} \times 100$$

2. Transient elastography (TE)—it can measure the speed of propagation of shear wave in liver. This method is affected by:
   i. Obesity
   ii. Ascites
   The measurement should be:
   i. Normal liver stiffness—4–6 kilopascals
   ii. In case of cirrhosis, it will be 12–14 kilopascals
   There is a positive correlation between measured liver stiffness and hepatic venous pressure gradient (HVPG)
3. Enhanced liver fibrosis (ELF) panel
4. Fibro test
   The above two methods—utilize the following to measure fibrosis:
   i. Algorithms of biochemical tests
   ii. Extracellular matrix components

Advantages of the above non-invasive methods:
   i. They reduce the necessity of liver biopsy to measure fibrosis
   ii. These can be done in different bleeding disorders
   iii. These are done in hepatitis C infection (chronic)

Disadvantages of the above non-invasive tests:
   i. Highly costly
   ii. Operator dependant
   iii. Not widely available
   iv. They require capital outlay

General management: Following co-morbid diseases may accelerate the progress of the disease and fibrosis:
1. HBV infection
2. HIV infection
3. Alcoholism
4. Obesity
5. Diabetes

6. Male gender
7. More than 50 years of age

So following advices should be followed:
  i. Prevention of intake of alcohol
 ii. Since parenteral route is the only route of transmission, blood donation must be prohibited.
iii. Vaccination should be done against HBV and HCV

Indications of treatment:
1. Patient with mild disease may not require treatment.
2. Patient with psychiatric comorbidities should be treated jointly with psychiatrist, because interferon treatment may deteriorate patient's psychiatric condition.
3. Patient with compensated cirrhosis is the ideal candidate. Decompensated cirrhotic patients may worsen with this therapy; hence liver transplantation is the method of choice in them.

Interferon Treatment

Nature and types: It is a type of protein, derived from multigene family. It has been classified into following types:
1. Type I IFN:
    i. IFN-α (leukocyte)
   ii. LFN-β (fibroblast)
  iii. IFN-ω (omega)
2. Type II IFN:
    i. Immune IFN
   ii. IFN-γ
   Recently IFN-γ has highly therapeutic potential

Mechanism of action:
It interferes with different stages of viral life cycle by inducing following enzymes:
  i. 2′ 5′ oligoadenylate synthatase
 ii. Double-stranded RNA dependent protein kinase
iii. RNase L
 iv. Mx protein GTPase

Mode of degradation:

It is excreted in urine
↓
Reabsorbed by proximal tubular cells
↓
Undergoes lysosomal degradation in these cells

Peak serum concentration is observed in 7–12 hours. Interferon unusually given subcutaneously once weekly.

Ribavirin: It is a guanosine nucleoside analogue.

Mechanism of actions: This drug must be transformed into mono-, di- and triphosphate nucleotides before commencement of action.

The mode of actions are:
  i. Perturbation of intracellular nucleoside triphosphate pool.
 ii. It interferes with the formation of 5′ cap structure of viral m-RNA by inhibiting guanylyltransferase and methyltransferase competitively.
iii. It directly inhibits viral m-RNA polymerase complex.
 iv. It enhances macrophage inhibition of viral replication.
  v. It induces mutation of hepatitis C genome.
    It is orally given and it enhances the activity of IFN.

Pegylated interferon: It is developed by covalent attachment of recombinant INF-α to polyethylene glycol moieties.

Advantages over standard interferon:
  i. It protects interferon protein from enzymatic degradation.
 ii. If reduces renal clearance.
iii. It has longer half life.

Dosage of interferon and RBV:
1. peg–interferon α-2b—1.5 mg/kg—weekly subcutaneously to maximum dose 180 mg/week, it is fixed dose.
2. RBV should be given according to body weight in genotype 1–6
    i. <65 kg body weight   -   800 mg/day
   ii. 65–85 kg body weight -   1000 mg/day
  iii. >85 kg body weight   -   1200 mg/day

    In patient with genotype 1 infection:
     i. <75 kg body weight   -   1000 mg/day
    ii. >75 kg body weight   -   1200 mg/day

In patient with genotype 2, 3 infection
Dose of RBV—800 mg/day

Duration of treatment:
1. For genotype 1 and 4—12 months
2. For genotype 2 and 3—6 months

Response to treatment:
1. In case of genotype 1—treatment should be discontinued in those patients who fail to show decline in HCV RNA level at least 2 log 10 after 12 weeks of therapy. After 24 weeks, if patient shows HCV RNA positive—treatment should be discontinued.
2. In case of genotype 2 and 3—since these are slow responder, HCV RNA should be checked at 24 weeks of treatment, if these are detectable, treatment should be continued for another 12 weeks.
3. In case genotype 4—the response is intermediate between 1 and 2 or 3.
4. For genotype 5—no data is available till date. Here SVR is—48%

Types of responses are following:
1. *Non-responders:* These patients do not show significant virological response, i.e. never become HCV RNA negative at any point of time of treatment.
2. *Relapsers:* Patients show virological response to treatment in the form of undetectable HBV RNA in serum till the end of treatment, but again relapse when the treatment will be discontinued.
3. *Break through:* Here patients show virological response before 24 weeks during treatment, but it is cannot be maintained till the end of the treatment.
4. *Sustained virological response:* Here HCV RNA becomes undetectable at the end of 24 and 28 weeks of antiviral treatment. Patient is being treated according to the genotype and this negative HCV RNA in serum will be maintained 24 weeks after completion of treatment.
5. *Rapid virological response:* Here HCV RNA becomes undetectable within 4 weeks of treatment.
6. *Partial early viral response:* Here HCV RNA is detected, but the level of decline will be by >2 log10 by 12 weeks of treatment.

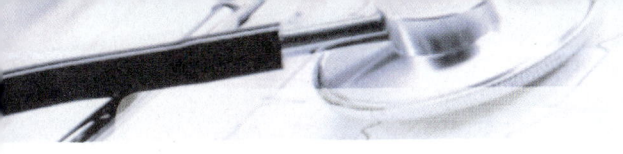

7. *Complete early viral response:* Here HCV RNA level will be undetectable by 12 weeks of treatment.
8. *Slow responder:* Here, there is gradual decline of HCV RNA level to become negative until after 12 weeks of treatment.

Side effects:

A. *Major early side effects:* Influence like syndrome:
    i. Chill
    ii. Fever
    iii. Backache
    iv. Malaise
    v. Headache
    These can be managed by paracetamol.
B. *Common side effects:*
    1. Headache
    2. Poor appetite
    3. Increased need for sleep
    4. Psychological effects
    5. Thrombocytopenic
    6. Hair loss
    7. Leucopenia
C. *Unusual and severe side effects:*
    1. Seizures
    2. Acute psychosis
    3. Bacterial infection
    4. Autoimmune reaction
    5. Thyroid disease
    6. Proteinuria
    7. Cardiomyopathy
    8. Skin rashes
    9. Interstitial lung disease
    10. Sarcoidosis
    11. Neuroretinitis—in this case, treatment must be stopped immediately.
D. *Major side effects:*
    1. Hemolytic anemia
    2. Myalgia
    3. Hyperuricemia
    4. Gastrointestinal upset
    5. Dyspepsia
    6. Cough
    7. Skin rash
    8. Irritability
    Uric acid and thyroid level monitoring should be done at 1 to 3 monthly intervals.
E. *Teratogenicity:* Due to chance of teratogenicity of RBV, there is need for contraception up to 6 months after completing treatment.

Abbreviated Treatment

1. In case of genotype 1, if:
    i. Viral load baseline is 600,000 IU/ml
    ii. RVR within 1 month by PCR
    Treatment can be stopped within 2 months.
2. In case of genotype 2 and 3, if:
    i. Viral load baseline is low
    ii. RVR
    Treatment should be stopped after 16 weeks.

Treatment of Nonresponders

The following factors are very important for predictive SVR in case of retreatment:

1. Genotype   2. Degree of fibrosis   3. Prior treatment.
    Genotype 2 and 3 show better response than genotype 1 regardless of prior responses.
    a. Peg-IFN plus RBV should be considered in case of non-responders or relapsers rather than standard IFN with RBV or IFN monotherapy.
    b. If the patient does not show SVR with retreatment with Peg-IFN plus RBV, this treatment can be stopped.
4. If the patients with cirrhosis or bridging necrosis do not respond to Peg-IFN with RBV treatment, maintenance therapy should not be given with these drugs.

Newer Treatments for HCV Chronic Infection

The drugs under trial are:

1. **NS3/4a protease inhibitors:**
    a. Linear class
        i. Telapovir
        ii. Boceprevir
        iii. Narlaprevir
    b. Macrolide class
        i. B1201335
        ii. Mk-7009
        iii. TMC 435
2. **NS5b polymerase inhibitors:**
    a. Nucleoside analogues
        i. IDX 184
        ii. PSI 7851
        iii. RG 7128
    b. Non-nucleoside inhibitors:
        i. Palm   I. ABT 333
                   II. ABT 072
        ii. Thumb I. VCH 759
                   II. VCH 916
3. **NS5a inhibitors**
4. **Immunomodulation**—Albuferon

Genotype-1
Ledipasvir—90 mg
+
Sofosbuvir— 400 mg
} × 12 weeks

Genotype-2
Sofosbuvir— 400 mg
+
Ribavirin
} × 6 months

Genotype-3
Sofosbuvir— 400 mg
+
Daclastavir—60 mg
} × 3 months

HEPATITIS D VIRUS

It is defective RNA virus (Fig. 4.20); it requires the help of HBV for assembly, release and transmission. Due to uniqueness of this virus, it has been classified as Delta virus.

It contains single-stranded negative circular RNA; within virus particle there is nucleocapsid—it is formed by RNA genome with HDAg. HDAg is present in two forms:
i. HDAg-S—it is essential for viral replication.
ii. HDAg-L:
    a. It contains isoprenylation motif at c terminal end
    b. It is essential for viral assembly
    c. It inhibits viral replication.
    Virus is coated by HBsAg
    The assembly and secretion of HDV depends upon:
    i. HBsAg level   ii. Sequence of natural HBsAg

The essential characteristic of HDV is its replication—since like all other RNA viruses, HDV lacks RNA polymerase, hence for replication of HDV requires host RNA polymerase II. In HDV, enzymatic activity is mediated by ribosomes.

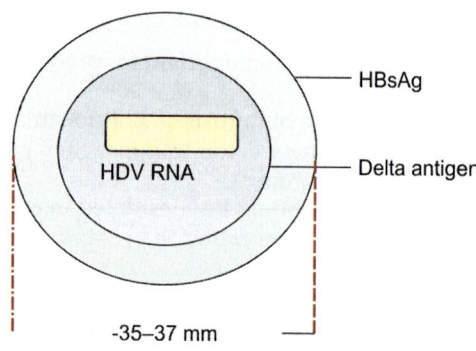

Fig. 4.20: Structure of HDV

Genotypes: HDV has high degree of heterogenicity. There are 8 genotypes. The distribution of genotypes is the followings:
1. Type-1—it is distributed worldwide.
2. Type-2 and 4—Far East.
3. Type-3—it is distributed in northern regions of South America.
4. Type-5, 6, 7, 8—it is distributed in West and Central Africa.

Epidemiology

1. It transmits simultaneously with HBV. If patient is anti-HBs antibody positive; he is not susceptible to HBV as well as HDV.
2. It can infect the chronic HBsAg carriers.
3. Routes of transmission:
   i. Perenteral route—through blood and blood products—either overtly or through interpersonal contact.
      HDV thus infects hemophiliacs, recipients of transfusion and health coworkers.
   ii. Intrafamily spread—in adults and children
   iii. Sexual transmissions through promiscuous groups—it is infrequent in homosexual men.
   iv. Vertical transmission—it is very rare.

Changes in the Epidemiology of HDV Infection

In last two decades, there is significant decline in HDV infection along with HBV infections. It is probably results of:
   i. Widespread HBV vaccination.
   ii. Improvement in the hygiene of the people.
   iii. Widespread campaign in AID program—which tells the danger of promiscuity and sharing syringes and needles.

However, immigration from different endemic parts of the world is recently producing new threats in Europe in the form of resurgence. Moreover survivals of HDV epidemic in 1970's and 1980's are the reservoir of HDV.

Pathogenesis of HDV Hepatitis

HDV is not directly cytopathic in liver tissue, but here the liver damage is mainly immune mediated. HDAg induces hepatic fibrosis through regulation of transforming growth factor β-induced signal activation.

The role of HDV genotypes in the pathogenesis of hepatitis is variable:
1. Genotype-1—is associated with broad-spectrum of infectivity.

2. Genotype-2, 4—are associated with milder form of acute and chronic hepatitis D.
3. Genotype-3—is associated with fulminant form of hepatitis in South American people. This genotype is exclusively associated with HBV genotype F.

Clinical Course of HDV Infection (Fig. 4.21)

Acute Hepatitis D

A. **Coinfection with hepatitis B virus:** In case HBV coinfection, disease course ranges from mild form to severe even, fulminant form. But the clinical picture is indistinguishable from HBV infection.

But the diagnostic clue is—biphasic rise in SGPT and SGOT levels occurring a few weeks apart. Here second rise is mainly due to HDV coinfection.

Course: 2% patients will enter into chronic phase, but rest will be recovered.

Simultaneous infection with HBV and HDV in acute hepatitis

B. **Superinfection with HDV in chronic HBsAg carrier:** In any patient with pre-existing HBV infection, it acts as a platform for full expression of HDV.

In case of pre-existing HBsAg positive chronic hepatitis, superinfection of HDV may produce acute severe form of hepatitis to fulminant hepatic failure.

But in case of HBsAg carrier, HDV infection produces acute hepatitis.

Again, since HBsAg carrier acts as a good platform for continuous replication of HDV, it may be responsible for chronically in 90% of cases.

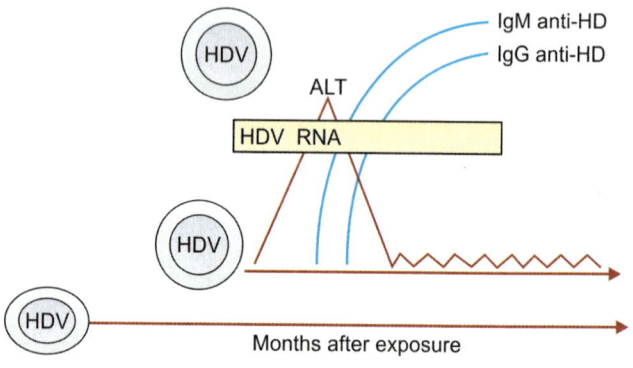

Fig. 4.21: Serological graph in HDV

Chronic Hepatitis D

Here the clinical presentation may vary in the following manner:
   i. Patient may be symptom free—can be diagnosed during routine medical checkup.
   ii. Patient may present with following symptoms, like:
      a. Fatigue
      b. Malaise
      c. Anorexia
      d. Right upper quadrant pain
      e. Dark-colored urine in advanced cases.
   iii. Patient may present with features of cirrhosis or its complications, like:
      a. Jaundice
      b. Ascites

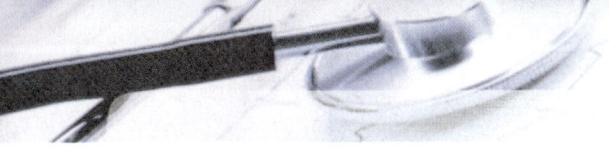

c. Encephalopathy
d. Portal hypertension

In chronic HDV hepatitis, there is persistently high serum aminotransferase level, but as the disease progresses; its level bends to decrease till late stage.

In this hepatitis—HBe antibody is high, low or undetectable HBV DNA. So here the liver fibrosis is mainly due to HDV infection.

Laboratory abnormalities are similar to HBV infection, except, there is high level of immunoglobulin.

There may be presence of varieties of antibodies against microsomal membrane of liver and kidney.

Hepatic Histology

1. **In acute HDV hepatitis:** Focal prominent intralobular lymphocyte and macrophage, degenerative eosinophilic infiltration. It leads to formation of acidophilic bodies in:
   a. Parenchyma
   b. Portal tract
2. **In severe or fulminant hepatitis:** There is drop out of most of the hepatocytes (massive necrosis)
3. **In chronic form of hepatitis:**
   a. Degree of periportal necrosis is more prominent
   b. Evidence of active micronodular or macronodular cirrhosis.

A special form of fulminant HDV hepatitis in Amazon Basin is—Microvascular steatosis of hepatocytes—which may lead to formation of morula cells.

Immunofluorescence or immunohistochemistry of liver cells show the presence of intranuclear HDAg, in acute or fulminant form of hepatitis, but not in chronic forms of disease.

Cause and Prognosis of HDV Infection

1. It is least common but most severe and rapidly progressive viral hepatitis.
2. In case of HDV-infected patients, 70–80% of them developed cirrhosis.
3. Risk of developing cirrhosis is threefold higher in HDV positive patients.
4. Cirrhotic patients become stable for many years, ultimately they develop complications of cirrhosis and hepatocellular carcinoma (2.6–2.8%), unless they undergo liver transplantation.
5. As the disease progresses, serum level of ALT and HDV replication rate gradually decrease.
6. Mean interval between primary infection and development of histological cirrhosis is one decade. Development of histological cirrhosis and maintenance of good quality of life interval is one decade. So the interval between primary infection and development of hepatic decompensation in cirrhosis is two decades.
7. In minority of cases, disease follows benign, non-progressive course.
8. In a few cases, disease resolution occurs with spontaneous clearance of HBsAg in HDV positive patients than HDV-negative HBsAg carriers.
9. Coinfection of HIV—cannot modify the chronic HDV disease course.

Diagnosis of HDV Infection

• In case of acute HDV hepatitis
• In case of coinfection with HBV virus

Most specific findings are:
a. High filter of anti-HBc IgM—indicates HBV infection.
b. HDAg—it may be detected transiently, before the appearance of anti-HD IgM.
c. Anti-HD IgM—it usually appears within 1–2 weeks of primary infection—persists for 5–6 weeks, in a few cases up to 12 weeks.
   i. Its disappearance indicates resolution of infection
   ii. Its presence indicates chronicity of infection.
d. Anti-HD IgG—it appears after the disappearance of anti-HD IgM
   i. It is present in convalescent period.
   ii. It disappears within months or years after recovery serological profile of HBV
      a. HBsAg
      b. HBeAg, or
      c. Anti-HBe antibody
      d. Anti-HBc antibody IgM.

Presence of HDAg indicates:
i. Active replication of virus
ii. Transient acute infection for a few days

In chronic hepatitis D: HDAg cannot be detected due to presence of antibody and antigen—antibody complexes formation.

Presence of HDV RNA indicates:
i. Active replication of virus.
ii. Transient acute infection.
iii. Chronic persistent infection.

Superinfection with HDV

1. In case superinfection: IgM anti-HBc will be present in low titer.
2. In case of HBV carrier state
   i. Presence of HBsAg
   ii. Presence of IgM anti-HBc
   iii. Presence of anti-HBe.

Superinfection with HDV is characterized by:
i. Presence of HDAg
ii. Presence of HDV RNA
iii. Increasing titer of IgM and IgG anti-HDAb.

In case of chronic hepatitis D:
1. High titer of IgM anti-HD
   i. IgM anti-HD—if pentameic (195) indicates primary infection.
   ii. IgM anti-HD—if monomeric (75)—indicates chronic infection.
   Level of IgM anti-HD indicates:
   i. Its presence indicates—chronic infection.
   ii. Its gradual disappearance—indicates gradual resolution of chronic infection.
2. In acute and chronic infection, due to sequestration of antigen–antibody complexes, detection of HDAg is not usually justified.

Detection of HDV RNA: The methods used to detect HDV RNA:

i. Quantitative detection of HDV RNA by reverse transcriptase polymerase chain reaction (RT-PCR), it can detect 10–100 copies viral genome per ml of serum.

ii. Qualitative detection of HDV RNA by real-time RT-PCR.

Importance:

i. It can investigate the molecular events during acute and chronic infection.

ii. It can monitor the response to antiviral therapy.

Treatment

Aim

i. Eradication of HDV and HBV

ii. Prevention of long-term sequelae of chronic infection:
  a. Hepatocellular carcinoma
  b. Cirrhosis.

HDV is difficult target for antiviral therapy because:

i. Lack of specific viral polymerase

ii. High pathogenic potential.

Acute Hepatitis D

i. Close monitoring of the clinical progression of the patient.

ii. Biochemical parameters in the form of liver function test at regular interval.

If the patient progresses to fulminant hepatic failure

i. Prompt transfer to liver unit

ii. Liver transplantation in the method of choice

Chronic Hepatitis D

α interferon therapy

Dosage: 9 million units thrice weekly
              Or   × 1 year
        5 million units daily

Response: Poor response to α interferon:

i. Coinfection with HIV and HDV

ii. Coinfection with HDV and HCV

iii. Children with chronic hepatitis D

New strategies to induce effective response with interferon

i. Long duration of treatment.

ii. Continuous therapy for 12 years

But drawback of the new strategies:

i. Relapse rate is very high.

ii. This type of therapy is poorly tolerated.

Response with 1 year therapy:

i. 10–20% chance of clearance of HDV

ii. 10% chance of HBsAg clearance

Pegylated interferon monotherapy:

i. It is well tolerated.

ii. More effective than standard interferon therapy

iii. It is more effective in non-responder of standard interferon therapy.

Combined therapy with standard and pegylated interferon has no significant advantage over interferon monotherapy.

Side effects of interferon: This is more common in high dose and prolonged course of therapy. The side effect is mainly psychiatric symptoms.

Hence continuous monitoring of medical and psychiatric symptoms is necessary to detect early and necessary management.

Nucleoside analogues like, lamivudine and famcyclovir have no or limited side effect on HDV replication in spite of presence of structural link between HDV and HBV.

Monitoring of antiviral therapy:

a. Full blood counts

b. Serum SGPT and SGOT levels

c. Quantification of HDV RNA—at:
  i. Baseline
  ii. 3 months
  iii. 6 months
  iv. 12 months of treatment
  vi. 6 months post-treatment.

d. Continuous medical and psychiatric monitoring

e. Quantitative detection of HBsAg level in serum

Major problem is—lack of commercial assays for quantitative and qualitative assessment.

Predictions of response of therapy: There is no biochemical or virological variables—which will predict the response to therapy. But follow predictors have been evaluated:

i. Patient without cirrhosis but not having chronic hepatitis D infection is most likely to respond.

ii. Negative PCR within 6 months of initiation of treatment shows sustained virological response.

But it is not possible to detect which patient will show sustained virological response or will relapse.

Current recommendations:

• Drug of choice is pegylated interferon

• Dose is once weekly administration for better compliance.

Indications for pegylated interferon:

i. Interferon native patient

ii. Previously non-responder to standard interferon

iii. In chronic hepatitis D without evidence of cirrhosis

In case of graft infection—risk of HDV infection can be lowered by continuous administration of immunoglobulin with lamivudine to prevent HBV infection.

Future antiviral agents: Since virological response to pegylated interferon is lower and patient may relapse after discontinuation of therapy, newer antiviral agents are being searched for. The probable newer agents are:

1. Prenylation inhibitor—it blocks essential step in HDV assembly

2. Antisense oligonucleotides.

3. Ribosomes.

4. Small interfering RNA.

NON-A-E VIRAL HEPATITIS

A. Hepatotrophic viruses
  a. Flaviviridae other than hepatitis C virus
    i. GBV-C/HGV
    ii. Yellow fever virus (YFV)

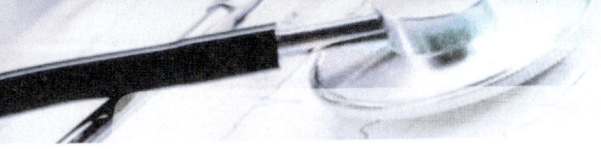

b. Circoviridae
   i. Torque tenovirus
   ii. Sanban, Yonban, SEN viruses
B. Systemic viral infections producing transient hepatic involvement
   a. Herpesviridae
      i. Epstein-Barr virus
      ii. CMV
      iii. HSV
      iv. Varicella-zoster virus
      v. Human herpes 6 virus.
   b. Severe acute respiratory disease syndrome/coronavirus
   c. Parvovirus B/9
   d. Measles
   e. HIV
   f. Lassa, Marburg, Ebola virus

G Virus

Hepatitis G virus has been detected by Linnel et al.

GB virus: It is an RNA virus with positive polarity. It contains 9400 nucleotides, one open reading frame; it encodes a polyprotein.

GBV—being a lymphotropic agent, it replicates in:
   i. Bone marrows
   ii. Spleen
   iii. Peripheral blood mononuclear cells
   iv. Vascular endothelial cells.

Fate of Virus Infection

   i. This virus may persist for many years without infection.
   ii. Spontaneous resolution occurs in 60–75% patients with development of antibodies (anti-E-2 antibodies).

Detection of HUBV-C antibody:
   i. Antibodies against E_2 glycoprotein of GBV-C by ELISA.
   ii. Detection of viral genome by real-time PCR.

Epidemiology

Transmission occurs through following routes:
   i. Blood-borne route
   ii. Sexual intercourse
   iii. Vertical transmission from mother to child
   iv. Intravenous drug users
   v. Hemodialysis
   vi. Blood and blood product transfusion
   vii. Homosexuals (13 to 63% male homosexuals, 14–25% female homosexuals)

Since the pathway of transmissions of GBV-C and HCV is common, correction rate is 20%.

Interactions with HIV

GBV-C interacts with HIV through following mechanisms:
   i. Viral interference
   ii. Upregulation of T-helper cells 1
   iii. Cytokine production
   iv. Downregulation of T-helper cell-2
   v. Inhibition of entry of HIV into target cells.

Clinical Features

GBV-C infection is usually acute, rarely chronic.

But childhood infection may become chronic.

Infection due to sexual transmission resolves spontaneously due to rapid clearance of virus.

There is no evidence of convincing liver damage in GBV-C infection unrelated to immune status of the patient.

There is no evidence of association of GBV-C and hepatocellular carcinoma.

ACUTE LIVER FAILURE

Definition and Classifications

This is a clinical syndrome characterized by severe impairment of liver function within 6 months of onset of symptoms.

Based on the time interval between the development of jaundice and onset of encephalopathy, it can be classified into:
   i. Hyperacute liver failure
   ii. Acute liver failure
   iii. Subacute liver failure

Alternative Classification of Acute Liver Failure

   i. Fulminant hepatic failure: Interval between jaundice and encephalopathy is less than 2 weeks.
   ii. Subfulminant hepatic failure: When the time interval is more than 2 weeks to less than 8 weeks.
   iii. Late onset hepatic failure: When the time interval is more than 8 weeks but less than 24 weeks.

Epidemiology

1. In Asia and developing countries—common cause is hepatitis B viral hepatitis, drug-induced liver failure is rare.
2. In western countries—viral hepatitis-induced liver failure is rare, whereas, paracetamol and idiosyncratic drug-induced liver injury are common.
3. In Spain, paracetamol is not readily available; here hepatitis B-induced liver failure is common.
4. In USA and UK—paracetamol self poisoning—45–60% of cases and idiosyncratic drug in 12% of cases.

Etiology

A. **Viral hepatitis**
   1. *Hepatitis A:* It is a rare cause of acute liver failure. Patient with chronic hepatitis due to hepatitis C virus if superinfected with hepatitis A virus—may produce acute liver failure. Indications of poor prognosis are:
      i. Serum creatinine >2 mg/d
      ii. SGPT less than 2600 IU/L
      iii. Those patients who need for ventilator support or pressor support.
   2. *Hepatitis B:*
      i. It is responsible for 1% case of liver failure. In fulminant case, IgM core antibody will be positive. In few cases, serology of hepatitis B will be negative.
      ii. In some cases, superinfection with hepatitis D may precipitate liver failure (4% cases).
      iii. Reactivation of hepatitis B virus along with replication in inactive B virus carrier who is under

chemotherapy or being treated with immuno-suppressive agents for organ transplantation—may be responsible for acute liver failure.

3. *Hepatitis C virus:* Here HCV RNA may be present in half of the cases. In case of super infection with hepatitis B virus, markers of B virus can be suppressed by acute HCV infection resulting erroneous contribution of liver failure to HCV virus alone.

4. *Hepatitis E virus:* It is a leading cause of hepatic failure in India. Pregnant women are more susceptible to HEV virus.

5. *Other viruses:*
   • Herpes simplex
   • Varicella zoster
   • Cytomegaly virus
   • Adenovirus
   • Epstein-Barr virus
   • Dengue fever virus.

B. **Drugs:**
   1. Paracetamol—characteristic pictures includes:
      i. Very high serum SGPT (~ 48000 IU/L)
      ii. Relatively low bilirubin level (4–6 mg/dl)
   2. Carbon tetrachloride
   3. Idiosyncratic drug relation
   4. Alcohol
   5. Mushroom poisoning—Amanita phalloides

C. **Ischemic causes ("shock liver"):**
   1. Cardiogenic shock
   2. Hypotension—in case of sepsis or cardiac events
   3. Heat stroke
   4. Cocaine

D. **Vascular:**
   1. Acute Budd-Chiari syndrome
   2. Sinusoidal obstruction syndrome after bone marrow transplantation. Vascular causes have poor outcome.

E. **Malignancy:** Massive infiltration of liver with tumor—lymphoma

F. **Other causes:**
   1. Wilson's disease—in this case, the associated pheno-menon
      i. Hemolytic anemia;   ii. Renal failure
      Ages are between 5 and 40 years.
   2. Autoimmune hepatitis

Clinical Features

Symptoms

   i. Nausea   ii. Vomiting
   iii. Malaise   iv. Jaundice
   v. Symptoms of encephalopathy—confusion, stupor, coma
   vi. Feature of hypoglycemia—like syncope, confusion
   vii. Features of metabolic acidosis—like, deep breathing
   viii. Feature of coagulopathy—like, bleeding from any sources.

Signs

   i. Tachycardia
   ii. Hypotension
   iii. Fever
   iv. Jaundice
   v. Signs of hepatocellular failure

vi. Shrunken liver due to loss of hepatic mass—which may be as small as 600 gm.

In patient with gradual onset of hepatic insufficiency (more than weeks)—may present with:
   i. Features of cerebral edema   ii. Ascites
   iii. Edema   iv. Renal failure

Differentiation from Chronic Liver Disease

A. **From history and signs:**
   i. History of liver disease
   ii. Duration of symptoms of liver disease
   iii. Presence of hard liver
   iv. Marked splenomegaly
   vi. Vascular spiders in the skin.

B. **Precipitating causes of hepatic decompensation:**
   i. Gastrointestinal bleeding
   ii. Infection
   iii. Dehydration
   iv. Sedative intake
   v. Alcohol intake

Investigations

Laboratory Tests

This is important for following reasons:
1. To establish the etiology
2. To defect severity of injury
3. To assess the prognosis, severity

A. **Hematology:** Complete blood count:
   i. WBC—elevated signifies infection
   ii. Hemoglobin—low:
      a. Wilson's disease
      b. Gastrointestinal bleeding
   iii. Platelet count—low.

B. **Biochemistry:**
   i. Glucose—low, may be severely low, responsible for altered mental status.
   ii. Sodium, potassium, phosphorus—low
   iii. Blood carbon dioxide low—indicates hyperventilation, due to metabolic acidosis.
   iv. Liver function tests:
      a. Serum bilirubin
      b. SGOT
      c. SGPT
      d. Alkaline phosphatase
      e. Total protein, albumin—abnormal
   Levels of amimotransferases—are of poor prognostic value, because, their level gradually fall in spite of patient's condition worsens or improves.

C. **Arterial blood gases:**
   i. PCO_2
   ii. PO_2
   iii. pH
   iv. Lactate—it is usually increased indicating metabolic acidosis.
   v. Ammonia—it is usually increased in case of hepatic encephalopathy.

D. **Viral serology:**
   i. HAV IgM antibody
   ii. HBsAg
   iii. Anti-HBs Abiv. anti-HIV antibody
   v. HEV IgM (in endemic areas)

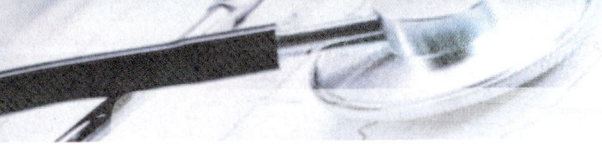

vi. HCV RNA
vii. HBV DNA
viii. HDV antibody if hepatitis B positive.
ix. HSV—PCR
x. CMV—PCR
xi. EBV—PCR
xiii. HIV.

E. Autoimmune markers:
  i. Antinuclear antibody (ANA)
  ii. Anti-smooth muscle cell antibody (ASMA)
  iii. Anti-liver/kidney microsome 1 antibody (ALKM1)
  iv. Immunoglobulin

F. Drugs and toxin
  i. Paracetamol
  ii. Alcohol
  iii. Acetaminophen

G. Metal
  i. Urinary copper
  ii. Serum ceruloplasmin is unhelpful

Ratio of ALP to bilirubin <4	these are the diagnostic of
Ratio of AST to ALT >2.2	Wilson's disease

H. Microbiology
  i. Blood culture—both aerobic anaerobic from both hands
  ii. Urine culture and microscopy
  iii. Sputum Gram strain, acid-fast stain, culture
  Regarding hepatoxicity due to paracetamol—one can use Rumack-Matthew normogram. But it cannot predict accurately the hepatotoxicity due to presence of following factors:
  i. If precise time of ingestion is unknown
  ii. If patient has taken multiple overdoses over time
  iii. If the patient has taken extended release tablets.
  iv. Paracetamol level will be elevated falsely if bilirubin level in blood will be more than 10 mg/dl
  Markedly elevated aminotransferases level of more than 3600 IU/L—it strongly suggests paracetamol over dose and toxicity.

I. EEG: Continuous EEG monitoring is case of hepatocellular failure shows (Fig. 4.22)—progressive increase in amplitude with decrease in frequency followed by progressive decrease in amplitude with little change in frequency which ultimately leads to no central activity.

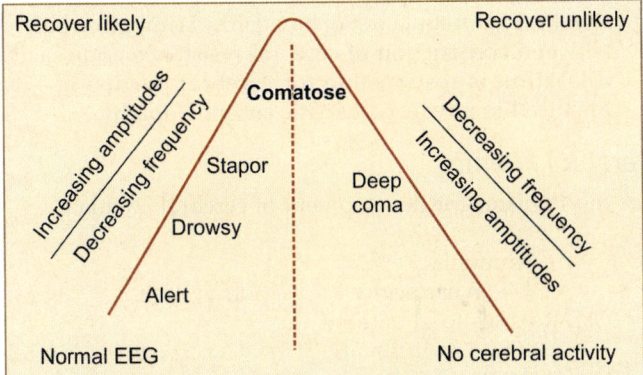

Fig. 4.22: Evaluation of EEG in hepatocellular failure

J. Computerized tomography: Non-contrast scan is useful to rule out evidence of cerebral infarction or hemorrhage. But:

i. The yield of this study is low
ii. It cannot justify the risk of moving critically ill patients

K. Abdominal imaging: It is helpful in following circumstances:
  i. Assess the vascular patients
  ii. To detect mass lesion
  iii. To detect hepatic nodularity—it is more common in acute setting—it confirms regenerative nodules
  iv. To detect liver site—it denotes severe hepatic necrosis.

Pathophysiology

Spectrum of Liver Damage

A. Parenchymal necrosis:
  1. Confluent necrosis with cell dropout and parenchymal collapse in zonal or nonzonal distribution
  +
  Activation of sinusoid lining cells, like, kupffer cells, stellate cells, and endothelial cells—in case of cell dropout in perivenular region—
  Etiology—i. drugs, ii. toxins, iii. ischemia, iv. viruses

  Hepatic necrosis—may be due to:
  a. Direct effect of etiological agents
  b. Activation of nonparenchymal cells with release of cytokines.
  2. In case of Budd—Chiari syndrome—venous out flow tract obstruction with sinusoidal dilatation and congestion.
  3. In case of Wilson's disease—since the liver is already cirrhotic, there will be superimposed parenchymal necrosis, collapse, steatosis, portoseptal inflammation.

B. Microvesicular steatosis: It occurs in absence of substantial hepatic necrosis.
  Etiology: i. Acute fatty liver of pregnancy
      ii. Mitochondrial toxins
      iii. Drugs—tetracycline

C. Malignant infiltration: It occurs in
    i. Lymphoma
    ii. Leukemia
    iii. Metastases

Molecular Mechanisms in Hepatocellular Failure

There are two pathways of liver cell death:
1. **Apoptosis:** It is characterized by shrinkage of nuclear and cytoplasm without the following:
    i. Disturbance of cell membrane integrity
    ii. Liberation of intracellular content
    iii. There is no secondary inflammation
2. **Necrosis:** This is characterized by—depletion of adenosine triphosphale (ATP), with resultant cell swelling and lysis, with resultant:
    i. Release of cellular content
    ii. Secondary inflammation

Apoptosis is triggered by two following mechanisms:
i. Extrinsic mechanism—this mechanism starts with the activation of death receptors present on cell-membrane.
ii. Intrinsic mechanism—this starts with oxidative stress of mitochondria and endoplasmic reticulum.
  Above two mechanisms activate a series of cysteine proteases—called capases.
  Types of proapoptotic signals dictate the type of capases to be activated, e.g.:

a. Capases 8 will be activated following stimulation of cytoplasmic death receptors.
b. Capase 9 will be activated as a result of oxidative damage of mitochondria

But if the mitochondrial damage is severe, it produces:
i. Depletion of ATP stores
ii. Inactivation of capases
The result is hepatocellular necrosis.
The following factors are the modulators of hepatocyte necrosis:
i. Cellular antioxidant
ii. Glutathione
iii. Nitric oxide
iv. Increasing number of tyrosine kinase
v. Transcription factors
vi. Cytokines
vi. Chemokines

Mechanisms of Hepatocellular Regeneration

Hepatocellular regeneration is more pronounced in hyperacute liver failure. Factors responsible for adequacy of regeneration (Fig. 4.23):
i. TNF-α
ii. IL-6
iii. Growth factors—hepatocyte growth factor (HGF)

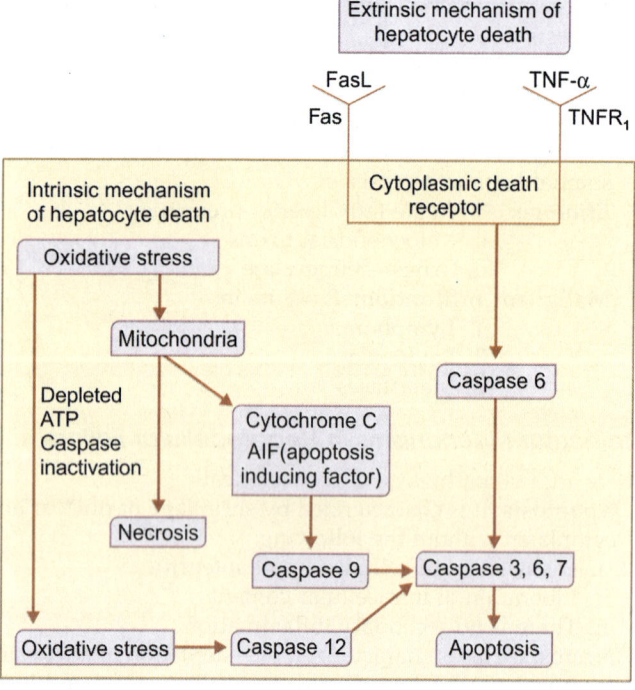

Fig. 4.23: Extrinsic mechanism of death of hepatocyte

Due to damage of extracellular matrix—following factors are elevated in serum:
i. Stimulatory HGF
ii. Inhibitory transforming growth factor-B.
Above two factors are activated by increased activity of fibrinolytic system.

Modulators of oxidative stress—pathway:
i. TNF-α, (+ve)   ii. Bile acid (+ve)
iii. Ceramide (+ve)   iv. CYP-450 (+ve)
v. Glutathione (–ve)

Modulators of caspase activity:
i. Nitric oxide
ii. Oxidative stress

Modulator or Fas/FasL pathway:
i. Hyperosmolarity (+ve)
ii. Copper (+ve)
iii. Oxidative stress (+ve)
iv. No (–ve)

Pathophysiology of Clinical Syndrome

Hemodynamic changes: This is characterized by:
i. Marked splanchnic vasodilatation
ii. Marked systemic arteriolar vasodilatation
iii. Hyperdynamic circulation
iv. Low arteriovenous oxygen difference

The factors responsible for vasodilatation and hypotension:
i. Elevated levels of IL-6 and IL-8.
ii. Adrenal insufficiency
iii. Increased activity of vasodilatory NO.

In case of sepsis-induced hepatocellular failure, the following factors are responsible for impaired tissue oxygen extraction:
i. Vasoactive amines
ii. Endothelial damage
iii. Generated oxygen free radicals
iv. Relative hypovolemia with reduced vascular resistance
There is evidence of microcirculatory plugging as a result of formation of microthrombi. *The factors responsible for formation of microthrombi are:*
i. Activation and consumption of platelet
ii. Increased adhesion of leukocytes to endothelium.

Hepatic Encephalopathy

Pathophysiological mechanisms responsible for hepatic encephalopathy are the following:
i. Accumulation of ammonia
ii. Dysregulation of central glutaminergic, serotonergic noradrenergic pathways
iii. Production of false neurotransmitters
iv. Activation of central γ-aminobutyric acid/benzodiazepine receptors
v. Altered cerebral metabolism
vi. Cerebral autoregulation of blood flow is impaired balance between constriction of cerebral resistance and reactive dilatation is responsible for cerebral perfusion—it is impaired in advanced hepatic encephalopathy.

Cerebral Edema

The mechanisms for development of cerebral edema:

1.   Ammonia
         ↓← In astrocytes
      Detoxifies to glutamine
                ↓
Accumulation of glutamine in brain cell
                ↓
Increased intracellular osmolarity
                ↓
         Cerebral edema

(Contd.)

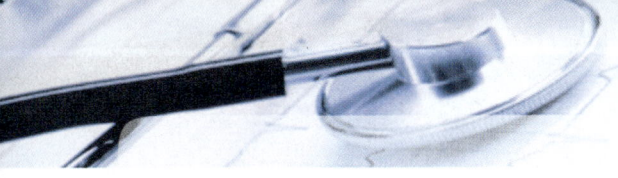

(Contd.)

Compensatory ability of astrocytes
↓
Looses osmolytes (myoinositol)
↓
Counter the osmotic effects of accumulated glutamine level
↓
Reduce the potency of cerebral edema
2. Locally generated glutamine and glutamate from ammonia
↓
Increased neuronal—derived nitric oxide level.
↓
Development of cerebral hyperemia
↓
Development of cerebral edema
3.   Ammonia
↓
It induces inhibition of α-ketoglutarate dehydrogenase
↓
Decreased entry of pyruvate to tricarboxylic acid cycle
↓
→ Increased production of lactate.
↓
Development of cerebral edema

Accelerated glycolysis
↑
Systemic inflammatory response syndrome
↑
Important mediators of SIRS like, proinflammatory cytokines such as tumor necrosis factor-α

Cerebral blood supply depends upon
Balance between—carotid arterial pressure and intracerebral pressure.
Cerebral perfusion pressure =
mean arterial pressure–Intracranial pressure

In fulminant hepatic failure

1. Loss of cerebral blood flow autoregulation
↓
Increase in cerebral blood flow
and
Increase in interstitial water
↓
Relative intracranial hypertension
2. Cerebral hypoperfusion and cerebral hypoxia due to systemic hypotension

Signs and Symptoms of Raised Intracerebral Pressure

1. **Systolic hypertension**—sustained or intermittent
2. **Increased muscle tone and myoclonus**—leads to:
   i. Myoclonus
   ii. Hyperpronation of arms
   iii. Extension of legs

   The above posture is called decerebrate posturing.
3. **Dysconjugate eye movements**—skew position of the eyes. If the disease progresses—there will be brainstem herniation
   i. Loss of papillary reflexes   ii. Respiratory arrest

Increased intracerebral pressure is uncommon in stage 1 and stage 2 encephalopathy. But it will start of stage 3 and will be high in stage 4 encephalopathy.

Renal Failure

It may be due to:
1. Acute liver failure itself (hepatorenal syndrome)
2. Acute tubular necrosis secondary to complications of acute liver failure:
   i. Sepsis
   ii. Hypotension
   iii. Bleeding
3. Use of nephrotoxic drugs
4. Use of paracetamol overdose producing hepatotoxicity

Hepatorenal syndrome results from:
   i. Hyperdynamic circulation
   ii. Low renal perfusion pressure
   iii. Activation of sympathetic nervous system
   iv. Increased synthesis of vasoactive mediators
   v. decreased glomerular capillary ultrafiltration

Metabolic Derangements

A. **Electrolytes:**
   1. *Hypoglycemic:* It may be persistent and intractable:
      Causes: i. Raised insulin levels due to reduced hepatic uptake
                 ii. Reduced neoglucogenesis
      Effect:
      i. Neurological deterioration
      ii. Death
   2. *Hypokalemia:*
      Causes:
      i. Urinary potassium losses
      ii. Inadequate replacement
   3. **Hyponatremia**
   4. **Hypophosphatemia**
   5. **Hypocalcemia**
   6. **Hypomagnesemia**
B. **Acid–base imbalance:**
   1. Respiratory alkalosis—due to hyperventilation—due to stimulation of respiratory center by toxic metabolites.
   2. Respiratory acidosis: Causes:
      i. Elevated intracranial pressure
      ii. Respiratory depression
      iii. Pulmonary complications
   3. Lactic acidosis—it is developed in stage-III encephalopathy causes:
      i. Inadequate tissue perfusion—related to hypotension
      ii. Hypoxia
   4. Metabolic acidosis—it occurs in paracetamol-induced acute liver failure.
C. **Coagulopathy:** Liver is the main site of synthesis of:
   i. All coagulation factors—except factor VIII
   ii. All inhibitors of coagulation
   iii. Proteins involved in fibrinolytic system

So coagulopathy in fulminant hepatic failure may be due to following mechanisms:
   i. Reduced hepatic synthesis of clotting factors
   ii. Reduced hepatic synthesis of anticlotting factors like, proteins c and anti-thrombin III

iii. Increased consumption of clotting factors and platelets due to disseminated intravascular coagulation:
iv. Qualitative platelet defect:
  a. Increased adhesiveness
  b. Impaired aggregation
v. Increased fibrinolytic activity.

The result of coagulopathy is:
i. Spontaneous bleeding from—mucous membrane in the gastrointestinal tract or into brain.
ii. Bleeding after invasive procedures—like after intracranial pressure monitor insertion.

Markers of Disease Progression

i. Decrease in platelet count day by day.
ii. Gradual progression of prothrombin time of INR. High INR in liver failure may over estimate the risk of bleeding. Its values vary from laboratory to laboratory.
iii. Gradual reduction of factor-V—since it has shortest half life, hence it is the most sensitive index of impaired clotting factor synthesis.

Pulmonary Complication

It occurs in following forms:
i. Coma with respiratory depression due to production of respiratory acidosis and hypoxia.
ii. Hypoxia may be due to intrapulmonary arteriovenous shunting.
iii. Acute lung injury—may be due to paracetamol-induced acute liver failure.
iv. Pulmonary edema—may be due to over administration of intravenous fluids.
v. Adult respiratory distress syndrome—may be the late manifestation.

Acute Pancreatitis

1. Patient may develop acute hemorrhage and necrotizing pancreatitis.
2. In 12% patient, hyperamylisemia may be developed. Of them, 9% patients develop clinical pancreatitis.
3. In comatose patient, acute pancreatitis may be very difficult to diagnose, but it may be a cause of death.

Management of Fulminant Hepatic Failure

Hepatic Encephalopathy

Since the main pathologic mechanism is due to absorption of toxic substances from intestine—which ultimately is responsible for development of cerebral edema and herniation. Level more than 150–200 mmol/L of ammonia is responsible for cerebral edema.

Symptoms and signs:
i. Sudden onset in the setting of liver disease
ii. Changes in personality
iii. Delusion
iv. Restlessness
iv. Asterixis
v. Fetor hepaticus—may be present.

Treatment:
1. Lactulose
2. Non-absorbable antibiotics—no enough evidence is found.

But in acute liver failure, lactulose may increase the risk of:
  i. Aspiration
  ii. Bowel distention.
3. L-ornithine L-aspartate (LOLA)—may increase muscle metabolism of ammonia.
4. Obtunded patient should be effectively treated by intubation for respiratory tract protection.
5. Sedative, like propofol, lowers the intracranial pressure.
6. Infection—should be effectively treated by proper antibiotics, because infection may trigger encephalopathy.

Prognosis:
i. In case of stage 1 and 2—prognosis is generally good.
ii. In case of stage 3 and 4—prognosis is poor.

Cerebral Edema

Diagnosis:
a. Invasive monitoring—insertion of ICP monitor.
  i. It is reliable in case of stage III and IV encephalopathy
  ii. It guides the management.

  In this method—the goal is:
  i. Cerebral perfusion pressure is above 50 mmHg
  ii. Intracranial pressure—below 25 mmHg
b. Non-invasive method:
  i. Infrared spectroscopy
  ii. Transcranial Doppler study
  iii. Jugular venous oxymetry

Treatment of Hepatic Encephalopathy with or without Cerebral Edema

The aim of neurological support:
i. Optimization of cerebral blood flow.
ii. Cerebral perfusion pressure optimization
iii. Decreased oxygen consumption
iv. Prevention of cerebral edema

In case of grade ½ encephalopathy:
i. Consideration regarding transfer the patient with acute liver failure to any liver transplant center.
ii. CT scan of brain to rule out other cases of decreased mental status.
iii. Avoid stimulation and sedation to prevent surge in ICP.
iv. Surveillance and proper treatment with antibiotics to prevent progress towards cerebral edema.
v. Lactulose—is helpful to prevent absorption of ammonia.

In case of grade ¾ encephalopathy:
1. Continuation the above treatment
2. Head end of the patient is to be elevated by 20° to 30°.
3. Endotracheal intubation under sedation, electric mechanical ventilation, minimal endotracheal suctioning, prevention of tactile stimulation.
4. Extradural pressure monitoring and insertion of transducer after achieving international normalized ratio of 2 or less and after giving platelet transfusion to achieve the count 50×10^9/L or more.
5. Inserted transducer should be removed within 5 days—to prevent infection.
6. Fall in cerebral perfusion pressure, difference between maximum arterial pressure (MAP) and intracranial pressure (ICP) to less than 50 mmHg must be managed properly.

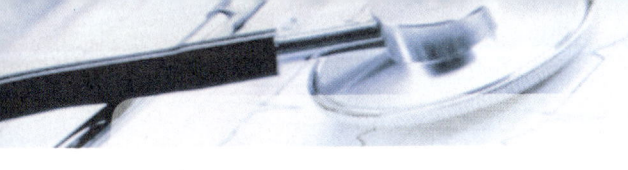

7. In presence of neurological signs or ICP of more than 25 mmHg for more than 10 minutes, bolus intravenous injection of mannitol (0.25–1 gm/kg, 20% solution) must be given immediately.

↓

This can be repeated, if the serum osmolarity does not exceed 320 mOsmol/L.

8. Renal replacement therapy should be started to remove the volume overload in the setting of renal impairment. 60% cases of intracranial hypertension responds to mannitol infusion.
9. Hyperventilation can be induced to produce:
   i. Cerebral vasoconstriction
   ii. Reduction in cerebral blood volume.
   This hyperventilation can prevent impending cerebral herniation.
10. In case of mannitol-resistant cerebral edema—following sedations can be introduced:
   i. Thiopental (5–10 mg/kg—bolus followed by 3–5 mg/kg per hour)
   ii. Phenobarbital (3–5 mg/kg bolus followed by 1–3 mg/kg per hour)
11. Intravenous indomethacin—25 mg bolus may be given in case of refractory intracranial hypertension. Risk is:
   i. Gastric toxicity
   ii. Cerebral ischemia
   iii. Renal toxicity
12. Hypothermia to 32°C–33°C—in case of:
   i. Uncontrolled increase in ICP through reduction in CBF
   ii. Uncontrolled increase in cerebral metabolism
   iii. Uncontrolled increase in glutamine synthesis

   Hypothermia prevents brain edema by following mechanisms:
   i. Decreasing arterial ammonia
   ii. Decreasing uptake of ammonia by brain
   iii. Reduction of cerebral blood flow
   iv. Re-establishment of cerebral autoregulation.

   Complications of hypothermia:
   i. Sepsis
   ii. Cardiac arrhythmias
   iii. Clotting problems.
13. Seizure activity resistant to phenytoin treatment may respond to diazepam but it should be avoided, because, it activates central gamma aminobutyric acid/benzodiazepine receptors and aggravates hepatic encephalopathy.

Treatment of Coagulopathy

The following options are:
1. Intravenous or subcutaneous vitamin K.
2. Fresh frozen plasmas, cryoprecipitate or platelets

   Indications:
   i. If INR is ≥1.5
   ii. Fibrinogen <100 mg/dl
   iii. Platelets <50000/mm³, if associated with active bleeding
   iv. Platelets <20000/mm², prophylactically
   v. Prior to invasive procedure

Blood transfusion should not be given, because it:
   i. Produces volume overload
   ii. Does not decrease the risk of bleeding
   iii. Obscures the trends of INR.
3. If fresh frozen plasma fails to correct coagulopathy, following factors can be given:
   i. Recombinant factor VII—but it can produce thrombosis.
   ii. Recombinant factor VIIa—it can be given prior to any invasive procedure.
4. Exchange plasmapheresis

Treatment of Renal Failure

1. Monitoring of fluid balance in the body.
2. Crystalloid or colloid—1 to 1.5 L—to be given rapidly to prevent prerenal azotemia.
3. Low dose dopamine infusion is not recommended because no benefit was demonstrated over other vasopressor.
4. Continuous renal replacement therapy (CRRT) with bicarbonate buffer is indicated in following conditions:
   i. Uncontrolled acidosis
   ii. Hyperkalemia
   iii. Fluid overload
   iv. Oliguria along with:
      a. Cerebral edema requiring mannitol administration
      b. Serum creatinine level >300 μmol/L

Continuous venovenous hemodiafiltration is better than intermittent hemodialysis because—hypotension may result in fall in CRP—which in turn exacerbate or precipitate cerebral edema.

Hemodynamic changes: The features of acute liver failure are:
   i. Hypotension
   ii. Decreased peripheral vascular resistance
   iii. Increased cardiac output

Possible mediators are:
   i. Nitric oxide
   ii. Prostaglandin
   iii. Tissue hypoxia producing lactic acidosis.

Treatments are the following:
1. Substantial volume of colloid or crystalloid infusion to improve cardiovascular filling pressure (pulmonary capillary wedge pressure 8 to 14 mmHg)
2. In case of hypotension refractory to volume supplementation, the vasopressor agent—should be the 1st choice—the specific aims are:
   i. Mean arterial pressure—more than 60 mmHg
   ii. Cerebral perfusion pressure—less than 50 mmHg.
      The drugs are: Epinephrine or norepinephrine
      But the drawback is—oxygen consumption will be decreased in spite of increase in arterial pressure—because oxygen delivery and oxygen extraction, both will be reduced.
      But extraction rate will be prevented by the simultaneously use of prostacycline.
   iii. Vasopressin, in absence of epinephrine or norepinephrine—may be given in patients with marked vasodilatation refractory to other drugs. The drug is terlipressin—because it is less likely to cause myocardial ischemia.

Caution: In grade IV hepatic encephalopathy—it may produce cerebral vasodilatation which in turn increases intracranial hypertension.

iv. In patient with persistent hypotension—the evaluation for adrenal insufficiency should be done.

In patient with sepsis, injection hydrocortisone 200–300 mg/day—intravenously has to be given.

Metabolic changes: Close follow up the measurements and regular monitoring of—glucose, potassium, sodium, magnesium, phosphate, metabolic acidosis.

Nutrition:
1. Daily calorie requirement—to meet resting metabolic demand—is 35–50 Cal/kg
2. Protein intake >1 g/kg required to maintain necessary nitrogen blank
3. 50% of non-protein calories are provided by lipid
4. Enteral nutrition is preferable with the aim to:
   i. Maintenance of integrity of the mucosa
   ii. Reduction in rate of bacterial translocation
   iii. Reduction in sepsis

Respiratory Complications

Management strategy include:
1. Continuous pulse oxymetry.
2. Daily chest X-ray.
3. Daily monitoring of infection.
4. If mechanical ventilation is needed, it can be administered in the form of—low tidal volume (6 ml/kg of body weight)
   +
Low positive pressure ventilation
The aims are:
   i. To minimize barotraumas
   ii. To minimize worsening of intracranial pressure

Specific Therapies

Paracetamol Toxicity

i. Toxic dose is—10 gm/day, but as low as 4 gm/day may produce hepatotoxicity.
ii. Raised aminotransferase level (3500 IU/L) and low bilirubin level—indicate paracetamol toxicity.

Treatment: N-acetylcysteine

Action: It can replete glutathione → it detoxifies toxic metabolite, N-aminoparaquinoneimine

It is active when it is administered with 10 hours of paracetamol toxicity.

It may produce benefit for 48 hours or more after ingestion.

Dose:
1. Orally—140 mg/kg—bolus dose followed by 70 mg/kg 4 hourly—for total 17 doses.
2. Intravenous injection

150 mg/kg in 5% dextrose bolus over 15 minutes
↓
50 mg/kg in 5% dextrose over 4 hour
↓
100 mg/kg over 16 hours

Toxicity—anaphylactic reaction—can be treated by:
i. Discontinuation of drugs
ii. Antihistamines
iii. Adrenaline

Mushroom Poisoning

Amanita phalloides is responsible for death in hepatic failure.
Toxic dose is—0.1–0.3 mg/kg—may produce hepatotoxicity even after cooking.

Treatment:
i. Gastric lavage with activated charcoal, if patient comes with nausea, vomiting, diarrhea after mushroom ingestion.
ii. Intravenous penicillin G—30000 to 1 million units/kg per day—it is most common antidote.
iii. Sillibinin—30–40 mg/kg/day oral or intravenous
±
N-acetylcysteine—may be of choice.

Hepatitis B

In case of serologically positive hepatitis B infection, lamivudine—100–150 mg/day.

Advantages:
i. It decreases the need for transplant.
ii. It decreases the risk of re-infection after transplantation.

Indications of antiviral therapy:
i. In HBsAg +ve hepatitis
ii. In HBsAg –ve, but anti-HBc antibody positive patients prior to organ transplantation to prevent reactivation of infection.

Herpes Simplex Virus Infection

1. It produces hepatic failure in:
   i. Immune compromised patient
   ii. Pregnant patient
2. Diagnosis:
   i. Detection of HSV DNA
   ii. Liver biopsy

Vesicular rash + high aminotransferase + immunosuppressed patient → indicates liver biopsy.

Drug of choice: Acyclovir—30 mg/kg/day
Prognosis: Poor

Autoimmune Hepatitis

1. Prednisolone—60 mg/day
2. Liver transplantation—in case of:
   i. Biopsy—multilobar collapse
   ii. Persistently elevated bilirubin
   iii. Failure to responds to steroid within 2 weeks.

Wilson's Disease

Diagnosis:
i. High bilirubin
ii. Low alkaline phosphatase
iii. High urinary copper
iv. Hemolysis

Treatment:
i. Penicillamine
ii. Trientine
   The above two drugs are ineffective in acute liver failure.
iii. Albumin dialysis
iv. CRRT
v. Plasmapheresis—or plasma exchange

The aims are:
i. To remove copper from circulation
ii. To prevent renal tubular damage

Prognosis:
1. Overall survival of grade I and II—65%
   Grade III and IV—20%
2. Transplant free survival of acute liver failure over 50% are seen in liver injury due to:
   i. Paracetamol
   ii. Hepatitis A
   iii. Pregnancy
   iv. Ischemia
3. *King's College criteria of prognostic tool for paracetamol and non-paracetamol-induced acute liver failure:* It has:
   i. Positive predictive value:
      • 80% for paracetamol
      • 70–90% for non-paracetamol
   ii. Negative predictive value—25 to 90%

Paracetamol-induced liver injury:
pH <7.30 (irrespective of grade of encephalopathy)
            Or
Prothrombin time >100 seconds (INR >7)
            and
Serum creatinine >300 mmol/L (>3.4 mg/dl)
(In patients with grade 3 and 4 hepatic encephalopathy)

Non-paracetamol-induced liver injury:
Prothrombin time >100 seconds (INR >7) (irrespective of grade of encephalopathy)
            Or
Any three of the following variables (irrespective of grade of encephalopathy):
1. Age <10 or >40 years
2. Etiology—Non-A–E hepatitis, viral hepatitis but no agent identified, halothane hepatitis, idiosyncratic drug reaction.
3. Duration of jaundice before onset of hepatic encephalopathy >7 days
4. Prothrombin time >50 seconds (INR >3.5)
5. Serum bilirubin >17.4 mg/dl (>300 mmol/L)

Clichy criteria for fulminant hepatic failure: It is based on presence of coma or confusion associated with:
• Factor V less than 20% in patients less than 30 years of age
• Factor V less than 30% in grade 3 or 4 encephalopathy

Mortality is high in above two criteria.

Other prognostic models are:
1. Factor VIII to factor V ratio
2. α-fetoprotein
3. Serial estimated prothrombin time
4. Hyperphosphatemia
5. GC-globulin levels
6. Acute physiology and chronic Health Evaluation scores APACHE II scores.
7. MELD (model of end stage liver disease) scores.

Since elevated ICP is responsible for the devastating consequences, it is necessary to measure ICP by following methods. *Four types of ICP catheters are usually used in encephalopathy:*

1. Epidural catheter—it is placed outside the dura mater. It is less invasive, so responsible for fewer complications.
2. Subdural catheter—it is placed just beneath the dura mater.
3. Parenchymal catheter—here, catheter is placed directly into the brain parenchyma.
4. Intraventricular catheter—here the catheter is placed within cerebral ventricles.

Three parameters are usually measured by ICP catheter:
1. Intracerebral pressure (ICP)
2. Cerebral perfusion pressure (CPP)
3. Cerebral oxygen consumption
   CPP = mean arterial pressure–ICP

Cerebral oxygen consumption = function of cerebral blood flow and oxygen gradient between arterial and jugular venous blood.

The goal of therapy:
1. ICP <20 mmHg
2. CPP <50 mmHg

Modified Parsons-Smith scale of hepatic encephalopathy:

Grade	Clinical feature	Neurological signs	Glasgow Coma Scale
0.	Normal	>Only seen during neuropsychometric testing	15
1.	Trivial lack of awareness shortened attention span	Tremor, apraxia, incoordination	15
2.	Lethargy, disorientation	Asterixis, ataxia	11
3.	Confusion, somnolence to semistupor, responsive to stimuli	Asterixis, ataxia, dysarthria	8-11
4.	Coma	± Decerebration	<8

Liver Transplantation

This should be considered in grade III and IV hepatocellular failure.

Survival is 20% with transplantation and 60 to 80% without transplantation.

But time for transplantation is very difficult to judge:
i. If transplantation will be done too early; lifelong immune suppression will be required.
ii. If transplantation is very late, transplantation may be unsuccessful.

Indications:
i. pH
ii. Age
iii. Etiology
iv. Time between the onset of jaundice and encephalopathy
v. Prothrombin time
vi. Serum bilirubin level
vii. Plasma factor V of less than 20% of normal

Etiology is important for grafting, because: Paracetamol-induced liver injury may be relatively well without grafting, but Wilson's disease or drug-induced liver injury require liver grafting for survival.

If there is a delay of 2 days or more between the onset of encephalopathy and finding of donor:
i. 9% will improve, and do not require transplantation
ii. 16% will die.

Contraindications:
A. Absolute contraindications:
  i. Severe infection
  ii. Malignancy outside the liver
  iii. Brain death
  iv. Severe cardiac disease
B. Relative contraindications
  i. Age over 70 years
  ii. Urgent requirement for vasopressor drugs
  iii. Under treatment for infection
  iv. Presence of psychiatric problem.

Serious neurological compromise means:
i. Fixed dilated pupil for more than 1 hour.
ii. Cerebral perfusion pressure less than 40 mmHg
iii. Intracranial pressure.

Intraoperative and postoperative care:

Intracranial pressure will be increased during dissection of liver and reperfusion of the graft

↓

The cerebral fluctuation can be prevented by veno-venous bypass grafting—but it is not routine procedure.

During this procedure, ICP monitoring is necessary for 10–12 hours post-transplant period—because if ICP will be more than 25 mmHg—it should be treated urgently.

Graft selection: In patient with stage IV encephalopathy:
i. Use of liver with incompatible blood group
ii. Use of liver with significant steatosis

The causes of primary graft non-function:
  i. Older donor age
  ii. Steatosis
  iii. ABO incompatibility

The types of graft rejections are:
  i. Primary graft non-function
  ii. Acute cellular rejection
  iii. Intrahepatic biliary strictures

Outcome:
1. Transplantation is more difficult in cirrhosis than FHF due to following factors:
  i. Cachexia
  ii. Portal venous collaterals
  iii. Adhesions
2. Mortality within 3 months of transplantation is due to following factors:
  i. If patient is critically ill before the procedure
  ii. Sepsis
  iii. Multiorgan failure before transplantation
3. Initial survival in post-transplant patient is less in acute liver failure than in cirrhosis.
4. Long-term survival is better in fulminant hepatic failure than cirrhosis.

5. Coagulation defects can be corrected by—transfusion of fresh frozen plasma and platelets.
6. In post-transplant patient for acute liver failure — if it is related to viral etiology, following outcomes may occur:
  i. If transplantation done in case of HBV-related FHF, post-transplant reduced recurrence of HBV infection than those with cirrhosis—which is HBV related.
    This may be due to clearance of HBV before this procedure.
  ii. There may be some evidences of recurrence of HIV in post-transplant patient with cirrhosis, but very little data are available regarding recurrence in FAF setting.
  iii. Recurrence of HAV infection in graft is occasionally described after transplantation for fulminant hepatic failure.
  iv. Recurrence of HEV infection is not observed in patients with organ transplantation for FHF.

Living Donor Liver Transplantation (LDLT)

This is an useful procedure, for children, where the outcome of left or left lateral lobe from living donor and whole graft from living donor is same.

But in case of adult, who requires right lobe, is more complicated.

But the main concern in this approach is—issue of informed consent from the donor in emergency situation under pressure. Because, here potential donor is unable to take a well-considered decision.

ALCOHOL AND LIVER

Absorption and Distribution

Alcohol after ingestion will be absorbed from duodenum and upper jejunum by simple diffusion.

Peak blood concentration will be achieved within 20 minutes.

Absorption of alcohol will be delayed by meal.

Alcohol absorption can be increased by increasing the concentration of alcohol.

After absorption, it will distributed in the entire highly vascular organ.
i. Brain rapidly equilibrates with the plasma level.
ii. Since alcohol is poorly soluble in lipids, hence high plasma concentration can be found in females than males.
iii. In the liver—obligatory oxidation of alcohol takes place.

Any healthy individual cannot metabolize >160–180 gm/day.

Alcohol Metabolism (Fig. 4.24)

Ratio of NADH/NAD is responsible for metabolic imbalances which is responsible for alcohol-induced fatty liver disease.

The induction of cytochrome P450 by alcohol—CYP2E1, this enzyme is responsible for hepatotoxicity by toxic metabolites of other drugs.

Accumulation of acetaldehyde in blood is mainly responsible for post-alcohol consumption flushing.

Pathogenesis

Following are the pathways through which alcohol can produce liver injury:

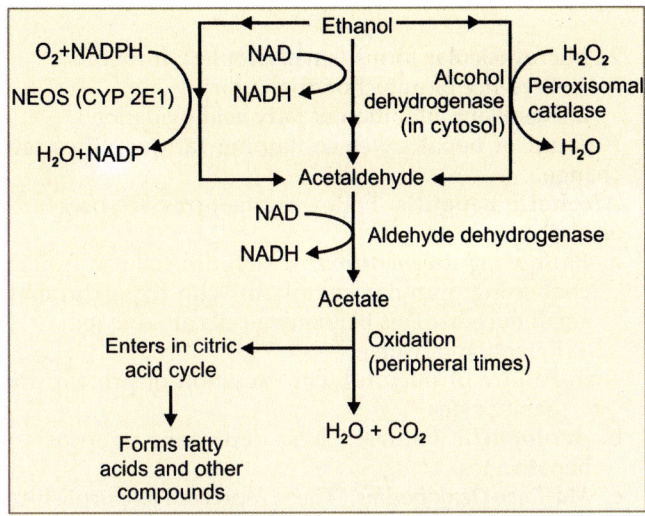

Fig. 4.24: Pathway of alcohol metabolism

Pathogenesis of Steatosis

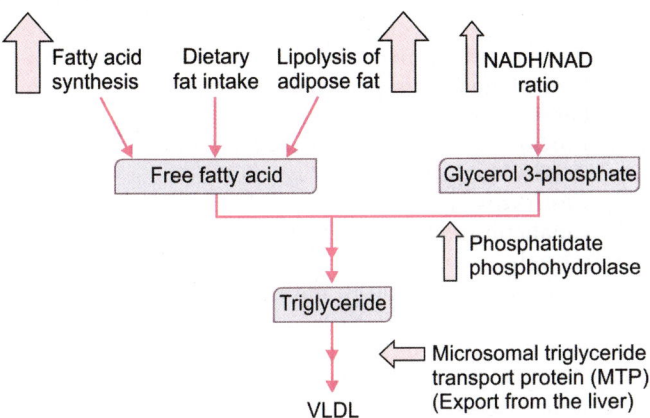

Fig. 4.25: Pathogenesis of steatosis

Hepatotoxic Effects of Acetaldehyde (Highly Toxic and Reactive)

i. Alteration of redox potential induces steatosis
ii. Induction of TNF-α-induced hepatocyte necrosis
iii. Binding of host proteins and:
  a. Formation of neoantigen
  b. Affection of microtubule function
  c. Induction of endoplasmic reticular stress—it induces:
   1. Further lipid synthesis
   2. Antioxidant depletion
   3. Ultimately apoptosis

Acetaldehyde binds to phospholipids, amino acids residue and sulphydryl groups.

↓

It unfolds protein and depolymerizes protein
↓
Accumulation of unfolded proteins in ER
↓
Production of ER stress

Oxidative stress and lipid peroxydation

1. Ethanol metabolism and activated phagocytes
↓
Generation of prooxidant
↓
Lipid peroxidation
2. Depletion of mitochondrial antioxidants in hazardous drinkers.

Endotoxins and Cytokine

{ Increased intestinal bacterial flora
Increased gut permeability
Reduced reticuloendothelial cell functions
↓
Endotoxemia
↓
Release of cytokines and reactive oxygen species from Kupffer cells
↓
Increased production of
  a. Tumor necrosis factor α
  b. Interleukin 8

TNF-α is involved in:
i. Induction of hepatic steatosis
ii. Production of reactive oxygen species
iii. Apoptosis of hepatocytes
IL-8 is involved in:
i. Recruitment of neutrophils
ii. Activation of neutrophils

Immunological Liver Damage

Protein adducts of alcohol metabolites and host protein
↓
Act as neoantigens
↓
Induction of B cell and T cell lymphocyte response
↓
Production of different antibodies against following:

i. Protein adducts derived epitopes
ii. Hydroxy-ethyl radical—CYP2E1 adducts
iii. Native CYP2E1

Role of Alcohol in Fibrosis

1. Kuffer cells proliferation and activation stellate cells
↓
Produces
  i. Transforming growth factor
  ii. TNF-α
  iii. ROS
↓
Induces collagen synthesis
↓
Induction of fibrosis
2. Hepatocytes ⟶
↓

(Contd.)

(Contd.)

Induce:
i. Production of ROS
ii. Apoptosis
Apoptotic hepatocytes
↓
Phagocytosed
↓
Activation of stellate cells

Role of Alcohol in Carcinogenesis

Alcohol produces cancer by following mechanisms:
i. Lipid peroxydation   ii. DNA mutagenesis
iii. Reduced DNA methylation   iv. Immune suppression

Following organs are involved in alcohol:
1. Mouth   2. Pharynx
3. Larynx   4. Esophagus
5. Stomach   6. Colon
7. Breast   8. Liver

Environmental Factors

A. **Alcohol:** Risk of developing alcoholic liver disease depends upon following factors
   1. Dose of alcohol—if 30 gm/day of ethanol. But significant risk develops when intake will be ≥80 gm/day.
   2. Duration of alcohol—it is usually >10 years
   3. Type of beverages:
      i. Beer and spirit intakes have higher risk than wine in-takers.
      ii. Mixed beverages have higher risk than mono-beverage
   4. Type of intakers or consumers—Daily consumers are at higher risk than intermittent consumers because in last case, liver gets opportunity to recover.
B. **Diet:** Following diets are the risk factors for ALD:
   1. High pork intake (high linoleic acid)
   2. Consumption of unsaturated fat
   3. Diet low in carbohydrate
   4. Obesity
   5. Hyperglycemia

Genetic Factors

Female are more susceptible to liver injury and more liable to relapse after treatment due to:
i. High intake of alcohol
ii. They present late stage of liver injury

Non-Gender Genetic Factors

1. Alcohol intake patterns is partially inherited.
2. Susceptibility to liver disease has a genetic component.
3. Concordance rate of ALD is three times higher in monozygotic twins than dizygotic twins.
4. Multiple polymorphism has also past contribution in ALD.

Histological Features in Liver

A. **Fatty liver:** Fat is predominantly distributed in zone 2 and 3. The fat is present in two forms
   1. Macrovesicular form (large droplet): It appears in hepatocyte within a few days of excess alcohol ingestion.
   2. Microvasicular forms (small droplet): It reflects:
      i. Presence of mitochondrial injury
      ii. Resultant inhibition of fatty acid oxidation
   Amount of hepatocytes containing fat quantifies fatty change.
B. **Alcoholic hepatitis:** Following features are present in alcoholic hepatitis
   a. *Ballooning degeneration:* It signifies cellular swelling containing granular cytoplasm with hyperchromatic small nucleus. This ballooning cells are due to:
      i. Retention of water.
      ii. Failure of microtubular excretion of protein from hepatocytes
   b. *Acidophilic bodies:* These represent apoptosis of hepatocytes.
   c. *Mallory-Denk bodies:* These represent as purplish-red cytoplasmic inclusions. Satellite of polymorph surrounds Mallory containing cells.
   d. *Giant mitochondria:* These are globular intracytoplasmic inclusions, can be seen by light microscopy.
   e. *Fibrosis:* Here collagen fibers deposit in perisinusoidal area of zone 3 enclosing normal or ballooned liver cells. As a result, porosity of sinusoidal liming will be diminished; this prevents exchange of substances between plasma and hepatocytes.
   f. *Portal zone:* Mild chronic inflammation in portal zone in advanced cases.
   g. *Cholestasis:* In all types of ALD cholestasis of bite canaliculi is a typical feature.
C. **Cirrhosis:** This is micronodular cirrhosis. Nodule formation is slow due to inhibitory effect of alcohol on hepatic regeneration.
   With the continuing hepatic necrosis and replacement by fibrosis, cirrhosis may progress from micronodular form to macronodular form.

Clinical Features

History, Examination and Early Recognition

1. For taking history regarding alcohol intake—AUDIT QUESTIONNAIRE
2. Symptoms related to digestion:
   i. Nausea
   ii. Anorexia
   iii. Diarrhea
   iv. Vague right upper abdominal pain
   v. Pyrexia
3. Symptoms related to alcohol:
   i. Social disruption   ii. Poor work performance
   iii. Accidents   iv. Violent behavior
   v. Fits   vi. Depression

Signs:
i. Tender hepatomegaly
ii. Prominent vascular spiders
iii. Associated features of CLD

Biochemical Tests

Liver Function Tests

1. Serum transaminase rarely exceeds 300 IU/L.
2. AST is usual higher than ALT with ratio 2:1.
3. Y-GT is raised—indicates heavy alcohol intake. It may be increased in other condition, like:

i. Drugs
ii. Non-alcoholic fatty liver disease
Raised YGT is due to:
 i. Enzyme induction
 ii. Hepatocellular damage
 iii. Cholestasis
Serum carbohydrate deficient transferrin level—it is a definite marker of excessive alcohol intake.
4. Serum alkaline phosphatase—It is four times the normal. It occurs in:
 i. Severe cholestasis
 ii. Alcohol-related hepatitis

Blood Levels

1. Serum IgA level—raised
2. Non-specific abnormalities are:
 • Raised:
   i. Uric acid
   ii. Lactate
   iii. Triglyceride
 • Low:
   i. Glucose
   ii. Magnesium
   iii. Phosphate
   iv. T_3 level (due to decreased hepatic conversion of T_4 to T_3)

Hematological Changes

1. Macrocytosis—due to direct effect of alcohol
2. Deficiency of folate or vitamin B_{12}—it occurs in malnourished person.
3. MCV—raised

Imaging Studies

1. **Ultrasound:**
 a. In early cases:
   i. Steatohepatitis
   ii. Early fibrosis
 b. In late cases:
   i. Shrunken liver with irregular edge
   ii. Portal hypertensions
   iii. Splenomegaly
   iv. Ascites
2. **CT or MRI of abdomen** demonstrates:
   i. Fatty liver
   ii. Irregular liver surface
   iii. Splenomegaly
   iv. Portal collateral circulation
   v. Ascites
   vi. Pancreatitis

Liver Biopsy

Indications:
 i. Staging of liver disease
 ii. To differentiate alcoholic hepatitis from decompensated cirrhosis.
 iii. To detect steatosis or steatohepatitis
 iv. To confirm cirrhosis
 v. To detect hepatocellular carcinoma
 vi. To exclude other treatable liver diseases

Clinical Syndrome

A. Fatty Liver

Symptoms:
 a. Mainly asymptomatic
 b. May present with following symptoms:
   i. Anorexia
   ii. Nausea
   iii. Vomiting
   iv. Right upper abdominal pain.
Signs:
 i. Usually not positive finding
 ii. These may be mildly enlarged smooth under from liver
Investigations:
 a. *Liver function test:*
   i. It may be normal in most of the cases
   ii. Transaminases and alkaline phosphatase may be mildly raised.
 b. *Ultrasonography:* Enlarge smooth liver can be demonstrated.

B. Acute Alcoholic Hepatitis

 a. **In most mild cases:** In asymptomatic chronic alcoholic patient with accidental detection of raised transaminase and macrocytosis—liver biopsy can only confirm it.
 b. **In more severe cases:** Patient may present with:
   i. Anorexia
   ii. Nausea
   iii. Vomiting
   iv. Weight loss
   v. Right upper abdominal pain
   vi. Fever
 Signs—tender hepatomegaly
 c. **In most severe cases:** Severe hepatic decompensation may be precipitated by:
   i. Vomiting
   ii. Diarrhea
   iii. Intercurrent infection
   iv. Ascites
   v. Hepatic encephalopathy
   vi. Bleeding manifestations
   vii. Blood pressure—low
   viii. Hyperdynamic pulse
   ix. Signs of vitamin deficiencies
   x. Gastric or duodenal erosions

C. Cirrhosis

It can present without any evidence of acute alcoholic hepatitis.
Signs and symptoms of hepatitis decompensation may be present.

Points in favor of alcoholic etiology include:
 i. History of intake of alcohol
 ii. Hepatomegaly
 iii. Extrahepatic manifestations of hazardous drinking
 iv. Splenomegaly

Extrahepatic Manifestation

1. Bilateral parotid enlargement
2. Gynecomastia, it may be complication of treatment with spironolactone

3. Testicular atrophy
4. Decline in sexual performance in men
5. Muscle wasting
6. Fall on ground followed by fracture may be due to alcohol-induced osteoporosis
7. Dupuytren's contracture
8. Signs of alcohol dependence:
   i. Loss of memory and concentration
   ii. Irritability
   iii. Hallucination
   iv. Convulsion
   v. Tremor
9. Hepatorenal syndrome
10. Cardiac abnormalities:
    i. Arrhythmia
    ii. Hypertension
    iii. Cardiomyopathy
    iv. Coronary artery disease
11. Cancer of:
    i. Oropharynx
    ii. Esophagus
    iii. Colon
    iv. Breast

Prognosis

Following histological pictures are unfavorable prognostic indicators
   i. Zone 3 fibrosis
   ii. Perivenular sclerosis
   iii. Alcohol related hepatitis
   iv. Cholestasis
   v. Pure fatty liver
   Following biochemical features are of bad prognostic indicators:
   i. Low serum albumin
   ii. Raised prothrombin time
   iii. Low hemoglobin level.
   Following signs are bad from the prognostic point:
   i. Hepatic encephalopathy
   ii. Esophageal varices
   Hepatic encephalopathy, persistent jaundice and azotemia is called as hepatorenal syndrome.

Management

General Management of Alcohol Dependence

1. Early and total abstinence from alcohol
2. Treatment of alcohol withdrawal syndrome (delirium tremens)
   i. Chlordiazepoxide—it is the first choice.
3. Less severely affected patient can receive "brief interventional counseling" from doctor.
4. More severely dependent patient may require psychiatric consultation.

Treatment of Acute Alcoholic Hepatitis

1. **Corticosteroids:** It suppresses the hepatic inflammatory response. But failure to drop bilirubin level after 7 days of therapy indicates the patient as steroid non-responders. These patients are prognostically poor.
   Maddery discriminant score for alcoholic cirrhosis/alcoholic hepatitis: $4.6 \times$ (prothrombin time of the patient—prothrombin time of control) + (serum bilirubin in µmol/L/17.1).

Table 4.8: Glasgow alcoholic hepatitis score

Items	Score		
	1	2	3
Age	<50	>50	–
White blood cell count	<15000	>15000	–
Urea (mmol/L)	<5	>5	–
Prothrombin time ratio	<1.5	1.5–2.0	>2.0
Bilirubin (µmol/L)	<125	125–250	>250

Women with ALD may survive for shorter time.
Patient with ALD and poor nutrition is most likely to die.

If the score is more than 32—it indicates poor prognosis and the patient is potential for steroid use.
   Life score for alcoholic cirrhosis/alcoholic hepatitis: $(3.10–0.101) \times$ (age in years) $+ 0.147 \times$ (albumin at day 0 in gm/L) $+ 0.0165 \times$ (evolution of bilirubin between day 0 and day 7 in µmol/L)$—0.206 \times$ (renal insufficiency, it is quoted if serum creatinine is more than 1.3 mg/dl and 0 in elsewhere)$—0.0065 \times$ (bilirubin at day 0 in µmol/L)$–0.0096 \times$ INR.
It is not known that all the alcoholic patients will respond to steroid but this score can detect the patients who will respond to steroid or not.
2. **Pentoxifylline:** It is indicated in case of steroid non-responders.
3. Protein and calorie malnutrition must be corrected.
4. **Colchicine:** It fails to show improvement in short time.

Treatment of Cirrhosis

Since treatment of cirrhosis cannot correct the disease, so, the treatment should be directed to correct the complications of cirrhosis like:
   i. Portal hypertension
   ii. Ascites
   iii. Encephalopathy

Propylthiouracil: It reduces zone 3 anoxic liver injury. But this therapy has not been accepted.

5-adenosylmethionine: It is under trial.

Phosphatidylcholine: This drug cannot show any benefit in human being.

Liver transplantation: ALD is 20–30% of all indications for liver transplantation. 5 years survival has been increased recently, but there is risk of recidivism.
   Hence ALD-related hepatitis is not an indication of liver transplantation.

NONALCOHOLIC FATTY LIVER DISEASE

Nonalcoholic fatty liver disease or "NASH"—was introduced by Ludwing, et al.
   Hepatic steatosis can be described by accumulation of fat (triglyceride, cholesterol and phospholipids) in excess of 5–10% of liver weight. But to diagnosis it, following disorders have to be exceeded:
   i. Viral hepatitis
   ii. Autoimmune liver disease

iii. Wilson's disease
iv. Hemochromatosis
v. ∝1-antitrypsin deficiency
vi. Drug-induced hepatitis
vii. Ethanol-induced liver injury.

Classification of Nonalcoholic Fatty Liver Disease

Accurate diagnosis of nonalcoholic fatty liver disease depends upon following "key" histological parameters:
i. Steatosis (mixed micro- and macrovesicular fat)
ii. Cellular ballooning
iii. Inflammation
iv. Fibrosis

Fibrosis ranges from—perisinusoidal fibrosis to bridging and fibrosis.

Working Classification of Nonalcoholic Fatty Liver Disease

Non-NAS fatty liver (NNFL)

Type-1 NAFLD: Simple steatosis without inflammation or fibrosis.
Type-2 NAFLD: Steatosis with non-specific lobular inflammation but without cell ballooning or fibrosis.

Non-alcoholic steatotic hepatitis (NASH)

Type-3 NAFLD: Steatosis with inflammation and variable degree of fibrosis.
Type-4 NAFLD: Steatosis, hepatocyte ballooning, inflammation and fibrosis or Mallory-Denk bodies.

Newer markers have been identified to diagnose the following:
i. Differentiation of NASH from NNFL
ii. Grading of NASH
iii. Severity of NASH
iv. Monitoring the response to therapy.

The newer markers (parameters) are the following:
i. Collagen-related metabolites—indicator of fibrosis.
ii. Adipocytokines—indicator of systemic fat metabolism.
iii. Insulin signaling ⎫ measures of apoptosis
iv. Cytokeratin 18 fragments ⎭ pathway activation

Clinical Features

There are two components of NASH:

A. Metabolic syndrome components (adult treatment programme III)

Risk factors	Defining level
1. Abdominal obesity	Waist circumference
Male	>102 cm (>40 inches)
Female	>88 cm (>35 inches)
2. Triglycerides	≥150 mg/dl
3. HDL cholesterol	
Men	<40 mg/dl
Female	<50 mg/dl
4. Blood pressure	≥130/≥85 mmHg
5. Fasting blood glucose	≥110 mg/dl

B. Insulin resistance

Tissue	Dysfunction
1. Liver	Failure to suppress glucose production and output by the process of gluconeogenesis and glycogenolysis.
2. Muscle tissue	Failure of glucose uptake which may be due to following reasons: i. Impairment of mitochondrial function ii. Increased myocytes iii. Increased lipid stores iv. Decreased translocation of GLUT-4 transporter.
3. Adipose tissue	i. Failure of suppression of hormone sensitive lipolysis. ii. Release of free fatty acids from triglyceride stores.

Usual age of occurrence:
i. In case of NASH—40–50 years
ii. In case of NASH-related cirrhosis—50–60 years
iii. But due to increasing obesity incidence, children may sometimes present with advanced fibrosis.

Family history: 20% patient may have family history of unexplained liver disease.

Other Disease Associations

i. Polycystic ovary syndrome
ii. Sleep apnea
iii. Small bowel bacterial overgrowth: These patients may present with vague abdominal pain:
  1. Most common presentation of NAFLD is—accidental defection of mildly elevated aminotransferase level, during routine biochemical examination.
    But the level of ammotransferase will gradually decline with progression of disease as steatosis is being replaced by progressing fibrosis.
    During this time, the patient may present with stigmata of cirrhosis, like:
    a. Firm palpable liver
    b. Cutaneous manifestations of cirrhosis like palmar erythema, spider angiomata.
  2. Sometimes cirrhosis can be accidentally diagnosed during gallbladder operation.
  3. Some patients may present with features of decompensation of previously unrecognized cirrhosis.

Other physical findings include:
i. Acanthosis nigricans: It is characterized by pigmentation with thickening of skin on prosterior neck and axillae—common in children
ii. Large dorsal pad of fat (buffalo hump)
iii. Lipodystrophy

Laboratory Investigations

1. Elevation of ALT and AST less than two times of normal. Ratio of AGT: ALT greater than 1—suggests more advanced fibrosis. This ratio is unreliable in patients on:
  i. Thiazolidinediones medication
  ii. Statin medication
2. Elevation of serum IgA levels due to:
  i. Oxidative injury
  ii. Neoantigen-induced biliary mucosal B cell response.

3. Hyperuricemia—due to:
   i. Abnormalities in ATP metabolism resulting ADP accumulation
   ii. Disposal of excessive purine.
4. Antinuclear antibodies—found in 20–30% of NASH
5. Abnormalities in thyroid hormone level
6. Abnormalities in lipoprotein profiles—hypertriglyceridemia
7. Insulin resistance measured by:
   i. QUICKI (quantitative insulin sensitivity check index) test
   ii. HOMA (homeostasis model assessment) test

Mitochondrial abnormalities may be found in NASH—which can be suspected, if there are following associations are present:
   i. Ophthalmoplegia
   ii. Neurodegenerative disease
   iii. Retinopathy
   iv. Neural deafness
   v. Severe lipomatosis

Epidemiology of NASH

1. NAFLD in responsible for one-third of cases of CLD.
2. In case of patients with abnormal transaminases levels 40–80% may be diagnosed as NASH, if there is coexisting diseases like:
   i. Obesity
   ii. Diabetes
   iii. Dyslipidemia
3. Three-fourths of type 2 diabetes patients have steatosis.
4. Incidence of diabetes in NAFLD patients is twice the prevalence of cirrhosis.

Ethnicity

Ethnicity influences the relationship between diabetes, obesity, hyperlipidemia and NAFLD. Example:
   i. African American people have significantly less steatosis in spite of prevalence of diabetes and obesity.
   ii. Hispanic American descents have high prevalence.
   iii. Northern European descents have intermediate prevalence.

   Familial association: Impaired skeletal muscle mitochondrial metabolism and insulin resistance in type 2 diabetic patient's offspring suggest genetic association.

Pathogenesis of NASH

The following mechanisms are involved in pathogenesis of NASH.

   Mechanisms of steatosis: Lipid accumulations in liver result from imbalance between overall calorie intake and overall calorie utilization.

Hepatic fat is derived from:
   i. Synthesis of new fatty acids from precursors of carbohydrate.
   ii. Uptake of circulating new non-esterified fatty acids—which is derived from adipose tissue lipolysis.
   iii. Uptake of diet-derived chylomicron remnants
   iv. Uptake of VLDL-derived LDL remnants.

Again hepatic fat can be disposed off by following mechanism:
   i. Oxidation   ii. Lipoprotein secretion, mainly VLDL
So, NAFLD results from:
   i. De novo lipogenesis
   ii. Uptake of non-esterified fatty acidy
   iii. Abnormal lipid export

Regulation of Lipid Synthesis

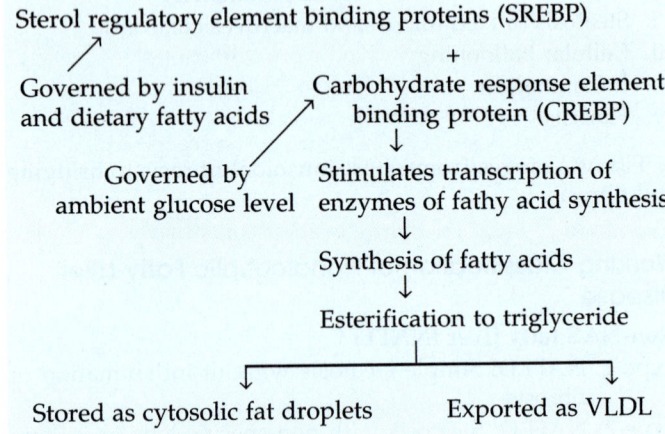

Steatosis in Human Being

In NAFLD:

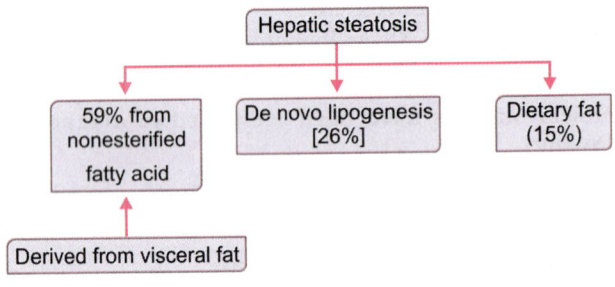

All fat will be transformed into triglyceride by the activity of acyl CoA: diacylglycerol acyltransferase 1.

Mitochondrial Dysfunction

In NASH as opposed to NNFL, mitochondria act as source of and target of prooxidant radicals (superoxide and hydroxyl radicals).
As a result, there in changes in mitochondria in the form of:
   i. Mitochondrial swelling
   ii. Presence of intramitochondrial crystals

   iii. Increase in mitochondrial cholesterol producing mitochondrial dysfunction and increased permeability.
   ↓
   Release of mitochondrial cytochrome c

Lipid Composition in NAFLD

Recent lipidemic analysis of hepatic fat shows:
1. Stepwise increase in ratio of
   i. Triacylglycerol: diacylglycerol
   ii. Free cholesterol: Phosphatidylcholine
   From Normal → NNFL → NASH patients
2. In NASH—low polyunsaturated fatty acids

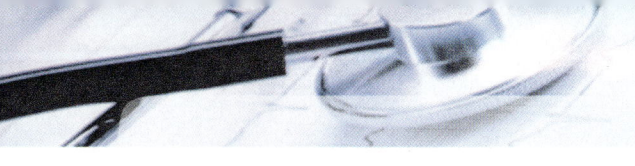

Eicosapentaenoic acid and docosahexaenoic acid.
↓
Elevated ratio of N6: N3
↓
Relative excess of proinflammatory fatty acids (arachidonic acid)

3. Increased concentration of ceramide, toxic intermediates in sphingolipid metabolism

Lipid Peroxidation in NAFLD

1. Superoxide radical derived from mitochondria
   ↓ ← Metabolized by superoxide dismutase
   Hydrogen peroxide
   ↓← In presence of Fe^{2+} via Fenton reaction
   Hydroxyl radical
   ↓
   It damages the following cellular constituents:
   i. Membrane fatty acids
   ii. Protein
   iii. DNA
2. Injury to fatty acids
   ↓
   Produces lipid peroxidation
   ↓
   Produces another free radical and lipid hydroperoxide
   ↓
   Catalyzed by iron to form lipid-based free radical

3. Oxidative injury to:
   i. Phospholipid bilayer of small fat droplet
   ii. Endoplasmic reticulum
   ↓
   Produces following events:
   i. Cellular ballooning
   ii. Disposal of toxic free fatty acids
   iii. Hepatic insulin resistance

Autophagy, Lysosomes, Fatty Acid Induced Injury and Apoptosis

Accumulated and injured fat droplets in the liver can be disposed of by lysosomes mediated autophagy

1. Impaired autophagy of small droplet
   ↓
   Accumulation of FFA
   ↓
   Leads to cellular lipotoxicity
2. Polymorphism of enzyme responsible for production of triglyceride is involved in the disposal of FFA
3. FFA → Alters the lysosomal permeability
   ↓
   Release of cathepsin (lysosomal proteases)
   ↓
   Responsible for changes in mitochondrial permeability
   ↓
   Release of mitochondrial cytochrome c
   ↓
   Activation of caspases
   ↓
   Further activation of proapoptosis pathways

Stress of Endoplasmic Reticulum, Activation of Inflammation, Fibrosis and Cellular Death

1. Activation of caspase 3
   ↓
   Fragmentation of cytokeratin 18 (this can be detectable in blood)
   ↓
   Leads to formation of Mallory-Denk bodies (in ballooned hepatocyte)
2. Accumulation of FFA and impaired function of ER associated Apo13100
   ↓
   Leads to ER stress
   and
   Accumulation of misfolded protein in ER
   Induction of proinflammatory cytokines (Interleukin 8)
   ↓
   Accumulation of inflammatory infiltrates
   and
   Activation of collagen producing stellate cells
   ↓ (Through activation of toll-like receptor)
   Fibrosis

Progression of fibrosis depends upon:
i. Altered repaired process with impaired replication of hepatocyte
ii. Increased activity of hepatic progenitor cells

Ballooning of Hepatocytes

These types of ballooned hepatocytes are associated with steatohepatitis. This ballooned hepatocyte consists of:
i. Accumulation of multiple small droplet
ii. Distorted mitochondria
iii. Dilated ER
iv. Mallory-Denk bodies

Final pathways:
i. Necrosis of cells
ii. Activation of apoptotic pathways

As a result, there is necroapoptosis of hepatocytes.

Natural History of NASH and NNFL

In early course, progression of NASH and NNFL is divergent.
But in case of NASH, progression to cirrhosis is more common and in case of NNFL, risk of hepatocellular carcinoma is similar to that of NASH.

Fibrosis of NASH can be staged in the following:
1. Stage-1   Pericentral vein or sinusoidal fibrosis zone-3.
2. Stage-2   Sinusoidal fibrosis zone-3.
             Periportal fibrosis zone-1.
3. Stage-3   Bridging fibrosis between zone 1 and zone 3
4. Stage-4   Cirrhosis
             NASH with cirrhosis.
             Cirrhosis with features suggestive of NASH
             Non specific cirrhosis (cryptogenic)

Clinical outcome of NASH will be influenced by:
i. Comorbid conditions
ii. Metabolic syndrome

But overall mortality diverges between NASH and NNFL.

Cryptogenic Cirrhosis

NASH usually progresses to cryptogenic cirrhosis with loss of hallmark of steatosis. The loss of fat may be due to following changes:

i. Sinusoidal blood flow
ii. Lipoprotein metabolism
iii. Fundamental changes in cellular metabolism

Management
Dietary Weight Loss

i. Drastic restriction of calorie may decrease the loss of fat within 11 weeks, but it is not sustainable.
ii. If the patient enters the stage of fibrosis—dietary restriction is of little value.

Fat loss from the liver depends upon:
i. Amount of weight loss
ii. Frequency and intensity of exercise
10–15% of weight reduction causes dissipation of fat from liver.

Type of Exercises

i. Structured exercise—offers some advantages
ii. Sustained exercise—improves glucose disposal from mitochondria of skeletal muscle—because it is impaired in diabetes.
iii. Exercise without weight loss—can also alter the hepatic histology.

Dietary Restriction

1. Avoidance of high fructose corn syrup—because this sweetner may aid in accumulation of triglyceride in liver.
2. Since ratio of N6–N3 is increased in NASH, hence supplementation of omega-3 fatty acids will be helpful.

Pharmacological Intervention

Pharmacological agents should be categorized into following:
1. Cytoprotective agents and antioxidants
2. Insulin sensitizers
3. Fat metabolism modulators
4. Modulators of specific intracellular pathways

Cytoprotective Agents and Antioxidants

i. Ursodeoxycholic acids—is a tertiary bile acid.
   No therapeutic benefit is seen when compared with placebo controlled trial.
ii. UDCA with vitamin E or isolatedly vitamin E may be responsible for demonstrated reduction in steatosis, but show no improvement in histological parameter in liver.

Insulin Sensitizers

Thiazolidinediones results reduction in:
i. Steatosis
ii. Inflammation
iii. Cell injury

But it has no effect on fibrosis.

It acts on PPAPγ receptor in adipose tissue and it is responsible for transfer of fat from liver to periphery.

Side effect: Peripheral weight gain.

But this side effect can be avoided, if during administration of this drug following should be continued as add on therapy:

i. Aerobic exercise
ii. Dietary modifications

Lipid modulating drugs:
A. Fibrate PPARα against it is responsible for fatty acid oxidation—it can be tried with promising results.
B. Statin—in statin treated NASH patient, level of serum aminotransferase is not a reliable indicator for assessment of drug-induced liver injury, because minor change in aminotransferase level will not lead to stoppage of statins.

Other pharmacological agents:
i. ARBS —telmisartan
ii. Grehlin—leptin pathway
iii. Antiplatelet agents—blocking profibrotic factors
iv. Agents modulating EP stress
v. Adenosine receptor blockers
vi. TNF antagonists

Bariatric Surgery

This surgery is reserved for the following:
i. Sever obesity (BMI >40)
ii. Sleep apnea syndrome with BMI >35 (obesity combined with diabetes)

Risk factors for surgery:
i. Portal hypertension in the late stage of NASH
ii. Advancing age

Liver transplantation:
1. Due to various stage of NASH at the time of diagnosis, it is very difficult to interpret the result of liver transplantation. But different comorbidities like, diabetes, obesity, may affect the procedure.
2. There may be chance of recurrence of NASH and NAFLD in liver transplant and it is progressive.

ASCITES

Definition

Collection of fluid in the peritoneal cavity is called ascites.

Etiology

A. **Portal hypertension:**
   i. Cirrhosis
   ii. Acute alcoholic hepatitis
   iii. Veno-occlusive disease
   iv. Budd-Chiari syndrome
   v. Massive liver metastasis
   vi. Congestive cardiac failure
   vii. Constrictive pericarditis
B. **Hypoalbuminemia:**
   i. Nephrotic syndrome
   ii. Protein loosing enteropathy   iii. Malnutrition
C. **Other disorders:**
   i. Myxedema
   ii. Ovarian tumor
   iii. Bile ascites
   iv. Pancreatic ascites
   v. Chilous ascites
   vi. Acquired immunodeficiency syndrome
D. **Peritoneal diseases:**
   i. *Malignant ascites:*
      a. Peritoneal carcinomatosis
      b. Peritoneal mesothelioma.

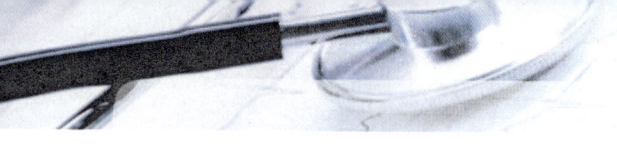

ii. *Infective:*
   a. Tuberculosis
   b. Fungal peritonitis
   c. Parasitic peritonitis
   d. *Candida albicans*
iii. *Other peritoneal diseases:*
   a. Sarcoidosis
   b. Barium peritonitis
   c. Starch granulomatous peritonitis
iv. *Vasculitis:*
   a. SLE
   b. Henoch-Schonlein purpura

Mechanism of Ascites Formation

1. Ascites will be developed when hepatic venous pressure gradient is more than 12 mmHg.
2. Ascites is unusual in case of surgical end-to-side or side-to-side portocaval shunt.

    Ascites disappears after insertion of stent and again reappears after blockage of stent.
3. Sinusoidal hypertensions—if portal pressure gradient is more than 12 mmHg.

Increased hydrostatic pressure in hepatic sinusoids:
i. Due to post-sinusoidal blockage of hepatic blood flow:
   a. Pericarditis
   b. Congestive heart failure
   c. Suprahepatic vena caval obstruction
   d. Budd-Chiari syndrome
   e. Hepatic veno-occlusive disease
ii. Due to blockage of hepatic blood flow at sinusoidal level:
   a. Cirrhosis with secondary development of regenerative nodule.
   b. Severe acute alcoholic hepatitis
   c. Fulminant or subacute viral hepatitis

Ascites will not develop in case of intrahepatic or extra-hepatic presinusoidal portal hypertension.

According to recent concept, ascites in cirrhosis will be developed from difference in permeability between hepatic and splanchnic peritoneal microcirculation.

Transmicrovascular fluid exchange in post-sinusoidal and prehepatic portal hypertension:
A. Hepatic sinusoid is lined by endothelial cells (main component), Kupffer cells and stellate cells (fat storing cells). Stellate cells together with a few collagen fibers and other particles are present in the space of Disse.

   In normal liver, there is free communication between the interstitial place of the portal and central venous area and space of Disse—here there are terminal lymphatic vessels.

   So in normal circumstances, concentration of protein in hepatic lymph is approximately 90% of that of plasma. Hence trans-sinusoidal oncotic pressure gradient in microcirculation is very low.

   In contrast, in case of splanchnic circulation, capillaries are less porous and have a basement membrane. So concentration of protein is less in splanchnic than in hepatic lymph (lymph to plasma ratio of proteins in case of intestine is 0.50, whereas 0.85 in hepatic lymph).
B. Capillary pressure in splanchnic circulation is auto-regulated but not in the liver.

Acute increase in hepatic venous pressure
↓
Completely transmitted back to hepatic sinusoids
↓
Increase in filtration coefficient in the sinusoids
Increased permeability to protein
↓
60% of acute increase in portal venous pressure
↓
Transmission back to capillary bed of small and large intestine
↓
Decrease in filtration coefficient

C. Compliance (relation between interstitial pressure and interstitial volume) is must lower in liver in comparison with intestine.
D. The presence of efficient lymphatic system in intestine is able to remove interstitial edema.

In case of Budd-Chiari syndrome and other suprahepatic portal hypertension:

Elevation in hepatic venous pressure
↓
Increased passage of fluid and protein concentration similar to that of plasma from sinusoidal lumen to space of Disse
↓
Marked enlargement of liver
↓
But due to less compliance in liver
And
Lymphatic system is less efficient to remove interstitial fluid
↓
Marked increase in interstitial pressure
↓
As a result, there is leakage of protein and lymph from liver surface into peritoneal cavity.
↓
Result is hepatomegaly and protein rich ascites.

Elevation of portal venous pressure
↓
Increased formation of lymph with **low protein** in stomach, colon, and small intestine.
↓
Formation of local edema of these organs

But there is no leakage of fluid into peritoneal cavity due to two following factors:
i. Increased filtration is rapidly counteracted by increase in oncotic pressure between capillary lumen and interstitial space.
ii. Ability of splanchnic circulation to return the excess lymph produced in stomach, small intestine or colon back to systemic circulation.

Transmicrovascular change of fluid and source of ascites in case of cirrhosis:

I. Transmicrovascular change of fluid and source of ascites in cirrhosis differ from that in presinusoidal and prehepatic portal hypertension

In cirrhosis

There is capillarization of sinusoid (continuous endothelial lining and absence of fenestra), deposition of collagen type 1 in basement membrane

↓

Decrease in permeability to albumin in hepatic microcirculation. But it varies from patient to patient **So, in cirrhotic patient**, hepatic lymph to plasma ratio for total protein ranges from 0.07 to 0.60.

II. **In cirrhosis**—there is autoregulation failure of capillary pressure and filtration coefficient in splanchnic microcirculation.

↓

Evidence of generalized splanchnic vasodilatation

↓

Forward transmission of high pressure to splanchnic capillaries

↓

Elevation of hydrostatic pressure in splanchnic capillaries

↑

Backward transmission of high portal venous pressure

↓

Fall in hepatic lymph to plasma ratio of protein (0.20 vs 0.50 to 0.60 in normal)

↓

Development of interstitial edema in all the layers of intestine.

III. **Lymph** from liver, pancreas, stomach, small intestines and colon drains into thoracic duct

↓

This drains into left subclavian vein or internal jugular vein. In normal person—thoracic duct lymph flow is 1 liter/day, whereas, in case of cirrhosis, it is about 8–9 liters/day to 20 liters/day.

It indicates large fluid filtration from hepatic to splanchnic microcirculation—then to interstitial space.

In cirrhosis, most of the fluid will be returned from lymphatic system into intravascular circulation, only less than 5% albumin leave the circulation into peritoneal cavity.

So in cirrhosis, ascites is the result of spillage of increased hepatic and splanchnic lymph formation.

Concentration of protein in ascitic fluid and thoracic duct is lower than that of hepatic lymph—it indicates significant contribution of splanchnic organ in the formation of lymph.

I. Sodium Retention

In cirrhosis, normal regulation of sodium balance will be lost. Again urinary sodium excretion is <5 mmol/day.

The net result is sodium retention even in absence of ascites.

ii. Vasodilator Theory

Increased production of nitric oxide, adrenomedullin carbon monoxide, endocannabinoids, prostacyclin, tumor necrosis factor alpha, urotensin (vasodilators).

↓

Peripheral arterial vasodilatation

↓

Decreased effective circulatory blood volume

↓

Activation of renin, angiotensin system
Activation of sympathetic nervous system

↓

Renin is produced from juxtraglomerular apparatus

↓

Angiotensinogen (produced in liver)

↓

Angiotensin I
Angiotensin-converting enzyme
Angiotensin II

↓

Stimulates secretion of aldosterone from adrenal cortex

↓

Aldosterone acts on collecting tubule
And
By cytoplasmic interaction

↓

Increased luminal uptake and basolateral passage of sodium

↓

Sodium retention

↓

Potent vasoconstriction of both venules and arteriole

↓

Stimulation of ADH from posterior pituitary

↓

Water retention ←

III. Overfill Theory

Hepatic insufficiency
Or
Sinusoidal hypertension

↓

Retention of sodium and water by kidney

Several factors has been suggested for this theory

i. Reduced hepatic synthesis of natriuretic agent
ii. Reduced clearance of sodium retaining hormone by liver
iii. 'Hepatorenal reflex' of unknown etiology.

↓

Increase in plasma volume

↓

Increase in cardiac output
Decreased systemic vascular resistance

↓

(Contd.)

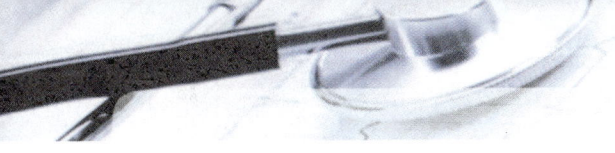

(Contd.)

Portal hypertension
↓
Overflow of fluid into peritoneal cavity
↓
Development of ascites

IV. Atrial Natriuretic Peptide (ANP)

Atrial natriuretic peptide is usually released from atria in response to expansion of intravascular volume.

In case of compensated cirrhosis, inspite of presence of antinatriuretic factors, ANP maintains sodium homeostasis.

But in case of decompensated cirrhosis, inspite of its high serum level, there is development of renal resistance; as a result, ANP will become ineffective.

V. Prostaglandins

The effective prostaglandins are PGI_2 and PGE_2.

These are responsible for maintenance of sodium and water homeostasis in following mechanisms
  i. Since they are potent vasodilators, they increase the sodium excretion through vasodilatation.
  ii. They have direct effect on loop of Henle.
  iii. They interfere with the action of ADH by inhibiting cyclic adenosine monophosphate synthesis.

But in case of cirrhosis, where there is reduced circulating blood volume, there is evidence of increased synthesis of prostaglandin.

This antagonizes the local effects of renin, angiotensin II, endothelin 1, vasopressin and catecholamines and counter-balances renal vasoconstriction.

But if NSAID will be given to cirrhotic patient
↓
Inhibition of prostaglandins
↓
Vasodilatory effect will be lost
↓
Renal blood flow will be reduced
↓
Reduction of glomerular filtration rate.

This renal dysfunction is due to unopposed vasoconstrictor action of renin, angiotensin.

Recirculation of ascitic fluid: Volume of ascitic fluid depends upon:
  i. Leakage of hepatic and splanchnic fluid into peritoneal cavity
  ii. Reabsorption of peritoneal fluid into intravascular component.

This reabsorption of ascitic fluid is done by subdia-phragmatic submesothelial lymphatic channels.

From subdiaphragmatic lymphatic channels
↓
To submesothelial lymphatic plexus
↓
Into deeper plexus of valved collecting vessels
↓

(Contd.)

Into parasternal trunk on ventral thoracic wall
↓
Into right lymphatic duct
↓
To right subclavian vein
Or
Internal jugular vein

There is constant circulation and recirculation of ascitic fluid. Rate of fluid reabsorption is 700–900 ml/day. Trans-peritoneal diffusion of water and water-soluble substances like antibiotics is very rapid in cirrhosis with ascites.

VI. Cardiac Dysfunction in Development of Ascites

In compensated cirrhosis:

Splanchnic and arterial vasodilatation
↓
Compensated by appropriate cardiac response

In the form of: i. Increase in heart rate
                 ii. Increase in left ventricular ejection fraction
                 iii. Increase in heart rate

In decompensated cirrhosis: Failure of compensatory mechanism (increase in arterial vasodilatation)—as a result—there are:
i. No increase in heart rate.
ii. Decrease in cardiac output.

So in this case, arterial pressure is solely dependent on endogenous vasoconstrictor systems:
i. Renin–angiotensin systems.
ii. Sympathetic nervous system.

The result is: There is decrease in renal perfusions and other organ perfusion—so there is sodium and water retention and ascites develops.

Clinical Features

Symptoms
  i. Increase in abdominal girth
  ii. Gradual increase in weight gain.
  iii. Gradual increase in fluid accumulation leads to:
    a. Elevation of diaphragm.
    b. Shortness of breath.
    c. Satiety.
    d. Generalized abdominal pain.

Physical Examinations

Ascites always indicates decompensated advanced stage of cirrhosis. So following manifestations are usually present.
a. Stigmata of cirrhosis:
    i. Spider nevi   ii. Palmar erythema
    iii. Muscle wasting
b. Jaundice
c. Signs of portal hypertension:
    i. Splenomegaly
    ii. Abdominal wall veins
    iii. Evidence of veins in the flanks from grain to costal margin.

(Contd.)

It may be due to: Inferior vena caval obstruction—due to secondary pressure on IVC by ascitic fluid in abdomen.

It will disappear after reduction of intra-abdominal pressure by peritoneal fluid drainage.

d. Detection of peritoneal fluid—peritoneal fluid must be at least 500 mL, so that it can be detected by normal examination:

  i. Flank fullness and flank dullness are the very sensitive signs for detecting ascites—in case of small amount of fluid

  ii. Shifting dullness—this sign is most sensitive finding as compared to abdominal distension.

  iii. Fluid thrill or fluid wave—it is less sensitive but highly specific.

e. In case of tense ascites:

  i. Liver and spleen may not be palpable.

  ii. Ballotable liver is a good indicator of ascites.

Associated Conditions

 i. **Umbilical hernias:** The factor responsible is increased intra-abdominal pressure. The hernial sites are:

  a. Inguinal

  b. Femoral

  c. Umbilical

  d. Abdominal incisions

   It may occur in 20% patient with ascites with cirrhosis. The risks of hernias are:

  a. Rupture

  b. Incarceration

   Incarceration occurs in following patients with reduction of ascites after:

  a. Paracentesis

  b. Peritoneovenous shunt

  c. Transjugular intrahepatic portosystemic shunt.

   After treatment of ascites, hernia should by repaired with permanent mesh.

ii. **Hepatic hydrothorax:** It is right-sided in 85%, left-sided in 13%, and bilateral in 2% patients.

   Cause: It usually occurs in ascites, but may occur without ascites.

   Ascitic fluid may enter into the pleural activity through a defect in the diaphragm.

   Diagnosis:

  a. Examination of ascitic and pleural fluid may not differentiate whether it may be due to local disease or may be due to hepatic hydrothorax.

  b. Intraperitoneal injection of technetium 99m-labeled sulfur colloid or macroaggregated serum albumin.

↓

   If, within 2 hours radiotracer can be detected in pleural cavity—**confirm hepatic hydrothorax.**

   Accumulation of large amount of pertinent fluid may produce discomfort. But collection of small amount of fluid (1–2 liters) in pleural cavity may produce respiratory distress.

Treatment—is usually—drainage or aspiration of peritoneal fluid.

iii. **Peripheral edema:** The factors are:

  a. Hypoproteinemia

  b. Block in inferior vena cava due to pressure of abdominal fluid.

   If edema is present without ascites—investigation should be done to detect cause.

Ascitic Fluid

Diagnostic paracentesis: Usually 30 ml fluid is recquired for diagnosis.

  i. It is a safe procedure

  ii. Very low incidence of serious complication, like, very large hematoma, which may require transfusion.

Appearance of fluid:

1. Clear
2. Green
3. Straw-colored
4. Blood-stained—indicates:

  a. Traumatic

  b. Malignancy

  c. Post-liver biopsy

  d. After transhepatic arteriography

Total protein in ascitic fluid:

High SAAG ≥1.1 gm/dl

1. Cirrhosis
2. Heart failure
3. Massive hepatic metastasis
4. Constrictive pericarditis
5. Budd-Chiari syndrome
6. Portal vein thrombosis

Low SAAG <1.1 gm/dl

1. Pancreatitis
2. Peritoneal tuberculosis
3. Nephrotic syndrome
4. Serositis
5. Peritoneal carcinomatosis

Ascitic fluid polymorphonuclear cells:

a. *If cell is >250/mm³*—indicates:

  i. Peritoneal infection

  ii. Intra-abdominal inflammatory conditions—like diverticulitis, cholecystitis

  iii. Malignancy

  iv. Subacute bacterial peritonitis.

b. *If cell is <100/mm³*—it indicates—cirrhosis—with predominance of mononuclear cells and low polymorphonuclear cells.

Ascitic fluid bacteriological culture:

1. Fluid should be sent for—aerobic or anaerobic culture. Culture is usually negative in 40% of patient with clinical features suggestive of SBP.
2. Direct inoculation of ascetic fluid into culture bottle at bed side—increases percentage of positivity.

Electrolyte concentration: Electrolyte concentration of ascitic fluid is similar to that of other extracellular fluid.

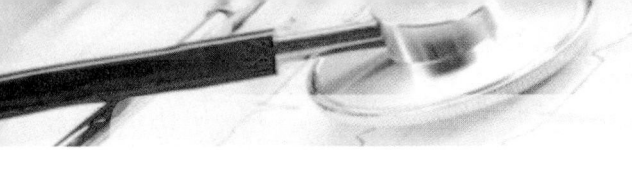

Rate of accumulation of ascitic fluid depends upon:
i. Dietary sodium intake
ii. Ability of kidney to excrete it

Radiological Features

1. Plain X-ray of abdomen
   i. Diffuse ground glass appearance of abdomen
   ii. Distended loops of bowel—looking like intestinal obstruction.
2. Ultrasound and CT scan of abdomen
   Space around the liver—it can detect very small amount of fluid.

Differential Diagnosis

A. **Malignant ascites:**
   i. Ascitic fluid protein—≤3 gm/dl
   ii. SAAG <1.1 gm/dl.
   iii. Lactate dehydrogenase or cholesterol—raised
   iv. Cytological examination is 60 to 90% accurate in diagnosis
   v. Immunocytochemical techniques—with monoclonal or polyclonal antibodies against tumor markers can differentiate malignant cells from atypical mesothelial cells
   vi. Hepatic venous pressure:
      a. WHVP—normal
      b. Free hepatic venous pressure (FHVP)—normal
      c. Hepatic venous pressure gradient (HVPG)—normal

B. **Postsinusoidal portal hypertension (cardiac failure, constrictive pericarditis):**
   i. Ascitic fluid protein >2.5 gm/dl
   ii. SAAG >1.1 gm/dl
   iii. Features of cardiac failure:
      a. Distension of internal jugular vein
      b. Edema
   iv. Features of constrictive pericarditis:
      a. Paradoxical pulse
      b. Radiological features of calcification in pericardium.
   v. Hepatic vein pressure:
      a. Wedged hepatic venous pressure—high
      b. Free hepatic venous pressure—high
      c. Hepatic venous pressure gradient—normal

C. **Tubercular ascites:**
   i. In malnourished alcoholic.
   ii. History of fever.
   iii. Palpable lump of matted omentum after paracentesis.
   iv. Ascitic fluid protein >3 gm/dl.
   v. SAAG <1.1 gm/dl
   vi. Culture of ascitic fluid for acid-fast bacilli
      a. It usually takes several weeks of incubation:
      b. It usually requires at least 1 liter of fluid for concentration and centrifugation before incubation
   vii. Deletion of DNA of *Mycobacterium tuberculosis* by polymerase chain reaction assay of ascitic fluid.
   viii. Peritoneal biopsy of the affected areas.

D. **Chylous ascites:**
   i. Presence of predominant chylomicrons, triglyceride in ascitic fluid—it is milky in color.
   ii. Causes of chylous ascites
      a. Primary abnormality in lymphatic vessels
      b. Obstruction of lymphatic systems by lymphoma
      c. Tuberculosis
      d. Sarcoidosis
      e. Pancreatitis
   iii. Triglyceride concentration >200 mg/dl
   iv. Most common non-surgical chylous ascites is cirrhosis
      It must be differentiated from: Pseudochylous ascites—where triglyceride concentration will be <110 mg/dl.

E. **Budd-Chiari syndrome:**
   i. SAAG in ascitic fluid >1.1 gm/dl
   ii. Ascitic fluid protein content is high
   iii. Ultrasonography and CT scan of abdomen showed:
      a. Inferior vena caval thrombosis
      b. Hepatic vein thrombosis
   iv. Hepatic stigmata
   v. Abnormal liver function test
   vi. Varices—in endoscopy

F. **Biliary ascites:**
   i. History of biliary surgery
   ii. Ascitic fluid color is green, exudative
   iii. Concentration of bilirubin in ascitic fluid high

G. **Pancreatic ascites:**
   i. History of acute pancreatitis
   ii. Ascitic fluid protein content is very high (>3 gm/dl)
   iii. High concentration of pancreatic enzymes (amylase) in ascitic fluid

Treatment

Indications for Treatment

1. **Symptomatic ascites**: It produces emotional and physical distress, hence requires treatment with diuretics and sodium restriction.
2. **Subclinical ascites** (diagnosed by ultrasound)—requires sodium restrictions, but if require diuretic.

   Over treatment may produce:
   i. Hypotension
   ii. Hyponatremia
   iii. Hypokalemia
   iv. Muscle cramps
   v. Dehydration
   vi. Renal dysfunction
3. **Large ascites:** Patient usually presents with abdominal distension, pain, and dyspnea. This patient requires abdominal paracentesis.
4. **Tense ascites:** It may be responsible for:
   i. Respiratory distress
   ii. Reversion and ulceration of umbilical hernia
   iii. Rupture of umbilical hernia
   iv. Shock
   v. Sepsis
   vi. Renal failure

   This patient requires urgent paracentesis.

Monitoring of Treatment

i. Daily weight measurement—to judge the progress of the treatment.
ii. Urinary electrolyte (sodium and potassium) measurement: It monitors— a. Dosage adjustment
   b. Response to treatment
   c. Complications of treatment

iii. Measurement of serum electrolytes two–three times per week
iv. Abstinence from alcohol
v. Mild case may be treated by diet alone
vi. Bed rest, because:
    a. It usually increases renal perfusion
    b. It increases portal blood flow

Diet

Patient with cirrhosis with ascites—with unrestricted sodium intake—shows:
i. <10 mmol/day (0.2 gm) in urine
ii. Extrarenal loss—0.5 gm/day
iii. Excess intake 0.75 gm/day

    1 gm sodium retains 200 ml of fluid.

So current recommendations are:
i. Use "no added salt" diet (1.5–2 gm/day)
ii. Use of diuretics in combination with above diet.
iii. Low sodium foods
iv. No addition of extra salt at the table.

Patients, who are the good responders may be:
i. Stable patient present with ascites and edema for the first time.
ii. Patient having normal creatinine clearance
iii. Patient having reversible liver disease like alcoholic hepatitis
iv. Patient in whom, some complications like infection, bleeding may precipitate ascites acutely.
v. Patients in whom, ascites is due to excessive sodium intake.

Diuretics

Increased renin–angiotensin activity and hyperaldosteronism are responsible for sodium retention and ascites. So diuretics are of choice. This diuretic has been divided into two main groups:
1. **Drugs inhibiting Na$^+$:K$^+$: 2Cl$^-$ (NKCC 2) cotransporters in ascending limb of loop of Henle are frusemide, bumetamide.** But these loop diuretics alone are inappropriate for treating ascites. Because remaining sodium in DCT and CT is reabsorbed by aldosterone due to hyperaldosteronism. So aldosterone antagonist should be given in combination with loop diuretics.
2. **Aldosterone antagonist**—spironolactone—amiloride, triamterine (inhibitors of sodium channel): These drugs prevent sodium absorption from distal tubule and collecting ducts. Since these drugs are potassium conservative, hence potassium supplement is not necessary.

    Moreover, this group of drug is of first choice in cirrhotic ascites.

Two therapeutic approaches:
A. *Spironolactone alone:*

Starting dose 50–100 gm/day
↓
If insufficient response after 3–4 days
(Weight loss <300 gm/day)
↓

(Contd.)

(Contd.)

Dose to be increased 100 gm/day at every 4th day up to 900 gm/day
↓
Lack of clinical response
↓
Check urinary sodium
↓
If the value is high
↓
Prevent the patient from taking high sodium in diet.

[**Caution:** Prevention of hyperkalemia]
B. *Combination of loop diuretics and spironolactone*
    Indications:
    i. If sufficient clinical response or no response to spironolactone alone (200 mg/day)
    ii. Presence of hyperkalemia
        Spironolactone—100 mg/day
        and
        Frusemide—40 mg/day

But in these patients, following monitoring are necessary:
• Daily weight recording is must.
• Daily ascitic fluid reabsorption—700–900 ml/day

    But if 2–3 liters/day diuresis occurs: Most of the fluid will come from:
    a. Edema fluid
    b. Intravascular component
    Sometimes, weight loss will be more than 2 kg/day, if there is presence of edema.

If it is continued even after disappearance of edema
↓
It may be responsible for renal dysfunction.

    So, recommendation is—daily weight loss 0.5 kg/day to maximum 1 kg/day.
    So, it is better to make weight loss of 0.5 kg/day to 1.0 kg/day in patient with edema.
    Administration of albumin along with diuretic increases natriuresis, but it is expensive.
    Long-term spironolactone may be responsible for painful gynecomastia. In this case—10 mg/day amiloride can be the replacement, though it is less effective.

Caution before diuretic therapy

1. 24 hours urinary excretion of sodium
↓
It is greater than prescribed dietary sodium intake
↓
The patient is non-complaint with sodium restriction.

2. Concomitant use of NSAID, and ACE inhibitor or ARBs.

Failure to respond to diuretics:
i. Patient with hepatocellular dysfunction
ii. Poor prognosis without liver transplantation

In those cases: Diuretics have to be withdrawn because of:
i. Hypotension
ii. Encephalopathy
iii. Intractable uremia

Complications:
1. *Rise in urea and creatinine:* This may occur due to:
   i. Contraction of extracellular volume
   ii. Reduced renal circulation (prerenal azotemia)
   iii. Hepatorenal syndrome

   Treatment:
   i. Reduction of diuretic therapy
   ii. Administration of plasma expansion with albumin
2. *Encephalopathy:* It usually occurs as a result of profound diuresis—it may be associated with:
   i. Prerenal azotemia
   ii. Hypokalemia
   iii. Hypochloremic acidosis.
3. *Hyperkalemia:* According to level of serum potassium, dose of spironolactone will be adjusted. If the level is not dangerous, loop diuretics can be added.
4. *Painful gynecomastia:* Since it is a complication of spironolactone, the dose of this drug should be reduced or can be replaced by amiloride.
5. *Muscle cramps:* It is a common complication of diuretic therapy:
   i. In this case, dose of diuretic should be adjusted
   ii. Quinine sulphate—300 mg at night

Follow-up advice:
1. Low sodium diet
2. Abstinence from alcohol
3. Bathroom scales have to be used to measure daily weight at same time of the day in nude or in same cloth.
4. Record of daily weight.
5. Dose of the diuretics should be adjusted according to
   a. Degree of ascites
   b. Severity of liver disease
6. Combination of spironolactone—100 to 200 mg/day

Or
Amiloride—10–20 mg/day
and
Frusemide—40–80 mg/day

7. Indications of improvement:
   a. Improvement in liver functions test
   b. Resolution of edema
   c. Resolution of ascites

Therapeutic Abdominal Paracentesis

Indications:
   i. Diuretic resistant ascites;
   ii. High dosage diuretic-related complications
   iii. Mobilization of ascitic fluid with diuretics is a slow process.

Advantages of therapeutic paracentesis:
   i. Considerable shortening of hospital stay.
   ii. Reduces the cost of treatment.
   iii. Reduces the incidence of complications.

Types of therapeutic paracentesis:
   i. Repeated large volume (4–6 liter/day) paracentesis until complete disappearance of ascites.
   ii. Total paracentesis—total removal of ascites in one session.

Advantages of total paracentesis:
   i. It is faster method of removing ascitic fluid
   ii. Reduction in incidence of complication.
   iii. Risk of leakage of ascitic fluid through punctured site is less—because very small amount of fluid will be left in abdomen.

Indication of total paracentesis: When flow of fluid through catheter will be intermittent inspite of mobilization of cannula within the peritoneal cavity even after mobilization towards left side.

Fate of peripheral edema after paracentesis: Mobilization of fluid from peripheral edema into abdominal cavity after total paracentesis will occur within 2 days of treatment.

Most of the pedal fluids will move into peritoneal cavity that is why, repeat paracentesis may be required.

To prevent leakage of fluid from punctured site—patient should be turned into opposite side of the drainage.

Postparacentesis without plasma expander administration:
a. No major changes in circulation like:
   i. Arterial pressure
   ii. Pulse rate
b. No change in serum creatinine.
c. No change in serum electrolytes.

Immediately after paracentesis—circulatory changes are:
a. Increase in cardiac output
b. Increase in stroke volume
c. Reduction in cardiopulmonary pressure
d. Suppression of renin–angiotensin system

Above changes will persist for 12 hours due to following factors:
   i. Reduction in intrathoracic pressure
   ii. Increase in venous return

The above events are followed by—opposing hemodynamic changes:
a. Reduction in cardiac output
b. Activation of renin–angiotensin system
c. Activation of sympathetic nervous system

Similarly—there will be improvement of renal function immediately after paracentesis followed by worsening of functions.

But according to different studies—there will be deterioration of circulatory function after paracentesis—it is mainly due to increased circulating levels of vasoconstrictors—angiotensin II and noradrenaline—these vasoconstrictors act by following mechanisms:
   i. Impair renal hemodynamics
   ii. Impair renal response to diuretics
   iii. Induce intrahepatic vasoconstriction, thus it:
      a. Reduces hepatic perfusion.
      b. Impairs hepatic functions.
      c. Increases portal pressure.

Administration of plasma expanders during paracentesis:
1. When ascitic fluid will be removed >5 liters—salt poor albumin 20% to be infused. At a rate of 6–8 gm/L of ascitic fluid.

   50% albumin has to be infused immediately after paracentesis and rest 50% of albumin to be infused after 6 hours.
2. When paracentesis is less than 5 liters—less costly plasma expander like polygeline (saline solution, 8 gm/liter fluid removed), dextran 70 (dextrose at solution 8 gm/liter fluid removed) can be used.

Refractory Ascites

Refractory ascites can be characterized by the following:
i. Ascites that cannot be mobilized.
ii. Where early recurrence cannot be prevented by medical therapy.

Refractory Ascites—Types

a. Diuretic resistant type: In this type, ascitic fluid cannot be mobilized in spite of maximum diuretic dosage (spironolactone 400 mg/day along with frusemide 160 mg/day)
b. Diuretic intractable ascites: This type of refractory ascites may be developed that preclude the use of effective dose of diuretics due to development of diuretics-induced complications as a result of increasing dose of diuretics—which are:
   i. Hepatic encephalopathy
   ii. Increased level of serum creatinine to a value of >2 mg/dl.
   iii. Decreased level of serum sodium to <125 mg/L.
   iv. Decrease in serum potassium level to <3 mg/L.

Recidivant ascites: This type of ascites develops in three or more occasions in 1 year period inspite of dietary sodium restriction and maximal diuretic dosage.

Most Important Mechanisms of Refractory Ascites

a. Inability of the diuretics to act on the effective sites on the tubular cells—owing to renal hypoperfusion.
b. As a result of reduced GFR and excessive sodium reabsorption, reduced amount of sodium will be delivered to ascending limb of loop of Henle and distal tubule. But one has to rule out the following factors during the diagnosis of refractory ascites:
   i. Inadequate sodium restriction
   ii. Use of NSAID

Treatment of Refractory Ascites

1. First line therapy : Serial therapeutic paracentesis Relapse is the rule.
2. Second line therapy : Transjugular intrahepatic portosystemic shunt
When:
   • Paracentesis >1 to 2/month
   • MELD (model for end stage liver disease) >15
3. Third Line : Peritoneovenous shunt—for candidates of non-LVP (large volume paracentesis) non-TIPS.

Treatment Options of Refractory Ascites

1. Large volume paracentesis (LVPs)
2. Transjugular intrahepatic portosystemic shunt (TIPs)
3. Peritoneovenous shunting—LeVeen shunt
4. Liver transplantation

1. Large volume paracentesis: Repeated large volume paracentesis every 2–4 weeks followed by reintroduction of diuretic treatment is the method—addition of diuretic lengthens the time of occurrence.

Advantages:
   i. It is inexpensive.
   ii. It is easy to perform.

   Drawback: It does act on the factor responsible for ascites formation.

2. TIPS: Side-to-side portacaval shunt is the treatment of choice in the management of refractory ascites. It usually corrects two principal factors responsible for the development of ascites. TIPS:
   i. Suppresses the endogenous vasoconstrictor system
   ii. Improves renal perfusion
   iii. Improves GFR
   iv. Increases the responses to diuretics
   v. Decompresses the splanchnic circulation
   vi. Decompresses the hepatic microcirculation—which may precipitate hepatic encephalopathy in absence of other factors.

Effects on cardiovascular systems: Since TIPS increases venous return due to presence of portacaval fistula—as a result:
   i. Increase in cardiac output
   ii. Decreased systemic vascular resistance
   iii. Elevation of right atrial pressure
   iv. Elevation of pulmonary artery pressure
   v. Elevation of pulmonary wedge pressure.

   In patient with cirrhosis with ascites, arterial pressure is maintained by:
   i. Over activity of renal angiotensin system
   ii. Sympathetic nervous system
   iii. Antidiabetic hormone.

   But in care of TIPS—there is vasodilatation associated with marked suppression of renin, noradrenaline, antidiuretic hormone. There is also impairment of renal circulation, but increase in urinary sodium excretion.

   40% cirrhotic patients after TIPS develop hepatic encephalopathy—this can be treated by:
i. Standard therapy
ii. Decreasing shunt size

Mortality:
   i. Early mortality (within 30 days of TIPS insertion)—is 12%.
   ii. Late mortality is 40%.

3. LeVeen shunt: Here a plastic intra-abdominal tube with multiple holes is placed in abdominal cavity. This type is connected through one wave pressure sensitive valve to another tube, which passes through subcutaneous tissue in the neck into internal jugular vein.
Tip of the tube will enter in superior vena cava near right atrium.

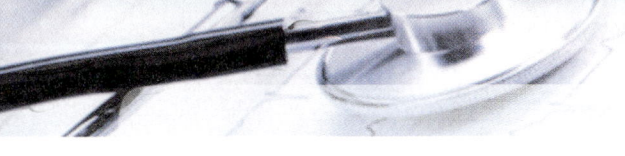

Caution:
  i. Drainage of most of the ascitic fluid before the tube to avoid massive passage of ascitic fluid into systemic circulation and produces:
    a. Pulmonary edema.
    b. Variceal hemorrhage.
    c. Severe intravascular coagulation.
  ii. Administration of prophylactic anti-staphylococcal antibiotic before and after surgery.

Advantages:
  i. Shunt expands the intravascular volume due to continuous passage of ascitic fluid from abdominal cavity into systemic circulation.
  ii. There is marked suppression of renin, norepinephrine and ADH.
  iii. There is increased response to diuretics

Complications:
  a. Obstruction in the cavity of shunt due to:
    i. Deposition of fibrin in the valve or around the catheter
    ii. Thrombotic obstruction of the venous limb of prosthesis
    iii. Thrombosis of superior vena cava.
  b. Long-term complication—small bowel obstruction—due to development of intraperitoneal fibrosis.

In case of obstruction of shunt, reoperation is needed.

AUTOIMMUNE HEPATITIS

Autoimmune hepatitis can be defined clinically, serologically as well as histologically as:
  i. Chronic relapsing hepatitis
  ii. Plasma cells infiltrate
  iii. Hypergammaglobulinemia
  iv. Positive autoantibodies
  v. Exclusion of:
    a. Negative viral studies
    b. Inherited metabolic disease
    c. Intake of over the counter drugs.

Determinants of the Disease

Hepatic immunological tolerance can be determined by the following:
  i. Priming of antigen in liver
  ii. Induction of sinusoidal tolerance
  iii. Regulatory T cell induction
  iv. Hepatic stellate cell-induced apoptosis of T cells

The loss of above tolerances due to interaction of different events is collectively responsible for hepatic injury.

Immunology

Following factors interact to develop loss of tolerance:
1. Genetic predisposition—related to HLA locus
2. Changes in T-regulatory cell function
3. Immune restricted response to autoantigens

Microscopical Findings

Portal mononuclear infiltrate involving the surrounding parenchyma to a variable degree is called interface hepatitis. The cells involve:

  i. Lymphocytes
  ii. Plasma cells
  iii. Macrophages.

This immune-mediated injury is done by:
  i. Cellular-cytotoxicity
  ii. Antibody-dependent cytotoxicity

The affected patients demonstrate:
  i. Reduced number of peripheral tags
  ii. Decreased proliferative activity in response to antigen.

In Type 2 Autoimmune Hepatitis

  i. Presence of LKM antibody titers correlates with Treg numbers.
  ii. Monocytic cell activation—may be responsible for chronicity.[1]

Three types of lymphocyte cells are responsible for interaction to produce this hepatitis. These are Th1, Th2, and Th17.

The actions these lymphocytic cells are following:
  i. Th1:
    a. It enhances expression of HLA—Class I antigen.
    b. It induces expression of class II molecules on hepatocyte.
  ii. Th2: It is responsible for autoantibody production through stimulation of B lymphocytes.
  iii. Th17: It is important for organ specific autoimmune inflammation.

Relation with HLA

In European and North American Caucasian people, the susceptible loci are:
  i. HLF A1-B8
  ii. HLA-DR 1*0301
  iii. HLA-DRB1*0401

Six amino acid sequence of 67–72 position of DRβ chain of class II molecules of MHO are encoded by HLA-DRB1*0301, HLA-DRB1*0401. Lysine of position DRB71 is the key[2].

Again, presence of HLA-DRB1*03 is associated with failure to respond to therapy in AIH.[3]

In different parts of the world, there are prevalence of above HLA loci, which are associated with AIH:
  i. In Japan, Argentina HLA-DR1*0405
  ii. In Brazil—HLA-DRB1*1301 and DRB3*1
  iii. In Mexican—HLA-DRB1*0404

Association with Non-HLA Loci

  i. Presence of autoimmune disease in any family—supports the contribution to the disease.
  ii. Genetic defect in autoimmune regulator type 1 (AIRE-1)—which is responsible for autoimmune polyglandular syndrome type 1.

Relation with Environmental Factors and Drugs

The following environmental factors may be the triggering factors:
  i. Nutritional supplements
  ii. Herbal chemical components
  iii. Drugs
  iv. Viral infections

Drugs may be responsible for:
  i. Immunologically medicated disease
  ii. Cholestatic liver disease

The bioactivated metabolites of the drugs produce:
a. Interaction with cellular macromolecules
b. Disruption of cellular signals

The result will be mitochondrial dysfunction.

In Immunologically Susceptible Individual

Apoptotic hepatocytes which contain the drug hapten—cytochrome P450—UDP glucuronosyltransferase complexes, are responsible for loss of tolerance, because they represent as autoantigen.[4]

In some cases:

Drugs bind to T cell receptors
↓
Mimic ligand receptor interaction
↓
Activation of MHC dependent T cell
↓
Production of AIH

Viral triggers: This can be evidence from the following:
 i. History of viremic symptoms prior to development of hepatitis.
 ii. Antigenic similarities between viral proteins and self proteins—which is responsible for autoimmunity.
 iii. Presence of inflammatory cytokines during viral infections.[5]

Clinical Presentation

AIH occurs in all ages and all sexes throughout the world, there are two types of AIH (Table 4.9):
 i. Type-I AIH
 ii. Type-II AIH

Symptoms and Signs of AIH

The patient may present with:
 i. Jaundice
 ii. Fatigue
 iii. Arthritis
 iv. Acne
 v. Amenorrhea
 vi. Anorexia
 vii. Nausea

Signs
 i. Hepatomegaly
 ii. Splenomegaly (here liver may not be palpable)
 iii. Features of liver failure as peripheral signs:
   a. Palmar erythema
   b. Telangiectesia

Other Disease Association
 i. Sjorgen's syndrome
 ii. Autoimmune rheumatoid arthritis
 iii. Autoimmune hemolysis
 iv. Autoimmune thyroid disease
 v. Ulcerative colitis
 vi. Idiopathic thrombocytopenic purpura
 vii. Celiac disease

In case of liver transplant:
 i. It can occur as alloimmune hepatitis.
 ii. It can recur in transplant which has been done for AIH.
 iii. There may be allograft dysfunction—mimicking autoimmune hepatitis.

Laboratory Features

A. **Liver biochemistry** (Fig. 4.26):
 1. *Aspartate transaminase:*
   i. <2 times upper limit of normal 10% patients
   ii. 2–10 times upper limit of normal in one-third of patients
   iii. >10 times upper limit of normal in half of the patients
 2. *Raised alkaline phosphatase:* If it is greater than 3 fold of normal—biliary investigation should be done.
 3. *Bilirubin*—raised

Table 4.9: Comparison of clinical presentation and serology in two types of hepatitis[6]

Item	Type-I	Type-II
1. Prevalence	>80% in western world	20% in Europe, 4% USA
2. Presence of autoantibodies	i. Antinuclear factor ii. Antismooth muscle cell antibody	i. Anti-liver kidney microsomal type-1 antibody
3. Age	i. Peak age—16–30 years ii. 50% patients are >30 years	i. Common in 10 years of age ii. In Europe, adults are affected
4. Sex preponderance	70% are female	Females are mainly affected
5. Other disease association	i. Thyroid disease ii. Synovitis iii. Ulcerative colitis	i. Diabetes ii. Thyroid disease iii. Vitiligo iv. Pernicious anemia v. IgA deficiency
6. Presentation	i. Slow insidious onset	i. Acute onset (bridging necrosis) ii. 30% cases silent, may present with chronic hepatitis or cirrhosis
7. Response to treatment	Response is excellent	Resistant to treatment.
8. Disease progression	i. 25% patients present with cirrhosis at presentation ii. 45% patients develop cirrhosis in later life.	i. 80% patients develop cirrhosis

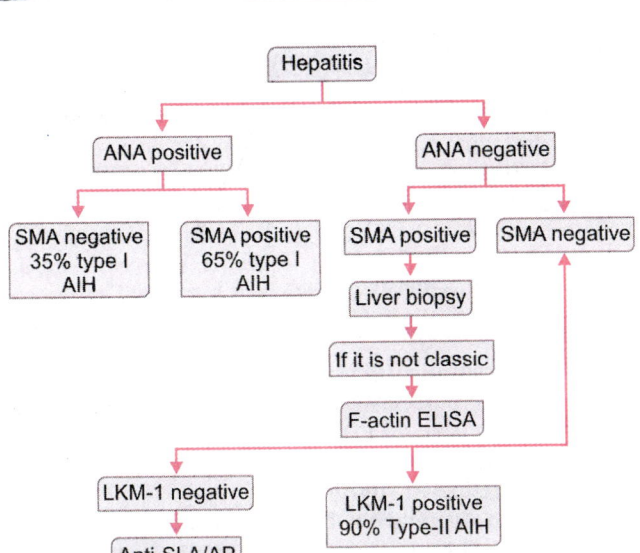

Fig. 4.26: Algorithm of diagnosis of autoimmune hepatitis

4. *Albumin*—low
5. *Prothrombin time*—low
B. **Evidence of hemolysis:** Investigations for Wilson's disease.
C. **Immunoglobulin:** IgG values—1.2–3 times of upper limit of normal
D. **Serology:**
   1. In type II AIH—i. ANA, ii. SMA
   2. In type II AIH—Anti-LKM-1 antibodies
   3. Usual titers of autoantibodies:
      i. 1 in 40 to 80 may be present in healthy individual. Titer may be increased in older age.

ii. Lower titer ≥ in 20 is significant in children.

Imaging Studies

It is useful for excluding:
   i. Budd-Chiari syndrome
   ii. Infiltrative disease
   iii. Unsuspected biliary abnormality

   Doppler ultrasound is the procedure of choice because it provides no radiation.

In acute or subacute hepatic failure, it can detect:
   i. Gross architectural collapse
   ii. Splenomegaly
   iii. Ascites

   MR cholangiography—to detect sclerosing cholangitis—because in childhood AIH, there may be overlap of biliary abnormalities.

   But careful interpretation is needed because in cirrhosis also there is biliary architectural distortion.
Periodic imaging is necessary to detect:
   i. Changes in spleen size
   ii. Increase in ascites.
      Because, it may necessitate variceal surveillance.

Liver Biopsy

Indications:
1. To identity the features of AIH
2. To exclude alternative liver disease
3. To estimate fibrosis
4. To predict the outcome of treatment
5. To confirm resolution of histological activity before stopping steroids.

   It is to be noted that histological activity lags behind the biochemical activity by 3–6 months.[7]

Name	Target site	Association with disease
Table 4.10: Following antibodies may be associated with AIH		
Origin from nuclei		
1. Antinuclear antibody	i. Nuclear membrane	i. Type I AIH
	ii. DNA	ii. Primary biliary cirrhosis
2 Histones	i. Nucleosomes	i. Type I AIH
		ii. PBC
3. P. ANCA	Neutrophil granules	i. Type I AIH
		ii. PBC
		iii. PSC
Microsomal origin		
LKM-1	Mitochondrial CYP 450 2D6	Type II AIH
Mitochondrial origin		
AMA	Antigen of inner-mitochondrial membrane	i. PBC
		ii. AIH
Smooth muscle		
1 SMA	i. Fibroblast actin	i. Type I AIH
	ii. Tubulin	ii. PSC
	iii. Intermediate filament	iii. PBC
2 Actin	i. Fibroblast actin	i. Type I AIH
Cytoplasmic origin		
1. SLA/LP	i. UGA repressor tRNA associated protest	AIH
2. Liver cytosol-1	i. Forminiotransferase cyclodeaminase	Type II AIH

Histological Features

These includes:

1. Lymphoplasmacytic interface hepatitis—evidence of mononuclear cell infiltrations invading the limiting plate.
2. Lobular hepatitis
3. Centrilobular necrosis

No specific feature will be present in autoimmune hepatitis. From history, viral and drug-induced liver injury has to be excluded.

Grading of AIH According to Histological Findings

1. Typical:
   i. Interface hepatitis: Lymphocyte/lymphoplasmacytic infiltrates in portal tract, extending into lobules
   ii. Emperipolesis—active penetration of one cell into and through a larger cell.
   iii. Hepatic rosette formation
   All the above features must be present in this grade.
2. Compatible with AIH: Chronic hepatitis with lymphocytic infiltration
3. Atypical: When signs of other diagnosis like, steatohepatitis, is present.

Biliary Lesions

In 10% of cases—it shows:
i. Bile duct destruction
ii. Lymphocytic infiltration of bile duct epithelium without ductopenia.[8]

It may be seen:
i. PBC or
ii. AIH—PBC overlap syndromes

So, all futures including clinical presentation, severity of underlying liver disease—should be considered to diagnose it as a case of AIH.

Evidences of Fibrosis

Fibrosis is always present, but with the progression of disease, following histological pictures are evidenced:
i. Periportal fibrosis
ii. Portal–portal bridges
iii. Portal–central bridges
iv. Nodular regeneration
v. Massive hepatic necrosis—which may be mistaken as cirrhosis.

Changes in Liver Cells

Following are evidenced:
i. Ballooning degeneration of hepatocytes
ii. Spotty hepatocyte necrosis
iii. Apoptotic bodies.
iv. Syncytial multinucleated hepatocyte giant cells seen in giant cell hepatitis, more common:
   a. Children
   b. Paramyxovirus infection
   c. Human herpes virus infection
   d. Occasionally in primary biliary cirrhosis
   e. Drug-induced liver disease

Drugs Involved in Autoimmune-Like Hepatitis

1. Minocycline
2. Nitrofurantoin
3. Statins
4. Indomethacin
5. Ramipril
6. Orlistat
7. Dihydralazine
8. Methyldopa
9. Halothane
10. Interferon-α

Dilemmas in Diagnosis (Table 4.11)

Autoantibody Negative Hepatitis

1. In ANA, SMA and LKM-1 antibody negative hepatitis, highly specific anti-SLA/LP antibody estimation should be considered.
2. Presence of ANA or SMA does not correlate with disease severity of AIH.
3. There is no correlation between antibody status and response to immunosuppressive therapy.
4. There is positive correlation between degree of hyper-gammaglobulinemia and disease severity of AIH.

Viral Hepatitis

In HBV or HCV hepatitis—there are evidences of various autoantibodies, not always in low filer (1:20 to 1:40).[9]

LKM-1 antibodies are present in 50–80% of German population and 1% western European population with HCV hepatitis.

Homology between cYP450 206 and HCV viral genome suggests molecular mimicry. Again patient with HCV hepatitis, if contains LKM-1 antibodies, this LKM-1 antibodies have less serological reactivity to recombinant CYP450 206. But if the patient is HCV negative, this LKM-1 antibody has high serological reactivity.

Hence, it has proved that LKM-1 antibodies in two types of patient are different.

It suggests, HCV and LKM-1 positive patient can be treated by interferon without any harm.

Table 4.11: Criteria for diagnosis of AIH

Items	Cut off	Points	Cut off	Points
ANA or SMA	>1:40	1	>1:80	–
LKM-1	–	–	>1:40	2
SLA	–	–	Positive	
IgG	>Upper limit of normal	1	>1.1 x Upper limit of normal	2
Histology	Compatible	1	Typical	2
Absence of viral hepatitis	–	–	yes	2

Additional points to be achieved for all autoantibodies—maximum 2 points:
Probable AIH ≥6 points
Definite AIH ≥7 points

Management of Autoimmune Hepatitis

Absolute Indications

1. Serum transaminases ≥10 times of upper limit of normal
2. Serum transaminases >5 folds, plus serum IgG >2 folds

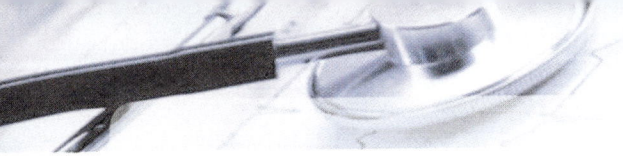

3. Histological evidence of multiacinar or bridging necrosis.

A. Table showing prednisolone (high dose therapy)

Weeks	Steroid with dose (prednisolone)
1st week	60 mg
2nd week	40 mg
3rd week	30 mg
4th week	30 mg
Maintenance till the end point	20 mg

B. Table showing initial monotherapy with prednisolone followed by addition of azathioprine

Week	Prednisolone	Azathrioprine
1st week	20–30 mg	x
2nd week	20–30 mg	x
3rd week	20–30 mg	x
4th week	20–30 mg	1–2 mg/kg if i. Patient is responding ii. Bilirubin <100 µmol/L
Maintenance	Tapering of the dose of steroid to 5–10 mg/day for 1 year	

Guidelines for maintenance dose:
i. Liver function test will be normal
ii. Serum IgG will be normal

Prednisolone dose should be decreased by 2.5–5 mg every 2–4 weeks.

C. Table shows combination therapy (prednisolone and azathioprine)

Week	Prednisolone	Azathioprine
1st week	30	50
2nd week	20	50
3rd week	15	50
4th week	50	50
Maintenance	10	50

Pretreatment during Steroid Alone/Plus Azathioprine Therapy

1. Stool for ova, parasites
2. Serum calcium and vitamin D estimation followed by supplementation
   i. Calcium 1000–1500 mg/day
   ii. Vit D_3—1000 IU/day
3. Calculation of bone mineral density with or without bisphosphonate prophylaxis.
4. Checking of blood pressure regularly and if blood pressure is present—antihypertensive.
5. Monitoring of blood glucose, and if required therapy.
6. Regular eye check up to see any evidence of cataract.
7. Prevention of infection, vaccination if required.
8. History taking to see any evidence of previous HBV hepatitis.
9. If treatment has to be given according to CAB status.

Discontinuation of Treatment

There is no concencious how long to treat particularly with azathioprine once prednisolone has been withdrawn.

Following factors predict the relapse:
1. Failure to maintain normal transaminase level during the course of therapy
2. Time of initial biochemical remission.
3. High immunoglobulin level
4. Marked plasma cell infiltration around portal areas

Relapses are less likely in following conditions:
1. Normal transaminase
2. Normal IgG.

Duration of treatment preceding withdrawal of prednisolone is main factor for predicting relapse.

If relapses, the patient responds quickly to same steroid. But this patient is at increased risk of relapse, if the steroid will be withdrawn.

In case of relapse:
1. Prednisolone has to be introduced to induce remission
2. The azathioprine has to be added lifelong.

Markers for Treatment Failure

i. Ethnicity
ii. Early age of onset
iii. Hyperbilirubinemia
iv. HLA DRB1*03
v. Model for end stage liver disease (MELD) score >12.

The alternative drugs used are:
1. Calcineurin inhibitors
2. Budesonide
3. Mycophenolate mofetil
4. Rapamycin
5. Cyclosporine as steroid sparing agents.

REFERENCES

1. Longhi MS, Mitry RR, Samyn M, et al. Vigorous activation of monocytes in juvenile autoimmune liver disease escapes the control of regulatory T cells. Hepatology 2009; 50:130–142.
2. Strettell MD, Donaldson PT, Yhomson LJ, et al. Allelic basis for HLA- encoded susceptibility to type 1 autoimmune hepatitis. Gastroenterology1997; 112: 2028–2035.
3. Czaja AJ, Strettell MD, Thomson LJ, et al. Associations between alleles of the major histocompatibility complex and type 1 autoimmune hepatitis. Hepatology 2000; 31:49–53.
4. Beaune P, Dansette PM, Mansuy D, et al. Human antiendoplasmic reticulum autoantibodies appearing in a drug-induced hepatitis are directed against a human liver cytochrome P-450 that hydroxylates the drug. Proc. Natl. Acad. Sci. U S A 1987; 84: 551–555.
5. Singh G, Palaniappan S, Rotimi O, et al. Autoimmune hepatitis triggered by hepatitis A. Gut 2007; 56:304.
6. Homberg JC, Abuaf N, Bernard O, et al. Chronic active hepatitis associated with antiliver/kidney microsome antibody type 1: a second type of 'autoimmune' hepatitis. Hepatology 1987; 1333–1339.
7. Murray-Lyon IM, Stern RB, Williams R. Controlled trial of prednisone and azathioprine in active chronic hepatitis. Lancet 1973; 1:735–737.
8. Czaja AJ, Carpenter HA. Autoimmne hepatitis with incidental histologic features of bile duct injury. Hepatology 2001; 34:659–665.
9. Cassani F, Cataleta M, Valentini P, et al. Serum autoantibodies in chronic hepatitis C: comparison with autoimmune hepatitis and impact on the disease profile. Hepatology 1997; 26:561–566.

CIRRHOSIS

Definition

Cirrhosis is a chronic, diffuse, progressive disease characterized by:

i. Degeneration of liver cells
ii. Excess collagen deposition leading to fibrosis
iii. Nodule formation
iv. Disorganization of normal vascular architecture—which intern produces hemodynamic alterations.

The inciting events produce parenchymal inflammation and necrosis followed by fibrosis by following mechanisms:

i. Directly
ii. Indirectly by immunologically.

Causes of Nodule Formation, Fibrosis and Cirrhosis

i. Fibrosis without nodule formation—congenital hepatic fibrosis.
ii. Fibrosis with nodule formation—cirrhosis
iii. Nodule formation without fibrosis—partial nodular transformation

Causes

1. Viral—hepatitis B, C, D
2. Alcohol
3. Non-alcoholic steatohepatitis
4. Metabolic:
   a. Iron overload hemochromatosis
   b. Copper overload—Wilson's disease
   c. α_1 antitrypsin deficiency
   d. Galactosemia
   e. Type IV collagen formation
   f. Tyrosinemia
5. Primary biliary cirrhosis
6. Primary sclerosing cholangitis
7. Hepatic venous outflow obstruction:
   a. Budd-Chiari syndrome
   b. Heart failure
8. Autoimmune hepatitis
9. Toxins:
   a. Methotrexate
   b. Amiodarone

Cofactors for Development of Cirrhosis

1. Alcohol—large number of people take large amount of alcohol daily, but only small proportion of patients develop cirrhosis.
2. Obesity—non-alcoholic steatohepatitis develops in a small proportion of obese patients.
3. Genetic factors—patient with α_1 antitrypsin deficiency may develop cirrhosis, if obese.
4. Age
5. Sex
6. Duration of the disease
7. Immunological status

Patient with hepatitis C may develop cirrhosis, if he is infected at older age.

Patient also is likely to develop cirrhosis, if he will suffer for long duration.

Diabetic, obese patient having insulin resistance or if he is immunosuppressed, may develop cirrhosis.

Pathology

Fibrosis to Cirrhosis

Fibrosis can be defined as formation of fibrotic tissue in the liver tissue where there will be a damage area in response to injury and necrosis. Scar tissue tries to encapsulate the area of damage.

Development of fibrosis followed by cirrhosis from normal liver is a very complex process, which involves:

i. Hepatic parenchymal cells
ii. Hepatic nonparenchymal cells
iii. Immune systems
iv. Cytokines
v. Proteinases and their inhibitors.

This development of fibrosis is not linear; it varies from individual to individual. Genetic determinants may be involved in this process.

Non-alcoholic steatohepatitis—ultimately produces cryptogenic cirrhosis which is end stage of NASH. It is more common in Hispanic American patients.

Recently single nucleotide substitution has been shown to be associated with different rates of progression to fibrosis.

Cellular and Molecular Features of Fibrosis

Anatomy of cellular architecture and sinusoids: Basement membrane having lining fenestrated endothelial cells separates sinusoid lumen from space of Disse. The other cells are:

i. Stellate cells in the space of Disse—which are attached to inner side of basement membrane.
ii. Kupffer cells are attached on the sinusoidal side of basement membrane.

Nutrients from sinusoidal lumen pass through the fenestrated area of basement membrane to basal surface of hepatocytes across the space of Disse

Extracellular matrix in normal liver tissue: The extracellular matrix in normal liver tissue is composed of:

i. Type IV collagen/non-fibrillary
ii. Glycoproteins—fibrinoactin and laminin
iii. Proteoglycans—heparan sulphate

As a result, the formed low density basement membrane in the space of Disse:

i. Separates sinusoidal lumen from basal surface of hepatocytes.
ii. Allows the transfer of solutes and growth factors between the sinusoidal lumen and hepatocytes.

Changes in extracellular matrix in case of liver injury:

i. Development of high density interstitial fibril forming collagen—type I and type III instead of type IV collagen
ii. Increased concentration of:
   a. Cellular fibrinoactin
   b. Hyaluronic acid
   c. Other matrix proteoglycans
   d. Glycol conjugates

As a result:

i. Eightfold increase in interstitial matrix
ii. Loss of endothelial cell fenestration
iii. Loss of hepatocyte microvilli
iv. Capillarization of sinusoids

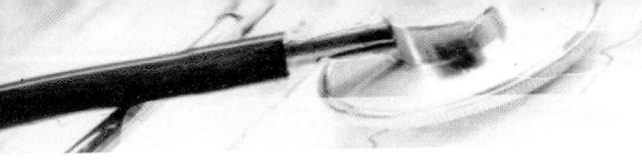

So there is impedance of exchange of metabolites between liver cells and blood in sinusoids.

Increased acumination of type 1 collages occurs due to:

i. Increased synthesis
ii. Decreased degradation

Stellate cells act a pivot role in the hepatic fibrogenesis.

Stellate cells are also known as lipocyte, fat storing cells, into cells and pericytes. It contains 40–70% of total body carotinoids. This cell is present in the space of Disse in direct contact with:

i. Endothelial cells
ii. Hepatocytes
iii. Inflammatory cells
iv. Nerve fibers

In normal state: Stellate cells produce type IV collagen—responsible for development of normal basement membrane.

In case of hepatic injury—there is phenotype changes in stellate cells called "activation" which is characterized by:

i. Loss of retinoid
ii. Cellular proliferation
iii. Increased number of endoplasmic reticulum
iv. Increased expression of muscle specific α-actin
v. Increased secretion of cytokines

This cell as a result of its phenotype change—produces:

i. Increased production of type I collagen which is responsible for development of high density basement membrane.
ii. Production of matrix degrading enzymes.

Activation of stellate cells occurs in two stages:

I. *Initiation phase:* In this early phase, as a result of changes in genetic and phenotypic expression, these cells are responsive to:
  i. Different types of cytokines
  ii. Oxidant stress (reactive oxygen metabolites)
  iii. Apoptotic bodies
  iv. Lipopolysaccharide
  v. Paracrine stimuli—this stimuli result from:
    a. Early changes in composition of extracellular matrix
    b. Alteration in homeostasis of sinusoidal endothelium of hepatocytes and Kuffer cells

II. *Perpetuation phase:* This phase is characterized by phenotypic changes through enhanced cytokine expression and responsiveness. They are:
  i. Enhanced stellate cell proliferation, contractility and fibrogenesis
  ii. Matrix degradation
  iii. Stellate cell chemotaxis
  iv. Direct interactions between stellate cells and immune system
  v. Secretion of proinflammatory mediators

So, if the initiating phase can be eliminated, then:

  i. Stellate cell reverts back to normal phenotype
Or ii. stellate cells are removed from liver through apoptosis or programmed death.

a. **Proliferations:** Proliferation of stellate cell occurs by the stimulation of a number of growth factors. These are:
  i. Platelet derived growth factor acting through its receptor β-PDGF.
  ii. Vascular endothelial growth factor (VEGF)
  iii. Thrombin

  iv. Endothelial growth factor (EGF)
  v. Transforming growth factor α (TGF-α)
  vi. Keratinocyte growth factor
  vii. Insulin like growth factor (IGF-1)

b. **Contractility:** During liver injury, stellate cell acquires the myogenic features like expression of smooth muscle cell action and myosin. These contractile properties of stellate cells are responsible for portal resistance—which is reversible.

But in advanced fibrosis, increased portal pressure is due to lobular distortion and increased septa. The factors responsible for controlling contractility are:

  i. Endothelin-1
  ii. Nitric oxide
  ii. Angiotensin II
  iv. Eicosanoids
  v. Atrial natriuretic peptide
  vi. Somatostatin
  vii. Carbon monoxide

c. **Fibrogenesis:** Stellate cell, after activation, produces type I collagen, the induction factors are:
  i. Tumor growth factor-β (TGF-β)—it is produced by sinusoidal cells, Kuffer cells and stellate cells during chronic liver injury.
  ii. CTGF
  iii. Fibroblast growth factor (FGF)
  iv. Vascular endothelial growth factor (VEGF)

d. **Chemotaxis:** In case of chronic liver injury, stellate cells become activated and encapsulate the area of injury; produce type I and III collagen, which in turn produce fibrosis. The chemotactic factors, which are responsible for the above incidences, are:
  i. PGDF
  ii. Monocyte chemotactic protein 1 (MCP-1)
  iii. CXCR3

Inflammatory Signaling

1. Stellate cells secrete proinflammatory cytokines like, MCP-1 and promote inflammation.
2. Stellate cells like dendritic cells present antigen to MHC-I and MHC-II restricted T cells and stimulate lymphocyte proliferation.
3. Toll like receptor-1 (TLR-4) helps in liver's immune response to injury.

Other Collagen Producing Cells

Stellate cells activation is the central to process of fibrosis in liver cell injury, similarly, other collagen producing cells take part in the process of fibrogenesis—which vary according to the etiology—like:

i. In biliary cirrhosis, portal fibroblasts are responsible.
ii. Conversion of hepatocytes and biliary epithelial cells to mesenchymal cells—which is known as epithelial mesenchymal transition.
iii. Liver sinusoidal cells initiate fibrogenesis through production of—cellular fibronectin extracellular domain A, and synthesize type I collagen.
iv. Fibrogenic cells derived from bone marrow may migrate to liver in chronic liver injury and initiates fibrogenesis.

Factors Influencing Fibrogenesis

i. **Interactions between** resident hepatic cells, infiltrating inflammatory cells, locally acting peptides (cytokines), extracellular matrix and cells interactions.

ii. **Cell-to-matrix and cell-to-cell interactions:**

Extracellular matrix proteins contain domains

↓

Domains interact with stellate cells and other cells through membrane e receptors like, integrins.

↓

Transduction of their effects through cytoplasmic signaling pathways

↓

Regulate collagen synthesis and metalloproteinase activity
Example fibrillary collagen

↓

Binds with tyrosine kinase receptor
discoidin domain receptor 2 on hepatic stellate cells

↓

Stimulate expression of matrix metalloproteinase 2

iii. **Cytokine:** Cytokines are the stimulators as well as mediators of fibrogenesis as a result of injury, inflammation. The cytokines are:
   a. Chemokines
   b. Interleukins
   c. Interferons
   d. Growth factors
   e. Angiogenic factors
   f. Soluble receptors
   g. Soluble proteases

   As a result of chronic inflammation—both stellate cells and infiltrating leukocytes are activated. The interactions of these cells are the key factors for determining the outcome of liver cell injury.

   Leukocyte derived cytokines stimulate stellate cells and thus fibrogenesis, similarly, stellate cells derived cytokines stimulate, recruit the leucocytes for fibrogenesis.

iv. **Immune interactions:** Immune mechanisms in the development of liver fibrosis are complex and depend on the etiology of the disease:
   a. Macrophages—plays an important role in fibrosis of liver. Depletion of macrophages is responsible for regression of fibrosis. This regression of fibrosis is further aided due to loss of macrophage—derived matrix proteases.
   b. Natural killer cells (NK cells)—suppresses fibrosis by killing activated myofibroblasts.
      NK cells also demonstrate profibrotic activity.
   c. **CD8 cell is more fibrogenic than CD4 cells**. So ratio of CD4/CD8 will be reduced in HCV and HIV mediated chronic liver injury.
   d. **B cells are responsible for matrix degradation.**

Methods of Matrix Production and Matrix Degradation

Chronic liver injury

↓

Activates the stellate cells

↓

(Contd.)

(Contd.)

Stimulation of fibrogenesis by TGF β_1/CTGF

↓

It consists of fibrillary collagen + matrix metalloproteinase like laminis, fibronectin and hyaluronic acid

Due to increased MMP ⟶ | Fibrinolysis
and decreased TIMPs | ⟵ changes in converting enzymes

↓

Increase in interstitial collagenase activity

[TIMPs—tissue inhibitors of MMPs]
[Converting enzymes are MT1-MMP and stromelysin]

But TIMPs act as a pivot role in liver fibrosis progression and regression—in the following ways:
i. Increased TIMPs levels:
   a. Decrease the degradation of type 1 collagen
   b. Persistence of activation of stellate cells
ii. Decreased TIMPs levels:
   a. Apoptosis of activated stellate cells
   b. Increases degradation of matrix

So the net result in hepatic fibrogenesis is:
i. Increased degradation of the normal basement membrane collagen
ii. Reduced degradation of interstitial type of collagen—which is due to increased TIMP-1 and TIMP-2 activity in comparison to MMP-1.

As a result of fibrinolysis—following two fragments are released into blood:
i. Glycoprotein fragment   ii. Collagen fragment

Classifications of Cirrhosis

The cirrhosis can be classified according to the size of the nodules.
1. **Micronodular cirrhosis:** Here nodule size is small (diameter is less than 3 mm and all the lobules are involved).
   Etiology:
      i. Alcoholic
     ii. Hemochromatosis
    iii. Cholestasis
     iv. Hepatic venous out flow obstruction
2. **Macronodular cirrhosis:** Here the diameter of the nodule is >3 mm and presence of normal lobule in larger nodules.
   Etiology: Viral hepatitis
3. **Mixed nodular cirrhosis:** Here there is transition between micronodular and macronodular cirrhosis.

So, alcoholic micronodular cirrhosis may transform into macronodular cirrhosis with the advance of liver damage.

Different serological markers can identify the etiology behind development of cirrhosis.

Reversible Cirrhosis

Normally cirrhosis is irreversible. But in following diseases, if the inciting events can be removed, fibrosis will be reversed.
   i. Hepatitis C
  ii. Iron overload
 iii. Biliary obstruction
  iv. Obesity

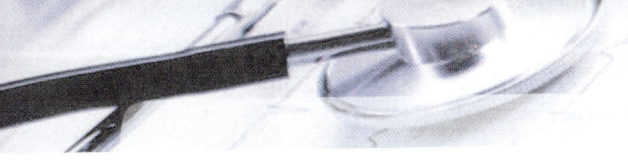

Compensated and Decompensated Cirrhosis

Compensated cirrhosis can be discovered during:
  i. Routine examination
 ii. Undergoing operation of other unrelated organ
iii. Routine biochemical examination

Cirrhosis may be suspected, if there is presence of:
   i. Vascular spiders
  ii. Palmar erythema
 iii. Unexplained epistaxis
  iv. Edema legs
   v. Enlarged firm liver mainly in epigastrium
  vi. Splenomegaly

If there is any suspicion by discovering any of the above signs, it should be confirmed by:
  i. Confirmatory biochemical tests
 ii. Ultrasound
iii. Liver biopsy

Compensated cirrhosis can be decompensated by any of the following initiating events:
  i. Bacterial infections
 ii. Trauma
iii. Medication
iv. Surgery

Decompensated cirrhosis: It means cirrhosis complicated by any one of the following features:
   i. Ascites—it appears first as a sign of decompensation.
  ii. Jaundice—when liver cells destruction exceed the liver cell regeneration.
 iii. Hepatic encephalopathy
  iv. Gastrointestinal bleeding—from varices or portal gastropathy
   v. Muscle wasting
  vi. Weight loss
 vii. Continuous mild fever—due to:
        a. Gram-negative bacteremia
        b. Ongoing alcoholic hepatitis
        c. Continuing hepatic cell necrosis
        d. Development of hepatocellular carcinoma
viii. Purpura in arms, shoulders and shins—due to low platelet count.
  ix. Liver may be enlarged or contracted and impalpable.
   x. Spleen enlarged.

Survival:
1. In case of compensated cirrhosis—10 year survival—50%
2. In case of decompensated cirrhosis—18 months survival—50%

Conversion:
  i. 10% cirrhotic patients are converted to decompensated cirrhosis per year.
 ii. Few decompensated patients again are converted into compensated cirrhosis with improvement of symptoms.

Vasodilatation and hyperdynamic circulation: Decompensated cirrhosis may be implicated by:
  i. Vasodilatation and
 ii. Hyperdynamic circulations. These are evidenced by:
        a. Flushed extremities
        b. Bounding pulses
        c. Capillary pulsation
        d. Relative arterial hypotension
        e. Increased peripheral arterial blood flow
        f. Increased portal venous blood flow
        g. Increased cardiac output with evidence of tachycardia and ejection systolic murmur
        h. Renal cortical perfusion will be decreased.
        i. Systemic and peripheral vascular resistance decreased.
        j. Arteriovenous oxygen difference will be reduced.
        k. In cirrhosis—there will be tissue hypoxia—due to:
            • Hyperdynamic circulation
            • Arteriovenous shunting

Arterial vasodilatation
↓
Fall in arterial volume
↓
Activation of renin–angiotensin system
↓
Sodium and water retention
↓
Development of ascites

Vasomotor tone is decreased in response to:
  i. Mental exercise
 ii. Valsalva maneuver
iii. Tilting the head from horizontal to vertical position
iv. Endogenous vasoconstrictor

Vasomotor tone will be decreased in response to autonomic neuropathy—it is an indicator of poor prognosis.

The abnormal openings of arteriovenous anastomoses (which are not normally present) are due to following reason.

Increased permeability of intestinal mucosa and evidence of portal systemic shunting
↓
Increased amount of endotoxins and cytokines (vasodilators) enters systemic circulation
↓
These are responsible for abnormal opening of portal–systemic circulation, vasodilatation and hyperdynamic circulation

The vasodilators are:
1. *Nitric oxide:* It is endothelium derived potent vasodilator. It is synthesized from L-arginine by the help of nitric oxide synthatase.
   This nitric oxide synthatase is inhibited by L-arginine analogue NG-monomethyl-L-arginine.
   Nitric oxide synthatase is induced by—various bacterial endotoxins.
2. *Gastrointestinal peptides:*
     i. Vasoactive intestinal peptide type-II—it has little effect on portal circulation.
    ii. Glucagon—acts as vasodilator
3. *Prostaglandins E_1, E_2 and E_{12}:* These are released into portal vein.

4. *Prostanoids*:

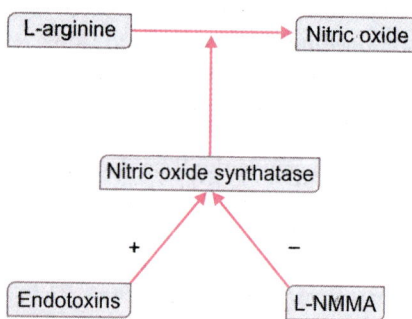

Prognosis in Cirrhosis

Poor prognosis in case of cirrhosis depends upon following factors:

i. Huge ascites
ii. Prolonged prothrombin time
iii. Increase age
iv. Huge gastrointestinal bleeding
v. High daily alcohol consumption
vi. High serum bilirubin and alkaline phosphatase
vii. Low albumin level
viii. Poor nutrition.

Child Classification (Grade A to C)

This classification depends upon:

i. Jaundice
ii. Ascites
iii. Encephalopathy
iv. Serum albumin
vi. Nutrition

Child-Pugh modification of Child classification—involves: Prothrombin time in place of nutritional status child's classification:

Group	A	B	C
1. Serum bilirubin mg/dl	<2	2–3	>3
2. Serum albumin gm/dl	>3.5	3–3.5	<3
3. Ascites	None	Easily controlled	Poorly controlled
4. Neurological disorder	None	Minimal	Advanced coma
5. Nutrition	Excelletant	Good	Poor-wasting

MELD Score

Full name is—Model for End stage Liver Disease score.

It can determine the prognosis in cirrhotic patient who is in the list of transplantation.

The factors which are involved in calculation are:

i. Prothrombin time
ii. Serum creatinine
iii. Serum bilirubin

New criterion—serum sodium has been added to the above criteria—hence it is called **MELD-Na**—as a result, its predictive ability is better.

UKELD: New criteria developed and used in UK is called UKELD. Here following criteria:

i. Serum bilirubin
ii. INR
iii. Serum creatinine
iv. Serum sodium

The predictive ability of UKELD is similar to that of MELD NA.

Disease Specific Scoring System

Maddrey's discriminant function (DF)—it is very helpful in case of alcoholic hepatitis. It can be calculated as follows

DF (discriminant function) =
Serum bilirubin (mol/L)/17 + prolongation of prothrombin time in seconds as compared to control x 4.6.

If DF >32—high mortality.

The clinical points are important in terms of prognosis:

1. *Etiology:* Prognosis can be improved by removal of etiological factors:
   a. Abstinence of alcohol—improves alcoholic cirrhosis
   b. Antiviral treatment—improves viral cirrhosis
2. *Precipitation of decompensation*: If correctable precipitating factor can be identified, correction of it improves prognosis—like alcohol, infection, hemorrhage.
   But if decompensation is spontaneous—prognosis is poor.
3. *Failure of response to therapy* within 1 month of initiation—prognostically poor.
4. *Persistent jaundice* is a serious sign.
5. *Neurological complications*—spontaneous or chronic encephalopathic signs are poor prognostic indicators.
6. *Ascites*—if resistant to diuretic therapy—prognostically poor.
7. *Liver size:* If liver is large—carries better prognosis but small carries poor prognosis. Because, large liver contains must more functioning cells.
8. *Portal venous pressure*—prediction of survival by Child-Pugh score is improved by adding portal pressure.
9. *Hemorrhages from portal varices*—in case of bleeding from portal varices, if the function of liver cell is good, this hemorrhage may be tolerated. But if, liver cell function is poor, prognosis is poor.
10. *Biochemical tests*—prognosis is grave, if:
    i. Serum albumin is <2.5 mg/dl
    ii. Diuretic unrelated hyponatremia <120 mmol/L
11. *Persistent hypotension* (if systolic BP <100 mmHg)—medical cause like, sepsis, should be searched because it is correctable.

Symptoms

A. **Some patients present with constitutional symptoms,** like:
   i. Weakness
   ii. Anorexia
   iii. Fatigue
   v. Weight loss
   v. Dyspepsia
   vi. Low grade fever
   vii. Raised liver enzymes

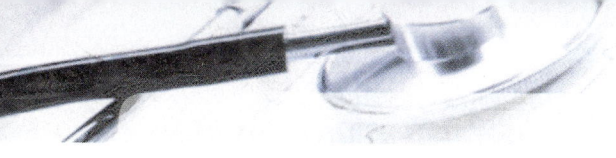

B. **Symptoms related to liver disease:**
  i. Spontaneous bleeding from gums
  ii. Easy bruising
  iii. Loss of axillary and pubic hair
  vi. Loss of libido in males
  v. Menstrual abnormalities in females
  vi. Gynecomastia
  vii. Jaundice
  viii. Pruritus
  ix. Arterial spider
  x. Parotid enlargement
  xi. Bleeding from gastrointestinal tract
  xii. Edema
C. **Symptoms related to nervous system:**
  i. Drowsiness
  ii. Irritability
  iii. Stupor
  iv. Coma
D. **Symptoms related to kidney:**
  i. Oliguria
  ii. Raised urea and creatinine
E. **Associated diseases:**
  i. Diabetes
  ii. Peptic ulcer
  iii. Symptoms related to gallstones
  iv. Psychiatric abnormalities

Physical findings in patient with cirrhosis are related to two major events:
1. *Hepatocellular failure*—it comprises of:
  i. Skin lesion
  ii. Disorder of protein metabolism—muscle wasting, hypothenar and thenar atrophy, ascites, edema
2. *Hematological abnormalities*—it comprises of:
  i. Splenomegaly
  ii. Esophageal varices
  iii. Abdominal collaterals
  iv. Ascites
  vi. Pulmonary complications.

Clinicopathological Correlations

Dermatological Manifestations

Vascular spiders
i. *Site*: In the area of superior vena caval distribution, but very rarely below nipple lines—in:
  • Necklace area
  • Face
  • Forearms
  • Dorsum of the hands
ii. *Description:* It consists of:
  a. Central arteriole, from which there are numerous radiating vessels
  b. Size—pinhead to 0.5 cm in diameter.
  c. If it enlarges in size, it can be felt to pulsate. This can be demonstrated by pressing a slide on it.
  d. Since central arteriole is the feeding arteriole, pressing on it with a pinhead, the whole lesion will be blanched.
iii. *Clinical importance:*
  a. It may disappear with improvement in liver function
  b. Appearance of fresh lesion—may suggest progression of liver disease

c. Multiple spiders along with clubbing of fingers—indicative of hepatopulmonary syndrome.
iv. *Disease association:*
  a. Alcoholic liver disease
  b. Transiently in viral hepatitis
  c. 2nd to 5th months of pregnancy
  d. Normal adults
  e. 38% children without liver disease—at least one nevus may be present.
v. *Associated lesions:*
  a. *Paper money skin:* It looks like smaller numerous vessels appearing on American dollar bills distributed in scattered fashion in the territory of vascular spider.
  b. *White spots:* These are present on arms and buttocks on cooling the skin, when the area is examined with the lens, there is early appearance of arterioles at the centre of white spot—which may be the beginning of spider.

Differential Diagnosis

Hereditary Hemorrhagic Telangiectasia (HHT)
1. It is found in upper body. Mucosal sites are:
  i. Tongue
  ii. Lips
  iii. Nose
  iv. Palate
  v. Pharynx
  vi. Esophagus
  vii. Stomach
2. It is also found in nail beds and palmar surfaces. HHT with liver angioma may produce high output heart failure.

Telangiectasia: It is an associated phenomenon of CREST syndrome—calcinosis, Raynaud's phenomenon, sclerodactyly, telangiectasia. The cirrhotic liver is due to primary biliary cirrhosis.

Campbell de Morgan's spot (cherry angioma): These are bright red flat or slightly elevated papules or macules present on front of the chest and arms and abdomen.
These will increase in size along with the age.

Venous stars:
i. These are present overlying the main tributary of veins of large size
ii. These are 2–3 cm in diameter.
iii. These cannot be obliterated by pressure.
iv. These are present on dorsum of foot, leg, buttock, lower border of ribs.

Hand Findings
1. **Palmar erythema:**
  a. Description:
    i. It is bright red in color. It blanches on presence and reappear as soon as pressure is relieved.
    ii. If a glass slide is pressed on the area, there may be flushing synchronously with pulse rate.
  b. Sites:
    i. Thenar eminences
    ii. Hypothenar eminences
    iii. Pulp of fingers
       Sole of the feel may be similarly involved.
  c. Symptoms—throbbing and tingling of palms
  d. Disease—alcoholic cirrhosis

Normal familial palmar flushing: It is usually seen in:
   i. Rheumatoid arthritis
  ii. Pregnancies
 iii. Chronic febrile illness
  iv. Leukemia
   v. Thyrotoxicosis.

Mechanism for skin changes: Traditionally, it has been attributed to estrogen excess. But in male cirrhotic patients, estradiol level may be normal, whereas, androgen level will be reduced. So ratio of estradiol to testosterone is more important than production of vascular spider—it is high in case of patient with cirrhosis.

2. **Dupuytren's contracture:**
   a. Pathology:
      i. There is flexion deformity of the fingers due to thickening and shortening of palmar fascia.
     ii. There may be knots and cords formation under the skin.
   b. Finger involved:
      i. The little finger and ring finger are most commonly involved.
     ii. The middle finger may be involved.
   c. It is found in:
      i. Alcoholic cirrhosis
     ii. Older adults
    iii. Smokers.
   d. Men are more likely to be involved than women.

3. **Nail changes:**
   a. *Muehreke's nails:* It is characterized by horizontal while bands separated by normal color across the skin.
   b. *Leuconychia:* It is characterized by presence of white lines or white spots on the nails—is of no significance.
   c. *Azure lunula:* This is characterized by white appearance of proximal two-thirds of nails and bluish-colored lunule—it is found in Wilson's disease.

4. **Clubbing:** This occurs in patient with cirrhosis complicated by cystic fibrosis or hepatopulmonary syndrome.

   Causes: It occurs due to plugging of capillaries along with release of platelet derived growth factor (PGDF) by aggregates of platelets after by passing pulmonary arterio-venous fistula.

5. **Asterixis (flapping tremor):** It is a rhythmical bilateral flapping tremor of wrist on extension (dorsiflexion).

   It may be asynchronous—due to interruption inflow of joint and other afferent information to rostral reticular formation.

   It is nothing but "negative myoclonus".

   Sites:
      i. Hand
     ii. Tongue
    iii. Skeletal muscles

Diseases involved:
   i. Hepatic encephalopathy—Asterixis may be reversible with the improvement of liver condition.
  ii. Respiratory failure
 iii. Renal failure
  iv. Electrolyte abnormalities
   v. Drugs intoxication—alcoholism, barbiturate phenytoin, primidone.

Endocrine Changes

1. **Testicular atrophy:**
   i. Here testes are small, soft.
  ii. Secondary sexual hair is lost.
   Cause: It is due to:
      a. Primary gonadal injury
   Or, b. Suppression of hypothalamic or pituitary function.
   Associated features:
   i. Infertility
  ii. Loss of sexual drive
 iii. Impotence
   Diseases involved:
   i. Alcoholic patient
  ii. Hypothalamic hypogonadism
   Importance: After liver transplantation, hypogonadism will be rapidly corrected.

2. **Gynecomastia:** This can be defined as enlargement of breast in male.

   It can be differentiated from lipomastia of obesity by its unique feature—i.e. palpable glandular tissue around the areola and the breast is tender.

   Causes: Increased ratio of free estradiol to free testosterone—which is responsible for associated following features also—loss of secondary sexual hair in male.

Disease associated:
   i. Alcoholic cirrhosis
  ii. Spironolactone therapy
 iii. Chronic autoimmune hepatitis

   Mechanisms: Liver has both types of receptors for estrogen and androgen. In cirrhosis—sensitivies to these hormones will be changed. As a result, androgen receptor concentration falls and esotrogen receptor concentrations rises.

   In partial hepatic resection or liver transplantation—there is increase in serum estrogen and decrease in serum testosterone, as well as increase in estrogen receptor concentration.

   In liver carcinoma, serum estrone level will be high and after removal of tumor, serum estrone level will come to normal. On examination of the biopsied liver tumor tissue, there is presence of trophoblastic tissue in the midst of abnormal liver tissue.

   In case of testicular atrophy—it may be due to either primary testicular failure or it may be secondary to pituitary–hypothalamic failure, if there is association with impaired released of luteinizing hormone along with gonadotropin hormone deficiency.

Eye Signs

Increased frequency of:
1. Lid retraction or
2. Lid lag—in absence of thyroid disease.

Muscle Cramps

It occurs in cirrhotic patients—and correlate with:
   i. Presence of ascites
  ii. Low mean arterial pressure

Nutrition

There is evidence of protein calorie malnutrition—which itself reduces the lifespan of the cirrhotic patients. The causes are mainly inadequate protein intake—which is responsible for reduced muscle mass and muscle wasting.

Another cause is increased resting energy expenditure.

Fat storage is also reduced.

Various dental and periodontal diseases supervene

This malnutrition mainly occurs in:
i. Alcoholic cirrhosis
ii. Child grade C—hepatic encephalopathy

Nutritional status can be measured by:
i. Triceps thickness
ii. Body mass index
iii. Mid-arm circumference
vi. Subjective global assessment.

Effects on Drug Metabolism in Cirrhotic Patients

Drug metabolism in liver disease is hampered mainly due to two causes:
1. Reduced overall hepatocellular mass, not the enzymatic activity.
2. Increased shunting of blood—in both portosystemic and intrahepatic circulation.

Other causes of disordered metabolism in cirrhosis are:
1. Drug absorption
2. Drug branding
3. Tissue distribution
4. Protein binding
5. Biliary excretion
6. Enterohepatic circulation
7. Target organ responsiveness

In case of increased shunting of blood—(high hepatic extraction ratio—high first pass effect)—predictability of the action of drug is very variable because of high degree of shunting.

But in case of reduced hepatocellular mass, the action of the drug can be predictable.

Infections

Liver is bacteriologically sterile and portal venous system contains no organism. But in case of cirrhosis, bacteria bypass, through:
i. Faulty hepatic filter
ii. Portosystemic circulation:
   a. So patients with ascites may develop spontaneous bacterial peritonitis.
   b. Patient with hydrothorax may develop bacterial empyema in absence of SBP.
   c. In febrile patient with coma, bacterial meningitis
   d. Nasal carriage of *Staphylococcus*.

Sepsis is suspected in cirrhotic patient with:
i. Unexplained pyrexia
ii. Gastrointestinal bleeding in child grade C

So antibiotic prophylaxis is always required after sending blood or urine for culture and sensitivity:
i. It reduces the incidence of sepsis.
ii. It increases the short term survival.

Sepsis is responsible for the terminal hepatocellular failure. The contributory factors for occurrences of septicemia are:

i. Impaired functions of Kupffer cells and polymorphs
ii. Reduction of following factors like:
   a. Fibronectin
   b. Opsonins
   c. Chemoattractants
   d. Complement cascade
iii. Scavenger functions of reticuloendothelial cells will be deteriorated due to endotoxemia of intestinal origin.
iv. Renal damage

Urinary tract infections is a common complication in cirrhotic patients, it is mostly gram-negative origin. Recurrent catheterization is an important factor.

Other infections common in cirrhotics are:
a. Pneumonia
b. Lymphangitis
c. Endocarditis

Hospital-acquired infections in cirrhotic patients—are due to:
i. Gram-positive organism
ii. In case of invasive investigations and treatment
   1. Methicillin resistant *Staphylococcus aureus*
   2. Vancomycin resistant enterococci
iii. Prophylactic treatment to prevent SBP may produce quinolone resistance.

Bad prognostic signs are:
i. Absence of fever
ii. Raised serum creatinine
iii. Marked leukocytosis
iv. Bacterial infections
v. Gastrointestinal bleeding

Fetor Hepaticus

It is characterized by sweetish, slightly fecal smell of breath just like freshly opened corpse or mice.

Causes:
i. It occurs in severe hepatocellular failure and extensive collateral circulation.
ii. The smell is of intestinal origin and it will be decreased after defecation.
iii. It may be due to alteration in gut flora as a result of broad-spectrum antibiotics.

Origin of gas: Gas is generated due to dimethyl sulphide and ketone in alveolar air.

Extrahepatic autoimmune diseases: These are:
i. Hemolytic anemia
ii. Thyroiditis

Other systemic diseases:
i. Chronic relapsing pancreatitis
ii. Pancreatic calcification
iii. Peptic ulcer disease.

Cardiopulmonary Conditions

Hepatopulmonary Syndrome

Definition: This disorder is characterized by pulmonary vasodilatation and defective oxygenation in absence of any detectable pulmonary disease in patient with chronic active liver disease.

Causes:

1. Advanced chronic liver disease
2. Arterial hypoxemia
3. Intrapulmonary syndrome
4. No primary cardiopulmonary disease

Pathophysiology:

i. PO_2 <80 mmHg
ii. Alveolar–arterial oxygen gradient >15 mmHg
iii. Intrapulmonary shunting is due to—marked dilatation of precapillary and capillary vessels. Result is:
   i. Diffusion limitation of capillary oxygenation
   ii. Ventilation—perfusion mismatch

Vasoactive substances responsible for pulmonary vasodilatation include:

i. Nitric oxide
ii. Endothelin-1
iii. Tumor necrosis factor-α

Diagnosis: The aims are:

i. Demonstration of pulmonary vasodilatation
ii. Increased alveolar—arterial oxygen gradient:
   a. *Contrast enhanced echocardiography:* It demonstrates: Passage of microbubbles through pulmonary circulation to left side of heart.
   b. *Technetium 99m (^{99m}Tc) macroaggregated albumin*—it is less sensitive.
   c. *Pulmonary angiography*—it detects—pulmonary arteriovenous shunts.
   d. *Transesophageal echocardiography*—it can exclude intracardiac shunt.

If hypoxemia is gradually increasing—liver transplantation is necessary.

After liver transplantation, hypoxemia will be resolved within weeks to months.

But if pulmonary arteriovenous shunt is very large, embolotherapy is to be done preceding transplantation.

Portopulmonary Hypertension

This can be defined as:

i. Portal hypertension
ii. Mean pulmonary artery pressure >25 mmHg
iii. Pulmonary vascular resistance >240 dynes/S/am^2
iv. Absence of other diseases associated with pulmonary hypertension.

The causes are:

i. Hepatic portal hypertension
ii. Perihepatic portal hypertension

Symptoms:

i. Asymptomatic
ii. Non-specific chest discomfort
iii. Dyspnea on exertion.

Physical examination reveals:

i. Right ventricular heave
ii. Loud 2dn heart sound

Investigations:

i. *Histometric study reveals:* Muscular pulmonary arterial wall will be thickened and artery will be dilated, occasionally presence of thrombi.
ii. *Plexogenic pulmonary arteriopathy*—it involves arteries having 10–200 mm in diameter. It is responsible for primary pulmonary hypertension.

Contraindication to liver transplant is mean pulmonary artery pressure >35 mmHg—because, it may be responsible for postoperative death due to right ventricular failure. If right ventricular systolic pressure is more than 30 mmHg—right heart catheterization is essential to confirm it.

Treatment: Oral sildenafil—reduces:

i. Mean pulmonary artery pressure
ii. Pulmonary vascular resistance

If the above parameter will be reduced, patient may undergo liver transplantation.

Pulmonary Changes in Chronic Liver Disease with Hepatocellular Failure

i. Hypoxia
ii. Intrapulmonary shunting
iii. Mismatched ventilation—perfusion
iv. Reduced transfer factor
v. Pleural effusion
vi. Raised diaphragm
vii. Basal atelectasis
viii. Primary pulmonary hypertension
ix. Portopulmonary shunting.

Cirrhotic Cardiomyopathy

Definition

The presence of one or more of the **following may help to diagnose a case of cardiomyopathy in alcoholic cirrhosis:**

i. Baseline cardiac output will be increased, but ventricular response to stimuli will be blunted
ii. Systolic and diastolic dysfunction
iii. Absence of overt left ventricular failure at rest
iv. Prolonged interval on electrocardiography

Major stresses responsible for overt cardiac failure are:

i. Sepsis
ii. TIPS
iii. Liver transplantation.

Major pathogenic mechanisms for cardiomyopathy are:

i. Defective cardiac muscle β signaling pathway
ii. Decreased fluidity of cardiac myocyte plasma membrane as a result of changes in lipid composition
iii. Negative effects of following substances:
   a. Nitric oxide
   b. Carbon monoxide
   c. Endocannabinoids in cardiac muscles.

Treatment

i. Diuretic and beta blockers—helpful
ii. Vasodilatation and digitalis—should not be given
iii. Successful liver transplant may improve the cardiac condition
iv. Long-term aldosterone antagonist—useful

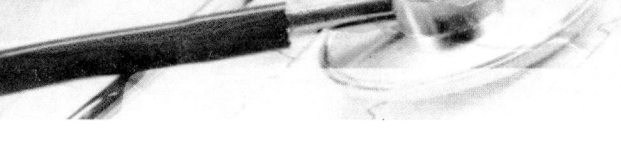

Laboratory Tests

Hematological parameters:

i. Normally normochromic normocytic anemia
ii. In alcoholic patient—macrocytic anemia
iii. In case of gastrointestinal bleeding—microcytic, hypochromic anemia
iv. In case of sepsis—leukocytosis
v. In case of hypersplenism—leucopenia associated with thrombocytopenia
vi. Prolonged prothrombin time—refractory to vitamin K therapy
vii. Bone marrow shows:
  a. Macronormoblastic
  b. Increased number of plasma cell due to hypergamma-globulinemia

Causes of hematological parameters

1. Anemia—causes:
  a. Blood loss
  b. Folate deficiency
  c. Alcohol toxicity
  d. Hypersplenism
  e. Bone marrow suppression
  f. Chronic disease inflammation
  g. Hemolysis
2. Leukocytosis—due to associated sepsis.
3. Leucocytopenia—due to hypersplenism
4. Thrombocytopenia—due to hypersplenism
5. Thrombocytopenia—due to:
  i. Sequestration in spleen—hypersplenism
  ii. Deficiency of thrombopoietin—which is produced in the liver

Biochemical tests: Liver enzymes:

i. *ALT*—it is most important screening tests for detection of:
  a. Metabolic liver injury
  b. Drug-induced liver injury.
ii. *AST/ALT ratio:*
  >2—Alcoholic liver disease
  <1—chronic hepatitis chronic cholestatic syndrome
iii. *AST/ALT ratio* >1—non-alcoholic cirrhosis
iv. *Serum albumin*—indicates hepatic synthetic function—level decreased in advanced liver disease.
v. *Serum globulin level*—increased due to:
  a. Poor reticuloendothelial cell function
  b. Increased blood levels of bacterial products
vi. *Serum alkaline phosphatase:*
  a. ~ 2 times normal—non-cholestatic liver disease
  b. >2 times normal—primary biliary cirrhosis, primary sclerosing cholangitis
vii. *Gamma glutamyl transpeptidase* (GGT) raised in alcoholic liver disease—this occurs due to—alcohol-induced hepatic microsomal GGT producing leakage of GGT. From hepatocytes, **in cholestatic cirrhosis**, there are parallel elevation of alkaline phosphatase and 5-neucleotidase along with GGT.
  GGT is also raised in:
  i. Barbiturates
  ii. Phenytoin

viii. *Serum bilirubin level:*
  i. Conjugated bilirubin is normal in compensated cirrhosis
  ii. In severe liver damage—bilirubin will be raised.
ix. *Cholesterol and triglyceride:*
  i. Raised in case of biliary obstruction
  ii. Low in nonbiliary advanced cirrhosis
x. *Other tests to detect synthetic function of liver:*
  i. Ceruloplasmin
  ii. Ferritin
  iii. α-1 antitrypsin
  iv. Lipoproteins

Serological, Immunological or Genetic Tests

I. **Serological tests for viral hepatitis**
  i. HBsAg
  ii. Anti-HBsAb
  iii. Anti-HCV
  iv. Anti-delta antibody
  v. HBV DNA
  vi. HCV RNA.
  Above serologies are helpful:
  i. To reveal etiology
  ii. To initiate antiviral therapy
    If HBsAg is positive—status of HBeAg should be evaluated.

II. **Autoantibody profile:** There are two types of auto-immune hepatitis—characterized by specific type of autoantibodies:
  1. Antinuclear antibody (ANA), anti-smooth muscle cell antibodies (anti-SMA), antiactin antibodies and/or a typical perinuclear anti-neutrophil cytoplasmic antibody (p-ANCA)—detect type 1 autoimmune hepatitis.
  2. Anti-LKM-1 and antiliver cytosol (anti-ALC-1) antibodies—detect type-2 autoimmune hepatitis.
    Importance of detection of autoimmune hepatitis—these patient can be benefited from—immunosuppressive and steroid treatment, with or without addition of methotrexate.

III. **For patient suffered from hemochromatosis:**
  i. Fasting transferrin saturation of 45%
  ii. Serum ferritin level   >300 ng/ml for men
                             >200 ng/ml for women
  iii. Analysis of HFE (HH) gene mutation
  iv. Liver biopsy to confirm

IV. **If patient is younger than 45 years with family history of cirrhosis:**
  i. Serum ceruloplasmin level—low (<20 mg/dl)
  ii. High basal 24 hours urinary copper secretion >100 μg (Normal 10–80 μg)
  iii. Low serum copper levels (80–60 μg is normal)—suggest Wilson's disease
  iv. Increased copper content in liver biopsy (>250 μg of copper per gram of dry weight).

V. **Test for α₁ antitrypsin deficiency**—useful is chronic hepatic injury in neonates.

Imaging

a. **In chronic liver disease**—following can be diagnosed by imaging:

i. Ascites
ii. Portal hypertension
iii. Hepatocellular carcinoma
iv. Portal vein thrombosis
v. Hepatic vein thrombosis.

b. **In case of cirrhosis**—ultrasound can demonstrate the following features:
   i. Altered echo pattern
   ii. Nodular surface
   iii. Irregular surface
   iv. Nodular liver edges
   v. Collateral vessels related to portal hypertension
   vi. Liver mass
   vii. Grade of steatosis
   Bright echo pattern with fibrosis—indicates the cause of cirrhosis as fatty liver.

c. **Doppler ultrasound demonstrates:**
   i. Vascularization of the lesion
   ii. Direction of blood flow through portal vein—whether centrifugal or centripetal
   iii. Blood flow in hepatic veins
   iv. Patency of portal and hepatic veins
   v. Localization of collaterals
   vi. State of collaterals

d. **Contrast enhanced CT scan:** Differentiate benign lesion from dysplastic nodule or hepatocellular carcinoma.

e. **Magnetic resonance imaging assesses:**
   i. Flow volume and direction of flow in portal vein
   ii. Portal vein thrombosis
   iii. Iron over load

In chronic liver disease—suppressor T lymphocyte functions will be depressed, as a result, there is reduction in suppression of B lymphocyte production—thus antibody production will be increased.

i. **In chronic liver disease**, intestinal antigen
↓
Bypass the liver through portal–systemic circulation developed around the liver nodules
↓
Enter the systemic circulation
↓
Enter the splenic circulation
↓
Production of antibody

ii. Similarly endotoxins enter the circulation in similar way.
iii. Polymeric IgA and IgA antigen may enter the systemic circulation bypassing the liver.
   [Grade-A score 5–6 (well compensated cirrhosis)
   Grade-B score 7–9 (significant functional compromise)
   Grade-C score 10–15 (decompensated disease)
   Grade-A 1 year survival 100%
   Grade-B 1 year survival 80%
   Grade-C 1 year survival 45%.]

Prognosis

Clinical cause and prognosis depend on the following:
i. Etiology of liver disease
ii. Severity of liver damage
iii. Complications of liver disease
iv. Co-morbid diseases—associations

Bad prognoses in cirrhosis are:
   i. Involvement of multiple agents in one patient:
      a. Obesity
      b. Alcohol
      c. Drugs
      d. Viral etiology
   ii. Advanced age
   iii. Severe ascites
   iv. Gastrointestinal bleeding
   v. Presence of peritonitis
   vi. Poor nutrition
   vii. Hepatic encephalopathy
   viii. Persistent hypertension

MELD score: This score is based on the following variables:
   i. Serum bilirubin
   ii. Creatinine
   iii. INR
   iv. Etiology of cirrhosis—to predict the mortality in hepatic failure.
   But etiology of cirrhosis has been removed from the scale, because it may create confusion.

The formula of MELD =
3.8 Ln serum bilirubin (mg/dl) + 11.2 {Ln x INR} + 9.6 {Ln serum creatinine (mg/dl)} + 6.4
Ln = natural logarithm

MELD can predict the prognosis in patient with chronic liver disease in following associated conditions:
   i. Alcoholic hepatitis
   ii. Hepatorenal syndrome
   iii. Sepsis
   iv. Surgical procedures

MELD score of 6–40 can prioritize the patient for organ allocation for liver transplantation.

The upper limit of MELD = 40
But in following condition, MELD can underscores the priority for transplantation:
   i. Hepatocellular carcinoma
   ii. Hepatorenal syndrome
   iii. Systemic metabolic acidosis.

Treatment of Cirrhosis

Basic Goals in the Treatment of Cirrhosis

   i. Treatment of the etiology to prevent further progression of liver disease.
   ii. Prevention of intake of substances, which are harmful to the liver
   iii. Prevention of complications of cirrhosis
   iv. Control of symptoms of cirrhosis
   v. Prioritization of a patient for liver transplantation.

Treatment of Etiology

1. To treat hepatitis C—ledipasvir, sofosbuvir, ribavirin, daclastavir
2. To treat hepatitis B—tenofovir, entecavir

All the above drugs:
a. Reduce inflammation
b. Reduce fibrosis
c. Prevent the development of hepatocellular carcinoma

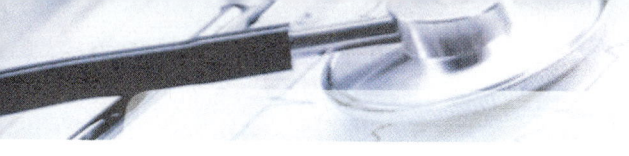

1. Antiviral therapy should be considered for decompensated cirrhosis infected with **hepatitis B**—either in combination of lamivudine or telbivudine

    +

    Adefovir or entecavir

    Then these patients should be referred for liver transplantation.
2. In case cirrhosis due **to hepatitis C**
    i. In compensated state:
       - Genotype 1—(Ledipasvir 90 mg + Sofosbuvir 400 mg) × 12 weeks
       - Genotype 2—(Sofosbuvir 400 mg + Ribavirin) × 6 months
       - Genotype 3—(Sofosbuvir 400 mg + Daclastavir 60 mg) × 3 months)
    ii. In decompensated state—no antiviral therapy will be considered if they are not the candidate for liver transplantation.
3. **In case of autoimmune hepatitis**—steroids and immunosuppressives.
4. **In case of Wilson's disease**—chelating agents—D-penicillamine or trientine.

    Once patient develops cirrhosis—the aim should be—prevention and management of its complications—like variceal bleeding, ascites, hepatic encephalopathy.

Avoidance of substances which many produce further harm to liver:
1. Alcohol abuse
2. Dose of vitamin A >25000 IU/day
3. Non-steroidal anti-inflammatory agents
4. Over the counter drugs

Following immunizations should be required:
1. Vaccination of hepatitis A
2. Vaccination of hepatitis B
3. Vaccination against influenza
4. Vaccination against pneumococcus

Nutrition requirement in cirrhosis:
1. Generally, low sodium, low fat, high proteins, high carbohydrate food is preferable. Energy requirement 25–35 Kcal/kg/day
2. In malnourished cirrhotic patient:
    - Energy requirement 35–40 Kcal/kg/day
    - Protein requirement 1–1.2 gm/kg/day
3. Cirrhotic patient in ICU or associated complication—protein requirement is 1.5 gm/kg/day.
4. Other supplementations are: Iron, vitamin B, virtamin K
5. Zinc supplementation—zinc sulphate 220 mg twice daily should be preferred—because it can stimulate appetite.
6. Raw seafood—since it may contain bacteria and produce life-threatening infection in cirrhotic patient, hence it should be avoided.

Treatment of Pruritus in Cholestatic Cirrhosis

1. It can be treated by antihistaminic.
2. Cholestyramine—since it is bitter in taste, should be given in a cup of fruit juice.
3. Other medications to give relief in pruritus are:
    i. Ursodeoxycholic acid   ii. Naltrexone
    iii. Rifampin   iv. Gabapantin
    v. Ondansetron.

4. In case of severe pruritus:
    i. Ultraviolet ray therapy   ii. Plasmapheresis.

The precipitating factors for hepatic encephalopathy:
    i. Constipation
    ii. Infection
    iii. Variceal bleeding
    iv. Subacute bacterial peritonitis
    v. Use of sedatives
    vi. Electrolyte imbalance in case of:
       a. Diarrhea   b. Vomiting.

Treatments are:
i. Lactulose—to prevent the buildup of ammonia.

In patient refractory to lactulose—non-absorbable antibiotic rifaximine should be used to reduce the intestinal bacterial count.

ii. To treat edema:
    a. Low sodium diet
    b. Spironolactone and frusemide combinations are usually used to reduce excess water and salt.
    c. Patient with refractory ascites
       Total paracentesis with 20% salt poor albumin.
    d. Albumin infusion at 1.5 gm/kg/day to reduce hypoproteinemia.

iii. To prevent hepatic encephalopathy: TIPS—acts as a bridge between liver transplantation and risk of hepatic encephalopathy.

iv. Treatment of hepatorenal syndrome:
    a. Vasoconstrictor and albumin
    b. TIPS
    c. Extracorporeal albumin dialysis molecular absorbents recirculation system (MARS)—in type 1 syndrome
    d. Liver transplantation will be future treatment of choice.

Following cirrhotic patients are at risk of developing hepatocellular carcinoma:
    i. Cirrhotic HBV carriers
    ii. Patients are in transplant list
    iii. Africans more than 20 years
    iv. Family history of HCC
    v. Patient with HBV carriers, living in endemic area for HBV and HCC.

In above patients, screening for HCC to be done at 6–12 months interval by:
    i. Ultrasound of upper abdomen
    ii. α-fetoprotein examination

Treatment of Hypogonadism

Patient with severe symptoms can get relief from topical testosterone preparations.

Cirrhotic patient many develop osteoporosis; again autoimmune hepatitis will get cortisteroids.

So, above patients may benefit from calcium as well as vitamin supplementation.

Cirrhotic patient should be screened for variceal bleeding by performing upper gastrointestinal endoscopy at regular interval (every 2 years).

To prevent bleeding from varices: Non-selective beta blocker (propranolol or nadolol)—can be administered to make 25% reduction in heart rate.

Surgical procedures in cirrhotic patients: All the operations in cirrhotic patient carry high risk and high mortality because of the following reasons:

i. Low serum albumin
ii. Presence of infection
iii. High prothrombin time.

Following operative procedures carry bad prognosis
i. Biliary tract operation
ii. Colonic resection
iii. Operation for peptic ulcer

PORTAL HYPERTENSION

Anatomy of Portal Venous System

Portal vein is formed by the union of superior mesenteric vein and splenic vein posterior to the head of pancreas at the level of 2nd lumbar vertebra.

Portal vein carries blood from:
i. Gastrointestinal tract
ii. Spleen
iii. Pancreas
iv. Gallbladder.

Portal vein near porta hepatis divides into two branches and enters the liver.

Course of Portal Vein

a. **Superior mesenteric vein:** It is formed by the branches from:
  i. Small intestine
  ii. Cecum
  iii. Right colon
  iv. Two-thirds of transverse colon
  v. Head of pancreas and
  vi. Stomach via right gastroepiploic vein

b. **Splenic vein:** It emerges from spleen hilum and runs medially. On its course, near the tail of pancreas, it joins with short gastric vessels to form main splenic vein.

The main splenic vein runs medially transversely in the body and head of pancreas, medially and in front of the hepatic artery. It receives tributaries from:
  i. Head of the pancreas
  ii. Left gastroepiploic vein.

c. **Inferior mesenteric vein:** It carries blood from:
  i. Left 1/3rd of transverse colon
  ii. Descending colon
  iii. Sigmoid colon
  iv. Rectum

It joins with splenic vein medially occasionally; it joins with splenic vein along with superior mesenteric vein.

Then portal vein runs slightly right of midline for distance of 5.5–8 cm to portal hepatis. Here, it is divided into right and left portal veins and run along the branches of hepatic artery and enters into the liver parenchyma.

- **Portal blood flow** = 1000–1200 ml/min.
- **Fasting arterio-portal oxygen differences** = 1.9 volume percent
- **Portal pressure**—7 mmHg.
- **Portal vein is responsible for 72% of oxygen supply** in the liver.

Streamlines in Portal Vein

No consistent hepatic distribution of portal inflow. Flow in streamline rather than turbulent.

Splenic flow will go to right or left branch of portal vein.

Collateral circulation: When the portal vein is obstructed in the liver or outside the liver, the blood will deviate from the portal vein to systemic collaterals.

Intrahepatic obstruction: In case of cirrhosis, only 13% of blood will be recovered from hepatic vein, the remaining 87% of blood will enter collateral circulation through **four main groups of collaterals.**

In all groups, portal systems anastomose with systemic veins.

Group-1: Here protective epithelium joins absorptive epithelium through following methods
1. *At the cardia of the stomach, portal systems consisting of:*
  i. Short gastric vein
  ii. Left gastric veins
  iii. Posterior gastric veins.
  Systemic veins consisting of:
  i. Intercostal veins
  ii. Diaphragm esophageal veins
  iii. Azygos min or veins.
  Result: Varicose veins develop in the submucosal layer at the lower and of esophagus and fundus.
2. *At the anus, portal system consisting of*—superior hemor-rhoidal vein.
  Systemic vein consists of—middle and inferior hemor-rhoidal vein.

  Result: Development of rectal varices

Group-2: Paraumbilical veins in falciparum ligament with the relics of **umbilical veins** of fetal life.

Group 3: In this group, collateral circulation will be developed where abdominal organs are in contact with retroperitoneal tissues.
1. Collateral veins run from liver to diaphragm
2. In splenorenal ligament and omentum: The involved veins are:
  i. Lumbar veins
  ii. Veins in the scar of previous operations
  iii. Veins of small or large bowel stomas.

In women specially, there are communications between ovarian vessels and iliac veins.

Group 4: Portal blood from:
i. Splenic vein
ii. Diaphragmatic vein
iii. Pancreatic
iv. Left adrenal
v. Gastric veins

Systemic vein: Left renal vein.

Blood from gastroesophageal vein and from other colla-terals via azygos and hemiazygos veins enters superior vena cava.

Blood from right branch of portal vein enters inferior vena cava through intrahepatic shunt.

Extrahepatic Obstruction of Portal Veins

In case of extrahepatic portal venous obstruction, **the blood bypasses** the block area and enters the portal vein at porta hepatis through other collateral veins involved are the following:

i. Veins at hilum
ii. Venae comitantes of portal vein and hepatic arteries
iii. Veins in suspensary ligament in the liver
iv. Diaphragmatic veins
v. Omental veins.

Effect of Portal Vein Obstruction

1. As a result of portal venous obstruction, portal blood will bypass the liver and enters the systemic circulation through collaterals; then liver has to depend on hepatic artery.

   As a result, liver will not get hepatotrophic factors like, glucagon, insulin of pancreatic origin, so damaged liver cells are unable to regenerate and liver shrinks gradually.
2. In case of extensive collateral circulation, there may be fall in portal pressure.
3. In case portal hypertension of short duration, there may be no evidence of collateral.
4. In case of large portal systemic shunt, there may be chance of hepatic encephalopathy, septicemia.

Pathology of Portal Hypertension

I. Spleen:
   i. It will be enlarged with oozing of blood on its surface (fibrocongestive splenomegaly)
   ii. Capsule will be thickened,
   iii. *Histologically:*
       a. Dilated sinusoid with thickened endothelium
       b. Occasional erythrophagocytosis with proliferating histiocytes.
       c. Periarterial hemorrhages—which may progress into siderosis and fibrotic nodules.
II. Splenic vein and portal vein:
   i. Aneurysmal dilatation with tortuosity
   ii. Endothelial hemorrhage
   iii. Mural thrombi
   iv. Intimal calcified or non-calcified plague.

Height of portal venous pressure correlates with the degree of nodularity, but does not correlate with degree of cirrhosis.

In case of esophageal varies, there are **4 zones** of venous drainage are involved in the formation of varices. These are:

i. **Gastric zone:** 2–3 cm below the gastroesophageal junction. At upper end of cardia of the stomach, veins meet and drain into—firstly:
   a. Short gastric vein
   b. Left gastric vein
   Then into splenic vein, then into portal vein.
ii. **Palisade zone:** 2–3 cm proximal to gastric zone into lower esophagus. In this zone, flow is bidirectional. Here veins communicate with periesophageal veins in the distal esophagus.

   This zone is known as dominant **watershed zone between systemic and portal circulations.**
iii. **Perforating zone**—this zone is proximal to palisade zone in the esophagus.

Network of esophageal submucosal veins.
↓
Connects with periesophageal veins
↓
Drains into azygos system of veins
↓
Then into systemic circulation

iv. **Truncal zone:** It lies proximal to perforating zone, 10 cm in length. This zone contains 4 longitudinal veins in lamina propriya of esophagus.

Esophageal varices: Blood supply of esophageal varices is left gastric vein—it has two branches:
i. Anterior branch drains into azygos vein
ii. Posterior branch communicates with varices below the esophageal junction and produces a bundle of thin parallel veins at the gastroesophageal junction and continuous with large tortuous varices at the lower third of esophagus.

There are four layers of vein in the esophageal wall:
i. *Intraepithelial veins:* It correlates with red spots on the esophageal wall found at endoscopic procedure
ii. *Superficial venous plexus:* This plexus drains into deep intrinsic veins.
iii. *Deep intrinsic veins*
iv. *Perforating veins:* These veins connect deep intrinsic veins with the adventitious plexus in the fourth layer.

Usually large varices arises from main trunk of deep intrinsic veins—these veins, in turn, communicate with gastric varices.

Gastric varices: These are supplied by short gastric veins and drains into deep intrinsic veins in the esophageal mucosa. Those gastric varices see more common in extrahepatic portal obstruction.

Colorectal varices: These are developed as association of splanchnic thrombosis.

Portal Hypertensive Intestinal Vasculopathy

In case of chronic portal hypertension: Patient may not develop varices, but there may be spectrum of intestinal mucosal changes due to abnormalities in microcirculation developed in these patients. The mucosal changes are:

a. *Portal hypertensive gastropathy:*
   i. This is usually seen in fundus, body and stomach in case of cirrhosis.
   ii. Histology revealed vascular ectasia.
   iii. Risk of bleeding is increased in patients taking NSAIDs.
   iv. These changes are usually found after sclerotherapy for varices
   v. This can be relieved only after reducing portal pressure.
b. *Gastric antral vascular ectasia:*
   i. This can be described by arteriovenous communication in between muscularis mucosae and dilated pre-capillaries and veins.
   ii. Here there will be increased gastric mucosal perfusion.
   iii. This is not directly related to portal hypertension but may be associated with liver dysfunction.
c. *Congestive jejunopathy and colonopathy:*
   i. This is characterized by increase in size and number of vessels in jejunal and colonic mucosa.
   ii. Histology of mucosa shows edematous, erythematous and friable mucosa.

iii. In case of congestive colonopathy—histology reveals dilated mucosal capillaries, thickened basement membrane, but no evidence of inflammation.

Classification of Portal Hypertension

Portal hypertension can be classified into three types:

A. Presinusoidal (Prehepatic)

a. **Extrahepatic:**
   1. Portal vein:
      i. Thrombosis
      ii. Portal vein invasion
      iii. Compression by tumor
   2. Splenic vein:
      i. Thrombosis,
      ii. Invasion of portal vein
      iii. Compression by tumor
   3. Increased blood flow:
      i. Idiopathic
      ii. Tropical splenomegaly syndrome
      iii. Arteriovenous fistula.
b. **Intrahepatic:** Portal vein involvement:
      i. Schistosomiasis
      ii. Early primary biliary cirrhosis
      iii. Chronic active hepatitis
      iv. Sarcoidosis
      v. Congenital hepatic fibrosis
      vi. Idiopathic portal hypertension
      vii. Toxins—vinyl chloride, copper, arsenic

B. Hepatic

a. **Sinusoidal:**
   1. Cirrhosis
   2. Non-cirrhotic portal fibrosis
   3. Acute alcoholic hepatitis
   4. Cytotoxic drugs
   5. Vitamin A intoxication
b. **Post-sinusoidal:**
   1. Veno-occlusive disease
   2. Alcoholic central hyaline necrosis.

C. Post-hepatic

a. **Hepatic veins:**
   i. Thrombosis
   ii. Web
   iii. Tumor
   iv. Invasion
b. **Inferior vena cava:**
   i. Webs
   ii. Tumor
   iii. Invasion
   iv. Thrombosis
c. **Heart:**
   i. Rise in atrial pressure
   ii. Constrictive pericarditis

Clinical Features of Portal Hypertension

From History

1. Relevant history to cirrhosis or chronic active hepatitis
2. History of alcoholism, blood transfusion, hepatitis B,C, sepsis—intra-abdominal or neonatal
3. History of use of oral contraceptives
4. History of myeloproliferative disorders
5. History of hematemesis:
   i. Number of episodes
   ii. Severity of bleeding
   iii. Whether the bleeding is associated with confusion or coma
   iv. Whether bleeding requires blood transfusion
6. History of melena:
   i. Whether it is associated with hematemesis or not
   ii. Whether it is associated with epigastric tenderness or dyspepsia
7. Any previous endoscopy done or not—if done—what was the previous finding?

Signs

1. Stigmata of cirrhosis:
   i. Jaundice
   ii. Vascular spindles
   iii. Palmar erythema
2. Signs of hepatocellular failure
3. Signs of hepatic encephalopathy
4. Abdominal wall veins
   a. **Site:**
      i. *In case of intrahepatic portal hypertension*—blood from left branch of portal vein will be deviated to umbilicus via paraumbelical veins—here, it reaches the vena caval system—so the veins appear around the umbilicus.
      ii. *In case of extrahepatic portal hypertension*—the tortuous and dilated veins appear in the flanks.
   b. **Direction:**
      i. *In case of intrahepatic portal hypertension*—prominent collateral veins are radiating away from umbilicus—termed as **caput medusae**—usually one or two veins are seen—in epigastric area—but it is rare.
      ii. *In case of inferior vena caval obstruction*—blood will flow below upwards to reach the superior vena cava from interior vena cava.
      iii. *In case of tense ascites*, there will be functional obstruction of inferior vena cava.
   c. **Murmurs:**
      i. Venous hum: Usually heard in xiphoid process and/or umbilicus. There may be associated thrill in that site. **It is due to** rushing of blood through a large umbilical or paraumbilical channel to be abdominal wall veins.
      ii. Venous hum can also be detected over the collaterals like, inferior mesenteric vein.
      iii. Arterial systolic murmur—indicates:
         a. Alcoholic hepatitis
         b. Primary liver cancer

Cruveilhier–Baumgarten syndrome: This is characterized by combination of:
i. Dilated abdominal wall veins
ii. Loud venous murmur at the umbilicus.

Causes:
i. Congenital patency of umbilical vein
ii. Well compensated cirrhosis

Paraxiphoid umbilical hum and caput medusae combination—indicates intrahepatic portal hypertension, because, here, obstruction is present beyond the origin of umbilical veins from left branch of portal vein.

Spleen:
  i. Splenomegaly is the single most indicator of portal hypertension.
 ii. Absence of palpability, or absence of enlargement in imaging may arise a doubt regarding the presence of portal hypertension
iii. Spleen will be enlarged along its axis, firm.
 iv. Splenomegaly is usually seen in young people having macronodular rather than micronodular cirrhosis.
  v. Presence of pancytopenia with splenomegaly—suggests secondary hypersplenism. It is usually due to reticuloendothelial cell hyperplasia rather than portal hypertension.

Liver:
  i. Soft liver—extrahepatic portal hypertension
 ii. Firm liver— cirrhosis
iii. Nodularity:
     a. Macronodular—viral related
     b. Micronodular—alcohol related
 iv. There may be nonpalpable liver

Ascites:
 i. In case of cirrhosis—ascites indicates portal hypertension.
ii. In this case, raised capillary filtration is the cause.

Rectum:
  i. Anorectal varices—found during sigmoidoscopy—found in 44% of patients.
 ii. They may be found in patient, bled from esophageal varices.
iii. This rectal varices must be differentiated from simple hemorrhoids because last one will not communicate with portal system.

Radiological Investigation

a. X-ray of abdomen: CT scan or ultrasound of abdomen: Linear, branched gas shadows near the peripheral branching of portal vein at the periphery of the liver—mainly occurs due to gas forming organism
  i. In adults with intestinal infarction
 ii. In infants with enterocolitis
 It may be associated with:
   a. Disseminated intravascular coagulation
   b. Suppurative cholangitis
b. X-ray of chest:
  1. Tomography of azygos vein: Enlarged azygos vein due to collaterals around azygos vein.
  2. Widened paravertebral shadow: Due to dilated hemiazygos vein producing lateral displacement of pleural reflection between aorta and vertebral column.
  3. Massive dilation of paraesophageal collaterals produces a shadow of retrocardiac posterior mediastinal mass.

Diagnosis of Varices by Endoscopy

A. Esophageal varices:
  Site: It can be seen as filling defects in lower third of esophagus—it may extend throughout the esophagus.
    There may be gross dilatation and widening of the esophageal cavity.

Size: Size may be ≤ 5mm in diameter or may be ≥5 mm in diameter.
  Appearance of the varices:
  1. Varices appear usually as white and opaque.
  2. *Red color*—due to flowing of blood through subepithelial or communicating veins—it occurs in case of large varices.
  3. *Raised cherry-red spots and red wheal markings*—due to dilated subepithelial veins (longitudinal white markings looking like whip marks)—these are present on the top of the vessels.
  4. *Hemocystic spots*—it is 4 mm in diameter. It occurs due to flow of blood from deep intrinsic veins directly straight outward through communicating veins to subepithelial veins.
    All the above signs are associated with severity of varices.

B. Gastric varices
  Site: It is usually seen in fundus of the stomach.
  Appearances:
  i. Looking like worm along the gastric folds in the stomach
 ii. Looking like lobulated mass in fundus—simulating gastric carcinoma

Portal Hypertensive Gastropathy

Sites: It usually occurs in antrum or fundus. But it may occupy throughout the stomach mucosa.

Description:
  i. Small polygonal reddish areas surrounded by whitish yellow depressed border
 ii. Red point lesions
iii. Cherry-red spots
 iv. Black-brown spots—due to intramucosal hemorrhage.
    If sclerotherapy is applied for esophageal varices, portal gastropathy will be aggravated.

Capsule endoscopy can diagnose
 i. Esophageal varices
ii. Portal hypertensive gastropathy where endoscopy is contraindicated

  If capsular endoscopy and upper GI endoscopy are contraindicated—platelet count/spleen diameter ratio is of choice.

| Positive likehood ratio | 2.77 |
| Negative likehood ratio | 0.13 |

Flow through azygos vein can be assessed by Doppler ultrasound probe passed through biopsy channel of standard gastroscope.

Imaging of Portal Venous System

A. Ultrasound: To detect portal venous system, following view are required.
  i. Longitudinal scan at subcostal margin
 ii. Transverse scan at epigastrium
    Normally portal vein and superior mesenteric veins are demonstrated. Normally tracing of splenic vein is difficult.
Mere presence of dilated portal vein is not diagnostic but associated collateral channel delineation is the diagnostic of portal hypertension.

B. Doppler ultrasound: It usually demonstrates anatomy of:
   i. Portal vein
   ii. Hepatic artery

   Color-coded Doppler improves visualization of the arterial or venous anatomy.

Clinical Uses of Doppler Ultrasound

a. Portal vein:
   i. *Patency of the vein*—any echogenic debris, thrombus
   ii. *Spontaneous hepatofugal flow* in portal, splenic and superior mesenteric veins—its presence indicates:
      a. Tendency towards hepatic encephalopathy
      b. Severity of cirrhosis
   iii. *Anatomical abnormalities* of intrahepatic portal veins—it is important in case of requirement of surgery.
   iv. *Demonstration of portal systemic shunt,* shunt patency and direction of flow. Shunts are:
      1. Surgical shunt
      2. Transjugular intrahepatic portosystemic shunt (TIPS)
      3. Intrahepatic portal systemic shunt
   v. Acute flow changes

b. Hepatic artery:
   i. Post-transplant patency
   ii. Anatomical abnormalities

   Delineations of hepatic artery is more difficult than hepatic vein because:
   i. Small size
   ii. Direction of vein
   So, **duplex Doppler** is useful for delineation of hepatic artery.

c. Hepatic vein: Screening of Budd-Chiari syndrome is required.

   Portal blood flow can be measured by real-time Doppler ultrasound—in the following method:

   Portal blood flow = Average velocity of blood flowing through the portal vein × cross-sectional area of the vein. Portal blood flow velocity has positive correlation with:
   i. Presence of esophageal varices
   ii. Size of esophageal varices
   If portal velocity <10 cm/second, indicates no portal hypertension.

Computerized Tomography

By this procedure, following abnormalities can be diagnosed:
   i. Portal vein potency
   ii. Retroperitoneal dilated veins
   iii. Perivisceral dilated veins
   iv. Paraesophageal varices
   v. Umbilical veins

   Esophageal varices can be diagnosed as—intraluminal enhanced protrusion after contrast.

   Gastric varices can be diagnosed as rounded structures, often which cannot be distinguished from gastric wall.

   CT arterioportography: This can be performed after injection of dye through superior mesenteric vein.
   Clinical uses:
   i. Focal lesions
   ii. Collateral circulation
   iii. Arteriovenous shunt

Magnetic Resonance Angiography

1. It is more reliable than CT scan
2. It is useful in following conditions:
   i. Portal vein patency
   ii. Portal vein morphology
   iii. Portal vein blood flow velocity

Portal Venography

When scanning procedures fail to detect patency of portal vein, portal venography will be the procedure of choice.

Clinical uses:
1. Patency of portal vein in case of:
   i. Diagnosis of splenomegaly in childhood
   ii. To exclude the invasion by hepatocellular carcinoma in patient with existing cirrhosis.
2. Anatomy of portal vein is very important before operation for shunt procedures like:
   i. Surgical shunt
   ii. Transjugular intrahepatic shunt
   iii. Hepatic resection
   iv. Hepatic transplantation
3. Diagnosis of large collaterals—in case of chronic hepatic encephalopathy.
4. Filling defect in portal vein.
5. Space occupying lesions in liver
6. Intrasplenic pulp pressure—it is index of portal hypertension

Venographic appearences:

In normal conditions:
   i. Only splenic and portal veins are filled, whereon no other vessels were outlined.
   ii. There is normal filling defect at the junction of splenic and portal vein—due to mixing of non-specified blood.
   iii. Within the liver there is gradual branching with gradual reduction in caliber of the portal vein.
   iv. Later on, the liver is becomes opaque due to filling of sinusoids.

In cirrhosis:
   i. There is large number of collaterals
   ii. Gross distortion of intrahepatic pattern with gradual attenuation of caliber of the vessels (tree in winter appearance)

In extrahepatic portal or splenic vein obstruction:
   i. From splenic vein, large number of vessels will go to:
      a. Diaphragm
      b. Thoracic cage
      c. Abdominal wall
   ii. Intrahepatic portal veins are usually not seen. But in some cases, paraportal vessels may bypass the lesion and reach the liver.

Visceral Angiography

New contrast material is nontoxic to kidney and other tissues and no evidence of hypersensitivity reaction seen.

Clinical uses:
   i. Demonstration of shunting of blood through collaterals
   ii. Evaluation of patients with hepatocellular carcinoma for radioactive bead therapy.
   iii. In case of liver transplantation, hepatic arterial problems.
   iv. Diagnosis of space occupying lesion in the liver

v. Detail anatomy of splenic and hepatic arterial anatomy is essential, if the patient requires surgery.
vi. Other space occupying lesions, like, hemangioma, aneurysms.

Portal vein may not be specified, if:
a. The flow is hepatofugal.
b. There is steal by the spleen.
c. There are large collaterals.

In this case, superior mesenteric angiography will reveal the portal vein structure.

Celiac artery is usually catheterized through femoral artery. The flow first will pass through splenic artery then to splenic vein ultimately into portal vein producing splenic as well as portal venography.

If contrast is injected into superior mesenteric artery—it will pass through superior mesenteric vein, ultimately to portal vein producing portal venography.

Digital Substraction Angiography

Selective arterial injection of the contrast
↓
Followed by subtraction of images.

The technique is very useful for:
i. Evaluation of parenchymal phase of hepatic angiography
ii. Diagnosis of vascular lesions
    a. Hemangioma
    b. Arteriovenous malformation

Splenic Angiography

Contrast materials injected into splenic pulp
↓
┌── Into splenic vein
│   ↓
↓   Into portal venous system
Collaterals can be delineated

Carbon Dioxide Occluded Venography

Injection of carbon dioxide in wedged hepatic venous position
↓
Delineations of hepatic and portal venous free

Portal Pressure Measurement

Balloon catheter is introduced into femoral vein or internal jugular vein, then into hepatic vein.

The pressures to be measured are (by inflating and deflating the balloon at the tip of the catheter)
i. Wedged hepatic venous pressure (WHVP)
ii. Free hepatic venous pressure (FHVP)

Hepatic venous pressure gradient (HVPG): WHVP—FHVP
HVPG is nothing by sinusoidal pressure (portal venous pressure)
FHVP is free hepatic venous pressure.

If the cause of portal hypertension is sinusoidal
WHVP = portal venous pressure

Normal HVPG = 5–6 mmHg
Significant portal hypertension = ≥10 mmHg—this is associated with:
a. Decompensated cirrhosis
b. Bleeding esophageal varies

Administration of beta-blocker (propranolol)
↓
Reduction of portal pressure >20% from the baseline
↓
There will be reduced risk of bleeding

Variceal Pressure

It can be measured by two methods:
i. Direct puncture of varices at the time of sclerotherapy
ii. Endoscopic balloon at the endoscopy tip

In cirrhotic patient, the pressure is 15.5 mmHg, which is significantly lower than the portal pressure (18.8 mmHg)

Estimation of Hepatic Blood Flow

A. Constant infusion method: Hepatic blood flow can be measured by following methods
    i. Constant infusion of indocyanine green
    ii. Catheterization of hepatic vein
B. Plasma disappearance method: Hepatic blood flow can be measured by:

Intravenous injection of indocyanine green
↓
Analysis of disappearance curve measured in peripheral artery.

Inference:
    i. If the extraction is 100%, hepatic blood flow can be measured by seeing the peripheral clearance—in normal patient. Here by there is no need of hepatic vein catheterization.
    ii. If the extraction is 20%, blood will not pass through the normal channel, hepatic extraction will be reduced. Here, hepatic vein catheterization is absolutely necessary to measure the hepatic blood flow.
C. Azygos blood flow: This can be measured by double thermodilution catheter method under fluoroscopy into azygos vein.

In alcoholic cirrhosis with history of bleeding varices azygos flow will be 600 ml/min. This flow will be reduced by administration of propranolol.

Extrahepatic Portal Venous Obstruction

a. **Infections:**
    i. In case of neonates or older children—infections spread from umbilical vein to left portal vein then to portal vein:
        1. Umbilical sepsis
        2. Acute appendicitis
        3. Peritonitis
    ii. Portal vein occlusion
        1. Neonatal dehydration
        2. Ulcerative colitis
        3. Crohn's disease

4. Wall stone with cholangitis
5. Primary sclerosing cholangitis

b. **Postoperative:**
   i. Splenectomy with normal platelet count
   ii. Surgical portosystemic shunt
   iii. Major difficult hepatobiliary surgery
      1. Repair of stricture
      2. Choledochal cyst

c. **Trauma:**
   i. Vehicle accident
   ii. Stabbing

d. **Hypercoagulable state:**
   i. Myeloproliferative disorder with or without presence of G20210A prothrombin gene mutation
   ii. Protein C deficiencies
   iii. Protein S deficiencies
   iv. Antithrombin III deficiencies

e. **Invasion and compression:**
   i. Hepatocellular carcinoma
   ii. Carcinoma of body of pancreas
   iii. Chronic pancreatitis—associated with splenic vein obstruction

f. **Congenital:**
   i. Congenital obstruction along the line of right and left vitelline veins.
   ii. In absence of portal vein, visceral venous return to systemic veins.

g. **Cirrhosis:**
   i. Invasion by hepatocellular carcinoma
   ii. Post-splenectomy thrombocytosis

h. **Miscellaneous:**
   i. Pregnancy
   ii. Oral contraceptives for long duration
   iii. Thrombophlebitis migrans
   iv. Other venous diseases
   v. Retroperitoneal fibrosis
   vi. Behcet's disease

i. **Unknown:** Associated with autoimmune disorders
   i. Hypothyroidism
   ii. Diabetics
   iii. Pernicious anemia
   iv. Dermatomyositis
   v. Rheumatoid arthritis

Clinical Features

A. **Present with underlying diseases like:**
   i. Polycythemia rubra vera
   ii. Primary liver cancer

B. **Variceal bleeding**—from esophageal varices

   i. In case of neonates—it starts at the age of 4 years
   ↓
   Increases in frequency between 10 and 15 years
   ↓
   Frequency decreases after puberty

   ii. In patients with portal venous thrombosis:
      a. Some patients may never bleed
      b. Some patients may bleed after 12 years of onset of disease

   iii. Intermittent minor blood loss—this can be diagnosed by:
      a. Fecal blood loss
      b. Iron deficiency anemia

Precipitating factors:
   i. Infections
   ii. Aspirin ingestion

Excessive exertion and swallowing large bolus of food do not precipitate bleeding.

Signs:

A. *Spleen*—Symptomless slpenomegaly is common in children.

B. *Periumbilical vein*—dilated abdominal wall vein in left flank.

C. *Liver:*
   i. It is normal in size.
   ii. Signs of hepatocellular disease—spider nevi, jaundice is usually absent
   iii. In elderly, due to hepatocellular deterioration, jaundice may appear.
   iv. In case of acute portal venous thrombosis—ascites appears early and it is transient. It will disappear after the appearance of collaterals.

D. *Hepatic encephalopathy:*
   i. Acute encephalopathy—uncommon in adult.
      Precipitating factors:
      a. Hemorrhage
      b. Infection:
      c. Anesthesia
   ii. In chronic encephalopathy—common in adult. Precipitating factors—large portal systemic shunt.

Investigations

A. **Imaging:**
   a. *Ultrasound*—echogenic thrombus in portal vein
   b. *Doppler ultrasound:*
      i. Slow flow velocity in cavernous collaterals
      ii. No portal signal
   c. *CT scan:*
      i. Non-enhancing filling defect within portal vein
      ii. Dilatation of many small hilar veins.
   d. *MRI:*
      i. Abnormal signal within the lumen of portal vein—appearing as isointense on T1-weighted image
      ii. More intense signal in T2-weighted image.

B. **Angiography:**
   i. In portal venous phase—as filing defect in portal vein
   ii. In case of extensive collaterals—portal vein may not be visualized.

Clinical hematology:

a. *Hemoglobin:*
   i. Normal usually
   ii. In case of blood loss—anemia

b. *Leukocytes:*
   i. Function—nomal
   ii. Leucopenia—in case of enlarged spleen with hypersplenism.

c. *Thrombocytes*—thrombocytopenia—in case of enlarged spleen with hypersplenism

d. *Blood coagulation*—normal

Serum biochemistry:
  i. Liver function test—is usually normal
  ii. Serum globulin—may be raised—which may be related to raised antigen, bypassing the liver through extensive collaterals.
  iii. Hypofunction of pancreas—which may be related to interruption pancreatic venous drainage

Prognosis

1. Prognosis depends upon underlying disease.
2. Prognosis is better than cirrhosis, because in this case, liver function test is normal.
3. Prognosis is better in child, if bleeding episode can be managed carefully.
4. Pregnant women may not bleed usually, but their babies are usually normal.

Treatment

A. Treatment of the etiology—like:
  i. In case of hepatocellular carcinoma—there may be a chance of invasion of portal vein by tumor tissue—hence, aggressive therapy for bleeding esophageal varices.
  ii. In case of polycythemia rubra vera
    a. Reduction of platelet count
    b. Anticoagulants may be required
B. Prophylactic treatment of varices: It is not usually required, because it will never rupture as, extensive number of collaterals will be opened up with progression in time.
  In case of acute portal vein thrombosis, anticoagulant administration results in:
  i. Recanalization of portal vein.
  ii. Prevention of the following events:
    a. Spreading of thrombosis
    b. Intestinal infarction
    c. Severe bleeding
  But alternate therapy is required for:
  i. Presence of ascites
  ii. Presence of splenic vein thrombosis
C. Avoidance of aspirin ingestion
D. Proper treatment of upper respiratory tract or other infections.
E. Adequate and compatible blood transfusion according to the need.
F. In case of massive bleeding:
  i. Balloon tamponade may be required.
  ii. Recurrent sclerotherapy mainly in children
  iii. Ligation
  iv. Glue injection in case of gastric varices
G. Shunt is not suitable in this condition because of the following factors:
  i. Normal looking vein in venography may be turn out to be poor condition due to extension of thrombotic process.
  ii. In children, veins are usually small and difficult to anastomose
H. If shunt is of 1st choice, following shunts can be done:
  i. Portacaval shunt
  ii. Mesocaval shunt
  iii. Splenocaval shunt

  iv. In children—mesentericoportal shunt—anatomizing patent left branch of portal vein, because:
    a. It improves growth
    b. Prevents bleeding
I. In case of exsanguinating patients in spite of massive blood transfusion—esophageal transection is the procedure of choice.

Splenic Vein Obstruction

Causes

  i. Pancreatic carcinoma
  ii. Pancreatitis
  iii. Pancreatic pseudocyst
  iv. Pancreatectomy

If the obstruction is distal to communication between left gastric vein and splenic vein

Blood flows through collaterals
↓
Bypass the splenic vein
↓
Through short gastric veins
↓
To left gastric vein and portal vein

Results: Development of varices in:
  i. Gastric fundus
  ii. Lower esophagus

Diagnosis

a. CT scan
b. MRI
c. Selective venous phase of angiogram.

Treatment

Splenectomy: It cures this condition by blocking the arterial inflow. It is usually curative.

Presinusoidal Intrahepatic and Sinusoidal Portal Hypertension

Portal Tract Lesions

a. **Schistosomiasis:** Here ova causes reaction in portal venous radicles.
b. **Congenital hepatic fibrosis:** Here deficiency of terminal branches of portal vein in fibrotic portal zones is responsible for portal hypertension.
c. **Myeloproliferative diseases:**
  i. Chronic myeloid leukemia
  ii. Myelosclerosis
  iii. Hodgkin's disease
  Mechanisms:
  i. Infiltration of portal zone by hemopoietic tissues
  ii. Thrombosis in minor or major portal vein radicles
  iii. Nodular regenerative hyperplasia
d. **Systemic mastocytosis:** Here portal hypertension is due to:
  i. Mast cell infiltration producing intrahepatic resistance
  ii. Increase splenic flow—due to:
    1. Arteriovenous shunting
    2. Increased histamine release
e. **Primary biliary cirrhosis**—fibrosis of portal zones
f. **Sarcoidosis**—due to massive fibrosis

Toxic Causes

> Injurious toxins
> ↓
> Taken up by the stellate cells in Disse's space
> ↓
> Minute portal vein radicals are obstructed and produces sclerosis
> ↓
> Intrahepatic portal hypertension

The agents are:
  i. Arsenic
 ii. Vinyl chloride
iii. Copper (angioscarcoma, may be a complication)
 iv. Vitamin A intoxication
  v. Cytotoxic drugs—methotrexate
 vi. 6 mercaptopurine
vii. Azathioprine

Hepatoportal Sclerosis

It can be termed as:
 i. Non-cirrhotic portal fibrosis
ii. Idiopathic portal hypertension

Causes:
  i. Infections, ii. Toxic (arsenic), iii. May be unknown

As a result of intrahepatic resistance, there is obstruction to hepatic blood flow.

In India, young males are mainly affected.

Liver biopsy:
  i. Sclerosis and obliteration of the intrahepatic venous bed
 ii. Minimal fibrosis
iii. Large veins near helium—thickened and narrow.
 iv. Perisinusoidal fibrosis.

Portal venography:
  i. Narrowed and spare portal vein radicles
 ii. Peripheral branches are irregular and in acute angle division
iii. 'Nonspecified large intrahepatic portal branches with increased very fine vasculature around them.

Hepatic venography:
 i. Confirmation of vascular abnormalities
ii. Vein to vein anastomoses

Hepatoportal sclerosis is characterized by:
  i. Splenomegaly
 ii. Hypersplenism
iii. Portal hypertension
 iv. Absence of any occlusion of portal and splenic veins
  v. No obvious pathology in the liver

Tropical Splenomegaly Syndrome

This is characterized by the following:
  i. It occurs in material area.
 ii. Splenomegaly
iii. Hepatic sinusoidal lymphocytosis
 iv. Kupffer cell hyperplasia
  v. Raised serum IgM and malarial antibody titer
 vi. Responds to prolonged antimalarial treatment
vii. Mild to morderate portal hypertension
viii. Rare variceal bleeding

Intrahepatic Sinusoidal Portal Hypertension

> Cirrhosis: Development in nodules
> ↓
> Obstruction to portal blood flow
> ↓
> Portal blood is diverted into collateral channels and some bypass the liver cells
> ↓
> Passes to hepatic venous radicles in fibrous septa
> ↓
> To hepatic vein
> ↓
> Hepatic vein will be displaced or further outward and lies in fibrous of septum—connected with portal venous radicles by pre-existing sinusoid.
> ↓
> Hepatic regenerating nodules will be devoid of portal blood supply
> ↓
> They will be nourished by hepatic artery.

One-third of total blood flow into liver tissue will bypass the liver sinusoid through collateral channels.

In cirrhosis—wedged hepatic venous pressure, as well as main portal venous pressures are identical.

Venous stasis must extend to portal inflow vessels.

In alcoholic patient:
  i. Due to excessive collagen deposition in space of Disse, sinusoids will be narrowed.
 ii. Swelled hepatocytes reduce the sinusoidal blood flow.

Again, regenerative nodules in cirrhosis compress the hepatic venous radicles—producing **post-sinusoidal portal hypertension**.

So in cirrhosis—portal vein obstruction occurs in the following levels:
  i. Presinusoidal level
 ii. Sinusoidal level
iii. Post-sinusoidal level

Normally:
 i. Hepatic artery supplies small volume of blood at high pressure
ii. Portal vein supplies large volume of blood at low pressure
    But equilibration occurs at hepatic sinusoid.

So hepatic artery, in normal person plays a little role in maintaining portal venous pressure.

But, in case of cirrhosis, there is hypertrophy of hepatic artery; as a result, there will be increased flow through hepatic artery to maintain normal sinusoidal perfusion.

Bleeding Esophageal Varices

In cirrhotic patient, first appearance of gastroesophageal varices followed by subsequent growth is ~ 7% per year after diagnosis of cirrhosis.

Precipitating Factors

  i. Inflammatory response to infection
 ii. Red signs on varices
iii. Size of the varices

iv. Degree of hepatocellular dysfunction—if it is moderate to severe, it is the sole predictor of bleeding irrespective of other factor.
v. Portal pressure
  a. >10 mmHg—is responsible for production of varices
  b. >12 mmHg—is responsible for variceal bleeding
vi. Alcoholic cirrhosis is at most risk.

Doppler sonography predict the bleeding from varices based on following factors:
i. Velocity of blood flow
ii. Diameter of portal vein
iii. Size of spleen
iv. Presence of collaterals

Child's grade of hepatocellular dysfunction correlates with severity of bleeding in following ways (Table 4.12):
i. Variceal size
ii. Presence of endoscopic red signs
iii. Response to emergency treatment

Table 4.12: Child's classification of hepatocellular dysfunctions in cirrhosis

Group	A	B	C
1. Serum bilirubin (mg/dl)	<2.0	2.0–3.0	>3.0
2. Serum albumin (mg/dl)	>3.5	3.0–3.5	<3
3. Ascites	None	Easily controlled	Poorly controlled
4. Neurological disorder	None	Minimal	Advanced coma
5. Nutrition	Excellent	Good	Poor (wasting)

Prevention of First Bleeding

A. **Improvement of liver function tests**
B. **Abstinence from alcohol**
C. **Avoidance of aspirin, NSAIDs**
D. **Beta-blockers**—the drugs are—propranolol, nadolol. These drugs reduce portal pressure by following mechanisms
  i. Splanchnic vasoconstriction
  ii. Reduction of cardiac output
  iii. Fall in blood flow through hepatic artery

The drug dose should be maintained to reduce the heart rate not below 55/minute.

But patients with advanced cirrhosis may not respond even with high dose of beta-blocker.

Hepatic venous pressure gradient (HVPG) below 12 mmHg or <20% of baseline is the ultimate aim.

Contraindications:
i. Chronic obstructive lung disease
ii. Diabetes adverse effect:
  a. Impotence
  b. Fatigue
  c. Mental depression
E. **Banding:** It is the treatment of choice, if there is contraindicative of using beta-blockers.

Diagnosis of Bleeding

A. Features of portal hypertension
B. Clinical features of gastrointestinal bleeding—like:

i. Sudden and massive hematemesis
ii. Slow oozing with melena
iii. Iron deficiency anemia—due to:
  a. Portal hypertension gastropathy
  b. Slow microscopic bleeding
  c. Massive collection of blood in large intestine or colon.

Liver cells are affected by injurious effects of bleeding varices due to following reasons:
1. Iron deficiency anemia—diminishing oxygen supply to liver cells.
2. Increased metabolic demand due to:
  i. Increased protein catabolism
  ii. Secondary stimulation of cytokines
3. Fall in blood pressure produces diminished flow through hepatic artery—resulting ischemic hepatitis
4. Diminished renal perfusion producing renal injury
5. Increased nitrogen absorption from intestine producing hepatic encephalopathy.
6. Deterioration of hepatic functions producing jaundice, ascites.

The non-variceal bleeding episodes occur due to:
i. Duodenal ulcer
ii. Gastric erosions
iii. Portal hypertensive gastropathy,
iv. Mallory-Weiss syndrome

Endoscopy is the procedure of choice within 12 hours of bleeding episode to detect the source of bleeding.

Criteria for Diagnosis of Bleeding by Endoscopy

i. Oozing of blood from an area within 5 cm of gastro-esophageal junction
ii. Venous spurt (active bleeding)
iii. White raised spot—indicating platelet plugging.

Prognosis: Severity of hepatocellular disease along with death within 6 weeks—occurs—in grade A 0–10% in grade C—20–40% survival score depends upon combination of variables like:
i. Severity of the liver disease
ii. Presence of active bleeding
iii. Encephalopathy
iv. Prothrombin time
v. Number of blood transfusion within 12 hours
vi. Abstinence from alcohol
vii. Patient surviving from chronic hepatitis
viii. Patients with primary biliary cirrhosis, if not jaundiced.

Management of Acute Variceal Bleeding

General management:
a. *Hemodynamic monitoring* by measuring central venous pressure
b. *Transfusion:*
  i. Blood transfusion—if hemoglobin ≤8 gm/dl.
  ii. Over transfusion and saline transfusion should be avoided.
    Systolic blood pressure should be maintained to ≥90 mmHg
  iii. Fresh frozen plasma and platelet transfusions are usually given to prevent worsening of coagulation.
c. *Vitamin K injection* must be routinely given.

d. *Acid suppression*—by:
   i. H$_2$ receptor antagonist, or
   ii. Proton pump inhibitor

   H$_2$ receptor antagonists have less risk of inducing *Clostridium difficile*.
   Stress-induced mucosal ulcer may be present.

e. Liver function tests, electrolyte balance and renal function should be properly monitored.

f. Prophylactic antibiotic:
   1. Third generation cephalosporin should be given to:
      i. Prevent infection
      ii. Reduce bleeding
      iii. Improve survival
   2. *During endoscopy*, pneumonia can be prevented by taking special care.
   3. *In patient with hepatic encephalopathy*—endotracheal intubation should be warranted.

g. *Administration of lactulose and phosphate* enema can prevent hepatic encephalopathy.

h. *Sedatives:*
   i. Usually it should be avoided.
   ii. If necessary, low dose **zopiclone**—can be given.
   iii. In alcoholics, to prevent delirium tremens—oral chlordiazpoxide or chlormethiazole usually given.

i. *In case of tense ascites*—cautious paracentesis with simultaneous administration of intravenous salt poor albumin and oral spironolactone.

Specific Therapeutic Options

Vasoactive drugs. It should be given:
1. Before admission in the hospital
2. Before diagnostic or therapeutic endoscopy

Drugs are:
i. Vasopressin
ii. Terlipressin

Actions: Constriction of splanchnic arterioles
↓
Increased resistance to the inflow of blood to the gut
↓
Lowering of portal venous pressure
↓
Control of variceal bleeding

Complications:
   i. Coronary vasoconstriction—so ECG must be done before administration of these drugs.
   ii. Abdominal colicky abdominal pain.
   iii. Evacuation of bowel
   iv. Facial pallor
   v. Myocardial ischemia or infarction
   vi. Intestinal ischemia or infarction.

Dosage:

Terlipressin—2 mg intravenously 6 hourly for 48 hours
↓
1 mg intravenously 6–8 hourly for 72 hours.

Somatostatin:

Actions: Constriction of splanchnic arterioles
Inhibition of number of vasodilatory peptides including glucagon
↓
Reduction of portal venous pressure

Its side effect is lower than vasopressin or terlipressin.

Dose: Bolus dose 250–500 µg intravenously.
↓
Infusion 6 mg/day for 5 days

Octreotide or vapreotide—synthetic analogue of somatostatin. They are less active.

Sengstaken-Blakemore tube: Nowadays, this tube is of less use after the advent of vasoactive drugs.

Description: It is a four luminal tube—has:
   i. Esophageal balloon
   ii. Gastric balloon
   iii. Aspirating channel from the stomach
   iv. Fourth lumen for continuous aspiration above the esophageal balloon.

Method of insertion:
1. Endotracheal intubation should be done first, if possible.
2. Before insertion, this tube has to be kept in ice box to make it harden, so that it may be easily inserted.
3. Stomach should be emptied.
4. New tested lubricated tube to be inserted into the stomach after passing through the mouth.
5. Gastric balloon should be inflated with 250 ml of air and doubly clamped.
5. The tube will be pulled upwards till the resistance can be felt at gastroesophageal junction.
6. Esophageal balloon will be inflated to make the pressure in the balloon 40 mmHg which will be greater than the expected portal pressure.
7. The tube should be taped at the corner of the mouth so that there will be a constant traction will be maintained in the esophagus
   i. If tractions less, gastric balloon will fall in the stomach cavity.
   ii. If the traction is too much, there will be retrosternal discomfort, reching and esophageal ulceration.
8. The position of the tube must be checked by X-ray.
9. Head end of the bed will be raised.

Follow-up:
1. Continuous low pressure suction and aspiration will be provided by esophageal balloon.
2. Tube traction and esophageal balloon pressure should be hourly checked.
3. After 12 hours, esophageal balloon will be deflated and traction will be released—to watch, if bleeding recurs.
4. If bleeding recurs, retraction and reinflation of esophageal balloon will be done until therapeutic endoscopy or TIPS can be performed.

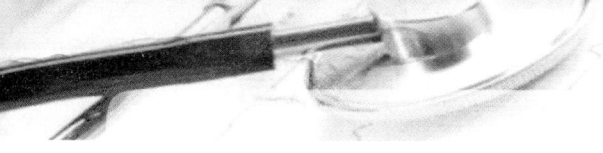

If bleeding will not be controlled, the following factors are responsible:
i. Tube will be slipped.
ii. Fundal varices will be the possible source.
iii. There may be another lesion.

Complications:
i. If gastric balloon deflates, the esophageal balloon will be migrated upwards to obstruct upper respiratory tract producing asphyxia.
In this case, esophageal balloon must be deflated or will be cut through.
ii. Prolonged and repeated use of esophageal balloon is responsible for esophageal ulceration.
iii. Aspiration of secretion can be prevented by continuous suction above the esophageal balloon.
iv. If gastric balloon will be inflated wrongly in esophagus— esophageal rupture may occur.
v. Esophageal tube is kept for more than 48 hours—it may produce esophageal ulceration.

Esophageal Stent

1. It is covered self-expandable stent, which can be removed endoscopically.
2. It can produce esophageal tamponade.
3. Patient drinks or eats.
4. In case of esophageal tear produced by Sengstaken tube— this stent will be the replacement.
5. Only expert can introduce this tube under radiological screening.

Endoscopic Banding and Endoscopic Sclerotherapy

Combination of vasoactive agents with endoscopic band ligation or sclerotherapy—is the treatment of acute variceal bleeding from esophageal varices and subcardial gastric varices.

1. Banding ligation is more preferable to sclerotherapy with 5% ethanol amine or 1% sodium tetradecyl sulphate or polydecanol—when there is no active bleeding.
2. In case of rebreeding, repeat emergency ligation or sclerotherapy should be done.
3. If several sessions of banding or sclerotherapy are required, then TIPS or injection of glue should be considered.
4. Before this procedure: Patient must be sedated or if required, intubated.
5. Double channel endoscopy should be preferred for continued suction and washing with normal saline before and during ligation.
6. In case of sclerotherapy, 2 ml of sclerosant solution should be infected into each varix, but never inject >4 ml of solution.
7. In case of esophageal ligation, 6 band ligator should be used. Banding should be started from gastroesophageal junction and should be confined to low 3–5 cm of esophagus.
8. Each band is applied to each varix in spiral fashion.
9. Complications of esophageal banding and sclerotherapy:
   i. Dysphagia
   ii. Retrosternal discomfort
   iii. Esophageal ulcer
   iv. Recurrence of bleeding

v. Aspiration pneumonia
Administration of sucralfate will aggravate healing and prevent bleeding.
10. In case of bleeding fundal varices, injection of cyano-acrylate glue is required.
Bleeding from fundal varices is more severe than bleeding from esophageal varices.

Variceal bleeding can be diagnosed by endoscopy based on following findings:
i. Spurting of blood from varices
ii. White nipple or clot adhered to varices
iii. No evidence of potential source of bleeding other than varices.

Significant indications of early re-bleeding risk:
i. Active bleeding in emergency endoscopy
ii. Gastric varices
iii. Low albumin
iv. High blood urea level
v. HVPG >20 mmHg

Most consistent death risk indicators:
i. Child-Pugh classification or its component
ii. Blood urea nitrogen
iii. Raised creatinine
iv. Age
v. Alcohol abuse
vi. Active bleeding found in endoscopy
vii. Bacterial infection
viii. HVPG >20 mmHg
ix. Hepatocellular carcinoma
x. Number of transfused units of blood.

Gastric Varices: Classifications

1. Gastric varices continuous with esophageal varices:
   i. Along the lesser curvature of stomach (GOV-1)—gastro-esophageal varices type-1
   ii. In the fundus (GOV2)
2. Isolated gastric varices:
   i. In the fundus (IGV-1)
   ii. In the rest of the stomach (IGV-2)

Gastric varices:
i. Is associated with lower portal venous pressure than esophageal varices.
ii. Is associated with spontaneous shunts (Gasto-renal shunt)
   a. between splenic vein (splenorenal shunt) through inferior phrenic vein and left renal vein through supra-renal vein.

Portosystemic Shunt

Transjugular intrahepatic portosystemic shunt: This is radiological procedure, where under general anesthesia or under local anesthesia:
i. Through internal jugular vein hepatic vein will be cannulated (usually middle right)
ii. Under ultrasonographic guidance, portal vein will be punctured through which a connection between hepatic vein and portal vein will be made.
iii. A self-expandable covered stent will be placed through that track—stent diameter is 10–12 mm.
iv. Caution must be taken upon following factors:
   a. Never encroach inferior venacava;
   b. Never too much encroachment into portal vein.

Above two encroachments render the future liver transplantation difficult.

Result:

Marked decrease in absolute portal pressure
And
Slight increase in inferior venacaval pressure
↓
Reduction PPG (<12 mmHg)
↓
Marked decrease in portal—collateral flow
↓
Reduction of bleeding

If there is shunt occlusion at portal vein or hepatic vein opening, there will be gradual increase in portal pressure gradient (PPL) to >12 mmHg.

Complications: Mortality during procedure <1%:

a. *Hemorrhage:*   i. Due to liver capsule puncture.
                  ii. Intrahepatic puncture.
   Both of which may result in intra abdominal bleeding or bleeding into biliary tract.

b. *Infection:*   It can be prevented by:
              i. Careful aseptic technique
              ii. Early removal of central line

c. *Intravascular hemolysis*—due to passage of erythrocytes through mesh of the stent.

d. *Hyperbilirubinemia*—in post shunt period it indicates poor prognosis.

e. *Shunt occlusion*—it can be treated by:
   i. Revision of shunt
   ii. Dilatation by Percuteneous catheterization
   iii. New shunt
   iv. distal spleno-renal shunt

Emergency Surgery

Indication:
i. It TIPS will fail
ii. If other measure will fail

Types of operations:
i. Portacaval shunt
ii. Esophageal transaction

Rebleeding and its Prevention

In case of variceal bleeding, rebreeding occurs in 70% of patients within 1 year—it is more common in child grade 3. The most effective therapy before discharge will be:
i. Endoscopic band ligation and
ii. Non selective beta blockers—titrated to such maximum dose where patient's pulse rate should never less than 55/minutes.

Repeat banding should be done at 2–3 weeks interval, because this interval is required for esophageal raw areas to heal. The indicators of stopping of band ligations are:
i. Total erradication of varices
ii. Varices are too small to band.
   Follow up endoscopy will be required at 6 months interval to watch the regrow the varices

Portacaval Shunts

Indications:
i. To reduce portal venous pressure.
ii. To maintain total hepatic blood flow.
iii. To maintain portal blood flow.
iv. To prevent high incidence of hepatic encephalopathy.

Shunt procedure: Main idea is to join portal vein with inferior vena cava. There are two procedures of joining:
i. End-to-side procedure with ligation of portal vein
ii. Side-to-side procedure to maintain continuity of portal vein.

Aims:
i. Fall in portal venous pressure
ii. Fall in hepatic venous pressure
iii. Increase is arterial flow

Drawback:
i. High incidence of post shunt encephalopathy
ii. Deterioration of liver function due to reduction of portal perfusion
iii. Subsequent hepatic transplantation will be difficult.

It is still useful in following conditions:
i. After control of bleeding episode
ii. In patients with good hepatic reserve
iii. Who cannot take get treatment in tertiary care hospital including TIPS.
iv. Patient who had bleeding episodes along with patent portal vein with following:
   a. Early primary biliary cirrhosis
   b. Congenital hepatic fibrosis
   c. Good hepatocellular function
   d. Portal vein obstruction at the hilum of the liver
v. Cirrhotic patient's age will be less than 50 years
vi. There is no history of hepatic encephalopathy
vii. Patient should be in child's grade A or B.

Mesocaval Shunt

i. Here shunt will be done between superior mesenteric vein and inferior vena cava with the help of Dacron graft.
ii. The technique is very easy.
iii. With time, shunt may be occluded followed by occurrence of rebleeding.
iv. Subsequent hepatic transplantation is usually possible.

Selective Distal Splenorenal Shunt

Procedure is:
i. Feeding veins to esophagogastric collaterals will be divided.
ii. Drainage of portal blood through short gastric veins and splenic veins to reach inferior vena cava through splenorenal shunt.

Results: Maintenance of portal perfusion pressure. But this shunt will be temporary for 1–2 years.

Complications:
i. Mortality is high.
ii. High incidence of hepatic encephalopathy.

Better results are found in:
i. Non alcoholic patient.
ii. Problem lies in gastric vein.

Results of portal-systemic shunt:
1. Bleeding from gastroesophageal varices will be reduced.
2. Varices will be reduced in size or will disappear within 1 year.
3. Decreased in blood pressure.
4. Hepatic function may deteriorate due to reduced hepatic arterial flow.
5. Ankle edema may appear due to:
   i. Low serum albumin.
   ii. Fall in portal venous pressure
6. Cardiac output may be increased to precipitate heart failure.
7. Transient hepatic encephalopathy with personality changes in one-third patients. It depends upon:
   i. Age of the patient
   ii. Size of the shunt
   iii. Child's grade
8. Rare neurological manifestations are:
   i. Paraplegia
   ii. Myelopathy
   iii. Parkinsonian cerebellar syndrome

TIPS

It is more effective than endoscopic therapy in the rebleeding point of view.

But in terms of survival, there is no difference, as there is more chance of hepatic encephalopathy.

TIPS Encephalopathy

It will decline after first 3 months of shunt due to cerebral adaptation.

It can be treated by:
i. Placing a smaller stent within intrahepatic shunt. Resistant encephalopathy can be treated by liver transplantation

Circulatory Changes in Shunt Procedures

i. Hyperdynamic circulation
ii. Systemic vasodilatation
iii. Increased cardiac output
iv. Increased systemic blood volume;
v. In patient with underlying cardiac problem—heart failure may be precipitated
vi. In alcoholics, unmasking of cardiomyopathy
vii. There may be development of pulmonary hypertension.

TIPS can be indicated in following conditions:
1. Ascites in child Grade B
2. Hepatic hydrothorax
3. Build-Chiari syndrome
4. Hepatorenal syndrome

Hepatic Transplantation

Indications

i. Occurrence of bleeding from varices in patients with end stage liver disease.
ii. At least two episodes of bleeding from varices in spite of proper therapy.

Previous surgical shunt may make transplantation more difficult.

But lienorenal shunt, mesocaval shunt and TIPS are not absolute contraindication.

Pharmacological Intervention to Control Portal Venous Pressure

Portal hypertension results from:
i. Hyperdynamic circulation
ii. Increased cardiac output
iii. Reduced peripheral resistance
iv. Changes in autonomic nervous system
v. Many hormonal factors.

Again, portal pressure can be reduced by:
i. Lowering cardiac output
ii. Reduction of inflow through splanchnic vasoconstriction
iii. Splanchnic venodilation
iv. Reduction of intrahepatic vascular resistance.

The aim is to reduce the portal pressure without decreasing hepatic arterial flow, because, liver function will be maintained.

Newer therapies:
i. Do not worsen systemic hemodynamics.
ii. acts specifically in hepatic microcirculation but do not reduce the portal flow.

The drugs are statin—this drug can be added with beta blocker.

Monitoring: This combination of therapy is required to maintain HVFG to less than 12 mmHg of 20% reduction from baseline.

Non-selective beta-blocker:
i. Reduces HVPG but to lesser extent
ii. Bacterial translocation will be reduced, so spontaneous bacterial peritonitis will not be developed.

This occurs due to following factors:
i. Increased intestinal transit
ii. Decreased mucosal congestion.

CONGENITAL LIVER DISEASES

Gilbert Syndrome

This disease is after the name of Augustine Gilbert, Parisian physician.

Definition

It is defined as:
1. Benign, familial, mild unconjugated hyperbilirubinemia.
2. No history of hemolysis.
3. Normal liver histology.
4. Normal liver function test.
5. Level of bilirubin is 1–5 mg/ml.

Jaundice is:
i. Mild and intermittent.
ii. Aggravated by infection, fasting, vomiting.
iii. It is associated with following symptoms:
   a. Nausea
   b. Malaise
   c. Pain in right upper quadrant of abdomen

Pathogenesis

There is deficiency in bilirubin glucuronidation. As a result, the bile contains mostly bilirubin monoglucuronide than bilirubin diglucuronide.

Genetic Basis

Promoter region [A(TA)$_6$TAA] of the gene encoding UGT1A1 (Uridine diphosphate glucuronoyl transferase) of this syndrome contains additional TA dinucleotide, as a result, promoter region will be changed to (A(TA)$_7$TAA).

There is also relationship between promoter region genotype and UGT liver enzyme activity, like:

i. Individual with genotype 7/7—have low enzyme activity.
ii. Individual with genotype 6/7—have intermediate enzyme activity.
iii. Individual with genotype 6/6—have normal enzyme activity.

Additional pathological finding may be—reduced hepatic uptake of bilirubin, which may be responsible for unconjugated hyperbilirubinemia. This can be evidenced by:

a. Impaired bromsulphthalein clearance.
b. Impaired Tolbutamide clearance.

Special Diagnostic Tests

1. Increased serum bilirubin on fasting.
2. Fall in serum bilirubin after taking phenobarbitone, because it induces hepatic conjugating enzyme.
3. Increase in serum bilirubin after administration of intravenous nicotinic acid, because, it raises osmotic fragility of red blood cells.

Prognosis

1. Patient has normal life expectancy.
2. Lifelong mild hyperbilirubinemia.

Crigler-Najjar Syndrome

It is autosomal recessive familial non-hemolytic jaundice, having high serum unconjugated bilirubin level. This syndrome has been divided into two types as follows.

Type I Syndrome

i. No bilirubin conjugating enzyme is present in the liver.
ii. Bile contains trace amount of bilirubin conjugates in the liver.

But serum bilirubin is ultimately stable, hence, there must be some other alternative pathways for bilirubin metabolism. Bilirubin level will be >350 µmol/L.

Genetic defect: The deficit lies on one of the five exons (1*1-5) of bilirubin UGT1A1 gene.

Complications:
1. Patient may develop kernicterus.
2. Bilirubin encephalopathy, which is characterized by:
    i. Central deafness.
    ii. Mental retardation.
    iii. Ataxia.
    iv. Choreoathetosis.
    v. Occulomotor palsy.
    vi. Seizures.
    vii. Spasticity.
    viii. Death.

Age of incidence:
i. It occurs in young patient.
ii. It may occur later in patient after prolonged period of fasting.

Treatment:
1. *Phototherapy:* It degrades unconjugated bilirubin into:
    i. Lumibilirubin (water soluble)—it is secreted into the bile.

    ii. Other degraded products
    ↓
Spontaneous revert to natural isomers of unconjugated of bilirubin.
    ↓
Administration of oral calcium salts prevents its reabsorption.

    Hence, administration of oral calcium salts makes the phototherapy more effective.
2. *Inhibitor of heme-oxygenase:* It prevents conversion of heam to bilirubin. The name of the inhibitor is tin protoporphyrin.
    It provides temporary decrease of unconjugated bilirubin in plasma for 5–7 weeks.
3. The definitive therapy is orthitopic liver transplantation.

Crigler-Najjar Syndrome Type II

The characteristics are:
1. Bilirubin conjugating enzyme is <10% of normal.
2. Serum bilirubin <350 µmol/L.
3. Age of incidence:
    i. It may occur in 1st year of life.
    ii. It may occur as late as 30 years of age.
4. It may be aggravated by
    i. Fasting.
    ii. Intercurrent illness.
5. Complication: Bilirubin encephalopathy.

Genetic analysis: Mutation occurs in exons 1*1-5 of UGT1A1 gene. The mutant shows some residual enzymatic activity, which is responsible for the presence of bilirubin glucuronides in bile.

Treatment:
1. Phototherapy.
2. Phenobarbitone—it reduces serum bilirubin level to <340 µmol/L.

Dubin-Johnson Syndrome

Definition

It is an autosomal recessive, chronic, benign, intermittent conjugated hyperbilirubinemia and bilirubinuria. It is most prevalent in Middle East areas.

Pathogenesis

The mutation is in gene encoding MRP-2. This gene is responsible for transport of conjugated bilirubin glucuronides across the canalicular membrane.

This transporter defect is also responsible for increased urinary excretion of coproporphyrin I.

Pathology

1. Macroscopically, the color of the liver is greenish black (black-liver jaundice).
2. Microscopically, black pigment is seen in the liver cells. It is not the bile pigment or melanin, but it is the result of impaired secretion of anionic metabolites of tyrosine, phenylalanine and tryptophan.
3. Electron microscopic finding shows dense bodies are related to lysozymes.

Clinical characteristics: Pruritus is absent.

Biochemically:
i. Normal alkaline phosphatase levels.
ii. Normal lysosomal levels.

Diagnosis

Delayed excretion of BSP—Initial fall followed by rise at 120 minutes. It is due to regurgitation of glutathione conjugates into circulation.

In this syndrome:
i. Contrast media for intravenous cholangiography is not transported into the bile.
ii. ^{99m}Tc-HIDA for biliary scintigraphy is normal.

Rotor Syndrome

This is a chronic autosomal familial disorder, characterized by conjugated hyperbilirubinemia like Dubin-Johnson syndrome. The differences between Rotor syndrome and Dubin-Johnson syndrome are the following:

1. Absence of brown pigment in Rotor syndrome.
2. Abnormalities of mitochondria and peroxisomes in electron microscopy.
3. Gallbladder can be opacified in cholecystography in Rotor syndrome.
4. No secondary rise in BSP excretion test in Rotor syndrome. Because, here there is defect in hepatic uptake of BSP.
5. ^{99m}Tc-HIDA excretion provides no visualization of liver, gallbladder or biliary tree.

HEPATIC ARTERY

Extrahepatic Anatomy

It originates from celiac axis
↓
It runs along the upper border of pancreas and reaches 1st part of duodenum
↓
It turns upwards in between the two layers of omentum. Here, portal veins lies posterior and common bile duct lies lateral to hepatic artery
↓
Hepatic artery reaches porta hepatis
↓
It divides into right and left branches

The branches of hepatic artery are:
i. Right gastric artery
ii. Gastroduodenal artery

Common hepatic artery after arising from celiac axis divides into **two main arteries**—one is **gastroduodenal artery** and other is **common hepatic artery**. Sometimes:

i. Accessory right hepatic artery originates from superior mesenteric artery.
ii. Accessory left hepatic artery arises from left gastric artery.
iii. Sometimes entire common hepatic artery arises from:
   a. Superior mesenteric artery
   b. Aorta

Intrahepatic Anatomy

Hepatic artery enters sinusoids adjacent to portal tract
↓
Here it produces capillary plexus around bile ducts.

Hepatic Arterial Flow

1. It supplies 35% of total hepatic blood flow
2. It supplies 50% of total liver oxygen
3. It regulates blood levels of:
   i. Nutrients
   ii. Hormones.
4. It regulates hepatic clearance of nutrients, hormones

If cirrhosis—there is increase of hepatic arterial flow, due to portal systemic shunting.

In case of tumor, it is the main source of blood supply.

Since portal vein and hepatic artery both supply oxygen to liver

In case of cirrhosis, there will be lowering of oxygen content of portal vein; as a result liver will be dependent on hepatic artery for its nutrition.

Hepatic Arteriography

It is helpful for the diagnosis of the following hepatic lesions:
i. Cyst
ii. Abscess
iii. Malignant tumor
iv. Benign tumor
v. Vascular lesions, like aneurysm, arterio venous malformations.

Embolization should be done through arterial catheter for the treatment of following lesions:
i. Hepatic tumor
ii. Hepatic trauma
iii. Arteriovenous fistula
iv. Arterial aneurysm

Hepatic arterial catheterization is required for:
i. Administration of cytotoxic drugs
ii. Administration of radioactive beads in case of hepatocellular carcinoma.
iii. Pump perfusion in case of hepatic metastasis from colorectal cancer.

Spiral CT scan is valuable in the diagnosis of:
i. Hepatic arterial thrombosis after liver transplant
ii. Variations in intrahepatic anatomy

Hepatic Artery Occlusion

The effect of hepatic artery occlusion depends on:
i. Site of occlusion
ii. Extent of collateral circulation
   1. If the occlusion is distal to the origin of gastric artery and gastroduodenal arteries:
     a. Patient may die
     b. If patient survives, collateral circulation develops.
   2. Slow thrombosis is better than rapid and sudden block.
   3. Simultaneous occlusion of portal vein and hepatic artery are fatal.

Size of infarct depends upon:
i. Rapidity of occlusion
ii. Extent of occlusion
iii. Extent of collateral circulation

Description of infarction:
i. Size is ~8 cm in diameter
ii. Pale center
iii. Surrounding hemorrhagic band
iv. In the infracted area, liver cells are jumbled up
v. In the liver cell—there is eosinophilic granular cytoplasm, but no glycogen or nuclei.

Subcapsular areas of liver will escape destruction due to presence of alternate blood supply.

Other causes of hepatic infarction other than occlusion:
i. Shock
ii. Cardiac failure
iii. Diabetic ketosis
iv. Toxemia of pregnancy
v. After liver transplant
vi. Systemic lupus erythematosus
vii. Polyarteritis nodosa
viii. Giant cell arteritis
ix. Embolism in patient with subacute bacterial endo-carditis.
x. Trauma to right hepatic artery or cystic artery in during laparoscopic cholocystectomy
xi. Gangrenous cholecystitis.

Clinical Features

i. Features of SLE, polyarteritis nodosa or subacute bacterial endocarditis.
ii. Sudden pain in upper abdomen
iii. Hypotension and shock
iv. Jaundice—progressively increase
v. Fever
vi. Tender hepatomegaly
vii. Hemorrhages
viii. If occlusion is major, patient may go into coma or die

Investigations

i. Leukocytosis
ii. Abnormal liver enzymes in hepatocellular damage
iii. Prothrombin time

Hepatic Arteriography

i. Obstruction in hepatic artery
ii. Intrahepatic collaterals arise in portal zones and sub-capsular area
iii. Extrahepatic collaterals are formed in suspensary ligaments and in adjacent structures.

Scanning

i. Infarcts are oval, round or wedge-shaped and centrally placed.
ii. In early case—lesions are hypoechoic.
iii. In CT scan:
   a. Low attenuated peripherally placed wedge-shaped lesion
   b. Occlusion of artery may be seen.
   c. In late phase—lesions may coalesce with distinct margin.

MRI Scan

1. T1-weighted images show low signed intensity.
2. T2-weighted images show high signal intensity

In case of large infarct, bile lakes are formed—these may contain gas.

Treatment

1. Treatment of etiology
2. Secondary infection may be prevented by antifungal or antibiotics.
3. Management of hepatocellular failure
4. Percuteneous arterial embolization in case of trauma to artery.

Aneurysm of Hepatic Artery

1. It is one fifth of all visceral aneurysm
2. It may be congenital or acquired.

Causes of acquired aneurysm:
i. Bacterial endocarditis,
ii. Polyarteritis nodosa
iii. Arteriosclerosis
iv. Polyarteritis nodosa.
v. Iatrogenic causes:
   a. Biliary tract surgery
   b. Liver biopsy
   c. Interventional radiological procedures.
3. Its size pin point to grape size

Causes of pseudoaneurysm:
i. Chronic pancreatitis with pseudocyst formation
ii. Bile—leaks

Clinical Features

Classical triad:
i. Jaundice
ii. Abdominal pain
iii. Hemobilia

Within 5 months of origination of abdominal pain, it many rupture—in to **following organ producing related clinical features:**
a. Peritoneum—hemoperitoneum
b. Biliary tract—hemobilia
c. Gastrointestinal tract—hematemesis/melena

Diagnosis

1. Ultrasonography
2. Hepatic arteriography
3. Contrast enhanced computerized tomography
4. Pulse Doppler ultrasonography—can exhibit turbulence in flow.

Treatment

i. Angiographic embolization
ii. Proximal and distal ligation of aneurysm of hepatic artery.

HEPATIC ENCEPHALOPATHY

Definition

This can be defined as a spectrum of neuropsychiatric manifestations ranging from subtle mental change at one end to clinically obvious changes in intellect, motor function, behavior and consciousness at other end as a result of hepatic dysfunction with or without portosystemic shunting.

Classifications

Overt Hepatic Encephalopathy

This is a neurological syndrome characterized by mental and motor disorders developing over period of hours to days occurred in previously stable cirrhotic patients. This type of encephalopathy occurs in two forms:

a. **Episodic overt encephalopathy:** This term denotes:
   i. Episodes occur intermittently or more frequently
   ii. In between the episodes patient becomes normal although some degree of mental or intellectual important remains.
b. **Persistent overt encephalopathy:** In it, there are persistent and stable neuropsychiatric abnormalities.

   These two types of overt encephalopathy have some common features:

   1. *Mental changes:* The changes in mental states are:
      i. Subtle alteration in personality
      ii. Alteration in intellectual capacity
      iii. Changes in cognitive function
      iv. Profound alteration in consciousness to deep coma to decerebrate posturing.
   2. *Personality changes:*
      i. Childness
      ii. Irritability
      iii. Loss of concern to their family.
   3. *Intellectual deterioration:* It ranges from slight impairment in mental function to gross disorientation. There may be disturbances in visual special agnosia, i.e.
      i. Constructional apraxia—this is characterized by inability to reproduce simple design, blocks or matches.
      ii. Inconsistent writing and oblivious of ruled lines.
      iii. Inability to differentiate objects of similar shape, size, functions
   4. *Altered consciousness:* This can be characterized by a series of manifestations:
      i. Reduction in spontaneous movement
      ii. Fixed share
      iii. Apathy
      iv. Slowness in movement
      v. Brevity of responses
      vi. Daytime somnolence
      vii. Night-time sleeping disturbances
      vii. Stupor
      ix. Coma
   5. *Fetor hepaticus:* It is characterized by sour, feculent, sweety smell like that of new corpse. This is due to presence of mercaptans. It has no relation with:
      i. Degree of encephalopathy
      ii. Duration of encephalopathy
   6. *Changes in motor function:* These include:
      i. Rigidity
      ii. Static tremor
      iii. Intention tremor
      iv. disordered speech production
      v. Choreoathetotic movements
      vi. Hyper- or hyporeflexia
      vii. Focal symptoms
   7. *In case of early hepatic encephalopathy:* Early extra-pyramidal symptoms, those which are less well identified are:
      i. Bradykinesia
      ii. Rigidity
      iii. Tremor at rest
   8. *Asterixis:* It is flapping tremor:
      i. It is caused by impaired inflow of joint and other types of afferent information to brain stem reticular formation—as a result there is arrhythmic loss of posture.
      ii. It is absent in rest, minimally visualized on movement and maximal in sustained posture;
      iii. It can be demonstrated by asking the patient to keep his both hand out stretched at arms, hyper extended at wrist, forearm fixed and separated digits. The movements seen in asterixis are:
         a. Flexion and extension movements at wrist and metacarpophalangeal joints.
         b. Lateral movements of the digits often can be seen.
      iv. The movement is usually bilateral, but may be unilateral in case, where one side is more involved than the other.
      v. Other sites of the body may be involved:
         a. Arm
         b. Jaw
         c. Neck
         d. Protruded tongue
         e. Tightly closed eyelids
         f. Gait.

         A sterixis may be seen in other following disorders:
         a. Respiratory failure
         b. Renal failure
         c. Severe cardiac failure
         d. Hypomagnesemia
         e. Diphenylhydantoin intoxication
   9. *Speech:* Usually slow and monotonous speech. But in stupor, it is always combined with perseveration.
   10. *Deep tendon reflexes:* In early stages of encephalopathy:
       i. Muscle tone are increased
       ii. Tendon reflexes are exaggerated
       iii. There may be ankle clonus

In coma:
i. Muscles become flaccid
ii. Loss of tendon reflexes
iii. Plantar reflexes—flexor

In case of deep coma: Plantar reflexes—extensor.

11. *Other reflexes:*
    i. Muscle twitching
    ii. Grasping reflexes
    iii. Suckling reflexes
12. *Visual disturbances:*
    i. Alteration in gaze deviation
    ii. Reversible cortical blindness
13. *Other abnormalities:*
    i. Impaired psychomotor performances
    ii. Disturbed neuropsychological performances
    iii. Altered cerebral neurotransmitter homeostasis
    iv. Reduction in cerebral blood flow
    v. Reduction in cerebral metabolism
    vi. Alteration in cerebral fluid homeostasis

Episodic Hepatic Encephalopathy

It usually occurs in previously stable cirrhotic patients. These patients undergo encephalopathy following some precipitating events. These are:
i. Gastrointestinal cause:
   a. Increase in intestinal nitrogen
   b. Dietary protein excess
   c. Constipation
   d. Bleeding
ii. Sepsis
iii. Constipation
iv. Electrolyte imbalance
   a. Hyponatremia
   b. Hypokalemia
v. Dehydration
   a. Fluid restriction
   b. Excessive diuresis
   c. Over enthusiastic paracentesis
   d. Diarrhea/vomiting
vi. Alcohol misuse—cerebral circulation can be compromised by:
   a. Infection
   b. Inflammation
vii. CNS—active drugs
viii. TIPS—transjugular intrahepatic portal–systemic shunt
ix. Surgery:
   a. Patient may return back to his clinical previous stable condition following an episode of encephalopathy, before the improvements in psychometric tests or electroencephalogram.
   b. But few patients with severe decompensated liver disease or patient having surgically or spontaneous parts systemic shunt.

Persistent Hepatic Encephalopathy

This type of encephalopathy occurs after extensive portal systemic shunting through either:
i. Multiple anatomic collaterals
ii. Major collateral shunt.

It may be—surgically created or after insertion of TIPS.

Clinical pictures may be variable—which may be worsening of previous stable conditions—like
a. **Prominence of Parkinsonian features:**
   i. Extensive rigidity
   ii. Fine tremor unaffected by intention
   iii. Staccato speech
   iv. Short shuffling gait
b. **Cerebellar features may be predominant:**
   i. Gait—cerebellar gait
   ii. Intention tremor
   iii. Truncal ataxia
   iv. Dysarthria
c. **Choreoathetoid movements:** In these patients, clinical, biochemical pictures may be present, equivocal or absent.

Hepatic Myelopathy

1. It occurs predominantly in men, having surgically created porto-systemic shunt. It is less common than hepatic encephalopathy.
2. It is characterized by:
   i. Spastic paraparesis
   ii. Progressive disease
   iii. No sensory impairment
   iv. No sphincter dysfunction
3. It occurs due to degenerative disease of spinal cord.

Minimal change hepatic encephalopathy: This can be defined as abnormalities of cognition and/or neuropsychological variable occurs in cirrhotic patients who are clinically normal.

Advantage of using this term: It helps hepatic encephalopathy as a single syndrome having quantitatively distinct clinical features.

Disadvantage: It cannot convey adequately that it may be without any detrimental consequences.

HE type	Nomenclature	Subcategory	Subdivisions
A	Encephalopathy with acute liver failure		
B	Encephalopathy with portal systemic bypass and no intrinsic hepatocellular disease.		
C	Encephalopathy with cirrhosis and portal hypertension/or portal systemic shunt.	Episodic HE	Precipitated spontaneous recurrent
		Persistent HE	Mild severe treatment dependent
		Minimal He	

Table 4.13: Nomenclature of hepatic encephalopathy

It may enter into the stage of overt hepatic encephalopathy.

Precipitated episodic HE: It can be precipitated by specific factors.

Spontaneous episodic HE: It can occur without any precipitations factor.

Recurrent episodic HE: It can be described as HE when two bouts of spontaneous or precipitated HE occur within 1 year period.

West Haven Criteria for Semiquantitative Grading in Mental Scale

Grade-1: Trivial lack of awareness, euphoria, anxiety, shortened attention space, hypersomnia, insomnia or invention of sleep rhythm, impaired performance of addition or subtraction.

Grade-2: Lethargy, or apathy minimal disorientation of place and time, personality changes, inappropriate behavior, obvious asterixis.

Grade-3: Somnolence to stuporos condition, but response to verbal stimuli, confusion, global disorientation.

Grade-4: Coma—unresponsive to verbal or painful stimuli.

Table 4.14: Glasgow Coma Scale

Variables	Scores
Eye open	
Spontaneously	4
To command	3
To pain	2
No response	1
Best motor response	
Obey verbal commands	6
Painful stimulus, localized pain	5
Painful stimulus, flexion/withdrawal response	4
Painful stimulus, abnormal flexion	3
Painful stimulus, abnormal extension	2
No response	1
Best verbal response	
Orientated and conversant	5
Disorientated and conversant	4
Inappropriate or words	3
In comprehensive sound	2
No response	1
Total score 3 worst. 15 best.	

Pathogenesis

The pathogenic mechanisms or hypotheses must explain the following points of clinical hepatic encephalopathy:

1. Broad-spectrum clinical pictures involving multiple cerebral systems.
2. Rapid evolution and rapid complete reversibility of the clinical syndrome.
3. The different pathogenic mechanisms by which different conditions precipitates diverse clinical pictures.
4. The mechanism of rapid restoration of clinical symptoms in responds to treatment.

Key Roles in Hepatic Encephalopathy

Two main factors play role in development of HE:
   a. Hepatocellular failure
   b. Portal systemic shunting

Portal systemic shunting in absence of hepatocellular disease may occur in portal vein thrombosis or schistosomal liver injury—here usually no evidence of encephalopathy seen.

Again, surgical shunts or TIPS insertion in chronic liver disease are usually associated with worsening or precipitation of neuropsychiatric changes.

So in presence of both above key-factors, hepatic clearance of gut derived neurotoxins will be impaired. As a result, following changes will occur:
a. Brain water homeostasis
b. Oxidative/nitrosative stress
c. Cerebral neurotransmission
d. Inflammation and infection
e. Astrocytes dysfunction

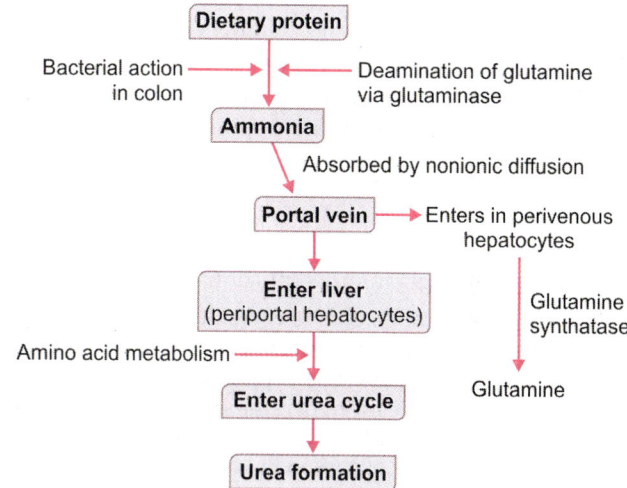

Fig. 4.27: Urea formation from dietary protein

These two systems work simultaneously to control blood ammonia concentration in hepatic veins.

But in cirrhosis of liver, blood ammonia concentration will be increased due to following factors:
   i. Increased concentration of urease containing bacteria in small bowel.
   ii. Enhanced absorption of ammonia through intestinal wall secondary to increased splanchnic blood flow in portal hypertension.
   iii. Presence of extensive extra- and intrahepatic portal systemic shunting.
   iv. In liver disease, reduction of functional hepatocyte mass.
   v. As a result of loss of muscle mass, ammonia metabolism in the muscles will be decreased.
   vi. In case of primary hyperventilation and hypokalemia, due to respiratory alkalosis, increase renal production of ammonia.

In cerebrum:
1. Cerebral intake of ammonia will be increased.
2. Blood–brain barrier is intact.
3. Permeability of surface area to ammonia is increased.

Since, there is no urea cycle in brain, following pathogenesis will occur in different parts of the brain

1. In astrocytes:

Ammonia
$\downarrow$ ← Amidation of glutamate via glutamine synthetase

Glutamine
$\downarrow$

In the brain, it produces deleterious effects in different levels.

As a result, following changes seen in astrocytes:
  i. Enlarged pale nuclei
  ii. Prominent nucleoli
  iii. Peripheral margination of chromatin
  iv. Accumulation of glycogen.

These changes are called Alzheimer type II astrocytosis. These changes occur in:
  i. Cerebral cortex
  ii. Basal ganglia
  iii. Cerebellum

2. **Direct effect of ammonia:**
  i. Affection in post-synaptic inhibitory potential
  ii. Activation of tricarboxylic acid cycle.

The **correlation between circulating blood ammonia and neuropsychiatry status** is poor due to following reasons:
  i. Technical difficulties associated with ammonia measurement
  ii. Difference in blood and brain ammonia concentration depending on pH in different compartments.

But there is definite positive **correlation between glutamine level and degree of neuropsychiatric manifestation**.

In case of congenital absence of enzymes involved in urea cycle may be responsible for hyperammonemia along with the features suggestive of hepatic encephalopathy, occasionally seizures, which is rarely observed in hepatic encephalopathy.

Other gut derived toxins responsible for hepatic encephalopathy are:
  i. *Indoles:* It is produced as a result of bacterial degradation of tryptophan.
  ii. *Mercaptans:* It is responsible for production of fetor hepaticus. It is sulphar containing compound.
  iii. *Phenols:* It is produced by bacterial degradation of phenylalanine and tyrosine.
  iv. Short and medium chain fatty acids.

γ-aminobutyric Acid Agonist

γ-aminobutyric acid receptors in brain are inhibitory neurotransmitter in brain.

Natural benzodiazepines, a group of non-pharmacological substances; bind to GABA—reception in brain and act as agonists or antagonists.

Against natural benzodiazepine are responsible for decrease in consciousness in HE.
  i. Ammonia directly or indirectly alters the affinity of natural ligands to GABA receptors.
  ii. Ammonia also increases the concentration of peripheral—type benzodiazepine receptors in astrocytic mitochondria—its activation results in synthesis of neurosteroids, a powerful ligands of neuronal GABA receptors.

Manganese

Raised level of manganese in blood in cirrhotic patient is responsible for parkinsonian manifestation through the mechanism that impairs the dopaminergic transmission in brain. Raised manganese level in blood may be developed for two reasons:
  i. Portosystemic shunting.
  ii. Reduction in biliary excretion.

Aromatic Amino Acids

In hepatic failure:
  i. Increased aromatic amino acid levels (tyrosine, phenylalanine, or tryptophan) level in blood
  ii. Decreased branched chain amino acid (valine, leucine and isoleucine) level in blood.

Above imbalance between AAA and BCAA
↓
Enhance the passage of AAA through neutral acid carrier into the brain in exchange of glutamine (generated from detoxification of amino acid)
↓
Excess AAA in the brain help in synthesis of false neurotransmitter (octopamine and phenylethanolamine), and serotonin (inhibitory neurotransmitter
↓
Responsible for HE

Brain water homeostasis

Influx of excess ammonia in the brain
↓
Result in accumulation of glutamine (osmotically active) in the astrocytes cells.
↓
Countered efflux of osmotically active compounds myoinositol, taurine and α-glycerophosphorylcholine from the brain
↓
Net result is in drawing of free water into the brain cells
↓
Development of low grade brain edema

This can be visualized in the following studies:
1. 'H-MRS studies—in cirrhosis with HE—show decrease in myoinositol peak and increase in glutamine/glutamate peak
2. Cerebral magnetization
3. Diffusion transfer magnetic resonance imaging

Other effects of ammonia-induced glutamine accumulation are:
  i. Hyponatremia   ii. Inflammatory cytokines

These also promote cerebral edema.

Abnormalities in γ-aminobutyric acid (GABA) neurotransmission (Fig. 4.28)

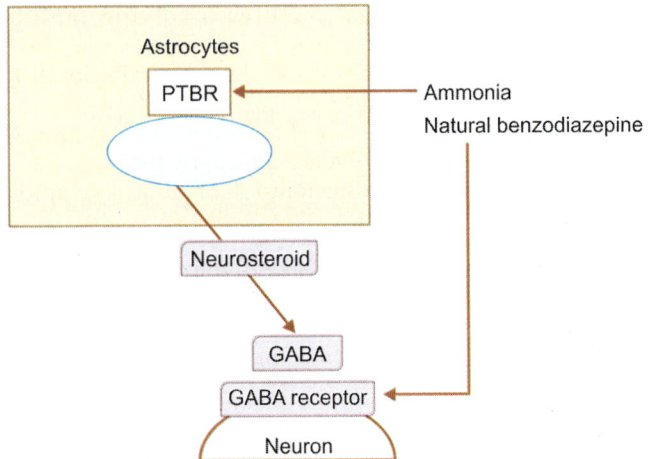

Fig. 4.28: Abnormalities in GABA transmission

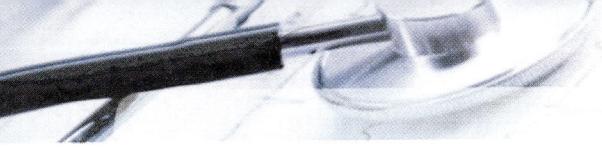

Oxidative/Nitrosative Stress

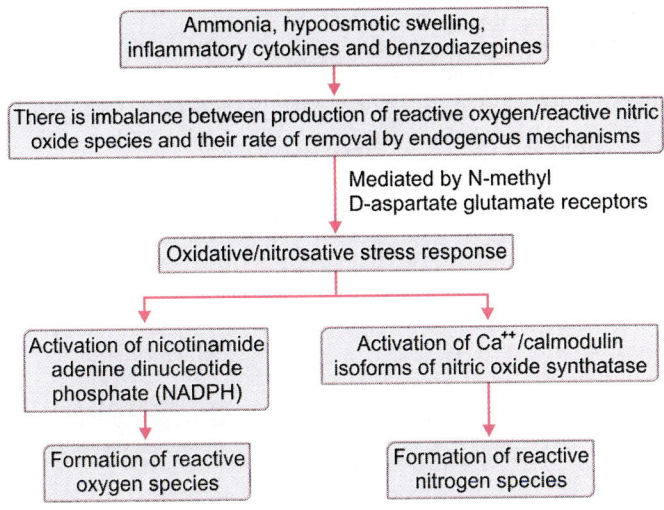

Astrocytes Dysfunction

Astrocytes swelling and oxidative/nitrosative stress

↓

Promote covalent modification of tyrosine residue in astrocytic protein (protein tyrosine nitration)

↓

i. Interferes with protein function.
ii. Interferes with intracellular transduction.

Astrocytes near the blood–brain barrier are usually affected. Since all the astrocytic protein not undergoes tyrosine nitration, hence, only selective alteration of blood–brain barrier is observed.

Oxidative stress

↓

Induce RNA oxidation

↓

Results in formation of defective or unstable proteins

↓

Result in multiple alterations in neurotransmitter receptor systems.

Nitrosative stress

↓

Promote mobilization of zinc from metallothionein and other proteins.

↓

Zinc affects

1. Activities of multiple enzymes and transcription factors
2. Augment GABA-nergic neurotransmission and decrease glutamate uptake

Ammonia produces direct toxic effect through following mechanism:

i. Alteration in gene expression
ii. Intracellular signal transduction transport
iii. Alterations in neurotransmitter processing
iv. Decreases synthesis of neurosteroids

The net results of above factors:

i. Disruption of glioneuronal communications
ii. Impairment of synaptic plasticity
iii. Slowing of oscillatory neuronal activity.

Alternations in cerebral neurotransmission: HE is associated with changes in neurotransmitter system—so hepatic encephalopathy is associated with—imbalance between inhibitory and excitatory neurotransmitter systems—favors inhibition. It may be due to any of the following factors:

i. Alteration of glutaminergic system
ii. Increase in GABAergic tone

Glutamate

It is principal excitatory neurotransmitter in brain synthesized in presynaptic nerve terminal and stores in the vesicles. From here, after release it activates receptor on the postsynaptic neuron. Astrocytic transporters remove this glutamate from synaptic cleft and push it into astrocyte, where it is converted into glutamine by addition of ammonia with the help of glutamine synthatase.

Again from here glutamine is then transported into presynaptic nerve terminal, where it is converted to glutamate.

But in cirrhosis (Fig. 4.29)—**dying from hepatic coma**, in presence of hyperammonemia, large amount of glutamine is being formed from glutamate, as a result, total brain level of glutamate is increased, whereas, glutamate concentration in CSF and extracellular spaces will be increased—this occurs due to following mechanisms:

i. Increased release of glutamate from astrocyte in response to cell swelling.
ii. Hyperammonemia mediated downregulation of astrocytic glutamate transporters prevents glial reuptake of glutamate.

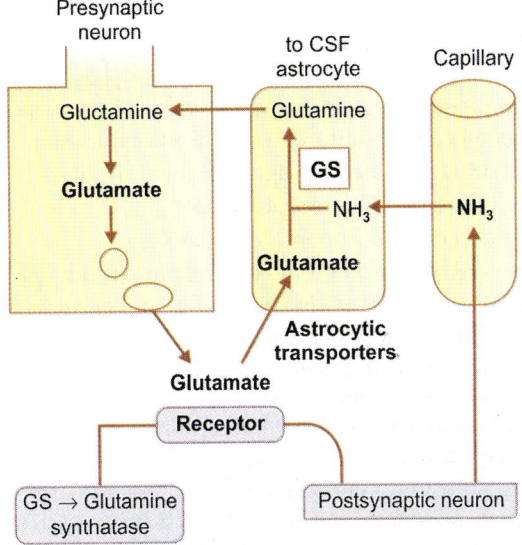

Fig. 4.29: Glutamate transmission in cirrhosis

γ-aminobutyric acid: Principal inhibitory neurotransmitter γ-aminobutyric acid is synthesized from glutamate with the help of glutamate dehydrogenase in presynaptic nerves and stored in presynaptic vesicles.

It binds to a **specific receptor in GABA receptor complex** which also contains binding sites of other molecules, like, benzodiazepines, barbiturates and neurosteroids. Binding of these legands **opens chloride channel,** through which influx of chloride ions enters the postsynaptic neurons and responsible for hyperpolarization of these cells (Fig. 4.30).

In hepatic encephalopathy, main neurotoxic compounds like, ammonia, benzodiazepine like legands, proinflammatory cytokines and neurosteroids activates the GABA receptor complex and increase the GABAergic tone.

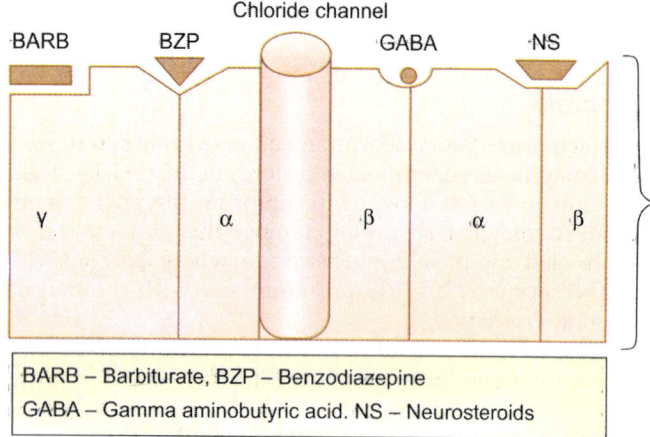

BARB – Barbiturate, BZP – Benzodiazepine
GABA – Gamma aminobutyric acid. NS – Neurosteroids

Fig. 4.30: Receptors in brain

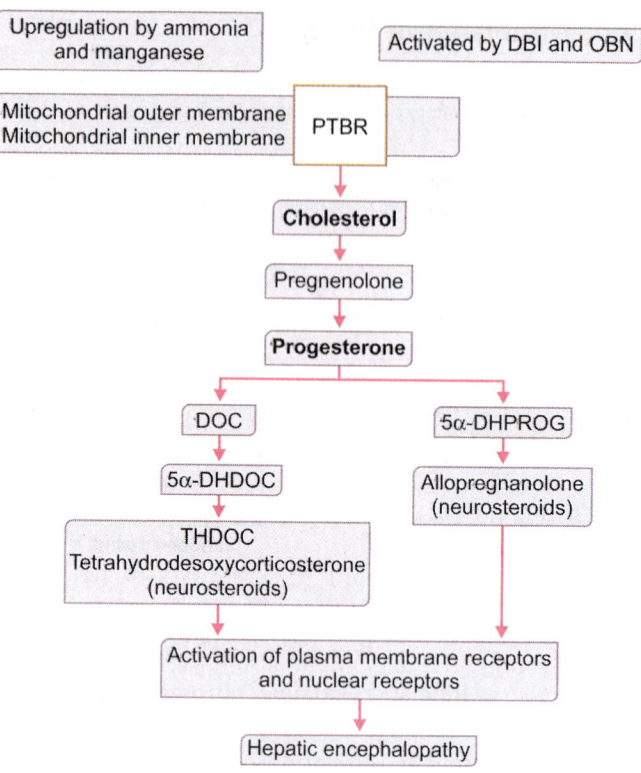

Fig. 4.31: Neurosteroids system

Neurosteroid System (Fig. 4.31)

A. Neurosteroid is synthesized in brain, (astrocytes)—via activation of peripheral type benzodiazepine receptor (PTBR). Its synthesis has no relation with steroid synthesis in gonads and adrenal.

   PTBR is present in outer-/inner-mitochondrial membrane and it is independent of central GABAergic complex receptors.

   In hepatic encephalopathy:
   1. Upregulation of PTBR is mediated by—ammonia and manganese, which accumulate in brain cells due to hepatocellular failure or portal–systemic shunting.
   2. PTBR is activated by–agonistic ligands, like:
      a. Diazepam like receptor (DBI)
      b. Octadecaneuropeptide (ODN)
   These are concentrated in cerebrospinal fluid:
   a. Allopregnanolone, in case of hepatic encephalopathy, modulate components of GABA A receptors.
   b. Again, this neurosteroid acts synergistically with ammonia, benzodiazepine like substances and barbiturates to activate GABA receptor complex and GABA nergic tone.
B. Neurosteroids, synthesized in peripheral organs, like kidney, adrenals and gonads, are increased in large concentration in case of liver failure. Since, these neurosteroids are lipophilic, hence they will cross the blood brain barrier easily and producing increased in GABA nergic tone.

   Neurosteroids also increase the function of serotonin, NMDA, glycine and opiod receptors in brain.

   Neurosteroids also bind to intracellular receptor which acts as transcription factors, thereby regulating expression of genes which are responsible for encoding brain proteins.

   Serotonin: This system is involved in control of cortical arousal thus consciousness of the patients.

   In patient with cirrhosis with hepatic encephalopathy—there are increase in:
   i. Activity of brain monoamine oxidase A—which responsible for serotonin metabolism.
   ii. Concentration of 5-HT metabolite, 5-hydroxy indole acetic acid.
   iii. Number of $5-HT_2$ receptors.

   The above changes are associated HE can be treated with 5-HT blocker ketanserin to treat portal hypertension.

   The above circumstances prove that there is association of serotonin system with hepatic encephalopathy.

   Dopamine: Dopamine, a catecholamine neurotransmitter, is responsible for—personality, behavior, cognition, working memory.

In patient with cirrhosis with hepatic encephalopathy:
i. The enzyme, responsible for dopamine degradation, monoamine oxidase A, will be increased.
ii. Homovanillic acid, metabolite of dopamine will be increased.
iii. Increased accumulation of manganese in globus pallidus, followed by neurodegenerative changes results in reduction in number of D_2 receptors—producing extra pyramidal manifestations.

Other Neurotransmitter Systems

Roles of histaminergic and opioidergic systems in the production are yet to be established.

Neuromodulatory Systems

There are two neuromodulators:

1.

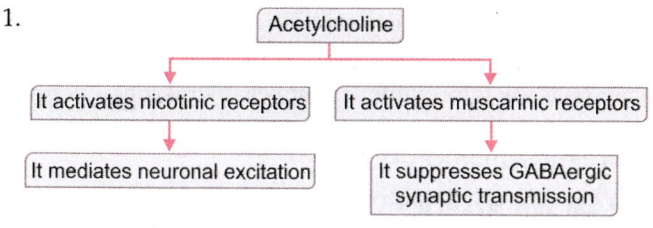

a. Nicotinic receptor density will be significantly lower in brains of these patients.
b. But affinity of acetylcholine for muscarinic receptors is reduced. Again, acetylcholine levels is reduced in cirrhosis with hepatic encephalopathy—because of increased activity of acetylcholinesterase enzyme.
   The net effect is—inhibitory neurotransmission.

2. **Adenosine:** Two receptors A_1 and A_{2A}—after activation, modulate neurotransmissions at presynaptic and post-synaptic levels.

   Activation A_1 receptors
   ↓
   Decrease in neurotransmitter release
   Activation of A_{2A} receptors
   ↓
   Facilitates release of
   i. Acetylcholine,   ii. Glutamate,   iii. GABA
   Activation of adenosine receptors
   ↓
   Control the dopamine receptors in basal ganglia.

   A_{2A} receptors either inhibit or neutralize the consequences of A_1 receptors after its activation at presynaptic level.
   But in patients with cirrhosis with encephalopathy, binding of A_1 and A_{2A} are reduced in brain.

Inflammation and Infection

Cirrhotic patients are at increased risk of infection—which may precipitate encephalopathy—because of following factors
1. Neutrophils and macrophages have reduced capability to phagocytose and thereby eliminate organisms.
2. There is evidence of translocation of bacteria from intestine producing endotoxemia.

   Infection means response to exogenous pathogens, whereas, inflammation is a biological response of body tissues to exogenous or endogenous stimuli, as a result, there is release of inflammatory cytokines.

   But both inflammation and infection may coexist. Astrocytic cells and endothelial cells in the blood brain banner.
   ↓
   Responds to inflammatory stimuli
   ↓
   Elicit inflammatory response involving neurotransmitter pathways.

Again, inflammation and infections synergistically alter the cerebral effect of ammonia in following manner:
i. It induces neutrophil dysfunction.
ii. It induces release of reactive oxygen species.

As a result
i. There is reduction in efficacy of the neutrophil to deal with the infection.
ii. There is increase in oxidative stress in astrocytic cells and systemic inflammation.

   Again, neutrophil dysfunction may produce its effect directly in producing hepatic encephalopathy:

Endothelial and neutrophil interaction in cerebral micro-circulation
↓ ← Enhanced by hyperammonemia and chronic endotoxemia
Increase migration of neutrophil across the blood–brain barrier.
↓
Increased production of chemokines, proinflammatory cytokines and ROS
↓
Increased oxidative stress in astrocytes

Diagnosis

There is no gold standard method in diagnosis of hepatic encephalopathy in patient with cirrhosis. There are number of methods—which in single or in combination can assess the cerebral functions. These are:
1. Mental state assessment
2. Psychometric analysis
3. Electroencephalography
4. Sensory evoked potential
5. Motor evoked potential
6. Neuroimaging

Mental Assessment

A. **Detailed careful history and physical examination should be done with attention to following:**
   a. Memory
   b. Concentration
   c. Cognition
   d. Consciousness
   e. Change in energy and activity
B. **Use of following scoring systems:**
   a. West Haven criteria on the basis of changes in consciousness, intellectual function and behavior.
   b. Glasgow Coma Scale
   c. Hodkinson mental state test
   d. Mini mental score test
C. **Comprehensive neurological examinations including subtle motor abnormalities**—like:
   i. Hypomania
   ii. Dysarthria
   iii. Increased tone
   iv. Reduction of speed of movement
   v. Ataxia
   vi. Alternating movements
   vii. Exaggerated deep tendon reflexes
   viii. Impaired postural reflexes

xi. Abnormal movements like:
  a. Tremor
  b. Asterixis
 x. Sensory changes
 xi. May be evidence of focal features.
D. **Exclusion of other causes producing similar neurological changes**—which include:
  a. Subdural hematoma
  b. Wernicke's encephalopathy
  c. Metabolic causes like:
    i. Renal
    ii. Diabetic
  d. Alcohol intoxication
  e. Drugs intoxication

Psychometric Performances

The neuropsychological tests should be performed to diagnose:
i. Minimal hepatic encephalopathy;
ii. Cognitive changes in persistant hepatic encephalopathy.

But following conditions should be assessed:
  i. It cannot be performed in patient with decreased arousal
 ii. Co morbidities
iii. Visual impairment
 iv. Cultural barriers

Patient with minimal HE may show deficit in:
  i. Attention
 ii. Visuospatial abilities
iii. Fine motor skills
 iv. Working memory.

Test batteries are better than any single tests because of better functional correlation with functional status.

For better diagnosis of minimal change encephalopathy—following tests can be used.

Five paper and pencil tests:
  i. Number connection test A
 ii. Number connection test B
iii. Line tracing test
 iv. Digital symbol tests
  v. Serial dotting

The above tests examine:
  i. Motor speed and accuracy
 ii. Visual perception
iii. Visual–spatial orientation
 iv. Visual construction
  v. Concentration
 vi. Attention
vii. Memory

Score:

SD ±	0 points
SD + 1	1 points
SD—1	–1 points
SD—2	–2 points
SD—3	–3 points

Subject could achieve in between + 6 to –18 points.
Subject with minimal HE = –4 points

Computerized psychometric tests—it helps in précised quantification of mental status. The test is—scan test—based on sternberg paradigm.

Neurophysiologic Testing

There are a number of neurophysiologic tests for:
i. Diagnosis and quantification of encephalopathy
ii. Response to treatment

For minimal change hepatic encephalopathy—these tests do not give any information about behavioral consequences.

Electroencephalography

In hepatic encephalopathy:
  i. Progressive slowing of normal alpha frequency of 8–13 Hz
 ii. Burst of theta activity (4–8 Hz) starting in temporal areas then over the scalp
iii. Slowing of delta wave (1–4 Hz)
 iv. Triphasic waves or arrhythmic delta activity in severe hepatic encephalopathy.
  v. Slow, low voltage delta activity with sequences of electrical silence—coma.

This generalized slowing of background EEG activities can also be evidenced in:
a. Metabolic encephalopathies (uremia, hyponatremia, hypocapnia)
b. Drug-induced encephalopathies (valproate, lithium baclofen)

These diagnoses can be confirmed by clinical background.
Sensitivity of EEG in diagnosis of HE varies with the type of analyses used.

Best result can be obtained by—spectral analysis based techniques.

Other techniques are:
i. Full automatic evaluation based on artificial neural network
ii. Technique for providing spatial and temporal information.

Evoked Potentials

1. **Sensory or exogenous evoked potential:**
  i. Here stimuli are provided by visual, auditory or peripheral nerve stimulation.
 ii. Information of brain stem and cortical activity are obtained.
    So abnormalities in functions of the above across of brain one can find in minimal or overt encephalopathy.
2. **Cognitive or endogenous evoked potential:** Here the triggering factor is cognitive activity.
    When the patient gets auditory, visual stimulus, potential will occur 300 ms after exposure to stimulus—hence it is called P300 latency. It is useful:
  i. For detection of minimal hepatic encephalopathy
 ii. For monitoring the status of mild to moderate encephalopathy

Critical flicker fusion frequency: This is based on the perception of light as flickering or fused as its frequency changes.

The importance:
i. This helps in diagnosis of hepatic encephalopathy
ii. This helps in monitoring the stages of hepatic encephalopathy

Disadvantage: This is not highly sensitive enough for diagnosis of minimal change hepatic encephalopathy.

Smooth persuit eye movements: This is characterized by conjugate eye movements which is used to track the smooth trajectory of small target.

Abnormality:
1. Clear disruption of smooth persuit—minimal HE
2. Complete loss of smooth pursuit or near complete loss—overt hepatic encephalopathy

This requires patient's co-operation.

Functional and Structural Cerebral Imaging

A. **Cerebral CT scan and MRI:** The findings are:
1. Cerebral and cerebellar atrophy—these changes are correlated with severity of liver dysfunction—which is mostly evidenced in alcohol abuse.
2. Hyperintensity of basal ganglia due to deposition of manganese in pallidum—which is the net result of total body increase in magnesium in patient with cirrhosis associated with:
   i. Presence of hepatocellular failure
   ii. Impaired biliary excretion
   iii. Presence of portal systemic shunting of blood.

This magnesium accumulation is responsible for upregulation of cerebral and peripheral benzodiazepine receptors which in turn act as a factor for development of hepatic encephalopathy.

So cerebral imaging except MRI does not provide any diagnostic information of the patient with hepatic encephalopathy.

But in case of MRI brain:
1. *Magnetization transfer and diffusion—weighed imaging:* Indirectly assesses the changes in cerebral water content and distribution.
2. *Functional MRI:* Measures the hemodynamic responses related to neural activity in the brain.

B. **Magnetic resonance spectroscopy (MRS):** It provides localized biochemical information of cerebral metabolic processes. This change is—relative changes in astrocyte volume. Homeostasis is due to following factors:
   i. Relative reductions in myoinositol and choline resonances.
   ii. Relative increase in composite glutamine/glutamate resonance.

Other recent techniques:
   i. Two-dimensional spectroscopy
   ii. Spectral editing
   iii. Use of higher magnetic field strengths.

C. **Radiotracer imaging:**
Importance: It provides direct pathophysiology of hepatic encephalopathy.

Disadvantage:
   i. It is highly costly.
   ii. It has no place in management of hepatic encephalopathy.

Activity: Access to:
   i. Metabolic process
   ii. Neuronal activity
   iii. Neurotransmitter system

D. **Blood ammonia:** When a patient with neurological changes of unknown origin with minimal signs of chronic liver disease and more or less normal liver function tests—blood ammonia is very important clue to the diagnosis of hepatic encephalopathy.

E. **Cerebrospinal fluid:**
   i. Clear
   ii. Normal pressure
   iii. Cell count—normal
   iv. Protein contest—increased
   v. Glutamine content—increased—it correlates with:
       a. Presence of hepatic encephalopathy
       b. Degree of hepatic encephalopathy

F. **Neuropathological changes in brain tissue:**
Most striking features:
   i. Proliferation of astrocytes
   ii. Changes in astrocytes
       a. Enlarged nuclei
       b. Prominent nucleoli
       c. Margination of chromatin
       d. Accumulation of glycogen
This is Alzheimer type II astrocytosis.
This pathology occurs in:
   i. Cerebral cortex
   ii. Basal ganglia
   iii. Cerebellum

G. **In case of persistent hepatic encephalopathy:**
1. Patchy cortical laminar and pseudolaminar necrosis and polymicrocavitation at:
   i. Corticomedullary junctions
   ii. Striatum
2. Uneven degenerations of neurons and medullary fiber in:
   i. Cerebral cortex
   ii. Cerebellum
   iii. Lentiform nuclei
3. In case of hepatic encephalopathy—demyelination of pyramidal tract

Current Guideline for Diagnosis in Hepatic Encephalopathy
1. Detailed clinical history and examinations to assess and exclude clinically apparent changes.
2. Psychomotor performance assessment using Psychometric Hepatic Encephalopathy Score (PHES)
3. Electrophysiological assessment by—EEG, or somato-sensory/cognitive EPs
4. Assessment of health-related life.

Management of Hepatic Encephalopathy
Management of hepatic encephalopathy varies according to type of encephalopathy.

General Measures
a. In case of minimal or stable persistent encephalopathy—management of hepatic encephalopathy.
b. In case of episodic/recurrent encephalopathy—precipitating factors must be looked after.

Management of Precipitating Factors

1. Gastrointestinal bleeding:
   i. Vasoactive drugs
   ii. Antibiotics
   iii. Endoscopic therapy
2. Anemia — blood transfusion
3. Blood pressure should be maintained to maintain
   i. Hepatic perfusion
   ii. Renal perfusion.
4. Infections are mainly—pulmonary, urinary and peritoneal—should be treated by antibiotics.
5. Electrolyte abnormalities:
   i. Correction of deficit
   ii. Discontinuation of diuretics
6. Decline in renal function can be treated by
   i. Stoppage of diuretics
   ii. Increase in circulating blood volume to maintain renal perfusion
   iii. Discontinuation of nephrotoxic drugs.
7. Stoppage of sedative drugs.
8. Other measures:
   i. Maintenance of intravenous lines
   ii. Monitor of vital signs
   iii. Maintenance of fluid balance
   iv. Maintenance of nutrition
   v. Avoidance of aspiration of pneumonia.
9. Large protein meals—cleaning of bowel.
10. Constipation—bowl cleaning, antibiotics.

Diet: The current recommendation is:
   a. Energy requirement—25.35 kcal/kg/day
   b. Protein requirement—1.2–1.5 gm/kg/day

Vegetable protein is better tolerated than animal protein.

Dietary fiber is required because:
   i. It decrease the transit time
   ii. It decreases intraluminal pH.
   iii. It increases fecal ammonia excretion.

Food intake has to be spreaded throughout the day to avoid excess protein load—into:
1. Six snacks—type meals
2. Three main meals

If hepatic encephalopathy persists for less than 2–3 days:
   i. Exclusive glucose supplements—as intravenous fluids.
   ii. After this period—diet will contain normal protein
   iii. Protein content—60–80 gm/day.

If hepatic encephalopathy persists for >2–3 days: Nitrogen supplementation in the form amino acid solution—70 gm/day—through enteral route.

Dietary deprivation should not be more than 24–36 hours because it may be harmful.

Enema:
1. *In acute encephalopathy:* Hyperosmolar enema should be given to encourage ammonia extraction.
   Both neutral phosphate and lactulose enema are used.
2. *In chronic persistant encephalopathy:* Daily enema is necessary as two to three time daily dose as an adjunct to oral therapy.

Specific Treatment

Non-absorbable disaccharides:
   i. Lactulose—discovered in 1966
   ii. Lactilol—introduced in 1980s

Mechanism of actions:

Both the above are not absorbed in small intestine because of absence of enzyme—disaccharidase.

↓

They enter in the colon in unchanged form

↓

They are metabolized extensively by colonic bacteria

↓

They breakdown into volatile fatty acids (VFA), hydrogen ± methane

↓

VFA are the suitable substrate for the bacterial growth

↓

As a result, there is bacterial overgrowth

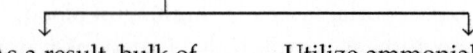

| As a result, bulk of the stool will be increased | Utilize ammonial nitrogen for incorporation into bacterial protein |

Beneficial effects of these drugs in hepatic encephalopathy:
a. *Cathartic effect of these drugs as a result of the following factors:*
   i. Decrease in intraluminal pH
   ii. Increase in intestinal gas formation
   iii. Increase in intraluminal osmolarity
   iv. Bulking effect of proliferating colonic bacteria
b. *Direct effect on ammonia in small intestine:*
   i. Interference with the uptake of glutamine and its metabolism in the small intestine—as a result ammonia production in small intestine will be reduced.
   ii. Incorporation of ammonial nitrogen into bacterial protein.

Lactulose:

Dose:
1. Orally—15–30 ml two to four times daily to maintain two semisolid motions per day.
2. Rectally—250 ml lactulose in 750 ml of water—enema.

Disadvantage:
   i. It can produce abdominal discomfort, anorexia, flatulence—but within a few days to months tolerance may develop.
   ii. Over enthusiastic administration may produce—severe diarrhea, dehydration and renal failure.

Effect:
   i. In acute case, improvement in neuropsychiatry status occurs in 80% patients of hepatic encephalopathy.
   ii. But in most severely decompensated patients—response may be doubtful.

Lactilol (β-galactosidosorbitol):
   i. It is produced usually in chemically crystalline form.
   ii. It is as efficacious as lactulose.

iii. Side effect is less.
iv. It is better tolerated.
v. Dose should be adjusted to produce two semisolid motion/day.

Antibiotics

Aim: The aim is to eliminate urease producing organisms, so that there will be less production of ammonia in the intestine.

The drugs are:

Neomycin:
i. It is poorly absorbable aminoglycoside.
ii. Dose is 4–6 gm/day.
iii. It should be used not more than a week
iv. Long-term use may produce:
   a. Nephrotoxicity
   b. Irreversible ototoxicity.

Small quantity of this drug will be absorbed from intestinal wall.

Rifaximin:
i. It is poorly absorbable (0.4%) synthetic antibiotic, closely related to rifamycin.
ii. It acts against gm +ve and gm –ve aerobic and anaerobic bacteria.
iii. It has an excellent safety profile and better tolerated.

Major risk factors: Long-term use of these antibiotics may be responsible for emergence of multidrug resistant organisms. Hence it can be prevented by:
i. Intermittent use of these antibiotics.
ii. During off period, use of probiotics.

Use of Combination of Non-Absorbable Disaccharides and Antibiotics

1. Non-absorbable disaccharides—actions depend upon the metabolism by colonic bacteria.
2. Non-absorbable antibiotics inhibit bacterial activity in colon.

So theoretically, there is no point of giving these combinations.

But in practice, these combinations can be given, who do not respond to either alone.

Bromocriptine: In cirrhosis with hepatic encephalopathy, there is deficit in dopaminergic neurotransmission.

So in chronic, stable, persistant hepatic encephalopathy, with prominent extrapyramidal features, who are resistant to treatment with other agents may get benefit from bromocriptine 2.5 mg/day.

Adverse effect: Ototoxicity, hence, at every 6 months, audiogram will be beneficial.

Caution: In well compensated chronic liver disease patient, its use in patient with ascites may develop SIADH.

L-ornithine-L-aspartate:

Mechanism of actions:
1. It stimulates residual hepatic urea cycle activity, thereby helps in hepatic removal of ammonia.
2. It promotes glutamine synthesis in skeletal muscles.

Dose: LOLA 6 gm/day—produce some benefit in grade II hepatic encephalopathy.

Its effect depends upon its route of administration—because orally administered LOLA will undergo transamination in intestinal mucosa.

So efficacy of the orally administered drug depends upon effect of ornithine moiety alone.

But in total, beneficial effects of LOLA is not strong.

Branched chain amino acids:

In cirrhosis with hepatic encephalopathy:
1. Plasma levels of branched chain amino acids (BCAA) are reduced.
2. Plasma levels of aromatic amino acid (AA) are increased.

As a result, there is change in neurotransmitter balance in case of hepatic encephalopathy.

If BCAA is administered orally or intravenously, there is significant increase in cerebral perfusion.

But in according to some study, BCAA is not effective for treatment of hepatic encephalopathy.

The nutritional beneficial effect of BCAA is through the following mechanism: Leucine is a potent stimulator of hepatocyte growth factor production by stellate cells by which it stimulates liver cell regeneration as compensation of death of liver cell.

Probiotics: It acts by increasing the population of non-urease producing bacteria.

It used in patients with hepatic encephalopathy, they may show neuropsychiatric improvement, as achieved by lactulose.

Sodium benzoate:

Mechanism of actions:
1. It fixes ammonia in alternate pathways for waste nitrogen excretion.
2. After conjugation with glycine, excess nitrogen will be excreted in urine as hippurate.

Dose: Recommended dose—5 gm twice daily.
          Patient may tolerate not more than 2 gm twice daily.

Zinc:
i. It is a trace element.
ii. It is a component of many metalloenzymes and metal protein complexes

Mechanism of actions:
a. It helps in nitrogen metabolism by increasing the activity of hepatic urea cycle.
b. It increases glutamate synthesis in muscles.

Zinc deficiency:
a. Impairs glutamate synthesis in muscles.
b. Decreases the hepatic urea cycle.

In cirrhosis with hepatic encephalopathy, serum zinc concentration is decreased.

Flumazenil:

In hepatic encephalopathy:
i. There is deficient GABAergic neurotransmission
ii. Increased benzodiazepine-like legands in circulation

Flumazenil is benzodiazepine receptor antagonist—when administered intravenously, is responsible for short-term improvement in hepatic encephalopathy.

Shunt Occlusion

The patients with persistent hepatic encephalopathy have:
  i. Significant portosystemic shunting.
  ii. Preservation of liver function tests.
  iii. Responds poorly to standard treatment.

These patients can be treated by—shunt occlusion by following mechanisms:
  i. Vascular embolization.
  ii. Vascular plugging with Amplatzer device.
  iii. Balloon occlusion.
  iv. Laparoscopic disconnection suitable for paraumbilical vein shunts.

TIPS may develop persistent disabling hepatic encephalopathy which is very difficult to treat, but, occlusion of TIPS may be beneficial sometimes.

Surgically created shunts may be responsible for debilitating hepatic encephalopathy—which may need surgical occlusion.

Liver Transplantation

Previously Model of End stage Liver Disease (MELD) was used to prioritize the patient in the list of liver transplantation which did not include neuropsychiatry status.

In patient with abnormal neuropsychiatry status but well preserved liver function, other causes of abnormal neuropsychiatry status has to be excluded.

Liver transplantation in patient with overt hepatic encephalopathy, may improve following:
  i. Major physical manifestations, like:
      a. Spastic paraparesis
      b. Parkinsonian features resistant to treatment.
  ii. Radiological features
      a. Cerebral MRI abnormalities
      b. Cerebral MRS abnormalities
      c. Cerebral PFT abnormalities
  iii. EEG
  iv. Cognitive functions—not completely

This may reflect:
  i. Unmasking of previously unrecognized abnormalities
  ii. Development of complications of transplant procedure like:
      a. Intraoperative hypoxia
      b. Osmotic stress
      c. Metabolic stress
  iii. Effects of immunosuppressive therapies
  iv. Presence and effect of comorbidities
      a. Diabetes
      b. Hypertension.

Neurological complications following liver transplantation is 10–47%. These are mainly due to:
  i. Preoperative neurological insult
  ii. Neurotoxic effects of immune suppressive agents

Artificial Liver Transport System

Decompensated cirrhotic patients with severe hepatic encephalopathy, not responding to conventional therapy are the patients—who require artificial liver transport system.

Molecular Adsorption Recirculating System (MARS) is the most extensively studied system. It purifies the blood by:
  i. Lipophilic albumin bound molecules
  ii. Water-soluble molecules

This process removes:
  i. Ammonia
  ii. Endotoxin
  iii. Inflammatory mediators

This process improves cerebral hemodynamics.

This system acts as a bridge between liver transplantation and the cirrhotic patients waiting for liver transplantation.

Colectomy Colonic Exclusion

The aim is—reduction of production of ammonia.
The method is—colectomy or colonic exclusion.
Operative mortality is very high.
These patients are the candidates of liver transplantation.

Potential Future Therapies

Like colon, small intestine, kidney and muscles are involved in metabolism of ammonia—so these are a future target for therapies of hepatic encephalopathies.

Small intestine is involved in uptake and breakdown of glutamine which is the major source of ammonia production. Non-absorbable disaccharides interferes with the above processes.

Ammonia is produced in intestine from:
  i. Dietary protein
  ii. Deamination of glutamine by glutaminase
  iii. Bacterial degradation in colon

Ammonia is produced in kidney from glutamine degradation by glutaminase.

In healthy individuals:
  i. Ammonia produced in intestine and kidney is metabolized in periportal hepatocytes to form urea—which is excreted in urine.
  ii. Small portion of ammonia is detoxified to glutamine by glutamine synthatase (GS) in perivenous hepatocytes.
  iii. Small portion of ammonia is detoxified in muscles and brain to glutamine by glutamine synthatase.
  iv. Glutamine produced in liver, skeletal muscles and brain are released into circulation—which ultimately enter in gut and kidney and undergo degradation to form ammonia.

In cirrhosis: Circulating ammonia level will be increased because:
  i. Liver's capacity for urea synthesis will be reduced.
  ii. Extensive portal—systemic shunting allows the blood to bypass the detoxification system in the liver.

But in presence of hyperammonemia: Glutamine synthesis is the only protective but temporary pathway of detoxification.
  i. Greater proportion of ammonia is generated in kidney and excreted in urine—thus reducing ammonia load in systemic circulation.
  ii. Additional amount of ammonia is detoxified in muscle to form glutamine, which in turn:
      a. Broken down to ammonia in enterocytes or
      b. Excreted in urine.
  iii. Small proportion of ammonia is detoxified in brain.

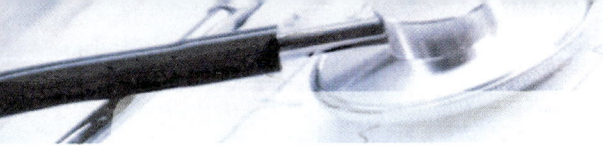

Phosphate activated glutaminase (PAG) is glutamine catabolizing enzyme present in small intestine (duodenum)—whose activity is four times greater in cirrhosis.

So the drug which can reduce the activity of PAG—may be of benefit in cirrhotic patients.

Ornithine promotes glutamine synthesis in muscles. **Phenylacetate** augments renal excretion of glutamine in the form of phenylacetylglutamine.

A number of **other important potential pathogenic mechanisms** have been detected—which offer us to initiate alternative methods of treatment.

A. **L-carnitine:** Protective effect is centrally mediated by:
   1. Activation of metabotropic glutamate receptors at the level of brain ammonia uptake.
   2. Mitochondrial energy metabolism.

   It treats hyperammonemia in:
   1. Children with urea cycle enzyme deficiencies
   2. Valproate-induced disease.

B. **Rivastigmine**

   Since in cirrhosis with hepatic encephalopathy
   ↓
   Reduction of acetylcholine level in brain

   Rivastigmine, a reversible cholinesterase inhibitor inhibits acetylcholine degradation, increasing the concentration of acetylcholine
   ↓
   As a result, psychomotor performance will be improved

C. **Endocarbinoids:** In hepatic encephalopathy

   In neural intoxication, there is cerebral energy flux disruption.
   ↑
   ←—— Endocarbinoids accelerates this process

   AMP activated protein kinase restores the cellular energy in response to metabolic injury

D. **Sildenafil:** In patient with hepatic encephalopathy:
   i. There is alteration in the function of glutamate—nitric oxide cyclic-GMP pathway.
   ii. Subsequent decrease in concentration of c-GMP in brain.

   As a result, intellectual capability and learning ability in patient with encephalopathy will reduced.

   Sildenafil, phosphodiesterase inhibitor, crosses the blood–brain barrier and restores the pathology.

   mGluR$_1$ antagonists: Alteration in glutaminergic transmission in substantia and par reticulate nigra is responsible for extrapyramidal features in hepatic encephalopathy.

   MGLUR$_1$ antagonists block this site and prevent the above features in these patients.

   Systemic inflammation: Anti-inflammatory agents modulate the systemic inflammatory response in patient with cirrhosis and prevent hepatic encephalopathy.

HEPATORENAL SYNDROME

This syndrome is characterized by functional renal failure in absence and renal pathology in patient with severe liver disease (Fig. 4.32).
i. In case of successful liver transplantation, renal function will come to normal.
ii. In case of death of cirrhotic patient, his kidney can be successfully transplanted to a normal patient.

Kidney functional changes may be due to:
i. Severest form of vascular changes
ii. Severest form of neurohumoral changes

Diagnostic Criteria of Hepatorenal Syndrome

1. Cirrhosis with ascites
2. Serum creatinine >1.5 mg/dl
3. No improvement in serum creatinine after:
   i. 2 days of diuretic withdrawal, and
   ii. Expansion of plasma volume with albumin (1 gm/kg of body weight up to maximum 100 gm/day)
4. Absence of shock
5. No history of current of recent treatment with nephrotoxic days or vasodilators
6. Absence of renal parenchymal disease as evidenced by:
   i. Proteinuria >500 mg/day
   ii. Microhematuria (>50 RBC/HPF), and/or
   iii. Abnormal renal ultrasonography

Classifications of Hepatorenal Syndrome

A. **Type 1 hepatorenal syndrome:**
   i. This is rapidly progressive (less than 2 weeks)
   ii. Reduction in renal function as indicated by rise in serum creatinine to >2.5 mg/dl.

   Recently proposed criteria of type 1 HRS: Evidence of acute kidney injury as evidenced by:
   i. Abrupt increase in serum creatinine ≥0.3 mg/dl
   Or, ii. Increase of more than 1.5-fold rise in serum creatinine from baseline value.

B. **Type 2 hepatorenal syndrome:**
   i. Slow progression of deterioration of kidney function
   ii. Relatively preserved renal function with refractory ascites.

Clinical Features

i. Features of advanced liver disease (median child pugh score 11.1)
ii. Refractory ascites.
iii. Hyponatremia—due to marked water retention.
iv. Features of marked hyperkalemia.
v. Death—may be due to liver failure.

Prevention of HRS

i. Careful use and monitoring of diuretic therapy
ii. Early recognition of any complication and its management like, bleeding, infection, electrolyte imbalance
iii. Avoidance of nephrotoxic drugs

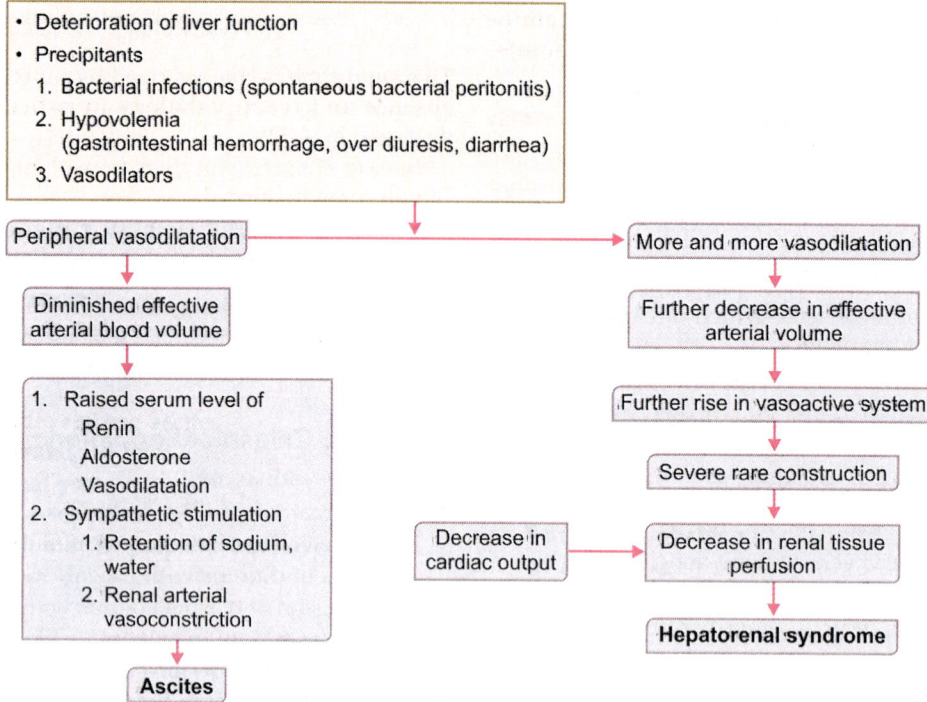

Fig. 4.32: Mechanism of hepatorenal syndrome

iv. Avoidance of large volume paracentesis
v. Worsening of HRS can be prevented by:
  a. Infusion of intravenous albumin
  b. Concomitant use of antibiotics—by this SBP can be present in those patients who did not experienced SBP previously.

Treatment

Since HRS is mainly due to development of hypovolemia, following will be the methods of choice:
  i. Stoppage of diuretics
  ii. Infusion of 20% human albumin—1 mg/kg up to maximum 100 gm
  iii. If after '1st administration of albumin, serum creatinine will not decrease—the above dose of albumin may be repeated—but provided CVP will be <10 mmHg.

After above treatment, serum creatinine will lower to normal then it can be diagnosed as prerenal azotemia.

Drugs to be avoided:
  i. Nephrotoxic drugs
  ii. Diuretics
  iii. Vasodilator drugs

Tissue Fluid Culture

If sepsis will be suspected, following will be of choice:
  i. Culture of:
    a. Ascitic fluid   b. Urine
    c. Blood   d. Cannula tips
  ii. Broad-spectrum antibiotic has to be administered after sending specimen for culture.

Renal replacement therapy in the form of:
  i. Continuous arteriovenous hemofiltration
  ii. Venovenous hemofiltration

Indications of renal replacement therapy:
  i. Severe volume overload
  ii. Metabolic acidosis
  iii. Hyperkalemia

Complication of renal replacement therapy:
  i. Hemorrhage   ii. Coagulopathy
  iii. Sepsis

Pharmacological Approaches

1. Vasodilator:
  a. Dopamine at its renal dose, it has not vasodilatory effect
  b. Prostaglandin—it does not produce any improvement in renal function.
2. Vasoconstrictors: Effects—administration for more than 3 days, they:
  i. Increase mean arterial blood pressure
  ii. Decrease serum creatinine level
  iii. Decrease plasma renin activity
  iv. Increase serum creatinine level

Drugs are:

> **Terlipressin**—0.5–1 mg intravenously 4–6 hourly
> ↓
> If no response after 2 days
> ↓
> Dosage can be doubled every 2 days up to 12 mg/day
> 2 mg every 4 hourly.

Stoppage of the above treatment in following conditions:
  i. Serum creatinine will not decrease by 50% after 7 days at its highest dose.
  ii. Serum creatinine does not reduce after 3–4 days of treatment.

If the treatment is successful.

Treatment should be continued till:
i. The serum creatinine will decrease to 1.5 mg/dl
ii. Treatment will be maximum up to 14 days
   A. Vasopressin—0.01–0.8 U/min (continuous intravenous infusion)
   B. Noradrenaline 0.5–3 mg/hour (continuous intravenous infusion)
   C. Octreotide + midodrine
      100–200 µg subcutaneously three times a day
      +
      7.5–12.5 mg orally three times day
      25 µg → 25 mg/hour (continuous intravenous infusion)
      +
      2.5 mg/day orally

Transjugular Intrahepatic Portosystemic Shunt (TIPS)

It should be considered:
i. If HRS recurs after discontinuation of vasoconstriction therapy and creatinine level will not come to normal values.
ii. If the patient is not fit for liver transplantation.
iii. If the patient has refractory ascites.

Extracorporeal Albumin Dialysis

If acts as a bridge between HRS and transplantation.

Liver Transplantation

It is the only definitive therapy for HRS—it can reverse HRS and improves survival.

If HRS can be reversed pre-transplantation—indicated by lowering of serum creatinine—post-transplantation outcome will be better.

In some cases, hemodialysis may be required in post-transplant patient.

Calcineurin inhibitor is the cause of renal function deterioration—following should be given till the commencement of diuresis (48–72 hours):

Azathioprine
+
Steroid or interleukin 2 receptor blocker

In case of type 2 HRS—after liver transplantation, renal functions return to normal in 90% of cases.

Prognosis

Prognosis is poor, if ascites develops in cirrhotic patients. Median survival:
i. In compensated cirrhosis ~ 9 years
ii. In decompensated cirrhosis ~ 1.6–1.8 years
   In patient with ascites, mortality 20% per years.

SPONTANEOUS BACTERIAL PERITONITIS

It is most common infection in cirrhotic patient with ascites.

It is called spontaneous because:
i. There is no contagious source of infection, like
   a. Intestinal perforation
   b. Intra-abdominal abscess
ii. There is no evidence of intra-abdominal inflammation:
   a. Abscess
   b. Acute cholecystitis
   c. Acute pancreatitis
   It is common in decompensated cirrhosis.

Pathogenesis

1. It is mainly blood-borne and monomicrobial.
2. Bacteria of gut origin are main isolated causative organisms.
3.

Enteric bacteria
↓
Migrate across the intestinal mucosa
↓   ↓
Extraintestinal   Bacterial translocation
sites   ↓
                    Systemic circulation

Sympathetic nervous system
↓
Slows the gut motility
↓
Stasis of bacteria
↓
Overgrowth of bacteria
↓
Bacterial translocation ⟶ **Extraintestinal sites**
↓
To systemic circulation

In cirrhosis, host defense is abnormal because:
i. Portosystemic shunting
ii. Impaired reticuloendothelial cell function
iii. Neutrophils are abnormal
iv. Decreased synthesis of protein—like
   a. Complements
   b. Fibronectin
v. Decreased adhesiveness
vi. Decreased phagocytosis

In ascitic fluid—bacterial growth depends upon opsonic activity of ascitic fluid which depends on the protein concentration of ascitic fluid, because, defective coating of bacteria makes it non-ingestible by polymorphs.

If ascitic fluid protein concentration is <1 gm/dl, and opsonic activity of ascitic fluid will be deficient, it leads to development of subacute bacterial peritonitis.

Precipitating factors for subacute bacterial peritonitis:
i. Gastrointestinal hemorrhage
ii. Hepatic encephalopathy
iii. Jaundice
iv. Invasive procedures, catheters
v. Previous history of subacute bacterial peritonitis

Clinical Features

i. Appearance of pyrexia
ii. Local abdominal pain
iii. Local abdominal tenderness
iv. Tachycardia

Laboratory Investigations

i. Leukocytosis
ii. Ascitic fluid examinations:
    a. Cell count >250/mm³
    b. Most of the cells are neutrophil
    c. Organisms:
        1. Mostly *Escherichia coli*
        2. Group D streptococci
        3. Rarely anaerobic bacteria
iii. Blood culture—50% positive for bacteria

Bacterascites—means:

i. Positive culture
ii. PMN <250/mm³

Fate of Bacterascites

i. If ascitic fluid opsonic activity is less—develops SBP
ii. If ascitic fluid opsonic activity is good—resolution of disease
    Patient with subacute bacterial peritonitis may develop renal complication—due to changes in systemic circulation as a result of inflammatory response to infection, generated by
a. Tumor necrosis factor
b. Interleukin 6.

Treatment

If ascitic fluid cell count >250 PMN/cc—following antibiotics can be given empirically and awaiting for the culture sensitivity report.
1. Cefotaxime—2 gm every 12 hourly
2. Amoxicillin and clavulanic acid combination

After getting c/s report—specific antibiotic should be started. Aminoglycosides should be avoided because of its renal toxicity.

Success Rate

i. In case of nosocomial infection—due to presence of multi-drug resistant organism—success rate is only 44%.
ii. In case of hospital acquired SBP: Broad-spectrum anti-biotics like, carbapenem, piperacillin/tazobactum should be given, mainly in those patient where:
    a. History of use of beta-lactam antibiotics during admission
    b. History of recent hospital admission
    c. Patient is on quinolone prophylaxis

Secondary bacterial peritonitis is suspected where the patient fails to respond to antibiotic therapy.

Prophylaxis

Long-term prophylaxis leads to development of resistant bacteria. But in following conditions prophylaxis should be provided.

In cirrhotic patient with history of upper gastrointestinal hemorrhage:
a. Norfloxacin—400 mg twice daily × 7 days
b. Intravenous ceftriaxone should he given in following conditions
        i. In the setting of high quinolone resistance
    Or, ii. Only two or more of the followings:
        • Malnutrition
        • Ascites
        • Encephalopathy
        • Serum bilirubin level >3 mg/dl

In case of recurrent subacute bacterial peritonitis:
i. Norfloxacin—400 mg/day
ii. This patient should be evaluated for liver transplantation.

Currently norfloxacin prophylaxis should be given in following conditions:
i. Low serum albumin level <1 gm/dl
ii. Advanced liver failure (Child-Pugh score >9 points) with following biochemical parameters:
        a. Serum bilirubin level >3 gm/dl
    Or, b. Impaired renal function
        • Serum creatinine >1.2 mg/dl
        • Blood urea nitrogen >25 mg/dl
iii. Serum sodium level <130 mEq/L

In following conditions, prophylaxis is not required:
i. Serum albumin level >1 gm/dl
ii. No past history of SBP.

HEPATOCELLULAR CARCINOMA

Epidemiology

It is the fifth most common cancer in the world and third most common cause of cancer death.

Risk Factors

1. **Liver disease:**
    A. *Non-cirrhotic causes:*
        1. Hepatitis B carrier
        2. Hepatitis C carrier
        3. Hereditary tyrosinemia
        4. Hepatic adenoma
    B. *Cirrhotic causes:*
        1. Hepatitis B
        2. Hepatitis C
        3. Alcoholic cirrhosis
        4. Non-alcoholic fatty liver disease
        5. Primary biliary cirrhosis
        6. Genetic hemochromatosis
        7. α1-antitrypsin deficiency
2. **Diabetes** is an independent risk factor
3. **Sex:** Males are more susceptible to be involved.
4. **Age:** It varies in different parts of the world:
    i. In Asia, age incidence is around 70 years.
    ii. In Africa, age incidence is 55 years.
5. **Exposure to aflatoxin in patients with chronic hepatitis B.**

Pathology

Several nodular lesions have been identified in liver in a case of hepatocellular carcinoma. These are:
1. **Dysplastic focus:** This is recognized by clusters of hepatocytes which is different from surrounding liver, size being <1 mm in diameter.
2. **Dysplastic nodules:** This is characterized by cluster of hepatocytes found in cirrhosis and often in the background of hepatocellular carcinoma, detected during ultrasound examination. Site is >1 mm in diameter. This has been subdivided into two forms:

a. Low-grade dysplastic nodule: This is composed of minimally abnormal hepatocytes surrounded by fibrous scar and is distinct from surrounding cirrhotic liver.

b. High-grade dysplastic nodule: This is composed of a typical clusters of hepatocytes, vague nodular appearance and indistinct fibrous margin, sometimes cannot be distinguished from hepatocellular carcinoma.

Small cell dysplasia is usually the precursors of HCC—because they have following characteristics:

I. There is evidences of expression of proliferation marker, like:
   i. Proliferation cell nuclear antigen
   ii. Increased labeling index of silver staining of the nucleolar organizing region
   iii. Evidence of expression of K1-67.
II. There is evidence of transition between small cell dysplasia and hepatocellular carcinoma (nodule in nodule appearance)

3. Large cirrhotic nodules: It shows least evidence of proliferation—which is also seen in small cirrhotic nodules.

Very Early Hepatocellular Carcinoma

i. Lesion is vaguely nodular, 40% lesions contain fat and altered nucleocytoplasmic ratio.
ii. Invasion of portal space by hepatocytes.
iii. Vascular invasion is absent.
iv. Margin is ill defined.
v. They have their own blood supply through unpaired arteries.
vi. Portal tracts will be reduced in number; as a result, overall blood supply will be reduced.
vii. Arterial phase—isointese/hypointense/hyperintense.
viii. Venous phase—isointense/hypointense.

Progressive HCC

Here the nodules are of three types:

i. **Well differentiated nodule:** It consists of plates of cord of hepatocyte like cells lined by endothelium. These cells have granular cytoplasm and nuclear pleomorphism.
ii. **Moderately differentiated nodule:** It contains glandular structures, bile stained, called pseudoacini.
iii. **Poorly differentiated nodules:** Here the cells are very large having multiple bizarre nuclei. Plate structures are absent.

Pathogenesis of HCC

1.
In case of viral hepatitis
↓
Repeated necrosis and regeneration
↓
Increased DNA mutations of rate
and
Decreased rate of repair of mutation
↓
Sufficient accumulation of mutations
↓
Development of HCC
2.
In case of hemochromatosis and α antitrypsin deficiency
↓

(Contd.)

(Contd.)

The injured cells give off the signals to neighboring cells
↓
These cells consequently divide
↓
There is risk of mutations
↓
Similar to that of viral hepatitis

3. Since HCC is a vascular cancer—arterial blood vessels proliferate enormously due to presence of angiogenic factors, VEGF.
4. There is evidence of three pattern of gene expression in HCC:
   i. In one-third cases—there is evidence of abnormalities in proliferative signals related to tyrosine kinase receptor pathway.
   ii. In one-third cases—activation of wnt/β-catenin pathway as a result of mutation in β-catenin gene.
   iii. In one-third cases—there is evidence of changes in gene involved in interferon signaling.
5. Genes related to prognosis—proliferative and anti-apoptotic gene, if over expressed in HCC, are related to poor prognosis.
6. **Biomarkers in HCC:**
   1. In early HCC—Glypican—3 is expressed in early HCC
   2. In progressive HCC—following biomarkers are present
      i. α-fetoprotein
      ii. Glycosylated AFP
      iii. Des-gamma carboxyprothrombin

Clinical Presentation

A. **Symptomatic presentation:** Patient usually presents with:
   i. Jaundice
   ii. Ascites
   iii. Variceal bleeding
   iv. Severe abdominal pain—which may be due to:
      a. Rupture of an HCC
      b. Bleeding into HCC
   v. Rupture of HCC may produce—hypotension or shock
   vi. Patient may present with weight loss
   vii. Patient may present with paraneoplastic syndrome like:
      a. Hypoglycemia—due to production of insulin like peptide
      b. Hypercalcemia
      c. Thrombocytosis
      d. Hypercoaguability with venous thrombosis
B. **Asymptomatic presentation:** Many patients can be diagnosed at early stage of the disease, when he presents with abdominal discomfort and sent for imaging studies.

Surveillance *(Fig. 4.33)*

Surveillance is necessary to detect this HCC at early stage, so that—more durable and care is possible. Following types of surveillance are used.

1. **Surveillance by biomarkers:**
   i. α-fetoprotein
   ii. Des-gamma carboxyprothrombin
   iii. AFP L_3/AFP ratio

All the above markers are elevated in patients with advanced cirrhosis.

2. Surveillance by ultrasonography:
It is of choice by ultrasonography—it can detect:
  i. Nodules—that is either cirrhosis
  ii. Dysplastic nodules <1 cm
  iii. Nodules >1 cm in diameter—which is suspicious of HCC

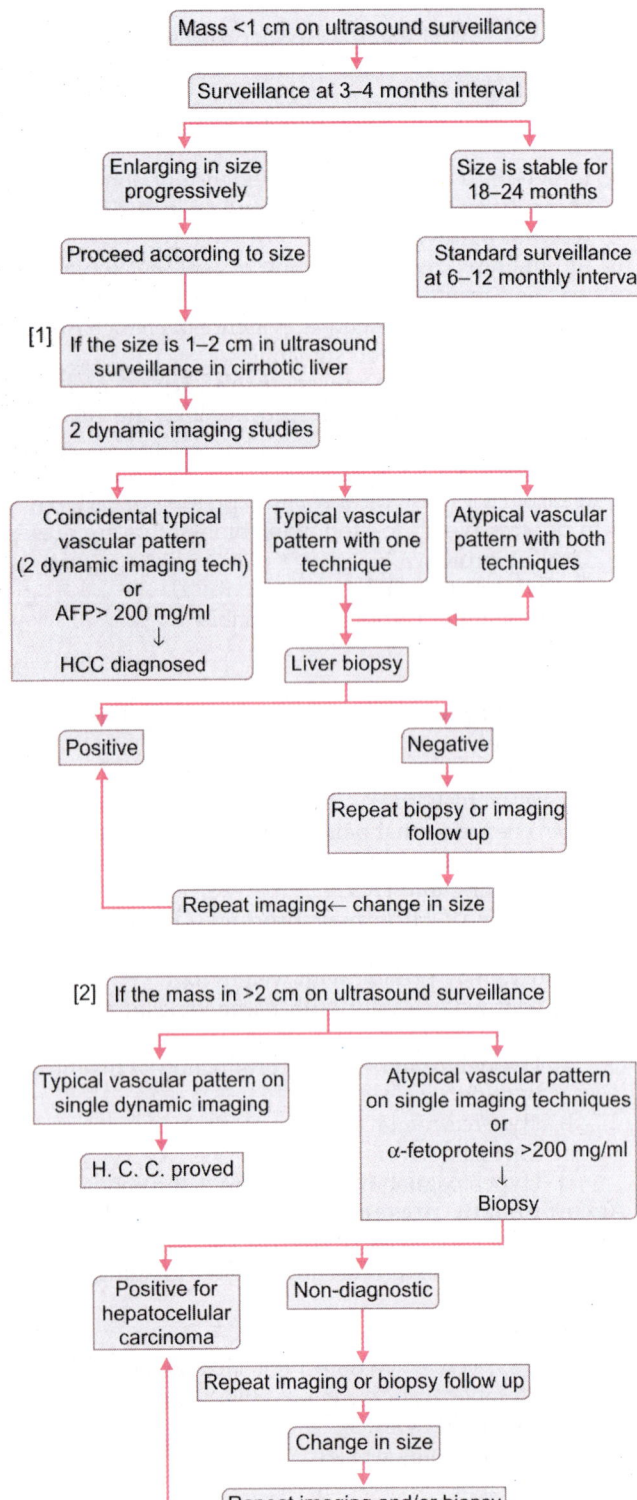

Fig. 4.33: Algorithm of surveillance of hepatic mass

Surveillance Interval

Ideal surveillance interval is unknown. Surveillance interval depends in:
  i. Growth rate of the tumor
  ii. Site of the tumor
    HCC doubling times ranges from 4 to 12 months.
    If the HCC is >2 cm in diameter, prognosis of HCC will be bad. So, surveillance time will be adjusted at frequently and as regular as possible till the size will be <2 cm in diameter.

Treatment

Preamble

Following are treatment techniques available for HCC:
a. Resection of liver
b. Liver transplantation
c. Hepatic artery ligation
d. Hepatic artery embolization
e. Chemoembolization
f. Internal radiotherapy
g. External beam radiotherapy
h. Various chemotherapeutic regimen
i. Local ablation with:
  a. Cold (cryotherapy)
  b. Heat (radiofrequency or microwaves)
  c. Corrosive substances (ethanol, acitic acids, hot saline)
  d. Targeted agents—raf kinase inhibitor or VEGE inhibitors

Hepatic Resection

  I. Best predictors of outcome of hepatic resection:
    i. Good liver function
    ii. Child's A cirrhosis
    iii. Normal bilirubin
    iv. Absence of portal hypertension, as measured by hepatic vein pressure gradient (<10 mmHg) or detected clinically
  II. In case of child grade B—overall result of liver resection is not good in spite of good liver function.
  III. In patient with macrovascular invasion, resection result is not good.
  IV. Most powerful predictors of postoperative recurrence:
    1. Presence of microvascular invasion
    2. Presence of additional tumor sites
  V. In cirrhotic patient, right lobectomy is more risky than resection of left lobe.

Liver Transplantation

Excellent results of liver transplantation in HCC occurs in following occasions (Milan criteria):
  i. Single HCC having <5 cm in diameter.
  ii. 2–3 nodules having <3 cm in diameter.

Most powerful predictors of post-transplantation recurrence:
  i. Absence of extrahepatic spread
  ii. Absence of microscopic vascular invasion
  iii. Poorly differentiated tumor

Staging of Hepatocellular Carcinoma (Fig. 4.34)

TNM classification is of less value in HCC because it does not capture the liver function test.
Barcelona cancer of liver clinic (BCLC) and model for end stage liver disease (MELD).

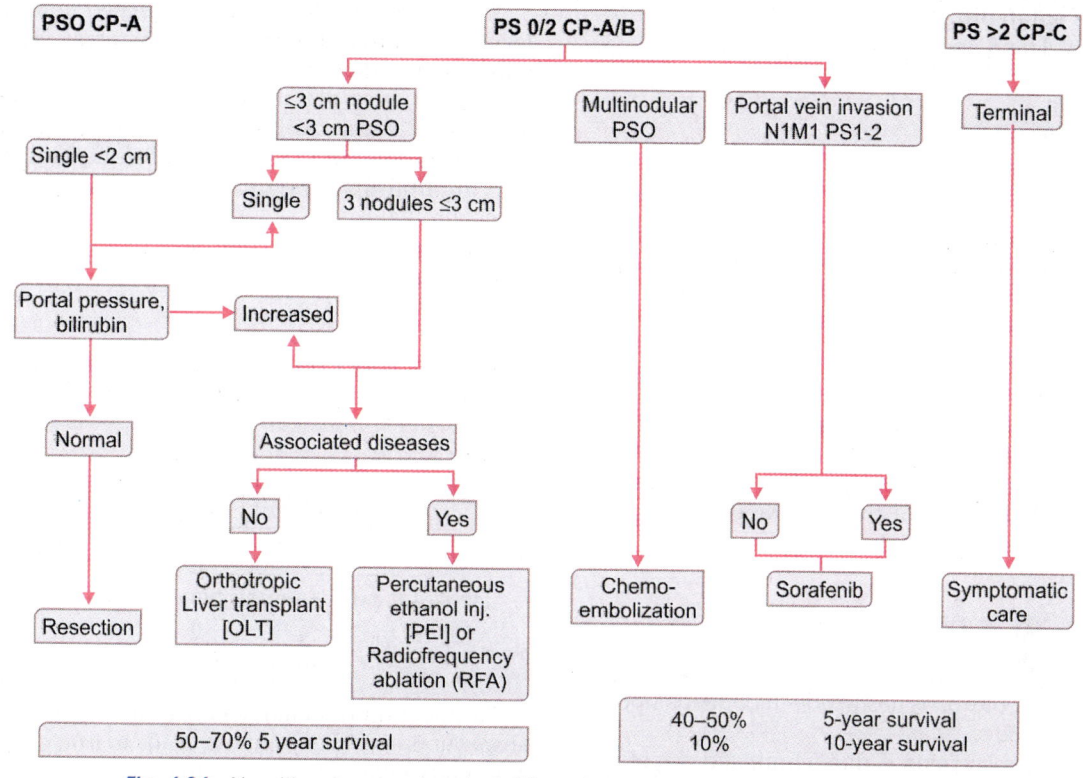

Fig. 4.34: Algorithm management of different stages of hepatocellular carcinoma

In absence of microvascular invasion, following two are the predictors:
i. Size of the largest lesion
ii. Number of the lesions

Ablation Therapy

Ablation by ethanol injection—produces complete necrosis in:
i. 90–100% patients with tumor <2 cm in diameter
ii. 70% with tumor having 2–3 cm diameter
iii. 50% with tumor having >5 cm in diameter

Radiofrequency Ablation

It should be done in HCC of less than 2 cm in diameter.

Drawback:
a. Higher cost
b. Higher rate of adverse events:
  i. Pleural effusion
  ii. Peritoneal bleeding

Following types of tumor are associated with non-suitability of RFA:
i. Subcapsular location of tumor
ii. Poor differentiation of tumor
iii. Close proximity of tumor to a large blood vessel

Embolic Treatment

Transarterial embolization: It should be done through hepatic artery to lobar and segmental branches, and then arterial flow has to be blocked through embolization.

The agents used commonly for embolization are:
i. Doxorubicin   ii. Cisplatin

Efficacy of TACE will be reduced by:
i. Limited hepatic function
ii. Presence of portal vein thrombosis

Contraindication for TACE: Complete portal vein thrombosis; because, there is risk of ischemic necrosis of that segment.

Side effect of TACE:
i. Chemotherapy-induced side effects:
  a. Nausea
  b. Vomiting
  c. Bone marrow depression
  d. Renal failure
  e. Alopecia
ii. Post-embolization syndrome
  a. Fever
  b. Abdominal pain
  c. Moderate degree of ileus
iii. Severe infection
  a. Hepatic abscess
  b. Cholangitis

Other agents used during TACE:
i. Gel foam pellets
ii. Gel foam powder
iii. Metallic coils
iv. Polyvinyl alcohol
v. Drug-eluting resin beads

Medical Therapy

The effective drug against HCC is sorafenib—a multikinase inhibitor. It inhibits cancer cell proliferation through different pathways including.
i. Angiogenesis through VEGF pathway
ii. Proliferation through RAF-MEK-ERK pathway

Side effects of sorafenib:
   i. Skin rashes: Hand–foot syndrome
  ii. Diarrhea
 iii. Fatigue
  iv. Hypertension

Other Therapies

A. **Intra-arterial radiotherapy using yttrium attached to microscopic glass beads**—Injected through hepatic artery. **Response is:**
   i. Tumor size reduction
  ii. Necrosis induction.

   However, this has not been tested.

   This procedure can be used in patient with portal vein invasion without fear of hepatic ischemic necrosis.

B. **Hepatic artery infusion therapy:** This process involves daily or weekly infusion of chemotherapeutic drug.

   This is under phase a trial.

IRON OVERLOAD STATES

Daily iron intake is 10–20 mg (90% is free, 10% is bound)

Of this, 1–1.5 mg of iron is absorbed—it depends upon the iron stores in the body.

The site of iron absorption is duodenum and upper small intestine.

The mechanism of absorption is controlled by following:
   i. HFE gene
  ii. Divalent metal transporter-1 (DMT-1)
 iii. Intracellular mechanisms for controlling expression of transport and storage protein, iron regulatory protein
  iv. Basolateral iron transporter
   v. Hepcidin (ferroportin)

In the intestine
↓

Ferric iron is reduced to ferrous form by ascorbic acid or ferriductase
↓

Thus it will be transported in the villus enterocytes by DMT-1. Expression of DMT-1 in enterocytes is controlled by intracellular iron by the interactions between IRP-1 and iron regulatory element of DMT-1.
↓

Then iron will be transported outside the cell through basolateral membrane with the help of a transporter, ferroportin.
↓

Here, the reduced iron will be oxidized to ferric iron and will be available for binding with transferrin.

Here this oxidation will be served by ceruloplasmin and hephaestin.

Regulation of Iron Absorption

HFE protein on the surface of the cells reacts with transferrin receptor TfR (1 and 2). As a result, affinity of TfR for transferrin will be reduced.

So the TfR/transferrin interaction controls uptake of iron into many cells.

Expression of TfR is inversely related to intracellular iron levels. So if intracellular iron level increases, expression of TfR will be reduced or vice versa.

There is inverse relationship between level of hepcidin and absorption of iron. So if hepcidin level is high, absorption of iron will be low, and vice versa. Hence hepcidin is responsible for maintaining pivot role in the development of hemochromatosis.

Hepcidin production is controlled by following:
1. Iron concentration
2. Hypoxia
3. Anemia
4. Inflammatory cytokines mainly interleukin-6
5. BMP through binding to hemojuvelin (HJV = HFE2)

Hepcidin is expressed on cells responsible for iron absorption.

Here it binds to ferroportin.
Normally if body iron is increased
↓
Hepcidin expression on hepatic cells will be increased
↓
Reduction of iron absorption

So hepcidin deficiency is responsible for increased iron absorption—which ultimately leads to iron overload in many hereditary hemochromatosis due to mutation of the following:
   i. HFE
  ii. Transferrin receptor-2
 iii. Hepcidin
  iv. Hemojuvelin.

Circulation of Iron

In the plasma
Transferrin synthesized in liver binds two ferric molecules.
↓
Binds to transferrin receptors present on reticuloendothelial cell and liver cell.
↓
Transferrin iron complex will be internalized
↓
Release of iron into the cells—(This process is returnable)
When the cell is saturated with iron—there will be down-regulation of transferrin receptor.
Normally 20–40% of total iron binding capacity will be saturated.
When transferrin will be fully saturated (overt hemochromatosis)
↓
Iron circulates in non-transferrin bound form along with low molecular weight chelator
↓
This iron will enter the cells by non-saturable process.

Storage of Iron

In the body, iron is stored in the form of ferritin. Ferritin is a combination of:
• Protein apoferritin (L and H subunits) and iron
• Each ferritin molecule contains 4500 atoms of iron.

The degradation product of ferritin is hemosiderin, which stains blue with ferrocyanide.

Lipofuscin, a non-iron containing yellowish brown material is also accumulated in iron overload.

This ferritin and hemosiderin are available for mobilization.

Normal total body iron is 4 gm. 3 gm iron is present in:
i. Hemoglobin
ii. Myoglobin
iii. Catalase
iv. Respiratory enzymes

Storage iron is 0.5 gm of which 0.3 gm is present in liver. Iron is mainly stored in liver absorbed from intestine, when storage capacity of liver is exceeded, excess iron will be stored in following areas:
i. Acinar cells of pancreas
ii. Cells of anterior pituitary gland.

Liver Damage due to Iron Overload

Hepatocellular damage is directly related to iron content of liver cell. Pattern of damage is similar whether due to:
i. Genetic origin.
ii. Multiple transfusion.

Severity of fibrosis is mainly in periportal areas.
In early form of storage disease—ferritin will be stored.
In late stage—the hemosiderin will be stored.

There are several mechanisms by which liver will be damaged:
1. Enhanced oxidative process associated with increased TGF-B, expression—as a result:

Lipid peroxidation of membrane organelles
↓
Increased lysosomal membrane fragility
↓
Release of hydrolytic enzyme in the cytosol
↓
Functional defect in mitochondria and microsomes

2. Hepatic stellate cell activation occurs due to release of cytokines from neighboring cells.

Genetic Hemochromatosis

This is an inborn error of metabolism.

It is autosomal recessive with mutation of gene in chromosome 6.
1. 85% of patients have single mutation in HFE gene.
   90% of Northern European patients are homozygous for mutation, whereas 65% of Southern European patient are homozygous for mutation.
2. There are also second type of mutation in HFE gen (H63D, also known as H si 63 asp).
3. Frequency of C282Y mutation is heterologous in 10% of patients of Northern population. In these patients, significant iron overload is rare, though serum iron and transferrin values are higher than normal.

Pathology

In liver:
i. Fibrosis in portal zone
ii. Deposition of iron in periportal liver cells and Kupffer cells

iii. Fibrous septa surround groups of lobules and irregular nodule (Holly leaf appearance)
iv. Ultimately development of macronodular cirrhosis
v. In cirrhosis, iron free areas are the foci of hepatocellular carcinoma.

In case of severe iron overload, following organs are involved.
1. Pancreas:
   i. Fibrosis of parenchymal cells
   ii. Iron deposition in:
      a. Acinar cells
      b. Macrophages
      c. Islets of Langerhans
      d. Fibrous tissue
2. Heart: Muscle fibres will be replaced by iron pigment within the sheath.
3. No deposition of iron is seen:
   i. Spleen
   ii. Bone marrow
   iii. Duodenal epithelium
   iv. Brain
   v. Nervous tissue
4. Varying amount of iron deposition with fibrosis seen in— endocrine glands:
   a. Adrenal cortex
   b. Anterior lobe of pituitary gland
   c. Thyroid
5. Testes are soft, small with germinal epithelium atrophy with evidence of iron overload.
6. Skin becomes flattened due to epidermal atrophy. Melanin content of basal layer is increased.

Association with alcohol: Combination of hemochromatosis with excess alcohol intake may be responsible for severely advanced liver disease.

In alcoholic liver disease, increased intestinal absorption of iron is responsible for deposition of iron in liver.

Clinical Picture

1. The patient may be symptomatic. In this case; diagnosis depends upon—high degree of suspicion in patient with hepatomegaly.
2. Age incidence:
   i. It is rarely diagnosed before the age of 20 years.
   ii. Peak incidence is between 40 and 60 years.
   iii. There is mean delay between presentation and diagnosis is 5–8 years.
3. Sex incidence:
   i. It is more common in males.
   ii. In female, the incidence is reduced due to following factors
      a. Presence of menstruation
      b. Pregnancy
   iii. In female it occurs, if there is evidence of the following:
      a. Scanty menstruation
      b. Hysterectomy
4. Skin pigmentation:
   i. Slaty grey in color
   ii. Sites—axillae, groins, genitila, old scar, exposed parts of mouth

iii. It occurs due to deposition of melanin in basal layer and can be seen due to atrophied epidermis.

Organ Changes

A. Hepatic changes:
  i. Right upper quadrant pain
  ii. Enlarged firm tender liver
  iii. Signs of hepatocellular failure, ascites—absent
  iv. Bleeding from esophageal varices—unusual
  v. Primary liver cancer:
    a. It may be the initial presentation.
    b. Sudden deterioration of clinical presentation in the form of:
      1. Rapidly developing ascites
      2. Rapidly enlarged liver
      3. Abdominal pain
      4. Raised α-fetoprotein.

B. Splenic changes: It may be palpable but never large.

C. Endocrine changes
  i. *Diabetes:*
    a. It may be insulin sensitive or insulin resistant.
    b. There may be family history of diabetes.
    c. There may be associated diabetes related complications, like:
      1. Nephropathy
      2. Proliferative retinopathy
      3. Neuropathy
      4. Peripheral vascular disease
  ii. *Sexual dysfunction:*
    a. Loss of libido in 35% patients
    b. Amenorrhea in 15% women
    c. Hypogonadism—due to:
      1. Hypothalamic dysfunction
      2. Pituitary dysfunction
      3. Gonadal dysfunction
      4. Combination of above three
  iii. *Pituitary dysfunction:* Gonadotropin-producing cells are mostly affected—producing hypogonadotropic testicular failure, characterized by:
      1. Impotence
      2. Loss of libido
      3. Testicular atrophy
      4. Skin atrophy
      5. Loss of secondary sexual hair
      6. Plasma testosterone is low, which can be raised to normal after given gonadotropin injection.
  iv. *Osteoporosis*—due to hypogonadism
  v. *Hypothyroidism*—rare.
  vi. *Adrenocortical insufficiency*—rare.

D. Cardiac changes: Cardiac presentation is due to iron deposition in myocardium and conductive system of the heart producing following features:
  i. Cardiac failure in young
  ii. Progressive right-sided cardiac failure
  iii. Dysrrhythmias
  iv. Sudden death.

E. Arthropathy:
  i. Aseptic arthropathy in metacarpophalangeal joint, it may also involve wrist joint and hip joint.
  ii. Radiologically:
    a. Hypertrophic osteoarthritis
    b. Chondrocalcinosis—in menisci, articular cartilage
  iii. Arthralgia may be presenting symptom.

Special Investigation

  i. Serum iron—increased
  ii. Transferrin concentration/total iron binding capacity—reduced
  iii. Normal transferrin level with raised serum ferritin level—suggests:
    a. Inflammation
    b. Metabolic syndrome
    c. Hepatic steatosis
    d. Alcohol excess
  iv. Serum ferritin: Serum concentration of ferritin is proportional to body iron store. It can asses body iron store, but it is unreliable in:
    a. Early diagnosis of precirrhotic stage
    b. Hepatic inflammation with raised transaminase level
       It is useful in follow-up of the treatment.
       Ferritin is also raised in following conditions:
      1. Hepatitis
      2. Alcohol excess
      3. Fatty liver
      4. Some cancers

Needle Biopsy of Liver

1. It is very important in C282Y homozygotes to assess the presence of cirrhosis or fibrosis.
2. Biopsy is not indicated in patients
   i. Without hepatomegaly
   ii. Normal serum transaminase level
   iii. Serum ferritin <1000 mg/L
3. But presence of any one of the above feature is the indication of biopsy.
4. Liver biopsy is not necessary following de-ironing treatment here serum iron is sufficient.

Imaging

A. Single energy CT scanning—It reveals hepatic attenuation which correlates with serum ferritin. It cannot detect hepatic iron overload <5 times the normal.
B. Dual energy CT scanning—accuracy is improved.
C. MRI scanning—in iron overload states—there is marked decrease in T_2 relaxation time.

Prognosis

Prognosis depends upon:
  i. Amount of iron deposition in tissues.
  ii. Duration of iron deposition in tissue.
  iii. Presence or absence of diabetes.
  iv. Stage in which treatment will be started.
  v. Whether the patient is continuously taking alcohol or not.

Bad prognoses in hemochromatosis are due to:
  i. Cardiac failure
  ii. Hepatic failure
  iii. Bleeding from esophageal varices
  iv. Cirrhosis with alcoholic

v. Development of hepatocellular carcinoma—risk is 200 times in patient with cirrhosis. This incidence is not reduced by de-ironing.

vi. In 15% of patient with non-cirrhotic hemochromatotic liver.

Treatment

A. **Venesection:** This can mobilize iron at rates of 130 mg/day.

500 ml of blood removes only 250 mg of iron. But tissue contains more than 200 times of that amount.

So to reduce iron store to normal, at least 2–45 gm iron should be removed from the body.

So by venesection in a co-operative patient, 500 ml of blood should be removed once or twice weekly to reduce ferritin level to its low normal range

Transferrin saturation will be gradually reduced till the patient become iron deficient.

Effects of venesection in a patient with hemochromatosis:
i. Well-being will be improved.
ii. Pigmentation will be reduced.
iii. Hepatosplenomegally will be reduced.
iv. Liver function test will be gradually improved.
v. Hypogonadism will be gradually improved in male patient of <40 years old.
vi. Cardiac function will be gradually improved—but it depends upon severity of cardiac muscle damage.
vii. Hepatic fibrosis will be improved—if the liver is cirrhotic, it is irreversible.

Maintenance therapy:
i. Venesection every 3–6 months should be done to prevent iron reaccumulation.
ii. Low iron diet—but it is not possible all the times.
iii. In that case, normal diet with intermittent venesection is of choice.

B. **Intramuscular depot injection of testosterone** should be given to treat gonadal atrophy.

C. **Human chorionic gonadotropin** can be injected to increase testicular volume and sperm counts.

D. **Diabetes**: It can be treated by:
i. Diabetic drugs
ii. Oral hypoglycemic or insulin injection

Liver Transplantation

Survival after liver transplantation in case of genetic hemochromatosis is low due to:
i. Cardiac complications
ii. Sepsis

Assessment of Body Iron Stores

There are many methods of detection and assessment of iron level in body stores:
A. Established methods:
i. Serum ferritin
ii. Liver concentration of iron in liver biopsy
B. Method under investigation:
i. Biomagnetic liver susceptometry (superconductive Quantum Interference Device, SQUID)
ii. Magnetic resonance imaging

Ferritin as a Marker

a. **Advantages:**
i. Easy to assess
ii. It is inexpensive
iii. Repeat measurement as a monitoring method to assess chelation therapy.
iv. It correlates with morbidity and mortality of patient.
b. **Disadvantages:**
i. It is an indirect method to assess iron burden in the body.
ii. Its level fluctuates with inflammation, metabolic deficiencies and abnormal liver function test.
iii. Serial measurement is necessary to monitor therapy.

Liver Content of Iron

a. **Advantages:**
i. It directly measures the liver iron content
ii. It is specific, quantitative
iii. It measures non-heme storage iron
iv. It usually provides information of liver cell status, evidence and extent of fibrosis.
v. It correlates with mortality and morbidity
b. **Disadvantages:**
i. There is risk of sample error.
ii. Skill of doctor and efficiency of laboratories are very important.
iii. Follow up is difficult.
iv. There is poor correlation with cardiac iron.
v. It is invasive and painful procedure.
vi. There may be chance of potential complications.

Advantages of magnetic iresonance imaging:
i. It is non-invasive.
ii. It can analyse the organ as a whole.
iii. It requires longitudinal follow up of the patients.
iv. Pathology of liver can be assessed.

Disadvantages:
i. Here measurement of liver iron is indirect.
ii. It requires images with dedicated imaging method.

Advantages of SQID:
i. It is noninvasive.
ii. Iron content measurement can be repeated.
iii. There is linear correlation with liver iron content found in biopsy.

Disadvantages of SQUID:
i. Highly expensive
ii. Low availability
iii. Indirectly measure liver iron content
iv. Underestimates liver iron content as compared with biopsy of liver.

Genetic Diagnostic Tests

1. C282Y/C282Y: It is homozygous for HFE type 1 hemochromatosis
2. C282Y/H63D: It is compound heterozygous for HFE type 1 hemochromatosis. In this case, severe iron overload occurs in only 15% of individual. In rest 85% patient iron overload is less severe.
3. H63D/H63D: It is homozygous for HFE type 1 hemochromatosis. In this case iron over load is unusual, with less chance of organ damage.

Genetic Screening

Indications:
1. Suggestive typical clinical presentation
2. Raised ferritin level with raised saturation of transferrin
3. When liver biopsy iron estimation as suggestive of iron overload.
4. When first degree relative is affected.

Advantages:
1. This can be done at any age
2. Parents of affected children can be screened

Disadvantages:
1. Both iron loaded and non-expressing homozygotes would be detected.
2. It is more expensive than phenotyping.

Family screening:
1. First degree relatives (parents, siblings and children) at risk carriers of HFE gene or inheriting the both copies of HFE gene of hemochromatosis.
2. Spouse should be tested if there are minor children to assess the risk.

PRIMARY BILIARY CIRRHOSIS

Clinical Presentation

Sex

90% patients are female—cause of disease prevalence is unknown. 10% patients are males.

Age

It usually occurs between 40 and 60 years of age. But it may occur in more than 80 years or less than 15 years.

Symptoms

1. **Jaundice versus pruritus:**
   i. Pruritus may develop without jaundice.
   ii. Jaundice or pruritus may develop simultaneously.
   iii. Pruritus may develop within 6 months to 2 years of onset of jaundice.
   iv. Onset of pruritus occurs during pregnancy, at that time, it may be confused with pregnancy-induced jaundice (cholestatic). But if it will persist after pregnancy, it is suggestive of primary biliary cirrhosis.
2. **Onset:** Onset is usually insidious.
3. **Fatigue:** It is frequent but non-specific symptom.
4. **Abdominal pain:** Vague right upper abdominal pain—it is chronic and non-progressive.

Signs

1. White shiny nails—suggestive of itching
2. Jaundice—it may or may not be present
3. Pigmentation present throughout the body
4. Liver—firm, enlarged non-tender
5. Spleen—palpable—if the patient is jaundiced.

In case of asymptomatic patient: Diagnostic points are:
   i. Raised alkaline phosphatase
   ii. Normal serum bilirubin or it may be minimally increased
   iii. Normal or mildly elevated serum cholesterol and transaminase

iv. If there is evidence of raised transaminase, there may be associated autoimmune hepatitis.

Abnormal physical signs are usually absent.

Associated Diseases

A. Collagen diseases:
   1. Sjorgen's syndrome with or without CREST
      C = Calcinosis
      R = Reynaud's phenomenon
      E = Esophageal dysfunction
      S = Sclerodactyly
      T = Telangiectesia
   2. Rheumatoid arthritis
   3. Dermatomyositis
   4. Mixed connective diseases
   5. SLE

B. Endocrinology:
   1. Autoimmune thyroiditis
   2. Graves' disease

C. Celiac disease

D. Hematological disorders:
   1. Autoimmune thrombocytopenia
   2. Autoimmune hemolytic anemia
   3. Risk of lymphoma

E. Renal complications:
   1. Distal tubular acidosis
   2. IgM associated membranous glomerulonephritis
   3. Asymptomatic bacteriuria
   4. Hyperuricosuria

F. Pulmonary abnormalities
   1. Lymphocytic interstitial pneumonitis
   2. Pulmonary hypertension
   3. Moderate to severe pulmonary hypertension with portal hypertension—indicates poor prognosis

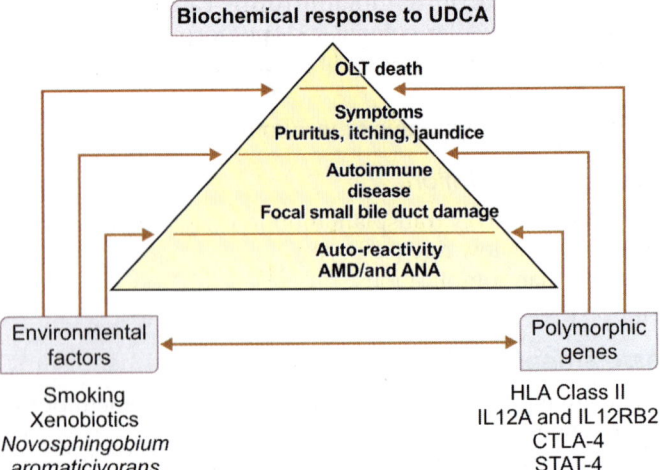

Fig. 4.35: Interrelations of factors in case of primary biliary cirrhosis

Natural History of the Disease

Different stages of primary biliary cirrhosis. This representation shows biochemical response to UDCA.

Progression of untreated primary biliary cirrhosis.

Stage

AMA	Biochemistry	Symptoms	Progression time
+	0	0	80% will progress
+	+	0	In 6 years 40% patients
+	+	+	In 10 years 70% patients

Natural history of histological changes in liver shows progression of primary biliary cirrhosis within 2 years. At that time, liver stiffness can be estimated by transient elastography.

Fatigue: It occurs in 60% of patients with PBC. Its presence indicates poor prognosis.

Abdominal pain may persist throughout the course.

Jaundice: When jaundice is obvious
i. Steatorrhea may be present
ii. Loss of weight—it may be acute or chronic progressive

Xanthoma: It may be present around the eyes, upper limb or lower limb.
a. If present in upper limb—it may present with pain in the fingers.
b. If present in lower limb—it may present with peripheral neuropathy.

Itching—escape area in chronic course of the disease, there is a butter fly area in the back—which escapes scratching—due to its inaccessibility of the fingers.

Osteoporosis: Its presence indicates:
i. Advancing age
ii. Severity of the disease
iii. Possible genetic component
There is increased risk of fracture.

Bleeding Esophageal Varices

i. It rarely develops before the generation of nodules—because in this case portal hypertension may be developed due to nodular regenerative hyperplasia.
ii. Varices are usually developed in case of advanced age with high serum bilirubin here prognosis is usually bad.
iii. Patients with platelet count of less than 1,40,000/ci may get benefit from endoscopy.
iv. In patient with varices, 1 year survival is 83% and 3 years survival is 59%.

Hepatocellular carcinoma: In case of molar with cirrhosis, risk of hepatocellular carcinoma is very high.

Mortality

In absence of liver transplantation terminal stage will last for 1 year. This may be characterized by:
i. Progressive deepening of jaundice.
ii. Disappearances of pruritus.
iii. Disappearances of xanthomas
iv. Low serum albumin and cholesterol
v. Development of edema and ascites

Terminal events may be:
i. Hepatic encephalopathy
ii. Uncontrollable bleeding
iii. Intercurrent infection
iv. Gram-negative septicemia

Biochemical Tests

1. Serum bilirubin—will be <2 mg/dl at the time of diagnosis
2. Serum alkaline phosphatase—raised
3. Serum γ-glutamyl transpeptidase—raised
4. Serum albumin—usually normal at onset, but will be low in late phase
5. Serum IgM—will be raised.

Serological Tests

A. Antimitochondrial antibodies—these antibodies are directed against 4 autoantigens of inner mitochondrial membrane:
  i. Dihydrolipomide acetyltransferase (E2) ⎫ Pyruvate
  ii. E3 binding protein ⎭ dehydrogenase complexes
iii. & iv. E2 components of other 2-oxo-acid dehydrogenase complexes.

B. Antinuclear antibodies—it is present in a few patients—with PBC. Here the antigens are (specific nuclear antigen)
  i. Glycoprotein of nuclear pore membrane
  ii. Nucleoporin P62
  iii. Interferon inducible nucleoprotein.

A few cases may be AMA –ve PBC, which can be mistakenly diagnosed as autoimmune cholangitis. But here, serum biochemistry, clinical presentation and liver histology will support the diagnosis of PBC.

In AMA negative make patient with inconclusive liver biopsy findings, MR visualizes the bite ducts.

In primary cholangitis, there is presence of bile duct irregularities.

Liver Biopsy

Liver biopsy should be done in case of AMA –ve patients. Histologically, the diagnostic lesion will be injured septal or interlobular bile ducts. This diagnosis may not be possible in case of needle biopsy unless the number of portal tracts is ≥10. Histometric examination shows:

A. Bile ducts:
  1. Destroyed bile ducts <70–80 μm is diameter
  2. Swollen and eosinophilic epithelial cells
  3. Irregular lumen of bite duct
  4. Disrupted basement membrane
  5. Cellular reaction involves—lymphocytes, plasma cells, eosinophils.
  6. Eventually bile ducts are destroyed and these sites are marked by lymphoid cell aggregates. Bile ductules begin to proliferate
  7. In zone 1, hepatic arterial branches are not accompanied by bile ductules.

B. Other areas of liver:
  1. Piecemeal necrosis
  2. Substantial amount of copper associated protein seen in the liver.
  3. Distortion of architecture of lobule by fibrous septa with the formation and regeneration of nodules.

Etiology

The following etiological factors are recognized.
1. Autoimmune process: Intolerance to mitochondrial autoantigen is main event in the progression of the disease. histologically, there is presence of 100-fold increases in

CD4+ and 10-fold increase in CD8+ cells surrounding damaged bile ducts.

CD4+ cells mature to differentiate Th1, Th2, Th17 or T-regulatory cells (treg).

These T-regulatory cells coil produce—interferon-γ, interleukin-17, tumor necrosis factor-α (TNF-α).

In PBC, there is evidence of few circulating treys and increased proportion of Th17 lymphocytes

2. **Xenobiotics:** It is a foreign compound complexes with native protein and change the molecular structure of that protein—which then is able to induce immune response.

In PBC, Xenobotic will be incorporated into major mitochondrial autoantigen and produce immune response.

3. **Antigenic similarity of infectious agents, mainly *E. coli*:** Antibody to mitochondrial autoantigen crossreacts with homologous E2 of *E. coli* in low titers.

Another candidate is *Novosphingobium aromaticivorans* which has antigenic mimicry with lipoyl domains with humans DDC-E2.

Epidemiology

1. All races in the world can be affected. Annual incidence is 0.7 to 49 cases per million population.
2. Cigarette smoking—has increased risk of fibrosis.
3. Family clustering
   i. Highest prevalence in mothers and daughters.
   ii. Concordance rate in monozygotic twins in 60%
   iii. Presence of AMA in 1st degree relatives
   iv. Major histocompatibility antigen (MHC) class-II molecule has been associated with PBC.
4. Cytotoxic T cell associated antigen 4 polymorphism is increasingly associated with PBC.
5. HL association: HLA Class II genes (DQ B1, DPB1, DRB1, and DRA) has been associated with PBC
6. Variants of multidrug resistance protein 3 and anion exchanger are associated with progression of PBC.

Treatment

Ursodeoxycholic acid (UDCA): It is non-hepatotoxic hydrophilic bile acid.

According to European and American Association for the study of liver, the dose is: 13–15 mg/kg body weight/day.

It is effective in stage I and stage II PBC, but less likely to respond in stage III or stage IV PBC.

This drug should be continued indefinitely. But following monitoring is required.

1. Serum bilirubin
2. Histological changes

Mechanism of Actions

i. It protects the cell membranes against detergent effect of hydrophilic bile acids
ii. It stimulates excretion of toxic bile acids
iii. It enhances the anion exchange in the liver
iv. It downregulates B cell activation and reduces the production of AMA
v. It induces expression of major antimicrobial peptide, cathelicidin in epithelial lining of biliary duct and responsible for epithelial cell inmate immunity.

Combination Therapy

1. Budesonide with UDCA—it improves liver histology. But it worsens osteopenia—it can be detected by monitoring bone mineral density.
2. Combination of fenofibrate with UDCA—it is under evaluation.

Management of Symptoms

1. Fatigue—it is responsible for day time somnolence. Modafinil—100–200 mg daily
2. Pruritus—it can be treated by
   a. Cholestyramine—starting dose is 4 gm/day can be increased up to 16 gm/day
      Since it interferes with the absorption of UDCA hence it should be taken 2–4 hours before intake of UDCA.
      Due to its unpleasant and bitter taste it should be taken with fruit juice.
   b. Rifampicin—can be used to get relief from pruritus
      Dose: To start with—150 mg/day and it can be increased up to 600 mg/day
      It many produce hepatotoxicity, hence monitoring of liver enzyme is necessary.
   c. Opioid antagonist—is also effective—it is difficult to start with because its withdrawal may be associated with withdrawal like reaction—which can be managed by intraveous naloxone—in the dose of –0.002 mg/kg/mm to 0.2 mg/kg/min over 3 days.
3. Vitamin A and D supplementation in case of Vit D deficiencies

Vitamin D_3—100,000 IU
   +   } 3 monthly
Vitamin A—50,000 IU intramuscularly
   +

Oral supplementation of calcium

4. Treatment of variceal hemorrhage.

Prognosis

1. As compared to general population, patient with PBC has 3 fold increases in mortality.
2. Prognosis also depends upon the biochemical response to UDCA
   i. Gradual lowering of ALP to normal in 1 year in response to UDCA has similar survival to age matched healthy population.
   ii. Biochemical response to UDCA in better than non responders.
3. Following factors predict the advent of ascites or other complications in PBC
   i. Age
   ii. Albumin
   iii. Log^{10} (bilirubin)

Liver transplantation is indicated in patients with end stage PBC. Model for end stage Liver disease (MELD) score should be used to predict survival.

MELD score of >16—indicates the survival benefit from liver transplantation.

Liver Transplantation in PBC

Indications:
 i. Intractable pruritus
 ii. Hepatic encephalopathy

iii. Spontaneous bacterial peritonitis
iv. End stage liver disease in PBC
Survival after transplantation for 1 year is >90%
For 5 years is >80%

After transplantation:
i. Pruritus will be resolved rapidly
ii. Fatigue will persist
iii. AMA will not be lost.

Recurrence of disease:
17% patients in 3.7 years

WILSON'S DISEASE

This is an autosomal recessive disorder of copper metabolism characterized by liver and neurological disease.
This disease was first defined by Kinner Wilson.

Molecular Genetics

This disease occurs due to mutations of gene ATP7B present on long arm of chromosome 13—this gene is mainly expressed in liver. The gene product is six copper binding unit "Wilson ATPase".

The roles of Wilson ATPase are:
1. Elemental copper is taken up by the sinusoidal membrane of hepatocyte by CTRI.
2. This elemental copper is taken up by ATOX1 and carried to trans-Golgi network where "Wilson ATPase" is present
3. Wilson-ATPase has two functions:
   i. Either it directs the copper to form ceruloplasmin
   ii. Or, it directs copper excretes into bile
   This action depends upon concentration of copper in bile.
   a. If the concentration of copper in bile will be low or normal: Wilson ATPase helps in production of holoceruloplasmin (Ceruloplasmin containing copper) in golgi apparatus and from there it will be secreted into blood.
   b. If the intracellular copper content will be high: Wilson's ATPase increases biliary excretion of copper by a process which involves COMMD1. Glutathione helps in biliary excretion of copper by MRP2.
      Mutation of "Wilson's ATPase" interferes with above process and responsible for Wilson's disease.
      Increased accumulation of copper in liver cells produces alteration in mitochondria and nuclei.

Pathology

Liver

There are spectrums of histologic findings—like:
a. Simple steatosis:
   i. Ballooned liver cells with glycogenated vacuolar nuclei.
   ii. In some cases, Malloy-Denk bodies like acute alcoholic hepatitis may be detected.
b. Periportal fibrosis
c. Macronodular cirrhosis—in a young with cirrhosis with no history of exposure—one has to exclude the possibility of Wilson's disease.
d. In case of fulminant hepatitis—submassive necrosis may occur.

Regarding presence of copper in liver—rhodamine stain is not reliable. In early case of Wilson's disease, since copper is present in cytoplasm, hence this may not detect copper. So absence of copper in liver biopsy cannot exclude the diagnosis of Wilson's disease.
In case cirrhosis copper can be detected in periportal area.

Electron microscope findings: Cystic dilatation of the tips of mitochondrial cristae along with the pleomorphism of mitochondria is the diagnostic.

Involvement of eye: Kayser-Fleischer ring—it occurs due to deposition of copper-containing pigment in Descemet's membrane at the periphery of the posterior surface of cornea.

Involvement of kidney: Copper deposition in proximal convoluted tubule occurs due to fatty as well as hydropic changes.

Clinical Picture

In case of child: Patient usually presents with liver disease (hepatic form). This is followed by neuropsychiatric manifestations (neurological form).

In case of adult: Predominant manifestation is neuro-psychiatric changes.

In a few cases: There may be overlap of two symptoms.

Kayser-Fleischer ring: This is characterized by greenish brown ring present at the periphery of iris—it can be visualized by slit lamp examination.
This ring is usually associated with neuropsychiatric changes. But in only 40–60% patient of hepatic form this ring may be present.
This type of ring may also be present in:
i. Prolonged cholestasis
ii. Cryptogenic cirrhosis.

Sunflower cataract: This is present on the posterior layer of capsule of the lens—color is grayish brown.

Hepatic Form

A. **Acute hepatic failure:** Patient may present with:
   i. Jaundice
   ii. Ascites
   iii. Features of hepatic failure
   iv. Features of renal failure—patient is usually child or young.
   v. Features of intravascular hemolysis due to destruction of RBC as a result of sudden flux of copper from necrotic hepatocytes.
   vi. K-F ring is usually absent.

   Biochemistry:
   i. Copper level in urine and serum are very high.
   ii. Usually serum ceruloplasmin is low but it may be high—since it is acute phase reactant.
   iii. Serum ammotransferase level is inappropriately low
   iv. ALP: TB (total bilirubin) = <4—highly suggestive
   v. AST: ALT >2.2

B. **Mimicry with autoimmune hepatitis:**
   i. Age incidence 10–30 years
   ii. Symptoms of acute or chronic hepatitis—jaundice

iii. Raised aminotransferase
iv. Hypergammaglobulinemia
v. Nonspecific autoantibodies
These patients should require necessary investigations related to Wilson disease.
C. **Cirrhosis:** The patient may present with well-compensated cirrhosis—the features include:
i. Vascular spider
ii. Splenomegaly
iii. Ascites
iv. Portal hypertension
v. Hepatic encephalopathy
These patients may respond to medical treatment.
This disease may not be associated with neurologic signs.
D. **Hepatocellular carcinoma:** Though it is uncommon, but may occur due to induction of hepatic metallothionein copper.

Neuropsychiatric Changes

This broad group has different subgroups—these are:
i. Parkinsonian
ii. Pseudosclerotic
iii. Dystonic
iv. Choreic
Two types of presentations:
a. **Acute and progressive:** Presentations are:
i. Flexion–extension tremor of wrist
ii. Grimacing
iii. Writing difficulty
iv. Drooling
v. Slurring of speech
vi. Slow deterioration of personality
b. **Chronic neurological changes:** It starts in early adult life. The findings are:
i. Wing-beating type tremor exacerbated by voluntary movement. Here there in no evidence of sensory loss or pyramidal tract involvement.
ii. Vacant expression
iii. Severe dystonia

EEG shows: Generalized non-specific changes.

Renal Changes

The following findings are evidence of renal tubular changes—as evidenced by:
i. Aminoaciduria
ii. Glycosuria
iii. Phosphaturia
iv. Uricosuria
Causes—deposition of copper in proximal convoluted tubules.

Other Changes

1. Eposides of hemolysis—evidence of gall stones.
2. Lunalae of nails—are lavender—it is due to deposition of copper.
3. Skeletal changes:
i. Demineralization
ii. Premature osteoarthritis
iii. Subarticular cysts
iv. Fragmentation of bone

4. Arthralgias
5. Muscle weakness
6. Cardiac disease—arrhythmias
7. Low fertility in women
8. Repeated abortion

Laboratory Investigations

a. **Serum ceruloplasmin:**
1. Low: Other causes of low ceruloplasmin:
i. Congenital aceruloplasminemia
ii. Advanced liver disease with synthetic failure
2. High—due to:
i. Inflammation
ii. Estrogen administration
iii. Oral contraceptive drugs
iv. Biliary obstruction
v. Pregnancy
b. **Basal 24-hour urinary copper excretion:** Increased (0.6 µmol/24 hour). Simultaneous measurement of urinary creatinine is required to validate the completeness of collection.
c. **Liver biopsy:** Copper content of liver tissue in gm of dry weight:
i. Normal—50 mg/gm of dry weight
ii. Wilson's disease ≥250 mg/gm of dry weight, but 70–100 mg/gm—may be found.
Elevated level may be found in:
i. Normal hepatic histology
ii. Long-standing cholestasis
iii. Indian childhood cirrhosis.

Imaging Studies

1. Computerized tomography of brain—enlargement of ventricle in patient with neuropsychiatric manifestations.
2. MRI of brain: The following findings may be found:
i. Dilatation of third ventricle
ii. Focal lesion in:
a. Thalamus
b. Putamen
c. Pallidum

Genetic Studies

i. Haplotype analysis—for cloning the gene in Wilson's disease.
ii. Recent method of sequencing of the entire ATP7B gene.

Treatment

A. Definite therapy for hepatic form of the disease—chelation therapy.
Definite therapy for neuropsychiatric manifestation—chelation therapy or zinc administration.
B. Maintenance therapy:
i. Reduced dose of chelators
ii. Reduced dose of zinc
C. Liver transplantation—Indications:
i. Fulminant hepatic failure
ii. Unresponsive to medical treatment

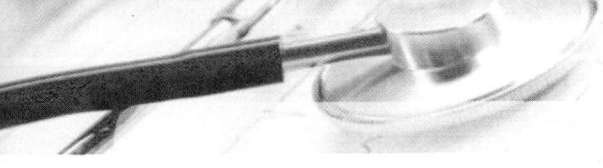

Drugs used in Definite Treatment

D-penicillamine:

Mechanism of actions:
 i. Chelation of copper
 ii. Increased excretion of copper in urine to 15–45 mmol/day.

 Dose in adult: 1–1.5 gm/day by mouth in three to four divided doses/day 1 hour before meals.

 Duration of treatment: Since improvement is slow, 6 months of continuous therapy should be required.

 Signs of improvement: In patient with neurologic disease—there is neurological deterioration followed by improvement. Following improvements are seen:
 i. Disappearance of K-F ring
 ii. Clearer speech
 iii. Rigidity and tremor will be lessened.
 iv. Hand writing will be progressively better
 v. Improvement in LFT
 vi. Liver biopsy showing slow reversal of cirrhosis.

Failure of improvement indicates:
 i. Irreversible tissue damage before starting the treatment
 ii. Non-compliance of treatment

 In case of non-improvement—dose should be increased to 2 gm/day

 Treatment failure: When there is no sign of improvement after 1–2 years of therapy it should regarded as treatment failure.

 After successful improvement, dose of D-penicillamine will be reduced to 750–1000 mg/day. Close follow-up is required to:
 i. Ensure continued improvement
 ii. Ensure stability of improvement
 iii. Monitoring of compliance

 Adverse reaction: It occurs in 30% patients with Wilson's disease. The reactions are the following
1. Hypersensitivity reaction—it occurs within first few weeks of treatment. Features are
   i. Fever
   ii. Rash
   iii. Leucopenia
   iv. Thrombocytopenia
   v. Lymphadenopathy
   This can be resolved by discontinuation of treatment.
   The treatment can be continued with administration of prednisone.
2. Proteinuria
3. SLE like syndrome
4. Aplastic anemia
5. Skin changes:
   i. Elastosis perforans serpiginosa
   ii. Cutis laxa (progeria wrinkling)—since it is dose related, hence long term treatment with dose >1 gm/day is not recommended.

Monitoring:
1. Whole blood cell and platelet count: Weekly then monthly for 6 months annually thereafter
2. Urine analysis for proteinuria
   Pyridoxin—25 mg/day to be given routinely.

 Trientine: It should be given in patient intolerant to D-penicillamine.

 Dose: 1000–1200 mg/day in two divided doses. Maximum dose is 1800 mg/day.

Side effects:
1. Fixed drug reactions
2. Rarely pancytopenia

 The drug should be taken at least 1 hour before taking food
 This drug should be kept in refrigerator to prevent its deterioration.

Zinc:

Mechanism of action: Zinc prevents absorption of copper through induction of intestinal metallothionein.

 Dose: 50 mg elemental zinc by mouth three times daily is empty stomach.

 Zinc is useful for maintenance therapy after initial treatment with chelators.

Side effects:
 i. Nausea
 ii. Vomiting
 iii. Gastric irritation

 Dimercaptopropanol (British anti-Lewisite): It is now rarely used, as an adjunct to available chelator in patient with refractory neurological/or psychiatric disease.

 Tetrathiomolybdate: It is an investigational agent.

Mechanism of actions:
 i. In the intestine it prevents absorption of copper
 ii. The drug after absorption, complexes copper with albumin.

 In blood and thus prevent copper from damaging the tissue.

 If it is used in patient with neuropsychiatric symptoms, it may initially worsen the neuropsychiatric symptoms.

Combination Therapy

It should be given in:
 i. Decompensated hepatic disease
 ii. Severe neurological symptoms

The drugs are:
 i. Trientine—500 mg in adults—as 1st and 3rd dose (6 AM and 6 PM)
 ii. Zinc—50 mg elemental—has to be given alternate with trientine, 5-6 hourly between administration as 2nd and 4th dose (12 noon and 12 mid-night)

 This combination should be continued for 3 months then treatment should be switched to monotherapy (trientine or zinc).
 If the patient with hepatic disease fails to respond with this treatment, Liver transplantation will be of choice.

Other Measurements

1. Physiotherapy—it should be done to improve patient's gait, writing and movement.
2. Diet:
   a. Copper containing drugs must be avoided. These are nuts, liver, shellfish, chocolate and mushrooms

b. Alcohol containing beverage should be stopped initially, but alter on, this should be customized.

c. Vegetarian should be under dietary supervision.

3. During pregnancy: Daily dose of D-penicillamine 750–1000 mg or trientine can be used in 1st two trimester of pregnancy.

Dose should be reduced to 500 mg/day in last trimester. The above drugs in pregnancy, if not used in patients with Wilson's disease, there is risk of hepatic insufficiency and death.

Hepatic Transplantation

Indications:

1. Fulminant hepatic failure
2. Young cirrhotic patient with hepatocellular decompensation who fails to show improvement after 2–3 months of optimal medical treatment.
3. If the patient develops severe hepatic failure after discontinuation of treatment.

Improvement after transplantation:

1. Hepatic metabolic defect will be corrected
2. Neurological improvement may occur very slowly.

Before transplantation, following should be corrected:

i. Renal failure and hemolytic anemia—should be treated by albumin dialysis.
ii. Acute hemolysis should be corrected by exchange transfusion.

Prognosis

Since most of the Wilson's disease cannot be diagnosed, the patient may die untreated.

1. In mimicking autoimmune hepatitis, treatment response may be poor due to presence of following ominous signs:
   i. Jaundice
   ii. Ascites
   iii. High serum bilirubin
   iv. Elevated aminotransferases
   v. Coagulopathy time
2. In children, a score is being made of following:
   i. Total serum bilirubin
   ii. AST
   iii. Albumin
   iv. INR
   v. Total WBC count
   This score may show the need for liver transplantation.
3. In acute neurological form
   i. Prognosis is poor
   ii. Basal ganglia cystic changes will be irreversible
4. In chronic neurological form—dystonia carries poor prognosis.

Common causes of death:

i. Chronic liver failure
ii. Variceal bleeding
iii. Intercurrent infections
iv. Bedridden neurological patients.

DISEASES OF PANCREAS

Pancreatic enzymes	Causes	Reasons
Amylase 1. Serum levels	Increased in pancreatic inflammation	Specific if the level is 3 times upper limits of normal Following causes should be excluded—gut perforation, gut infarction It will be elevated within 24 hours of onset of pain; it will remain raised for 3–7 days and returns to normal within 7 days. It will remain raised in following condition: i. Pancreatic ductal disruption, ii. Pancreatic ductal obstruction, iii. Pancreatic pseudocyst The value may be normal in following conditions: i. There is a delay (2–5 days) before taking blood samples. ii. Presence of underlying chronic pancreatitis iii. Presence of hypertryglyceridemia
2. Urinary level	Urinary level and ratio of urinary amylase/creatinine ratio—increased	It is no more specific and sensitive

3. Ascitic fluid	It occurs in:
	i. Disruption of main PD
	ii. Leakage of pseudocyst
	iii. Abdominal disorders:
	  a. Intestinal obstruction
	  b. Intestinal infarction
	  c. perforated peptic ulcer
		False positive elevation occurs in abdominal disorders

4. Pleural fluid	It occurs in i. Acute pancreatitis, ii. Chronic pancreatitis	False positive tests occurs in i. Carcinoma of lung, ii. Esophageal perforation
Lipase	In case of acute inflammation of pancrease	It is positive in 70–85% of cases

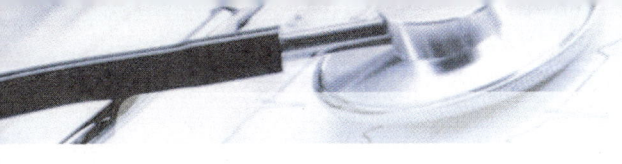

Amylase is present in following organs other than pancreas:
1. Salivary gland
2. Fallopian tube
3. Lung
4. Thyroid
5. Tonsils
6. Various tumors of:
   - i. Lung
   - ii. Esophagus
   - iii. Breast
   - iv. Ovary

Causes of hyperamylasemia other than pancreatic causes:
1. Renal insufficiency
2. Salivary gland
   - i. Mump
   - ii. Irradiation
   - iii. Calculus
3. Tumor
   - i. Lung
   - ii. Esophagus
   - iii. Breast
   - iv. Ovary

Table 4.15: Radiological investigations

Name of the test	Causes	Interpretations
Plain straight X-ray of abdomen	May be abnormal in: i. Acute pancreatitis ii. Chronic pancreatitis	It is usually normal in >50% of cases
Ultrasonography	Following information can be obtained: i. Edema ii. Inflammation iii. Heterogeneous echogenic shadow iv. Calcification v. Cyst formation vi. Mass lesion	**In acute pancreatitis:** Enlarged heterogenous appearance **In chronic pancreatitis:** Presence of calcification **In pancreatic pseudocyst:** Presence of smooth round fluid collection. **In pancreatic carcinoma:** Mass lesion >3 cm in diameter Following may interfere with USG of pancreas: i. Obesity ii. Small or large bowel gas
CT scan of abdomen	Aim: i. Evaluation of suspected pancreatic disorder ii. Evaluation of complications of acute and chronic pancreatitis Most lesions are characterized by i. Enlarged pancreatic outline ii. Distortion of pancreatic contour iii. Different attenuation co-efficient of fluid present in pancreas	It is useful in the diagnosis of: i. Pancreatic calcification ii. Dilated pancreatic duct iii. Pancreatic tumor: It cannot distinguish between inflammatory and neoplastic lesions.
Dynamic CT scan (IV administration of contrast)	It estimates: i. Extent of pancreatic necrosis ii. Morbidity, and mortality	
Spiral CT scan	i. It provides clear image more rapidly ii. It negotiates the artifact produced by patient movement	
Endoscopic ultrasound	It is useful for following purpose: i. Information of pancreatic parenchyma ii. Information of pancreatic duct iii. Detection of CBD stones iv. Biopsy from pancreatic mass	It can detect: i. Acute pancreatitis ii. Chronic pancreatitis It can assess: i. Chronic pancreatitis, ii. pancreatic carcinoma
Endoscopic retrograde cholangiopancreatography	It can visualize: i. Luminal narrowing ii. Alternate dilatation and constriction of PD iii. Blockage of PD by calcific deposits	It can diagnose 60–80% of cases. But chronic pancreatitis may not be differentiates from pancreatic carcinoma
Magnetic resonance cholangiopancreatography (MRCP)	It can detect: i. Common bile duct ii. Pancreatic duct iii. Pancreatic parenchyma. Secretin enhanced MRCP in under current investigation	Three dimensional turbo—spin—echo technique produces super MRCP images
Biopsy of pancreatic tissue by US or CT guidance	It can diagnose pancreatic masses	High diagnostic yield. But technical skill is essential

Table 4.16: Exocrine pancreatic function test

A. Direct stimulation of pancreas secretin—pancreozymin test Normal value: i. Volume >2 ml/kg/hour ii. Bicarbonate >80 mmol/L iii. Bicarbonate output >10 ml.L in 1 hour	Secretin produces—increased secretion of: i. Bicarbonate ii. Pancreatic juice CCK produces: Increased output of pancreatic enzymes This secretion depends upon—functional pancreatic tissue	i. It can detect occult disease ii. It involves duodenal intubation and fluoroscopy iii. In chronic pancreatitis, there may be abnormally low HCO_3 output. So, secretin test measures secretory capacity of ductular epithelium
Endoscopic secretin—CCK test	It negates the needs for tube placement in duodenum	

Table 4.17: Measurement of intraluminal digested products

1. **Stool microscopy for detection of meal fibers and fat**	Due to absence of proteolytic and lipolytic enzymes, there is decreased digestion of meat fibers and triglycerides	It cannot detect milder pancreatic deficiency
2. **Quantitative estimation of stool fat**	Due to absence of lipolytic enzyme, fats are not digested	It cannot differentiate between maldigestion and malabsorption. But markedly reduced lipolytic enzyme may produce steatorrhea
3. **Estimation of fecal nitrogen**	This occurs due to lac of proteolytic enzyme in stool	i. It cannot differentiate between maldigestion and malabsorption ii. It has low sensitivity
4. **Measurement of pancreatic elastase**	This enzyme is not degraded intestine	It is highly sensitive to detect severe pancreatic exocrine insufficiency in case of: i. Chronic pancreatitis ii. Cystic fibrosis But stool must be solid, not liquid.

4. Burns
5. Macroamylasemia
6. Diabetic ketoacidosis
7. Pregnancy
8. Trauma to brain
9. Abdominal disorders (other than pancreas):
   i. Biliary causes:
     a. Cholecystitis
     b. Choledocholithiasis
   ii. Intra-abdominal causes:
     a. Peptic perforation
     b. Intestinal obstruction
     c. Intestinal infarction
     d. Peritonitis
     e. Aortic aneurysm
     d. Chronic liver disease

Physiology of Pancreatic Exocrine Secretion

Daily pancreatic fluid secretion: 1500–3000 ml iso-osmotic alkaline (pH >8) fluid. It contains 20 enzymes.

Regulation of Pancreatic Secretion

The following factors are responsible:
A. Hormonal systems
B. Neural system

A. Hormonal systems:

Gastric acid
↓
Stimulates secretion of secretin from the duodenum
↓
Stimulates pancreatic ductal cells to secrete water and electrolytes
Long chain fatty acids
And
Amino acids (tryptophan, phenylalanine, valine, methionine)
↓
Stimulates release of CCK from duodenum and proximal jejunum
↓
Stimulates enzyme-riched secretion from pancreatic acinar cells

B. Nervous system

Parasympathetic system (vagus nerve) → increased release of VIP
↓
Control release of secretin and CCK
↓ ↑
Control release of enzyme

Pancreatic exocrine function is influenced by following inhibitory neuropeptides:
  i. Somatostatin
  ii. Pancreatic polypeptide
  iii. Peptide YY
  iv. Neuropeptide Y
  v. Encephalin
  vi. Pancreastatin
  vii. Calcitonin—gene-related peptide
  viii. Glucagon
  ix. Galanin

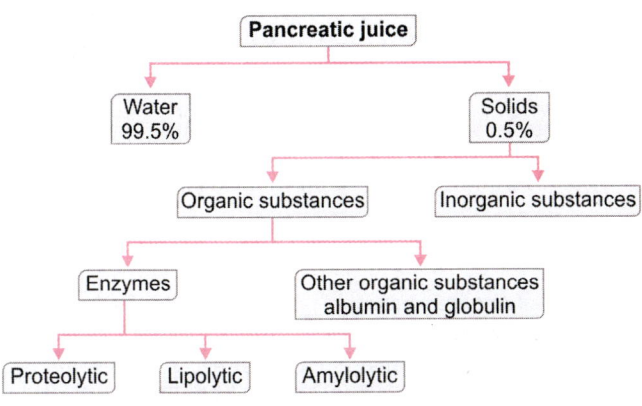

Neurologic stimulation is cholinergic. It involves:
  i. Extrinsic innervation by vagus nerve
  ii. Innervation by intrapancreatic cholinergic nerves
Stimulatory neurotransmitters:

  i. Acetylcholine   ii. Gastrin-releasing peptides

Neurotransmitters
↓
Activate calcium dependent second messenger systems
↓
Release of zymogen granules

Stimulates

VIP
↑
Intrapancreatic nerves

Autodigestion of pancreas can be prevented by packaging consisting of:

1. Precursor of pancreatic proteases
2. Synthesis of protease inhibitors
   ↓
   It binds to trypsin → inactivates trypsin
3. Mesotrypsin, chymotrypsin c, enzyme y

   ↘ ↓ ↙
   Lyse and inactivate trypsin

These protease inhibitors are found in:
  i. Acinar cells
  ii. Pancreatic secretions
  iii. α1 and α2 globulin
4. Low calcium concentration in acinar cell cytoplasm of normal pancreas destroys spontaneously activated trypsin.

So, loss of any of the above protective mechanism will be responsible for activation of zymogen granules which may lead to development of acute pancreatitis.

Enteropancreatic Axis and Feedback Inhibition

Following are the methods of stimulations of pancreatic enzymes as well as feedback inhibitions:

1. Phenylalanine perfusion in duodenal lumen
   ↓ Stimulates
   Increased plasma level of CCK, chymotrypsin and other enzymes
   ↑
2. Trypsin perfusion in the duodenal lumen
3. Perfusion of duodenal lumen with protease inhibitions
   ↓
   Hypersecretion of pancreatic enzymes
4. A peptide, CCK releasing factor present in duodenal lumen ↑   ↓ (+)
   Inhibit | (-) stimulation of CCK release
5. Serine protease inhibitor
6. Acidification of duodenal contents
   ↓

Table 4.18: Enzymes in pancreas

Enzymes	Activators	Substrate	End products
Trypsin	Enterokinase Trypsin	Protein	Proteases and polypeptides
Chymotrypsin	Trypsin	Proteins	Polypeptides
Carboxy-peptidases	Trypsin	Polypeptides	Amino acids
Nucleases	Trypsin	RNA and DNA	Mononu-cleotides
Elastase	Trypsin	Elastin	Amino acids
Collagenase	Trypsin	Collagen	Amino acids
Pancreatic lipases			
Pancreatic lipase	Alkaline medium	Triglycerides	Monogly-cerides + Fatty acids
Cholesterol ester hydrolase	Alkaline medium	Cholesterol esters	Cholesterol + Fatty Acids
Phospholipase A	Trypsin	Phospholipid	Lysophos-pholipid
Phospholipase B	Trypsin	Lysophos-pholipid	Phosphoryl choline + Free fatty acids
Colipase	Trypsin	Facilitates Trypsin	
Pancreatic amylase		Starch	Dextrin maltose

Release of secretin
↓
Stimulation of vagal and other neural pathways
↓
Stimulation of pancreatic ductular cells
↓
Stimulation of bicarbonate secretions
↓
Neutralization of duodenal acid content

Dietary protein
↓
Binds with proteases
↓
Increase in free CCK releasing factor through neural pathways
↓
Release of CCK in circulation in physiological concentration
↓ Through neural pathways
This leads to acetylcholine-mediated pancreatic enzyme secretion.
↓
These enzymes are continued to be secreted till all the proteins will be digested

ACUTE PANCREATITIS

Definition

This is characterized by varying degrees of inflammation along with injury to pancreatic tissue along with its dysfunction as well as dysfunction of adjacent organ or organs distant to pancreas.

Incidence

It is 5–73 per 100000/year. The incidence is due to several reasons:
  i. This incidence varies in different population and different ethnic groups due to presence of precipitating factors like, alcohol abuse, and gallstone disease.
 ii. Histological confirmation can be found in few cause of acute pancreatitis.
iii. Some patients do not come into the medical attention because of mild disease.

Classifications

According to International Symposium in Atlanta, acute pancreatitis has been subdivided into two forms:
1. **Acute mild pancreatitis**
   i. Absence of local and systemic complications
  ii. Uneventful recovery
 iii. No need of medical and surgical interventions
  iv. Only supportive care is sufficient.
2. **Acute severe pancreatitis**
   i. Presence of local and systemic complications
  ii. Need for urgent medical and surgical interventions
 iii. Significant mortality rate.

Major pathobiologic processes responsible for acute pancreatitis are the interactions of intracellular and extracellular events (Fig. 4.36).

Intracellular events are:
 i. Activation of digestive enzymes
ii. Inhibition of secretion—occurring during acute pancreatitis

Extracellular events are:
 i. Vascular response
ii. Neural response

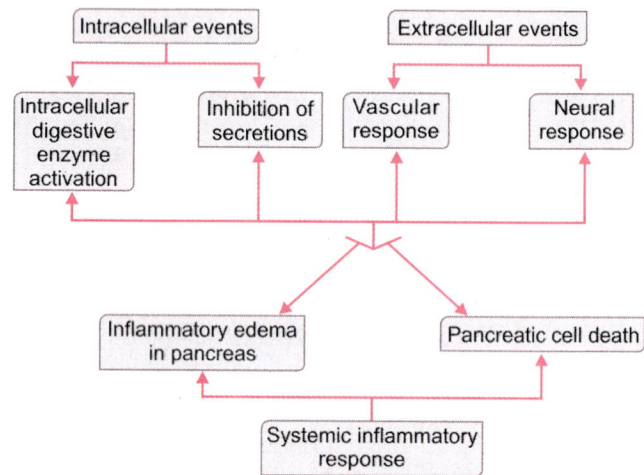

Fig. 4.36: Events in acute pancreatitis

Alcohol metabolism in pancreas

In the liver — By oxidative system of metabolism:
Alcohol
↓ ← Alcohol dehydrogenase
Acetaldehyde
↓ ← Acetaldehyde dehydrogenase
Acetate

In pancreas — By esterification systems:
Alcohol
↓ ← Different enzymes in pancreas
Fatty acid ethanol esters (FAEE)

As compared to liver, FAEE synthesis is greater in pancreas. Following are the significant pathophysiological effects in pancreas produced by FAEE (Fig. 4.37):
1. Activation of proinflammatory transcription factors responsible for inflammatory response

2. Increased lysosomal fragility
↓
Activates intracellular digestive enzymes
↓
Increased incidence of cell death

3. Increased cytosolic and mitochondrial calcium levels
↓
Activates cell death pathways

In this way, there is chance of development of acute pancreatitis in case of alcohol abuse.

Inflammation and edema (Fig. 4.38):

Causative noxious stimuli to pancreatic acinar cells

↓

Alcohol feeding

> Upregulation of intracellular signaling system like:
> i. Nuclear factor Kβ
> ii. Activating protein-1
> iii. P-38 mitogen—activated protein kinase

↓

↳ Upregulation of production of cytokines, chemokines and growth factors from pancreatic acini

↓

These are responsible for inflammatory response in acute pancreatitis

Proinflammatory cytokines and chemokines include:
 i. Tumor necrosis factor (TNF-α)
 ii. Platelet activating factor (PAF)
 iii. Interleukin-6, 8, 1β
 iv. Monocyte chemotactic protein-1
 v. Macrophage migration inhibitory factor
 vi. Nitric oxide synthatase
 vii. Intercellular adhesion molecule-1

↓

Systemic inflammatory response producing adult respiratory distress syndrome

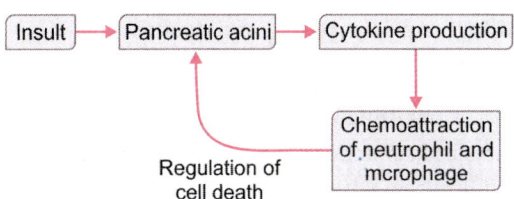

Fig. 4.37: Effect of inciting events on pancreas

Cell Necrosis

Pancreatic necrosis is always associated with severe pancreatitis and poor outcome. Two major categories of cell death in case of acute pancreatitis:

A. **Apoptosis:** It is called programmed cell death. This is required for:
 i. Normal development   ii. Tissue homeostasis
 iii. In some pathological conditions

In case of apoptosis, following morphological changes will occur:
 i. Shrinkage of cells and their organelles
 ii. Condensation of nuclear chromatin
 iii. Translocation of phosphatidyl serine from inner layer to outer layer of plasma membrane.

This apoptotic body or apoptotic cells with externally located phosphatidylserine is phagocytosed by mcrophages followed by its removal from pancreatic tissue.

B. **Necrosis:** This occurs in extremely pathological situations. It represents the extreme response to injury. In necrosis, following events will occur:

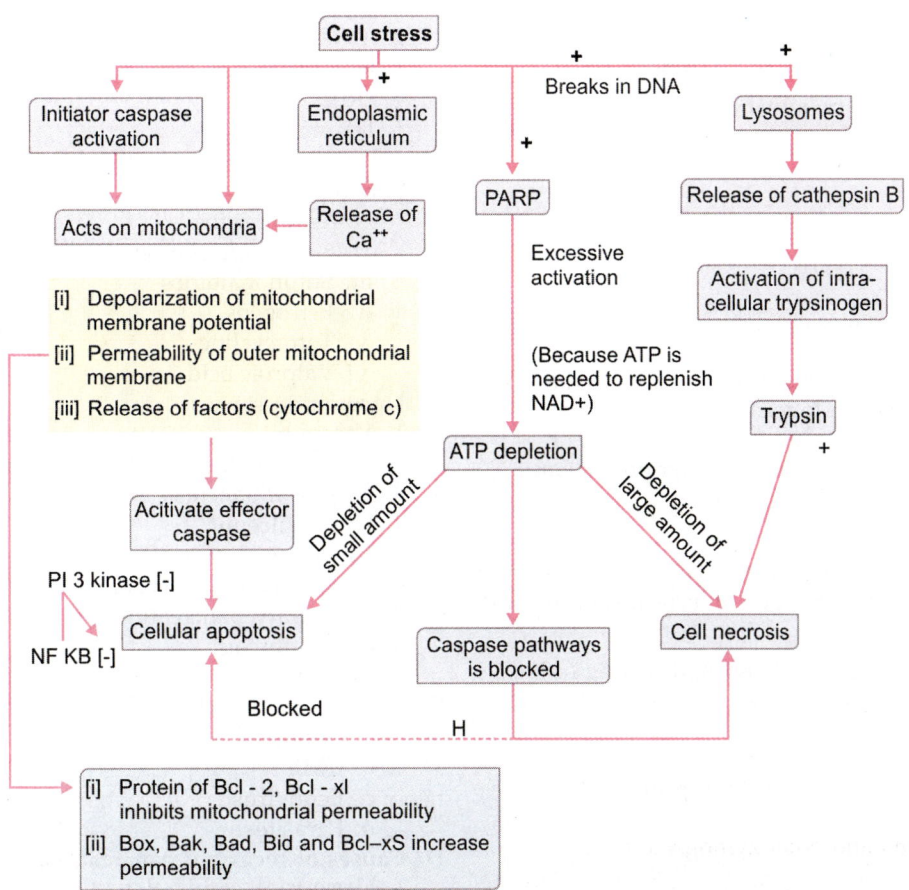

Fig. 4.38: Algorithm of inflammatory response in acute pancreatitis

i. Mitochondrial swelling and dysfunction
ii. Rupture of plasma membrane
iii. Release of intracellular constituents to extracellular spaces resulting acute inflammatory response.

ATP acts as key steps in the caspase pathway.

ATP is necessary for maintaining ion pumps—which is responsible for cellular integrity.

Nuclear enzyme poly (ADP-ribose) polymerase (PARD)
↓
Catalyzes poly-DP—ribosylation of DNA binding protein

Inhibitors of apoptosis are responsible for pancreatic necrosis in acute pancreatitis. So grades of apoptosis direct the severity of acute pancreatitis

Alcohol → FAEES $\xrightarrow{+}$ release of $\begin{cases} \text{ATP depletion} \\ \text{Necrosis} \\ \uparrow\uparrow \text{Mitochondrial uptake} \end{cases}$

Metabolized in   Calcium from ER
pancreas

Intracellular Activities of Digestive Enzymes

Intracellular activation of enzymes occurs in early course of acute pancreatitis.

In normal state, pancreatic acinar cells protect themselves from their damaging effects by following mechanisms
i. Synthesis of enzymes as inactive zymogens
ii. Trypsin inhibitor packed in zymogen granule
iii. Segregation of enzymes in membrane—bound compartments
iv. Enterokinase restricted to small intestines

Digestive enzymes are synthesized and stored in zymogen granules as:
a. Trypsinogen
b. Chymotrypsinogen
c. Procarboxypeptidase
d. Proelastase
e. Prophospholipases

Normally these proenzymes are delivered into duodenum
↓
Here, brush border enzyme enterokinase activate trypsinogen to form trypsin
↓
Trypsin catalyzes the activation of other proenzymes

In case of acute pancreatitis: There is activation of proenzymes in pancreatic acinar cells

In case of hereditary pancreatitis: There is mutation of trypsinogen genes leads to activation of trypsinogen enzymes in pancreatic acinar cells.

In case of acute pancreatitis: Abnormal sorting of lysosomal cathepsin B and digestive enzymes in common compartment
↓
Cathepsin B converts trypsinogen to trypsin
↓
Trypsin activates itself and other zymogens
↓
Pancreatic necrosis

Inhibition of Secretions

Inhibition of activated enzymes from the acinar cells occurs due to derangements of apical actin cytoskeleton which is responsible for exocytosis.

Vascular Response

Microvascular circulation is seriously affected in acute pancreatitis. These are:
i. Increased and homogenous microperfusion in mild edematous pancreatitis.
ii. Increased vascular permeability may be responsible for edema formation.
iii. Progressive decrease in capillary perfusion in necrotizing pancreatitis—it is the key feature for development of severe pancreatic necrosis.

Microvasculature plays following roles in inflammatory response in acute pancreatitis:
i. Expression of adhesion molecules results adhesion and migration of leukocytes from intravascular space into parenchyma.
ii. Vascular response are maintained by:
  a. Endothelin-1
  b. Cytokines/chemokines
  c. Endothelial nitric oxide synthatase

Etiology of Pancreatitis

A. Common causes:
  1. Gallstones:
    i. Macrolithiasis
    ii. Microliithisis
  2. Alcohol abuse
  3. Hypertriglyceridemia
  4. ERCP
  5. Trauma
  6. Dysfunction of sphincter of Oddi
  7. Drugs:
    i. Azathioprine
    ii. 6-mercaptopurine
    iii. Sulphonamides
    iv. Estrogens
    v. Tetracycline
    vi. Valproic acid
B. Uncommon causes:
  1. Vasculitis
  2. Thrombotic thrombocytopenic purpura
  3. Cancer of pancreas
  4. Hypercalcemia
  5. Pancreatic division
  6. Periampullary diverticulum
  7. Hereditary pancreatitis
  8. Cystic fibrosis
  9. Renal failure
C. Rare causes: Infections:
  a. Mumps
  b. CMV
  c. Echovirus
  d. Parasites
D. Causes of recurrent pancreatitis:
  1. Hypertriglyceridemia
  2. Pancreatic divisum

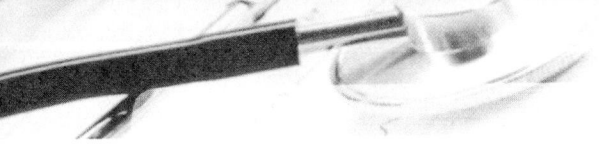

3. Carcinoma pancreas
4. SOD
5. Cystic fibrosis

Gallstone-Induced Pancreatitis

1. Increased risk in men 14–35-fold, in women 12–25-fold.
2. Predisposing factors:
   i. Small gallstones <5 mm
   ii. Large cystic duct
   iii. Large common channel in the ampulla
   iv. Metabolic factors—hyperlipidemia—manifested by delayed chylomacron clearance
3. In patient with hyperbilirubinemia and pancreatitis—incidence of recovery of gallstone is 85%. Passage of stone into the duodenal lumen mainly occurs on 1st day of attack of gallstone-induced pancreatitis.
4. Presence of stones in CBD or in ampulla—indicate severity.

Microlithiasis: It means crystals aggregates in bile—it may present with recurrent bout of pancreatitis in absence of gallstones. It can be identified by:
i. Abdominal ultrasound
ii. Endoscopic ultrasound

It looks:
i. Amorphous, layering nonshadowing material—it is sludge.
ii. Brightly echogenic cholesterol crystals in gallbladder
iii. By bile examination:
   a. Birefringent cholesterol, monohydrate crystals
   b. Reddish brown calcium bilirubinate granules

Materials for examination:
i. Bile aspiration during ERCP
ii. Bile aspiration from duodenum after slow intravenous administration of CCK or octapeptide.

Sphincter of Oddi Dysfunction

It is composed of complex muscular structure—it regulates flow of pancreatic and bile secretions independently and functionally.
a. Effect of CCK on sphincter of Oddi:
   1. It causes both components of sphincter to relax and allow the flow into duodenal cavity.
   2. It directly acts on sphincter to contract.
b. Other factors responsible for sphincter of Oddi relaxation:
   1. Vasoactive intestinal peptide:
   2. Glucagon
   3. Nitric oxide
   4. Secretion—it produces—increase in phasic contraction followed by relaxation of sphincter

Suspicion of pancreatic duct stenosis may come into mind in presence following factors:
1. Dilated pancreatic duct
2. Poor pancreatic drainage
3. Difficulty in passage of ERCP catheters through papilla over pancreatic guide wire.

Pancreatic manometry during ERCP may diagnose pancreatic duct hypertension.

Treatment of SOD

A. Surgical therapy:
1. Endoscopic pancreatic sphincterotomy
2. Pancreatic duct stenting—it may produce pain in patients and may be responsible for chronic pancreatitis. (in case of prolonged placement of stents)

B. Medical therapy:
1. Calcium channel blocker
2. Intraampullary botulinum toxin injection

Pancreatic Divisum

During fetal development, dorsal and ventral pancreatic buds form duct which enters into duodenum.

Ventral pancreatic bud rotates around the duodenum and fuses with dorsal bud. Ventral duct drains through major papilla (duct of Wirsumg)

Dorsal pancreatic duct drains through minor papilla (duct of Santorini)

If the two above ducts fuse partially or do not fuse—dorsal duct drains the secretion of most of the pancreas through minor papilla—it is called pancreatic divisum.

Pancreatic divisum can be subdivided into two types:
a. Complete type: Here ventral and dorsal pancreatic ducts never communicate.
b. Incomplete type: Here diminutive duct joins ventral and dorsal pancreas.

But most of the exocrine secretion occurs through minor papilla.

In both cases, dorsal papilla will be dominant.

In case of pancreatic divisum:
1. Incidence of acute pancreatitis is 5%. It usually occurs due to relative obstruction of minor papilla.
2. Diagnostic tests for stenosis of minor papilla—pancreatic duct imaging before and after intravenous secretin injection.
   a. In normal person: Pancreatic duct dilates transiently after injection of secretion—it return to 1mm or baseline within 15 minutes.
   b. In patient with pancreatic divism: There is evidence of prolonged pancreatic duct dilatation following intravenous secretin injection.

Imaging should be done through:
i. Ultrasound
ii. Endoscopic ultrasound
iii. MRI

Occasionally dorsal duct dilatation occurs terminally—called santorinicele.

Treatment

Minor papilla sphincterotomy:
i. Responds in 50–70% of patients—some of these patient may relapse.
ii. Patient with chronic pancreatitis less likely to responds.
iii. Patient with abdominal pain but no history of pancreatitis has short term symptomatic improvement.

Following patients are less likely to benefit from endoscopic intervention:
i. Cystic fibrosis transmembrane receptor (CFTR) mutations with pancreatic divisum.
ii. CFTR mutation with idiopathic pancreatitis.

Injection of botulinum toxin into minor papilla may be given in patient with pancreatic divisum with recurrent pancreatitis.

Alcoholic Pancreatitis

Alcoholic pancreatitis may present after bout of alcohol ingestion. Incidence is surprising low.

Mechanisms for development of alcoholic pancreatitis:
i. Spasm of sphincter of Oddi
ii. Plugging of small pancreatic ductules by proteinous sludge
iii. Direct toxic and metabolic effects of alcohol
iv. Stimulation of pancreatic functions through cholinergic pathways.
v. Sensitization of pancreatic tissue to different insults through production of proinflammatory cytokines.
vi. Conversion of digestive enzymes to their activated terms
vii. Activation of intracellular death pathways.

Mechanisms of proteinous plug formation:
i. Change in concentration and composition of protein secreted by pancreas—results in formation of protein plugs—blocking small pancreatic ductules—as a results, pancreatitis occurs
ii. Increased viscosity as well as increased protein concentration of pancreatic secretions—results in plugs formation.
iii. Formation of rigid, insoluble protein structure secretory proteins like, lithostathine and glycoprotein-2 responsible for formation of protein plug.

Drugs Responsible for Acute Pancreatitis

The drugs can be classified according to relationship with pancreatitis.
A. **Fully related:**
  1. Azathioprine
  2. Didanosine
  3. Estrogens
  4. ACE inhibitors
  5. 6-mercaptopurine
  6. Valproate
B. **Probably related:**
  1. Protease inhibitors
  2. Acetaminophen
  3. Furosemide
  4. Isoniazid
  5. Procainamide
  6. Rifampicin

Production of acute pancreatitis by scorpion venom by following mechanisms: Toxin polypeptides tityustoxin:
i. Acts through cholinergic pathways—stimulates pancreatic secretion.
ii. It directly stimulates pancreatic secretion
iii. It induces spasm of sphincter of oddi
iv. It alters the blood flow.

Hypertriglyceridemia

It may be produced by acute pancreatitis; again, it may be responsible for precipitation of acute or chronic pancreatitis, when serum level will be 2000–3000 mg/dl.

High level of triglyceride in serum of pancreatic capillary bed
↓
Lipase acts on triglycerides
↓
Generation of toxic free acid radicals in serum
↓
It acts on endothelial lining of small pancreatic blood vessels
↓
Damage of small blood vessels
↓
Recruitment of inflammatory cells and development of thrombosis
↓
Development of acute pancreatitis

Following types of hypertriglyceridemia may be responsible for acute pancreatitis:
i. When intravenous lipid administration raises serum level to 500 mg/dl
ii. Development of hypertriglyceridemia after fatty meal.
iii. Hypertriglyceridemia due to therapy with estrogen, retinoid derivatives and HIV protease inhibitory.

Its treatment includes:
1. Good supportive care
2. Monitoring of serum triglyceride level in case of parenteral nutrition.
3. If serum triglyceride level >10,000 mg/dl—plasmapheresis.
4. After recovery from acute pancreatitis—low fat diet.

Viruses Causing Acute Pancreatitis

1. Coxasackie B virus.
2. Hepatitis B virus
3. Influenza A and B virus
4. Enteroviruses
5. Cytomegalovirus
6. Rubellavirus
7. AIDS virus
8. Opportunistic infections:
   i. *Mycobacterium avium*
   ii. *Cryptococcus*
   iii. *Toxoplasma gondii*
   iv. *Histoplasma*
   v. *Mycobacterium tuberculosis*
   vi. *Candida*.

Bacteria producing acute pancreatitis:
1. *Salmonella species*
2. *Shigella*
3. *Campylobacter species*
4. Hemorrhagic *E. coli*
5. *Legionella* species
6. *Leptospira*

Autoimmune Pancreatitis

Lymphoplasmocytic Sclerosing Pancreatitis

1. **Symptoms:**
   i. Acute or subacute symptoms of pancreatitis
   ii. Evidence of obstructive jaundice
   iii. Recurrent symptoms

2. **In imaging studies:**
   i. Diffusely enlarged "sausage shaped" pancreatic mass without surrounding inflammatory changes
   ii. CT scan of MRI studies

   Gland appears to have capsule—like edge
3. **Pancreatography shown:**
   i. Irregular narrowing of main pancreatic duct
   ii. Pancreatic duct stricture simulating malignancy
   iii. Biliary involvement is usual by may present with
      a. Intrapancreatic bile duct stricture
      b. Hilar stricture simulating malignancy
      c. Intrahepatic biliary ductular changes similar to sclerosing cholangitis
4. **Histological changes:**
   i. Lymphoplasmocytic infiltrates involving g small duct and venules.
   ii. IgG_4 positive inflammatory infiltrate.
5. **Laboratory abnormalities:**
   i. Elevated autoantibody levels
   ii. Elevated IgE concentrations
   iii. Main characteristics—Raised serum IgG_4 level
   iv. Generalized hypergammaglobulinemia.

IgG_4 disease includes:
   i. Retroperitoneal fibrosis
   ii. Peritonitis
   iii. Biliary disease
   iv. Occular disease
   v. Renal disease

Treatment

Oral glucocorticoids:
   i. Resolution of pancreatic swelling.
   ii. Resolution of pancreatic obstruction.
   iii. Decrease in IgG_4 level.
   iv. Resolution of pancreatic insufficiency.

Genetic

The disease produced by genetic abnormality is hereditary pancreatitis—it usually progresses to chronic pancreatitis. Genes responsible are
1. Mutation at Arg 117—it makes trypsin resistant to proteolytic degradation.
2. Mutation in pancreatic secretory trypsin inhibitor gene
3. Mutation in cystic fibrosis transmembrane regulator gene responsible for two patterns of pancreatic disease.
   i. Pulmonary disease with pancreatic insufficiency rarely pancreatitis, elevated sweat sodium chloride level and diminished CFTR function in nasal mucosa — is called classical cystic fibrosis.
   ii. Second type is pancreatic phenotype—it is not associated with pulmonary disease. In these patients
      a. Sweat sodium chloride level—normal.
      b. CFTR function in nasal mucosa present but diminished
      c. Though there is mutation of CFTR gene—but it is heterogenous.
      d. There may be partial loss of CFTR function—it is adult onset.

ERCP-Induced Pancreatitis

Chance of developing ERCP-induced pancreatitis is:
a. **Procedure related:**
   i. Skill and experience of endoscopist
   ii. Risk is high if pancreatic duct will be visualized
   iii. Hydrostatic pressure given during injection of dye injection.
   iv. Volume of fluid injected into pancreatic duct.
   v. Number of attempts are done to visualize the PD.
   vi. Visualization of pancreatic parenchyma by injected contrast.
   vii. Pancreatic outflow tract obstruction due to periampullary edema or spasm.
   viii. After percuteneous biliary drain are advanced through ampulla into the duodenum.
   ix. Endoscopic sphincterotomy by:
      a. Thermal injury
      b. Ampullary edema
   x. Measurement of sphincter of oddi manometry.
b. **Patient related factors:**
   i. Sphincter of Oddi dysfunction, undergoing sphincterotomy without pancreatic duct stenting
   ii. Patient with small bile duct
   iii. Younger age
   iv. Obesity
   v. Patient with chronically exposed pancreatic duct.
   vi. History of contrast allergy—it can be prevented by:
      a. Use of steroid
      b. Non-ionic control media.

Diagnosis

   i. Abdominal pain—developed 2–6 hours post-ERCP—it is a poor predictor of subsequent pancreatitis.
   ii. Elevation of serum amylase or lipase to three fold upper limit of normal on the day of procedure. Because amylase or lipase may be slightly raised in the serum after ERCP.

   Normal serum amylase or lipase is strong negative predictor of post-ERCP pancreatitis when measured within 2 hours of procedure.

Prevention:
1. Avoid ERCP
2. Pharmacological and endoscopic strategies to prevent post-ERCP pancreatitis:
   i. A protease inhibitor gabexate mesilate inhibits proteolytic activities of pancreatic enzymes.
   ii. Somatostatin—decrease the incidence of pancreatitis when it will be given 12 hours intravenous infusion or bolus injection immediately before papilla cannulation.
   iii. Temporary pancreatic duct stenting decrease the incidence of post sphincterotomy pancreatitis.

   Postoperative period: In this case, pancreatitis may be due to following:
   i. Hypotension
   ii. Medications
   iii. Pancreatic trauma
   iv. Administration of calcium during cardiac bypass surgery
   v. Pancreatic ischemia during cardiac bypass surgery.

Unexplained Pancreatitis

10% patients of acute pancreatitis are unexplained pancreatitis in-spite of following invegetations:

i. History
ii. Physical examination
iii. Laboratory tests
iv. Transabdominal ultrasound
v. CT scan

Process of Diagnosis in Case of Unexplained Pancreatitis

History:
i. Alcohol
ii. Medications
iii. Male infertility—absence of vas deferens—suggest decreased CFTR functions indicates genetic basis

Laboratory investigations (Fig. 4.39):
i. Serum triglyceride—to be measured just after beginning of symptoms.
ii. Hypercalcemia—it can be diagnosed after recovery from symptoms—because during pancreatitis serum calcium level will be lowered.
iii. Serum IgG_4 level—will be increased.

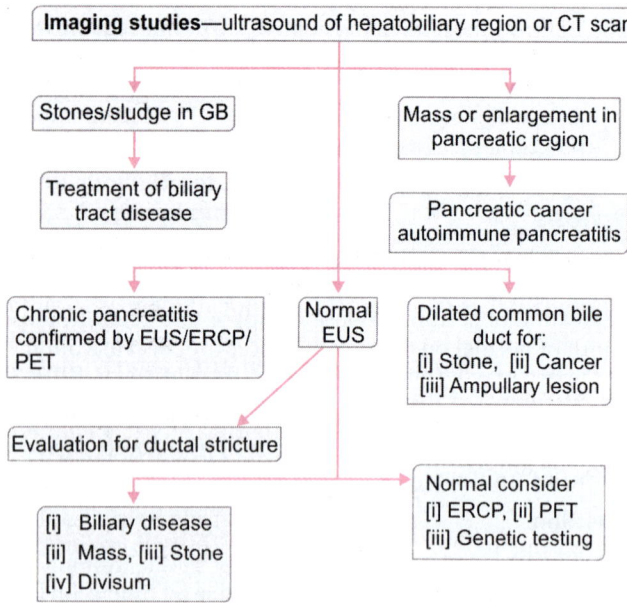

Fig. 4.39: Imagining studies for acute pancreatitis

Symptoms:
1. Pain:
   a. It is dull aching
   b. Location—in the epigastrium and umbilical region
   c. Radiation—to lower thoracic region and back
   d. Timing—it does not reach its peak for 30 minutes to several hours
   e. Duration—it lasts for hours to days
   f. Relieving factors: In sitting and leaning forward or curling up on the left side.
2. Nausea
3. Vomiting—it cannot relieve pain.

Signs:
1. Fever:
   i. Low grade fever—in 60% patient
   ii. High grade fever in:
      a. Cholangitis
      b. Sterile or infected necrosis.
2. Tachycardia, hypotension—it occurs in case of:
   i. Intravascular volume depletion
   ii. Hemorrhage
   iii. Enhanced vascular permeability
   iv. Vasodilatation
3. Abdominal tenderness and guarding
4. Bowel sound—decreased or absent
5. Pleural effusion—usually it is found in left or it may be bilateral
6. Mild jaundice
   But if bilirubin is >4 mg%, it suggests:
   i. Extrahepatic obstruction
   ii. Underlying liver disease
7. Dark discolouration on the flank—Cullen sign
8. Dark discoloration on periumbelical region—Turner sign

Laboratory Tests

Regarding enzyme measurement, following factors are responsible for alteration of serum markers in pancreatitis:
1. Serum level of pancreatic enzymes = Tissue enzyme production + release of enzyme into the blood + clearance of enzymes through urine. So in case of renal failure, serum enzymes will be elevated.
2. Measurement of enzyme activities can be influenced by several factors like, hyperlipidemia—because, it reduced routine serum enzyme determination.
3. The enzymes may be produced by non pancreatic tissues.
4. Standard enzyme assays cannot give information regarding severity of pancreatitis.

Amylase

Since there is no circulating inhibitors of amylase activity, amylase level is reliable in acute pancreatitis.

Though amylase is secreted by many tissues in the body, but—most of the amylase is secreted by pancreas and salivary gland.

There are two isoamylases:
i. P isoamylase—it is secreted by pancreas
ii. S isomylase—it is secreted by salivary gland, fallopian tubes and lung.

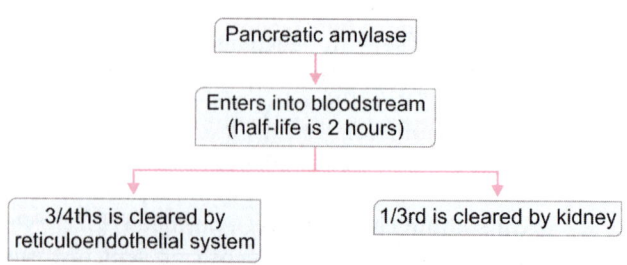

In case of acute pancreatitis—raised amylase level is due to:
i. Increased release into the blood
ii. Decreased renal clearance.

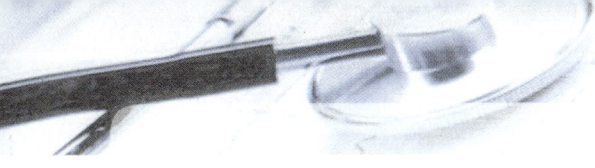

In case of acute pancreatitis:

Serum amylase and lipase level will raise within 1st hour.
↓
The serum amylase falls rapidly than lipase
↓
Serum amylase level returns to normal but serum lipase level will be raised—so it will be the indication of acute pancreatitis.

Serum amylase level will be less in the following conditions:
i. Alcoholic pancreatitis
ii. Pancreatic cancer
iii. Penetrating ulcers

Value of measuring P isoamylase is valuable in case of acute pancreatitis, by this value may be compromised in following conditions:
a. Assay may inaccurately measure small amounts of this isoform.
b. The following conditions may raise the value of this isoform
1. Biliary tract disease
2. Intestinal perforation
3. Intestinal obstruction
4. Intestinal ischemia
5. Ruptured abdominal aortic aneurysm

Level of S isoamylase will be raised in following conditions:
i. Chronic alcoholic
ii. Postoperative states
iii. Lactic acidosis
iv. Anorexia nervosa
v. Bulimia
vi. Esophageal perforation
vii. Bronchogenic carcinoma
viii. Gastric carcinoma
ix. Breast carcinoma
x. Myeloma

Macroamylasemia: Persistent elevation of serum amylase in absence of symptoms related to pancreas occurs in an uncommon condition—it is macroamylasemia.

Molecular weight of macroamylase is 250 kDa. In this condition, the ratio of pancreatic to salivary amylase is normal.

Antibody complex with amylase to form amylase polymer. This macroamylase is unable to enter the renal tubule, as a result, it will be accumulated is serum.

It can be diagnosed by the following methods:
i. Amylase to creatinine ratio <1% to ceonfirm it moleceular weight of the serum amylase will be determined
ii. Immunological studies.

Acquired macroamylasemia occurs in lymphoproliferative disorders.

Lipase

Serum lipase activity is generated in number of following tissues
i. Pancreas
ii. Intestine
iii. Liver
iv. Biliary tract
v. Lingual tissue
vi. Gastric tissues

Following conditions indicate the importance of lipase as important indicator of acute pancreatitis:
i. It will be raised for several days even after value of amylase comes to normal.
ii. Its level will be normal in case of macroamylasemia.
iii. Its level will be normal in diabetic ketoacidosis.
iv. L_2 pancreatic lipase is more specific for acute pancreatitis.

Other pancreatic enzymes are:
i. Serum trypsin
ii. Chymotrypsin
iii. Catalase
iv. Ribonuclease
v. Phospholipase A_2.

Urinary enzyme level: Following enzyme levels in urine will be raised in acute pancreatitis:
i. Urinary trypsinogen 2
ii. Urinary levels of activated peptide of carboxypeptidase B.
iii. Urinary amylase level.

Trypsinogen activation peptide: The peptide removed during activation of trypsinogen to trypsin is called trypsinogen activation peptide (TAP). The level of TAP has been reported to be increased in case of mild to severe form pancreatitis.

Inflammatory markers: Leukemoid reaction is present in acute pancreatitis in absence of infection. Following inflammatory markers are present in acute pancreatitis.
1. Neutrophil specific elastase:
   i. It is released by inflammatory cells
   ii. It will be detected within 12–24 hours of pancreatitis.
2. Interleukin-6: It is released by macrophages.
3. Acute phase reactants: C-reactive protein:
   a. It is induced by interleukin-6.
   b. It is increased during the 2nd day of acute pancreatitis

Those markers are prognostically significant.

Markers of biliary tract involvement in acute pancreatitis:
1. Elevation of raised SGPT and alkaline phosphatase are very sensitive test for biliary tract involvement—which will fall following improvement of gall stone induced pancreatitis.
2. Fluctuation is seen in patient with CLD having baseline elevation of SGPT and SGOT.
3. Serum amylase >200 IU/L—suggest acute pancreatitis, if associated with raised LFT.
4. Ration of lipase to amylase is greater in alcoholic pancreatitis.
5. Hyperbilirubinemia is associated with high incidence of bile duct stones and acute pancreatitis.

Imaging

A. Radiography

1. Straight X-ray of abdomen in erect and supine position to exclude intestinal perforation. The findings are:
   i. Evidence of generalized paralytic ileus
   ii. Isolated dilated loop of small intestine overlying pancreas—it is sentinel loop.
   iii. Accumulation of air in right colon and transverse colon with sudden termination at splenic flexure—colonic cut off sign.
   iv. Loss of psoas margin
   v. Increased separation between stomach and colon
   vi. Pancreatic calcification
   vii. Calcified gallstones—suggest biliary cause.

2. Straight X-ray of chest—left-sided or bilateral pleural effusion.

B. Ultrasonography

Common findings are:
i. Hypoechoic shadow in sonography—it may be due to increased water in the parenchyma
ii. Gallstones—visualization—sensitivity—95%

Limitations:
1. Intestinal gas   2. Adipose tissue—in 30–40% patients
   Non-visualization of CBD stones due to presence of intestinal gas.

It may miss following findings:
i. Focal masses in pancreas
ii. Peripancreatic focal fluid collection

C. Computerized Tomography

The findings are:
i. Diffuse pancreatic enlargement
ii. Effacement of usual lobulated contour of the pancreas
iii. Inhomogenicity of pancreatic parenchyma
iv. Fluid infiltration of parenchyma
v. Detection of focal masses in pancreas

Last two are better visualized by CT scan than ultrasonography: Dynamic CT scan during bolus administration of intravenous contrast—shows poorly perfused or non-perfused areas in the pancreas—this can be interpreted as pancreatic necrosis—which is of greatest significance from prognostic point of view.

D. Helical CT Technique

It can detect the bile duct stones more efficiently, because presence of sufficient amount of calcium is required for its detection in CT scan.
   Helical CT without contrast detects stone by the presence of bright rim around the periphery of stones.

E. Magnetic Resonance Imaging

i. By giving intravenous gadolinium—it can demonstrate poor perfusion in or around the pancreas.
ii. It can demonstrate solid debris in the collected fluid in the pancreas

Disadvantages:
i. Expensive
ii. Cumbersome
iii. It is difficult to perform MRI quickly
iv. Failure to detect pancreatic calcifications

Contraindication:
i. Pregnancy,   ii. Contrast allergy

F. Secretion Stimulated MRI

Its role:
i. Diagnosis of functional pancreatic duct outlet obstruction
ii. Traninvasive diagnosis of pancreatic duct disruption and/or leakage.

G. MRCP

It can diagnose the following with 95% of sensitivity:
i. Diagnosis of vascular complications
ii. Persistent bile duct stones in acute pancreatitis

H. Endoscopic Retrograde Cholangiopancreatography

i. In case of acute pancreatography, there may be normal pancreatogram
ii. It can diagnose the following:
   a. Ductal stricture
   b. Ductal stores
   c. Pancreatic divisum
   d. Recurrent pancreatitis
   e. Sphincter of odds dysfunction

I. Endosonography

It can diagnose following:
a. Detection of persistent bile duct stones
b. Detection of persistent ampullary stones
c. Differentiates unexplained acute pancreatitis, because it can demonstrate biliary sludge and stones.
d. Detection of small pancreatic tumor
e. Detection of ampullary tumor
f. Detection of pancreatic divisum.
g. Detection of chronic pancreatitis
h. Detection of complex material within pancreatic fluid.
i. Guide during endoscopic pseudocyst drainage

Complications of Acute Pancreatitis

According to ATLANTA Definition

A. Local complications:
   a. Acute fluid collection—it occurs early, there is no wall.
   b. Necrosis—presence of nonviable parenchyma
   c. Acute pseudocyst—collection of pancreatic juice encysted by wall
   d. Pancreatic abscess—collection of pus
B. Organ dysfunctions:
   a. Shock—systolic blood presence <90 mmHg
   b. Lung—PaO_2 <60 mmHg
   c. Renal failure—creatinine >2 mg/dl, inspite of proper hydration.
   d. Gastrointestinal—gastrointestinal blood loss >50 ml/24 hours
   e. Hematological:
      i. Platelet <100000/mm^3
      ii. Fibrinogen <1 gm/L
      iii. Fibrin degradation product > 80 mg/dl
   f. Metabolic—Serum calcium >7.5 mg/dl

According to MODS Criteria

Organ dysfunction:

a. Shock	Pressure adjusted heart rate >15
b. Lung	$PO_2/FiO_2 \leq 225$
c. Renal	Creatinine level > 2.26 mg/dl
d. Hematological	Platelet $\leq$ 80000/cc
e. Neurological	Glasgow coma cell $\leq$ 12.

Laboratory Tests to Detect Severity of Acute Pancreatitis

a. Detection of biomarkers:
   i. Neutrophil elastase: These are elevated
   ii. Monokine interteukine-6   within 24 hours
   iii. C-reactive protein—it will be elevated within 48 hours, because it is induced by IL-6.

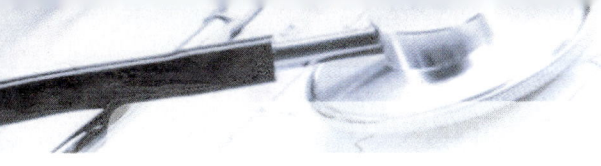

b. Hematological parameters:

1. *Hematocrit:* Detection of pancreatic necrosis:
   a. Hematocrit level > 44% at the time of hospital admission
   b. Failure to decrease hematocrit in first 24 hours of admission.
   So aggressive fluid administration after admission can prevent pancreatic necrosis.
2. *Trypsinogen activation peptide (TAP) assay:* It can measure indirectly the amount of active trypsin. So TAP will be raised in case of acute pancreatic necrosis.

Severity of Acute Pancreatitis According to Computerized Tomography (Severity Index According to CT Scan)

A. Grade of acute pancreatic necrosis:	*points*
1. Normal pancreas	0
2. Pancreatic enlargement	1
3. Inflammation confined to pancreas and peripancreatic fat	2
4. One peripancreatic fluid collection	3
5. Two or more fluid collection	4

B. Degree of necrosis:	
1. No necrosis	0
2. Necrosis of one third pancreas	2
3. Necrosis of one half of pancreas	4
4. necrosis of more than one half of pancreas	5

So, severity index will be: Grade points + degree of necrosis

Assessment of Acute Pancreatitis

Ranson criteria

A. On admission:

1.	Age	>55 years
2.	WBC count	>16000/cc
3.	LDH	>350 IU/L
4.	Glucose	>200 mg/dl
5.	AST	>250 IU/L

B. Within 48 hours of admission:
1. Hematocrit decrease by >10%
2. BUN increased be >5 mg/dl
3. Serum calcium > 8 mg/dl
4. Arterial PO_2 <60 mmHg
5. Base deficit >4 mEq/L
6. Estimated fluid sequestration >6 liters

Systemic inflammatory response syndrome (SIRS) is an early definite predicator of multiorgan dysfunction syndrome in case of acute pancreatitis, if SIRS persists >48 hours. The SIRS are:

1.	Temperature	>38° or <36°C
2.	Heat rate	> 90 beats/min
3.	Respiratory rate	>20/minutes
4.	WBC count	>12000/cc or <4000/cc

Local Complications

A. Acute fluid collections:

i. It is usually formed in or around the pancreas in the early course of acute pancreatitis, having no wall around it.
ii. It may be simple, having uniform CT density, like that of water.
iii. It may be complex having multiple CT densities and poorly defined margin.
iv. In MRI or EUS, it may show multiple locules.

Fate of acute fluid collection:
1. It may resolve spontaneously
2. It may develop pseudocyst—factors are:
   i. Not completely understood
   ii. Due to disruption of pancreatic duct disruption followed by its drainage into fluid collection.

Course and treatment:
i. Some may advocate the drainage of fluid—but there is no benefit.
ii. Best method is observation—for the following evidences:
   a. The rapid expansion of collected fluid
   b. Absence or presence of infection because it is the main but uncommon complication

In case of suspected infection, following procedure of management should be done:

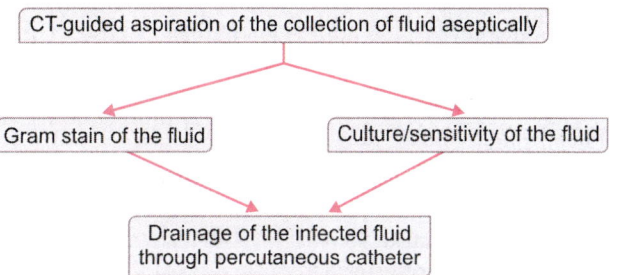

B. Necrosis and infected necrosis:

1. Pancreatic necrosis: It is the severe form of disease. It occurs due to following factors:
   i. Ischemia
   ii. Marked inflammation of pancreas
2. It may be diffuse or may be foul smelling.
3. The necrotic areas is usually separated from viable tissue
4. Histological picture shows:
   i. Devitalized pancreatic tissue along with necrosis of the tissue
   ii. Evidence of vessel damage
   iii. Evidence of hemorrhage and fat necrosis.
5. It can be diagnosed clinically and dynamic contrast enhanced CT

Scan: It shows—Areas of nonenhanced pancreatic tissue having well margin around it.

Laboratory predictors of pancreatic necrosis include:
i. Serum level of C-reactive protein >150 mg/L at 48 hours
ii. Ranson score ≥3
iii. APACHE II score >7

Complications of pancreatic necrosis:
a. Early in the coarse:
   i. Systemic inflammatory response syndrome along with increased capillary permeability
   ii. Sepsis-like syndrome
   iii. Organ failure syndrome—it occurs when necrosis involves 50% of pancreas
b. Late in the course—infected pancreatic necrosis.

Since there is no fibrotic wall or capsule to contain infection in it, the infection may spread to adjacent tissue.

Infected pancreatic necrosis: It is a leading cause of death in acute pancreatitis. Infection occurs due to translocation of bacteria from intestine into the portal venous system and seedling of the necrotic tissue.

Clinical manifestations:
  i. High fever
 ii. Sudden increase in abdominal tenderness
iii. There may be subtle presentation in patient receiving prophylactic antibiotics.
 iv. There may be associated organ failure inspite of ongoing supportive care

Laboratory investigations:
1. Marked leukocytosis
2. Bacteremia
3. Blood culture—negative blood culture does not exclude the diagnosis.
4. CT guided fine needle aspiration cytology—and to be examined for:
    a. Gram stain
    b. Fungal stain
    c. Culture and sensitivity
    Organisms:
     i. Polymicrobial gram-negative organism
    ii. Anaerobic organism
5. Inflammatory markers:
    a. Serum procalcitonin
    b. IL-6 level—these are raised.

Fate of necrosis:
  i. Gradual disappearance of necrotic tissue with residual inflammation and scar.
 ii. Gradual organization of pancreatic necrosis.
iii. Persistent sequestrum of pancreatic necrosis—it may be responsible for persistent organ failure inspite of prolonged supportive care.
In this case, drainage of sterile pancreatic necrosis is advisable.

Organized pancreatic necrosis: This is characterized by the following:
  i. The necrotic region is 4 weeks old
 ii. Walled off the necrotic areas
iii. It still contains necrotic material

Treatment:
  i. It can be drained endoscopically using transmural gastric or duodenal approach.
 ii. Percuteneous approach

Complications: Necrosis is often accompanied by disruption of pancreatic duct. If disruption occurs in the mid portion of pancreatic duct, there is gradual expansion of necrotic region due to drainage of pancreatic juice from viable pancreatic tail. This is called "disconnected duct syndrome".

Treatment of complications:
  i. Resection of disconnected tail with islet cells autotransplantation.
 ii. Creation of fistula to the intestine may be an option.

Pseudocyst

This can be defined as collection of pancreatic fluid surrounded by fibrotic wall or granulation tissue. Here epithelial living is absent.

Pancreatic fluid contains:
1. Pancreatic enzymes.
2. Particulate matter.

Pseudocyst commonly occurs in following conditions:
  i. Commonly in alcoholic pancreatitis
 ii. Particulate matter
iii. 30% cases of gallstone pancreatitis

Presenting symptoms:
1. Abdominal pain—it is postprandial or constant
2. Early satiety
3. Nausea with or without vomiting due to gastric outlet obstruction.

Fate of pseudocyst:
1. Rapid enlargement
2. Rupture
3. Hemorrhage
4. Leaking of pancreatic fluid
5. Obstruction of biliary tract
6. Compression on inferior venacava
7. Erosion to surrounding structure
8. Extension into mediastinum
9. Infection

Risk of complication varies with:
  i. Site of pseudocyst
 ii. Age of the pseudocyst

Indications of drainage of pseudocyst:
  i. Progressive enlargement of the pseudocyst
 ii. Infected pseudocyst
iii. Large pseudocyst—that fails to shrink with time.

Pseudocyst can be drained:
  i. Percutaneous drainage
 ii. Endoscopic drainage
iii. Surgical drainage

Surgical drainage will be required when the lesion may be suspected as cystic lesion or pancreatic cystic neoplasm. In that case, during surgical drainage, large piece of cavity wall must be taken for histological examination.

The choice of procedure depends upon:
  i. Location of pancreatic cyst
 ii. Relationship of pseudocyst with the pancreatic duct

In this case, pancreatography is required to delineate:
  i. Ductal obstruction
 ii. Ductal communication with pseudocyst:
    a. If there is no communication of pancreatic duct with pseudocyst—procedure of choice is internal or external drainage.
    b. If there is communication or disruption of pancreatic duct with pseudocyst—procedure is internal drainage.
    c. If the pseudocyst resolves slowly when drained externally—procedure of choice is internal drainage
    d. If percutaneous drainage leads to pancreaticocutaneous fistula—procedure of choice is internal drainage.

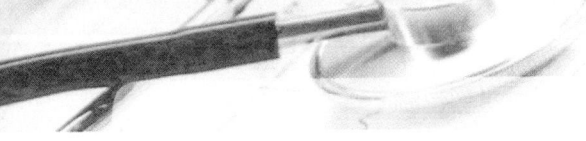

There are two types of endoscopic drainage into stomach and duodenum:
1. Transpapillary drainage
2. Transmural drainage

This is followed by placement of internal stent.

Pseudocyst of pancreatic head can be treated by transpapillary drainage.

EUS is helpful in case of pseudocyst drainage in following conditions
i. When there is no obvious buldge seen endoscopically.
ii. When there is presence of various venous collaterals.

Incomplete drainage of pseudocyst by endoscopic or percutaneous means—produces: Infection of pseudocyst—it is more common in case of "organized pancreatic necrosis".

Prior to drainage: EUS or MRI should be done to assess the solid material in the cystic cavity.

If solid material is present in cystic cavity, endoscopic or percutaneous drainage is absolutely necessary.

Following factors are responsible for importance of examination of drainage sample:
i. Amylase content of pancreatic fluid—if it is high, it reflects persistent communication between pancreatic duct and pseudocyst—it suggests poor outcome of external drainage.
ii. Symptoms of pseudocyst infection may be indolent—it can be sent for bacterial or fungal culture.
iii. Cystic lesson like cystic neoplasm can be mistaken as pseudocyst.

Pancreatic Abscess

This can be defined as—collection of pus in a circumscribed area in or around the pancreas—having little or no necrotic material in it.

Time of occurrence: It usually occurs more than 4 weeks after the asset of acute pancreatitis.

Signs and symptoms—of pancreatic abscess is usually rise in temperature with mild tenderness in epigastric region

Macroscopically:
i. The collection is walled off
ii. Surrounding pancreatic is not involved.
iii. No evidence of spread of infection to surrounding tissue

Diagnosis:
i. CT scan
ii. MRI

Treatment:
i. Endoscopic transpapillary drainage—if the abscess cavity communicates with pancreatic duct.
ii. Percutaneous drainage
iii. Surgical drainage

Pancreatic Ascites

Accumulation of fluid rich in pancreatic enzymes is called pancreatic ascites.

Causes of pancreatic ascites:
i. Peritoneal inflammation resulting from chemical peritonitis
ii. Associated chronic liver disease
iii. Communication of pancreatic duct with pseudocyst and peritoneal cavity.

Signs of pancreatic ascites:
i. Gradual increase in abdominal girth
ii. There may be associated subcutaneous fat necrosis
iii. Peritonitis is uncommon, since pancreatic enzymes in the ascetic fluid are inactive.

Diagnosis of pancreatic ascites can be suspected when:
i. Ascites fails to respond to diuretic therapy
ii. Persistent elevated serum amylase level
iii. Marked elevation of pancreatic amylase level
iv. Ascitic fluid protein concentration >3 gm/dl.

Diagnosis:
i. CT scan
ii. MRI
iii. MRCP

Treatment:
i. Endoscopically placed pancreatic stents would be to bridge the ductal disruption.
ii. Parenteral nutrition with administration of somatostatin or octreotide
iii. Surgical drainage
iv. Endoscopic therapy is better than medical therapy.

Pancreatic Fistulae

Causes of pancreatic fistulae:
i. After a bout of alcoholic pancreatitis.
ii. Pancreatic pseudocyst
iii. Pancreatic trauma
iv. Acute pancreatic duct disruption
v. Percutaneous catheter placement
vi. Pancreatic surgery

Anterior pancreatic duct disruption is responsible for ascites, posterior pancreatic ductal disruption is responsible for pancreatic fistulae.

Tract or fistulae:
i. Through retroperiteneum to skin.
ii. Through esophageal or aortic hiatus into plural cavity producing pleural effusion or mediastenal collection
iii. To colon
iv. To gallbladder
v. To small bowel
vi. Fistulae to vascular structure like portal vein.

Investigations:
A. Fluid from pancreatic fistula
    i. High protein
    ii. High amylase content
B. Fistulogram—it reveals external fistula
C. ERCP—It is highly beneficial test for identification of internal fistula
D. CT scan—it can identify the communication of fistula into thoratic cavity.

Treatment:
1. Spontaneous healing in more common in case of cutaneous fistulae.
2. Drainage of fluid by thoracocentesis or peracentesis may help in heating of fistulae

3. Administration of somatostatin analogues helps in reduction of pancreatic secretion—which intern helps in resolution of fistulae.
4. Stenting of pancreatic duct may recover pancreatic duct disruption.

Vascular Complications

A. Thrombosis

Pancreatitis or pancreatitis pseudocyst is responsible for thrombosis of the following vessels—splenic vein thrombosis—effects are:
a. Mesenteric venous congestion
b. Bowel ischemia
c. Bowel edema

Treatment: Thrombolytic therapy

Risk of therapy: Retroperitoneal hemorrhage in patient with ongoing pancreatitis.

B. Hemorrhage

1. Pseudocyst eroding—pancreatic artery—production of pseudoaneurysm whose wall is partially formed by artery and partially by pseudocyst
2. Pseudocyst in the pancreatic body or tail erodes splenic artery.
3. Pseudocyst in the head of the pancreas involving:
   i. Gastroduodenal artery or
   ii. Branches of pancreaticoduodenal artery
4. Communication of pseudocyst with pancreatic duct producing.
   i. Hemosuccus pancreaticus or
   ii. Bleeding into duodenum

Diagnosis:
1. CT scan
2. Angiography

Treatment:
1. Embolization of bleeding artery
2. Surgical ligation of bleeding artery
3. Occasionally broad surgical resection

After control of bleeding, treatment of pseudocyst is strongly recommended.

Extension of pseudocyst into the spleen produces—splenic hematoma, splenic rupture.

Presenting symptoms:
1. Abdominal pain radiating to left shoulder
2. Fever
3. Abdominal mass

Diagnosis:
1. Ultrasonography
2. CT scan
3. Arteriography may demonstrate splenic artery pseudoaneurysm.

Treatment:
1. Emergency splenectomy—in case of splenic rupture
2. Prophylactic splenectomy may be advocated in case asymptomatic splenic pseudocyst

Gastrointestinal Obstruction

Following types of gastrointestinal obstruction occur in acute pancreatitis:
1. Compression of duodenum
2. Gastric outlet obstruction
3. Bile duct obstruction
4. Extension of inflammation to transverse colon and splenic flexure, producing spasm and edema producing classical colonic cut off sign.

   To prevent colonic perforation in a case of colonic obstruction along with proximal colonic dilatation—cecostomy can be done.
5. Extension of inflammation produces:
   i. Colonic stricture
   ii. Colonic fistulae
   iii. Colonic perforation
6. Erosion of colonic blood vessels—producing acute lower gastrointestinal hemorrhage

Systemic Complications

Causes are:
1. Direct toxicity of activated pancreatic enzymes
2. Systemic inflammatory response to pancreatic necrosis
3. Circulating endotoxins due to bacterial translocation arising from the gut
4. Combination of above factors.

Following are signs of failure:
1. Respiratory insufficiency
2. Shock
3. Sepsis-like syndrome
4. Disseminated intravascular coagulation
5. Renal failure
6. Gastrointestinal bleeding
7. Confusion
8. Coma
9. Multiorgan dysfunction syndrome

   Organ failure is uncommon in interstitial pancreatitis.
   It is common in 56% cases of pancreatic necrosis.
   Early mortality in acute pancreatitis is mainly due to organ failure.
   Late mortality is mainly due to infection.

Multiple Organ Dysfunction Syndromes

The causes of MODS:
1. High levels of circulating tumor necrosis factor
2. IL-6
3. Systemic activation of mcrophages and complement system.

Common complications are:
   i. Respiratory complications
   ii. Vascular complication
   iii. Renal failure

Predictors of MODS are:
1. Admission APACHE II score
2. Serum CRP level at 48 hours
3. Presence pancreatic necrosis
4. Presence of SIRS

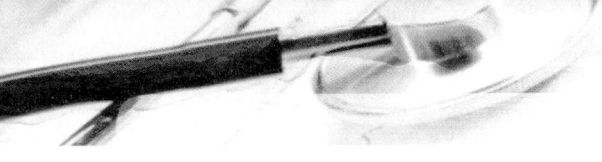

The mortality of acute pancreatitis depends upon the duration of MODS:
   i. If organ dysfunction restores with 1st week, mortality rate will be low.
   ii. If organ dysfunction takes several weeks to deteriorate, mortality rate will be >50%.
   iii. Persistence of SIRS is associated with development of MODS.

Respiratory Failure

a. Adult respiratory distress syndrome: There is evidence of hypoxemia. It is associated with the following:
   i. Normal pulmonary venous wedge pressure.
   ii. Decreased pulmonary compliance
   iii. Pulmonary capillary injury
   Associated risk factors:
   i. Obesity
   ii. Hypertriglyceridemia
b. Pleural effusion
c. Decreased diaphragmatic movement due to:
   i. Ascites
   ii. Retroperitoneal inflammation

Fat Necrosis

Fat necrosis usually occurs in the region distant from pancreas. It results from:
   i. Pancreatic enzymes may initiate injury.
   ii. Cleavage of adipocyte plasma membrane glycerosphingotipids by phospholipase

Adipocyte associated lipase activity in the circulation
↓
Enter the cells
↓
Converts triglycerides to monoglyceride and toxic free fatty acids
↓
It is responsible for fat necrosis

Cutaneous Fat Necrosis

This is characterized by disseminated raised erythematous tender nodules having diameter >2 cm.
   Symptoms: Fever with eosinophilia

Fate of nodules:
   i. It may resolve within days to weeks.
   ii. It may rupture followed by healing with hyperpigmentation.
   iii. It may affect marrow cavity which is followed by:
      a. Vascular damage
      b. Bone infarction:
         1. It occurs at the end of long bones like femur
         2. It is painless, osteolytic
         3. It occurs within 3–6 weeks of acute pancreatitis
   iv. It may involve synovial fat—it is associated with arthritis.
   v. It may affect middle ear.

Other Complications

1. Confusion and coma—is due to cerebral edema
2. Gastrointestinal hemorrhage—is due to:
   i. Mucosal erosion
   ii. Ulcerations
   iii. Gastric varices
   iv. Colonic varices
   v. Pancreatic pseudoaneurysm
3. Temporary blindness—it is due to retinal ischemia with leukocyte emboli.

Treatment of Acute Pancreatitis

Treatment is mainly supportive. This supportive care involves:
1. Aggressive fluid replacement
2. Management of pain, nausea and vomiting
3. Prompt identification and treatment of complications
4. Proper nutritional support
5. Prophylaxis and proper treatment of infection
6. Nasogastric tube intubation will be reserved for patient with:
   i. Persistent emesis
   ii. Colonic obstruction
7. Regular assessment of vital signs
8. Regular assessment of oxygen saturation
9. Parenteral narcotic administration:
   a. Meperidine:
      i. It does not cause acute pancreatitis
      ii. It does not significantly alter the sphincter of Oddi dysfunction
      iii. It is less effective analgesics than other narcotics.
      iv. Complication due to accumulation of its metabolites:
         • Paranoia
         • Psychosis
         • Seizures
   b. Morphine: It should not be used because:
      i. It may produce acute pancreatitis
      ii. It produces spasm of sphincter of oddi

Fluid and Electrolyte Replacement

Main cornerstone of the therapy is adequate volume replacement. In case of acute pancreatitis:

There is evidence of third space accumulation of fluid
↓
Intravascular volume depletion
↓
Worsening of pancreatic perfusion
↓
Exacerbation of acute pancreatitis
↓
Development of pancreatic necrosis

So volume should be repleted adequately by monitoring urine output and other vital signs
Signs of inadequate fluid replacement:
   i. Elevated hematocrit
   ii. Evidence of renal insufficiency
   iii. Central venous pressure monitoring

Metabolic Abnormalities

Hyperglycemia: It is present in patients with acute pancreatitis so tight glycemic control (80–100 mg/dl)—may be responsible for:
   i. Decreased rate of organ dysfunction
   ii. Infection

Serum calcium level: In case of acute pancreatitis, the serum calcium level will be decreased. Following factors are responsible for hypocalcemia:

i. Sequestration of calcium by free fatty acids—which has been generated due to peritoneal fat necrosis.
ii. Dilution of intravenous administration of calcium poor liquids
iii. Hypoalbuminemia—results in low serum calcium in spite of normal serum ionized calcium.
iv. Parathormone resistance
v. Hypermagnesemia
vi. Hypersecretion of calcitonin and glucagon

Intravenous calcium should be given to treat hypocalcemia.

Hyperlipidemia: Hypertriglyceridemia may be responsible for acute pancreatitis. It may be accompanied by alcoholic pancreatitis.

Treatment:
i. Antilipidemic therapy
ii. Plasmapheresis

Inhibition of enzymes, secretion and inflammation: Following methods limit the acute pancreatitis:

i. Inhibition of active pancreatic enzymes
ii. Inhibition of pancreatic secretion
iii. Interruption of inflammatory cascade

The drugs responsible for inhibiting pancreatic enzymes—gabexate mesilate. This drug is not available in United States.

Following drugs are responsible for inhibiting pancreatic secretions:

i. Somatostatin
ii. Octreotide

The above drugs reduce the mortality rates but do not reduce the complication rates.

Treatment of Mild Acute Pancreatitis

In this case, main therapy is supportive care. It includes:
i. Bowel rest
ii. Intravenous hydration, with crystalloid
iii. Analgesia

Oral intake can be started in following conditions:
i. Patient is free of pain in absence of providing analgesics
ii. No history of nausea and vomiting
iii. Presence of normal bowel sounds
iv. Patient is hungry

Oral diet to be started with

Clear or full liquid diet
↓
Followed by low fat solid diet.

If patient is discharged in spite of continued pain with intolerance to sold diet—there will be high chance of getting admitted for recurrence.

Again in patient with gallstone-induced pancreatitis; laparoscopic cholecystectomy should be recommended in the same admission to prevent recurrence.

Severe Acute Pancreatitis

Following factors are at increased risks of severe acute pancreatitis:

i. Obesity
ii. Azotemia
iii. Hemoconcentration

Following factors are responsible for favorable response to fluid resuscitation in case of acute pancreatitis:
i. Decrease in hematocrit
ii. Fall in blood urea nitrogen by 5 mg/dl.

Enteral and parenteral nutrition: Early parenteral nutrition may be responsible for following complications:

i. Sepsis
ii. Pancreatic infection
iii. Intravenous lipid infusion may be responsible for hyperlipidemia—which in turn may trigger acute pancreatitis.

Enteral feeding should be started as soon as possible and is preferable to parenteral nutrition. Because:
i. It stimulates pancreatic secretion.
ii. It maintains the gut barrier integrity thus it prevents bacterial translocation.
iii. It decreases systemic immune response
iv. It reduces bacterial translocation

There are two routes of enteral nutrition:
i. Nasogastric route
ii. Nasojejunal route—it bypasses stomach and duodenum and responsible for less pancreatic secretion

If the patient with acute necrotizing pancreatitis starts oral feeding:
i. Pancreatic enzyme supplementation should be given to digest fat.
ii. Proton pump inhibitor should be given to reduce gastric acid hypersecretion, because pancreatic bicarbonate secretion will be reduced.

Through nasojejunal tube—isotonic full strength formula should be started at a rate of 25 ml/hour. Then it should be increased at 4 hourly intervals till patients target will be met.

It is successful even in presence of ileus

Antibiotic prophylaxis: Infections in case of acute necrotizing pancreatic may be responsible for death which can be prevented by:
i. Systemic antibiotic prophylaxis
ii. Selective decontamination of gut.

Following drugs has excellent penetration in pancreas:
i. Third generation cephalosporin
ii. Metronidazole
iii. Quinolones
iv. Imipenam—cilastatin
v. Mezlocillin.

Following drugs has poor penetration in pancreatic tissue:
i. Ampicillin
ii. Aminoglycosides

The good penetrating drugs are responsible for lowering incidence of pancreatic infection.

Common bacterial isolates from pancreatic necrosis include:
i. Enteric organism
ii. *Staphylococcus epidermidis*
In both groups, mortality is similar.

The prophylactic antibiotics should be given in following conditions in demand:
i. Patient with SIRS
ii. Patient with multiorgan dysfunction syndrome

iii. Patient with documented infection.
iv. Clinical suspected infection

The prophylactic drugs should be started:
i. Within 48 hours of admission
ii. It should be continued for 2–3 weeks
The drug—imipenam cilastatin—500 mg 3 hourly.

Since necrotizing pancreatitis is susceptible to fungal infection, fluconazole can be administered.

Luminal antibiotics can be administered to prevent translocation of gut bacteria.

Probiotics may be helpful in the management of acute pancreatitis.

Treatment of Infected Pancreatic Necrosis

1. Prompt surgical debridement to remove the infected necrotic material.
2. If required, re-exploration can be done for further debridement. Mortality rate in this treatment is 20 to 60%.
3. Percutaneous drainage of infected necrosis is inadequate, because this procedure may be inadequate to drain solid material.

On the other hand, this catheter may introduce infection into the necrotic areas.

So techniques to remove this material are:
1. Introduction of large bore (28 French) multiple tubes
2. Frequent bedside catheter irrigation.
3. Periodic vigorous manual irrigation under fluoroscopy
4. Endoscopic placement of percutaneous catheter

Instruments for removing necrotic material:
i. Forceps
ii. Snares
iii. Jet irrigation

Complications are:
i. Hemorrhage from retroperitoneal vessels
ii. Persistent pancreatic sepsis.

Endoscopic drainage of organized pancreatic necrosis (which will be developed within 2–3 weeks after the onset of acute pancreatitis)—it allows adequate debridation of the necrotic tissue.

This process may be repeated daily or weekly depending upon the amount of necrotic tissue present in that area.

Drainage of sterile necrosis: This process is required in patient with sterile necrosis associated with deteriorating course in spite of proper supportive care and prolonged organ failure or ongoing systemic inflammatory response.

This process is required also in case where gastrointestinal obstruction occurs due to necrotic collection.

Urgent ERCP for removal of gallstones: Persistent gallstones are responsible for recurrent pancreatitis. So, prompt removal of gallstones in CBD or in ampullary area is necessary for prevention of future pancreatitis. Clear indication of urgent MRCP followed by ERCP and stone extraction is:
i. The presence of sepsis
ii. Severe pancreatitis who fails to improve over 12–24 hours of observation.

Elective ERCP followed by sphincterotomy is being considered in following conditions:
i. Persistent biliary duct obstruction
ii. Incipient biliary duct obstruction

iii. Poor candidate for cholecystectomy
iv. In patient with strong suspicion of CBD stones after cholecystectomy
v. Pancreatic duct disruption which occurs as a part of inflammatory process.

Sphincterotomy: It eliminates common channel between bile duct and pancreatic duct which enters in duodenum in different locations. It prevents recurrence of pancreatitis. But the complications of this process are:
i. Biliary obstruction
ii. Cholangitis
iii. Acute cholecystitis
These complications occur within 6 months of pancreatitis or later.
iv. Stenosis at sphincterotomy sites.

CHRONIC PANCREATITIS

According to Marseiller classification—pancreatitis can be subdivided into two forms:

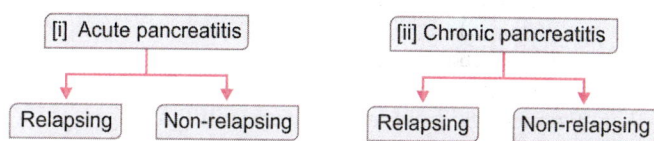

In chronic pancreatitis, there is evidence of permanent and progressive morphological and functional damage of pancreatic duct.

Chronic pancreatitis can be subdivided into two forms:
1. Chronic obstructive pancreatitis—it is characterized by
   i. Dilatation of the ductal system
   ii. Diffuse atrophy of acinar parenchyma
   iii. Uniform fibrosis
2. Other form of chronic pancreatitis is characterized by:
   i. Absence of intraductal plugs or stones

Based on morphology, biochemistry, molecular biology and epidemiology, Sarles classified chronic pancreatitis into four groups

1.
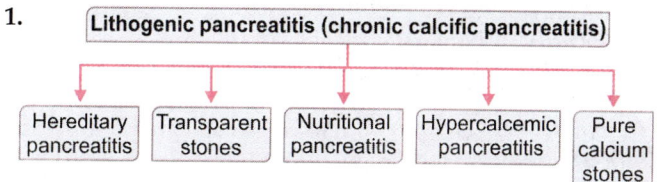

2. **Obstructive pancreatitis**—due to obstruction of pancreatic duct with uniform distribution of the lesion beyond the obstruction.
3. **Inflammatory pancreatitis**—it is characterized by:
   i. Diffuse fibrosis
   ii. Destruction of exocrine parenchyma
   iii. Infiltration of mononuclear cells.
4. **Pancreatic fibrosis:** It is characterized by silent diffuse perilobular fibrosis.

Classification

Recent classification is TIGAR-6 system of classification:
A. Toxic—metabolic:
   i. Alcoholic
   ii. Tobacco smoking

iii. Hypercalcemia
iv. Hyperlipidemia
v. Chronic renal failure
vi. Medications—phenytoin abuse
vii. Toxins.

B. Idiopathic:
   i. Tropical
   ii. Early onset
   iii. Late onset

C. Genetic:
   i. Autosomal dominant
   ii. Cationic trypsinogen
   iii. Autosomal recessive
   iv. CFTR mutation
   v. SPNK 1 mutation
   vi. α-1 antitrypsin deficiency

D. Autoimmune:
   i. Isolated autoimmune chronic pancreatitis
   ii. Association with:
      a. Primary sclerosing cholangitis
      b. Sjorgen's syndrome
      c. Primary biliary cirrhosis
      d. Type 1 diabetes mellitus

E. Recurrent and severe acute pancreatitis:
   i. Postnecrotic (severe acute pancreatitis)
   ii. Vascular disease ischemia
   iii. Postradiation exposure

F. Obstructive:
   i. Pancreatic divisum (controversial)
   ii. Sphincter of Oddi dysfunction (controversial)
   iii. Obstruction of pancreatic duct by tumor
   iv. Periampullary duodenal wall cysts
   v. Post-traumatic pancreatic duct scars.

Incidence

1. In autopsy studies, prevalence rate of chronic pancreatitis is 0.04 to 5%.
2. According to different epidemiological studies, incidence varies in different areas of the world, because due to low alcohol intake in Japan, the prevalence of chronic pancreatitis will be low.
3. Environmental and hereditary factors may also influence the incidence of alcohol related chronic pancreatitis.

Etiology

1. Alcohol—commonest—70%
2. Idiopathic (tropical)—20%
3. Other causes—10%:
   i. Hereditary factors
   ii. Hyperparathyroidism
   iii. Hypertriglyceridemia
   iv. Autoimmune causes
   v. Obstruction
   vi. Trauma
   vii. Pancreatic divisum

Alcohol-induced pancreatitis: To develop alcohol-induced pancreatitis, genetic, anatomic, environment cofactors are required.

There is linear relationship between logarithm of risk of development of chronic pancreatitis and mean daily consumption of alcohol.

Risk of chronic pancreatitis in alcoholic depends upon:
i. Amount of daily consumption of alcohol
ii. Duration of alcohol intake (6–12 years)

There is no or doubtful relationship with chronic pancreatitis:
i. Type of alcoholic beverages
ii. Pattern of drinking (weekend or daily)

Pattern of attack of chronic pancreatitis in alcoholic:
1. In early period, bouts of recurrent attacks abdominal pain lasting for 5–6 years.
2. This is followed by development of exocrine insufficiency of 13 years from the onset.
3. Development endocrine insufficiency of 20 years from the onset.

All the patients with alcohol-induced pancreatitis will not enter into the state of chronic pancreatitis, cause in unknown.

Alcoholics consuming high fat and protein diet are at major risk of developing chronic pancreatitis.

In alcoholics, following factors are responsible for developing chronic pancreatitis:
i. High fat and high protein diet
ii. Group B coxsackie virus infections
iii. Genetic predisposition
iv. Cigarette smoking

Coxsackie virus produces chronic pancreatitis in alcoholic by the following mechanism: Lack of tissue repair, which is associated with preferential activation of M_1 macrophages and T helper T_1 cells, rather than M_2 macrophages and T helper T_2 cells.

Alcohol:
i. Potentiates virus-induced injury
ii. Impairs pancreatic regenerations
iii. Helps in viral replication

It depends upon:
i. Duration of alcohol intake
ii. Dose of alcohol intakes/day.

Genetic Susceptibility

Following genetic mutations are responsible for developing chronic pancreatitis:
i. Mutations of the serine protease inhibitor, kazar type 1 (SPINK1) gene
ii. Association of cystic fibrosis transmembrane conductance regulator gene mutation with idiopathic and alcoholic chronic pancreatitis.

In case of chronic alcoholic pancreatitis, high protein, low bicarbonate and low volume pancreatic secretions due to chronic alcohol consumption produces protein precipitates in secondary pancreatic ducts with sparing of main pancreatic duct.

Lithostatin, a protein is capable of inhibiting the formation of insoluble calcium salts. It is found it pancreatic tissue. In case of chronic pancreatitis, lithostatin is decreased in pancreatic juice in alcoholic patient, it induces the formation of pancreatic calcification.

In case of chronic pancreatitis:

There is increased viscosity of pancreatic juice
↓
Increased concentration of protein, hydrolytic enzymes, hexosamine
↓
Decreased flow of pancreatic juice
↓
It contributes to the formation of protein precipitates
↓
Blockage of small ductules in random fashion
↓
There in progressive damage of ducts and acinar tissue
↓
Development of chronic pancreatitis
Alcohol interferes with intracellular transport and discharge of digestive enzymes.
↓
Causes co localization of digestive and lysosomal hydrolase
↓
Autodigestion of pancreatic tissue
↓
Formation of chronic pancreatitis

Biochemical Mechanism for Formation of Chronic Pancreatitis

Pancreatic stellate cells (PSCS) are derived from vitamin A containing cell, and are perivascular. PSCS are stimulated by the following:
  i. Transforming growth factor-β
  ii. Basic fibroblast growth factor
  iii. Fibrogenic cytokines
    a. Tumor growth factor-α
    b. TGF-β
    c. Interleukin-1
    d. Interleukin-6
  iv. Ethanol
  v. Oxidative metabolite acetaldehyde
  vi. Mono-oxidative ethanol metabolites
  vii. Fatty acid ethyl esters

Activated PSCs
↓
Secretes extracellular matrix proteins
↓
Tissue restitution followed by fibrosis.

General strategies which will be directed toward pancreatic stellate cells are:
  i. Inhibiting or inactivating PSCs
  ii. Elimination of PSCs by induction of apoptosis
  iii. Providing PSCs to phagocytose inflammatory cell thus reducing inflammation.

Major proteins of therapeutic targets are: Mitogenic peptide—TGF-α, TGF-β. They are involved in cellular proliferation and cellular differentiation

Cigarette smoking is associated with:
  i. Risk of acute or chronic alcoholic pancreatitis
  ii. Early onset of alcoholic chronic pancreatitis

  iii. Accelerated progression of alcoholic chronic pancreatitis
  iv. Accelerated progression of late onset idiopathic chronic pancreatitis.

Tropical (Nutritional) Pancreatitis

It is a major disease of juvenile and young adult in African and Asian countries.
The natural history as summarized by Gee Varghese:
  i. Recurrent abdominal pain in childhood
  ii. Diabetes in puberty
  iii. Death at the prime time of life.

Diabetes usually occurs a few years after the onset of abdominal pain—it is brittle due to marked blood glucose fluctuation. Straight X-ray of abdomen—usually shows marked pancreatic calculi.

Histology shows:
  i. Dilatation of duct.
  ii. Pancreatic lithiasis.
  iii. Infiltration with chronic inflammatory cells.
  iv. Parenchymal atrophy

Etiopathogenesis

1. Toxic products in nutritional components (cassava)— contain 65 mg of toxic glycosides/100 gm
↓
Glycosides react with gastric hydrochloric acid
↓
Liberation of hydrocyanic acid
↓
The enzyme rhodase acts on hydrocyanic acid
↓
Production of thiocyanate in presence of adequate amounts of methionine and cysteine
↓
Cyanogens impair number of enzymes (superoxide dismutase)—this acts on free radicals
↓
These free radicals are responsible for pancreatic cellular injury.

Other nutritional deficiencies like zinc, copper and selenium
↓
Impair the detoxification of cyanogens
↓
Accumulation of free radicals
↓
Pancreatic cellular injury

2. Generic factors:
  i. Mutation of gene CFTR, reg1A101, PRSS1
  ii. Mutation of SPINKI gene—impair the trypsin inhibitor

As a result, trypsin enzyme will be activated and it will lead to pancreatitis.

Hereditary Pancreatitis

It is an autosomal dominant disease. It begins in childhood and incidences in both sexes are equal.

Etiology

Mutation in the gene for cationic trypsinogen
↓
There is failure of cleavage
↓
Presence of persistent trypsin activity
↓
Autodigestion of pancreatic tissue

Another form begins in 3rd or 4th decade.
Mutation at codon 16, 22, 23 in trypsinogen gene is associated with chronic pancreatitis.

Clinical Picture

1. Recurrent attack of severe upper abdominal pain
2. Overt diabetes occurs 8–10 years after the onset of pain.
3. Gross steatorrhea in 15–20% cases.

2–3 members of same family will be affected by acute or chronic pancreatitis in absence of alcohol consumption or other causes.

These patients are very much prone to develop pancreatic carcinoma.

Autoimme Pancreatitis

Epidemiology

1. It is reported in 2 to 8% of non-US population
2. It affects in elderly (mean age 63–68 years)
3. Males are predominantly affected (>80%)

Clinical Features

1. Mild abdominal pain
2. Pancreatic mass lesion

Uncommon presentations are:
1. Features of pancreatitis
2. Steatorrhea
3. Calcifications
4. New onset diabetes mellitus
5. Features of obstructive jaundice due to stenosis of common bile duct

Diagnosis

1. Ultrasonography or computerized tomography:
    i. Diffusely enlarged pancreas
    ii. Sausage shaped appearance of pancreas
    iii. Capsule-like rim having low density in CT scan
    iv. Calcification occurs in 50% of patient.
    v. May be presence of pseudocyst.
2. ERCP:
    i. Diffuse or segmental narrowing of main pancreatic duct.
    ii. Extrinsic stenosis of intrapancreatic portion of common bile duct, as a result proximal CBD will be dilated.

According to Japanese criteria:
    i. Diffuse pancreatic enlargement
    ii. Diffuse or segmental pancreatic duct narrowing
    iii. Abnormal serological tests

Histological changes: Diagnostic histological changes are:
    i. Fibrotic changes in the pancreas
    ii. Infiltration of plasma cells, lymphocytes, eosinophils around the pancreatic duct.
    iii. Obliterative phlebitis
    iv. Cholangitis
    v. Edema

The above features are named on lymphoplasmacytic sclerosing pancreatitis.

The lymphocytes are:
i. CD4+ cells
ii. HLA—DER+ T cells

Less common variant is: Idiopathic duct centric chronic pancreatitis: It is characterized by lobular inflammation with predominant neutrophilic infiltration without phlebitis.

There may be presence of associated disease:
    i. Primary sclerosing cholangitis
    ii. Ulcerative colitis
    iii. Sjorgen's syndrome
    iv. SLE
    v. Primary biliary cirrhosis

Patients have following antibodies:
    i. Antinuclear antibody
    ii. Antilactoferrin antibody
    iii. Anticarbonic anhydrase antibody
    v. Rheumatoid factor
    vi. Antismooth muscle cell antibody

Recently IgG_4 related autoimmune pancreatitis have been identified where, there is evidence of increased serum level of β-globulin of IgG_4 levels.

Clinical Features

A. Abdominal Pain

1. Site: Epigastric
2. Character—dull aching, constant rather than colicky
3. Radiation—radiates to both upper quadrant, occasionally to lower quadrant.
   It radiates to back directly—it is the characteristic feature.
4. Aggravating factors:
    i. Supine posture
    ii. Ingestion of food
    iii. Ingestion of alcohol
5. Relieving factors:
    i. Sitting posture with trunk bent forward
    ii. Lying down in prone position.

Pain may vary according to type of chronic pancreatitis:
1. At the beginning of disease in case of alcoholic chronic pancreatitis (75%)
2. 50% patients with late onset idiopathic chronic pancreatitis
3. All patients with early onset idiopathic chronic pancreatitis.

There are two major patterns of pancreatic pain:
1. Type A pain: It is characterized by: Short episodes of pain of less than 10 days duration, it will be separated by pain free interval of months to years.
2. Type B pain: It is characterized by daily constant pain occurring 2 or more days per week for at least 2 months. This type of pain occurs due to presence of local complication like; pseudocyst, obstructive cholestasis which is amenable to surgical correction.

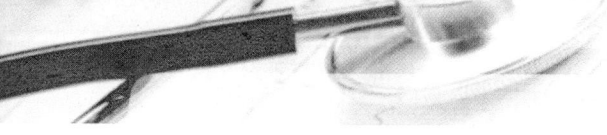

This disease may be painless in 15% of patients chronic idiopathic pancreatitis is more likely to be painless than alcoholic chronic pancreatitis.

B. Weight Loss

It may occur due to:
i. Fear of intake of food to prevent aggravation of pain induced by ingestion of food.
ii. Malabsorption
iii. Nausea with vomiting
iv. Anorexia
v. Uncontrolled diabetes

So, chronic upper abdominal pain with rapid weight loss—should suggest the possibility of chronic pancreatitis.

C. Malabsorption

This occurs in the form of:
i. Diarrhea
ii. Steatorrhea
iii. Anorexia

This occurs due to pancreatic exocrine deficiency.

All types of malabsorption occur in this disease. Fecal weight will contain less fecal water.

Again stool may be bulky but formed. Low fecal water in pancreatic insufficiency may be due to better absorption of carbohydrates (disaccharides)

Sometimes the patient may complain of steatorrhea, which is oily slicky stool and floats in water. But in pancreatic steatorrhea, absorption of vitamin A, D, E and K will not be hampered like that of celiac sprue. But total body stores of these vitamins will be reduced in chronic pancreatitis.

Pancreatic Diabetes

Common symptom in early chronic pancreatitis is glucose intolerance—again it may be the only presentation in a few cases of chronic pancreatitis.

But ketoacidosis and diabetic nephropathy are very uncommon. On the other hand, retinopathy and neuropathy are common.

Other presentations:
i. Jaundice—due to bile duct compression by pancreas
ii. Ascites and/or pleural effusion due to leakage of pancreatic secretions from disrupted pancreatic duct or pseudocyst in to peritoneal or pleural cavity respectively.
iii. Painful nodules in the extremities due to test necrosis.
iv. Polyarthritis involving small joints of the hand.

Physical examination in abdomen shows:
i. Epigastric tenderness—it ranges from mild to marked.
ii. Involuntary guarding or rebound tenderness

Complications

i. Pseudocyst
ii. Ascites
iii. Pleural effusion

Abdominal pain is due to:
i. Pancreatic inflammation
ii. Increased intrapancreatic pressure
iii. Microvascular ischemia

iv. Neural inflammation
v. Extrapancreatic causes:
   a. Common duct stenosis
   b. Duodenal stenosis
   c. Pseudocyst.
vi. Peripancreatic inflammation involving duodenum and retroperitoneum

The involved mediators of inflammation and fibrosis are:
1. Cytokines—interleukin-6, interleukin-8.
2. Chemokines—Mob-1, tumor necrosis factor-α

The cells responsible for pancreatic inflammation and fibrosis are pancreatic stellate cells—because of their:
i. Perivascular locations
ii. Their contractile potentiality.

Several neuropeptides and downstream receptor signaling are responsible for pain in chronic pancreatitis. These are:
i. Over expression of nerve growth factor in pancreas
ii. Over expression of substance P and CGRP in dorsal root ganglion.
iii. 3–5-fold increase in mast cells—and their degranulation products (nerve growth factor).
   ↓
   a. Stimulates proalgesic receptors

   b. Stimulates channels—like:
     i. Tyrosine kinase A
     ii. Receptor potential family V receptor (TRPV1)

Laboratory Diagnosis

Routine Laboratory Testing

1. Leukocytosis—due to exacerbation of inflammation
2. Anemia—usually absent in pancreatic malabsorption it will be present, if there is associated celiac disease
3. Megaloblastic anemia—rare
4. Fat soluble vitamin deficiency—like hypocalcemia, hypoprothrombinemia—rare
5. Cholestasis—due to varying degree of compression of common bile duct by pancreatic fibrotic process:
   i. Raised alkaline phosphatase
   ii. In severe compression—bilirubin will be raised.

So in patient with pancreatitis, findings of cholestatic liver functions—usually requires extensive radiological studies.

Specific tests for diagnosis of chronic pancreatitis: It has been divided into two categories:
a. Chemical measurement of pancreatic function
b. Radiological procedures required

Following factors prevent true sensitivity and specificity of the tests:
1. Biopsies from pancreas are not obtained in patients with chronic pancreatitis.
2. Results of specificity and sensitivity depend upon the extent and duration of pancreatic damage. In long-standing pancreatitis—the entire test will be positive, whereas in early pancreatitis sensitivity will fall.
3. Associated comorbid conditions of the patients—in patients with diabetes mellitus, celiac disease and cirrhosis may have subnormal level of pancreatic secretions.

Serum Pancreatic Enzymes

1. In acute pancreatitis, the serum level of the enzymes will be very much high.
2. In case chronic pancreatitis, the serum enzyme levels will be mildly elevated, normal or low.
3. In acute exacerbation of chronic pancreatitis—serum enzyme level will be moderately elevated.

Tests for Pancreatic Exocrine Functions

These tests can be subdivided into following categories:

I. **Direct test of pancreatic exocrine functions:** Since the basal level of pancreatic secretion is variable, hence stimulated pancreatic secretion will be helpful. This can be done by:
   i. Secretin
   ii. CCK
   iii. Standard meal (Lunch test)
   Direct measurement for pancreatic juice components:
   i. Concentration of bicarbonate
   ii. Concentration of enzymes:
      a. Amylase
      b. Lipase
      c. Trypsin
   All the enzymes and bicarbonate levels will be depressed in chronic pancreatitis.

II. **Indirect tests of pancreatic secretion:** Most of the stimulatory tests measure the compounds absorbed which are being digested by pancreatic enzymes before being absorbed. But positivity of these tests occurs, only when the pancreatic juice will be 10% of normal. Hence these tests cannot detect chronic early pancreatitis.

Bentriomide test: It is used rarely.

Ingestion of N-benzoyl tyrosyl-p-aminobenzoic acid
↓
Digested by chymotrypsin
↓
Para-aminobenzoic acid will be released
↓
It is absorbed by small intestinal mucosa
↓
Excreted by kidney in urine
↓
Quantity of it will be measured in urine.

Sensitivity is:
i. 100% in very severe disease
ii. 50% in minor damage to pancreas

Disadvantage: Reduced PABA excretion occurs in:
i. Diabetes mellitus
ii. Renal insufficiency
iii. Liver disease
iv. Malabsorption states
   a. Celiac sprue
   b. Crohn's disease
   c. Postgastrectomy state

So, this test is of value in determining the extent of pancreatic in sufficiency.

Demonstration of malabsorption of vitamin B₁₂

Patient ingests:
[^{57}Co] coblamin bound to intrinsic factors
+
[^{57}Co] coblamin bound to R protein
+
Excess intrinsic factor
+
Cobalamin analogue which saturates all empty R—protein binding site
↓
Patient with pancreatic insufficiency absorbs cobalamin bound to intrinsic factors not cobalamin bound to R protein.

Nowadays, this test proves to be very poorly sensitive.

Measurement of Fecal Chymotrypsin

Total fecal chymotrypsin output 24 hours fecal collections provide little advantage over much simple measurement of chymotrypsin concentration in random fecal sample. Again, false positive test occurs in:
i. Celiac sprue
ii. Crohn's disease
iii. Postgastrectomy states.

Measurement of Fecal Elastase

Both monoclonal and polyclonal enzyme linked immunosorbent antibody fecal elastase 1 test—it is very less sensitive and less specific for diagnosis of exocrine pancreatic insufficiency.

14CO₂ Breath Test

Administration of [14c] olein
↓
Hydrolysis of triglyceride + absorption of [14c] oleate
↓
Production of 14CO₂
↓
Pulmonary excretion of 14CO₂
↓
Measurement of breath 14CO₂

It can measure normality of hydrolysis of labeled triglyceride. This test is negative in early chronic pancreatitis.

Imaging Studies

A. **Plain X-ray of abdomen:** Calcification within the pancreas
   i. Alcoholic pancreatitis
   ii. Tropical pancreatitis
B. **Ultrasound:**
   a. In case of severe chronic pancreatitis:
      i. Dilatation of pancreatic duct >4 mm
      ii. Cavities >1cm in diameter,
      iii. Calcifications
   b. In case of less severe chronic pancreatitis:
      i. <4 mm dilatation of main pancreatic duct
      ii. Small cavities
      iii. Reduction in echogenicity in pancreatic parenchyma
      iv. Irregular contour of the gland.
   This test has sensitivity >70% specificity >90%.

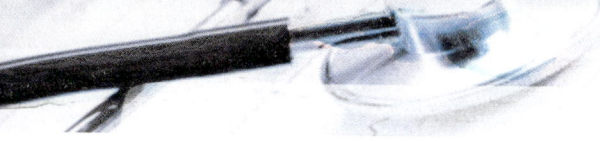

C. CT scan of abdomen: The findings include:

i. Ductal dilatation
ii. Ductal calcification
iii. Cystic lesions
iv. Enlargement or atrophy of pancreatic gland
v. Heterogenous density of pancreatic parenchyma

This can differentiate chronic pancreatitis from pancreatic carcinoma by virtue of following findings:

In case of pancreatic carcinoma—dilated duct will be smooth or breaded.

In case of chronic pancreatitis—duct is calcified and irregular.

Drawback: It in rates exposure to radiation.

D. ERCP: This is gold standard method in diagnosis of chronic pancreatitis.

Cambridge classification of chronic pancreatitis is usually based on changes in main pancreatic duct (Table 4.19).

Table 4.19: Cambridge classification of chronic pancreatitis

Grade	Main pancreatic duct	Side branches
1. Normal	Normal	Normal
2. Suggestive	Normal	< 3 abnormal
3. Mild	Normal	≥ 3 abnormal
4. Moderate	Abnormal	> 3 abnormal
5. Severe	Abnormal and at least one of the i. Large cavity ii. Duct obstruction iii. Dilatation or irregularity iv. Intraductal filling defects	

ERCP is generally reserved in patients where therapeutic interventions can help to recover the patient.

E. MRCP: It helps in direct visualization of pancreatic duct without radiation exposure, but less sensitive in evaluation of sick branches.

So, it can be used in pregnant women or in patient with allergy to contrast.

It is less sensitive in mild pancreatitis.

Secretion is helpful to enhance visualization of both main pancreatic duct and its side branches.

Endoscopic Ultrasound

Endosonographic criteria of chronic pancreatitis include two types of changes as shown in Table 4.20.

By this procedure, 5 or more criteria are required for diagnosis of acute pancreatitis.

It is more beneficial in differentiating, cystic lesion from neoplastic lesion in the background of chromic pancreatitis.

Pancreatic Function Testing

Administration of secretin intravenously
↓

A. Aspiration of duodenal juice through duodenal lumen (Dreiling tube)—every fifteen minutes for 1 hour.

If peak bicarbonate concentration <80 mEq/L—is the diagnostic of chronic pancreatitis.

Table 4.20: Endosonographic criteria of chronic pancreatitis

Features	Implication
A. Ductal changes:	
1. Duct size >3 mm	Ductal dilatation
2. Tortuous pancreatic duct	Ductal irregularity
3. Intraductal echogenic foci	Stones and/or calcification
4. Echogenic duct wall	Ductal fibrosis
5. Side branch ectasia	Periductal fibrosis
B. Parenchymal changes:	
1. Heterogenous echo pattern	Edema
2. Reduced echogenic foci (1–3 mm)	Edema
3. Enhanced echogenic foci	Calcification
4. Prominent interlobular septae	Fibrosis
5. Outer lobular margin	Fibrosis glandular atrophy
6. Large echo-poor cavities (>5 mm)	Pseudocyst

B. Combined EUS—endoscopic pancreatic function testing. Administration of secretin
↓
Duodenal fluid collection through EUS—ePFT—15, 30, 45 and 60 minutes interval

Gene Testing

Following genetic alterations are responsible for development of chronic pancreatitis:

i. Mutations of cationic trypsinogen gene PRSSi1 (it is risk factor for pancreatic cancer)
ii. Cystic fibrosis transmembrane conductance regulator (CFTP, an apical membrane chloride channel)
iii. Serine protease inhibitor, Kazal type 1 (SP1NK1)

Complications

1. Pseudocyst
2. Biliary ductal or duodenal obstruction
3. Pancreatic ascites
4. Pleural effusion
6. Splenic vein thrombosis
6. Pancreatic fistulae
7. Pseudoaneurysm
8. Increased risk of pancreatic cancer

Treatment of Pseudocyst

Indications for operations of pseudocyst:
1. Persistent abdominal pain
2. Enlargement of pseudocyst (>6 cm in diameter)
3. Complications of pseudocyst

Effective Treatment

Excision and external or internal drainage: Mature cyst with mature cystic wall and size >6 cm in diameter—treated by:

a. Anastomosis of cyst with gastric wall (cystogstrostomy)
b. Anastomosis of cyst with duodenal lumen (cystodudenostomy)
c. Anastomosis of cyst with jejunal lumen (cystojejunostomy)
The cyst wall will be collapsed within 1 week.
Success rate is 62–34%.

Complications of Endoscopic Treatment

1. Gastric hemorrhage
2. Infection of pseudocyst

External drainage through abdominal wall is indicated in following conditions:
a. Infected pseudocyst
b. Immature wall of the pseudocyst, it cannot hold the rupture effectively.

CT guided percutaneous transabdominal catheter drainage of chronic pseudocyst—it is preferred alternative to surgical treatment in the management of pseudocyst.

Medical Treatment

1. Somatostatin, a potent inhibitor of pancreatic secretion can be used in case of pancreatic pseudocyst.
2. Octreotide may be used prior to surgery in case of pseudocyst.

Pancreatic Ascites

Incidence is <1% of chronic pancreatitis.

Causes

It is due to leakage of pancreatic enzyme secretion into
i. Pseudocyst
ii. Pancreatic duct

It occurs in case of alcoholic with cirrhosis.

Presentation: Mild to moderate abdominal pain due to abdominal distension.

Diagnosis

Elevation of following in ascitic fluid:
i. Pancreatic enzymes
ii. Total protein
iii. Albumin

Treatment

A. **Medical treatment**
   1. Subcutaneous octreotide 100–250 µg every 4 hours to suppress pancreatic secretion. In one-third of patients, ascites may be resolved spontaneously.
   2. Parenteral nutrition should be provided to improve their nutritional status.
B. **Surgical treatment:** Most patients need it. But prior to operation, ERCP should be done to identity the site of leak.

Pancreatic Fistula

The causative factors:
1. Operative or percuteneous drainage of pseudocyst
2. Following pancreatic biopsy
3. Leakage of pancreatic anastomosis

Clinical suspicion occurs when there is evidence of leakage of clear fluid from any cuteneous fistula.

Diagnosis: Estimation of amylase in fistula fluid

Medical Treatment

Conservative:
a. Electrolyte replacement
b. Nutritional support
c. Raise amylase content of fistula fluid
d. Eradication of infection

Surgical Treatment

First, fistulogram should be done prior to surgery to identity the tract. If there is any ductal obstruction seen between the site of leak and the duodenum, surgery is necessary.

Splenic Vein Thrombosis

Splenic vein runs long the posterior surface of pancreas. It is usually obstructed due to:
i. Peripancreatic inflammation during acute exacerbation of chronic pancreatitis;
ii. Pancreatic pseudocyst, formation along with extension.
So it is an extrahepatic splenic vein thrombosis with portal hypertension.

Treatment

If the patient is symptomatic and is undergoing surgery for chronic pancreatitis, in that case, splenectomy will be considered.

Treatment of Chronic Pancreatitis (Fig. 4.40)

Aim of Treatment

i. Control of pain
ii. Correction of malabsorption
iii. Adequate replacement of pancreatic enzymes

Treatment of Pain

Causes of pain in chronic pancreatitis:
i. Recurrent tissue inflammation
ii. Necrosis
iii. Pancreatic ductal hypertension
iv. Increased interstitial pressure
v. Pancreatic ischemia
vi. Fibrotic encasement of sensory nerves.

So, treatment should be aimed at:
i. Analgesia
ii. Reduction of inflammation
iii. Reduction of intrapancreatic pressure
iv. Alternation in neural transmission

Another cause of pain in chronic pancreatitis is narcotic bowel syndrome. This is characterized by—abdominal discomfort in patient with chronic pancreatitis receiving high dosage of narcotics, but cannot be explained by the disease process itself.

Causative factors and pathway for pain in chronic pancreatitis over expressed in acinar cells:
1. Upregulation of pain mediators
   a. Substance P
   b. Calcitonin gene related peptides
2. Nerve growth factor—dependent nociceptors, TrKA
3. High affinity receptor for a nerve growth receptor
4. Brain derived neuro trophic factor
5. Proteinase activated receptor-2

Two terms in pain in chronic pancreatitis include:
1. *Mechanical allodynia:* Here pain being sensed even in absence of noxious stimuli, which are being given by prior sensitization of nociceptive system.
2. *Inflammatory hyperalgesia:* This is characterized by intense pain induced by minor inflammation of pancreas, if it is already primed pancreatic nociceptors.

According to WHO, there should be stepwise approach in management of pancreatic pain.

Inflammation and pancreatic pressure: This can be achieved by following methods:
i. Cessation of smoking
ii. Trial of total parenteral nutrition
iii. Enteral feeding
iv. Surgery for obstructive pancreatitis
v. Corticosteroid for autoimmune pancreatitis.

Method of reduction of pancreatic pressure: This can be done by suppression of secretion by:
i. Proton pump inhibitors
ii. Enzyme therapy
iii. Octreotide therapy

Avoidance of alcohol: It decreases frequency and severity of abdominal pain in chronic pancreatitis.

If patient has significant exocrine secretory function, alcohol may act as triggering factor for further secretion. In that case, avoidance of alcohol is necessary. But if the patient has no exocrine secretory function, avoidance of alcohol has no role in mechanism of pain.

Analgesics: It is the main method of reducing pain in chronic pancreatitis. These are:
a. Non-narcotic analgesic
  i. Salicylates
  ii. Acetaminophen
b. It should be given prior to meal to prevent post-prandial exacerbation of pain.
c. Lowest effective dose should be prescribed
d. Dosage of the drugs should be increased according to increasing severity of pain.

Modification of Neural Transmission

1. Endoscopic ultrasonographic guidance celiac axis block by alcohol injection.
2. Bilateral thoracoscopic splanchnicectomy
3. Transcranial magnetic stimulation

All the above procedures produces short term relief of pain but there is high rate of relapse in long term follow up.

Exocrine Deficiency

Intraluminal action of pancreatic protease enzymes regulates pancreatic enzymes secretion.

Diversion of pancreatic juices stimulates CCK release, whereas, intraduodenal administration of pancreatic enzymes inhibits CCK release.

So CCK releasing factors secreted by proximal small intestine is responsible for enhanced CCK release.

Trypsin in small intestine
↓
Cleaves the CCK releasing factors and inactivates it
In chronic pancreatitis
Less amount of enzymes are secreted in small intestine by pancreas
↓
Results in increased secretion of CCK releasing factors
↓
Enhanced secretion of CCK
↓
Responsible for pain in pancreatitis

So, effective enzyme replacement produces:
i. Reduction of pancreatic stimulation
ii. Decrease in intraductal pressure
iii. Decease pain

Treatment by Octreotide

Somatostatin exerts its beneficial response through following mechanisms:
i. Inhibits pancreatic secretions.
ii. It has cytoprotective actions.
iii. Beneficial effects on reticuloendothelial system.
iv. It has antinociceptive activity.
v. It has beneficial effects in inflammatory conditions through inhibition of cytokine release.
vi. It reduces secretion of interleukin 1 and interleukin 8 from intestinal epithelial cells.
viii. It reduces secretion of interferon y from activated peritoneal macrophages.

Octreotide, a synthetic analogue of somatostatin inhibits:
i. Basal release of pancreatic enzymes
ii. Neural stimulated pancreatic enzymes

It has long duration of action.

Long-term use of octreotide may be responsible for production of gallstones.

Dose: Subcutaneously—40–200 µg three times daily.

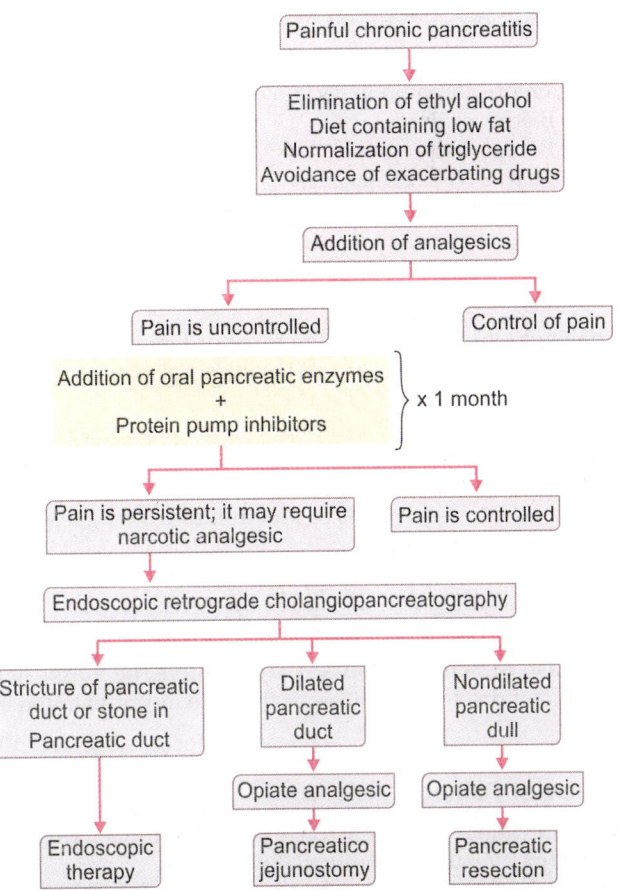

Fig. 4.40: Algorithm of treatment of painful alcoholic chronic pancreatitis

Long-acting octreotide—it consists of octreotide acetate microcapsulated by biodegradable polymer.

Slow cleavage of the polymer followed by release of drug occurs through fluid hydrolysis.

After single intravenous injection, drug level will be constant for 3–4 weeks.

Obstruction

It there is ductal obstruction due to—stricture, stone or pseudocyst—endoscopic intervention or surgical exploration is necessary.
1. In case of ductal stones
    i. Endoscopic clearance of stones
    ii. Surgical therapy
    iii. Extracorporeal shock wave lithotripsy
2. In case of large symptomatic pseudocyst
    i. Percuteneous drainage
    ii. Endoscopic drainage
    iii. Surgical drainage

Surgical options in chronic pancreatitis:
i. Lateral pancreatic-jejunostomy for decompression of dilated main pancreatic duct.
ii. Removal of diseased area through
    a. Whipple procedure
    b. Resection of tail
    c. Total pancreatectomy

TUMOR OF PANCREAS

Epidemiology

i. It is more common in men than women.
ii. It is more common in certain ethnic and racial groups
    a. Blacks
    b. Polynesians
    c. Native New Zealanders
iii. It occurs in patients more than 45 years of age, most common in seventh decade.

Pathology

In pancreas, tumor occurs from three different cells:
i. Acinar cells—80% of total volume of pancreas, 1% of exocrine tumor
ii. Ductal cells—10–15% of total volume of pancreas. 90% of tumor occurred in pancreas.
iii. Endocrine cells—1–2% of total volume pancreas
                        1–2% of total tumors of pancreas

In case of ductal tumors:
i. 70% of tumors in head of pancreas
ii. 5–10% of tumors in the body of pancreas
iii. 10–15% of tumors in the tail of pancreas

In case of acinar tumors: Large pancreatic mass—with evidence of distant metastasis at the time of presentation can be seen.

Molecular Pathogenesis

Pancreatic tumor develops from—small intraductal precursor lesions (pancreatic intraepithelial neoplasia)

Though exact mechanism and sequence of genetic mutation in the development of pancreatic neoplasia is unknown, but genetics alteration can be classified into three groups:

1. **Activation of oncogenes:** Mutation of k-ras oncogene—is irresponsible for 90% cases of pancreatic adenocarcinoma.

    It may occur also in case of chronic pancreatitis.
2. **Inactivation of tumor suppressor genes:**

    Inactivation and loss of function of tumor suppressor genes

    ↓

    It results in disruption of cell cycles—involving:
    i. Cellular differentiation
    ii. Growth inhibition
    iii. Regulation of transcription
    iv. DNA repair
    v. Apoptosis

    The genes involved:
    i. CDKN2A (95%)
    ii. P53
    iii. OPC4 (50%)
    iv. BRCA2
    iv. STK11

    In a few cases, germiline mutation of BRCA2 gene is responsible for hereditary pancreatitis.
3. Defect of DNA mismatch repair gene—mutation of following mismatch repair genes is responsible for pancreatic tumor:
    i. MLH1
    ii. MSH2

Hereditary Risk Factors

1. **Family history of pancreatic cancer:**
    a. Genetic predisposition is greatest risk factor
    b. 8–10% patients have 1st degree relative with this disease. These patients present at early age and smoking is the contributory factor.
2. **Hereditary chronic pancreatitis:** This autosomal dominant condition may be a risk factor for future pancreatic cancer. These patients present with recurrent attack of pain of acute pancreatitis in early life, which may progress into chronic pancreatitis—upon which carcinogenesis usually comes into play. It occurs at 70 years of age and occurs mainly in smokers.
3. **Other associated factors:** Pancreatic cancer may develop in certain conditions:
    i. Peutz-Jeghers syndrome
    ii. Ataxia telangiectesia
    iii. Familial adenomatous polyposis
    iv. Lynch syndrome II

    Association with diabetes mellitus: It may occur within 2 years of onset of diabetes mellitus. It may be due to high serum concentration of glucose and insulin along with evidence of insulin resistance.
4. **Environmental risk factors:**
    a. *Cigarette smoking*—it is the commonest environmental risk factor—relative risk is 2.5. The incidence depends upon—number of cigarette smoked.

        It returns to baseline 15 years after cessation of smoking.
    b. *Diet* i. Diet risk in fat is associated positive risk
            ii. Diet risk in fruits and vegetables has protective effect

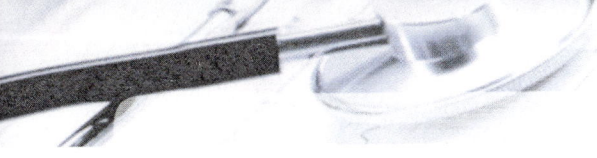

iii. Diet with low level of selenium, and lycopene are associated with pancreatic cancer.
c. *Obesity:* It is associated with increased risk of cancer
d. *Helicobacter pylori*—cag A strain has been associated with increased risk of gastric cancer
e. Coffee, alcohol consumption, aspirin ingestion—association with pancreatic cancer is conflicting.
5. **Non-hereditary risk factors:** In case of non-hereditary pancreatitis, risk of pancreatic carcinoma is high 20 years after onset.

Signs and Symptoms

Late diagnosis in case of pancreatic tumor is mainly due to lack of characteristic signs and symptoms of this disease. Hence after surgical resection with negative margins, 5 years survival rate is 10–25%.

Characteristic pain dull aching sensation radiating to back, it occurs mainly due to—invasion of:
i. Celiac plexus
ii. Superior mesenteric plexus

Associated symptoms are:
i. Weight loss
ii. Nausea
iii. Vomiting
iv. Anorexia
v. Weakness
vi. Diarrhea

Symptoms and signs can be dictated by location of tumor in pancreas:
a. **Tumor in the head of pancreas:**
i. Early symptoms
ii. Painless jaundice due to compression on CBD by tumor
iii. Palpable nontender gallbladder—Courvoisier's signs

This finding can be seen in following conditions:
i. Cholangiocarcinoma
ii. Duodenal carcinoma
iii. Carcinoma of ampulla of Vater
b. **Tumor in body and tail of pancreas**
i. Symptoms are non-specific, like abdominal discomfort
ii. It is usually diagnosed after the development of metastasis.

Obstruction of pancreatic duct is responsible for:
1. Exocrine insufficiency producing steatorrhea and malabsorption
2. Endocrine insufficiency in the form of diabetes mellitus after the age of 50 years in case of:
i. Absence of family history of diabetes
ii. Pancreatic carcinoma

Other uncommon presentations are:
i. Signs of acute pancreatitis.
ii. Thrombophlebitis
iii. Psychiatric disturbances
iv. Pruritus
v. Cholestasis
vi. Signs of gastrointestinal bleeding—due to invasion with erosions of duodenal wall by pancreatic growth.

Laboratory Findings

Following levels are raised:
i. Alkaline phosphatase 4–5 times of upper normal limit
ii. Bilirubin—mainly conjugated part

iii. Mild elevation of transaminases
iv. Lipase and amylase, in case of pancreatic duct obstruction—it usually presents with features of acute pancreatitis.

Tumor Markers

CA-19-9 is helpful in both diagnosis and monitoring treatment. Specificity and sensitivity of this test has been greatly elevated if the cut off value will be 37 units/mt.

But in case of common bile duct obstruction due to non malignant cause—CA-19-9 can be elevated to high level.

Imaging Studies

A. Computerized tomography:
i. It can detect pancreatic moss with the pancreas
ii. Detection of involvement of adjacent organs
iii. Detection of vascular invasion.
B. Endoscopic ultrasound:
i. It may be superior in diagnosis of pancreatic tumor
ii. EUS-guided fine needle aspiration may increase the accuracy up to 86%
iii. It is safe procedure
iv. There is minimal risk of seeding.
v. It can diagnose superior mesenteric vein and superior mesenteric artery invasion with less accuracy.
C. Endoscopic retrograde cholangiopancreatography:
i. Stricture of pancreatic duct or bile duct
ii. Stricture of pancreatic duct and bile duct called "double duct" sign. Helical CT make ERCP as unnecessary test.
Major limitations:
i. Limited ability to obtain tissue diagnosis in bile duct obstruction
ii. It provides no information about
a. tumor extent,
b. Vascular invasion
c. Involvement of lymph nodes,
d. Risk of complications
1. Pancreatitis
2. Perforation
D. Magnetic resonance imaging: It is as sensitive as ERCP in the diagnosis of pancreatic cancer.
E. Positron emission tomography: It is useful in the diagnosis of pancreatic recurrence after pancreatic resection.
F. Laparoscopy: It is useful in case of following:
i. Peritoneal invasion
ii. Hepatic metastasis
iii. Tissue diagnosis from peritoneum

Staging of Pancreatic Tumor

TNM Staging

Primary tumor (T):
Tx   Primary tumor cannot be assessed
To   No evidence of primary tumor
Tis   Carcinoma in situ
T_1 Tumor limited to pancreas: ≤2 cm in largest diameter
T_2 Tumor limited to pancreas: ≥2 cm in largest dimension
T_3 Tumor extends beyond the pancreas: No involvement of celiac axis and superior mesenteric artery.
T_4 Tumor involvement of celiac axis and superior mesenteric artery

Lymph node involvement (N):

Nx   Regional lymph node cannot be assessed
No   No involvement of regional lymph node
Ni   Regional lymph node involvement.

Metastatis (M):

Mx   Evidence of metastasis cannot be assessed
Mo   No evidence of distant metastasis
M1   Distant metastasis

Staging

Stage 0   Tis, N0, M0
Stage 1A   T1, N0, M0
Stage 1B   T2, N0, M0
Stage IIA   T3, N0, M0
Stage IIB   T3, N1 M0
Stage III   T4, N0 or N1, M0
Stage IV   Any T, and N, M1

Treatment

Depending upon the extent of involvement of the disease pancreatic cancer can be subdivided into following three categories:

1. Tumor confined to pancreas only 15–20% cases
2. Locally advanced disease—40% of cases
3. Metastasis outside the pancreatic tissue—40% of cases.

Resectable Disease

Surgical reaction is of choice

a. Whipple pancreaticoduodenectomy—when tumor is located in pancreatic head. The procedure involves— removal of
   i. Gastric antrum
   ii. Pancreas
   iii. Duodenum.

   Associated removal of regional lymph node is not associated with improved survival. Here the 5% survival rate is 10–25%.

b. In case of tumor located in pancreatic body and tail: The procedure of choice is subtotal pancreatectomy with splenectomy.

Endoscopic stent placement in common bile duct to relieve jaundice prior to surgery is not at all recommended.

Locally Invasive Disease

Treatment should be chemotherapy with radiation, this procedure may be associated with modest survival.

In case of tumor involving pancreatic head, the common complications are:
 i. Obstructive jaundice
ii. Gastric outlet obstruction

In case of tumor involving pancreatic body and tail, abdominal pain is the main presenting symptoms.

Treatment of Obstructive Jaundice

If the patient is not considered for surgical treatment, in that case to relieve bile duct obstruction by tumor compression, endoscopically metal stent will be considered.

Metal stent in considered over plastic stent because, this may be chance of occlusion of stent and it requires repeated and frequent stent placement.

Treatment of Gastric Outlet Obstruction

Gastric outlet obstruction usually occurs due to extension of pancreatic tumor. So it can be treated by:
 i. Gastrojejunostomy
ii. Endoscopically placement of self-expandable metal stent.

Treatment of Abdominal Pain

1. Narcotic medication
2. Blocking of celiac plexus (chemical blood) by:
   i. Percutaneous approach
   ii. EVS
3. Radiation

Metastatic Disease

1. Chemotherapy—for palliation therapy
2. Gemcitabine based combination therapy—it is the treatment of choice, it is responsible for:
   i. Better pain control
   ii. Decreased weight loss
   iii. Improvement of performance status.

Hematology

IRON METABOLISM AND IRON DEFICIENCY ANEMIA

1. Most of the iron in the body is contained in hemoglobin of circulating red cells.

Destruction of mature and senescent RBC by
Reticuloendothelial system (spleen)
↓
Iron released into plasma bound to transferrin
↓
Return to bone marrow for preparation of hemoglobin

2. Small amount of iron is lost from the body in epithelial cells sloughed from skin and gastrointestinal tract.
3. Loss from menses.
4. Small amount is lost through feces, sweats, and urine.

To balance this loss:
1. Adult male absorbs 1 mg of iron per day.
2. Menstruating female absorbs 2 mg iron per day.
3. Almost 3–4 mg of iron is absorbed each day enough to produce 3–4 ml of RBC—this is maximum.
4. In contrast, 40–60 mg of iron can be transferred from ferritin to transferrin per day to produce 40–60 ml of RBC—this is maximumm.

Body iron distribution has been shown in Fig. 5.1.

Methods of Iron Absorption in the Body (Fig. 5.2)

Ferric form of iron is not soluble in alkaline pH of duodenum so it cannot be absorbed
↓
So it must be solubilized in acidic mucosa of stomach by forming loose complex with amino acids and ascorbate.
↓
In this form, it enters in the duodenum
↓
Ferric reductase in duodenal mucosa reduces iron to divalent state (ferrous state)
↓
Ferrus form enters into the intestinal wall through transporter protein (DMT_1)
Heme containing iron is taken up through heme receptor (HCP_1)
↓

(Contd.)

(Contd.)

In the enterocytes, iron is complexed with a protein apoferritin to form ferritin.
Rest of the iron is transported to basal side of enterocytes and from there, it passes to other side through a transporter called ferroportin.
↓
Ferrous form will be oxidized to ferric form by ferroxydase.
↓
Ferric form is bound to transferring and then released into circulation.

Factors Preventing Absorption of Iron (Fig. 5.3)

1. Achlorhydria
2. Iron chelators—a. Tannin, b. phytates

Medicinal iron is already in ferrous state, so its absorption cannot be interfered by above factors.

Release of iron from duodenal enterocyte is enhanced by exporter—ferroportin. It is regulated by the hormone hepcidin. It acts as fence:
i. When concentration of hepcidin is high—iron will be trapped in enterocytes.
ii. When concentration of hepcidin will be down—iron enters the circulation.

So concentration of hepcidin correlates inversely with the activity of erythropoiesis, e.g.
i. If erythropoietic activity is high, hepcidin concentration will be low.
ii. Hepcidin concentration will be high in chronic inflammation due to increased activity of interleukin-6.

Progression of Laboratory Abnormalities in Absolute Iron Deficiency

1. **Serum ferritin:** Iron stores in the body in this form. When iron has been lost from the body—stainable bone marrow iron (hemosiderin) and serum ferritin begin to decrease.
   Serum ferritin will be increased inflammation, because inflammation:
   i. Stimulates ferritin synthesis independent of amount of storage iron
   ii. Releases ferritin from injured hepatocytes
   So: i. *In absence of inflammation*—serum ferritin level <20 ng/dl—suggests absolute iron deficiency.

(Contd.)

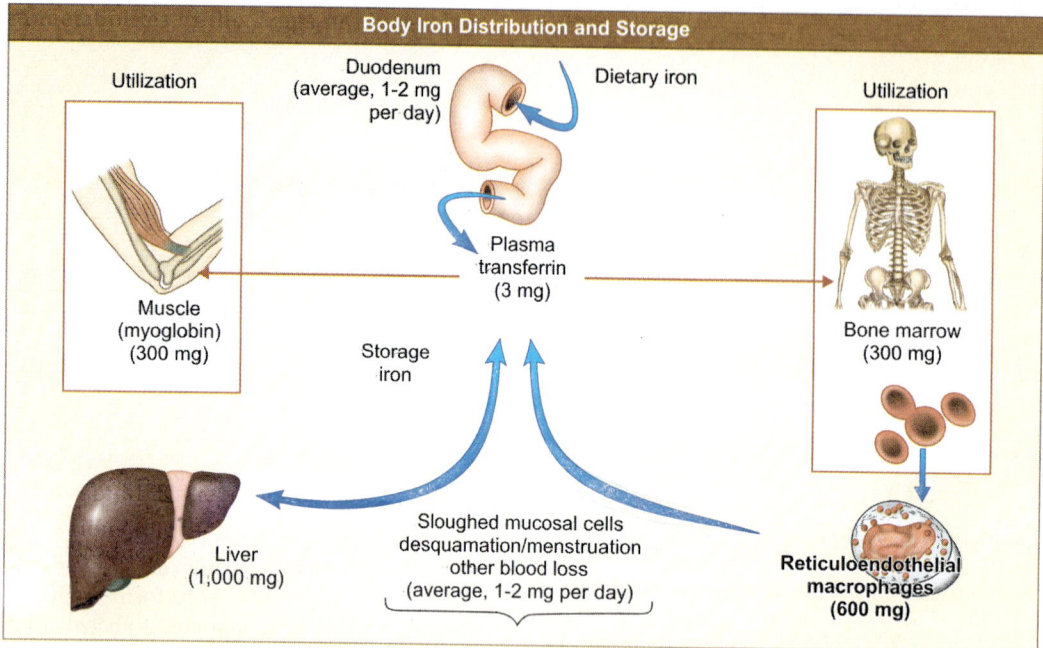

Fig. 5.1: Body iron storage

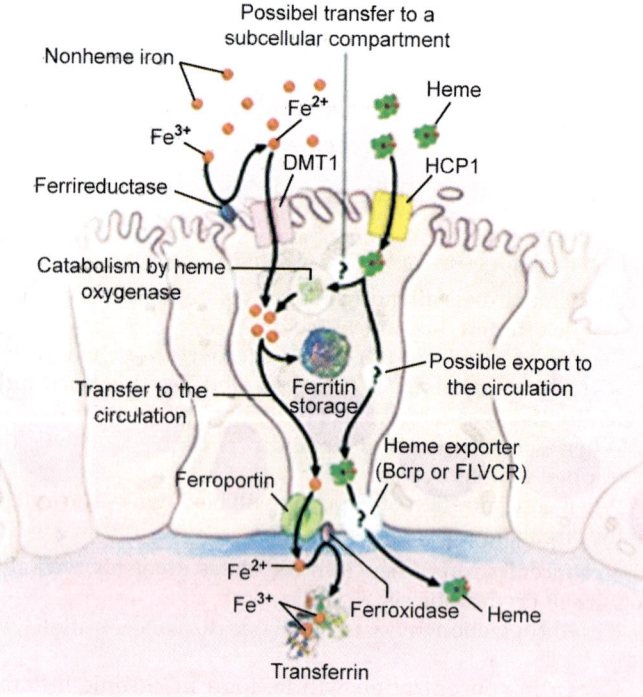

Fig. 5.2: Methods of iron absorption: Iron absorption across the gut wall

   ii. *In presence of inflammation or liver disease*—cut off value will be 100 ng/ml.

2. **When storage iron has been depleted:**
   i. Serum iron and transferrin saturation begin to drop.
   ii. Serum transferrin concentration usually rises.

3. **As a result, supply of iron to developing RBC** becomes rate limiting—red cell count begins to decrease in number and size.

4. **New iron deficient red blood cells are smaller than the older** ones → so red cell distribution width begins to increase.

5. **MCV falls below normal**—typical when hemoglobin concentration reaches <10 gm/dl.

Causes of Iron Deficiencies

1. **Gastrointestinal tract**—any type of bleeding from stomodium to proctodium—ulcer, cancer, polyp, congenital arteriovenous malformation
2. **Malabsorption**—celiac disease, atrophic gastritis, gastrectomy.
3. **Physiological**—growth spurts, pregnancy
4. **Dietary**—vegans, elderly (Fig. 5.4)
5. **Genitourinary system**—hematuria
6. **Other**—Paroxysmal nocturnal hemoglobinuria
7. **Worldwide**—hookworm manifestation

Assessment

   i. **Clinical history**—review of potential sources of blood loss especially gastrointestinal loss
  ii. **Menstrual loss**
 iii. **Other sources of blood loss**—hemoptysis, epistaxis, hematuria
  iv. **Drug history**—intake of NSAID, corticosteroid may cause gastrointestinal bleeding
   v. **Past medical history** of gastric surgery (malabsorption)
  vi. **Pica**—craving for eating unusual substances—clay, ice, starch, hair, etc.
 vii. **In children**—poor attention, retardation of behavior
viii. **In elderly**—restless leg syndrome.

Examination

   i. **Assessment of mucous membranes**—pallor, glossitis, stomatitis
  ii. **Look for possible sources of blood loss**—retinal hemorrhage and exudates—in severely anemic (Hb% — <5 gm%).
 iii. **Abdominal examination**
  iv. **Rectal examination**—seek for source of bleeding
   v. **Per vaginal examination**—to look for source of bleeding

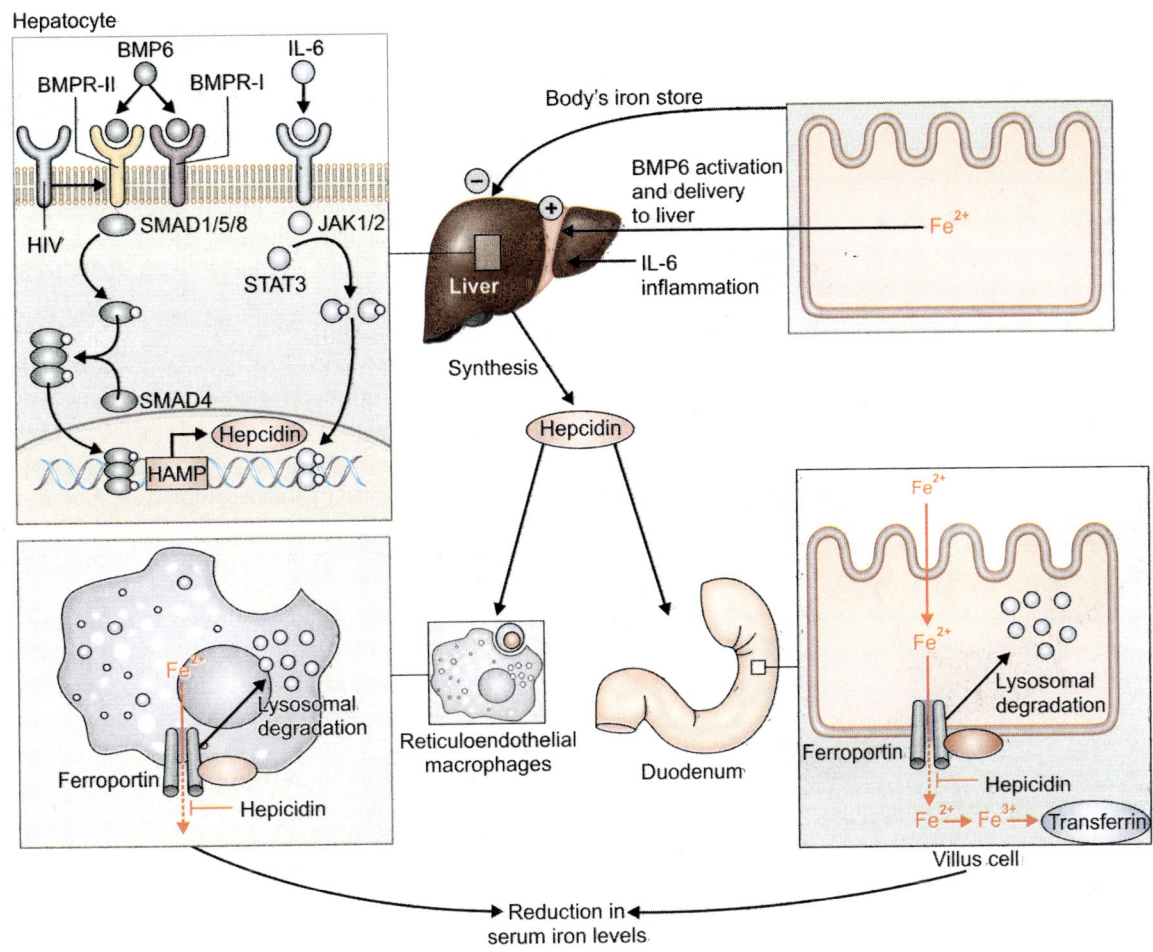

Fig. 5.3: Role of hepcidin in iron absorption

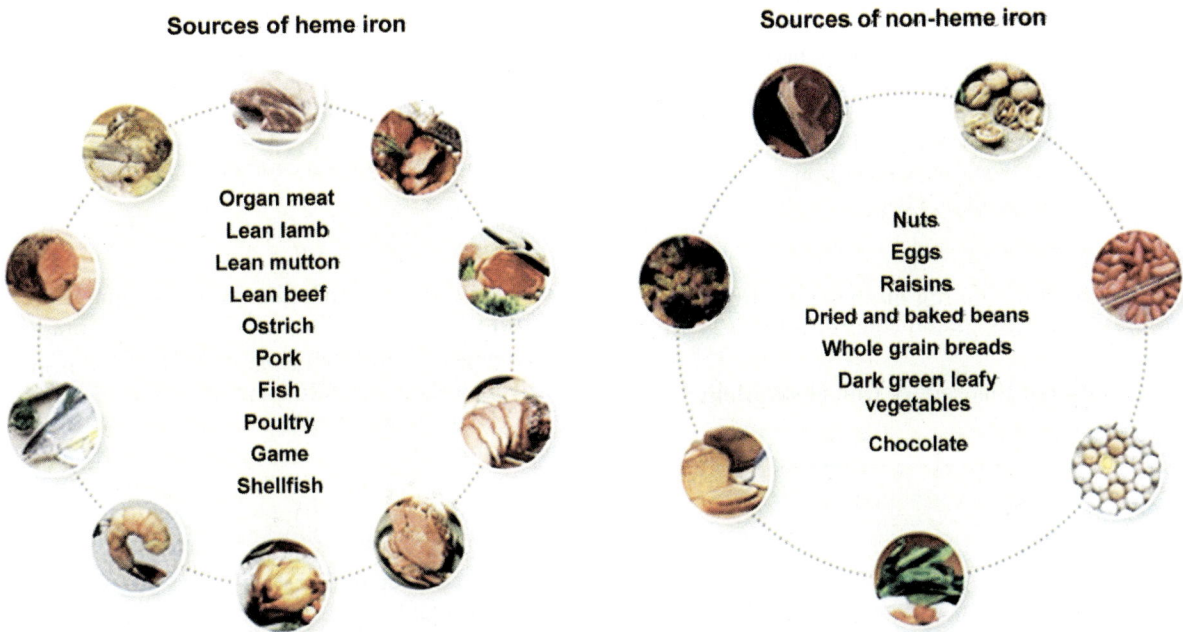

Sources of heme iron

Organ meat
Lean lamb
Lean mutton
Lean beef
Ostrich
Pork
Fish
Poultry
Game
Shellfish

Sources of non-heme iron

Nuts
Eggs
Raisins
Dried and baked beans
Whole grain breads
Dark green leafy vegetables
Chocolate

Fig. 5.4: Sources of iron

vi. **Hair loss**—may be consequence of low ferritin.
vii. **Mucosal atrophy in laryngopharynx** leads to web formation in the post-cricoid region—giving rise to dysphagia (Paterson-Kelly syndrome or Plummer-Vinson syndrome).
viii. Nail: Koilonychias (Fig. 5.5).

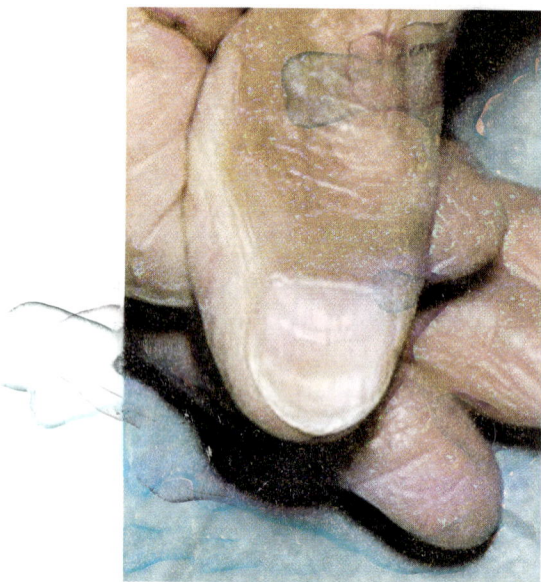

Fig. 5.5: Koilonychia

Laboratory Test

Hematology:
1. Hb% low—men—13.5 gm%, women—11.5 gm%.
2. Mean corpuscular volume (MCV) <76 fl
   ↓ MCV in thalassemia and chronic disease
3. MCHC—low(32.5 ± 2.5 gm/dl).
4. Red cell distribution width (RDW)—increased
5. Serum ferritin—in absence of chronic inflammation <20 mg/ml—but in presence of chronic inflammation <100 mg/ml (this is cut-off value)
6. Soluble transferrin assay—is useful where ESR is raised (rheumatoid arthritis and chronic disease)
7. Hypochromic RBC—percentage will be increased in iron deficiency anemia, thalassemia and CRF on erythropoietin therapy with insufficient amount of iron.
8. Reticulocyte count—will be raised.

Treatment

A daily supplement of 200 mg of elemental iron provides marrow to raise the hemoglobin concentration 0.25 gm/dl/daily.

Medications and food that reduce iron absorption:
1. Antacids
2. H_2 blocker
3. Proton pump inhibitor
4. Doxycycline
5. Bisphosphonates
7. Cholestyramine
8. Calcium supplement
9. Tea
10. Dairy product

Oral iron therapy:
1. Ferrous gluconate or ferrous fumerate
2. Oral dose of elemental iron of 150–200 gm/day
3. Side effects 10–25% patients develop gastrointestinal intolerance—abdominal distension, pair, and constipation

Response to treatment:
   i. Rise in hemoglobin—2 gm/dl over 3 weeks
   ii. Mean corpuscular volume—raised
   iii. Reticulocyte count will be raised initially in 3–4 days.

Duration of treatment:
   i. Generally 6 months
   ii. After normalization of Hb% and MCV—this therapy should be continued for at least 3 months

Failure of response:
1. Iron deficiency anemia may be wrong—consider anemia of chronic disease or thalassemia
2. Any additional complicating illness
3. Is the dose is correct or adequate or formulation is correct
4. Is the blood loss is being continued
5. Is there any associated continued malabsorption
6. Is there any associated folate or vitamin B_{12} deficiencies

Intravenous Iron Therapy

Indication:
1. Intolerance to oral iron therapy
2. Problem with compliance
3. Need to replace the store rapidly
4. Prior to major surgery

The drugs are:
1. Ferric gluconate with sucrose
2. Iron sucrose (ferric hydroxide with sucrose)
3. Iron dextran (ferric hydroxide with dextran).

These can be administered in two ways:
   i. Administration of total dose of iron required to correct hemoglobin deficit and provide the patient with 500 mg of iron stores
   ii. Administration of repeated small dose of parenteral iron over a protracted period—this is common in dialysis center, where it is not unusual to give 100 mg of elemental iron weekly for 10 weeks to augment the response of erythropoietin therapy. The amount to be given in a patient according to his need can be calculated by using following formula:

   Body weight (kg) × 2.3 × (15–patient's hemoglobin gm/dl) + 500 or 1000 mg (for store)

Complications of newly discovered preparation:
i. Arthralgia,   ii. Skin rash,   iii. Low grade fever

Method of administration: If >100 mg of iron dextrose to be given, it should be diluted in 5% dextrose or 0.9% NaCl and to be given over 60–90 minutes period.

Iron infusion should be stopped, if in early infusion period:
1. Chest pain
2. Wheezing
3. Fall in blood pressure.

Various oral preparations:
1. Ferrous sulphate—325 (65 elemental iron)
2. Ferrous fumerate—325 (107 elemental iron)
3. Ferrous gluconate—325 (39 elemental iron)

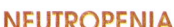

NEUTROPENIA

Defined as neutrophil count $<2 \times 10^9/L$

Causes of Neutropenia

A. Decreased Production

1. **Drug-induced:**
   i. Alkalyting agent
   ii. Antimetabolites (methotrexate, 6-mercaptopurine)
   iii. Antibiotics (chloramphenicol, penicillin)
   iv. Phenothiazines
   v. Anticonvulsants
   vi. Antithyroid drugs
   vii. Anti-inflammatory agents
2. **Hematologic diseases:**
   i. Aplastic anemia
   ii. Cyclic neutropenia
   iii. Idiopathic
3. Tumor invasion
4. Myelofibrosis
5. Nutritional deficiency—vitamin B_{12}, folate deficiency
6. Infection—tuberculosis, typhoid fever, measles, malaria, infectious mononucleosis, viral hepatitis

B. Peripheral Destruction

1. Anti-neutrophil antibodies
2. Autoimmune disorders—Felty's syndrome, rheumatoid arthritis, SLE
3. Polyangitis—Wagener's granulomatosis
4. Drugs (as haptens): Phenothiazines, phenylbutazone ∝-methyldopa

C. Peripheral Pooling

1. Over whelming bacterial infections
2. Cardiopulmonary bypass

D. Hereditary Neutropenia

1. Kostmann's syndrome $<100/\mu L$—mutation of anti-apoptosis gene
2. Severe chronic neutropenia—$300–1500/\mu L$—due to mutation in neutrophil elastase
3. Shwachman–Diamond syndrome associated with pancreatic insufficiency

Lymphocytosis

i. Lymphocytosis $>4 \times 10^9/L$
ii. Normal infants and young children <5 years
iii. Acute infectious lymphocytosis—seen in children
iv. Infectious mononucleosis—these lymphocytes are often large and atypical—diagnosis confirmed by heterophil agglutination test
v. In CMV infection and hepatitis A infection
vi. Brucellosis, tuberculosis, secondary syphilis
vi. CLL, ALL

Hepcidin binds to *ferroportin* and triggers its lysosomal *degradation*, leading to a reduction in iron release from enterocytes (and macrophages). Hepcidin may also inhibit DMT1 directly. Hepcidin *gene expression* is upregulated during infection and inflammation by proinflammatory cytokines—mainly IL-6 (involving JAK-dependent activation of STAT3). Hepcidin levels are correlated with the body's iron stores. BMP regulates hepcidin

by sensing enteric iron status. *Iron absorption* in enterocytes leads to activation of BMP6 expression and, subsequently, to the delivery of BMP6 to the liver. In the liver, BMP6 binds to type I and II receptors (BMPR1 and BMPR2) and to the coreceptor HJV leading to phosphorylation of SMAD1, SMAD5 and SMAD8, and complex formation with SMAD4. This complex translocates to the nucleus to activate the HAMP gene promoter, leading to synthesis of hepcidin. (Abbreviations: BMP, bone morphogenetic protein; DMT1, divalent cation transporter 1; HJV, hemojuvelin; IL-6, interleukin 6).

MEGALOBLASTIC ANEMIA

This is a heterogeneous group of disorders—that share common morphologic characteristics. Morphological hallmark is megaloblast. **Megaloblastosis** is a generalized disorder involving most rapidly growing cells, e.g. gastrointestinal and uterine cervical mucosal cells.

Pathophysiology

Common features of megaloblastosis is:
1. Defect in DNA synthesis in rapidly dividing cells
2. Defect in RNA synthesis
3. Defect in protein synthesis

Common Causes of Megaloblastosis

Cobalamin and folate deficiencies

Cobalamin

1. **Sources**—fish, meat, dairy products
2. Natural active forms—5-deoxyladenosylcobalamin, hydroxycobalamin and methyl cobalamin

Uptake of cobalamin:

Dietary cobalamin binds nonspecifically to protein
↓
Gastric digestion at low pH releases cobalamin from these proteins.
↓
Cobalamin binds to R-proteins
↓
R-protein–cobalamin complex in duodenum
↓
Degraded by pancreatic enzyme release cobalamin
↓
Free cobalamin binds to intrinsic factor (IF) produced in gastric fundus and cardia
↓
Stabilizes the cobalamin transport throughout jejunum and reaches it to terminal ileum
↓
Cobalamin—IF complexes are processed by receptors in terminal ileum
↓
Cobalamin is released and absorbed and enters into the circulation
↓
Cobalamin in circulation binds to transcobalamin II
↓
Transcobalamin II carries cobalamin to cells
↓
Cobalamin enters the cells and helps in DNA synthesis

Transcobalamin I helps in storage of cobalamin in water soluble form.

Transcobalamin I is increased in CML.

3 mg of cobalamin is stored in the body of which 1 mg is stored in liver.

Folate

1. Sources—vegetables, fruits, animal proteins
2. Both monoglutamate and polyglutamate forms exist in nature.

Uptake of folate:

i. Uptake of folate is receptor mediated.

ii. Uptake occurs throughout the small intestine.

Folate derivatives are essential cofactors in thymidylate synthesis—it is the rate limiting step in DNA synthesis.

Metabolic pathways: Cobalamin is necessary in the pathway leading to synthesis of S-adenosyl methionine—if the only donor of methyl groups for numerous reactions in brain involving proteins, membrane phospholipids and neurotransmitters.

Causes of Vitamin B$_{12}$ Deficiency

1. **Gastrointestinal:**
   - i. Gastric atrophy
   - ii. Bariatric surgery
   - iii. Gastrectomy
   - iv. Gastric bypass
   - v. Terminal ileum resection
   - vi. Extensive celiac disease
   - vii. Crohn's disease
   - viii. Bacterial overgrowth
2. **Medications**
   - i. Large doses of vitamin C
   - ii. PPI
3. **Increased utilization**
   - i. Pregnancy
4. **Fish tapeworm**
   - i. *Diphyllobothrium latum*
5. **Malabsorption disorder**
   - i. Tropical sprue
   - ii. Celiac disease
6. **Dietary deficiency**
   - i. Strict vegetarian

Requirement of Folate

1. **Normal daily requirement**—0.1–0.2 mg
2. **Body folate stores**—10–15 mg

Causes of Folate Deficiency

1. **Decreased intake** — Poor nutrition, e.g. poverty, old age, alcoholic
2. **Increased requirements**
   - i. Pregnancy
   - ii. Increased cell turnover
     - a. Hemolysis
     - b. Exfoliative dermatitis
     - c. Renal dialysis
3. **Malabsorption**
   - i. Coeliac disease
   - ii. Tropical sprue
   - iii. Crohn's disease
4. **Drugs**
   - i. Antifolate drugs
     - a. Methotrexate
     - b. Trimethoprim
   - ii. Anticonvulsant
   - iii. Oral contraceptive
   - iv. Nitrofurantoin
5. **Alcohol**

Clinical Presentation

1. In some patients, anemia develops insidiously—so they may be asymptomatic.
2. Some patients may present with weakness, fatigue, respiratory distress, tinnitus—due to severe anemia.
3. Some patients may present with gastrointestinal symptoms, e.g. anorexia, weight loss, nausea and constipation, canker sores, macroglossia, sore tongue (Fig. 5.6).
4. May present with lemon-colored complexion—due to intramedullary hemolysis.
5. Many present with spectrum of mental changes—from personality changes to psychosis.
6. Peripheral neuropathy—pain, tingling, numbness, burning sensation in feet.
7. Ataxia, unsteadiness in gait, loss of balance, speech impairment—suggestive of subacute combined degeneration.
8. **History findings to identify folate deficiency are:**
   - i. Poor nutrition, excessive heating of food
   - ii. Chronic alcoholism
   - iii. History of IBD, gluten sensitivity
   - iv. Increase in folate consumption, e.g. pregnancy, lactation, hemolytic anemia, exfoliative dermatitis
   - v. Hyperalimentation
   - vi. Drugs—affecting metabolism or absorption of folate.
9. **History findings to identify vitamin B$_{12}$ deficiency:**
   - i. Abdominal discomfort, early satiety, abdominal bloating
   - ii. Pernicious anemia—patients have also other signs of autoimmune disorders, e.g. thyroid disorder, type 1 diabetes, Addison's disease
   - iii. History of gastrectomy
   - iv. Conditions affecting terminal ileu, e.g. IBD, tropical sprue, extensive ileal resection
   - v. Exposure to fish—*Diphyllobothrium latum*
   - vi. H/o megaloblastosis since childhood—suggestive of hereditary cause of cobalamin deficiency.

Physical Examinations

1. Evidence of anemia—pale conjunctiva
2. Lemon-yellow hue of skin due to combination of anemia and increased indirect bilirubin level (due to intramedullary hemolysis)
3. Glossitis—due to loss of papillae—cobalamin deficiency

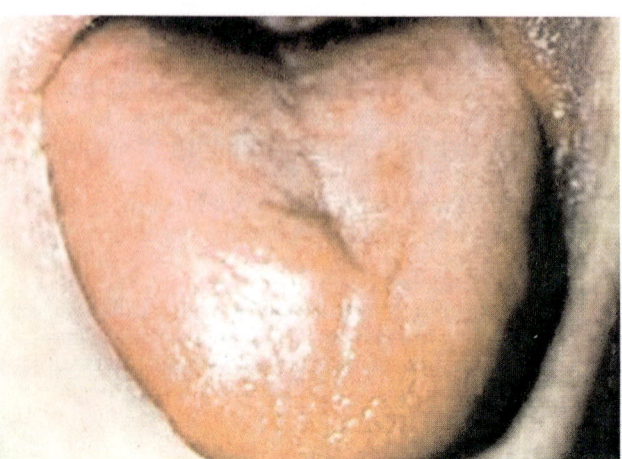

Fig. 5.6: Sore tongue

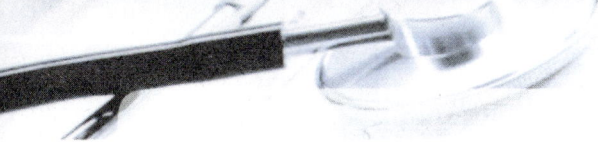

4. Dermatologic sign—hyperpigmentation of skin and abnormal pigmentation of hair—due to increased melanin synthesis.
5. Wide range of mental changes
6. Signs of peripheral neuropathy
7. Abnormal gait, loss of balance, speech impairment, loss of proprioceptive and vibratory senses—suggestive of subacute combined degeneration of spinal cord.
8. Abdominal scars—suggest blind loop syndrome due to gastric surgery.
9. Evidences of malabsorption (tropical sprue, celiac disease), weight loss, abdominal distension, diarrhea, steatorrhea
10. Children with inborn error of folate and vitamin B_{12} deficiency—have signs of these hereditary disorders.

Megaloblastic Anemia Workup (Fig. 5.7)

1. **Complete blood count—RBC picture:**
   i. Macrocytic anemia (MCV>110 ft)
   ii. Anisopoikilocytosis.
   iii. Basophilic stippling
   iv. Howell-Jolly bodies
   v. Circulating megaloblast

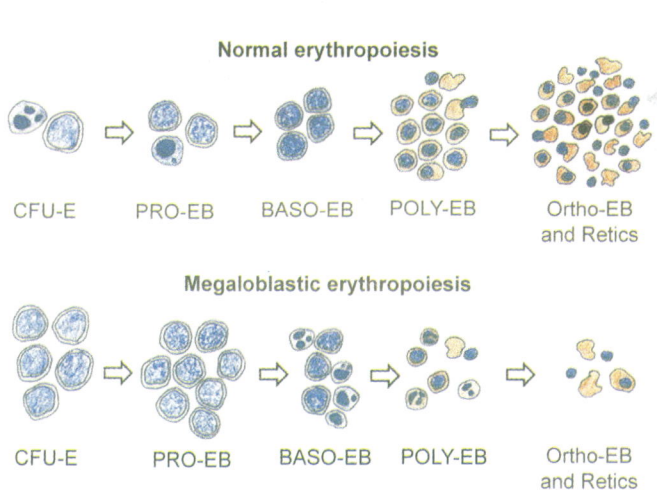

Fig. 5.7: Megaloblastic erythropoiesis

WBC shows: Hypersegmented neutrophil (Fig. 5.8) containing 5 or more lobes (normal neutrophil contains 3–4 lobes)

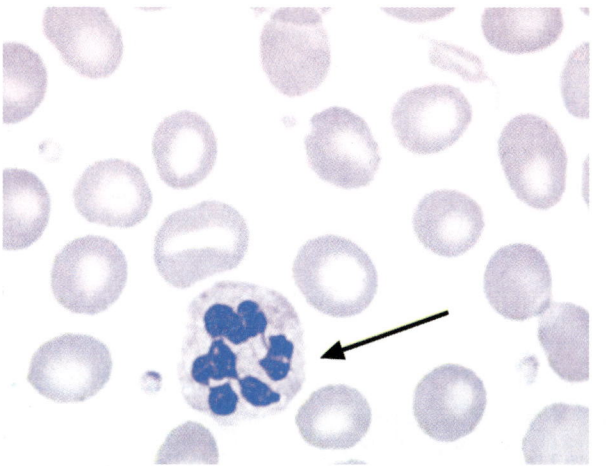

Fig. 5.8: Hypersegmented neutrophil

In case of associated iron deficiency anemia: Microcytosis may be masked by hypersegmented neutrophil.
Count may show:
   i. Leucopenia
   ii. Thrombocytopenia
2. **Bone marrow shows** (Fig. 5.9):
   i. Megaloblastic changes of RBC.
   ii. Marked erythroid hyperplasia, with predominance of early erythroid precursors.
   iii. Open atypical nuclear chromatin pattern
   iv. Mitotic figures
   v. Giant metamyelocytes

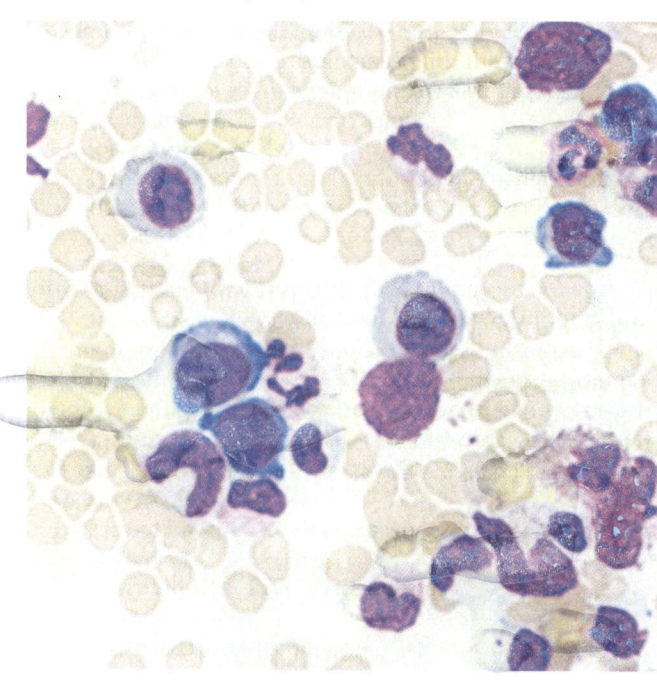

Fig. 5.9: Bone marrow picture

3. **Reticulocyte count** low despite hemolysis—this is characteristics of intramedullary hemolysis.
4. **Serum LDH**—is markedly increased in megaloblastic anemia—reflecting ineffective erythropoiesis.
5. Serum **vitamin B_{12} and folate level** low.
6. **Ferritin** is increased.
7. **RBC folate level** is normal or increased because it is not affected by diet, since folate content is established early in RBC development.
8. **Serum homocysteine and methylmalonic acid levels:**
   i. Serum homocysteine and methylmalonic acid level are elevated in vitamin B_{12} and folate deficiency.
   ii. Serum methylmalonic acid level is elevated in vitamin B_{12} deficiency.
9. **Autoantibodies:** i. Parietal cell antibodies are present in 90% cases of pernicious anemia; ii. Anti-intrinsic factor antibodies—are highly specific for pernicious anemia—found in 55% of pernicious anemia.
10. **Schilling test**—this test is usually not done nowadays.
11. **Other tests to diagnose the cause of vitamin B_{12} and folate deficiency**
   i. Abdominal radiograph
   ii. Upper and lower gastrointestinal series
   iii. Computerized tomography
   iv. Endoscopy of upper gastrointestinal tract

v. Colonoscopy with terminal ileoscopy
vi. Double balloon enteroscopy with biopsy
vii. Capsule endoscopy

Management of Megaloblastic Anemia (Fig. 5.10)

I. Cobalamin Deficiency

1. Parenterally cobalamin (100–1000 µg)—daily for 2 weeks then weekly until the hematocrit value is normal, then monthly for life.
2. Oral cobalamin (1000–2000 µg)—can also be administered.

The following are the indications of IV cobalamin:

i. Oral therapy is indicated in patient, with hemophilia to avoid intramuscular bleeding.
ii. In case of parenteral therapy, absorption of cobalamin are bypassed.
iii. It is practical to administer vitamin B$_{12}$ parenterally followed by oral therapy.

II. Folate Deficiency

i. 3–5 mg folate—orally daily, if it is difficult, comparable dose can be administered parenterally.
ii. It can be administered prophylactically during pregnancy, lactation, perinatal period, chromic hemolytic anemia, exfoliative dermatitis, psoriasis, during extensive hemo-dialysis.

Supportive therapies:

i. Bedrest
ii. Moist O$_2$ inhalation
iii. Transfusion should be avoided, but 2 units of concentrated RBC may be given in severely anemia patient.

Response to therapy:

i. In 3–5 days—reticulocyte count will be >10%.
ii. Normoblastic conversion of bone marrow within 12–24 hours.
iii. Bone marrow morphology appears normal within 2–3 days.

Continuation of treatment: Oral vitamin B$_{12}$—50–150 mg/day between meals.

Follow-up:

i. Pernicious anemia patient requires long-term follow-up with annually blood count, and thyroid function test.
ii. Broad-spectrum antibiotics should be given to suppress bacterial over growth in blind loop syndrome
iii. Prophylactic treatment with folate in—pregnancy, prematurity.

MAIN GROUPS OF ANEMIA CLASSIFIED ACCORDING TO THE UNDERLYING CAUSES

I. Reduced red cells production:
1. Defective precursor proliferation
2. Defective precursor maturation
3. Defective precursor proliferation and maturation

II. Increased red cell destruction: Hemolysis

III. Loss of red cells from circulation: Bleeding.

Main Causes of Anemia Due to Defective Production of Red Cells

I. Reduced proliferation of precursors:
1. Iron deficiency anemia
2. Anemia of chronic disorder

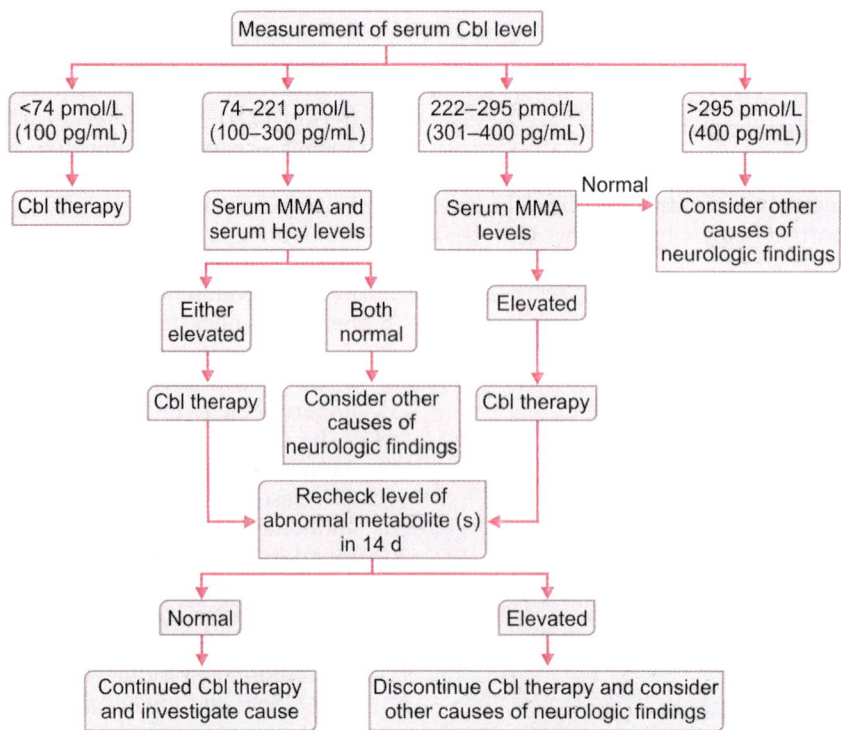

Fig. 5.10: Algorithm showing response to therapy

a. Infection
b. Malignancy
c. Collagen diseases
3. Reduced erythropoietin production: Renal disease
4. Reduced oxygen requirement:
   a. Hypothyroidism
   b. Hypopituitarism
5. Reduced oxygen affinity of hemoglobin
6. Primary disease of bone marrow:
   a. Aplastic anemia
      i. Primary
      ii. Secondary to drugs, irradiation, chemicals, toxins, etc.
7. Pure red cells aplasia
8. Infiltrative disorders:
   a. Leukemia
   b. Lymphoma
   c. Secondary carcinoma
   d. Myelofibrosis

II. Defective maturation of precursors:
1. Nuclear maturation:
   a. Vitamin B_{12} deficiency
   b. Folate deficiency
   c. Erythroleukemia
2. Cytoplasmic maturation:
   a. Iron deficiency
   b. Disorder of globin synthesis
   c. Disorder of heme and/or iron metabolism
   d. Disorder of porphyrin metabolism
3. Other mechanisms:
   a. Congenital dyserythropoietic anemia
   b. Myelodysplastic syndrome
   c. Infection
   d. Toxins
   e. Chemicals

Main Causes of Anemia Classified According to the Associated Red Cell Changes

I. Hypochromic–microcytic (reduced MCV, MCH, and MCHC)
   a. Genetic:
      1. Thalassemia
      2. Sideroblastic anemia
   b. Acquired:
      1. Iron deficiency
      2. Sideroblastic anemia
      3. Chronic disorders
II. Normochromic–macrocytic (increased MCV)
   a. With megaloblastic marrow:
      1. Vitamin B_{12} deficiency
      2. Folate deficiency
   b. With normoblastic marrow:
      1. Alcohol
      2. Myelodysplasia
III. Polychromatophilic–macrocytic (increased MCV) hemolysis
IV. Normocytic–normochromic (normal indices):
   a. Chronic disorders:
      1. Infection
      2. Malignancy
      3. Collagen disease

b. Renal failure
c. Hypothyroidism, hypopituitarism
d. Aplastic anemia
e. Pure red cell aplasia
f. Primary disease of marrow:
   1. Leukemia
   2. Lymphoma
   3. Myelosclerosis
   4. Other tumors
V. Leukoerythroblastic (indices are usually normal):
   a. Myelosclerosis
   b. Leukemia
   c. Metastatic carcinoma

Functional Iron Deficiency

This is a condition characterized by—hypoferremia despite seemingly adequate or increased iron stores.

It occurs in:
i. Chronic infection
ii. Inflammation
iii. Neoplastic diseases
iv. Patient with maintenance HD and starts receiving EP.

In this case, response to erythropoietin will be blunted until iron is adequately supplied.

Characteristic blood picture:
1. *MCV*—usually normocytic, but may be microcytic.
2. *Serum iron and transferrin saturation* will be low suggestive of absolute iron deficiency.
3. *Serum transferrin concentration* is low or normal
4. *Serum ferritin*—elevated
   Chronic inflammation reduces transferring level but elevates ferritin.

Most reliable diagnostic parameter to identify the absolute iron deficiency in patient with chronic inflammation is—ratio of serum transferrin receptor concentration (mg/L) to the log of serum ferritin concentration.

Treatment of Functional Iron Deficiency

1. Treatment of underlying cause
2. Supplementation of iron to raise the hemoglobin level 10–12 gm/dl. Hemoglobin concentration above this level may increase the risk of:
   i. Cardiovascular events
   ii. Thromboembolic events
   iii. Increased tumor progression
3. Administration of erythropoietin at the same time of iron supplementation.
4. These patients may respond well to parenteral iron than oral iron.

AUTOIMMUNE HEMOLYTIC ANEMIA

Pathophysiology

RBC membrane acts as autoantigen
↓
Reacts with developed autoantibody ± complement (IgG)
↓
Recognized by Fc receptors on reticuloendothelial macrophages
↓

(Contd.)

(Contd.)

Phagocytosis of RBC → RBC will be completely destroyed (where complement is involved)

↓

If phagocytosis is incomplete

↓

Remaining portion of RBC continue to circulate in blood as spherocytes

↓

Destroyed in splenic pulp

Types of Hemolytic Anemia

Warm Antibody Hemolytic Anemia

1. **Causes:**
   a. Idiopathic
   b. Lymphoproliferative disorders—CLL, NHL
   c. Autoimmune disease—SLE
2. **Epidemiology:** Predominantly >50 years of age.
3. **Clinical features:**
   a. Ranges from asymptomatic to severely anemia
   b. Anemia
   c. Jaundice
   d. Splenomegaly
4. **Diagnosis** (Figs 5.11 and 5.12):
   a. Hb% 8–10 gm%
   b. ↑ Bilirubin—unconjugated
   c. Spherocytes in peripheral blood film
   d. Reticulocyte ↑↑
   e. Neutrophilia
   f. Direct antiglobulin test with daunorubicin +ve for RBC coated with IgG
   g. Autoantibody—i. anti-E antibody, ii. Anti-D antibody
   h. ↑ LDH in serum
   i. Decreased serum haptoglobin.
   j. Bone marrow picture of lymphoma
   k. Autoimmune profile—to exclude SLE or other connective tissue disorder.

Treatment

1. Prednisolone—1 mg/kg orally for 1–2 weeks—produces remission promptly.
2. If no response—immunosuppression, e.g. azathioprine or cyclophosphamide.

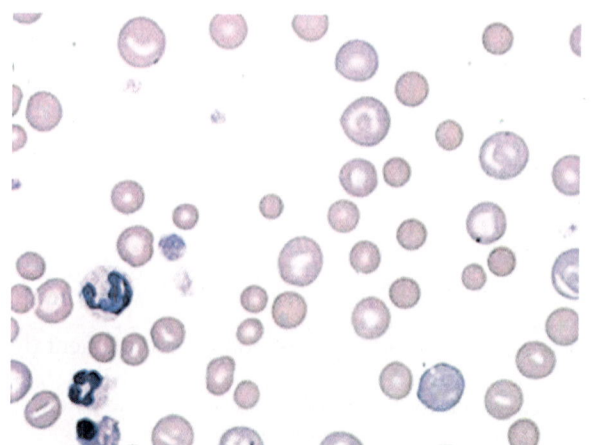

Fig. 5.11: Spherocytes

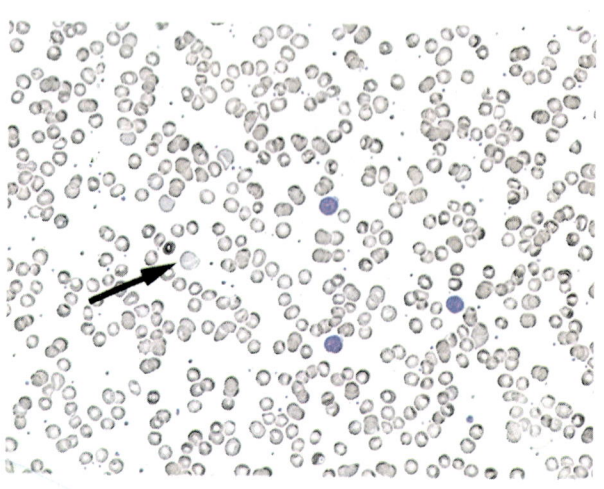

Fig. 5.12: Hemolytic anemia

3. Third line of treatment: Anti-CD-20 antibody or splenectomy.

Indications

1. Who do not respond to prednisolone or immunosuppressive therapy.
2. Who have relapsed.
3. Who require >15 mg/day prednisolone to prevent relapse.

CD-20 antibody is better than splenectomy because:
1. Splenectomy does not cure the disease.
2. Rituximab produces remission up to 80% of patients.
3. Rituximab can be used repeatedly.

Dreaded Side Effect of Rituximab

Progressive multifocal leukoencephalopathy

Splenectomy—removes major site of hemolysis, thus reducing the need for therapies and improves anemia

→ Complement	→ Complement activation with formation of membrane attack complex	→ destroyed red cell membrane and free hemoglobin
↓ Reticuloend-othelial system		
Mononuclear phagocytic cell	IgG1 or IgG3 antibody complex	
CMPC	Fc receptor	
Phagocytosis	Fragmentation	Antibody dependant Cytotoxicity (ADCC)

Mechanism of antibody-mediated immune destruction of red cells.

FANCONI ANEMIA

1. It is **most common constitutional** aplastic anemia.
2. It is **autosomal recessive or X-linked.**
3. It is found in **all races, mainly in children.**
4. Genetics—mutation can occur in 13 genes—amongst **those FANCA—is most common.**

5. **Chief criteria**—i. Pancytopenia, ii. hyperpigmentation, iii. malformation of skeleton, small stature, iv. hypogonadism.

6. **Clinical features:**
    i. Hypo- or hyperpigmented skin lesion (Fig. 5.13)
    ii. Short stature (café-au-lait spot)
    iii. Abnormalities in thumb, radius, genitourinary tract
    iv. Characteristic facial feature—broadened nasal base, epicanthic fold, micrognathia
    v. Anemia.

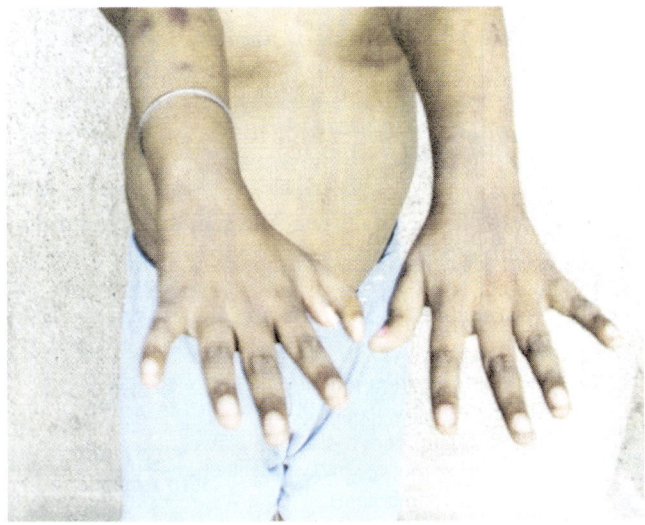

Fig. 5.13: Hyperpigmented skin

7. **Diagnostic test:** Chromosome breakage test by Mithramycin C. 40% of positive MMC test is normal appearing, may undergo unnoticed—unless family history is taken.

8. **Hematological abnormalities:**
    i. Pancytopenia—may be preceded by leucopenia or thrombocytopenia—it typically worsens with time.
    ii. Macrocytic erythropoiesis.
    iii. Bone marrow may show fatty hypocellularity sometimes dyserythropoiesis or dysplasia.

9. **Patient may develop myelodysplastic syndrome or acute myeloid leukemia.**

10. **Solid organ malignancies**—particularly esophageal, head and neck cancers.

11. **Treatment:**
    i. Allogenic bone marrow transplant from HLA matched sibling donor—is the only curative therapy. Since these patients are radio- and chemosensitive, hence dosage of chemotherapy should be adjusted.
    ii. Androgen induces hematologic response in 50% of patients. This therapy is initiated with platelet count <30,000/cc and/or hemoglobin level <7 gm/dl.

Oxymethalone—started with 2–5 mg/kg/day
+
Prednisolone—5–10 mg at alternate day

They counterbalance anabolic properties of oxymethalone and catabolic properties of corticosteroids.

Dyskeratosis Congenita

1. This is characterized by mucous membrane leukoplakia, dystrophic nails, reticular hyperpigmentation and aplastic anemia in childhood (Fig. 5.14).

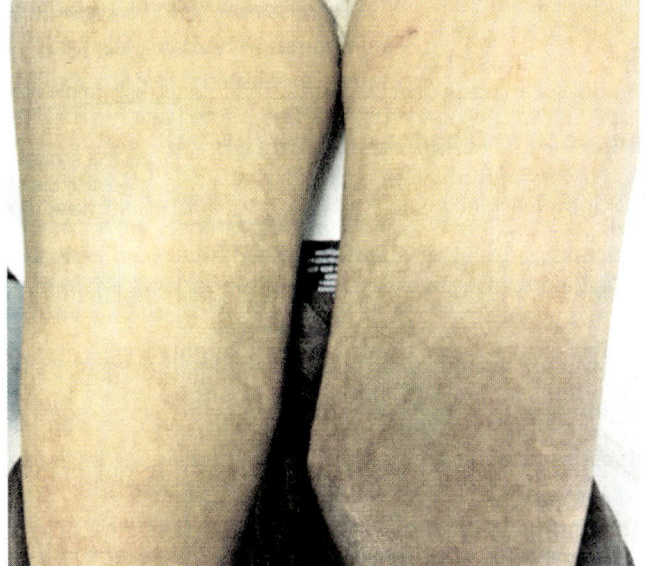

Fig. 5.14: Reticular hyperpigmentation

2. It is X-linked disease: Mutation in DKC1 (dyskerin) gene (Fig. 5.15).

3. In unusual autosomal dominant type—mutation in TERC gone—which encodes RNA template

TERT gene—which encodes reverse transcriptase

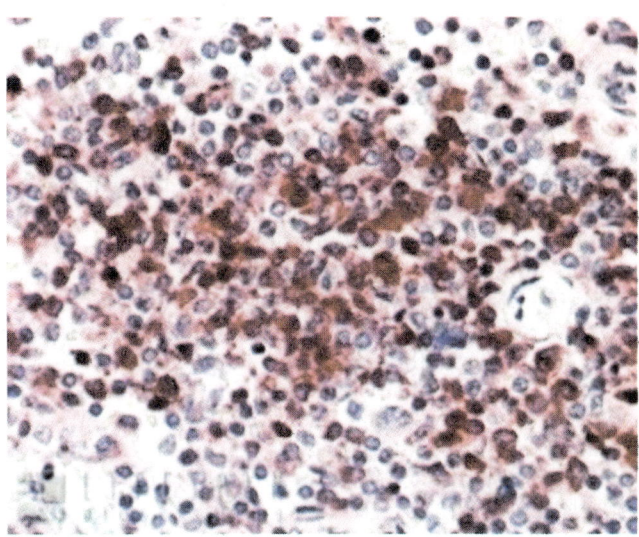

Fig. 5.15: Bone marrow picture in Shwachman-Diamonded syndrome

Shwachman-Diamond Syndrome

1. **Third most common constitutional marrow** failure syndrome.

2. **Autosomal recessive**, presents in infancy.

3. **Clinical features:**
    i. Exocrine pancreatic insufficiency
    ii. Short stature
    iii. Bone abnormalities (Fig. 5.15)
    iv. Immune dysfunction
    v. Liver disease
    vi. Renal tubular defect

vii. Hematologic abnormalities—neutropenia, raised fetal hemoglobin, anemia, thrombocytopenia, impaired neutrophil chemotaxis.

viii. It can transform into acute myeloid leukemia or MDS.

Approach to Diagnosis

1. History and physical examination
2. Complete blood count, reticulocyte count, examination of blood film.
3. Marrow aspiration and biopsy.
4. Marrow cell cytogenetics to evaluate clonal myeloid disease.
5. Fetal hemoglobin level and DNA stability test as markers of Fanconi anemia.
6. Immuno-phenotyping of red and white cells, especially for—CD55, CD59 to exclude PNH.
7. Direct and indirect Coomb tests to rule out immune cytopenia.
8. Serum lactate dehydrogenase (LDH) and uric acid—if increased may reflect neoplastic cell turnover.
9. Liver function test to assess evidence of any recent hepatitis virus exposure.
10. Screening tests of hepatitis virus B, C and A.
11. Screening tests for Epstein-Barr virus, cytomegalovirus and HIV virus.
12. Serum B-12 and red cell folic acid levels to exclude megaloblastic pancytopenia.
13. Serum iron, iron binding capacity and ferritin as a baseline prior to chronic transfusion therapy.

Initial Management of Aplastic Anemia

1. Discontinue any potentially offending drug and use of an alternative class of agents, if essential.
2. Anemia—transfusion of leukocyte depleted, irradiated red cells as required for very severe anemia.
3. Very severe thrombocytopenia or thrombocytopenic bleeding, consider å-amino caproic acid, transfusion of platelet is required.
4. Severe neutropenia—take infect ion precautions.
5. Fever (suspected infection), microbial culture—broad-spectrum antibiotics, if specific organism not detected. Granulocyte stimulating factor (G-CSF) in severe cases.
6. If child or young adult with profound infection (e.g. Gm-negative bacteria, fungus, persistent blood cultures)—consider neutrophil transfusion from a G-CSF pretreated donor.
7. Immediate assessment for allogenic stem cell transplantation, histocompatibility testing of the patients, siblings. Search databases for unrelated donor, if appropriate.

HEMOLYTIC ANEMIA

Hemolytic anemia can be defined as accelerated destruction of RBC—producing decreased level of circulating erythrocytes (anemia).

Normally, RBC in circulation is exposed to:

i. Turbulence in blood flow
ii. Endothelial damage
iii. Age-related catabolic changes

Two types of RBC destruction produce hemolytic anemia:

i. Damaged RBCs are taken up by reticuloendothelial systems and destroyed—**extravascular hemolysis.**
ii. Damaged RBCs are destroyed in circulation.

Intravascular hemolysis: Normal RBC lifespan is 120 days. In case of hemolytic anemia, lifespan of RBC will be reduced to <100 days.

When sufficient numbers of RBCs are destroyed
↓
Oxygen delivery to tissues are impaired
↓
Tissue hypoxia leads to increased release of erythropoietin
↓
This stimulates bone marrow to produce more and more RBC
↓
Increased number of reticulocytes in peripheral blood

Causes of Hemolysis (Fig. 5.16)

Intrinsic Causes of Hemolysis

1. **Abnormal hemoglobin:**
   a. Alfa and beta thalassemia
   b. Other hemoglobinopathies
   c. Unstable hemoglobin's
2. **Membrane defect:**
   a. Hereditary spherocytosis
   b. Hereditary elliptocytosis
   c. Hereditary acanthocytosis
   d. Hemolytic uremic syndrome
   e. Macleod syndrome
   f. PNH
3. **Enzyme deficiency:**
   a. Glucose-6-phosphate dehydrogenase deficiency
   b. Pyruvate kinase deficiency
   c. Hexokinase deficiency

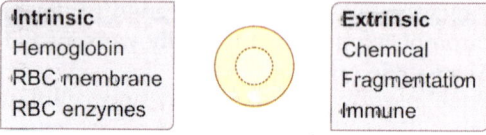

Fig. 5.16: Causes of hemolysis

Extrinsic Causes of Hemolysis

1. **Immune hemolytic anemia:**
   a. Transfusion-induced alloantibody
   b. Hemolytic disease of newborn
   c. Autoimmune syndrome
2. **Infection:**
   a. Malaria
   b. Babesosis
   c. Bartonellosis
   d. *Clostridium perfringens*
3. **Chemicals:**
   a. Oxidants   b. Snake venom
   c. Lead   d. Arsine gas
4. **Fragmentation:**
   a. Heart valves (prosthetic)
   b. DIC
   c. TTC
   d. HUS
   e. Hemodialysis
   f. Burns
   g. Drowning

h. Malignant hypertension

i. Marathon/March hemoglobinuria

5. Other causes:

a. Liver disease

b. Hypersplenism

Clinical Approach to Patients with Suspected Hemolysis

I. History:

1. Onset and duration of hemolytic anemia
2. History of fatigue
3. History of jaundice
4. Abdominal pain/cholelithiasis (chronic hemolysis)
5. Medications (may exacerbate enzyme deficiencies)
6. Travel (consider infection)
7. History of current or recent infection
8. Vascular/cardiac surgery
9. Blood loss or sequestration (increased reticulocytes in absence of hemolysis)
10. Discolored urine (intravascular hemolysis)
11. Complete family history
    i. Jaundice, ii. Gallbladder disease, iii. Splenectomy, iv. Hereditary anemia, v. Other inherited disease

II. Physical examination:

1. Pallor
2. Increased temperature
3. Rapid high volume pulse
4. Jaundice (chronic hemolysis)
5. Mechanical click from heart valves
6. Splenomegaly

III. Rule out blood loss from any sources

IV. Screening of laboratory evaluation:

a. *Complete blood count*—confirm diagnosis of anemia

b. *Review of smear* (Table 5.1)

c. *Absolute reticulocyte count:* Absolute reticulocyte count [ARC] =

$$\frac{\text{Reticulocyte percentage}}{100} \times \text{RBC count/}\mu\text{l.}$$

Normal ARC = 25,000—75,000/μl

In patient with hemolysis = >100000/μL

Normal value of reticulocyte count in newborn—2.5–6.5%

In adult—0.5 to 1.5%

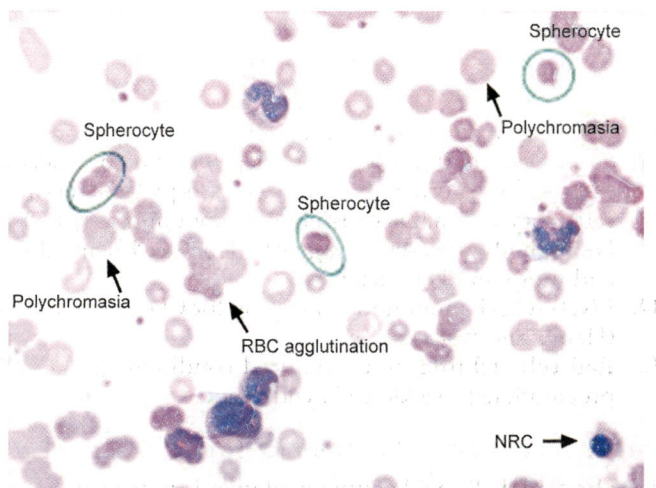

Fig. 5.17: Different shapes and character of RBC

Table 5.1: Review of smear (Fig. 5.17)

		Intrinsic	*Extrinsic*
1.	Acanthocytes	Glutathione peroxidase def. Hereditary choreoacanthocytosis Abetalipoproteinemia McLeod syndrome LCAL deficiency	Liver disease Asplenia
2.	Basophilic stippling	Hemoglobinopathies In effective erythropoiesis	Lead poisoning 5' nucleotidase deficiency
3.	Elliptocyte	G6PD deficiency Hereditary elliptocytosis Glycophorin c deficiency Pyropoikilocytosis	Malaria
4.	Heinz bodies	G6PD deficiency Thalassemia Unstable hemoglobin	Drug induced injury
5.	Parasites	x	Malaria Babesosis Bartonellosis
6.	Pyropoikilocytes	Hereditary pyropoiekilocytosis α spectrin mutation	Burns
7.	Schistocytes	x	Microangiopathic hemolytic anemia
8.	Sickle cells	Hemoglobin SS Hemoglobin SC Hemoglobin Sβ-thalassemia	x
9.	Spherocytes	Hereditary spherocytosis Ankyrin-spectrin deficiency Hemoglobin C disease Band 3 defects Protein 4.2 defect	Immune mediated hemolysis Infections Chemical injuries
10.	Stomatocyte	Hereditary stomatocytosis Rh-null disease	Alcohol intoxication Liver disease
11.	Target cell	Thalassemia Hemoglobin C disease Unstable hemoglobin	Liver disease

Stressed erythropoiesis associated with hemolysis causing release of large polychromatic reticulocytes with decreased area of central pallor are released into circulation called **shift cell.**

d. *Serum lactate dehydrogenase (LDH)*—released from hemolysed red blood cells—increased.

e. *Serum haptoglobin*—decreased because free hemoglobin is attached with haptoglobin—and taken up by liver cells.

f. *Methemoglobin*—Free hemoglobin, not bound with haptoglobin—will be oxidized to methemolglobin so its concentration will be raised in circulation.

g. *Hemoglobinuria* As the capacity of renal tubular cells is limited, excess hemoglobin filtered through glomerulus producing hemoglobinuria.

h. *Hemosiderinuria* Renal tubular cells containing hemosiderin when shed— produces hemosiderinuria, urine hemosiderin in absence of urine hemoglobin— suggest subacute or chronic intravascular hemolysis

i. *Red blood cell survival* (chromium Cr51 survival)—it can definitively demonstrate shortened RBC survival (hemolysis).

Discriminate Diagnostic Features

1. **Direct antiglobulin test**: If positive:
   a. Serum IgG specific reagents suggest warm antibody.
   b. Serum C3 specific reagents suggest cold antibody.
   c. Red cell alloantibody
2. **Cold antibody:** Examination of agglutination:
   i. Check MCV on initial blood count
   ii. Check MCV again after incubation at 37°C
      a. Mycoplasma—IgM antibody (anti-I antibody)
      b. Serology for Epstein-Barr virus (anti-I antibody)
      c. Presence of Donath-Landsteiner antibody (cold reacting IgG antibody with anti-P specificity)
3. **Warm antibody** (Fig. 5.18): IgG +ve direct antiglobulin test—examine film for spherocytes, lymphocytosis or abnormal lymphocytes—suggest myeloproliferative disorders.

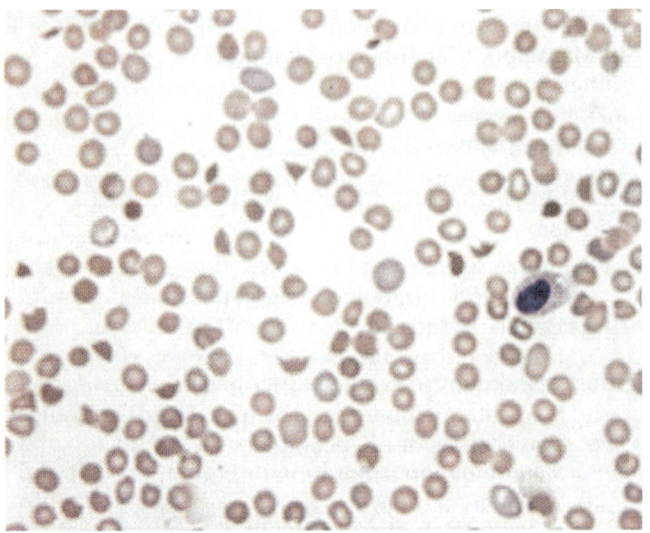

Fig. 5.19: Peripheral blood picture in HUS

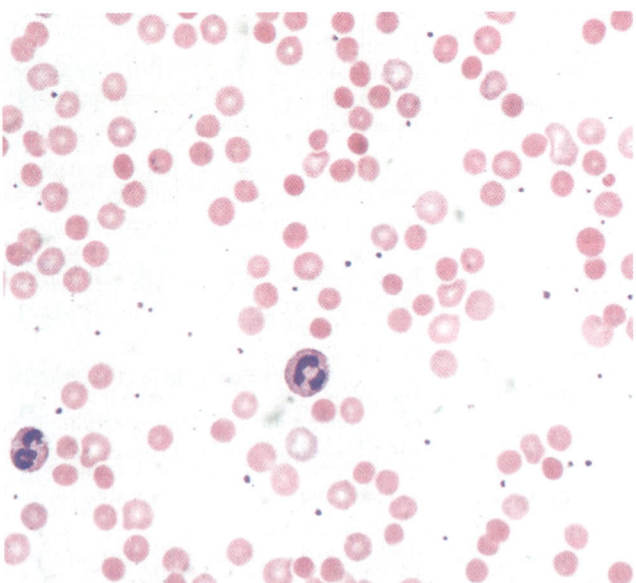

Fig. 5.18: Warm antibody hemolytic anemia

4. **Check urinary hemosiderin**—Schumm's test
5. **Sepsis**—Blood culture, urine culture
6. **Malaria**:
   i. Examination for dual antigen
   ii. Thick and thin blood film
7. **Liver abnormality**—hepatomegaly, splenomegaly, abnormal LFT
8. **Renal abnormality**—serum urea, creatinine, eGFR
9. **Low platelets**—TTP/HUS (Fig. 5.19).

10. **Hemoglobinopathy**—check hemoglobin electrophoresis
11. **Red cell membrane abnormality** (Fig. 5.20):
    i. Family history
    ii. Red cell fragility test

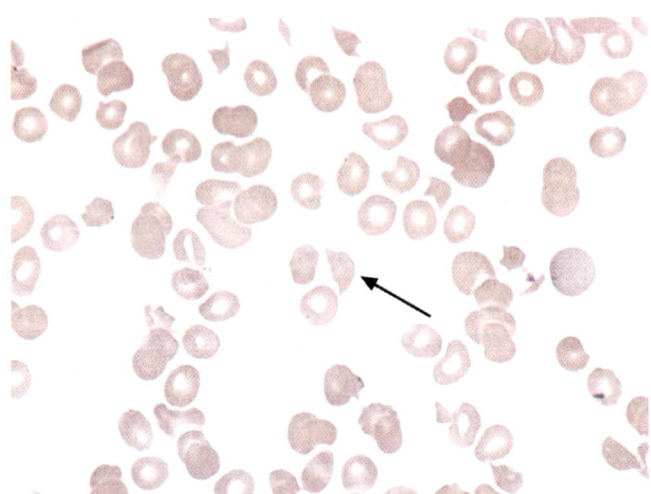

Fig. 5.20: Microangipathic hemolytic anemia

12. **Red cell enzyme disorder:** Family history
13. **G-6-PD screening**—detect deficiency of this enzyme, but results can be normal if reticulocytosis is present. (Because reticulocyte contains considerable amount of G-6-PD) **Heinz body**—present—suggests denatured hemoglobin and thus G-6-PD deficiency
14. **PNH**—check immunophenotyping for CD 55 and CD 59. (Ham's and lysis test)
15. **Red cell sickling** under reduced conditions (sickle cell preparations)—sickle cell syndrome.

Treatment of Hemolytic Anemia (Figs 5.21 and 5.22)

1. **Folic acid**: Folic acid supplementation is indicated.
2. **Corticosteroid**—in autoimmune hemolytic anemia.

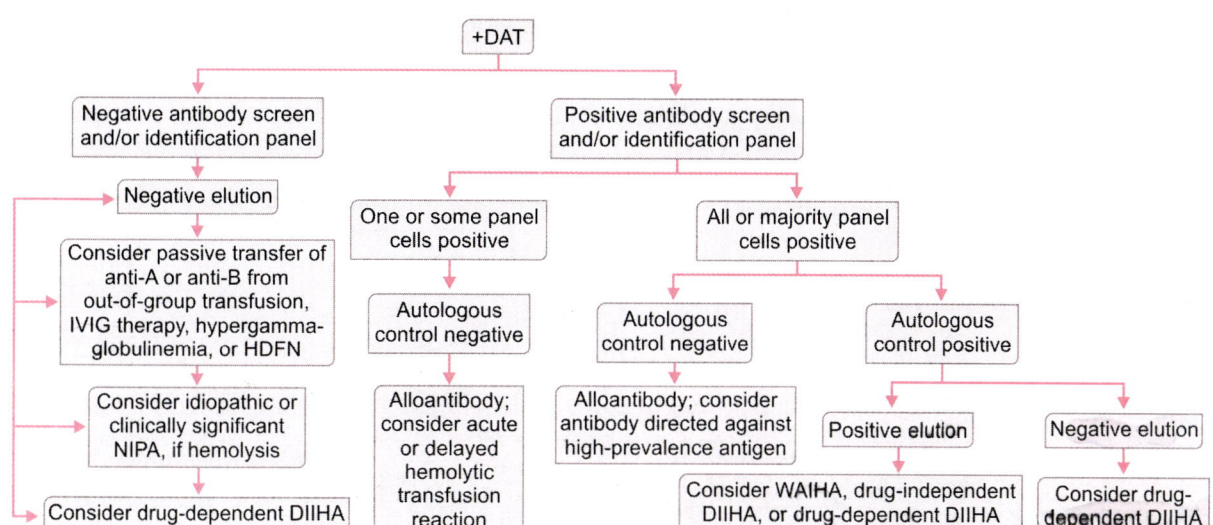

Fig. 5.21: Algorithm of drug-induced hemolytic anemia

3. **Intravenous immunoglobulin** G (IVIG)—given in patient with autoimmune hemolytic anemia—but response has been transient.
4. **Transfusion therapy:** Always avoid unless it is absolutely necessary. Transfusion is essential in patients with:
   i. Angina
   ii. Severely compromised cardiopulmonary status

   So packed RBC should be given to avoid cardiac stress.

In case of autoimmune hemolytic anemia:

i. Crossmatching is difficult. So least incompatible blood transfusion is indicated.
ii. Risk of destruction of transfused blood is high—it depends upon the rate of blood transfusion.

   So, half units of packed RBC should be transfused to avoid destruction of transfused blood.

   Iron overload due to multiple transfusions can be treated by:
1. Oral iron chelator—desferasirox, deferiprone
2. Parenteral iron chelator—desferoxamine

Discontinuation of offending drugs:
1. Penicillin   2. Cephalothin   3. Ampicillin
4. Methicillin   5. Quinine   6. Quinidine
7. Sulfa drugs in patient with G-6PD deficiency

Iron therapy:
i. Iron therapy is contraindicated in case of hemolytic anemic because as a result of hemolysis released iron will be reused.
ii. Iron therapy is indicated in patients with severe intravascular hemolysis—in which substantial iron loss occurs through hemoglobinuria.

   So before iron replacement—serum iron studies and bone marrow iron stores should be done.

Splenectomy: It is indicated in:
1. Hereditary spherocytosis
2. Autoimmune hemolytic anemia

   It is not recommended in—cold agglutinin hemolytic anemia

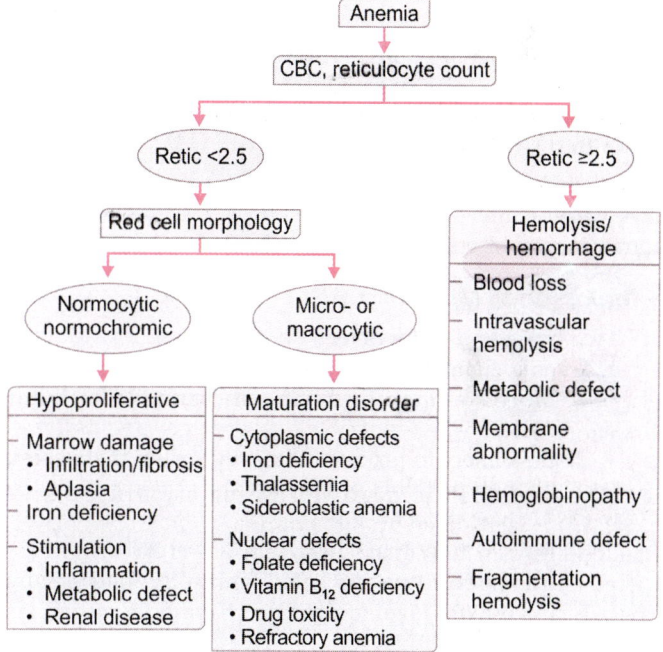

Fig. 5.22: Algorithm of anemia

THALASSEMIAS

Two types of thalassemia:
i. α thalassemia
ii. β thalassemia

α Thalassemia (Figs 5.23 and 5.24)

These are four α globin genes—two in each chromosome 16. These are designated as αα/αα.—So α thalassemia becomes more heterogeneous than β thalassemia.

α thalassemia syndromes result from deletion of a large globin gene segment from unequal crossing over or recombination or mutation.

1. Deleted segment if involve one gone (-+/++)—**silent carrier**
2. Deleted segment if involve two genes—(--/++) or (- +/- +)—α **thalassemia minor**

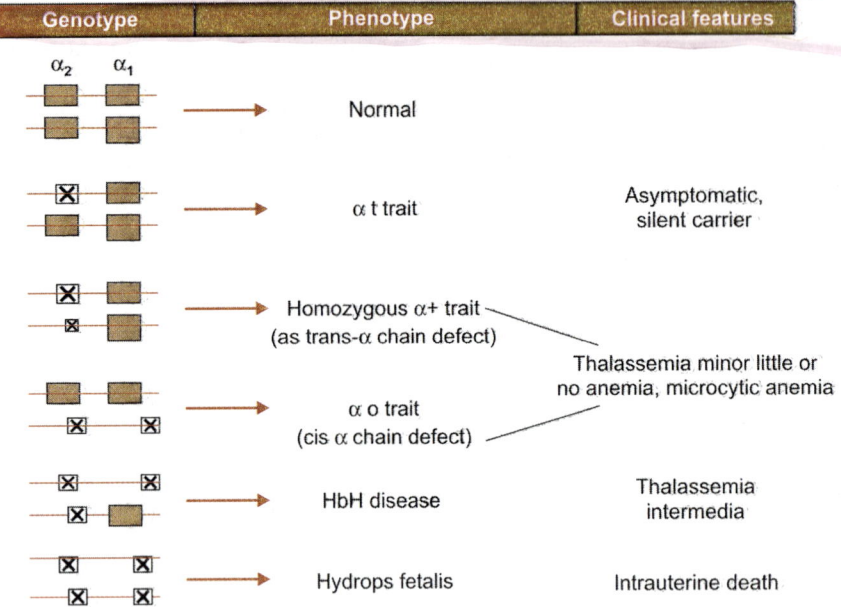

Fig. 5.23: Genotype and phenotype with clinical features in α thalassemia

3. Deleted segments—if involve three genes (--/-+)-**HbH (β4)** - It is unstable form of hemoglobin.
4. Loss of all 4 genes (--/--)—produce **hydrops fetalis with Hb Bart's (ϒ4)**

Silent carrier:
i. Asymptomatic
ii. In minority of patients ↓ MCV ↓MCH

α Thalassemia Minor *(Fig. 5.25)*

i. Two types of α chain defect:
  a. Trans-α chain defect (-+/-+)
    1. More common in Asian—Indian subcontinent. Africa
    2. Less likely to produce clinically severe thalassemia phenotype (HbH or Hb Bart's)
  b. Cis-α chain defect (--/++)
    1. More common in China, South East Asia
    2. Most likely produce clinically severe thalassaemia phenotype
ii. Elevated RBC number
iii. Normal or borderline HbA2
iv. MCH <25 pg
v. MCV <78 micron
vi. Requires no therapy

Hemoglobin H Disease

i. **Three α genes are deleted**, only one functional copy of α globin chain/cell
ii. **Clinical pictures**—variable:
  a. Anemia
  b. Jaundice
  c. Hepatosplenomegaly
  d. Chronic leg ulcers
  e. Recurrent infection
  f. Drugs treatment and pregnancy may worsen anemia.
iii. **Blood film shows:**
  1. Hypochromia
  2. Target cells

3. Increased reticulocytes.
4. Brilliant cresol blue stain will show—Hb H inclusions (tetramer of β globin β_4).
5. Hb pattern consists of 2–40% HbH (β_4) with some HbA, HbA_2 and HbF.
6. Peripheral blood smear in HbH disease—can be stained with cresol blue to show HbH precipitates in erythrocytes and reticulocytes

iv. **Treatment:**
  1. Prompt treatment of infection
  2. Regular folic acid supplementation
  3. Regular monitoring—may require blood transfusion
  4. May require splenectomy

Hemoglobin Bart's Hydrops Fetalis *(Fig. 5.26)*

i. Deletion of all 4 α genes occurs (Yu)
ii. Yu chain binds oxygen very tightly—resultant poor tissue oxygenation
iii. Fetus is either stillborn (at 34–40 weeks of gestation) or dies after birth
iv. **Clinical features:**
  a. Pale, distended
  b. Jaundice
  c. Marked hepatosplenomegaly
  d. Ascites
v. **Blood picture:**
  a. Hemoglobin is 6.0 g/dl
  b. Film shows:
    1. Hypochromic RBC
    2. ↑ reticulocytes
    3. Target cells
  c. Neucleated reed cells
  d. Hemoglobin electrophoresis—shows:
    1. Hb Bart's
    2. Absent HbA
    3. Absent HbA_2
    4. Absent HbF.

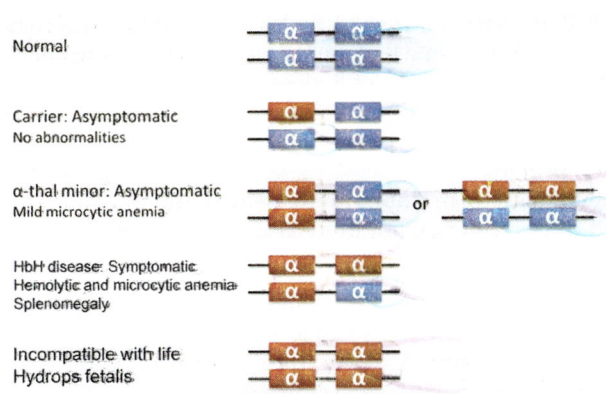

Fig. 5.24: Alpha-thalassemia—genetics and clinical consequences

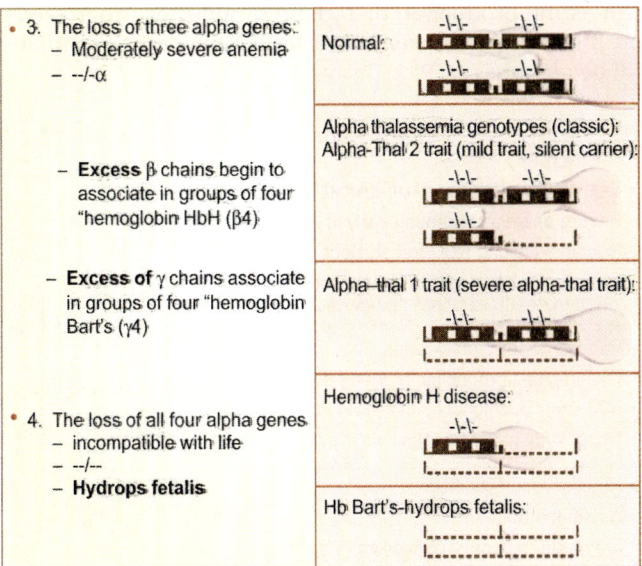

Fig. 5.25: α-Thalassemia

β Thalassemia

There are only two β genes—one on each chromatid of chromosome 11.

1. Abnormality in one β globin gene—results β thalassemia trait or β thalassemia intermedia—here synthesis of β chain is reduced to half, no accumulation of excess ∝ chain
2. Abnormality in both β globin gene results in β thalassemia major (Cooley's anemia)

β Thalassemia Minor

1. **Prevalent** in Mediterranean region, Middle East, India, Pakistan and South-East Asia.
2. **Carrier state**
3. **Blood picture:**
   i. Hb% <10.0 gm/dl.
   ii. MCV—63–77 fl
   iii. MCH <25 pg
   iv. Reticulocyte count ↑
   v. *Blood film*—microcytic hypochromic RBC target cell Basophilic stippling
   vi. *Hemoglobin electrophoresis:* ↑ HbA2 ($\alpha_2\Upsilon_2$)—useful diagnostic test for β thalassemia trait
   vii. *Serum iron and ferritin*—normal or increased
   viii. *Bone marrow*—6x the number of erythroid precursor
   ix. *Free erythrocyte porphyrin* (FEP) test is useful in situation, where the diagnosis of beta thalassemia is unclear. Because:
       a. FEP is normal in beta thalassemia trait
       b. FEP is elevated in iron deficiency anemia and leads poisoning.
   x. Mentzer index (defined as mean corpuscular volume per red cell count) less than 13 suggest thalassemia trait, more than 13 suggest iron deficiency anemia.
4. **Treatment**—not usually required

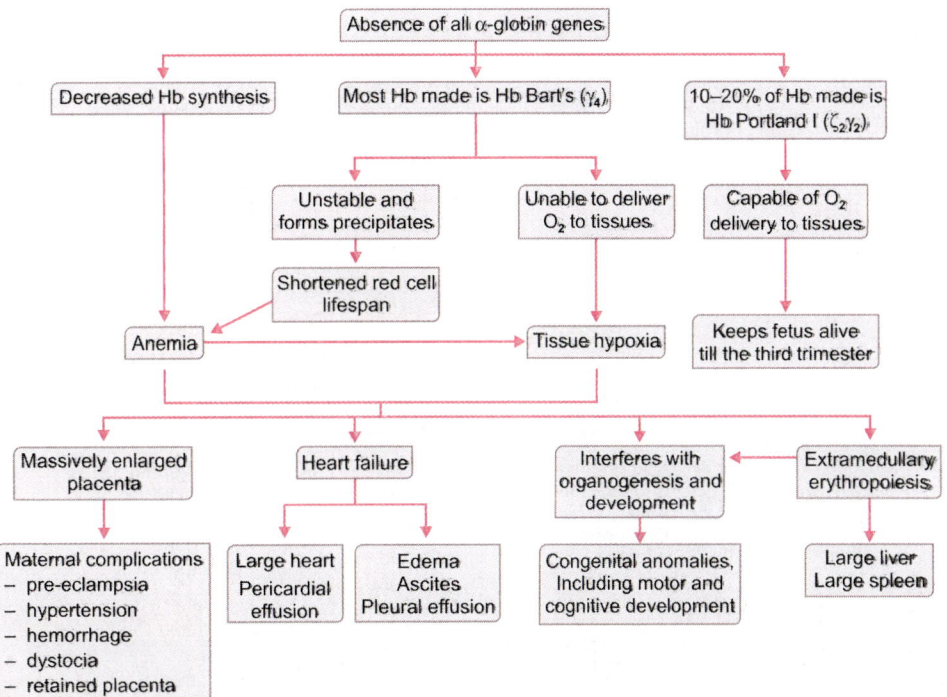

Fig. 5.26: Algorithm of loss of all alfa globin chains

β-thalassemia Intermedia

1. Symptoms like β thalassemia major but with moderate degree of anemia (10–12 g/dl).
2. Hepatosplenomegaly
3. Features of iron overload
4. Severe anemia in some cases, although not requiring regular blood transfusion.
5. Impaired growth
6. Skeletal deformities
7. Chronic leg ulceration

Blood picture:

 i. Elevation of HbF
 ii. Coinheritance of α thalassemia
 iii. Coinheritance of β thalassemia with Hb Lepore
 iv. Hb <6 gm/dl
 v. MCV ↓
 vi. MCH—normal or low

Treatment: Depends on severity, patient may require:

 i. Intermittent blood transfusion
 ii. Fe chelator
 iii. Folic acid supplementation
 iv. Prompt treatment of infection

β-thalassemia Major *(Figs 5.27–5.29)*

There are **two copies of β globin gene** in each cell. β thalassemia affects both β globin genes.

Defect can be complete absence of β globin protein **(β° thalassemia)** or **severely reduced synthesis of β globin** protein **(β plus thalassemia)**

Genetic defect may be (Fig. 5.30):

 i. Missence or nonsense mutation in beta globin gene, or
 ii. Genetic deletion of β globin gene and surrounding regions.

In β thalassemia minor (β thalassemia trait or heterozygous carrier type)—one β globin gene is defective—results in 50% decrease in synthesis of β globin protein.

In β thalassemia major (homozygous β thalassemia), both globin genes are defective—so severely impaired synthesis of β globin protein.

In β thalassemia minor, no excess α chain.

In β thalassemia major, there is excess α chain

This α-globin chain precipitates in developing RBC and damage the wall and results in intravascular hemolysis
↓
Premature destruction of erythroid precursors results in intramedullary ineffective erythropoiesis.

At birth, there is excess production of ϒ chain. But after birth as the production of ϒ chain diminishes progressively, and β globin production increases, so the effect of mutation will be obvious.

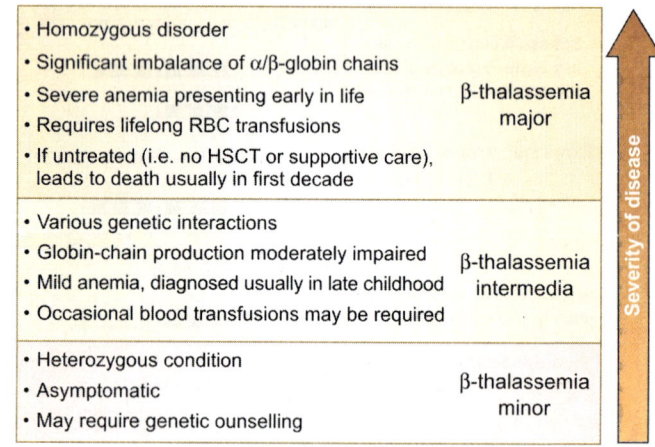

Fig. 5.27: Clinical classification of beta thalassemia

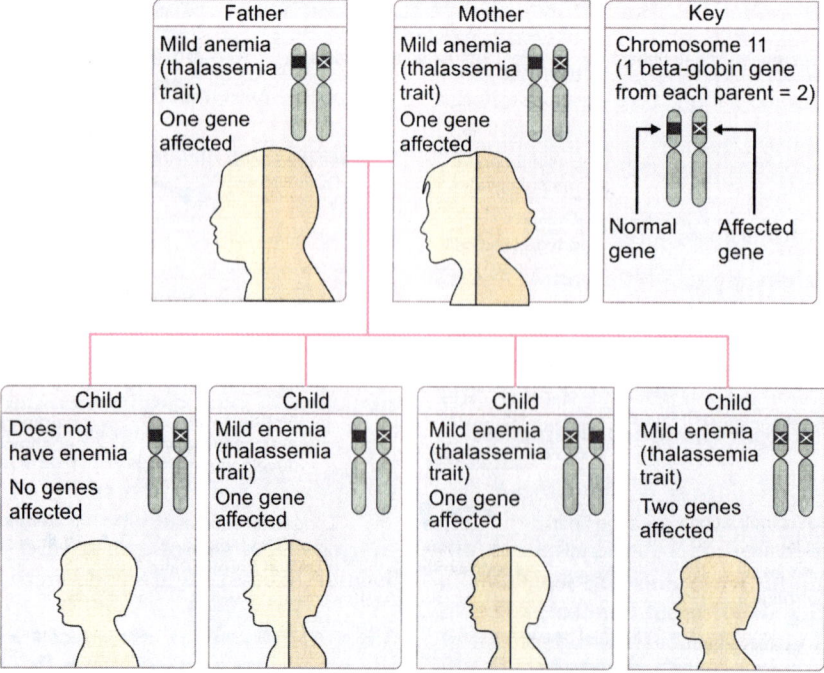

Fig. 5.28: Inheritance of beta thalassemia

Patients with coinheritance of α thalassemia have a milder clinical course—because they have less severe α-β chain imbalance.

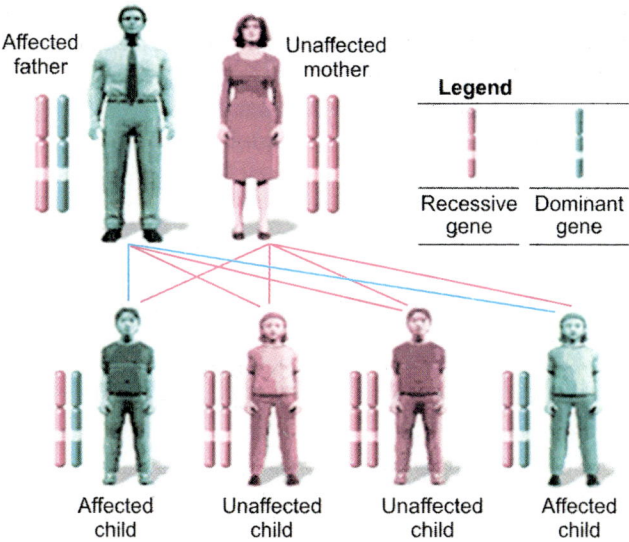

Fig. 5.29: Inheritance of beta thalassemia

Epidemiology

1. This disease is found must commonly in Mediterranean region, Africa, Southeast Asia.
2. Patients of Mediterranean area are β thalassemia trait. But African patients are β thalassemia.
3. Manifestations of the disease may not be apparent until a complete switch from fetal to adult hemoglobin synthesis.

Physical Examination

1. Skin—pallor from anemia, jaundice from hyperbilirubinemia
2. Skull—flat bones and other bones may be deformed secondary to erythroid hyperplasia with intramedullary expansion and cortical bone thinning.
3. Skull radiograph shows 'hair on head' appearance—reflecting intense marrow activity of skull bones.
4. Cardiac examination—may reveal—cardiac failure and arrhythmia—due to severe anemia and iron overload.
5. Abdominal examination reveals:
   i. Hepatomegaly—due to:
      a. Extramedullary hematopoiesis
      b. Multiple blood transfusion
      c. Chronic iron overload
   ii. Splenomegaly—due to:
      a. Extramedullary hematopoiesis
      b. Hypertrophic response to extravascular hemolysis
   iii. Gallbladder contains bilirubin stones
6. Endocrine dysfunction: Iron overload can produce dysfunction of:
   i. Pancreas
   ii. Testes
   iii. Thyroid
7. Portal hypertension due to transfusion induced CLD

Investigations (Fig. 5.31)

1. Blood picture shows:
   i. Moderate to severe anemia 3–6 gm%
   ii. ↓ MCV, <70 fl. MCH <25 pg.
   iii. Increased reticulocytosis

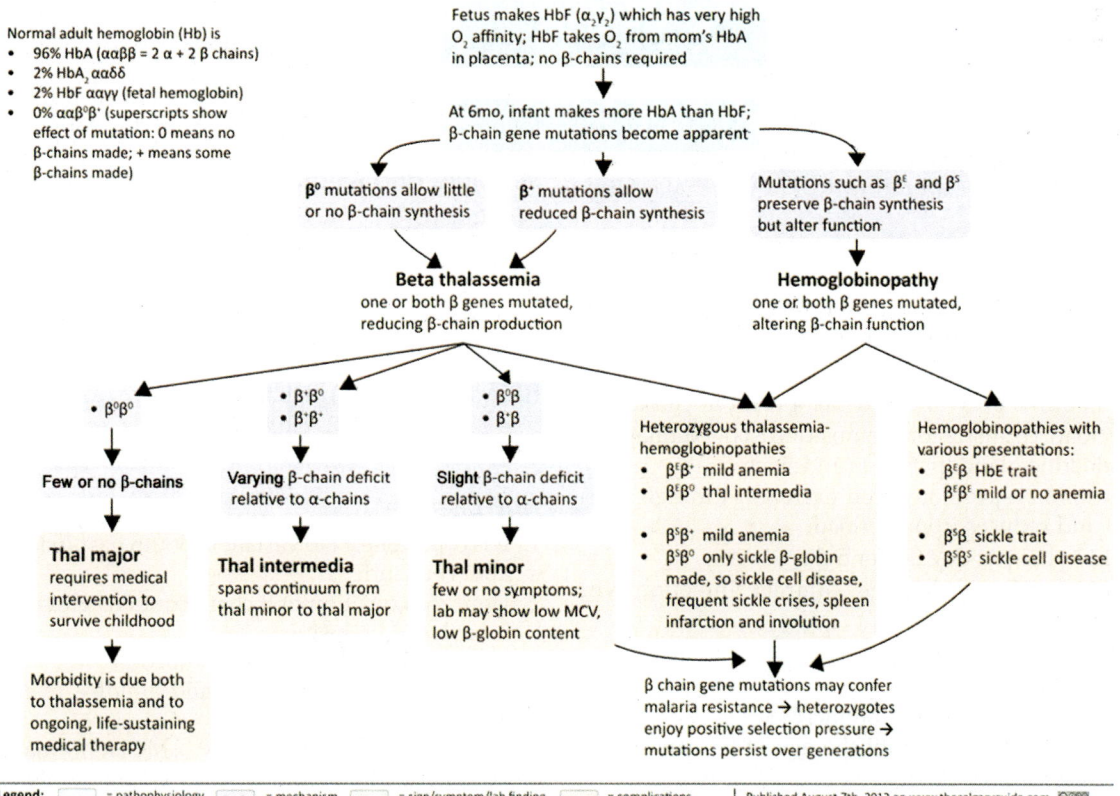

Fig. 5.30: Pathogenesis of beta thalassemia and associated hemoglobinopathies

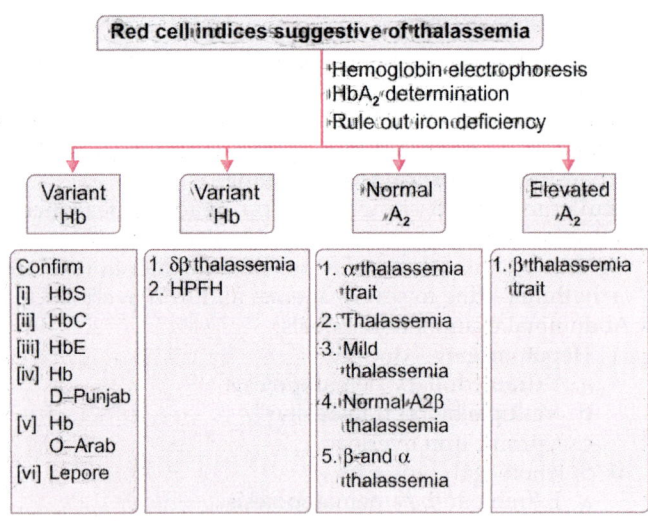

Fig. 5.31: Diagnostic scheme of thalassemia

2. Blood film shows:
   a. Anisocytosis
   b. Poikilocytosis
   c. Target cells
   d. Nucleated red blood cells
3. Methyl violet stain shows RBC inclusions containing precipitated α globin
4. Hemoglobin electrophoresis shows: Mainly HbF ($\alpha_2 \Upsilon_2$) 4–7%, no Hb A.
   In some β thalassemia, there may be little HbA ($\alpha_2 \beta_2$).
   HbA2 may be mildly elevated ($\alpha_2 \delta_2$) >3.5%.

Prenatal Diagnosis

1. Analysis of DNA obtained via chorionic villi sampling at 8–10 weeks of fetal gestation.
2. Amniocentesis at 14 to 20 weeks of gestation.
3. DNA is amplified using the PCR assay test, then is analyzed for the presence of thalassemia mutation using oligonucleotide probes corresponding to known thalassemia mutation.

Management

1. Regular lifelong blood transfusion (every 2–4 weeks) to maintain hemoglobin level at 9–10 gm/dl—it:
   i. Suppresses ineffective erythropoiesis
   ii. Allows normal growth and development in childhood
2. Iron overload (transfusion hemosiderosis)—damages—heart, endocrine gland, pancreas and liver.
   Desferrioxamine—promotes iron excretion through urine and stool and reduces iron overload.
   Dose: 8–12 hours per day SC for 5 days/week
   Complications: Renal damage, cataract, infection with Yersinia species.
3. **Splenectomy**—Indications:
   i. Massive splenomegaly
   ii. Increasing transfusion requirements
   But it should be avoided until the age of 5 years due to increased risk of infection.
4. **Bone marrow transplantation**—allogenic using sibling donor, HLA matched

Good results in young patient with β thalassemia major. Mortality and morbidity:
   i. Procedure related
   ii. GVHD
5. **Increase in HbF using 5 azacytidine or hydroxycarbamide should ameliorate symptom**.

Iron chelation therapies:
A. **Desferrioxamine**—parenteral painful, complain problem
   Side effects:
   1. GI symptoms
   2. Raised creatinine
   3. Cytopenia.
B. **Deferiprone:** Orally given in three divided doses.
   Side effect:
   1. Arthralgia   2. Nausea
   3. Other GI symptoms   4. Derangement of LFT
   5. Leukopenia
   6. Zinc deficiency desferrioxamine

GENETIC CONTROL OF HEMOGLOBIN PRODUCTION

Hemoglobin comprises 4 protein subunits—each unit linked to heme group.

Globin chain genes are located in chromosomes 11 and 16.
All related to α globin are located in chromosome 16.
All related to β globin are located in chromosome 11.

The sequences in which they are produced during development reflect their physical order on chromosomes, e.g.

ζ is the 1st α like globin to be produced in life.
   ↓
When ζ globin production stops—α chain starts production.

On chromosome 11, arrangement of β like globin is as follows: ε → Υ - δ - β starting from development.

Structure and Quantity of Normal Hemoglobin

I. Embryo	1. Hb Gower 1	$\zeta_2 \epsilon_2$	
	2. Hb Gower 1	$\alpha_2 \epsilon_2$	
	3. Hb Portland	$\zeta_2 \Upsilon_2$	
II. Fetus	1. HbF	$\zeta_2 \Upsilon_2$	– 85%
	2. HbA	$\alpha_2 \beta_2$	– 5–10%
III. Adult	1. HbA	$\alpha_2 \beta_2$	– 97%
	2. HbA$_2$	$\alpha_2 \zeta_2$	– 2.5%
	3. HbF	$\alpha_2 \Upsilon_2$	– 0.5%

HbE Disease

1. It is commonest Hb variant in South East Asia, India, Burma, and Thailand.
2. Here 26th position of β chain contains glutamic acid which is replaced by lysine.
3. May produce thalassemia syndrome.
4. Clinical features—anemia, mild jaundice, liver and spleen—normal
5. Blood picture shows: ↓MCV, ↓MCH, normal reticulocytes
6. Peripheral blood picture shows: Target cells, hypochromic and microcytic red cells
7. Treatment is not usually required.

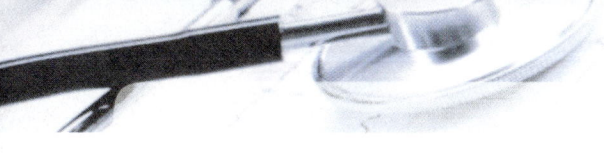

HbD Disease

1. It is found in North West India, Pakistan, and Iran
2. Here glutamic acid in 21st position of β chain is replaced by lysine.
3. Film shows—target cells

HbC Disease

1. It is found in West Africa
2. Here glutamic acid at 6th position of β chain will be replaced by lysine
3. Anemia, splenomegaly—common
4. Gallstones are recognized complication.
5. Hematological investigation
   i. Mild decrease in Hb
   ii. MCV, MCH ↓
   iii. Reticulocyte count ↑
6. Blood film—i. prominent target cells, ii. HbC crystals
7. Hemoglobin electrophoresis—HbC and some HbF. HbA—is absent.
8. Care should be taken during anesthesia.

Unstable Hemoglobin

It is congenital Heinz body hemolytic anemia caused by—point mutation in globin genes.

Here precipitate in red blood cells during oxidative stress—producing Heinz bodies.

In normal hemoglobin, there are non-covalent bonds maintaining hemoglobin structure. During stress, loss of bonds leads to hemoglobin desaturation and precipitation.

As a result of production of Heinz bodies and precipitation, there is deformity of RBC and reduction of lifespan.

It is predominantly **autosomal dominant**. It mainly affects β chain.

Clinical Features

i. Well compensated hemolysis
ii. Hb% may be normal
iii. Jaundice, splenomegaly
iv. Hemolysis exacerbated by infection and oxidant drugs.

Investigation

i. Hb—normal or mildly low.
ii. MCV ↓
iii. *Film:* Hypochromic RBC, polychromatic RBC, basophilic stippling
iv. Heinz bodies seen post-splenectomy
v. Reticulocyte ↑
vi. Demonstrable unstable Hb with heat and stress
vii. Hemoglobin electrophoresis—normal
viii. Estimation P_{50} is helpful

Management

i. Mostly benign course
ii. Recommended regular folic acid supplementation
iii. Splenectomy is helpful in some patients with severe hemolysis
iv. Avoidance of stress

Hb Lepore

i. It is caused by fused globin chain consisting of N-terminal half of δ chain and C-terminal half of β chain.

ii. It is typical present in Greeks or Italian.
iii. It can occur alone or associated with β-thalassemia.

Hb Constant Spring

i. It is caused by point mutation in the stop codon of ∝ chain mRNA leading to an elongated α china ($∝^{cs}$)
ii. Because synthesis of $∝^{cs}$ is reduced—Hb constant spring behaves like α chain deletion.

DRUG-INDUCED HAEMOLYTIC ANEMIA

This type of hemolytic anemia is either immune or non-immune. **The following mechanisms are:**

I. **Some drugs interfere with lipid component** of RBC membrane
II. **Oxidation and denaturation of hemoglobin**—mainly in G6PD deficiency subjects: Dapsone, sulfasalazine
III. **Hapten mechanism**—describes interactions between certain drugs and RBC membrane components acting as antigen which stimulate antibody production: Direct antiglobulin test is +ve.

   Drugs are:
   • Penicillin
   • Cephalosporin
   • Tetracycline
   • Tobutamide

IV. **Antibody-mediated hemolytic anemia**—warm antibody-mediated hemolysis—direct antiglobulin test +ve

   The drugs are: Quinine, quinidine, rifampicin, tetracycline, melphalan, probenacid, cefotaxim.

Laboratory Diagnosis

Findings of autoimmune hemolytic anemia, low hemoglobin, increased reticulocyte.

Treatment

1. Discontinue offending drugs
2. In DAT +ve with hemolysis no need to stop unless hemolysis
3. Blood transfusion in case of severe hemolysis or patient is symptomatic

METHEMOGLOBINEMIA

Ferrous form of iron is able to bind oxygen. But ferric form of iron (oxidized form)—called methemolgobin (Fig. 5.32) is unable to bind O_2 leading to poor tissue oxygenation. In healthy individual, methemoglobin should be <3% of total hemoglobin. It may be congenital or acquired.

Congenital

1. **HbM**—due to α and β globin mutation, iron becomes stabilized in ferric form.
2. **Met Hb reductase deficiency:** Clinical features: cyanosis from infancy. PaO_2 is normal.

Acquired

When RBC is exposed to oxidizing agent producing methemoglobinemia.

The drugs are: Phenacetin, lignocaine, inorganic nitrates. Patient may experience severe tissue hypoxia.

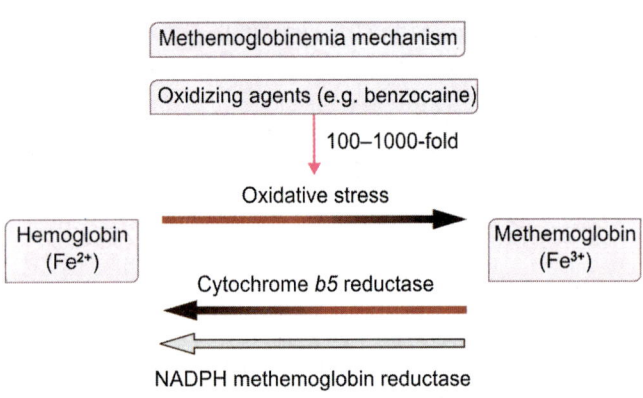

Fig. 5.32: Process of conversion to methemoglobin

Symptoms

Symptoms of methemoglobinemia are described in Table 5.2.

Table 5.2: Symptoms of methemoglobinemia		
Methemoglobin concentration	*% Total hemoglobin**	*Symptoms^*
<1.5 g/dl	10%	None
1.5–3.0 g/dl	10–20%	Cyanotic skin discoloration
3.0–4.5 g/dl	20–30%	Anxiety, lightheadedness, headache, tachycardia
4.5–7.5 g/dl	30–50%	Fatigue, confusion, dizziness, tachypnea, tachycardia
7.5–10.5 g/dl	50–70%	Coma, seizures, arrhythmias, acidosis
>10.5 g/dl	>70%	Death

*Assumes hemoglobin = 15 g/dl. Patients with lower hemoglobin concentrations may experience more severe symptoms for a given percentage of methemoglobin level

^Patients with underlying cardiac, pulmonary, or hematologic disease may experience more severe symptoms for a given methemoglobin concentration

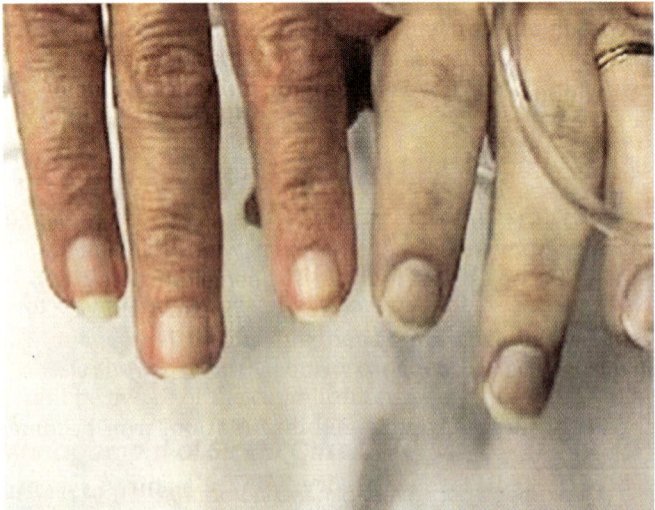

Fig. 5.33: Nail condition in methemoglobinemia

Diagnosis

1. History of exposure to oxidant drugs or chemicals
2. Spectrophotometry or hemoglobin electrophoresis will demonstrate methemalbumin (Fig. 5.34).

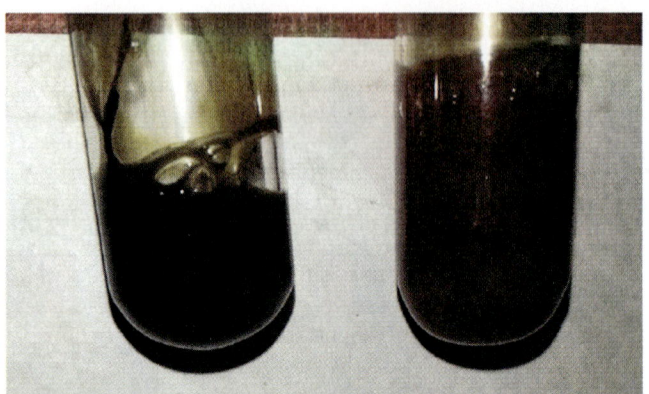

Fig. 5.34: Color of blood in methemoglobinemia

Treatment

1. **Congenital HbM disease**—can be treated by:
   i. Ascorbate
   ii. Methylene blue
2. **Acquired HbM disease**—can be treated by:
   a. Removal of oxidant drugs
   b. Administration of methylene blue (Fig. 5.35)
   c. Exchange blood transfusion in severely affected patients.

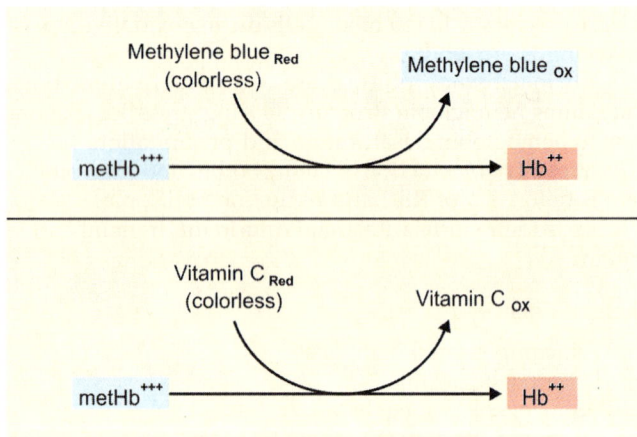

Fig. 5.35: Administration of methylene blue

GLUCOSE-6-PHOSPHATE DEHYDROGENASE DEFICIENCY

Pathophysiology

G-6-PD is involved in pentose phosphate shunt pathway. It generates NADP and NADPH and glutathione—which maintain integrity of RBC membrane.

In absence of G-6-PD, there is oxidant damage to RBC components.

Epidemiology

i. It is X-linked.
ii. Affect predominantly males, females are carrier.

Features

i. In response to oxidants and infection—hemolysis
ii. With exposure to Faba beans—acute episodes of hemolysis
iii. Methemoglobinemia
iv. Neonatal jaundice

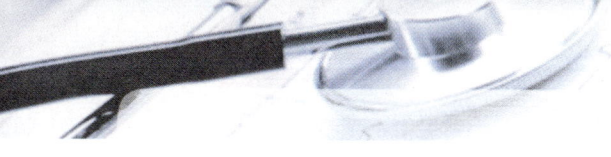

Three main forms of diseases, those associated with:
1. Acute intermittent hemolytic anemia
2. Chronic hemolytic anemia
3. No risk of hemolytic anemia

Mechanisms

Oxidants
↓
Hemoglobin is denatured
↓
Methemoglobin
↓
Heinz bodies
↓
Precipitates in RBC
↓
RBC less deformable
↓
Trapped in splenic pulp
↓
Hemolysis

Enzymes—two types:
1. G-6-PD-B normal, most prevalent, worldwide
2. G-6-PD-A differs from B in one amino acid
3. G-6-PD-A mutant variety—two types:
   i. G-6-PD-A (+) normal activity—in black individual
   ii. G-6-PD-A (–) defective—African origin
   Drugs involved in hemolysis due to G-6-PD deficiency

Definite Risk

A. Antimalarial drugs:
   i. Primaquine
   ii. Pamaquine.
B. Analgesic:
   i. Aspirin
   ii. Phenacetin
C. Others:
   i. Dapsone
   ii. Methylene blue
   iii. Nitrofurantoin
   iv. Quinolone—ciprofloxacin, nalidixic acid
   v. Sulphonamide—co-trimoxazole

Possible Risk

A. Chloroquine
B. Probenecid
C. Quinine and quinidine

Drug-induced Hemolysis in G-6-PD Deficiency

1. Begins 1–3 days after ingestion of drugs
2. Anemia—most severe 7–10 days after ingestion
3. Low back and abdominal pain
4. Dark or sometimes black urine
5. Red cell shows Heinz body inclusion
6. Self-limiting hemolysis
7. Severity is dose related

Hemolysis due to Infection or Fever

1. Begins 1–2 days after onset of infection
2. Mild anemia
3. More common in pneumonic illness

Neonatal Jaundice

1. May develop kernicterus—possible permanent brain damage
2. Rare in A(–) variants
3. More common in Mediterranean or Chinese variants

Laboratory Investigations

1. In steady state—RBC normal in site and shape
2. In drug induced hemolysis—Heinz bodies in RBC
3. Spherocytes and RBC fragments in film (in severe hemolysis)
4. ↑ Reticulocytes
5. ↑ Uncojugated bilirubin LDH, urobilinogen
6. ↓ Haptoglobin
7. Direct antiglobulin test –ve

Management

1. Avoid oxidant drugs
2. Blood transfusion in severe hemolysis.
3. IV fluid to maintain normal urine output
4. Exchange transfusion in infants
5. Folic acid supplements
6. Splenectomy in severe recurrent hemolysis.

CRYOGLOBULINEMIA

Classifications and Pathogenesis

Three types are:
1. **Type-1** i. Single monoclonal IgM, less often IgG
              ii. Associated hematological disorders
2. **Type-2** i. Polyclonal IgG + monoclonal IgM
              ii. Rheumatoid factor activity (anti-IgG)
3. **Type-3** i. Polyclonal IgG and IgM
              ii. Small monoclonal component

Types 2 and 3 are called mixed cryoglobulinemia.

Mixed cryoglobulinemia is associated with:
i. HCV infection
ii. B cell clonal expansion leading to lymphoproliferative disorder.

This cryoglobulinemia is associated with:
i. Lymphoproliferative disorder
ii. Hematological disorder
iii. Autoimmune diseases
iv. Infections
v. Renal disorders
vi. Liver disorders

Clinical Features

1. **Type-1 associated with:** Signs of peripheral vessel obstruction and hyperviscosity (Fig. 5.36):
   a. Purpura
   b. Acrocyanosis
   c. Raynaud's phenomenon
   d. Leg ulcers
   e. Gangrene
   f. Dystrophic manifestation
   All above signs are due to precipitation of paraprotein at low temperature.

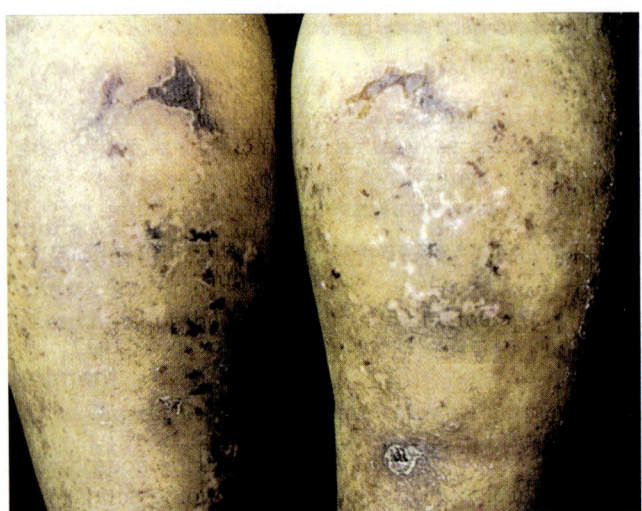

Fig. 5.36: Clinical picture in cryoglobulinemia

2. **Mixed cryoglobulinemia**—characterized by (Fig. 5.37):
   a. Purpura
   b. Arthralgia with multisystem involvement like—chronic hepatitis, glomerulonephritis, peripheral neuropathy.

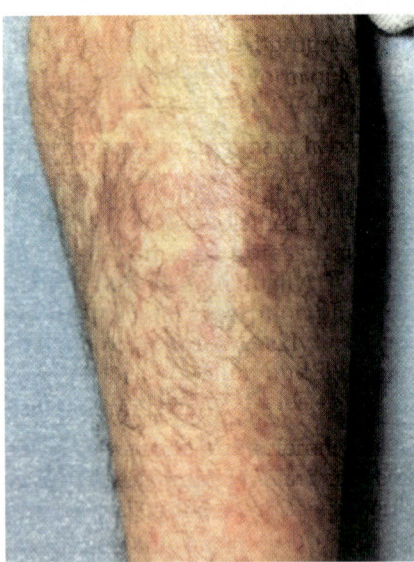

Fig. 5.37: Purpuric rash of lower extremities

Diagnosis

Precipitation of protein at 2–4°C in serum prepared from blood collected and allowed to clot at 37°C.

Treatment

1. Type-1—treat underlying MM, WM or CLL avoid cold
2. HCV related MC—Interferon ± ribavirin to eradicate HCV
3. Non-HCV related MC—Low dose prednisolone and analgesia—mild symptoms
   Severe symptoms—CTX ± prednisolone ± plasmapheresis

COLD HEMAGGLUTININ DISEASE

This disease is characterized by—acrocyanosis in cold weather due to agglutination antibody and RBC complex in the blood vessels in the skin.

Pathophysiology

RBC combines with antibody at temperature <32°C
↓
Complement is activated
↓
Lysis of RBC
↓
Hemoglobinemia
↓
Hemoglobinuria

Risk factors: Mycoplasma infection, Epstein-Barr virus infection.

Clinical Pictures

1. Elderly are involved.
2. Acrocyanosis—in cold conditions
3. Splenomegaly

Diagnosis

a. Anemia
b. ↑Reticulocytes
c. Neutrophilia
d. Hemoglobinemia
e. Hemoglobinuria
f. Direct antiglobulin test—with C_3 complement +ve
g. Immune electrophoresis—IgG or IgM
h. Specific antibody to detect etiology
   i. Anti-I   *Mycoplasma pneumoniae*
   ii. Anti-I   Infectious mononucleosis
i. ↑ LDI+
j. ↓Serum haptoglobin

Treatment

i. Warm environment
ii. Cyclophosphamide or chlorambucil—in case of etiology—lymphoma
iii. Plasma exchange in some cases
iv. In case of emergency—exchange transfusion
v. Splenectomy—in a few cases
   Liver is main site of RBC sequestration of C3b-coated RBCs.

HEREDITARY ELLIPTOCYTOSIS (Fig. 5.38)

It is heterogeneous group of disorders with elliptical RBCs. Three major groups are:
   i. Hereditary elliptocytosis   ii. Spherocytic HE
iii. South East Asian ovalocytosis.

Pathophysiology

Partial, complete deficiency or structural abnormality of protein 4.1 or absence of glycophorin C.
   Mutations occur in α-spectrin, β pectrin and band 4.1 genes

Clinical Pictures

1. May be asymptomatic
2. Few patients have chronic symptomatic anemia
3. In homozygous state, haemolysis may be lifelong and exacerbated by acute or chronic illness.
4. In heterozygous state—persons are asymptomatic

Diagnosis

1. May have positive family history
2. Blood film shows—increased elliptical or oral RBCs
3. Reticulocytosis
4. Increased LDH
5. Increased uncojugated bilirubin, urinary urobilinogen
6. Decreased haptoglobin in blood
7. Osmotic fragility test—normal
8. Direct antiglobulin test with daunorubicin –ve.

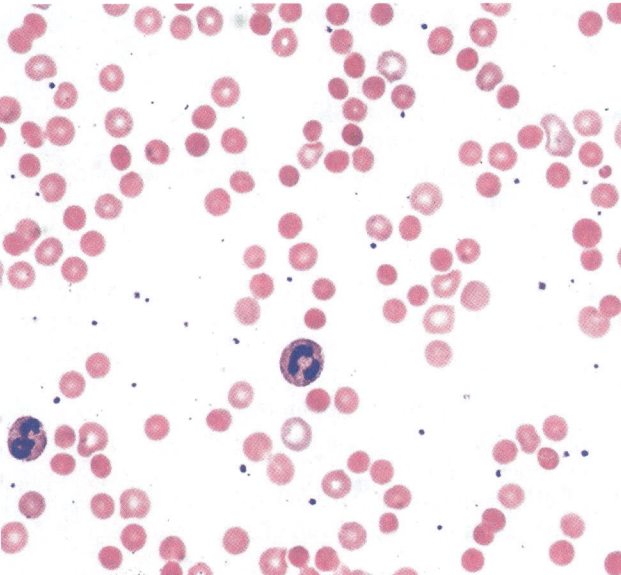

Fig. 5.39: Spherocytes

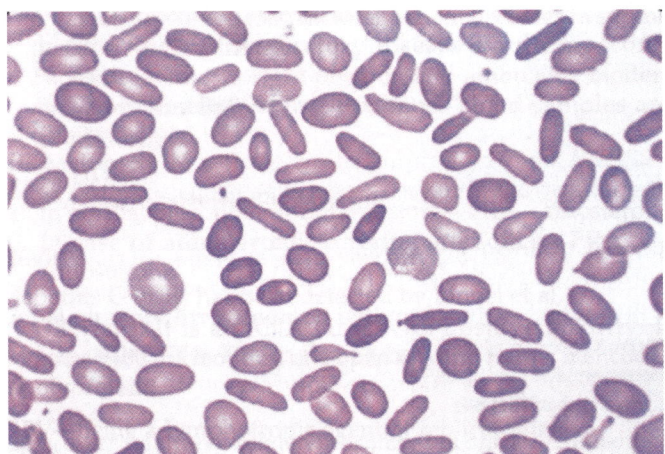

Fig. 5.38: Elliptocytosis

Complications

i. Gallstone formation
ii. Folate deficiency

Treatment

1. Supportive treatment—control of infection, folate supplementation.
2. Curative—splenectomy

HEREDITARY SPHEROCYTOSIS

Most common inherited defect in RBC membrane characterized by:
1. Variable degree of hemolysis
2. Spherocytic RBC (Figs 5.39 and 5.40)
3. Increased osmotic fragility

Pathophysiology

Mutation of gene that encodes the components of erythroid cytoskeleton—(α and β spectrin, ankyrin, band 3, protein 4.2)
↓
Loss of lipid layer from RBC membrane
↓
RBC becomes spherical with reduced surface area
↓
Get trapped in splenic cord
↓
RBC have reduced life span

RBC membranes have increased sodium permeability (loss of intracellular Na⁺)

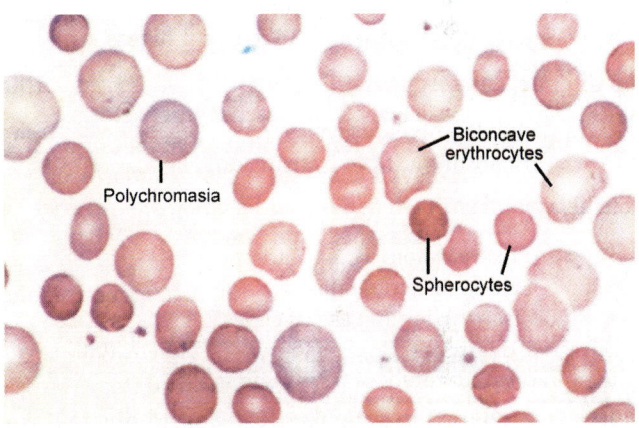

Fig. 5.40: Spherocytes (high magnification)

So RBC uses more energy to restore the Na⁺ balance hence RBCs are less deformable than normal.

Epidemiology

i. Usually autosomal dominant, but autosomal recessive inheritance has been reported.
ii. Mostly occurs in northern European descent

Clinical Presentation

1. Present at any age
2. Spectrum of presentation having asymptomatic at one end of spectrum and severe anemia at other end
3. In 60% of patients—positive family history has been reported.
4. Patients are usually present in child hood.
5. Clinical trial of: i. Anemia, ii. Jaundice, iii. Splenomegaly
6. Aplastic crises may occur with parvovirus B19 infection.

Diagnosis

1. Positive family history
2. Blood film shows ↑↑ spherocytic RBCs
   Spherocytic RBC can be identified by: i. Small size, ii. Central pallor absent.

3. Anemia, increased reticulocytosis.
4. Increased LDH
5. Uncojugated bilirubin
6. Urobilinogen in urine is increased
7. Decreased haptoglobin
8. **Osmotic fragility test:** Positive in near isotonic concentration, where as normal RBC can show simply swelling in this concentration of saline.
9. **Autohemolysis test:** Since spherocytic RBC uses more glucose than normal RBC (to maintain normal shapes), incubation of RBC in serum for 48 hours show—lysis and release of large amount of hemoglobin than normal RBC.
10. **Cryohemolysis test:** Although positive, but this test is not specific for Hereditary spherocytosis.
11. **SDS-PAGE:** Can be used to defect deficiency in RBC membrane protein
12. **Genetic analysis:** DNA-based assays to defect mutations within genes for RBC membrane protein

Complications

1. Aplastic crises—due to parvovirus infection
2. Megaloblastic changes and folate deficiency.
3. Increased hemolysis during intercurrent illness
4. Gallstones
5. Leg ulcers
6. Extramedullary hematopoiesis
7. Iron overload in multiple transfusion.

Treatment

1. Supportive treatment
   a. Folic acid supplementation
   b. Blood transfusion in case of crises
2. Curative treatment: Splenectomy—In patient with severe anemia or moderately severe anemia.

It is best avoided in patients <10 years old due to risk of increased fatal infection post-splenectomy.

Prerequisite—pneumococcal vaccine—Pneumovax 23 to be taken before splenectomy.

PAROXYSMAL COLD HEMOGLOBINURIA

1. It monthly occurs in children.
2. It is triggered by viral infection.
3. It is self-limited.
4. The involved antibody—Donath-Landsteiner antibody. Its unique serological features:
   i. It has anti-P specificity
   ii. It binds to RBC at low temperature (at 4°C)
   iii. At 37°C temperature—lysis of RBC takes place in presence of complement.
5. Supportive treatment—blood transfusion.

PAROXYSMAL NOCTURNAL HEMOGLOBINURIA

This is a clonal disease of bone marrow produces clinical triad of:
   i. Intravascular hemolysis
   ii. Venous thrombosis
   iii. Aplastic anemia.

Etiopathology

Mutation of **PIG-A gene** occurring in hemopoietic stem cell.
↓
Deficient synthesis of glycoprotein moiety glycosylphosphoinositol GPI)
↓
Lack of surface protein linked to GPI on RBC membrane
↓
Absence of one protein CD 59 on erythrocyte cell
↓
Susceptibility to complement
↓
Intravascular hemolysis.

PIG-A gene containing mutant cell may be present in normal marrow—but their clonal expansion is unusual. But it occurs in:
   i. Aplastic anemia (40–50%)
   ii. Myelodysplastic syndrome (20%)

But which GPI—anchored protein is responsible is not known.

Clinical Features

1. Evidence of intravascular hemolysis—dark-colored urine sometimes patient may unotice or suppress it.
2. Feature of anemia—weakness, lethargy, ringing in ear's shortness of breath.
3. Features of venous thrombosis—acute abdominal/pain—which may recurrent—mesenteric vein thrombosis, hepatomegaly, ascites—hepatic vein thrombosis—Budd-Chiari syndrome.

Course of the Disease

   i. Without treatment median survival is 8–10 yrs.
   ii. Most common cause of death is:
      a. Venous thrombosis
      b. Intractable infection secondary to severe neutropenia.
      c. Hemorrhage from thrombocytopenia.
   iii. It may turn into aplastic anemia
   iv. It may terminate into acute myeloid leukemia.
   v. Full spontaneous recovery has been documented but—rare.

Laboratory Investigations

A. RBC:
   i. Normocytic or macrocytic anemia.
   ii. MCV it high (macrocytosis)—denotes reticulocytosis
   iii. Reticulocyte count high—20% (4,00,000/μL)
   iv. Microcytic—if chronic urinary blood loss through hemoglobinuria.
B. Blood biochemistry:
   i. Uncojugated bilirubin—raised
   ii. LDH—markedly elevated
   iii. Haptoglobin—undetectable
C. Urine—routine:
   Hemoglobinuria—it is the telltale sign of intravascular hemolysis. Since, hemoglobinuria varies from day to day and hour to hour—so serial sample of urine is usually required to confirm it.

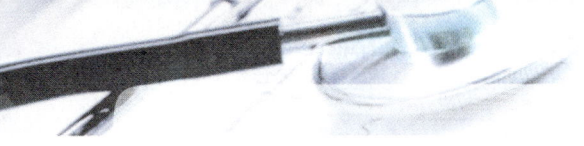

D. Bone marrow:
  i. Normocellular with massive erythroid hyperplasia.
  ii. Later on with its turn into aplastic variety—marrow becomes hypocellular.
E. Definitive diagrams of PNH: To see the hemolysis of clone of red blood cells deficient in CD59 and CD 55—on RBC surface because they are complement sensitive. The following test can be done:
  1. Sucrose hemolysis test
  2. Acidified serum (HAM) test
  3. Gold standard test—flow cytometry—can be carried out on granulocyte and red blood cells.

Bimodal distribution of cells with discrete population—CD59 and CD 55 in diagnostic of PNH.

Treatment

A. Supportive treatment:
  1. Transfusion of RBC in the form of packed cell or filtered red cells to raise the hemoglobin level.
  2. Folic acid supplementation (3 mg/day) is mandatory.
  3. Iron supplementation should be appropriate.
  4. Long-term glucocorticoid therapy is not indicated in chronic hemolysis, rather it may produce dangerous side effects.
B. Definitive treatment:
  Eculizumab: It is monoclonal antibody directed against active complement (C5).
  Benefit:
    i. Clinical improvement is evident.
    ii. Reduce the requirement of blood transfusion.
    iii. Raise the hemoglobin level.
    iv. Reduce the risk of clinical thromboembolism.

But in 50% of cases:
1. Anemia remains sufficiently severe to give blood transfusion.
   This drug should be given intravenously for 14 days.

2. **Bone marrow transfusion:** Allogenic transplant from HLA matched sibling donor is the treatment of choice for complete cure in younger patient, if available.

SICKLE CELL DISEASE

It is an inherited disorder in parts of India, Middle east and Africa.

Pathogenesis (Figs 5.41 and 5.42)

a. Normal glutamic acid is substituted by valine in the sixth codon of β globin chain

↓

It favors bonding of hemoglobin molecules

↓

Hemoglobin S (HbS) is less soluble in deoxygenated conditions.

↓

Morphologic change in RBC to crescent shape

↓

The wall of sickled RBC wall is very rigid

↓

As it passes through the vessel

↓

Rigid RBC becomes precipitated within the vessel.

↓

Obstruction of vessels produced by clumps of sickled cells

To start with, sickling process occurs in deoxygenated condition, but increased oxygen tension reverse the sickle shape to normal.

But repeated sickling and unsickling processes leads to irreversible formation of sickled cell—these cells are called **irreversibly sickled cells.**

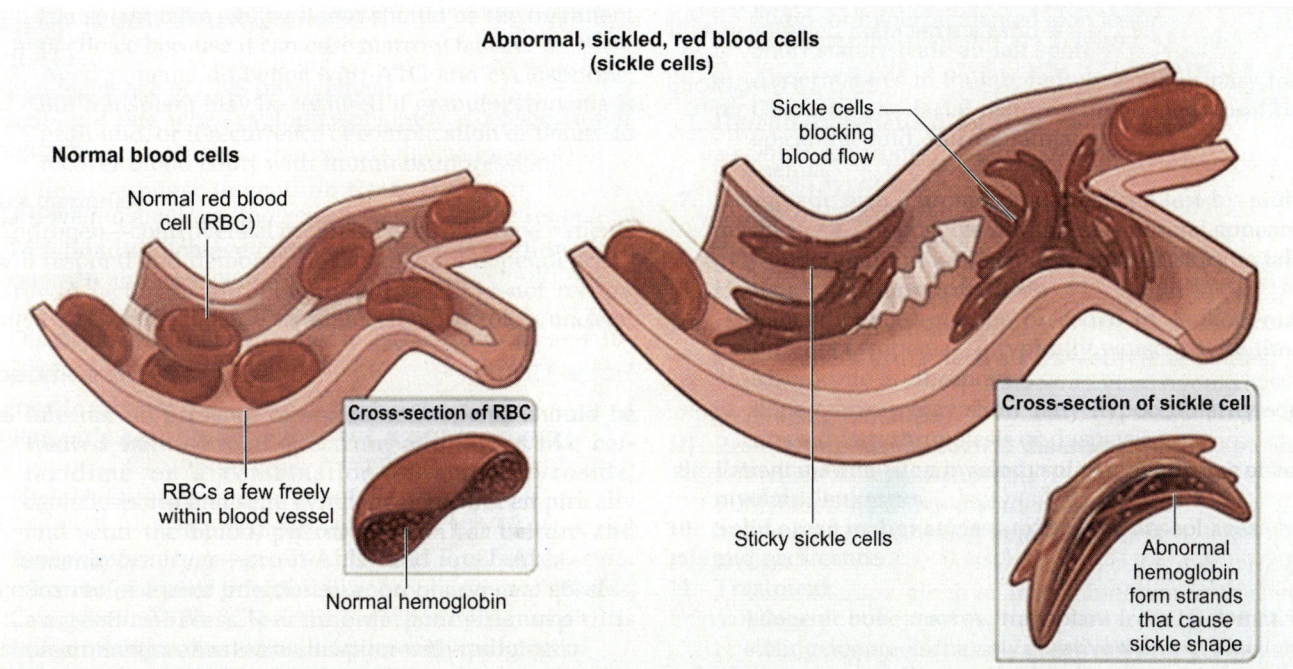

Fig. 5.41: Passage of sickled cells through vessel (*Source:* National Heart, Lung and Blood Institute)

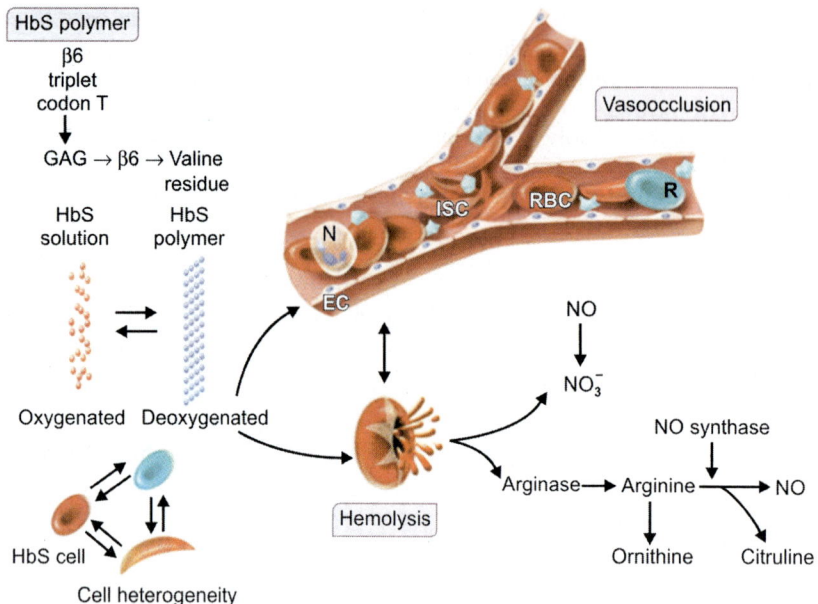

Fig. 5.42: Pathophysiology of sickle cell anemia

The rate and extent of polymerization depends upon:
1. Intracellular hemoglobin concentration
2. Presence of hemoglobin other than HbS
3. Blood oxygen saturation
4. Blood pH
5. Temperature
6. 2, 3, DPG

b. **Microvascular occlusion by sickled cells is favored by:**
1. Prolonged transit time through the microcirculation
2. Rapid deoxygenation
3. Increased number of dense sickled cells containing polymer even at normal O_2 saturation.

c. **Sickled cells are adherent to vascular endothelium**
↓
Leads to endothelial damage
↓
Exposure of molecules, e.g. thrombospondin, laminin, and fibronectin
↓
i. Activation of blood coagulation
ii. Enhanced thrombin generation
iii. Hyper-reactivity of platelets

d. **Scavenging of nitric oxide (NO):** NO has antiplatelet, vasodilatory and anti-inflammatory activity. But released free hemoglobin as a result of hemolysis consume NO. As a result, there is endothelial dysfunction and promote vasoconstriction.

e. **Inflammation:** In this anemia due to chronic hemolysis, there is abnormal leukocytosis, abnormal activation of leukocytes and platelets, released of inflammatory mediators, e.g. TNF-α, IL-6, IL-1β, thrombin, platelet activating factors.

f. **Activation of coagulation system** due to elevation of initiator of coagulation.

g. **Chronic vasculopathy:** Large vessel intimal proliferation and smooth muscle cell proliferation seen.

h. **Cellular dehydration:** Due to activation of calcium activated potassium channel (Gardos channel)—intracellular potassium is lost along with water—as a result there will be intracellular dehydration.

Clinical Features

Patient may presents with a spectrum of symptoms having very few symptoms at one end and severe symptoms with frequent crisis organ damage at other end.

HbF plays an important role in ameliorating symptoms having inverse relationship with symptoms severity.
1. **In infancy**—due to high HbF level in the blood protection of symptoms present till 8–20 weeks of life.
   But symptoms start with gradual fall of HbF levels. They are susceptible to malaria infection.
2. **Infection:** The patients with sickle cell anemia are susceptible to following infections:
   i. Pneumococcal septicemia (*Streptococcus pneumonae*)
   ii. Meningitis—(*Neisseria meningitidis*)
   iii. *Escherichia* coli
   iv. *Haemophilus influenzae*
3. **Anemia:** Adult or children will suffer from well compensated haemolytic anemia (Hb 6.0–9.0 gm %) but will be symptomatic during decompensation (infection).

Figure 5.43 shows the genetic modulation in sickle cell anemia.

Sickle Crises

1. **Vaso-occlusive crises:** This produces:
   a. **Dactylitis:** Mainly occurs in children. Bones involved are:
      i. Metacarpals   ii. Metatarsals
      iii. Back of the hands   iv. Feet
      Features: Swollen and tender joints—recurrent episodes produces permanent radiological deformities.
   b. **Acute chest syndrome:** More in children, but severe in adult.
      Features—chest pain, shortness of breath, fever—similar features like pulmonary infarction. They are very prone to infection.

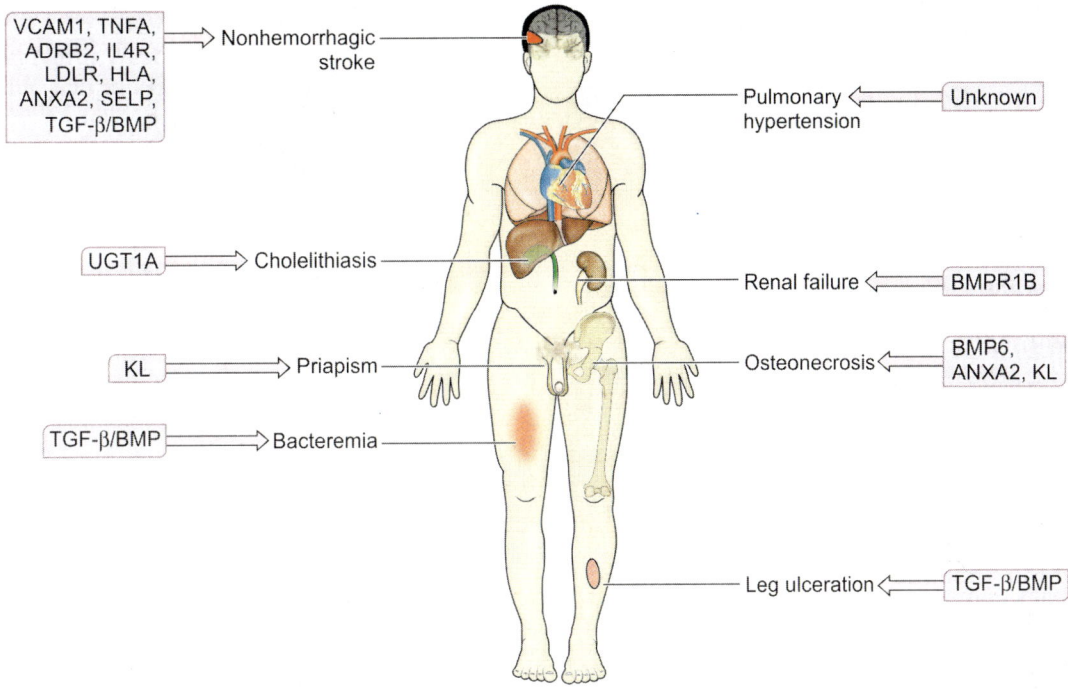

Fig. 5.43: Genetic modulation of sickle cell anemia

c. **Girdle syndrome:** Patient may present with pain in girdle area.
Provocating factors:
  i. Infection
  ii. Dehydration
  iii. Alcohol
  iv. Menstruation
  v. Cold
  vi. Temperature changes
2. **Aplastic crisis:** Sudden decreased marrow production due to parvovirus B19 infection infecting developing RBC. This is self limiting. After 1–2 weeks, marrow will start normal functioning.
3. **Hemolytic crises:** Markedly reduced lifespan of RBC due to:
  i. Malaria infection
  ii. Drug induced
  iii. Associated G6PD deficiency.
4. **Sequestration crises:** In children <6 years of age or following viral infection—sequestration of large volume of blood in spleen produce severe hypotension, profound anemia and death.
5. **Other problems:**
  a. *Growth retardation*—mainly in children, sexual maturation will be delayed.
  b. *Locomotor systems:*
    i. Avascular necrosis of head of the femur or humerus
    ii. Arthritis
    iii. Osteomyelitis
    iv. Chronic leg ulcers.
  c. *Genitourinary:*
    i. Renal papillary necrosis—hematoma, renal tubular defect; inability to concentrate urine
    ii. Priapism,
    iii. Frequent UTI in women

d. *Spleen:* Pain in left upper abdomen due to splenic infarction. Repeated infarction produces hyposplenism in 9–12 months.
e. *Gastrointestinal:*
    i. Gallstones is common
    ii. Derangement of LFT (due to hepatitis B, hepatitis C)
f. *CVS:*
    i. Hemic murmur due to anemia
    ii. Tachycardia
g. *Eye:*
    i. Proliferative retinopathy
    ii. Blindness
    iii. Retinal artery occlusion
    iv. Retinal detachment
h. *CNS:*
    i. Conversion
    ii. TIA
    iii. Stroke
    iv. Sensory hearing loss.
i. **Psychological**—depression

Laboratory Investigation

I. **Hematological:**
  1. Anemia—Hb 6–9 gm/dl, Hb SS—have much lower Hb
  2. Reticulocytes—10–20% due to intense bone marrow production of RBC.
    Anemic symptoms are usually low in HBS—because HbS has low O_2 affinity.
  3. *Blood film shows* (Fig. 5.44):
    i. Sickle cells
    ii. Target cells
    iii. Basophilic stippling
    iv. Howell-Jolly bodies
    v. Pappenheimer bodies (hyposplenic picture in infancy)

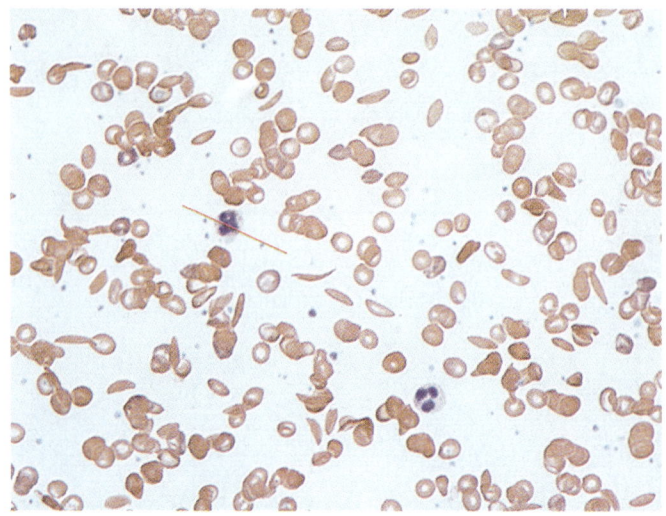

Fig. 5.44: Peripheral blood picture

4. *Sickle cell test* (e.g. with sodium dithionate) will be positive
5. *Serum bilirubin*—raised due to excess red cell breakdown.

II. **Confirmatory test:** Hemoglobin electrophoresis or high performance liquid chromatography—shows:
   i. 80–90% HBS
   ii. No normal HbA
   iii. HbF may be elevated to about 15%.

III. **Screening** (Fig. 5.45):
   i. Pregnant woman at risk should be screened in 1st trimester of pregnancy.
   ii. If both parents of fetus are carrier, offers prenatal diagnosis.

IV. **Prenatal diagnosis:** Should be carried out in:
   i. 1st trimester (chronic villous sampling from 10 weeks gestation.
   ii. 2nd trimester (fetal blood sampling from umbilical cord or trophoblast DNA from amniotic fluid)

V. **Neonatal screening programme:** By dry blood spots used with HPLC or IEF.

Management

a. **General:**
   i. Lifelong prophylactic penicillin 250 mg orally
   ii. Folate supplement
   iii. Pneumovax – 23
b. **Management during pregnancy and anesthesia**—anesthesia should be carried out by experienced anesthetist who will be aware of the complications.

Management of Sickle Crises

1. **Rest to patient**
2. **IV fluid and oxygen** supplementation (for recovery from dehydration through poor oral intake of fluid and excess loss due to fever.
3. **Empirical antibiotic** (especially after sending blood, urine or sputum for culture) with cephalosporin followed **by definite antibiotics**—according to culture sensitivity report, if patient is not recovered.

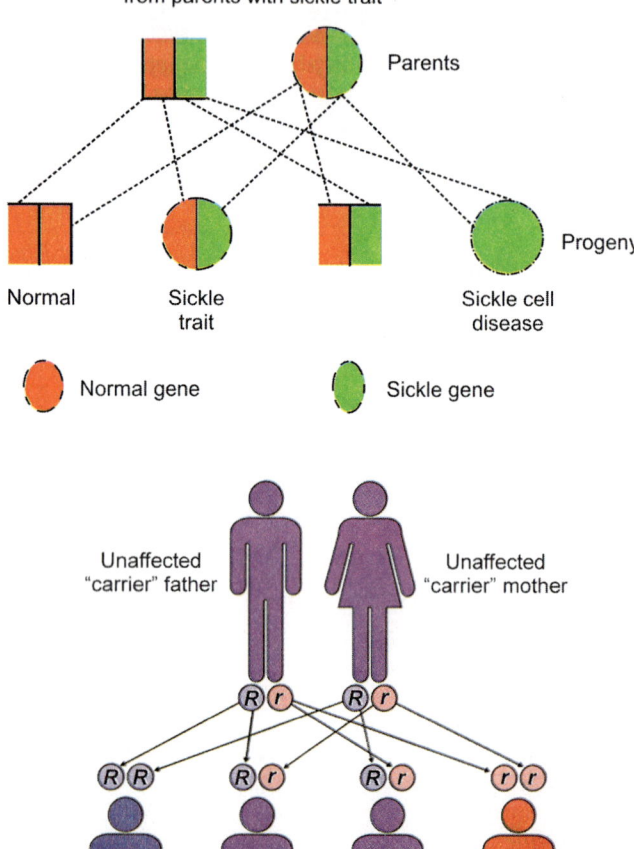

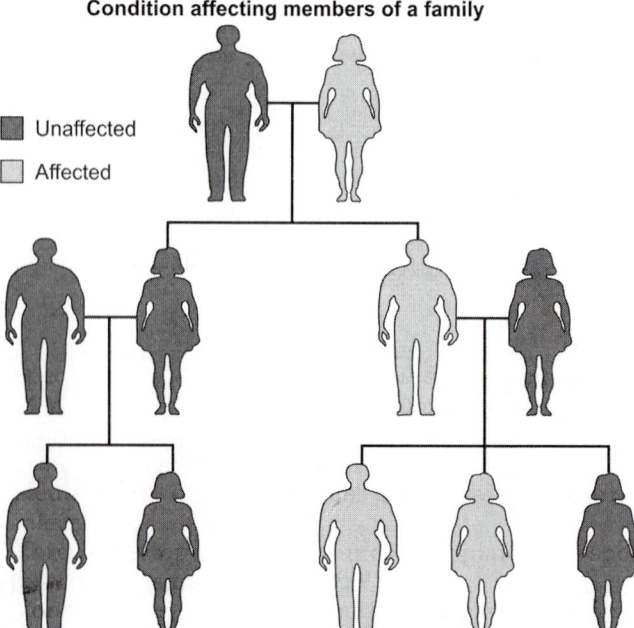

Fig. 5.45: Screening for sickle cell disease

4. **Analgesia**—opiates (morphine) IV followed by oral analgesics when initial crises abates
5. **In case of neurological manifestation**—consider blood exchange transfusion. Aim is to reduce HbS
6. **Exchange transfusion** if PaO_2 <60 mmHg on air.
7. **∝ Adrenergic** stimulation for priapism
8. **Regular blood transfusion,** if:
   i. Anemia is severe.
   ii. Crises is frequent.
   iii. Patient had CVA or abnormal brain scan.
9. **Top-up transfusion,** if Hb <4.5 gm/dl.

Management of Chest Syndrome

1. O_2 supplementation
2. Antibiotics
3. Monitor fluid balance
4. Implementation of pain management
5. Bronchodilator therapy
6. Red cell transfusion—indicated in
   i. Sudden anemia in children
   ii. Parvovirus infection—B19

Newer Therapies

I. **Agents that elevate HbF levels:** Aim to raise HbF level—to ameliorate—β thalassemia and sickle cell anemia.
   i. It reduces HbS polymerization
   ii. HbF level >10% reduces episodes of aseptic necrosis
   iii. HbF level >20% reduces painful crisis.
   The drugs are:
   a. *Hydroxycarbamide:*
      i. Raises HbF level
      ii. Low risk of malignancy with prolonged use.
      iii. At myelosuppressive dose—highest elevation of HbF
      iv. Reduces number of neutrophil, monocytes, reticulocytes
   b. *Erythropoietin:*
      i. Raises the level of HbF
      ii. Additive effect when alternated with hydroxycarbamide
   c. *Azacytidine:*
      i. Inhibitors of methyltransferase, prevent methylation of ϒ Globin gene—leads to raised HbF
      ii. Risk of malignancy
   d. *Short chain fatty acid:* Elevation of butyrate analogues concentration and other fatty acids in diabetic mothers responsible for persistently elevated HbF.
II. **Membrane active drugs:** Clotrimazole and magnesium salts.
   i. These reverse cellular dehydration
   ii. Some drugs block cat ion transport channel
III. **Bone marrow transplantation:** There is gross reduction of sickle cell disease from 30 to 70% with the advent of hydroxyurea therapy—BMT is usually not required now a days.
IV. **Gene therapy:** Globin gene transfer has been attempted with variable results nowadays.

Sickle Cell Trait

These patients have **one abnormal βˢ gene and one normal β gene.**

Clinical Features

   i. Carriers are not anemic and have no abnormal clinical feature.
   ii. Sickling is rare unless O_2 concentration falls below 40%.
   iii. Occasionally renal papillary necrosis, hematuria, inability to concentrate.

Laboratory Findings

Hematological:
   i. Hb%, MCH, MCV, MCHC—normal (unless ∝ thalassemic trait)
   ii. HbS level 4–35%
   iii. Film shows—microcytic and target cell.
   iv. Sickle cell test +ve (Hb SS and HB AS)

Carrier detection:
By Hb electrophoresis or HPLC
Hb%—50%, HbS—50%

BONE MARROW FAILURE SYNDROME

Bone marrow failure syndrome is characterized by inadequate blood cell production leading to low red blood cell, white blood cell and platelet in peripheral blood.

Bone marrow failure may occur with relatively cellular marrow—because of:
   i. Ineffective erythropoiesis.
   ii. Associated cytogenic abnormalities
   iii. Genetically altered cell as in PNH.

Aplastic anemia: Characterized by:
i. Pancytopenia
ii. Hypocellular or empty bone marrow.

Aplastic anemia may be classified in following categories:
A. *Constitutional:*
   1. Fanconi's anemia (Fig. 5.46)
   2. Dyskeratosis congenita (Fig. 5.47)
   3. Shwachman-Diamond syndrome.
   4. Amegakaryocytic thrombocytopenia.
   5. Familial aplastic anemia.
   6. Non-hematologic syndrome: Down, Sickle, etc.

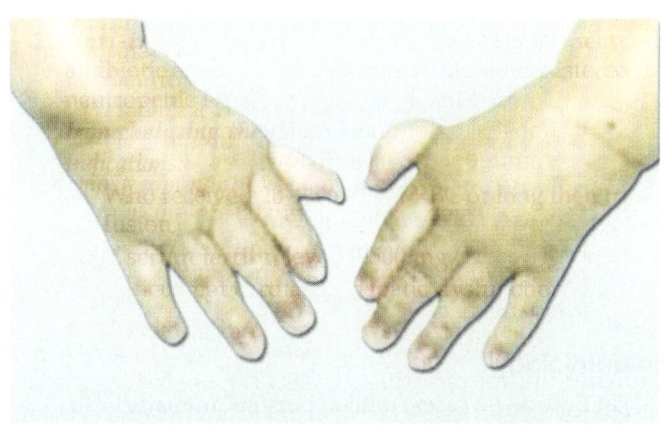

Fig. 5.46: Clinical features of Fanconi's anemia

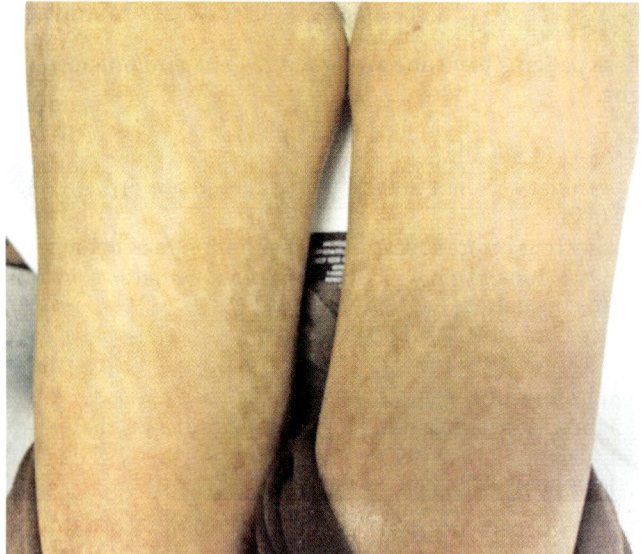

Fig. 5.47: Dyskeratosis congenita

B. *Acquired:*
 i. Drugs:
   a. NSAID—butazones, indomethacin, piroxycam, diclofenac.
   b. Antibiotics—sulphonamides, chloramphenicol.
   c. Antithyroid drugs—methimazole, methylthouracil, propylothlounacil.
   d. Cardiovascular drugs—furosemide.
   e. Antiprotozoals—quinacrine, mepacrine, chloroquine.
   f. Anticonvulsant—hydantoin, carbamazepine, phenacemide.
   g. Heavy metals—gold, arsenic, mercury
   h. D-penicillamine
   i. Allopurinol.
   j. Sedatives—chlorpromazine, chlordiazopoxide.
   k. Chemotherapeutic agents.
 ii. Radiation
 iii. Chemicals—benzenes
 iv. Infections:
   a. Hepatitis—must common preceding infection. Post-hepatitis bone marrow failure—5% of etiologies—(seronegative hepatitis)—so yet no etiological agent is identified.
   b. Epstein-Barr virus—(infectious mononucleosis)
   c. Parvovirus-B19. (Transient aplastic crisis)
   d. HIV–I
 v. Immunologic diseases:
   a. Transfusion related graft versus host disease—after transfusion of non-irradiated blood products to an immunodeficient individual.
   b. Eosinophilic fasciitis.
   c. Hyperimmunoglobulinemia
 vi. Paroxysmal nocturnal hemoglobinuria
 vii. Pregnancy.
 vi. Idiopathic.

Epidemiology
 i. In Europe—2 cases/million persons annually.
 ii. In East Asia—2–3-fold increased incidence annually.

 iii. Male: Female ratio—equal.
 iv. Age distribution—biphasic—major peak in teen or twenties and second peak in older adults.

Radiation

Denatures DNA, so tissues dependent on active mitosis are susceptable.

Power plant workers, employees in hospital, laboratories and innocents exposed to stolen, misplaced and misused sources may be involved by nuclear accident.

Radiation dose can be approximated by the rate and degree of decline of blood counts.

Dosimetry by reconstruction of exposure can help to:
 i. Estimate the patient's prognosis
 ii. Protect the medical personnel from contact with radiation tissues and excreta.

Clinical Features

May be of abrupt in onset or insidious onset.

History

1. **Features of anemia:** Lassitude, weakness, fatigue, shortness of breath, ringing sensation in ears.
2. **Features of thrombocytopenia**—bleeding is most common early symptom. Easy bruising, bleeding from gum, epistaxis, menorrheagia, petechie. Intracranial bleeding is the most catastrophic symptoms.
3. **Infection** may occur in the setting of neutropenia. Striking features of aplastic anemia is the restriction of symptoms to hematologic system, patients look well in spite of dramatically reduced blood court.
4. **History includes:**
   a. Prior drug ingestion
   b. Exposure to radiation or chemicals
   c. Preceding viral illness.
5. **Family history** of hematologic disorders, pulmonary or liver disorders (fibrosis)

Physical Examination

 i. Petechiae
 ii. Echymoses
 iii. Gum bleeding without hypertrophy
 iv. retinal hemorrhages.
 v. Pelvic and rectal examination if done, with great gentleness to avoid trauma—show blood in stool or blood in cervix.
 vi. Pallor of skin and mucous membranes.
 vi. Café-au-lait spot, short stature—suggest Fanconi's anemia.
 vii. Peculiar nails and leukoplakia—suggest dyskeratosis congenital.

Laboratory Studies

Peripheral Blood Studies

1. **Red blood cell**—large erythrocytes—MCV—increased, MCHC—reduced, reticulocyte—absent or law.
2. **Platelet** count—low, with normal morphology. Giant platelet suggestive of peripheral destruction is not evident
3. White blood cell court—low with normal morphology.

Bone Marrow

1. Aspirated bone marrow material is dilute, grossly pale containing fatty tissue (Fig. 5.48)
2. In severe aplasia—aspirated material shows only few Red cells, residual lymphocytes, plasma cells, mast cells and stromal cells.
3. Biopsy >1 cm length shows fat under microscope with 25–30% of marrow space occupying hematopoietic cells excluding lymphocytes.
4. Biopsy material shows few pockets of hypercellularity so-called hot-spots.
5. Myeloblast and megakaryocytes are almost always absent.
6. Marrow cytogenetics should be normal.

In moderate aplastic anemia—iliac crest biopsy is usually done. If iliac crest specimen is inadequate, sterna biopsy in usually needed.

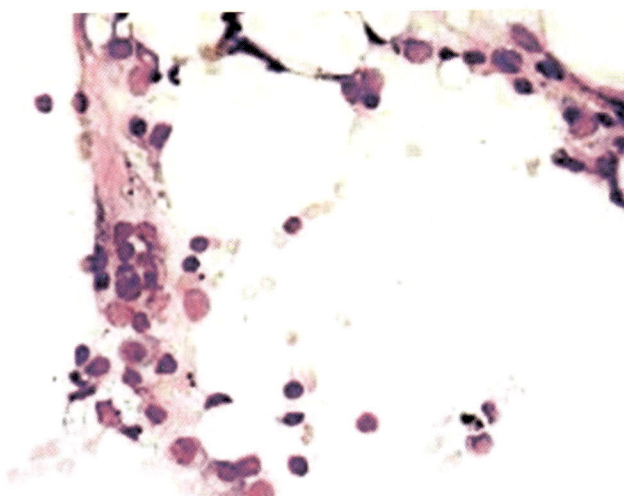

Fig. 5.48: Bone marrow picture of bone marrow failure syndrome

Differential Diagnosis of Pancytopenia

A. **Pancytopenia with hypocellular marrow:**
   1. Inherited aplastic anemia.
   2. Acquired aplastic anemia.
   3. Aleukemic leukemia
   4. Some myelodysplastic syndrome.
   5. Some acute lymphoblastic leukemia
   6. Lymphoma of bone marrow.
B. **Hypocellular marrow with or without cytopenia:**
   1. Q fever.
   2. Legionnaires disease.
   3. Anorexia nervosa, starvation.
   4. Mycobacteria.
   5. Tuberculosis
C. **Pancytopenia with cellular marrow:**
   1. *Primary bone marrow disease:*
      a. Myelodysplastic syndrome
      b. Paroxysmal nocturnal haemoglobinuria.
      c. Myelofibrosis.
      d. Myelothisis
      e. Hairy cell leukemia
      f. Bone marrow lymphoma.
   2. *Secondary to systemic disease:*
      a. SLE
      b. Hypersplenism.

c. Vitamin B_{12} and folic acid deficiency
d. Brucellosis.
e. Alcoholism.
f. Sarcoidosis.
f. Tuberculosis.
h. Overwhelming infection.

Ancillary Studies

1. **Chromosome breakage studies** of peripheral blood using mitomycin C shows—should be done in children or young adult to exclude Fanconi's anemia.
2. **Chromosomal studies of bone marrow cells**—reveal MDS negative in aplastic anemia.
3. **Flow cytometry**—sensitive diagnostics for PNH
4. **Seronegativity** in hepatitis.
5. **Serological test**—Paul-Bunnel test—Epstein-Barr virus. Western Blot test—HIV.
6. **CT scan or MRI**—shows splenomegaly.
7. **MRI**—to estimate fat content of a few vertebrae—distinguish aplastic anemia from MDS.

Diagnosis

Diagnosis of aplastic anemia is:
1. Pancytopenia   2. Fatty bone marrow

It should be a leading diagnosis in pancytopenia in adolescent or young adult.

The criteria of severe aplastic anemia include:
1. Marrow biopsy showing <25% of normal cellularity, or showing <50% of normal cellularity in which <30% of the cells are hematopoietic.
2. At least 2 of the 3 following features:
   i. Absolute reticulocyte count <40,000/cmm.
   ii. Absolute neutrophil count <500/cmm.
   iii. Absolute plate count <20,000/cmm.

The criteria of very severe aplastic anemia are all the above except the absolute neutrophil count—500/cmm.

Figure 5.49 demonstrates algorithm of differential diagnosis of hypocellular pancytopenia.

Prognosis

1. In case of server aplastic anemia—rapid deterioration and death.
2. Major prognostic determinant is blood count.
   i. Historically—severe disease can be defined by the presence of two of three parameters
      a. Absolute neutrophil court <500/il.
      b. Platelet count <20,000/il.
      c. Absolute reticulocyte court (automated) <60,000/uL. Or corrected reticulocyte count <1%.
   ii. In the era of immunosuppressive therapies—following are the better prognostic markers of response to treatment:
      a. Absolute reticulocyte count > 25,000/iL.
      b. Lymphocyte count > 1000/iL.

Treatment of Aplastic Anemia

Definite Treatment

It consists of:
A. **Allogenic hemopoietic stem cell transplantation:**
   i. This *is best therapy for younger patient* with fully histocompatible sibling donor.

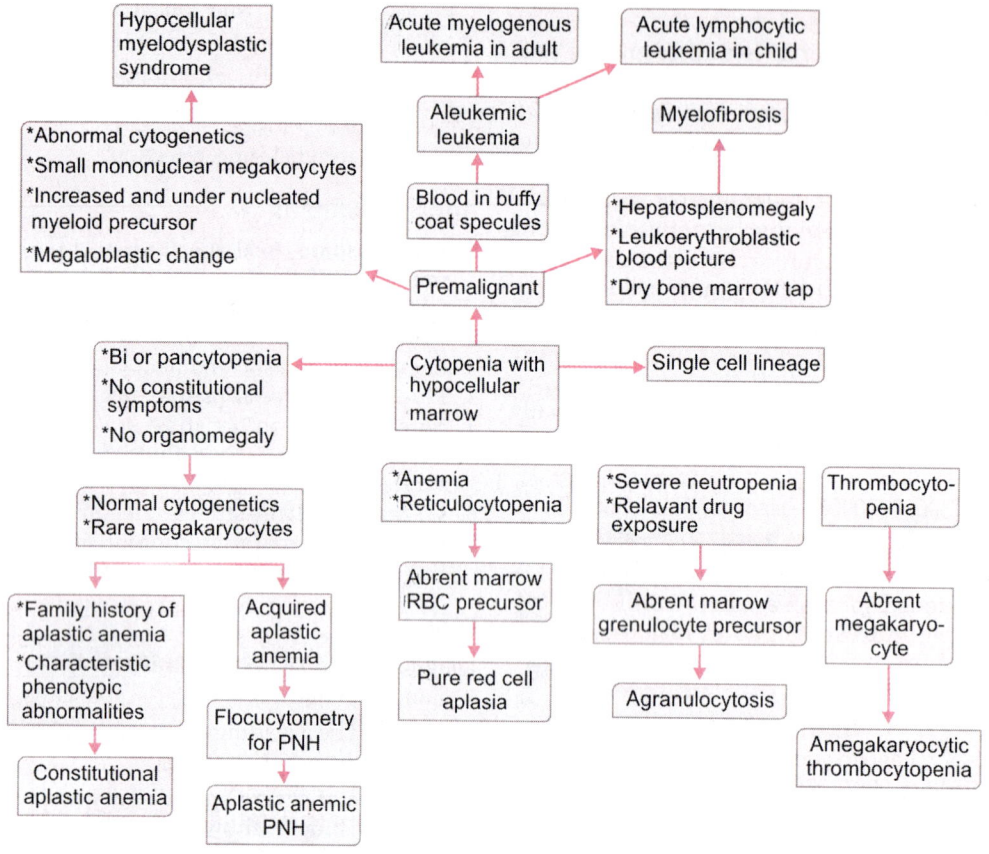

Fig. 5.49: Differential diagnosis of hypocellular pancytopenia

ii. *Soon after diagnosis has been established,* HLA antigen typing and matching should be ordered.

iii. *Before HSCT*—no blood transfusion to be given to patient from his family member to prevent sensitizations to HLA antigen.

iv. *For allogenic HSCT* from fully matched siblings, survival rate in children is 90%.

v. *But in case of adult,* mortality and morbidity are increased due to high risk of graft versus host disease. (GVHD).

vi. *In case of non-availability of fully matched sibling donor,* full phenotypic matched either unrelated but histocompatible donor or closely but not perfectly matched family member may be selected as donor.

Matched unrelated donor bone marrow transplantation may be considered when patient fulfils the following criteria:
1. <40 years of old and have fully matched (at DNA level for both class I and class II antigen. donor.
2. Have severe aplastic anemia and have no evidence of active infection and acute bleeding at the time of bone marrow transplantation.
3. For adult, have failed at least two course of ATG and cyclosporin and , for children, at least one course.

In this case, survival can be improved by:
a. High resolution matching at HLA.
b. More effective conditioning regimen.
c. Graft versus host disease prophylaxis.

If radiation is used as a method of conditioning—risk of cancer in future will be increased.

B. Immunosuppression:

Indications of immunosuppressive therapy:
1. Patients with non-SAA, who are dependent on red cell and/or platelet transfusions.
2. Patients with SAA or very SAA, who are >30–45 years of age.
3. Patients with SAA or very SAA, disease who lack an HLA—compatible sibling donor.
   Therapy of choice is:

   *ATG—combination with cyclosporine—*induces hematologic response in 60–70% patients in following manners:
i. Improvement in granulocyte number in 3 months to resist infection.
ii. Bone marrow cellularity recovered very slowly if at all.

The following things will remain:
i. MCV will remain raised.
ii. Some degree of blood cell depression.

Complications after therapy:
i. Relapse of pancytopenia (recurrent pancytopenia) is frequent—mainly after withdrawal of cyclosporine therapy.
   a. Some of above patients respond to reinstitution of cyclosporine therapy—so they require continued cyclosporine administration.
   b. Some may not respond to reinstitution of cyclosporine therapy.
ii. Some patient develop myelodysplastic syndrome with cytogenic abnormalities (15%) not invariably associated with pancytopenia mainly in trisomy 8 and monosomy 7.

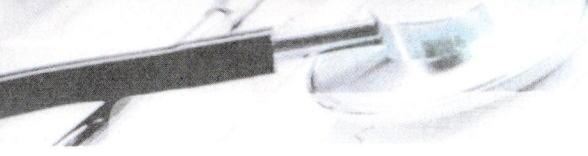

iii. Some patients develop leukemia.

iv. Some recovered patients may develop hemolysis, if their PNH clone expands.

Antithymic globulin: Daily intravenous infusion over 6–8 hours.

a. ATG of Horse –20–40 mg/kg/day for 4 days.

One vial of horse ATG, lymphoglobulin, contains 250 mg of protein.

b. ATG of rabbit—3.75 mg/kg/day for 5 days.

One vial of rabbit ATG, lymphoglobulin, contains 25 mg of protein.

Toxicities:

i. ATG binds to peripheral blood cells—hence peripheral platelet and granulocyte number are further decreased during active treatment.

ii. Serum sickness with characteristic cutaneous eruption

iii. Arthralgia

These start after two days of initiating a treatment.

Methylprednisolone—1 mg/kg/day for 2 weeks may recover the patient from above toxicities.

But extended use of steroid—produces avascular joint necrosis.

c. Cyclosporine—to begin with:

10 mg/kg in adult and 15 mg/kg in children

Adjust the dose to maintain a blood level of 200 mg/ml.

Important side effects are:

i. Hepatotoxicity

ii. Nephrotoxicity

iii. Hypertension

iv. Seizure

v. Opportunistic infection, (*Pneumocystis carinii*)—in this case prophylactic treatment with pentamidine is required)

vi. Gingival hypertrophy:

1. Most patients with aplastic anemia—treatment of choice is immunosuppression.

2. But in case of children and young adult, allogenic transplant from sibling donor should be the treatment of choice because it can cure marrow failure.

3. Aged patients do better with ATG and cyclosporine, but transplant may be required if granulocytopenia is profound, or if recurrence of complication or failure to recover blood court with Immunosuppression.

Other therapies:

1. Androgen—controversial in clinical trial, but some patients will respond and demonstrate blood count dependence.

2. Growth factor (erythropoietin and G-CSF)—not recommended as initial therapy, as adjunct therapy role is unclear.

Supportive Cares

i. Infection in presence of severe neutropenia should be treated with—broad spectrum antibiotics like ceftazidime or a combination of aminoglycoside, cephalosporin and semi synthetic penicillin empirically and send the blood, pus or sputum for culture and sensitivity.

ii. Search for foci of infection like, oropharyngeal abscess, anorectal abscess, pneumonia, sinusitis, typhlitis (necrotizing colitis) in association with radiologist.

iii. If indwelling catheter infection is suspected, send urine for culture, catheter tip for culture and add vancomycin.

iv. Persistent or recrudescence of fever give clue to suspicion of fungal infection specially *Candida* and *Aspegillus*—add antifungal drugs intravenously.

v. Granulocyte colony-stimulating factor addition is required in case of severe overwhelming infections or refractory infections.

vi. To pervert spread of infection—examiners and nurses should use sterile gloves, mask and cap and slipper.

vii. HLA matched platelet transfusion is effective in patient with refractoriness to randomly used platelet.

viii. Rational regimen of platelet transfusion is required once or twice weekly to maintain platelet count >10000/ìl, because oozing from gut and other vascular bed increases when platelet will be <5000/ìL.

ix. Menstruation should be stopped hay oral estrogen or nasal follicle stimulating hormone/LH.

x. Aspirin and NSAID should be stopped.

xi. Packed RBC—2 units every 2 weeks—will replace normal losses in patient without functional marrow—to raise the hemoglobin 7 gm/dl and 9 gm/dl in the patient with cardiac and pulmonary disease.

xii. In chronic anemia—iron chelating agent desferoxamine and desferasirox—should be added at 50th transfusion to prevent secondary haemochromatosis.

Fanconi Anemia

1. It is **most common constitutional** aplastic anemia.

2. It is **autosomal recessive or X-linked.**

3. It is found in **all races, mainly in children.**

4. Genetics—mutation can occur in 13 genes—amongst **those FANCA—is most common.**

5. **Chief criteria:**

i. Pancytopenia

ii. Hyperpigmentation

iii. Malformation of skeleton, small stature

iv. Hypogonadism.

6. **Clinical features:**

i. Hypo- or hyperpigmented skin lesion

ii. Short stature (café-au-lait spot)

iii. Abnormalities in thumb, radius, genitourinary tract

iv. Characteristic facial feature—broadened nasal base, epicanthic fold, micrognathia

v. Anemia.

7. **Diagnostic test:** Chromosome breakage test by mithramycin C. 40% of positive MMC test is normal appearing, may undergo unnoticed—unless family history in taken.

8. **Hematological abnormalities:**

i. Pancytopenia—may be preceded by leukopenia or thrombocytopenia—it typically worsens with time.

ii. Macrocytic erythropoiesis.

iii. Bone marrow may show fatty hypocellularity sometimes dyserythropoiesis or dysplasia.

9. **Patient may develop myelodysplastic syndrome or acute myeloid leukemia.**

10. **Solid organ malignancies**—particularly esophageal, head and neck cancers.

11. **Treatment:**

i. Allogenic bone marrow transplant from HLA matched sibling donor—is the only curative therapy. Since these patients are radio- and chemosensitive, hence dosage of chemotherapy should be adjusted.

ii. Androgen induces hematologic response in 50% of patients. This therapy is initiated with platelet count <30,000/hi and/or hemoglobin level <7 gm/dl.
Oxymethalone—started with 2–5 mg/kg/day

+

Prednisolone—10 mg at alternate day

They counterbalance anabolic properties of oxymethalone and catabolic properties of corticosteroids.

Dyskeratosis Congenita

1. This is characterized by mucous membrane leukoplakia, dystrophic nails, reticular hyperpigmentation and aplastic anemia in childhood.
2. It is X-linked disease: Mutation in DKC1 (dyskerin) gene.
3. In unusual autosomal dominant type—mutation in TERC gone—which encodes RNA template

   TERT gene—which encodes reverse transcriptase

Shwachman-Diamond Syndrome

1. **Third most common constitutional marrow** failure syndrome.
2. **Autosomal recessive**, presents in infancy.

Clinical Features

i. Exocrine pancreatic insufficiency
ii. Short stature
iii. Bones abnormalities
iv. Immune dysfunction
v. Liver disease
vi. Renal tubular detect
vii. Hematologic abnormalities—neutropenia, raised fetal hemoglobin, anemia, thrombocytopenia, impaired neutrophil chemotaxis.
viii. It can transform into acute myeloid leukemia or MDS.

Approach to Diagnosis

1. History and physical examination.
2. Complete blood count, reticulocyte count, examination of blood film.
3. Marrow aspiration and biopsy.
4. Marrow cell cytogenetics to evaluate clonal myeloid disease.
5. Fetal hemoglobin level and DNA stability test as markers of Fanconi's anemia.
6. Immunophenotyping of red and white cells, especially for—CD55, CD59 to exclude PNH.
7. Direct and indirect Coomb tests to rule out immune cytopenia.
8. Serum lactate dehydrogenase (LDH) and uric acid—if increased, may reflect neoplastic cell turnover.
9. Liver function test to assess evidence of any recent hepatitis virus exposure.
10. Screening tests of Hepatitis virus B, C and A.
11. Screening tests for Epstein Barr virus, cytomegalo virus and HIV virus.
12. Serum B-12 and red cell folic acid levels to exclude megaloblastic pancytopenia.
13. Serum iron, iron binding capacity and ferritin as a baseline prior to chronic transfusion therapy.

Initial Management of Aplastic Anemia

1. Discontinue any potentially offending drug and use of an alternative class of agents, if essential.
2. Anemia—transfusion of leukocyte depleted, irradiated red cells as required for very severe anemia.
3. Very severe thrombocytopenia or thrombocytopenic bleeding, consider ε-aminocaproic acid, transfusion of platelet is required.
4. Severe neutropenia—take infect ion precautions.
5. Fever (suspected infection), microbial culture—broad-spectrum antibiotics, if specific organism not detected. Granulocyte-stimulating factor (G-CSF) in severe cases.
6. If child or young adult with profound infection (e.g. Gm-negative bacteria, fungus, persistent blood cultures)—consider neutrophil transfusion from a G-CSF pretreated donor.
7. Immediate assessment for allogenic stem cell transplantation, histocompatibility testing of the patients, siblings. Search databases for unrelated donor, if appropriate.

MYELODYSPLASTIC SYNDROME

Definition

Myelodysplastic syndromes (Fig. 5.50) are a heterogenous group of clonal stem cell disorders characterized by:
i. Ineffective erythropoiesis
ii. Variable tendency to progress to acute myelogenous leukemia

Epidemiology

i. Disease of adult—median age is 60 years
ii. MDS can be seen in association with:
   a. Aplastic anemia
   b. PNH
   c. T-large lymphocyte lymphoproliferative disorder MDS progresses to AML

Risk Factors

I. **Prior cancer therapy:**
   i. Radiotherapy
   ii. Alkalyting agents—chlorambucil, cyclophosphamide, melphalan 4–10 years after therapy.
   iii. Epipodophyllotoxin (etoposide, teniposide, peaks at 5 years)
   iv. Autologous transfusion (20% in patient with NHL)
II. **Environmental toxins**—benzene and other solvents, petroleum products, fertilizers.
III. **Genetic:**
   i. Fanconi anemia
   ii. Children with Schwachman-Diamond syndrome
   iii. Type 1 neurofibromatosis

Pathophysiology

1. Clonal hematopoietic stem cell disorder characterized by stepwise genetic progression possibly due to combination of genetic predisposition factors and environmental factors.
2. Early mutation produces differentiation arrest and followed by dysplasia followed by later mutations leading to proliferation and expansion and development of acute myeloid leukemia.

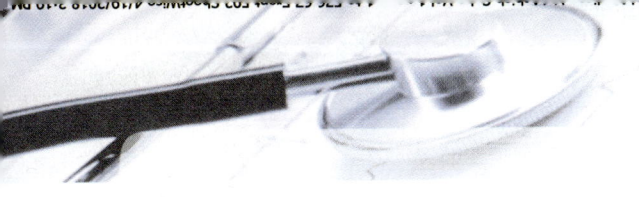

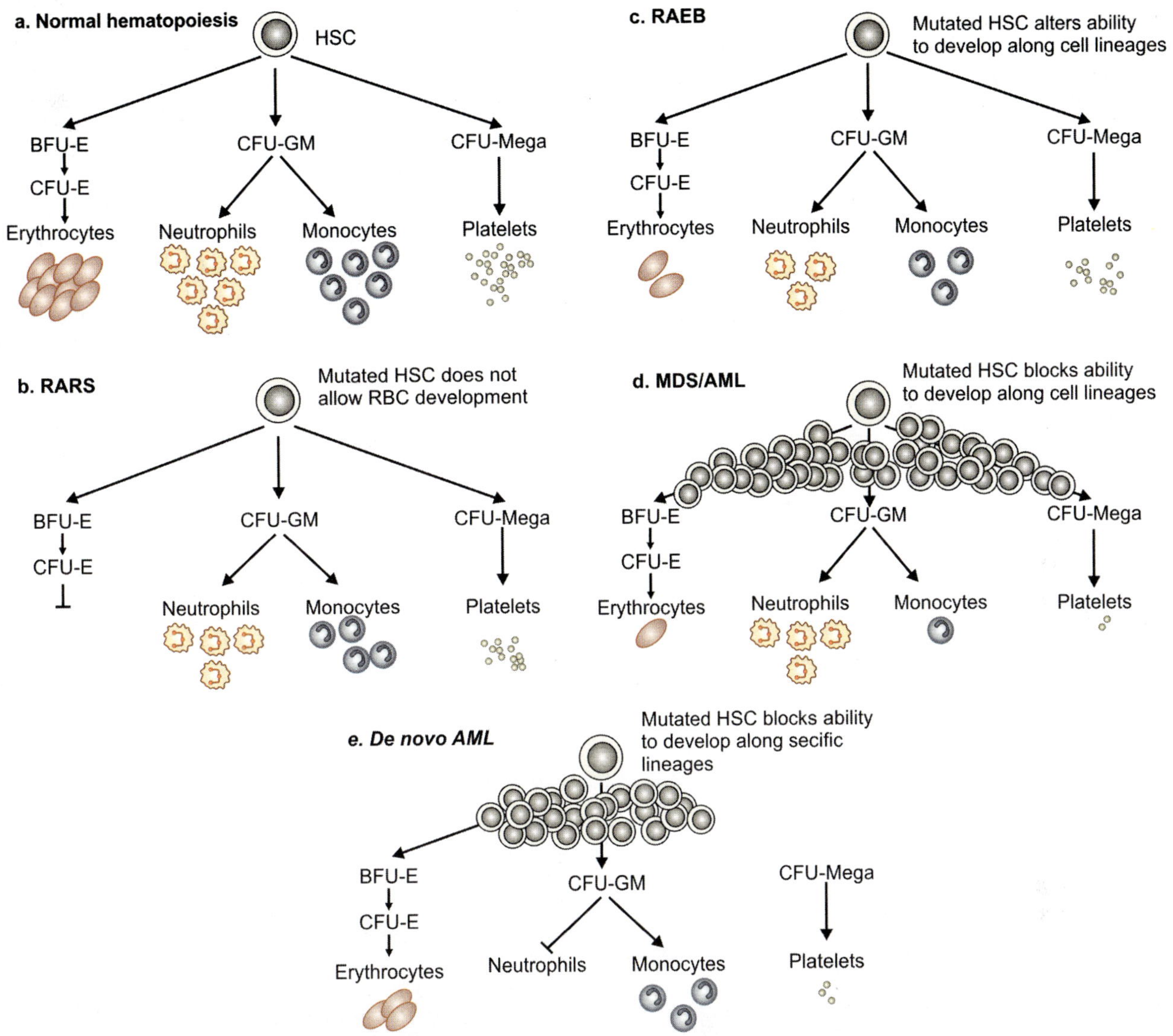

a. Normal hematopoiesis

HSC

BFU-E
CFU-E
Erythrocytes

CFU-GM
Neutrophils   Monocytes

CFU-Mega
Platelets

b. RARS — Mutated HSC does not allow RBC development

BFU-E
CFU-E

CFU-GM
Neutrophils   Monocytes

CFU-Mega
Platelets

c. RAEB — Mutated HSC alters ability to develop along cell lineages

BFU-E
CFU-E
Erythrocytes

CFU-GM
Neutrophils   Monocytes

CFU-Mega
Platelets

d. MDS/AML — Mutated HSC blocks ability to develop along cell lineages

BFU-E
CFU-E
Erythrocytes

CFU-GM
Neutrophils   Monocytes

CFU-Mega
Platelets

e. De novo AML — Mutated HSC blocks ability to develop along secific lineages

BFU-E
CFU-E
Erythrocytes

CFU-GM
Neutrophils   Monocytes

CFU-Mega
Platelets

Fig. 5.50: MDS: The myelodysplastic syndromes (MDS): Cell clone can suppress normal hematopoiesis (**a**) directly or indirectly through stroma. Stem-cell defects can result in single-lineage deficiency (refractory anemia and ringed sideroblasts (RARS), (**b**) multiple-lineage deficiencies (refractory anemia with excess blasts (RAEB), (**c**) MDS stem-cell diseases, (**d**) might seem like *de novo* acute myeloid leukemia (AML), however, the two are distinguishable. For example, (**e**) cytopenias in *de novo* AML can be more restricted owing to a failure in differentiation. HSC, hematopoietic stem cell.

3. MLL gene at 11q23 is up regulated in significant number of patient with MDS.
4. Aberrant cytokine production in marrow micro environment and altered stem cell adhesion.
5. MDS marrow stem cells show lower apoptotic threshold to TNF-α, IFN-α etc.

Classifications

Two systems of classifications are usually used.

FAB Classification System

i. Morphology based classifications
ii. Defines 5 subtypes
iii. Requires dysplastic changes in ≥ 2 lineages
iv. Useful for predicting prognosis

1. **Refractory anemia:**
   i. Normocellular or hypercellular marrow with dysplasia ≥ 2 lineages
   ii. <1% peripheral blood blast
   iii. <25% BM blasts

2. **Refractory anemia with ring sideroblast:** Constitution >15% nucleated red blood cells.

3. **Refractory anemia with excess blasts:**
   i. Cytopenia in ≥2 peripheral blood lineages
   ii. Dysplasia of all 3 bone marrow lineages
   iii. <5% peripheral blood blasts
   iv. 5–20% bone marrow blasts

4. **Refractory anemia with excess blasts in transformation:**
   i. Cytopenia ≥2 peripheral blood lineage
   ii. Dysplasia of all 3 bone marrow lineages
   iii. >5% peripheral blood blasts
   iv. 21–30% bone marrow blasts or Auer rods in blasts

5. **Chronic myelomonocytic leukemia:**
   i. Peripheral blood monocytosis (>1 × 10^9/L)
   ii. <5% peripheral blood blasts
   iii. <20% bone marrow blasts.

World Health Organization (WHO) Classification

1. **Refractory anemia** (Fig. 5.51):
   a. Anemia, no or rare blasts in peripheral blood
   b. BM shows:
      i. Erythroid dysplasia only
      ii. <5% blast
      iii. <15% ring sideroblast.

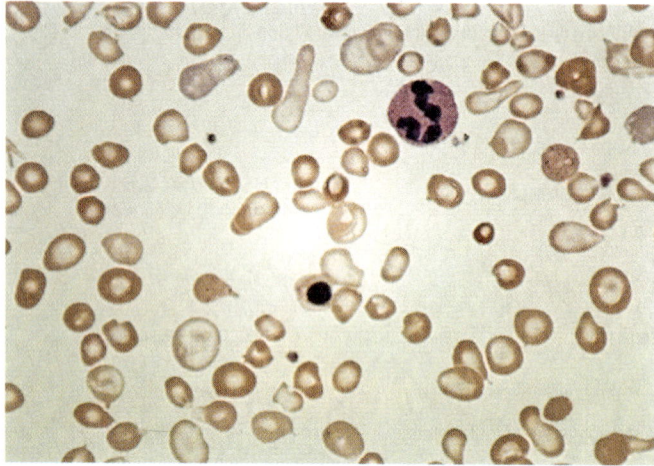

Fig. 5.51: Refractory anemia

2. **Refractory anemia with ringed sideroblast** (Fig. 5.52):
   a. Anemia, no blast in peripheral blood
   b. BM shows:
      i. ≥15% ringed sideroblast
      ii. Erythroid hyperplasia
      iii. <5% blasts

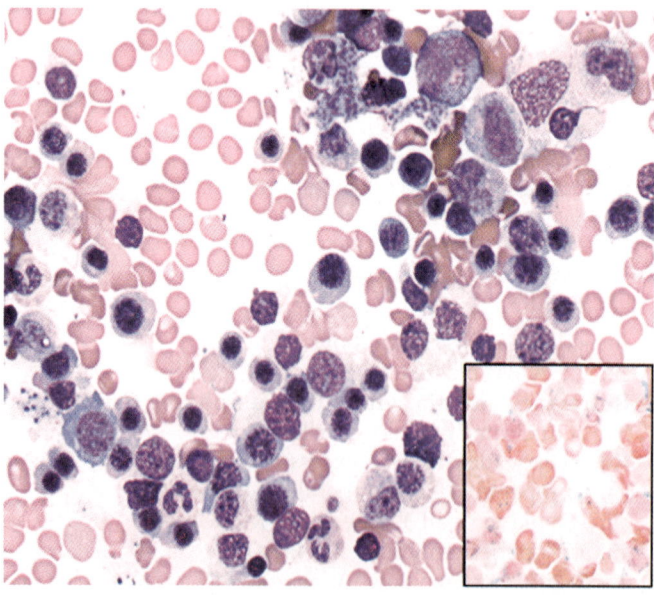

Fig. 5.52: Refractory anemia with ringed sideroblast

3. **Refractory cytopenia with multilineage dysplasia:**
   a. Bi or pancytopenia, no blast or auer rods in peripheral blood
   b. BM shows:
      i. Dysplasia in >10% cells
      ii. ≥ 2 myeloid cell lines
      iii. <5% blasts
      iv. <15% ring sideroblast

4. **Refractory cytopenia with multilineage dysplasia and ringed sideroblast**

5. **Refractory anemia with excess blasts** (Fig. 5.53):
   a. <5% blasts, no auer rods, $<1 \times 10^9$/L monocytes in peripheral blood.
   b. Uni- or multilineage dysplasia, 5 to 9% blasts no Auer rod in peripheral blood

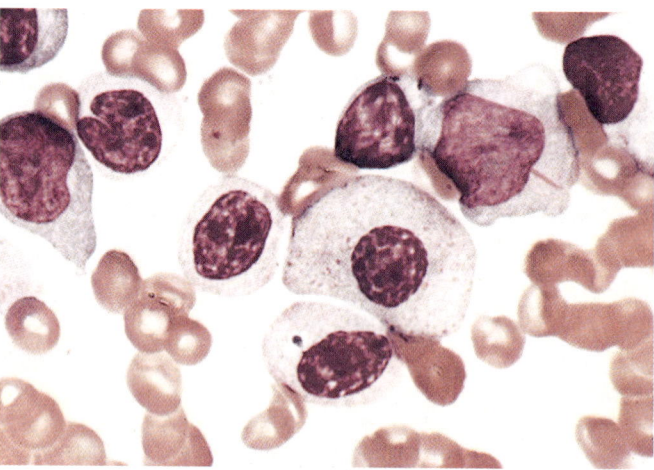

Fig. 5.53: Refractory anemia with excess blast

6. **Refractory anemia with excess blasts** (Fig. 5.54):
   a. 5–19% blasts and ± Auer rod, $< 1 \times 10^9$/L monocytes in peripheral blood
   b. 10–19% blasts ± Auer rods in bone marrow.

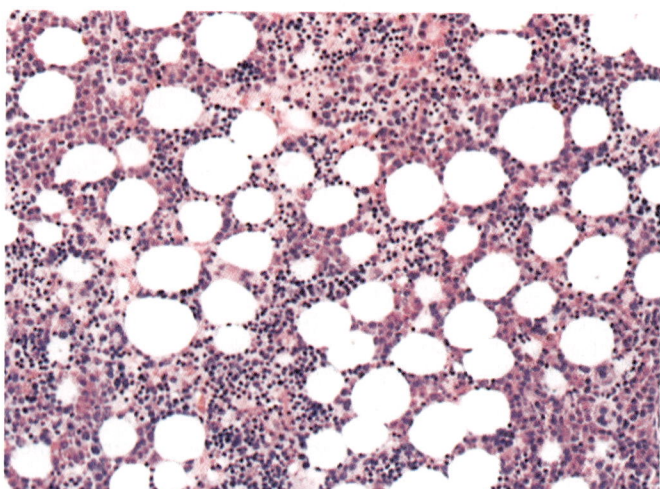

Fig. 5.54: Refractory anemia with excess blast (10–19% blast cells)

Clinical Pictures

1. Spectrum ranges from mild anemia to severe pancytopenia. Mild anemic patient may be asymptomatic
2. Symptoms of anemia—fatigue, shortness of breath, exacerbation of cardiac symptoms.
3. Neutropenia or dysfunctional granulocytes—recurrent infection.
4. Thrombocytopenia or dysfunctional platelets—spontaneous bruising, bleeding gum
5. Constitutions symptoms—anorexia, weight loss, fever, sweating
6. On examination—splenomegaly, purpuric spots, bruise

Investigations

I. **FBC:** Macrocytic/normocytic anemia ± neutropenia ± thrombocytopenia ± neutrophilia ± monocytosis ± thrombocytosis

II. **Blood film:**
   i. Dimorphic red cells ± peppenheimer bodies in RARS, basophilic stippling in RBC
   ii. Dysplastic granulocytes
   iii. pseudo-Pelger forms
   iv. Hypersegmented neutrophils
   v. Hypogranular neutrophils
   vi. Dysmorphic monocytes ± blasts

III. **Chest X-ray, ECG, LFT**—to assess comorbidity

IV. **Serum ferritin, vitamin B₁₂, folate**—normal

V. **Bone marrow aspirates** (Fig. 5.55):
   i. >10% dysplastic cells in >1 lineage
   ii. Megaloblastoid erythropoiesis
   iii. Nuclear cytoplasmic asynchrony in myeloid/erythroid precursors
   iv. Dysmorphic megakaryocytes, or micromegakaryocytes, increased monocytes.
   v. Increased storage iron >15%
   vi. Ring sideroblast in RARS or RCMD-RS.

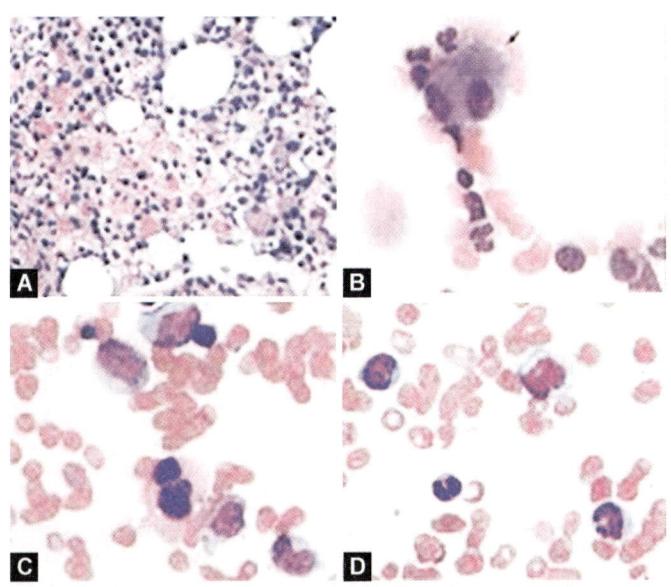

Fig. 5.55: Bone marrow aspirates: **A. and B:** Abnormal megakaryocytes with multilobulated or hyperlobulated nuclei; **B.** Dyserythropoiesis' **C.** Nuclear hypolobulation (Pseudo Pelger-Huet nucleus of granulocyte (arrow), and **D.** A blast (arrow-head).

VI. **Immunohistochemistry:** Minimum CD-34, CD-31, 42 or 61 (megakaryocytes) and tryptase (mast cells) recommended in all cases.

VII. **Bone marrow cytogenetics:** Demonstrate, clonal chromosomal abnormality
   a. Confirm diagnosis
   b. Provide prognostic information
   c. Exclude Fanconi anemia, dyskeratosis congenital

VIII. **HLA typing**

IX. **CMV serology**

X. **HIV serology**

XI. **Flow cytometry**—in selected cases to exclude PNH

XII. **HLA-DR 15** screening

XIII. **Clonal studies**—to establish diagnosis in difficult cases

Diagnostic Criteria—Minimal Diagnostic Criteria in MDS

A. **Prerequisite criteria:**
   I. *Constant cytopenia in ≥1 of the following cell lineage:*
      i. Erythroid (Hb <11 gm/dl)
      ii. Neutrophilia (ANC <1.5 × 10⁹/L) or
      iii. Megakaryocytic (platelet <100 × 10⁹/L)
   II. *Exclusion of all other hematopoietic or non-hematopoietic disorders*

B. **MDS-related criteria:**
   I. *Dysplasia in >10% of all cells in one of the following lineage in bone marrow smears:*
      i. Erythroid, neutrophil or megakaryocytic or
      ii. >15% ring sideroblast on Fe stain
   II. *5–19% blast cells in bone marrow smear.*
   III. *Typical chromosomal abnormality* (by conventional karyotyping or FISH)

The diagnosis can be established when both prerequisite criteria and at least 1 decisive criteria are fulfilled.

Therapy Strategy

1. **Low risk MDS**—Observation + Supportive care (only indicated)
2. **Low/Int-1 risk MDS**—Low intensity therapy + Supportive care
3. **Int 2/high-risk MDS**—Intensive therapy (who can tolerate it)
4. **Int 2/high-risk MDS—who are ineligible for intensive therapy**—palliative or investigational therapy to maintain the quality of life.

A. **Supportive care:**
   1. *Transfusion*—aim to maintain adequate peripheral count to prevent and to treat infections.
      i. *Leukodepleted platelet transfusion* to maintain platelet count >10 × 10⁹/L.
      ii. *Tranexamic acid* 0.5 1 gm thrice daily in useful to treat bleeding refractory to platelets or with profound thrombocytopenia
      iii. Pure red cell transfusion to be instituted in patient of MDS to maintain hemoglobin level >9 gm/dl.
   2. *Anti-infective therapy:* Empirical broad-spectrum antibiotic and/or antifungal should be administered for neutropenic sepsis.
   3. *Iron chelating therapy*
      Indications:
      i. Who received 20–25 units of RBC or long then transfusion
      ii. If serum ferritin level >2500 mg/L.
      iii. Concurrent cardiac or hepatic dysfunction.

   Drugs used:
   a. *Desferrioxamine*—.20–40 mg/kg by 12 hour subcutaneously 5–7 nights/week—reduced to 25 mg/kg when ferritin level <200 mg/L
   b. *Desferasirox* 20–30 mg/kg orally.

B. Treatment aimed at improving bone marrow function:
1. Growth factors (erythropoietin, G-CSF, GM-CSF)
2. Immunosuppression (ATG, cyclosporine)
3. Anticytokine approaches (thalidomide and analogs)
4. Antiapoptosis

C. Treatment directed at the abnormal clone:
1. Low intensity chemotherapy (hydroxyurea, melphalan, low dose Ara-c, VP-16)
2. Induction regimen (anthracycline/Ara-c combination, FLAG, ADE)
3. DNA—methyltransferase inhibitors (5-azacytidine, decitabine)
4. Famesyltransferase inhibitor
5. Remission induction/autologous stem cell transplant
6. **Antiangiogenesis** (arsenic trioxide, anti-VEGF, thalidomide)

D. Curative attempts (stem cell transplantation)
1. Myeloablative transplantation
2. Reduced intensity conditioning

ADE: Adriamycin (daunorubicin, cytarabine, etoposide)
ATG: Antithymic globulin
FLAG: Fludarabine, cytarabine, granulocyte colony-stimulating factor
RTK: Receptor tyrosine kinase inhibitor
VEGF: Vascular endothelia and growth factor

Low Intensity Therapy

Erythropoietin (EPO) + G-CSF:
1. *For patients with refractory anemia (RA): Refractory anemia with excess blasts with symptomatic anemia,* transfusion requirement <2 units/month, basal EPO level <200 IU/L. **Consider:**
   a. EPO—10000 U/day or 40,000–60,000 U 1–3 X per week for 6 weeks.
   b. *In nor responders,* consider adding daily G—CSF (1–2 mg/kg/day or 1–3 x/week) sc
   In responders—reduce the dose of G-CSF to 3 weekly and EPO in steps to lowest maintenance dose
2. *For patients with refractory anemia with ring sideroblast (RARS) with symptomatic anemia,* transfusion requirement <24 months, basal EPO level <500 IU/L—combined therapy with EPO and G-CSF should be started from outset:
   i. *In nor responders* EPO dose should be increased after 6 weeks
   ii. *If no response* after 2–3 months—treatment failure
   iii. *In responders*—doses and frequency as tolerated
3. *Hyperglycosylated long-acting EPO derivative* (darbepoetin alfa 150–300 µg/week) is an effective alternative with response up to 60%.
4. *G-CSF is useful for patient:*
   a. With neutropenia and recurrent infection
   b. With neutropenia and antibiotic resistant infection. Not recommended for chronic prophylaxis

Lenalidomide:
1. It achieves major clinical response and cytogenic response in 5q-syndrome, by directly suppressing 5q-clone
2. It may alter the natural history of MDS with durable responses.
3. Improve overall survival (10 year estimate of 78% for cytogenic responders
4. Reduces AML transformation at 10 years.

Thalidomide:
i. Inhibits angiogenesis
ii. Interfere with cellular adhesion
iii. Alters inflammatory cytokine profiles
iv. Capable of producing hematological responses in 20% of transfusion dependant patients.

DNA methyltransferase inhibitor:
The agents are: Azacitidine and decitabine
Mode of action: They inhibit DNA methyltransferase
Reduce DNA methylation and
Reactivate abnormally suppressed gene expression.

In such way, they:
i. Ameliorate anemia
ii. Decrease the risk of leukaemic transformation and improve overall survival.

These agents are currently approved for use in patients with all FAB subjects.

Dose and frequency: Optimal dose and duration of therapy is yet not established.

But low dose or high dose—intensity regimen may be the best.

Side effect: Rash and vomiting more frequent with azacitidine but only after several months.

Response: Minimum 3 cycles required before evaluation of response. Response duration <1 year for both drugs

Immunosuppression:
A. *Horse antithymic globulin*—40 mg/kg/day × 4 days produces hematological response in 1/3rd of patients **with low-risk MDS.**
   Responders are:
   i. <50 years of age, shorter duration of RBC transfusion dependence
   ii. Who are HLA DR 15+
B. *Cyclosporin A*—(5 mg/kg/day for 3 months then tapering the dose thereafter) effective in **MDS patients who are HLA DR 4 positive.**
C. *AIG + Cyclosporin A combination*

Non-Intensive Chemotherapy

Indication:
i. Elderly patient with transformed or transforming MDS
ii. Transient reduction in blast counts may be the at the price of increased cytopenia
iii. Transfusion dependence

Drugs are:
a. *Hydroxycarbamide:*
   i. Control monocytosis in CMML
   ii. Titration of dose to achieve optimum control of myeloproliferation with minimum additional cytopenia
   iii. More preferable to oral etoposide
b. *Low dose melphalan:* Best response in hypoplastic MDS.

High Dose Therapy and Stem Cell Transplantation

Sibling allogent SCT are indicated in:
1. Patients <50 years with IPSS intermediate-1 and sibling donor.

2. IPPS—intermediate-2/high-risk patient >60 years for best overall survival.

SCT should be delayed for: Low/intermediate-1 MDS patient until progression.

Factors for decision to transplant and its outcome:
  i. Age
  ii. Comorbidity
  iii. Disease stage
  iv. Non-transplant chemotherapy
  v. Type of donor
  vi. Source of stem cell
  vii. Conditioning regimen

5 years disease free survival:
  i. IPSS—low/intermediate-1—60%
  ii. Intermediate-2—36%
  iii. high risk—28%

Matched unrelated donor allogenic SCT:
  i. Lower disease free survival (<30% in 2 years)
  ii. Higher treatment related mortality (>50%)
  iii. Lower relapse rate (<15%)
  iv. High mortality associated with patient age.

Autologous SCT is less indicated because:
  i. Adequate stem cell numbers achieved in only 40–60% patients
  ii. Lower treatment related mortality but higher relapse rate
  iii. Higher relapse rate than allograft
  iv. Disease free survival in only 15% patient.

ACUTE LYMPHOBLASTIC LEUKEMIA

Epidemiology

  i. 25% of childhood cancer today.
  ii. Peak age of incidence is 2–9 years
  iii. There is male predominance
  iv. Caucasians have two fold increased incidence.

Etiology

1. Predisposition in congenital diseases:
   i. Down syndrome
   ii. Bloom's syndrome
   iii. Klinfelter's syndrome
   iv. Fanconi syndrome
2. Acquired chromosomal diseases
   i. Aneuploidy, ii. Hyperdyploidy, iii. Translocation
3. Chemicals
4. Pollution
5. Viruses
6. Radiation exposure

Clinical Features

Acute presentation is common—due to bone marrow failure:
  I. **Anemia**—weakness, lethargy, breathlessness, light-headedness, palpitations
  II. **Infections**—chest, mouth, perianal skin, (*Staphylococcus, Haemophilus influenzae, Pseudomonas, HSV, Candida*)
  III. **Fever**, malaise, night sweat
  IV. **Hemorrhage**, purpura, menorrhagia, epistaxis, bleeding gum, rectal and retinal bleeding
  V. **Signs of leukostasis**—hypoxia, retinal hemorrhage, confusion, diffuse pulmonary shadow.
  VI. **Bone and joint pain**—more common in children
  VII. **Mediastinal involvement**—superior vena caval syndrome—in T-ALL.
  VIII. **CNS involvement**—cranial nerve palsy—facial nerve, sensory disturbance and meningium
  IX. **Signs**:
    i. Hepatomegaly 45%
    ii. Splenomegaly
    iii. Lymphadenopathy—55%
    iv. Orchidomegaly.

Classification

I. FAB morphology:
  • L_1= Small monomorphic, → small homogenous blasts, single inconspicuous nucleolus, regular nuclear outline, minimal cytoplasm, commonest subtype in children.
  • L_2= Large heterogenous type → large blast cells, more pleomorphic and multiple nucleoli, irregular clefted nuclei with conspicuous nucleoli, commonest in adult.
  • L_3= Burkitt cell type → large homogenous blasts, prominent nucleoli, basophilic cytoplasm, prominent vacuolization.

II. Bone marrow classification:
  M_1 = <5% blasts (Fig. 5.54)
  M_2 = 5–25% blasts
  M_3 = >25% blasts

Cerebral Fluid Cytological Classification

CNS-1 = No blast cell
CNS-2 = WBC <5/μL, with blast cells
CNS-3 = WBC ≥ 5/μL, with blast cells

Immunological Classification

A. B-lineage—85%:
  1. **Pro – B – ALL** = HLA DR +VE, TDT +VE, CD 19+VE
  2. **Common ALL** = HLA DR +VE, TDT +VE, CD 19+VE, CD 10+VE
  3. **Pre-B-ALL** = HLA DR+VE, TDT+VE, CD 10+VE, CD-10±VE, cytoplasmic IgM+VE .
  4. **B cell ALL** = HLA DR+VE, TDT+VE, CD 19+VE, CD 10±VE, surface IgM+VE

B. T-lineage—15%
  1. **Pre-T-ALL** = cytoplasmic CD3+VE, CD7+VE
  2. **T-cell ALL** = cytoplasmic CD3+VE, CD 1A/2/3+VE, CD5+VE

Investigations

1. Complete hemogram, peripheral blood picture
2. Bone marrow aspirate ± trephine biopsy (Fig. 5.55)
3. Bone marrow cytogenetics and nuclear analysis
4. Immunophenotyping of blood or marrow blasts
5. Total WBC count is high with blast cells on film, but low—aleukemic leukemia
6. Hemogram—Hb%, neutrophil and platelet—low, clotting—deranged
7. Bone marrow infiltrated with ≥ 20% blast cells
8. CT scan of chest and abdomen—abdominal and mediastenal lymph adenopathy
9. Lumbar puncture is mandatory to detect CNS involvement—but it should be done after reduction of peripheral blast cell count (Figs 5.56 and 5.57)

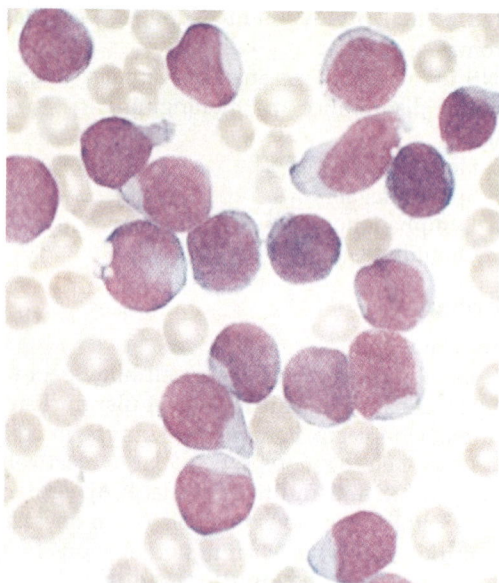

Fig. 5.56: Blast cell in the bone marrow

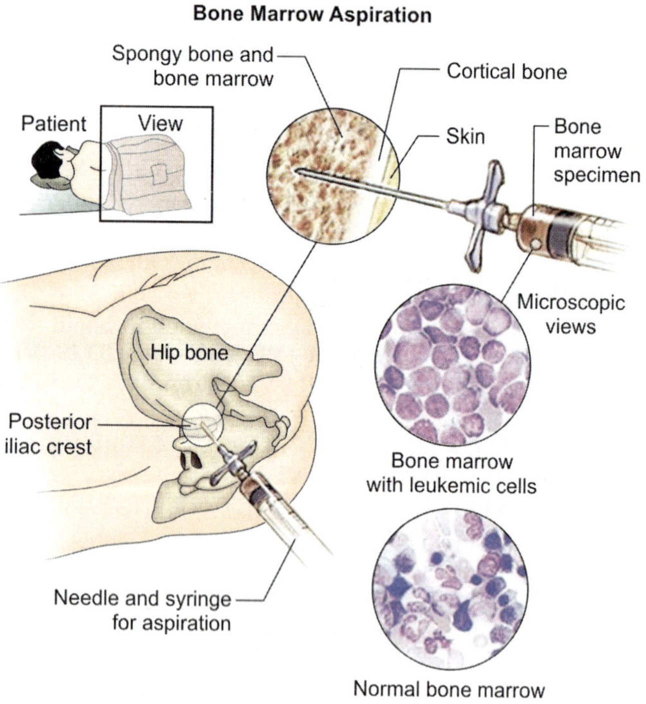

Bone Marrow Aspiration

Fig. 5.57: Method of collection of bone marrow

Treatment

I. Emergency treatment:
1. Cardiovascular and respiratory resuscitation—septic shock and massive hemorrhage
2. Empirical broad-spectrum antibiotics for neutropenic sepsis.
3. Leukopheresis—if blast cell count is high or signs of leukostasis (retinal hemorrhage, reduce conscious level diffuse pulmonary shadow).

II. Supportive treatment
1. Similar to that of AML
2. Hydration should be started to get urine output >100 ml/hour throughout induction therapy

3. Allopurinol should be started to prevent hyperuricemia. Interaction with 6MP—discontinue allopurinol or reduce the dose of 6-MP.

Chemotherapy—complete hematological remission (CR) can be defined by:
1. Normal bone marrow cellularity—blast cells <5% normal trilineage hematopoiesis.
2. Normalination of peripheral blood count, no blast cells
   i. Neutrophil >1.5×10^9/L
   ii. Platelet count, >100×10^9/L
   iii. Hb% >10 gm/dl

Treatment of ALL consists of:

Remission induction: Drugs are (standard risk):
   i. Prednisolone—40–60 mg/m^2/day × 21–28 days
   ii. Vincristine—1.5 mg/m^2/dose IV weekly × 4 doses (Days 0, 7, 14 and 21)
   iii. *E. coli*-L-asparaginase—6000–10000 IU/m^2/dose IM × 6–9 doses—3 days per week × 2–3 weeks.

   (Four drugs—high risk)
   In addition to drugs described above
   iv. Doxorubicin 25–30 mg/m^2/dose
       Or   } IV weekly × 4 doses
   Daunorubicin 25–45 mg/m^2/dose } (days 0,7,14,21)

   (Five drugs—highest risk)
   In addition to above four drugs
   v. Cyclophosphamide—800–1200 mg/m^2/dose IV × 1 dose (day 0)

Response evaluation:
Day-14—Bone marrow
   M$_1$—Rapid early responder
   M$_2$ to M$_3$—Slow early responder
Day-28—Bone marrow
   M1—remission, continue as below.
   M2–M3—Induction failure, reinduction is required.

CNS prophylaxis:
   i. Cranial irradiation with 18–24 Gy in 12 fractions in 2 weeks.

+

   Intrathecal (IT) chemotherapy with
   a. CNS-1—methotrexate every two weeks × 2 doses (days 0,14)
   b. CNS-2 or CNS-3—weekly × 4 doses (days 0,7,14,21)
   ii. Intrathecal chemotherapy should be **continued in consolidation and maintenance phases.**
   Simultaneous administration of IT methotrexate and IV vincristine must be avoided because it is fatal.

Consolidation phases—indication:
   i. To further reduce tumor burden
   ii. To reduce the risk of relapse
   iii. To prevent development of drug resistant cells

Pretreatment criteria:
   i. Neutrophil count ≥ 750/mL
   ii. Platelet count > 75000/mL
   iii. ALT <20 times of upper limit of normal
   iv. Serum creatinine is normal for age
   v. No active infection or organ dysfunction

Drugs are (from 5th week):
   i. Cyclophosphamide—1000 mg/m^2/dose IV × 2 doses (days 0,14)
   ii. Mercaptopurine—60 mg/m^2/dose × 28 days (days 0–27)

iii. Vincristine 1.5 mg/m²/dose × 4 doses (days 14, 21, 42, 49)
iv. Cytarabine—75 mg/m²/dose IV (days 1–4, 8–11, 29–32, 36–39)
v. *E. coli*—asparaginase 6000 IV/m²/dose IM × 12 doses every other day—3 days/week.
vi. IT—Methotrexate—weekly × 4 doses

Maintenance therapy (2–3 years): It is necessary for patients who do not proceed to SCT

Drugs are:
i. Daily 6-mercaptopurine—75 mg/m²/dose once daily.
ii. Weekly methotrexate, orally—20 mg/m²/dose once weekly
iii. Cyclical vincristine—1.5 mg/m²/dose IV every 4 weeks.
iv. Oral prednisolone—40–60 mg/day
v. IT methotrexate—every 4–12 weeks × 1–2 years.

Stem Cell Transplantation

1. **Allogenic/SCT**—option for adult:
   i. Adult <50 years.
   ii. Compatible siblings
   iii. Leukemia free survival superior after 1st remission
   iv. Treatment related mortality 30%.
   Option for younger patients:
   i. Younger patients <40 years
   ii. Matched unrelated donor
   iii. Used in very high-risk diseases
   v. Treatment-related mortality–48%
2. **Autologous SCT:**
   i. Adult >60 years
   ii. No compatible donor
   iii. Treatment-related mortality—8%
   iv. No clear advantage of survival over maintenance therapy.

BCR-ABL—ALL:
1. Limatinib mesylate should be added to the above regimen
2. Eligible patient should receive SCT.

T-cell ALL:
1. High incidence of CNS involvement
2. High cure rate when cyclophosphamide is added to this regimen

Prognosis

i. 75% of adult achieve complete remission with modern regimen and good supportive care
ii. Median duration of remission is 15 months
iii. Disease free survival in adult is <30% in 5 years and 10–20% in >50 years of age.

Prognostic factors:
i. *Patient's age*   < 50 years   CR >80%
                      > 50 years   CR <60%
ii. *High leukocyte count*   > 30 × 10⁹/L
             B precursor ALL—100 × 10⁹/L—poor risk
iii. *Immunophenotype*—pro-B-ALL—and Pro-T-ALL—poor outcome—so poor prognosis..
iv. Cytogenetics—Ph BCR—ABL+ve—poor prognosis
v. Longer the time to reach CR—poorer the prognosis
vi. High minimal residual volume of blast cell—after induction (>10⁻³)

CNS leukemia:
i. Incidence is high in T cell-ALL and high blast count.
ii. Patient may present with headache, vomiting, lethargy, neck rigidity, cranial and peripheral nerve dysfunction.
iii. On clinical examination—papilledema, meningism, neurodeficit, lumbar puncture shows—blast cells in CSF
iv. Treatment—intensified intrathecal triple therapy, if methotrexate + cytarabine + hydrocortisone 2–3 times weekly × 3–4 weeks, or until 2 consecutive CSF samples are –ve
v. If relapse—requires systemic reinduction
vi. Poor prognosis.

Transfusion

To decrease transfusion associated complications specialized products should be used.
i. To prevent bleeding platelet count should be maintained >10000/ml.
ii. Higher level is required prior to invasive procedure—lumbar puncture and reduce the risk of leukostasis included CNS hemorrhage.
iii. RBC transfusion should be avoided when WBC count is >100000/mt.
iv. To increase hemoglobin and hematocrit slowly small aliquots of packed RBC are given.
v. To reduce risk of GVHD, all cellular products must be irradiated.

ACUTE MYELOID LEUKEMIA

It is heterogeneous group of disorders characterized by uncontrolled proliferation of myeloid progenitor cells gradually replacing the normal hemopoiesis in bone marrow and infiltrates the blood and other tissues.

Epidemiology

1. Age—15–20% incidence in children and adolescents, 90% in adult. Most patients are >65 years of age at presentation.
2. Age adjusted male female ratio is 4.3: 2.9.

Etiology (Fig. 5.58)

I. **Hereditary/genetic disorders:**
   a. Down syndrome
   b. Bloom syndrome
   c. Fanconi anemia
   d. Ataxia telangiectesia
   e. Kotsmann syndrome
   f. Klinefelter syndrome.
II. **Environmental exposure:**
   a. Benzene and its derivatives—ethylene oxides, herbicides
   b. Ionizing radiation
III. **Pre-existing hematological disorders:**
   a. Myelodysplastic syndrome
   b. Myeloproliferative disorders
   c. Paroxysmal nocturnal hemoglobinuria
IV. **Drugs:**
   a. Radiotherapy alone or in combination with chemotherapy
   b. Alkalyting agents—these drugs can produce leukemia 4–6 years after exposure. Affected persons have chromosomal aberrations in 5 and 7.

Normal blood cells

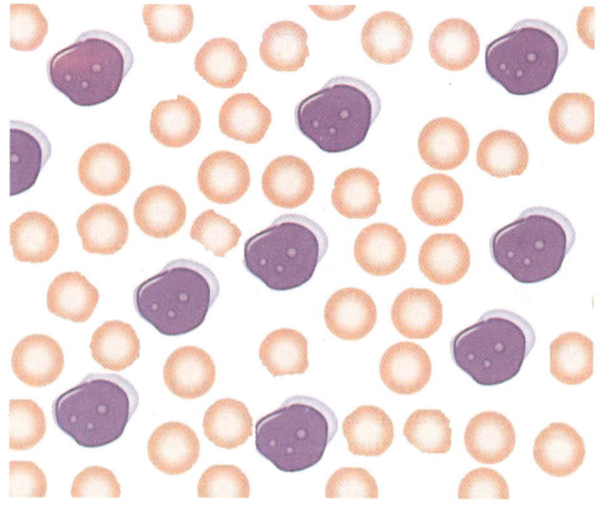

Fig. 5.58: Dynamics of epigenetic modifications in leukemia

d. Other drugs—chloramphenicol, phenylbutazone, chloroquine—can produce bone marrow failure and evolve into AML.

Classifications

Two commonly used classifications in AML.

1. Older Classification

French-American-British (FAB) classification based on:
  i. Morphology
  ii. Cytochemical staining
  iii. Immunohistochemistry and immunophenotype of predominant cells

AML is divided into eight subtypes:
1. M_0—*minimally differentiated AML* (Fig. 5.59):
   i. Negative peroxidase reaction
   ii. Flow cytometry shows two or more myeloid markers
   iii. Complex cytogenic abnormalities.
   iv. Poor prognosis
2. M_1—*AML without maturation* (Fig. 5.60): Less than 10% promyelocytes or more matured form.

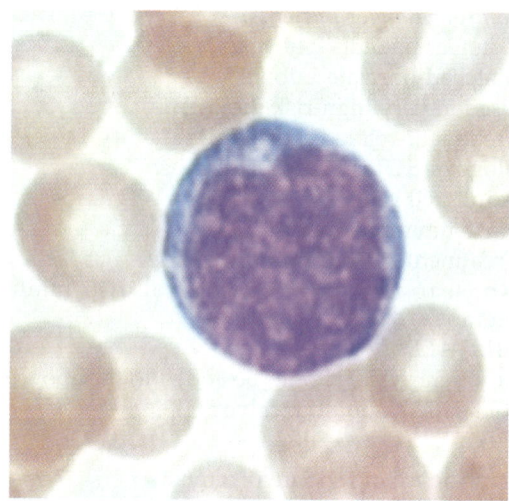

Fig. 5.60: M_1—AML without maturation

3. M_2—*AML with maturation* (Fig. 5.61):
   i. Subtype has translocation at t (8:21)
   ii. Favorable prognosis.

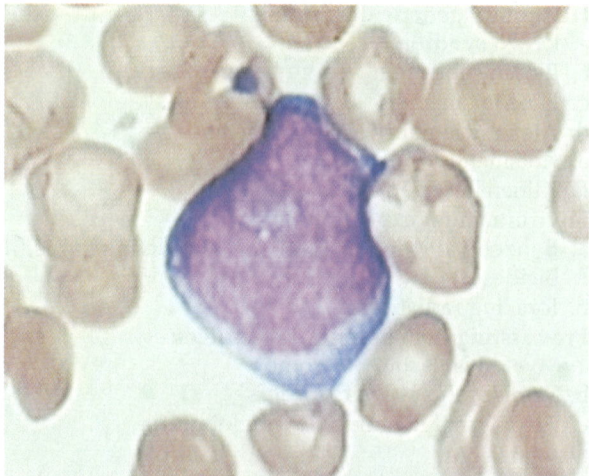

Fig. 5.59: M_0—minimally differentiated AML

c. Topoisomerase II inhibitors—leukemia occurs 3–7 years after exposure to these drugs and have chromosomal aberration at 11q, 23.

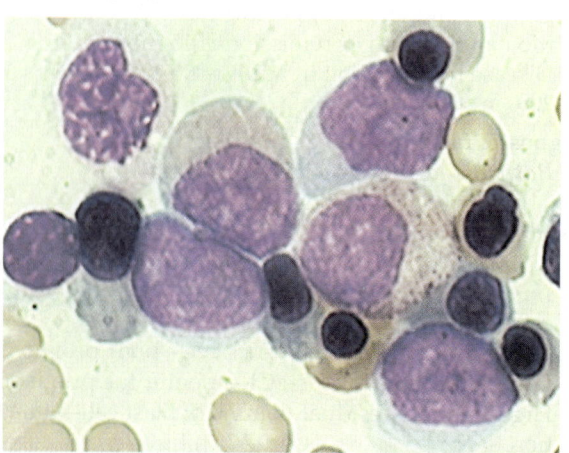

Fig. 5.61: M_2—AML with maturation

4. **M_3—acute promyelocytic leukemia (APL)** (Fig. 5.62):
   i. Heavy granulation and bilobed nuclear contour.
   ii. Microgranular variant with inconspicuous granules.
   iii. Most cases have translocation at t (15:17)
   iv. Favorable prognosis

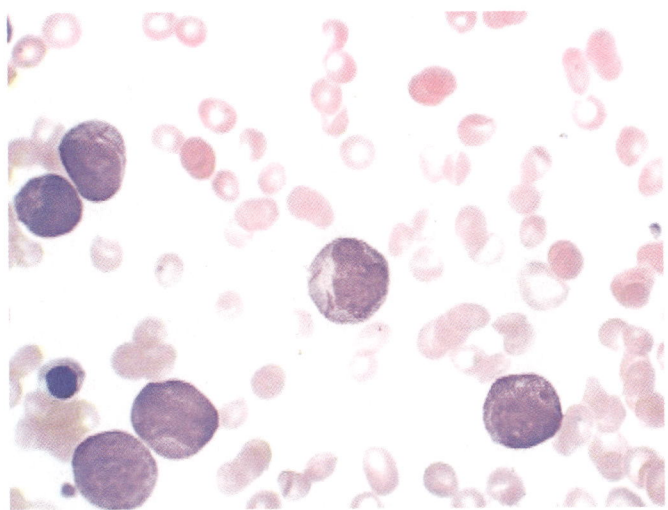

Fig. 5.62: M₃—acute promyelocytic leukemia

5. **M_4—acute myelomonocytic leukemia:**
   i. In marrow >20% monocytes and promonocytes
   ii. M_4E_o variant—contain >5% abnormal eosinophils
   iii. Inv (16) cytogenic abnormality
   iv. Favorable prognosis
6. **M_5—acute monocytic leukemia** (Fig. 5.63):
   i. 80% or more cells are monocytes, monoblast or promonocytes
   ii. Non-specific esterase stain is positive.
   iii. Associated with extramedullary disease
   iv. Abnormalities of long arm of chromosome 11.

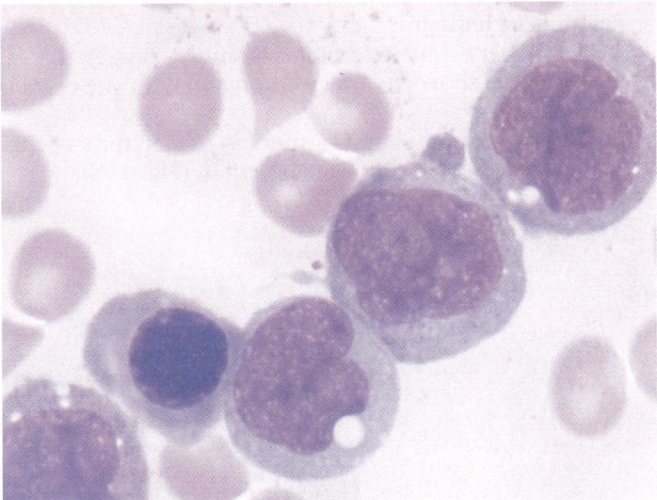

Fig. 5.63: M₅—acute monocytic leukemia

7. **M_6—acute erythroleukemia** (Fig. 5.64):
   i. More than 50% cells in bone marrow are erythroid cells
   ii. Erythroblasts are strongly PAS +ve and glycophorin positive

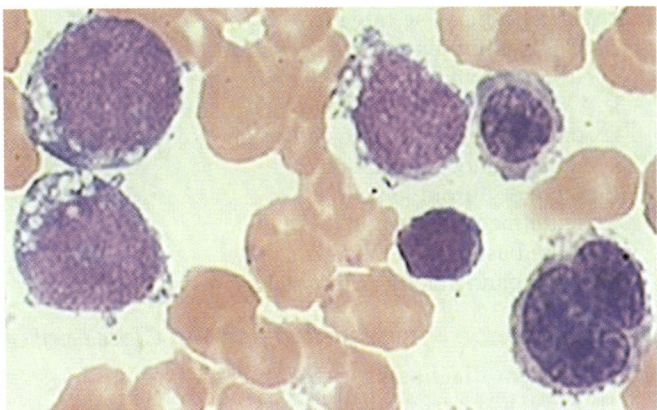

Fig. 5.64: M₆—acute erythroleukemia

8. **M_7—acute megakaryocytic leukemia** (Fig. 5.65):
   i. Bone marrow has micromegakaryoblast.
   ii. Confirmed by immunohistotyping (CD41) or electron microscopy (platelet peroxidase).

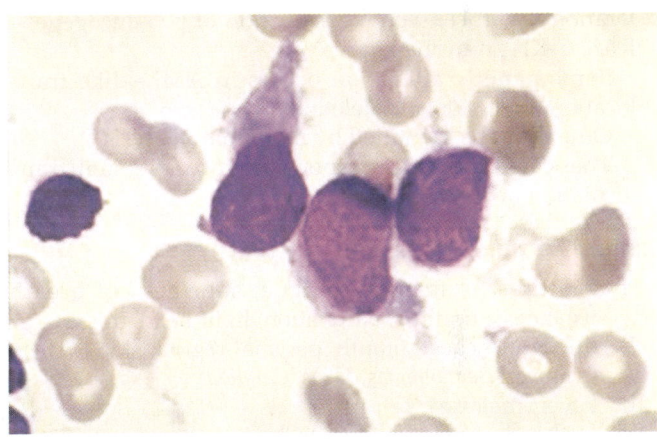

Fig. 5.65: M₇—acute megakaryocytic leukemia

Second Classification

WHO classify AML based on:
   i. Molecular genetics
   ii. Therapy-related leukemia
   iii. Biphenotypic leukemia

A. AML with recurrent cytogenic translocations
   1. AML with t (8:21) (q22; q22)
   2. AML with t (15:17) (q22; q11) + variants = APL (M₃)
   3. AML with abnormal marrow eosinophils Inv (16) (p13q22) or t (16:16)(p13;q11)
   4. AML with 11q23 (MLL) abnormalities

B. AML with multilineage dysplasia:
   1. With prior myelodysplastic syndrome
   2. Without prior myelodysplastic syndrome

C. AML and MDS; therapy related:
   1. Alkalyting agent related
   2. Epipodophyllotoxin-related
   3. Others

D. AML not otherwise categorized:
1. AML with minimal differentiation
2. AML with maturation
3. AML without maturation
4. Acute myelomonocytic leukemia
5. Acute monocytic leukemia
6. Acute erythroid leukemia
7. Acute megakaryocytic leukemia
8. Acute basophilic leukemia
9. Acute panmyelosis with myelofibrosis.

Major Difference Between WHO and FAB Classification

Blast cutoff for diagnosis of AML:
- 20% in WHO classification
- 30% in FAB classification

Pathogenesis

This is a multistep process—results from the interaction between two different classes of mutations:
1. **First class mutations**—impairs cell differentiation resulting in clonal expansions of myeloid progenitors.
2. **Second class mutation**—produce abnormal cell proliferation—with consecutive activation of pro-oncogenes—RAS, C-KIT, tyrosine kinase

Some **genetic alteration** occurs in AML—like translocation, inversion and deletion.

Others can be identified by molecular analysis.

These mutations are responsible for malignant transformation of blood cells.

Clinical Features (Fig. 5.66)

I. Features of anemia—fatigue, shortness of breath, weakness, tinnitus, palpitation, light headedness
II. Infection—chest, mouth, perianal region, skin (*Staphylococcus, Pseudomonas*, HSV, *Candida*)
III. Fever, malaise
IV. Hemorrhage (M_3 due to DIC)
V. Leukostasis and hyperviscosity producing organ dysfunctions (confusion, visual impairment, shortness of breath)
VI. Leukostasis producing hemorrhage in retina, brain lung and other organs.
VII. Purpura, epistaxis, menorrhagia, gum bleeding—thrombocytopenia.

VIII. Gum hypertrophy (Fig. 5.67)—(M_4 and M_5)
IX. 20% cases—hepatomegaly, 24% splenomegaly—it may suspect the conversion from CML to AML
X. Rarely
   i. Skin rash with neutrophilic infiltration in the dermis—sweet syndrome
   ii. Chloroma—tumor of myeloid blast cells.

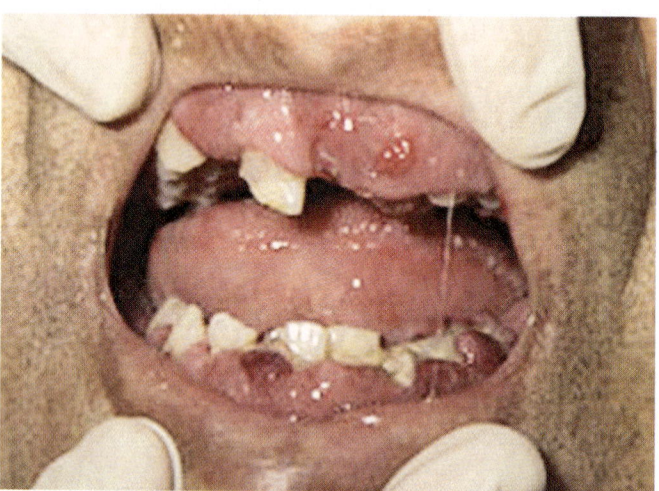

Fig. 5.67: Gum hypertrophy with bleeding

Investigations

A. Hematological investigations:
a. *Anemia:* i. Normocytic normochromic—due to decreased erythropoiesis.
b. *Reduced reticulocyte count:* If there is hemorrhage—hypochromic and microcytic.
c. **White blood cell count:**
   i. Medium presenting count 15000/cc
   ii. 25 to 40% patient <5000/cc
   iii. 20% patients have 100000/cc
   iv. <5% patients have no leukemic cells in blood

Features of leukemic cell:
i. Cytoplasm contains primary granules
ii. Neucleus shows fine, lacy chromatin with one or more nucleoli.
iii. Abnormal rod-shaped granules—Auer rods—when present—myeloid lineage is certain (Fig. 4.68).

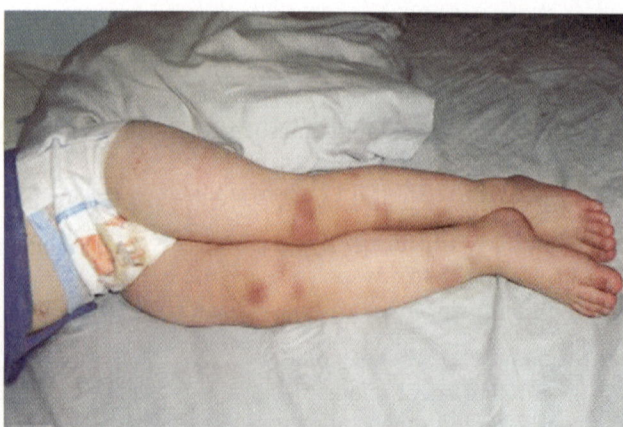

Fig. 5.66: Brusing in AML

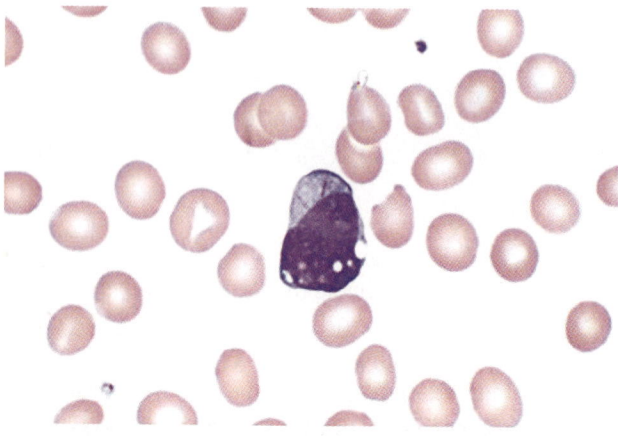

Fig. 5.68: A single blast cell containing Auer rods

Poor neutrophil functions are characterized by:
  i. Impaired phagocytosis
  ii. Impaired migration
  iii. Morphologically abnormal lobulation and deficient granulation.
  d. *Platelet count:*
    i. 75% patients have <100000/cc
    ii. <25% patients have <25000/cc
Abnormal platelets are characterized by:
  i. Large and bizarre-shaped platelet
  ii. Abnormal granulation
  iii. Inability of platelet aggregation and adhesion.
B. **Biochemical investigation**
  i. Hyperuricemia
  ii. Elevated blood urea nitrogen and creatinine (urate nephropathy)
  iii. High LDH
  iv. Hypokalemia (tumor dysfunction)
  v. Lactic acidosis (leukostasis)
  vi. Hypercalcemia
  vii. Hyperuricemia, hyperphosphatemia, hypocalcemia, hypokalemia—tumor lysis syndrome.
C. **Imaging studies:**
  i. Chest X-ray and CT scan of thorax
  ii. CT scan of brain—intracranial hemorrhage
  iii. MRI—thickened nerve sheets.
D. **Coagulation profile:**
  i. Prothrombin time
  ii. Activated partial thromboplastin time
  iii. Fibrinogen
  iv. D-dimer
E. **Evelution of liver function**
F. **Evaluation of renal function**
G. **Serologies of:**
  i. Hepatitis B virus
  ii. Herpes simplex virus
  iii. CMV
  iv. HIV
H. **Bone marrow aspirate for:**
  i. Morphology
  ii. Cytochemistry
  iii. Cytogenetics
  iv. Flow cytometry
I. **HLA typing of patient's siblings, if younger than 55 years.**
J. **Lumbar puncture delayed until blasts cells cleared** from blood in patients for high risk of CNS involvement—CNS symptoms, elevated leukocyte count, extramedullary disease and monocytic morphology FAB M_4 and M_5.
K. **Evaluation of cardiac function**—ECG, echocardiogram.
L. **Intervention for specific patient**
  1. *Dental evaluation* in case of poor dentition
  2. *Lumbar puncture*—for those with symptoms of CNS involvement
  3. *Screening of spine* in MRI (for patient with back pain, lower extremity paresthesia)
     Immunotype
     Immunocytochemistry

Treatment

Emergency Treatment

  i. **In case of massive hemorrhage or septic shock—cardio-vascular and respiratory resuscitation**
  ii. In **case of sepsis**—Empirical broad-spectrum antibiotic treatment.
  iii. **Leukopheresis:**
    a. If blast cells are high, >100 × 10^9/L (risk of early death)
    b. Signs of leukostasis—but not in APL
  iv. **Intensive hydration + alkalization of urine—to prevent acute tumor lysis syndrome**, if peripheral blast cell count is very high >100 × 10^9/L.

Supportive Treatment

  i. **Explain diagnosis and counseling**—regarding the disease and prolonged chemotherapy.
  ii. **RBC transfusion**—continued throughout the treatment
  iii. **Platelet transfusion:** To maintain count:
    a. >10 × 10^9/L—if not septic or not on antibiotics
    b. >20 × 10^9/L—if patient is hemorrhagic or other hemostatic abnormality.
    c. >50 × 10^9/L—in bleeding acute promyelocytic leukemia.
  iv. **Prophylactic regimen for neutropenic patient:**
    a. Isolation procedures—strict handwashing of contacts, visitor restriction, gloves, apron, gown, masks, caps full reverse barrier
    b. Drinks—use of boiled water or sparkling mineral water. Avoid unpasturized milk and fresh juice
    e. Food—avoid cream, ice-cream, cheeses, live yoghurt raw eggs, mayonnaise.
    f. General mouth care
    g. Antimicrobial prophylaxis
       Ciprofloxacin 250 mg twice daily
       Or
       Cotrimoxazole 480 mg twice daily
       Or
       Colistin 1.5 MU thrice daily + neomycin 500 ml 4 times daily.
    h. **Antifungal prophylaxis:** Fluconozole—100 mg orally daily
    i. **Antiviral prophylaxis**—acyclovir is most important drug for preventing herpes infection, 400 mg twice daily prevents HSV reactivation.

Chemotherapy

There are two stages of chemotherapy:
A. **Induction of remission:** To achieve complete remission.
   Complete hematological remission can be defined as:
   i. Normal bore marrow cellularity (blast cell <5%, and normal trilineage hematopoiesis.
   ii. Normal peripheral blood count and no blast cells:
     a. Neutrophil >1.5 × 10^9/L
     b. Platelet ≥ 100 × 10^9/L
     c. Hb >10 gm/dl.

Drugs most commonly used are:
i. *Daunorubicin*—45–60 mg/m² IV × 3 days
                        +
Cytarabine 200 mg/m²/day IV infusion over 12 hours × 7 days.
   The above combination (3 days + 7 days regimen) results in complete remission in 60 to 80% patients younger than 55 to 60 years of age.
   Addition of etoposide may improve complete remission (CR) duration.

Assess the bone marrow response at 14th and 21st day of remission period.

ii. *If blast cell persist >10% in bone marrow,* 2nd identical course of above region should be applied here.
Cytarabine for 5 days and daunorubicin for 2 days. Idarubicin is superior to daunorubicin.

In spite of above two courses:

i. A few patients become resistant to drugs—called drug resistant leukemia.
ii. A few patients develop fatal complication of bone marrow aplasia or impaired recovery of normal stem cells.

Induction treatment-related mortality depends on:

i. Increasing age
ii. Have prior hematological disorder—myelodysplastic syndrome
iii. Chemotherapy treatment for another malignancy.

In the patient with CR after two induction courses should be treated with allogenic hemopoietic stem cell trans plantation, if appropriate donor exists.

Higher dose of cytarabine is better than standard dose because: More cytarabine enter the cells and saturate the cytarabine inactivating enzymes and increase the intracellular levels of active metabolite—and increase the inhibition of DNA synthesis.

Higher doses of cytarabine toxicity: i. Myelodepression, ii. Occasionally cerebellar toxicity.

B. Post-remission treatment

Aim:

i. To reduce leukemic burden further
ii. Reduce the risk of relapse

Strategies are:

1. Low dose maintenance therapy—is not generally helpful
2. Intensive consolidation therapy improves survival of younger patients
3. Marrow ablative therapy with autologous stem cell rescue
4. Allogenic stem cell transplantation

Course: Cytarabine—2 to 3 gm/m²/day continuous infusion per day on days 1, 3 and 5.

Optimal number of course have not been determined, but two to four courses are reasonable:

i. Patient with age <55 years with favorable cytogenetics with core binding factor mutation (t 8: 21 and inv 16) responds well with this therapy.
ii. Patients with >60 years do not respond to this therapy.

Hematopoietic Stem Cell Transplantation

Two types of transplantation are:
A. Autologous SCT
B. Allogenic SCT
  1. Autologous SCT requires collection of stem cell from patient in complete remission.
  Allogenic SCT requires stem cell from HLA-matched siblings or unrelated donor or cord blood.
  2. Relapse rate following allogenic SCT is low but treatment-related toxicity is very high. Toxicity includes:
     i. Veno-occlusive disease
     ii. Graft versus host disease
     iii. Infections.

Toxicity following autologous transplant is low, but relapse rate is very high because:

i. Absence of graft versus leukemia effect in this therapy
ii. Possible contamination of autologous stem cells with residual tumor cells
3. Allogenic SCT can be administered in patients aged <70–75 years with high-risk cytogenetics.
Autologous SCT should be administered in younger and older patients with poor risk as intensive consolidation therapy.

Prognosis

1. 70–80% patients aged <60 years achieve complete remission with modern intensive regimen, supportive care, consolidation regiment and reduce the risk of relapse.
2. Relapse rate at 5 years:
     i. <60 years with favorable risks   29–42%
     ii. <60 years with intermediate risks   9–60%
     iii. <60 years with poor risk   68–90%
3. 50–60% patients with age >60 years will have complete remission with induction therapy, but relapse rate is 80–90%, due to presence of associated comorbidity, myelodysplasia.

Prognostic Factors

Following factors are responsible for subsequent relapse

1. Age <50 years—favorable, >60 years unfavorable.
2. Presence of cytogenic abnormality—classified as—poor, intermediate and favorable risk factors.
3. Failure of complete remission after 1st induction dose predicts subsequent relapse.
4. Mutation of FLT3 gene predicts poor outcome in all cytogenic subtypes.
5. History of antecedent myelodysplastic syndrome or leukemogenic therapy—unfavorable.
6. Presenting blast cell count $<25 \times 10^9/L$—favorable $>100 \times 10^9/L$—unfavorable.
7. FAB subtype $M_3 M_4 E_O$—favorable
FAB subtype $M_0, M5_a, M5_b, M_6, M_7$—unfavourable

Management of Relapse

1. 50% patient in CR will relapse.
2. Most relapse will occur in first 2–3 years.
3. Younger age and longer duration of first CR (>6 months)—are good prognostic factors for achieving 2nd CR.
4. 50% patients achieve 2nd complete remission with the dose of cytarabine therapy (FLAG—fludarabine + cytarabine + G-CSF), 10% survive >3 years without transplant.
5. Allogenic SCT is the treatment of choice in younger patient (<45 years) who achieve complete remission with 2nd dose.
6. Autologous SCT is restricted to older and younger patients.
7. In younger patient, refractory to 2 cycles of conventional chemotherapy—allogenic SCT can achieve prolonged disease free survival in 20% of patients.

Treatment of AML in Pregnancy

1. Chemotherapy should be avoided in 1st trimester of pregnancy because there is chance of malformation.
2. Chemotherapy in 2nd and 3rd trimesters of pregnancy is associated with increased risk of abortion, premature delivery, IUGR, neonatal pancytopenia.
3. Single agent, ATRA is the safest approach for APL in 2nd and 3rd trimesters.

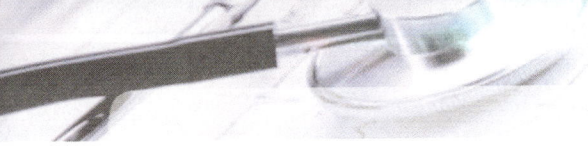

Treatment of Acute Promyelocytic Leukemia

APL (FAB M₃) requires separate treatment approach because:

i. *Risk of DIC prior to and during initial therapy* due to release of thromboplastins from leukemic cells—is an indication for urgent treatment.

ii. *Rapid confirmation of PML-RARA fusion protein* by PML—immunofluorescence test or fluorescence in situ hybridization (FISH) analysis predicts favourable response with all trans retinoic acid (ATRA) or arsenic oxide

iii. *Variant PLZF-RARA fusion protein* confers resistance.

Mode of action of ATRA:

i. ATRA helps in differentiation of abnormal clone of cells by overcoming molecular block resulting from t(15,17) translocation.

ii. It reduces the risk of DIC.

Mode of therapy:

In **induction period**: ATRA + cytarabine—70% patients cured

In **consolidation phase**: Cytarabine therapy

Complication of ATRA therapy:

i. Marked neutropenia
ii. Fever
iii. Pulmonary infiltrate
iv. Hypoxia
v. Fluid overload

Treatment of Complication

1. Discontinue ATRA treatment
2. Dexamethasone 10 mg IV twice daily

Incase of relapse (persistence of abnormal PML-RARA fusion protein)—Arsenic oxide should be given for 2nd CR.

But in consolidation phase—SCT is required.

CHRONIC MYELOID LEUKEMIA

Epidemiology

i. Rare 1–1.5 in 100,000
ii. Incidence increases with age—median age of diagnosis is 66 years, rare in children.
iii. Male predominance 1.5:1
iv. Worldwide distribution
v. Ionizing radiation is the only causative factor; leukemia develops 6–8 years after exposure.
vi. No known genetic factors responsible for CML.

Natural History

1. Biphasic or triphasic disease—characterized by chronic phase, accelerated phase and blast crisis, occasionally chronic phase to blast crisis.
2. Duration of chronic phase is 3–6 years
3. Transformation is least likely in 2 years, immediately after diagnosis.
4. Accelerated phase is characterized by—blood count and organomegaly becoming refractory to therapy
5. Blast phase is characterized by >20% blasts and promyelocytes in bone marrow and rapidly fatal

WHO Criteria of Accelerated Phase

1. Blast—10–19% of WBC in peripheral blood and/or nucleated bone marrow cells

2. Peripheral blood basophils >20%
3. Persistent thrombocytopenia (<100 × 10⁹/L) unrelated to therapy or persistent thrombocytosis (>100 × 10⁹/L) unresponsive to therapy.
4. ↑ spleen size and increased WBC count unresponsive to therapy.
5. Cytogenic evidence of clonal evolution.

WHO Criteria of Blast Phase

1. Blasts ≥20% of peripheral blood WBC in or of nucleated bone marrow cells.
2. Extramedullary blast proliferation
3. Large foci or clusters of blasts in bone marrow biopsy.

Clinical Symptoms and Signs

1. 30% patients are asymptomatic, can be diagnosed after complete hemogram and peripheral blood picture.
2. Fatigue, lethargy, weight loose, sweats
3. Early satiety left upper quadrant pain or mass—due to splenomegaly and splenic infarction.
4. Symptoms of platelet dysfunction—bleeding, thrombosis.
5. Symptoms of granulocyte dysfunction—infection.
6. Present with leukostatic manifestations—vaso-occlusive disease, cerebrovascular accidents, myocardial infarction, venous thrombosis, priapism, visual disturbances, pulmonary in sufficiency.
7. Patients with P230^BCR-ABL positive CML, have more indolent course.
8. Progressing of chronic myeloid leukemia is associated with following symptoms:
   i. Significant weight loss
   ii. Increase in dose for controlling the disease
   iii. Joint pain, bleeding, thrombosis, infections—suggestive of transformation to accelerated or blast phases.
9. Pruritus, diarrhea, flushing—secondary to histamine release.
10. Clinical signs include:
    i. Moderate to huge splenomegaly
    ii. Mild hepatomegaly
    iii. Persistent splenomegaly despite continued therapy—sign of blast crisis.

Investigations

1. Complete hemogram shows (Fig. 5.69):
   i. Raised WBC >25 × 10⁹/L 100–300 × 10⁹/L.—predominantly both mature and immature granulocytes, basophilia, sometimes eosinophilia, <5% blast cells, majority of cells being metamyelocytes, myelocytes and band forms.

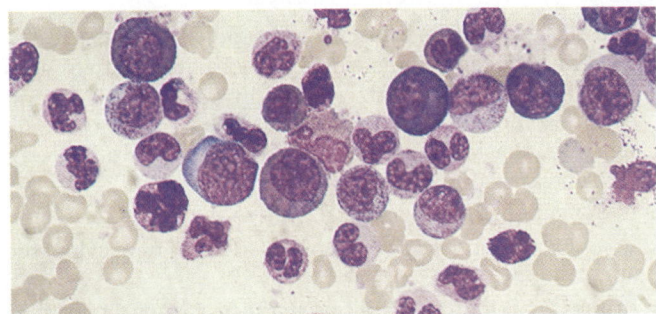

Fig. 5.69: Peripheral blood picture in CML

2. Platelet count—mostly elevated
3. Anemia—mild degree of normocytic, normochromic
4. Neutrophil alkaline phosphatase is low in CML cells.
5. Decreased ESR in absence of infection
6. LDH level and urate level raised.
7. Raised histamine secondary to basophilia
8. Bone marrow trephine biopsy shows (Fig. 5.70)
   i. Bone marrow cellularity is increased with increased myeloid: erythroid ratio
   ii. Blasts <10% in chronic phase
   iii. >20% in accelerated phase.
   iv. It assesses the amount of marrow fibrosis—diagnosed by reticulin stain.

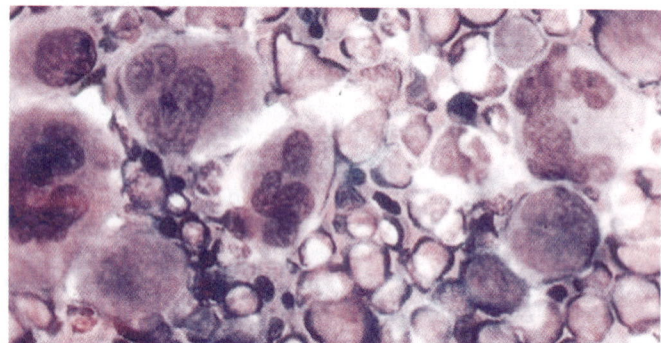

Fig. 5.70: Bone marrow picture in CML

Accelerated phase is defined by one or more of the following:
   i. Development of increasing degree of anemia
   ii. Cytogenic clonal evolution
   iii. Bone marrow blast cells between 20% and 50%
   iv. Blood or bone marrow basophila—≥ 20%
   v. Platelet count <100,000/μL
   vi. Organomegaly
   vii. Leukocytosis basophilia, thrombocytosis or thrombocytopenia in patient previously controlled by therapy
   viii. Myelofibrosis with tear drop cells in blood smear and increased bone marrow reticulin

Blast crisis can be defined by
   i. Features of acute leukaemia
   ii. Bone marrow blast cells > 50%
   iii. Hyposegmented neutrophil may appear (Pelger-Huer anomaly)
   iv. Blast cells can be classified as—myeloid, lymphoid, erythroid or undifferentiated cells.
   v. Cytochemical and immunologic features

Cytogenic and Molecular Analysis

1. In >80% patient has Ph chromosome—reciprocal translocation between chromosome 9 and 22 involving two genes BCR and ABL—producing fusion gene BCR-ABL on chromosome 22. This produces an aberrant 210 kDa protein, which is constitutively active and has greater activity of tyrosine kinase.
2. In 8% patient, there is Ph –ve CML
3. In accelerated phase, there is acquisition of new cytogenic abnormalities
4. In blast crisis there are additional copies of Ph chromosomes 8+ and i(17q).

Prognostic Factors

1. Sokal score—based on age, spleen size, platelet count, and % of blast cells in blood—can identify the patient's prognosis
   i. Low risk <0.8
   ii. Intermediate risk = 0.8–1.2
   iii. High risk >1.2
2. Based on interferon ∝ treatment Hasford calculation has been developed—It identified the effect of basophilia and eosinophilia at diagnosis with above Sokal scores.
3. Above two score can predict cytogenic response to imatinib 400 mg once daily in newly diagnosed patient in chronic phase.

Treatment of Chronic Phase of CML

I. **Imatinib—400 mg** orally once daily is the treatment of choice in newly diagnosed CML—chronic phase.
   i. *It signals transduction inhibitor*—targeting BC-ABL fusion gene and other tyrosine kinase.
   ii. *Responses:*
      a. 96% complete hematological response (CHR)
      b. 87% major cytogenic response (MCyR)—within 6 months of therapy and lower risk of relapse.
      c. 76% complete cytogenic response (CCyR)
      d. 50% major molecular response
   iii. *Commonest side effects:* a. Myelosuppression, b. Edema, c. Nausea, d. Rash, e. Cramps, f. Fatigue, g. Diarrhea, h. Headache, i. Arthralgia, j. Abnormal liver function tests
   iv. *Addition of:*
      a. *Granulocyte colony-stimulating factor (G-CSF)* to maintain neutrophil count >1 × 10⁹/L or stop the therapy or reduce the therapy to 300 mg/day
      b. It platelet count <50 × 10⁹/L—stop the therapy or reduce the dose of imatinib
      c. If anemia—therapy should be discontinued or dose should be reduced and addition of erythropoietin
      d. In case of grade two Hepatotoxicity—reduction of dose of stoppage of imatinib is required.
      e. In case of rash—topical or systemic corticosteroids
   v. *In case of toxicity:* Therapy can be changed to dasatinib, nilotinib

II. **Dasatinib—100 mg/day—orally**
   Nilotinib—400 mg twice daily—orally
      a. Above two drugs are given in chronic phase—intolerant to imatinib or offer resistance to imatinib
      b. Food restriction is required before and after dosing
      c. Both of them are more effective than imatinib as a first line of treatment in newly diagnosed CML patient
      d. *Complications:*
         1. Plural effusions in 22% of patients in dasatinib treated patients
         2. Sudden death in Nilotinib treated patients.

III. **Other new agents approved for therapy in CML:**
   Hydroxycarbamide: It is used to:
   1. Control leukocytosis and thrombocytosis
   2. Normalize full blood count
   3. Reduce spleen size in chromic phase

   It is used in elderly.

   Side effect: Skin rash, mouth ulcers, diarrhea

   Maintenance: 1–1.5 gm orally once daily.

Interferon **α:** It is given at a dose of 3 million, subcutaneously, three times weekly:

1. Corrects hematological response
2. 10–15% cytogenic response
3. 15–30% major cytogenic response
4. Longer survival and longer time to progression than hydroxycarbamide.

Side effects: i. Malaise, ii. Febrile reaction, iii. Anorexia, iv. Weight loss, v. Reduce the quality of life

Other drugs to be added with imatinib:

1. Allopurinol—300 mg daily orally until blood count normalize.
2. Hydroxyurea 1–2 gm daily for patients with leukocyte count over 100,000/cc with massive splenomegaly

Complete hematological response:

1. Platelets $<450 \times 10^9$/L
2. White blood count $<C6 \times 10^9$/L
3. Differential— no immature granulocyte, and <5% basophils
4. Non palpable spleen

Monitoring: 2 weekly check up until complete hematological response, then confirmed twice, then every 3 months: 2 weekly check up until complete hematological response, then confirmed twice, then every 3 months

Cytogenic response (examination of ≥ 20 marrow metaphase):

1. Complete cytogenic response (CCyR)—Ph +ve metaphase 0%
2. Partial cytogenic response (PCyR)—Ph +ve 1–35%
3. Major cytogenic response (MCyR)—CCyR + PCyR
   Minor: Ph + 36 65%
   Minimal: Ph + 66–95%

Monitoring: Every 6 monthly check up until CCyR achieved and confirmed twice then at every 12 months.

Failure of imatinib treatment:

 i. No hematologic response in 3 months.
 ii. No cytogenic response in 6 months (Ph >95%)
 iii. Less than partial cytogenic response (Ph >35%) in 12 months
 iv. No complete cytogenic response (any Ph detected) in 18 months
 v. Loss of previously achieved response—loss of complete hematologic response, complete cytogenic response.

Suboptimal response to imatinib treatment:

 i. No complete hematological response in 3 months.
 ii. Less than partial cytogenic response (Ph >35%) in 6 months
 iii. No complete cytogenic response in 12 months
 iv. No major molecular response in 18 months
 v. Loss of previously achieved response, loss of major molecular response.

Allogenic stem cell transplantation:

1. HLA matched sibling donor related SCT—is treatment of choice for patient <45 years
2. Treatment related mortality—20%
3. Survival:
   i. Incase of early phase of chronic myeloid leukemia—50%
   ii. In case of late chronic myeloid leukaemia—20%

Complications:

1. Increased risk of infection, by atypical organism
2. Progression to blast crisis

3. Lymphoid blast crisis (25%)—treatment with tyrosine kinase inhibitor followed by SCT
4. Myeloid blast crisis—refractory to conventional therapy. Survival—2 to 5 months, may respond briefly with tyrosine kinase inhibitor or SCT

Treatment of Accelerated Phase

 i. Imatinib—600–800 mg orally daily
 ii. Allogenic stem cell transplantation from fully or partially matched sibling donor (HLA identical donor)
 iii. In case of imatinib resistant cases—second generation tyrosine kinase inhibitors are effective.
 iv. Alternatively interferon in combination with cytosine arabinoside can achieve disease control

Treatment of Blast Crisis

 i. A proportion of patients with BC phase responds to imatinib 600–800 mg orally daily, but response duration is short (<10 months)
    Hence associated SCT should advisable
 ii. In imatinib refractory patient—second generation BCR-ABL inhibitors—dasatinib or nilotinib
 iii. **In case of ALL type blast crisis:**
    1. Daunorubicin—45 mg/m^2/day in day 1 and 2
    2. Vincristine—2 mg/m^2 weekly
    3. Prednisolone 60 mg/m^2 daily for 3 weeks
 iv. In **case blast phase—AML type:**
    1. Daunorubicin 50 mg/m^2 × 2–3 days
    2. Cytosine arabinoside 200 mg/m^2 × 5–7 days
 v. **Patient with lymphoid blast crisis:** Prophylactic meningeal treatment to prevent meningeal leukaemia
 vi. **Allogenic SCT** may be associated with significant mortality in patient having blast phase

A significant number of patients develop prolonged cytopenia after successful irradiation of blasts cells. For this reason moderate intensity remission induction chemotherapy should be used.

In chronic myeloid leukemia, if leukostasis occurs, though uncommon—it suggests leukocyte count >3,00,000/cc

In above case:

1. First few sessions of large volume apheresis to lower the leukocyte count.
   Apheresis should be associated with
   i. High dose hydroxyurea—(up to 4 mg daily) or
   ii. Cytosine arabinoside 1 gm/m^2 with allopurinol 300 mg/day
2. Adequate hydration
3. Imatinib—may be started once daily once leukocyte count will be under control

Blood film: Hall mark of CML is basophilia—basophil count often exceeding 1000/cc.

CHRONIC LYMPHOCYTIC LEUKEMIA

Definition

CLL is characterized by mature appearing, functionally incompetent, long-lived B lymphocytes in peripheral blood, bone marrow, lymph node, spleen, liver and in other organs.

Epidemiology

i. Age—CLL incidence increases with ages
ii. Male female ratio = 2:1
iii. Commonest leukemia in western adult

Etiology

i. Unknown. There is no relationship with radiation, chemicals or viruses.
ii. May be familial—as occurs in 1st or 2nd degree relatives of CLL patients.
iii. Genetic—more common in Japanese even after migration
iv. Molecular mechanism:
   a. High expression of anti-apoptotic molecules such as BCL-2, or
   b. Defect in pro-apoptotic molecules

Clinical Presentation

1. Patient may present with asymptomatic lymphadenopathy
2. Patient may present with abdominal fullness, fatigue, and reduced exercise tolerance
3. Features of anemia
4. In advanced stage—patient may come with recurrent infections, weight loss
5. Patient may come with bleeding disorder
6. Patient may present with gastrointestinal bleeding
7. Respiratory distress due to lung involvement or pleural involvements
8. Signs are:
   i. Anemia, ii. Thrombocytopenia, iii. Bilateral symmetrical (often) non-tender lymphadenopathy, iv. Hepatomegaly because of malignant cell infiltration, v. Splenomegaly—frequent, vi. Signs of lung parenchyma or pleural involvement.
9. Autoimmune phenomenon occurs:
   a. Warm antibody hemolytic anemia
   b. Autoimmune thrombocytopenia.
10. Clinical staging is shown in Table 5.3.

Diagnosis

1. **Peripheral blood picture shows** (Fig. 5.71):
   i. Small mature appearing lymphocytes with round nuclei, clumped chromatin, scanty cytoplasm
   ii. Smudge cells, bar and nuclei—that appear squashed "smear cells"—classic feature of CLL
   iii. Lymphocytosis $>5 \times 10^9/L$ to $>20 \times 10^9/L$
   iv. Anemia, thrombocytopenia, neutropenia—absent in early stage but present in late stage.
   v. If features of autoimmune hemolytic anemia—spherocytes, polychromasia, increased reticulocyte count.
   vi. If features of idiopathic thrombocytopenia—decreased thrombocytes.
   vii. In 15% patients—promyelocytes, medium sized cells with prominent nucleoli
2. **Bone marrow picture:**
   i. >30% mature lymphocytes
   ii. Trephine biopsy—provides prognostic information
      a. Nodular variety—favorable
      b. Interstitial, mixed, diffuse—unfavourable
3. **Lymph node biopsy:** It can distinguish CLL from lymphoma

Table 5.3: Clinical staging: Rai clinical staging system

Level of risk		Stage		Median survival
1	Low	0	Lymphocytosis alone	>13 years
2	Intermediate	I	Lymphocytosis + Lymphadenopathy	8 years
		II	Lymphocytosis + Splenomegaly Or Hepatomegaly	5 years
3	High	III	Lymphocytosis + Anemia (Hb <11 gm/dl)	2 years
		IV	Lymphocytosis + Thrombocytopenia (<100/10⁹L)	1 year

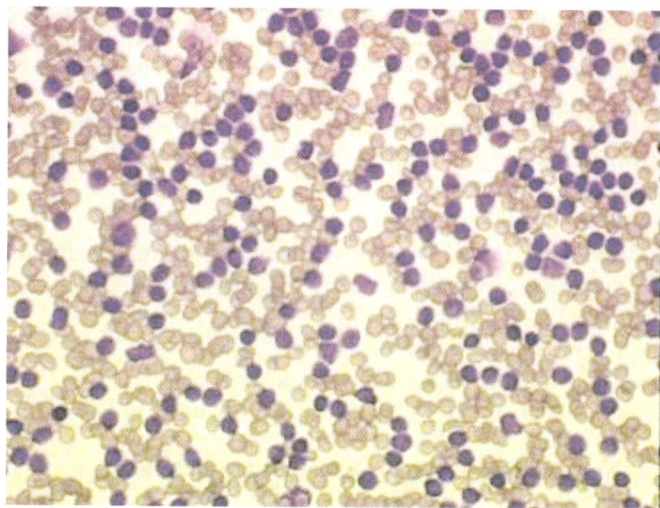

Fig. 5.71: Peripheral blood picture in CLL

4. **Flow cytometry and immunotyping:** This study is most helpful to confirm the diagnosis of CLL and differentiates from other lymphocytoses. CLL characteristically:
   a. CD2 and FMC7 –ve
   b. CD5, CD10 and CD23 +ve
   c. Smig, CD22, CD796 weak, d. CD 38 → Poor outcome
5. **Immunoglobulin:**
   i. Immunoparesis (hypogammaglobulinemia)
   ii. Monoclonal paraprotein (IgM) <5%
6. **Cytogenetics:** Fluorescence in situ hybridization (FISH) can identify following abnormalities which are of variable prognostic value:
   i. 11q -, 17q -   → very unfavorable
   ii. 6q -   → Intermediate
   iii. Isolated 13q - → favorable
7. **Other necessary tests:**
   i. Direct antiglobulin test—autoimmune hemolytic anemia

ii. Reticulocyte count—increased in AIHA
iii. Uric acid in serum
iv. Liver function test,
v. β_2 microglobulin
vi. LDH
8. **Radiological investigation:**
   i. Chest X-ray
   ii. CT scan of abdomen and thorax
   iii. Ultrasound

Prognostic Factors

Following are the poor prognostic factors:
1. Male sex
2. Advanced clinical stage
3. Initial Lymphocytosis $>50 \times 10^9/L$
4. >5% prolymphocytes in blood film
5. Diffuse pattern of infiltrate on trephine biopsy
6. Blood lymphocyte double time <12 months
7. Cytogenic abnormalities 11q -, 17q
8. P53 mutations—correlates with refractory CLL.
9. Unmutated IgΥH gene—progressive advanced disease
10. Serum β_2 microglobulin—poor response to therapy
11. Increased serum LDH
12. Poor response to therapy

Treatment of CLL (Fig. 5.72)

Patients with asymptomatic lymphocytosis should be observed.

Monitoring of CLL—Rai stage I and II—with:
i. Periodical clinical evaluation
ii. Basic laboratory testing 3–6 months interval

Consensus treatment indications:
1. Constitutional symptoms due to CLL
   i. >10% wt loss in 6 months
   ii. Fever >38°C
   iii. Extreme fatigue
2. Symptomatic massive (>10 cm) lymphadenopathy

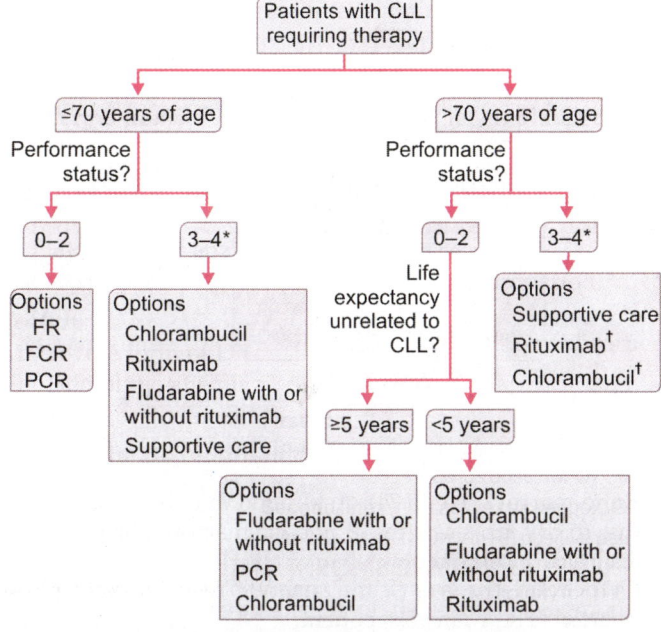

Fig. 5.72: Treatment plan of CLL

3. Symptomatic massive splenomegaly (>6 cm below costal margin)
4. Progressive marrow failure—worsening of anemia and thrombocytopenia
5. Rapidly progressive lymphocytosis (lymphocyte doubling time <6 months)
6. Autoimmune cytopenias (ITP, AlHA) poorly responsive to corticosteroid treatment.

Definite Therapy

I. **Chlorambucil** 6–10 mg/day or 0.1–0.2 mg/kg/day Orally 7–14 days in 28 days cycle × 6–12 cycles
   Effect: It shrinks spleen, lymph nodes—complete response
   Side effects: i. Myelosuppression, ii. increased risk of myelodysplasia, iii. 2nd degree leukemia

II. **Combination regimen**—cyclophosphamide, prednisolone vincristine ± anthracycline (CVP ± H). This combination induces more rapid and higher response compared with chlorambucil.

III. **Purine analogue:** Dose—40 mg/m²/day—orally × 5 days in 28 days cycle for 6–8 cycles
   Overall response is 70–80% for 2 years.
   Side effect: 1. Myelosuppression, 2. Lymphopenia, 3. Opportunistic infection, 4. Precipitation of autoimmune hematologic complications
   To prevent opportunistic infection—cotrimoxazole (160–800 mg)—1 tab daily orally as prophylaxis.

IV. **Monoclonal antibodies:**
   a. *Rituximab*—CD20 chimeric monoclonal antibody
      Dose: 375 mg/m²/wk × 4 weeks
      It can induce short lived response in 50% patients.
      If added to purine analogue or purine analogue + cyclophosphamide—shows better response.
   b. *Alemtuzumab:* Humanized anti-CD52 monoclonal antibody—it is approved for fludarabine refractory **CLL, 17b—CLL**
      Dose: 300 mg/m² IV or subcutaneously three times per week. It eliminates CLL from blood, marrow and spleen.
      Side effects: 1. Cytokine release syndrome, 2. Neutropenia, 3. Pronounced neutropenia, 4. Increased risk of opportunistic infections—it requires cotrimoxazole prophylaxis

2nd Line and Subsequent Treatment

This treatment and response are determined by:
   i. Stage at which it begins
   ii. Adverse prognosis factors
   iii. Number, quality and duration of response to prior treatment

Drugs are:
1. *Chlorambucil*—prior responders respond on one or more occasions.
2. *Fludarabine*—according to NICE guidelines—it is used as 2nd line therapy in patients who failed or intolerant to chlorambucil therapy. Not recommended in patient with AlHA.
3. *Fludarabine+ chlorambucil*—this combination can be used in patients who are resistant to fludarabine

4. *High dose methylprednisolone* (1 gm/m^2/day × 5 day in 28 days cycle): It should be used in patient with:
   i. Refractory to fludarabine
   ii. Bulky lymphadenopathy
   iii. P53 mutations
   Contraindication: active peptic ulcer disease
   Cautions: i. Diabetes, ii. Congestive cardiac failure
5. **Alemtuzumab:** It should be used in:
   i. Refractory to fludarabine
   ii. P53 mutations
   iii. Combination with fludarabine can be used in patient resistant to either drugs
6. **Rituximab:** It can only be used with fludarabine + cyclophosphamide (FCR)—with high response compared with use as single therapy.

Stem Cell Transplantation

I. **Autologous stem cell transplantations:** It can be given in younger patient (<55 years of age) after high dose chemotherapy ± total body irradiation with advanced or poor risk CLL

It is not curative.
Complications:
   i. Increased risk of malignancy
   ii. Myelodysplastic syndrome.
II. **Allogenic stem cell transplantation:**
   i. It is given in younger symptomatic patients with high risk of CLL.
   ii. It is prepared from HLA matched siblings or unrelated donors.
   iii. High treatment related morbidity.

Treatment of Complications

1. **Infections:** It occurs mostly in case of:
   i. Elderly   ii. Advanced stage of disease
   iii. During fludarabine treatment.

   So prophylaxis with cotrimoxazole to be started during treatment.
2. **Autoimmune cytopenia:**
   i. Autoimmune hemolytic anemia and idiopathic thrombocytopenic purpura should be treated with corticosteroid, IV immunoglobulin, chemotherapy, rituximab or splenectomy may be tried.
   ii. Pure red cell aplasia patient—test for parvovirus infection—can be treated by corticosteroid, or ATG or cyclosporine
3. **Radiotherapy:** It is required in:
   i. Patients with bulky lymphadenopathy
   ii. Huge splenomegaly—not fit for splenectomy
4. **Splenectomy:** It should be done in:
   i. Massive splenomegaly
   ii. Hypersplenism
   iii. Refractory cytopenia
5. **Lymphomatous transformation** (Richter's syndrome):
   i. It occurs in 10% of patients in all stages
   ii. Median interval for diagnosis—24 months
   iii. Abrupt onset and progressive

Prognosis

1. CLL is a incurable disease with current therapy except in a few allografted patients.

2. Most patients in early stage may die due to unrelated causes.
3. Infection is a major cause of mortality and morbidity
4. Patients in advanced stages develop refractory disease and bone marrow failure.
5. Some refractory patients may develop prolymphocytic transformation
6. Malignancy of skin and colon occurs in 20% cases.

HAIRY CELL LEUKEMIA

Definition

Low grade B cell lymphoproliferative disorder associated with:
   i. Splenomegaly
   ii. Pancytopenia
   iii. Typical hairy cells in peripheral blood film and bone marrow.

Epidemiology

   i. Male: female—4:1
   ii. Present in middle age >45 years
   iii. 8% of Lymphoproliferative disorder.

Clinical Features

   i. Non-specific symptoms—asthenia, malaise, fatigue, weight loss
   ii. Infection—by atypical organism
   iii. Bleeding, bruising
   iv. Hepatosplenomegaly
   v. Lymphadenopathy
   vi. Vasculitic polyarthritis and visceral involvement

Investigation

1. **Peripheral blood:**
   i. Moderate to severe pancytopenia;
   ii. Hairy cell in 95% kidney shaped nuclei, clear cytoplasm, irregular cytoplasmic projections (Fig. 5.73)
   iii. WBC—differential neutropenia

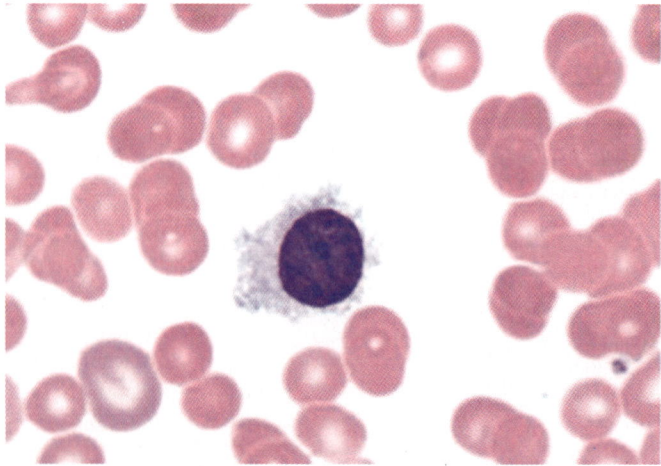

Fig. 5.73: Peripheral blood picture in hairy cell leukemia

2. **Bone marrow** (Fig. 5.74): Aspiration may be unsuccessful due to dry tap—as a result of bone marrow fibrosis. Trephine biopsy shows—hairy cells.
3. **Cytochemistry** → +ve for tartarate resistant acid phosphatase (TRAP) in 95% patient.

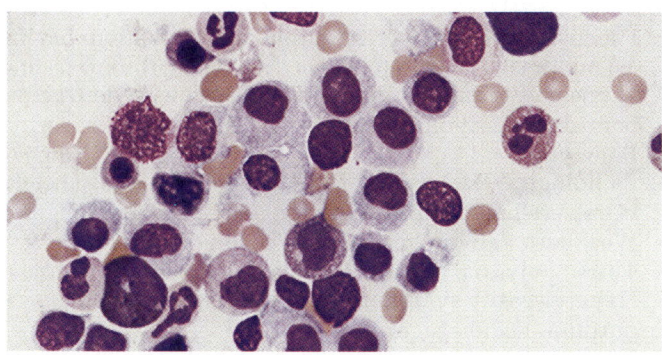

Fig. 5.74: Bone marrow pictures in hairy cell leukemia

Prognostic factors:
i. Response to therapy is probably best prognostic indicator.
ii. Bulky abdominal lymphadenopathy at diagnosis correlates with poor response to 1st line of therapy.

Management

Therapy is required in patient when:
i. Hb% <10 gm/dl
ii. Neutropenia <1.0 × 10⁹/L
iii. Thrombocytopenia <100 × 10⁹/L
iv. Symptomatic splenomegaly
v. Recurrent infection
vi. Extralymphatic involvement
vii. Autoimmune complication
viii. Progressive disease

Treatment

1. Supportive treatment
2. Cladribine (purine analogue)—continuous infusion—0.1 mg/kg/day × 7 days—produces temporary myelo-suppression
3. Deoxycoformycin—alternative purine analogue—4 mg/m²/IV. bolus every 2 weeks to maximum response plus 2 cycles.
4. Granulocyte—colony-stimulating factor in case of severe neutropenia.
5. In profound cytopenia—Interferon may be initial therapy for 2–4 months before purine analogue
6. Allopurinol—to prevent sour
7. Splenectomy—rarely required

Second line and subsequent therapy:
i. Interferon—3 million units SC thrice weekly and 12–18 months
ii. Rituximab 375 mg/m²/wk IV × 4–12 doses.

PARAPROTEINEMIAS

This is characterized by a heterogeneous group of disorders as evidenced by:
i. Deranged proliferation of single clone of plasma cells or B lymphocytes and usually associated with
ii. Detectable monoclonal immunoglobulin (paraprotein or M-protein) in serum or urine.

Condition-Associated Paraprotein Production

A. Stable production
   1. Monoclonal gummopathy of undetermined significance (MGUS)

2. Smoldering myeloma
3. Cryoglobulinemia

B. Progressive production:
   1. Multiple myeloma:
      i. Complete immunoglobulin (IgG, IgA, or IgD, rarely IgM or IgE)
      ii. Free light chain K (Bence Jones proteinuria)
      iii. Non-secretory
   2. Plasma cell leukemia
   3. Solitary plasmacytoma of bone
   4. Extramedullary plasmacytoma
   5. POEMS syndrome
   6. Walderstorm's macroglobulinemia
   7. CLL
   8. Malignant lymphoma
   9. Heavy chain disease

Multiple Myeloma

Definition

Multiple myeloma is a clonal B cell malignancy **characterized by plasma cell proliferation**—that mainly accumulate in bone marrow and usually secrete monoclonal IgM or IgG light chain—it may be associated lytic bone lesion, pathological fracture (Fig. 5.75).

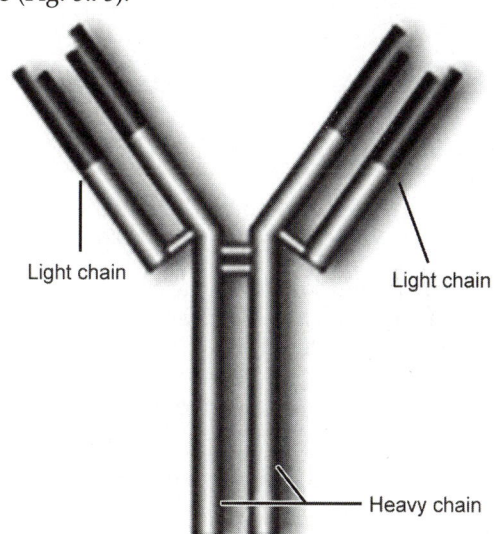

Light chain · · · Light chain · · · Heavy chain

Fig. 5.75: Light and heavy chain (*Source:* Reproduced with permission from the Multiple Myeloma Research Foundation Web site, Available at: http://www.multiplemyeloma.org/about_myeloma/index.html)

Epidemiology

i. Median age—60 years
ii. Male: female = 1:1.5
iii. Incidence is mostly occurs is African followed by: Caucasians, lowest in Asians

Risk Factors

i. Family clusters have been reported
ii. Exposure to radiation, benzene, pesticides.

Pathology

Multiple myeloma arises from post-germinal centre B cell.
   Two mutually exclusive pathogenic pathways have been postulated.

i. **Hyperdiploidy** (48–75 chromosomes) typically with multiple trisomies involving chromosome 3, 5, 7, 9, 11, 15, 19 and 21

ii. **Non-hyperdiploid** (<48, >75 chromosomes) here somatic hypermaturation may contribute to neoplastic transformation.

Two early events have been described:

i. **Loss of chromosome** 13 or 13q 14 deletions

ii. **Dysregulation of a cyclin D gone** → level of cyclin D ↑↑

Other genetic abnormalities may occur, but it is usually late event.

Pathophysiology

Plasmoblast from post-germinal center B cells
↓
Migrate to bone marrow
↓
They differentiate into long lived plasma cells
↓
In case of optimal environment in bone marrow MM cells adheres to stromal cells
↓
It enhances MM cell growth survival and confesses protection against drug-induced apoptosis.

A.   **MM cells activate stroma**
↓

i. Helps in secretion of range of cytokines and growth factors.
IL-6 is the major growth and survival factor in MM and confers resistance to dexamethasone.

ii. Vascular endothelial growth factor—enhances MM cell growth, migration and survival.

iii. Angiogenesis is altered.

iv. Increased marrow microvascular density—leads to progression of disease and poor prognosis.

B.   **MM cells and stroma**
↓
Produce variety of osteoclast activation factors
↓
Proliferation and activation of osteoclast and inhibition of osteoblast
↓
Produces punched out lytic bone lesion and hypercalcemia and normal alkaline phosphatase

C. **Due to dysregulation of genetic factors**—there are decrease number of osteoblast cells—decrease bone formation.

D. **Bone marrow infiltration produces anemia.**

E. **Immunophoresis of normal Ig production** predisposes to infection, and different types of paraprotein formation which determine:

i. Amyloidal deposition

ii. Renal damage

iii. Hyperviscosity

Clinical Features

1. Patient may present with **spectrum of presentations** having asymptomatic paraproteinemia detected on routine testing at one end to rapidly progressive illness with destructive bone diseases at other end.

2. **Bone pain**

3. **Pathological fracturen** (Fig. 5.76)—kyphosis, loss of height from vertebral compression

4. **Weakness, fatigue, recurrent** infection (10%)

5. **Thirst, polyuria, nocturia, edema** due to renal impairment

6. **Hyperviscosity symptoms**—mental slowing, visual upset, purpura, hemorrhage

7. **Neuropathy, spinal cord compression** (Fig. 5.77).

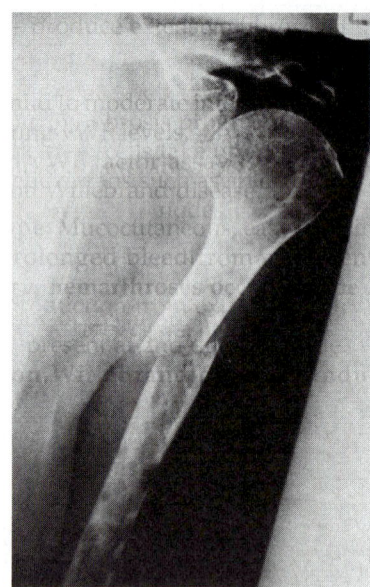

Fig. 5.76: Pathological fracture

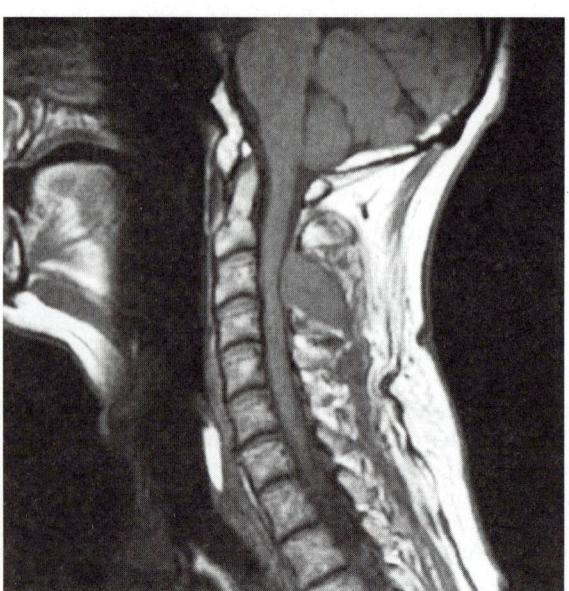

Fig. 5.77: Spinal cord compression by myeloma tissues

Investigations of Patients with Suspected Myeloma

a. Screening tests:

1. FBC and film	Normochromic, normocytic anemia
2. ESR or PV	Raised, not in light chain, non secretary multiple myeloma
3. Urea, creatinine, electrolyte	To detect renal impairment
4. Uric acid	Increased
5. Serum albumin, calcium phosphorus, alkaline phosphatase	Low albumin, hypercalcemia, normal alkaline phosphatase
6. Serum protein electrophoresis	Detect serum paraprotein
7. Serum immunoglobulin	To detect immunoglobulin
8. Serum protein light chain	To detect light chain
9. Routine urine analysis	To detect proteinuria
10. Urine electrophoresis	To detect Bence Jones protein
11. 24 hours urine collection	For creatinine clearance and 24 hours proteinuria to detect renal damage
12. X-ray of bone	Pathological fracture, lytic bone lesion

b Diagnostic tests:

1. Bone marrow	Monotonous sheets of plasma cells (Fig. 5.78)
2. Radiological skeletal survey	Lytic bone lesion, pathological fracture, osteoporosis (Fig. 5.79)
3. Paraprotein immunofixation and densitometry	Characterizes and quantifies paraprotein IgG, IgA, IgD, IgM (Fig. 5.80)

c. Tests to establish tumor burden and prognosis:

1. Serum β_2 microglobulin	Measure of tumor burden
2. Serum CRP	Surrogate measure of IL-6 which correlates with tumor aggression
3. Serum LDH	Raised in plasmablastic MM measure tumor aggression
4. Serum albumin	Hypoalbuminemia, correlates with poor prognosis.
5. Bone marrow trephine biopsy	Light chain restriction, extent of infiltration and hematopoietic reserve

d. Tests which may be useful:

1. MRI	i. Spinal cord compression
	ii. Whole spine in staging solitary plasmacytoma of bone to exclude occult disease
2. CT scan	i. To detect localized plasmacytoma of bone
	ii. To detect bone fracture
	iii. CT guided biopsy
3. PET scan	It may clarify extent of extramedullary disease

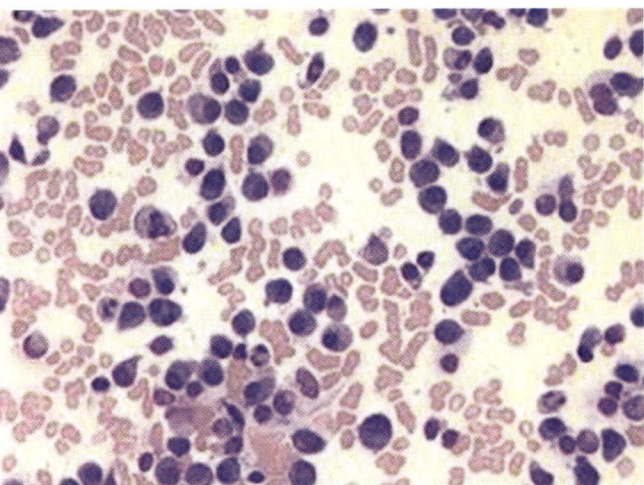

Fig. 5.78: Monotonous plasma cells in the bone marrow

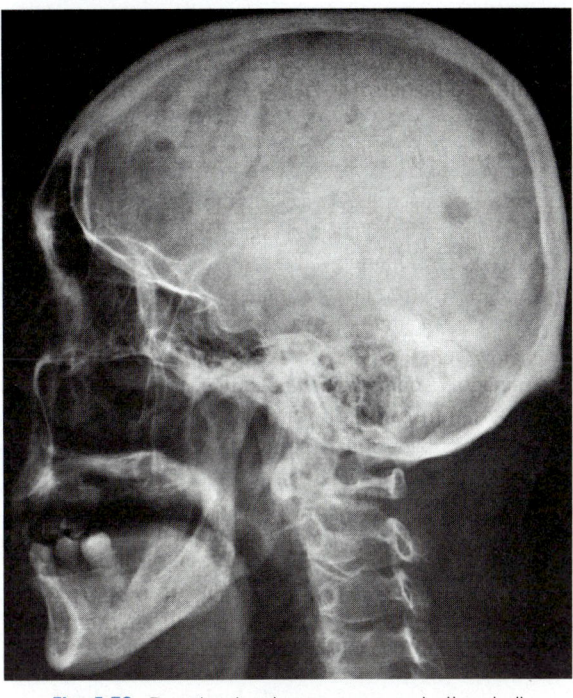

Fig. 5.79: Punched out appearance in the skull

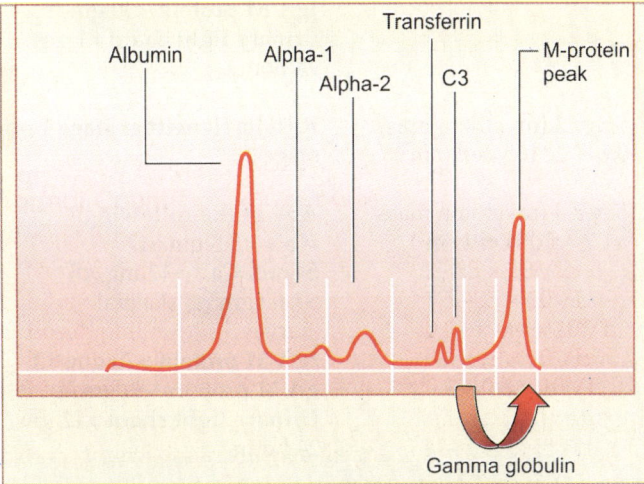

Fig. 5.80: M band in protein electrophoresis

4. Bone marrow flow cytometry
   i. Confirm monoclonal plasmacytic infiltration.
   ii. To detect solitary plasmacytoma or extraosseous plasmacytoma

5. Tissue biopsy
   i. To defect solitary plasmacytoma or extraosseous plasmacytoma

Diagnostic Criteria of Multiple Myeloma

WHO—criteria:

I. *Major criteria:*

a. Bone marrow plasmacytosis >30%
b. Plasmacytoma on biopsy
c. Presence of monoclonal protein (M protein) in serum and urine
   i. Serum IgG > 3.5 gm/dl or
   ii. Serum IgA > 2 gm/dl or
   iii. Urine Bence-Jones protein >1 gm/24 hours

II. *Minor criteria:*

a. Bone marrow plasmacytosis 10 to 30%.
b. M protein present, but less than major criteria concentration.
c. Presence of lytic bone lesions.
d. Reduced normal immunoglobulin to <50% of normal.

Diagnosis of multiple myeloma requires a minimum one major and one minor critera or three minor criteria, including the presence of bone marrow plasmacytosis and the presence of M protein.

Staging System of Multiple Myeloma

Durie-Salmon system:

1. *Stage 1* (myeloma mass <0.6 × 10^{12} cells/m^2)

   All the following:
   Hb% >10 gm/dl,
   Serum Ca^{++} <12 mg/dl.
   ≤1 lesion on skeletal survey;
   IgG M protein <50 gml,
   IgA M protein <30 gm/L,
   urinary light chain <9 gm/ 24 hours

2. *Stage 2* (myeloma mass 0.6–1.2/10^{12} cells/m^2)

   Results fit neither stage 1 nor stage 3

3. *Stage 3* (myeloma mass >1.2 × 10^{12} cells/m^2)

   Any of the following:
   Hb% <8.5 gm/dl,
   Serum Ca^{++} >12 mg/dl
   >1 lesion on skeletal survey,
   IgG M protein >70 gm/LI
   gA M protein >50 gm/L
   Urinary light chain >12 gm/ 24 hours

Sub-classification A — **Serum creatinine <2 mg/dl**
Sub-classification B — **Serum creatinine ≥ 2 mg/dl**

International staging system:

		Median survival
Stage-1	β$_2$ microglobulin <3.5 mS/L Serum albumin >3.5 gm/dl	62 months
Stage-2	Neither stage 1 nor stage 3	44 months
Stage-3	β$_2$ microglobulin >5.5 mg/L	29 months

Treatment of Multiple Myeloma

I. *Definite treatment:* Initial therapy for patients eligible for stem cell transplantation:

A. ***High dose dexamethasone:*** It reduces thrombotic, neurotoxic and infective complications.

B. ***Thalidomide + Dexamethasone:*** Thalidomide 200 mg/day orally + Dexamethasone 20 mg/m^2/day orally × 4 days—repeated every 8 days—(days 1–4, 9–12 and 17–20)—3 cycles.
   Toxicity: Thromboembolism—prophylaxis with enoxaparin

C. ***CTD:*** *Cyclophosphamide* 500 mg orally once weekly, + (*thalidomide*, 200 mg/day orally + *dexamethasone* 40 mg orally × day 1–4, and day 15–18). × 4–6 courses.

D. ***VAD:*** *Vincristine*—0.4 mg/day continuous IV infusion for 4 days (day 1–4)
   Adriamycin—Doxorubicin 9 mg/m2/day IV infusion for 4 day (day 1–4)
   Dexamethasone 40 mg/day orally for 4 days—repeated every 8days (day 1–4, 9–12, 17–20)
   Cycles repeated every 25 days.
   Toxicity: GI intolerance, myelotoxicity.

E. ***Lenalidomide + Dexamethasone:*** Lenalidomide 25 mg orally 4 times daily × 1–21 days + Dexamethasone 40 mg/day orally × 4 days—repeated every 8 days (1–4, 9–12, 17–20 day) in 28 days cycle.

F. ***Bortezomib + Dexamethasone*** Bortezomib 1.3 mg/m^2 IV bolus × 2/week for 2 weeks—day 1, 4, 8 and 11 in 21 days cycle + Dexamethazone 40 mg/day orally × 4 day—to be repe4ated every 8 days.

II. Initial therapy of patient not eligible for stem cell transplantation

A. ***Melphalan + Prednisolone***
   Melphalan—10 mg/m^2/day orally × 4 days (d-1–4)
   +
   Prednisolone—60 mg/m^2/day orally × 4 days (d-1–4) – (every 4–6 weeks cycle duration)

B. ***Melphalan + Prednisolone + Thalidomide***
   Melphalan—10 mg/m^2/day orally × 4 days (d-1–4)
   Prednisolone—60 mg/m^2/day orally × 4 days (d-1–4)
   Thalidomide—100 mg/day orally
   Cycle duration—4–6 weeks
   Toxicity—Peripheral neuropathy. Thromboembolism.

C. ***Cyclophosphamide + Thalidomide + Dexamethasone— 28 days cycle***

D. ***Bortezomab + Melphalan + Prednisolone***

E. ***Melphalan + Prednisolone + Lenalidomide***—28 days cycle for 9 cycles

Other Therapy

1. **Bisphosphonates: Action**
   Inhibits osteoclast activation—so less bony lesions—less pain and fracture

Dose: Chlodronate daily orally 1600 mg or monthly pamidronate

Contraindication restriction:
i. 50% dose reduction—if creatinine clearance 10–30 ml/min
ii. No administration, if creatinine clearance <10 ml/min.

2. **Thromboprophylaxis to reduce the frequency of VTE:**
   i. Warfarin in full dose reduces the risk (INF 2–3.0)
   ii. Low molecular weight heparin
   iii. Aspirin (75–325 mg/day)

   Risk factors:
   i. High tumor therapy
   ii. Hyperviscosity
   iii. High dose dexamethasone
   iv. Old age
   v. Obesity
   vi. Infection
   vii. Diabetes

   Duration of treatment: 4–6 months—or during the duration of treatment with thalidomide and lenalidomide

3. **Radiotherapy:**
   i. *Local radiotherapy*—8–30 cy at the site of lytic bone lesion
   ii. *Urgent radiotherapy*—in case of cord compression
   iii. *Hemi body irradiation*—in case of multiple wide spread lesion

Symptomatic Therapy

1. **Pain control:**
   i. *Mild to moderate pain*—paracetamol
   ii. *Moderate pain*—week opiod
   iii. *Severe pain*—strong opiod
   iv. *Local radiotherapy*—extremely effective
   v. **Spinal support corset** other helpful
   vi. *Neuropathic pain*—by non-analgesic adjuvant

2. **Renal impairment:**
   i. *Vigorous rehydration with high fluid input* (3–4 litre/day) to maintain urine output >3 liter/day
   ii. *Plasmapheresis* in case of cast nephropathy
   iii. If renal failure will not improve within 48 hours, *peritoneal or hemodialysis.*

3. **Hypercalcemia:**
   i. *Vigorous rehydration* 3–6 liter/day
   ii. *Loop diuretics*—increases Ca^{++} excretion
   iii. *IV bisphosphonates*
   iv. *IV corticosteroids* or *calcitonin*, if refractory

4. **Bone disease:**
   i. *Local radiotherapy* for localized pain
   ii. *Fixation of fracture* followed by radiotherapy
   iii. *Vertebroplasty* in patients with persistant back pain
   iv. *Long-term bisphosphonate* prophylaxis.

5. **Infection:**
   i. *Prompt and vigorous broad-spectrum antibiotic* therapy
   ii. *Prophylactic trimethoprim + sufamethoxazole* therapy

6. **Anemia:**
   i. *Blood transfusion* for symptomatic anemia
   ii. *EPO therapy* if Hb is persistently <10 gm/dl

7. **Hyperviscosity**—due to mainly IgA >IgG—producing cerebral, pulmonary and renal manifestation.
   Plasmapheresis followed by chemotherapy.

8. **Cord compression:**
   i. *Urgent MRI scans* to define lesion
   ii. *Oral dexamethasone* stat (8–10 mg/day)
   iii. *Local radiotherapy*
   iv. *Surgery* 1% indicated and feasible

9. **Hemorrhage:** Heparin like anticoagulants

Table 5.4: Cytogenetic abnormalities associated with "high-risk" multiple myeloma

Conventional karyotyping
Deletion of chromosome 13
Hypodiploidy
Fluorescence in situ hybridization (FISH)
Abnormalities of chromosome 1
Del(77p)
t(4; 14)
t(14; 16)
Information from references 9, 42

MONOCLONAL GUMMOPATHY OF UNDETERMINED SIGNIFICANCE

Definition

It is an asymptomatic premalignant disorder characterized by:
i. Limited monoclonal plasma cell proliferation
ii. The presence of stable monoclonal paraprotein in serum or less commonly in urine
iii. Absence of clinicopathological evidence of multiple myeloma, Walderstorm's macroglobulinemia, amyloidosis or another lymphoproliferative disorder.

Epidemiology

i. Median age 72 years
ii. More common in male
iii. More frequent in USA

Pathophysiology

MGUS appears to arise from a pre-germinal centre cell whose progeny pass through the germinal centre and undergo mutation. Stimulators are:
i. Autoimmune
ii. Infections
iii. Inflammatory disorder

Natural History

i. 50% die of unrelated causes
ii. 1% per annum progresses to MM, WM, AL
iii. 5% patients do not progress
iv. Actual rate of progression 17% at 10 years 39% in 25 years

Clinical Features

i. Typically asymptomatic and an incidental finding on investigation of—ESR of—globulin on routine LFT.
ii. No abnormal physical findings (end organ damage)

iii. Lack of progression and absence of additional evidence of progressive plasma cell or β cell lymphoproliferative malignancy.

Investigation

i. **FBC**—anemia or cytopenia
ii. **Chemistry**—hypercalcemia
iii. **Immunoglobulin electrophoresis**—quantifies IgG—70%, IgM—15%, IgA—12%, biclonal—3%
iv. **Skeletal radiology**—No bone lesion
v. **Serum β_2 microglobulin** level normal
vi. **Bone marrow aspirates** <10% plasma cells

Risk Factors for Progression

1. **Paraprotein type**—IgM > IgA > IgG
2. **Bone marrow plasma cells** >5%
3. **Circulating plasma cells** by immune fluorescence
4. **Bone marrow angiogenesis**, presence of urinary para-protein

Management

1. No treatment
2. **Long-term follow-up** and review of clinical and laboratory finding to see evidence of progression.

Diagnostic criteria for MGUS—all 4 criteria must be met:
1. *Serum monoclonal protein* <30 gm/L
2. *Bone marrow plasma cells* <10% (IgM MGUS—Lympho-plasmacytic cells <10%)
3. *No evidence of other B cell lymphoproliferative disorders*.
4. *No myeloma*—related end organ or tissue impairment, e.g. lytic bone lesions, anemia, hypercalcemia, renal failure.

SMOLDERING MULTIPLE MYELOMA

Smoldering or asymptomatic multiple myeloma patients with:

i. Paraprotein >30 gm/dl
ii. Bone marrow >10% plasma cells
iii. Natural history is that of MGUS rather MM
iv. No clinical evidence of complications associated with MM

Pathogenesis

i. All have either translocation involving IgH or hyper-diploidy
ii. BM angiogenesis is greater than in MGUS but less than MM

Clinical and Laboratory Features

i. Absence of **symptoms** and **physical signs** of MM
ii. **Hb%** >10 gm/dl, Normal **serum Ca^{++}**
iii. Normal **β_2 microglobulin**, or minimally raised
iv. **Bone marrow** >10% plasma cells
v. **Skeletal radiology**—no lesion

Diagnostic Criteria

1. Serum monoclonal protein >30 gm/L and/or bone marrow plasma cell ≥10%
2. No evidence of other B cell LPD.
3. No myeloma related end organ or tissue impairment, e.g. lytic bone lesions, anemia, hypercalcemia or renal failure

Risk Factors for Early Progression of Asymptomatic MM

1. Serum paraprotein >30 gm/L
2. IgA paraprotein type
3. Urinary Bence Jones proteinuric >50 mg/day
4. Bone marrow plasmacytosis >25%
5. Abnormal MRI

Management

Observation and assessment of risk factors at regular interval at every 3–4 months

MYCOSIS FUNGOIDES

This is characterized by **leukemic phase of low grade cutaneous mature T cell lymphoma.**

Incidence

i. Male female ratio 2:1
ii. Median age 52 years

Clinical Features (Fig. 5.81)

i. Patient may present with exfoliative erythroderma.
ii. Classically progresses through eczematoid plaque stage, infiltrative plaque stage and overt tumor stage.

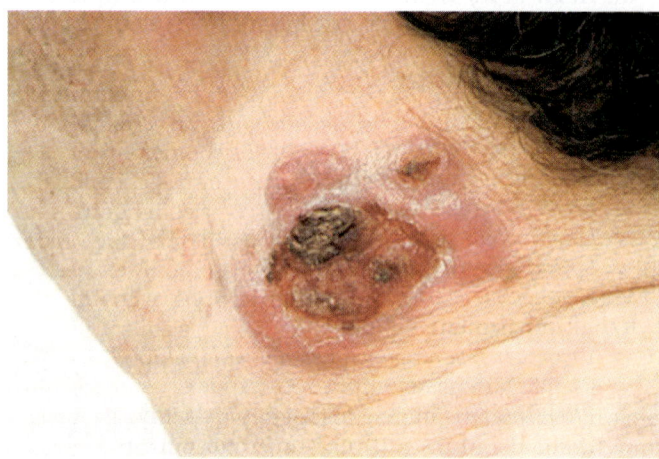

Fig. 5.81: Cutaneous lesion

Investigation and Diagnosis (Figs 5.82 and 5.83)

1. **Full blood count**—moderate leukocytosis (>20 × 10^9/L) Hb% platelet normal
2. **Peripheral blood films**—Large numbers of large lymphoid cells with characteristic 'cerebriform' folded nucleus.
3. **Skin biopsy from lesion**: Epidermotropism and Pautrier's microabscesses.
4. **Immuno-phenotyping**: CD2+, CD3+, CD4+, CD5+, CD7-, CD8-, CD25- T cells

Management

A variety of treatment have been reported for limited stage of disease—but respond to therapy is unknown.

Topical Treatment

Topical gel formation:
1. Combining **methotrexate** and **laurocapram** and **topical nitrogen mustard**.

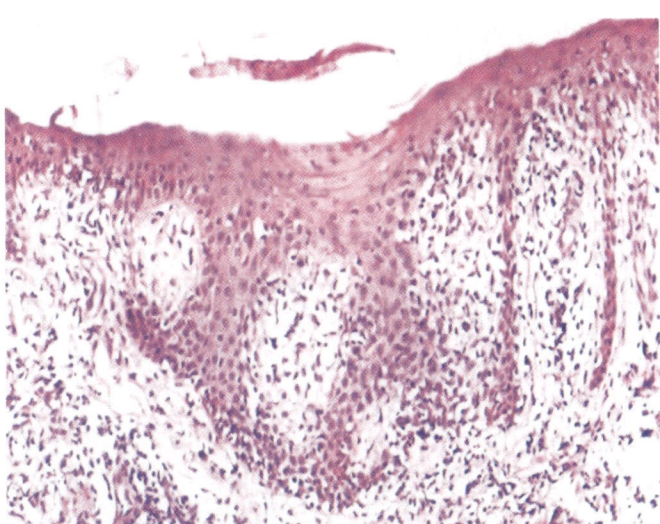

Fig. 5.82: Histology of skin

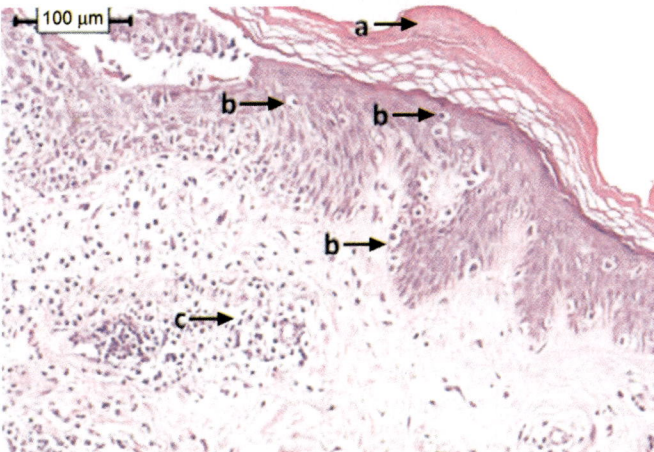

Fig. 5.83: This skin biopsy section shows: Parakeratosis **(a)**; Lymphocytes at all levels of the epidermis, including the basal cell layer **(b)**; Upper dermis lymphocytic infiltrates **(c)**

2. Low dose oral **methotrexate** and topical **bexarotene gel**.
3. Combined modality of therapy including

Subcutaneous **interferon-α** and oral **isotretinoin** followed by total skin **electro-beam** therapy

↓

Long term maintenance therapy with **topical nitrogen mustard and interferon-α**

HODGKIN'S LYMPHOMA

Definition

Classical Hodgkin's lymphoma is characterized by the presence of multinucleated giant cell of B cell origin, known as Reed-Sternberg cells in the background of numerous reactive lymphocytes.

Epidemiology

1. Most common malignancy in young adult.
2. Bimodal age incidence—major peak between 20 and 29 years and minor peak at 60 years. Median age 35 years.

3. Higher incidence in male.
4. Histological subtype—nodular sclerosis is most common subtype in young adult.

Pathological Classification

WHO Revised European American Lymphoma Classification

I. **Classical Hodgkin's lymphoma:** Reed-Sternberg giant cells are only 1–2% of cellularity of the lymph node. Predominant cells are infiltrate of lymphocytes, plasma cells, eosinophils and histiocytes containing scarred neoplastic cells and variable degree of fibrosis. There are 4 histological subtypes
   1. *Nodular sclerosis* (*classical Hodgkin's lymphoma*) (Fig. 5.84):
      i. Nodular growth pattern
      ii. Broad band of fibrosis
      iii. Lacunar cells—a variant of RS cells.

   This variety has been graded according to:
      a. Presence of neoplastic cells
      b. Presence of necrosis
      c. Depletion of lymphocytes.

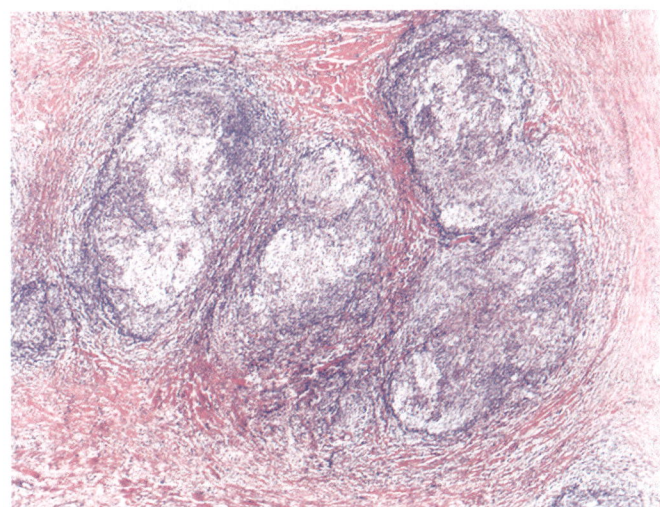

Fig. 5.84: Nodular sclerosis

   2. *Mixed cellularity HL* (Fig. 5.85)—characterized by:
      i. Numerous classic RS cells
      ii. Fine reticulin fibrosis
      iii. Mixed infiltrate of lymphocytes, eosinophils and histiocytes
   3. *Lymphocyte depleted HL* (Fig. 5.86): Rare variety, characterized by:
      i. Diffuse hypocellular infiltrate
      ii. Necrosis
      iii. Fibrosis
      iv. Sheets of RS cells
   4. *Lymphocyte rich HL* (Fig. 5.87): Uncommon. Characterized by:
      i. Cellular milieu rich in normal lymphocytes
      ii. Paucity of malignant cells
      iii. Scanty RS cells

   This variety is present in older individual.

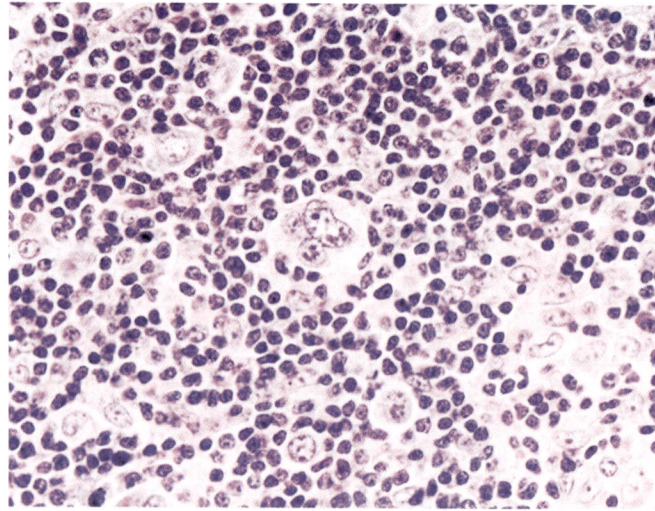

Fig. 5.85: Mixed cellularity HL

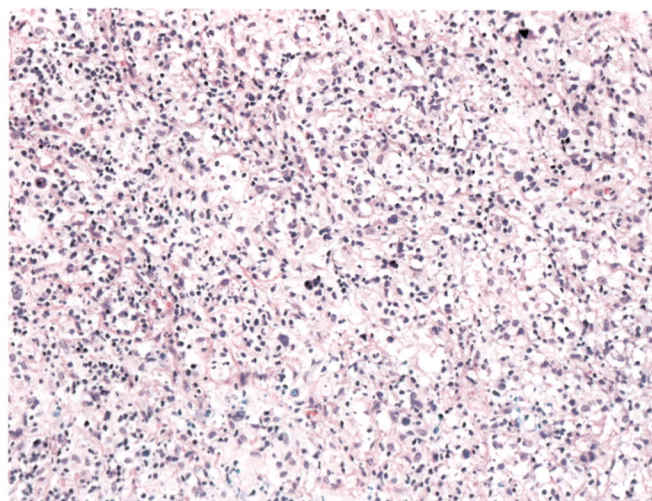

Fig. 5.86: Lymphocyte depleted HL

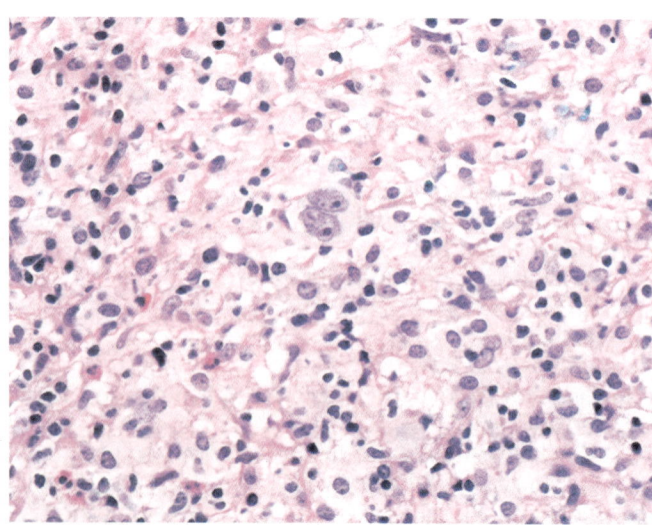

Fig. 5.87: Reed-Sternberg giant cell

II. Nodular lymphocyte predominant HL (Fig. 5.88): It differs from classical HL:

    i. Its immunophenotype profile
    ii. Histological characteristic
    iii. Clinical behavior
    iv. Absence of RS cells

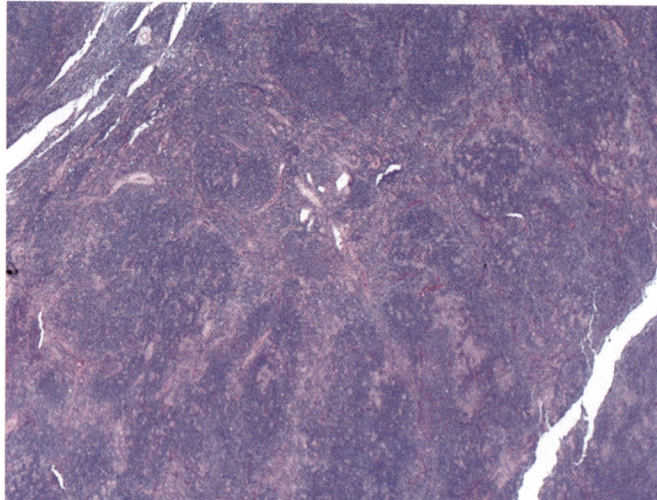

Fig. 5.88: Nodular lymphocyte predominant HL

    v. Neoplastic cells or popcorn cells (Fig. 5.89)—they cluster within the nodule associated with lymphocytes and histiocytes (L and H), they are large B cells.

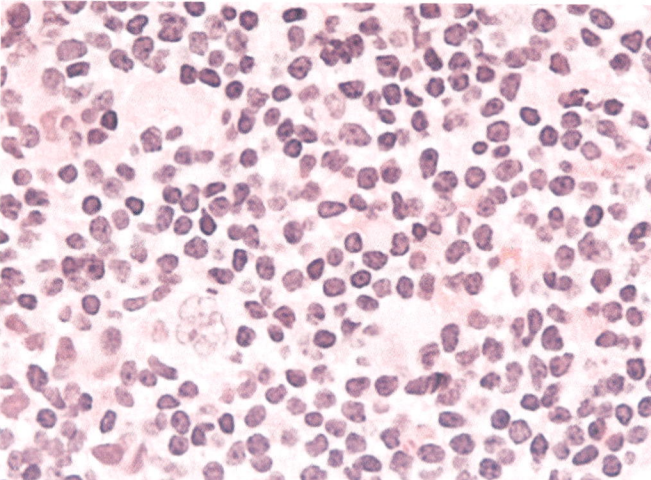

Fig. 5.89: Popcorn cells in nodular lymphocyte predominant HL

Pathophysiology

Both forms of HL are B cell originated lymphoma:

1. Reed-Sternberg cell in classical HL appears to be transformed post-germinal center B cell.
2. L and H cells of nodular lymphocytic predominant HS— are neoplastic germinal center B cells.

Risk Factors

1. It is associated with high socioeconomic status in childhood (NS in young adult).
2. Familial aggregations are frequently reported.

i. Increased risk in identical twins

ii. Increased risk for siblings of young adult

iii. There is genetic and environmental predisposition.

3. Four times increased risk in individual with history of infectious mononucleosis. Epstein-Barr virus encoded RNA is detected in RS cells.

4. HIV-infected patient has 8 times increased risk of developing HL.

Clinical Features

1. Patient usually presents with painless rubbery supra-diaphragmatic lymph node enlargement mainly cervical region (Fig. 5.90).

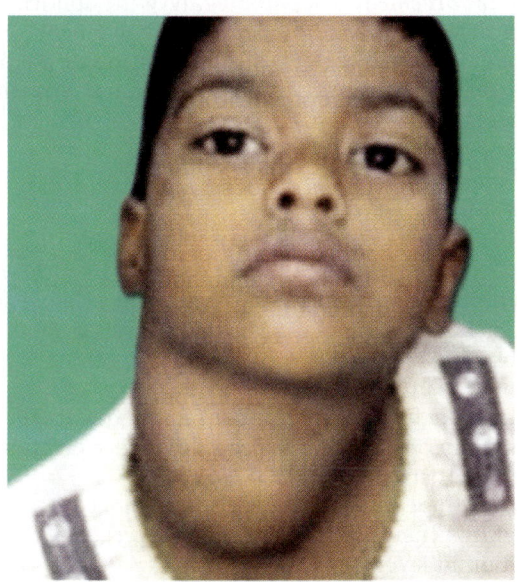

Fig. 5.90: Cervical node enlargement

2. Contagious nodes are also involved by contagious spread—like auxiliary nodes, supraclavicular nodes.

3. Waxaning and waning of lymph node0

4. Splenomegaly (1–30%), hepatomegaly (5%):

i. Abdominal lymphadenopathy is unusual without splenic involvement

ii. Disease restricted to subdiaphragmatic area is unusual except in NHL.

5. Mediastenal and hilar lymphadenopathy—may produce local symptoms, like: Superior vena caval syndrome

6. Direct extension to pleura (plural effusion), pericardium (pericardial effusion), lung (collapse, consolidation)

7. Extranodal involvement, through bloodstream:

i. Bone marrow

ii. Lung

iii. Liver

8. Constitutional symptoms:

i. Weight loss >10% body weight in last 6 months

ii. Unexplained fever

iii. Drenching night sweat.

The above constitutional symptoms correlate with:

a. Disease extent

b. Disease bulk

c. Prognosis

Other constitutional symptoms are:

i. Pruritus

ii. Alcohol-induced pain in lymph node

9. Patients having defect in cell-mediated immunity are very prone to develop virus, bacterial, tubercular and fungal infection.

10. **Young adult having stage I/II nodular sclerosis** variety are:

i. Prognostically good,

ii. Disease is localized to cervical, supraclavicular or mediastenal.

11. **Mixed cellularity HL variety involve children and older persons**—are in advanced stage, prognosis is intermediate.

12. **Lymphocytic depleted variety involves older age group**—disease extensive, prognosis is poor.

13. **Lymphocytic rich variety**—is localized disease and favorable prognosis.

14. **Nodular lymphocytic predominant** variety

i. More frequent in male

ii. Localized at presentation

iii. Indolent symptoms

iv. Relapse occur

v. Median age—35 years.

Investigations

Hematological

1. Complete blood count:

i. Normochromic normocytic anemia

ii. Reactive lymphocytosis

iii. Eosinophilia

iv. Mild reactive lymphocytosis.

2. ESR—raised

3. Urine—routine

4. LFT

5. Serum uric acid—raised

6. LDH—raised

Radiological

1. Chest X-ray

2. CT scan of thorax, abdomen to see evidence of nodal and extranodal involvement

3. Positron emission tomography often combined with CT scan

4. Isotope bone scans

Interventional/Invasive

1. Bone marrow trephine biopsy—to exclude marrow involvement in patient with stage IB/IIB or stage III/IV—it may show reactive lymphocytosis.

2. Lymph node excision biopsy, because fine needle aspiration may be inadequate. Image guided core needle biopsy, mediastinoscopy or mediastinotomy may be required.

3. Biopsy from liver

Other Test

1. Pregnancy test in pregnant woman

2. Fertility counseling

Staging of Hodgkin's lymphoma (Fig. 5.91)

Ann Arbor Staging, Cotswold Modification

1. **Stage-I:** Involvement of single lymph node region or lymphoid structures (spleen, thymus, waldeyer's ring) or, Involvement of a single extra nodal site (E)

2. **Stage-II:** Involvement of two or more lymph node regions, on the same side of diaphragm (II) which may be accompanied by localized contagious involvement of any extranodal organ or site (E). Number of anatomic sites may be indicated by numeric subscript.
3. **Stage-III:** Involvement of lymph node regions on both sides of diaphragm (III) which may also be accompanied by localized involvement of an associated extra-lymphatic organ or site (IIIE), by involvement of the spleen (IIIS) or both (III E+S).
4. **Stage-IV:** Disseminated involvement of one or more extra-lymphatic organs, with or without associated lymph node involvement, or isolated extra-lymphatic organ involvement with distant (non regional) nodal involvement.

Each stage is subdivided into A and B categories. B for those with defined systemic symptoms and A for those without systemic symptoms.

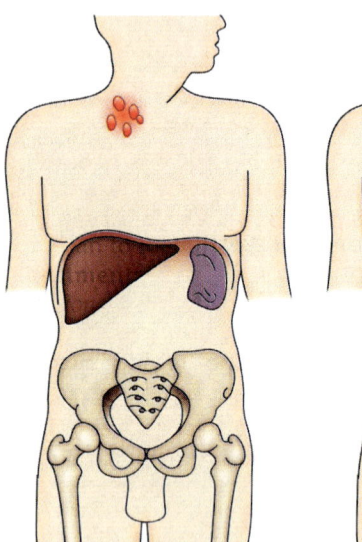 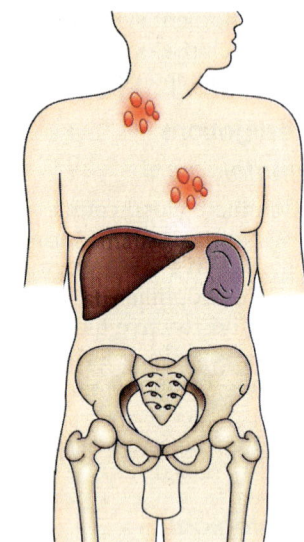

Stage I
Involvement of single lymph node or group of nodes

Stage II
Involvement of two or more sites on same side of diaphragm

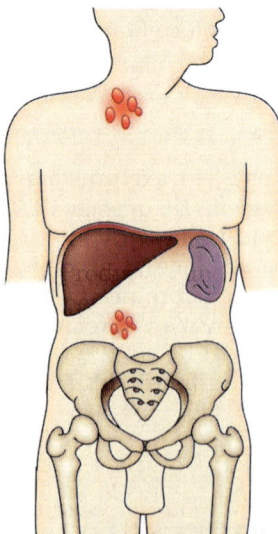 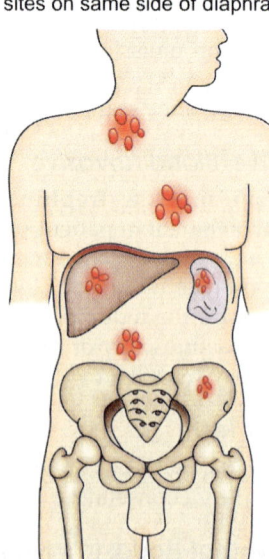

Stage III
Disease on both sides of diaphragm. May include spleen or localized extranodal disease

Stage IV
Widespread extralymphatic involvement (liver, bone marrow, lung, skin)

Fig. 5.91: Staging in Hodgkin's lymphoma

Systemic symptoms (B)
Fever >38°C
Weight loss >10% in last 6 months
Drenching night sweats
X = A mass >10 cm or a mediastinal mass larger than one-third of the thoracic diameter.
E = Involvement of a single extranodal site contagious to a known nodal site.

Clinical imaging criteria:
1. *Lymph node involvement* >1 cm on CT scan is considered abnormal.
2. *Splenic involvement*—splenomegaly may be reactive, filling defect on CT or ultrasound—confirm involvement.
3. *Liver involvement*—hepatomegaly with abnormal LFT, filling defect on imaging—confirm involvement.
4. *Bulky disease* >10 cm in largest dimension or mediastinal mass greater than one-third by maximal intrathoracic diameter.

Prognostic Features

I. **Favorable prognostic features:**
 1. ESR <50 cm/1st hour
 2. Age <50 or younger
 3. Lymph node predominant or nodular sclerosis variety in histology
 4. Absences of associated B symptoms.
 5. Fewer than 3 sites of involvement
 6. No bulky adenopathy, including mediastinal disease, less than one-third of the chest diameter on chest X-ray or tumor size <10 cm.
II. **International prognostic factors project on advanced Hodgkin's lymphoma prognostic score:**
 1. Albumin level <4 gm/dl
 2. Hemoglobin level <10.5 gm/dl
 3. Male sex
 4. Age ≥45 years
 5. Stage IV disease
 6. WBC >15000/mm^3
 7. Absolute lymphocyte count <600/mm^3 or lymphocyte count that was less than 8% of total WBC count.
    5 years survival rate:
    i. Factor 0–84%
    ii. Factor 1–77%
    iii. Factor 2–67%
    iv. Factor 3–60%
    v. Factor 4–51%
    vi. Factor ≥5–42%

Treatment

Two types of treatment are available.

Radiation Therapy

In adult Hodgkin's lymphoma:
 i. Appropriate dose of radiation is 2500 to 3000 cGy to clinically uninvolved sites.
 ii. 3500–4400 cGy to the region of initial nodal involvement.

Toxicities of radiation treatment:

Long-term complications:
 i. Breast cancer in young women
 ii. Lung cancer in patients with history of smoking
 iii. Thoracic irradiation accelerates coronary artery disease

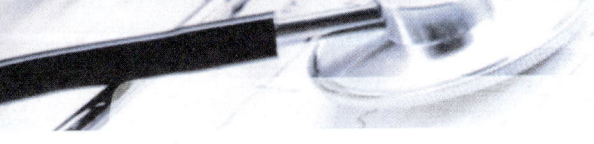

iv. Cervical irradiation increases the risk of carotid athero-sclerosis and stroke.

v. Patient receiving thoracic radiotherapy eventually develops hypothyroidism.

vi. Lhermitte's syndrome—as a consequence of thoracic radiotherapy—this is characterized by:

"Electric shock" like sensation in the lower extremities on flexion of the neck.

vii. Infertility—in both women and men, this is age-related younger patients more likely to recover fertility.

Radiotherapy is usually delivered in three major fields

1. Mantle field;
2. Para-aortic field
3. Pelvic or inverted Y field

Extended field refers to: Inclusion of adjacent clinically negative nodal sites.

Involved field irradiation	Subtotal nodal irradiation including mantle and spade fields
Mantle field irradiation	Inverted field irradiation

Chemotherapy

1. Patients with all stages of Hodgkin's disease are treated initially with chemotherapy.
2. Patient with localized disease or good prognostic disease receives a brief course of chemotherapy followed by radiotherapy to the sites of involvement.
3. Patient with more extensive disease or those with B symptoms, receive a complete course of chemotherapy.

The most popular chemotherapy regimen include the following:

A. ABVD:

1. Doxorubicin 25 mg/m^2/dose—IV for 2 doses (Day 1 and day 15)
2. Bleomycin 10U/m^2/dose IV push for 2 doses (Day 1 and Day 15)
3. Vinblastine 6 mg/m^2/dose IV push for 2 doses (Day 1 and Day 15)
4. Dacarbazine 375 mg/m^2/dose IV infusion for two doses (day 1 and day 15)

Treatment cycle—every 28 days.

B. MOPP:

1. Mechlorethamine—500 mg/m^2/dose I.V. push for 2 doses (day 1 and day 8)
2. Vincristine—1.4 mg/m^2/dose IV push for 2 doses (day 1 and day 8)
3. Procarbazine—100 mg/m^2/day orally for 14 days (day 1—day 14)
4. Prednisolone—40 mg/m^2/day orally for 14 days (days 1—days 14)

Treatment cycle repeat after every 28 days.

C. Combination of 4 ABVD + MOPP—every 28 days

D. BEACOPP:

1. Bleomycin—10 mg/m^2 (day 8)
2. Etoposide—100 mg/m^2 (days 1–3)
3. Doxorubicin—25 mg/m^2/dose (day–1)
4. Cyclophosphamide—650 mg/m^2/dose (day 1)

5. Vincristine—1.4 mg/m^2 (day 8)
6. Procarbazine—100 mg/m^2 (days 1–7)
7. Prednisolone—40 mg/m2 (days 1–14)

Regimen was repeated on day 22.

E. Increased dose BEACOPP:

1. Bleomycin—10 mg/m^2 (day 8)
2. Etoposide—200 mg/m^2 (day 1–3)
3. Doxorubicin—35 mg/m^2/dose (day 1)
4. Cyclophosphamide—1250 mg/m^2 (day 1)
5. Vincristine—1.4 mg/m^2/dose (day 8)
6. Procarbazine—100 mg/m^2 (day 1–7)
7. Prednisolone—40 mg/m^2 (day 1—14)

Regimen repeated on day 22.

G-CSF starting on day 8 until count recovery.

F. Stanford V:12 weeks of chemotherapy comprising of 3 cycles of 28 days followed by 2–4 weeks by 36 Gy IFRT in patients with disease >5 cm or splenomegaly.

1. Mustard—500 mg/m^2/dose IV weeks 1, 5, 9
2. Vincristine 1.4 mg/m^2/dose IV weeks 2, 4, 6, 8, 10, 12 (maximal dose 2 mg)
3. Prednisone—40 mg/m^2/day orally every other day, weeks 1–9, then taper.
4. Doxorubicin—25 mg/m^2/dose IV weeks 1, 3, 5, 7, 9, 11
5. Bleomycin—5U/m^2 IV weeks 2, 4, 6, 8, 10, 12
6. Vinblastine—6 mg/m^2/dose IV weeks 1, 3, 5, 7, 9, 11
7. Etoposide—60 mg/m^2 IV daily for 2 days weeks 3, 7, 11
   - Taper prednisolone by 10 mg of total dose (every other day) on weeks 10 and 11.
   - Reduce the dose of Vinblastine to 4 mg/m^2 on weeks 9 and 11 for patients over the age of 50 years.
   - Reduce the dose of vincristine to 1 mg/m^2 on weeks 10 and 12 for patients over the age of 50 years.

Complications:

A. *Early complications:*

1. Nausea, 2. Vomiting, 3. Alopecia, 4. Myelosuppression, 5. Infection

B. *Late complications:*

1. Sterility (primarily with MOPP—based regimen)
2. Neuropathy (primarily with vincristine)
3. Cardiomyopathy (doxorubicin)
4. Pulmonary fibrosis (Bleomycin)
5. Secondary leukemia (MOPP ± radiation)

Treatment of Hodgkin's Lymphoma in Relapse

1. Patients who relapse after primary therapy of Hodgkin's disease can frequently be cured.
2. Patients who relapse after initial treatment with only radiotherapy have an excellent outcome when treated with chemotherapy.
3. Patients who relapse after an effective chemotherapy regimen are usually not curable with subsequent chemotherapy administered at standard dose.

Follow-up and Monitoring for Late Complication

1. **Review and check full blood count, blood biochemistry** every 2–4 months for 1–2 years → then every 3–6 months for 3–5 years.

   Thyroid stimulating hormone annually, if radiotherapy to neck.

2. **Chest X-ray**—every 3–6 months for first 2–3 years then annually.
3. **Annual mammography/**breast MRI starting from 5–8 years post-therapy or age 40 years if earlier, if RT above the diaphragm.
4. **Annual blood pressure, serum glucose, lipid** screen after 5 years.
5. **Pneumococcal vaccination** every 5–7 years, if splenic RT or splenectomy.
6. **Consider spiral CT** of 5 years if increased risk of lung cancer.
7. **Baseline exercise test/ECG** of 10 years then annually.

Treatment Modalities

A. Classical HL, favorable stage (I/II), no risk factor:
Treatment of choice:
Combined modality treatment (CMT): ABVD—2–4 cycles + involved field radiotherapy (20–30 Gy) (Avoid high cervical region when possible and axilla in women) Expected outcome >90%

Alternative regimen:

i. Stanford V × 2 cycles for 8 weeks
↓
IFRT (30 Gy) within 3 weeks of last chemotherapy

ii. Subtotal lymphoid radiation—(36–40 Gy mantle ± para-aortic-spleen or inverted Y)—in patient, intolerant to chemotherapy
B. Stage 1A patients with subdiaphragmatic disease: Chemotherapy ± involved field radiotherapy avoiding extended pelvic/abdominal fields—that are myeloablative and sterilizing in women.
C. Classical HL unfavorable stage I/II ≥1 risk factor: ABVD × 6 cycles + IFRT (bulky disease 30–36 Gy non-bulky disease—20–30 Gy) is widely used. Expected outcome >85%

Alternative regimen:
1. Stanford regimen – × 3 cycles (12 weeks)
+
IFRT within 3 weeks of last chemotherapy (36 Gy to initial sites >5 cm or involved spleen, 30 Gy to other involved sites)
D. Classical HL—advanced stage: Chemotherapy ABVD/MOPP

Alternating regimen:

1. Stanford regimen × 3 cycles
↓
Followed for IFRT (36 Gy) to sites of bulky disease
2. Extended BEACOPP

Nodular Lymphocytic Predominant HL

A. Early stage non-bulky NLPHL:
i. With unilateral high cervical or epitrochlear lymphadenopathy—by IFRT
ii. localized inguinal or femoral NLPHL—by regional radiotherapy only. Survival ≅ 90% at 10 years.
Most of them die due to radiotherapy related toxicity.
B. Stage III/IV NLPHL:
i. Standard HL regimen   or
ii. CHOP ± rituximab

NON-HODGKIN'S LYMPHOMA

It is a group of histologically and biologically heterogeneous clonal malignant diseases arising from lymphoid system.

Epidemiology

Annual incidence in western countries is 14–19 cases per 100000 populations.

There is steady increase in incidence. 3–4% per annum. It is mainly due to AIDS.

Other causes are increased exposure to environmental carcinogen.

Incidence ratio in male: female = 3:2

The difference between NHL due to AIDS and non-AIDS: Diffuse large B cell lymphoma (DLBCL)—30% in non-AIDS and 70 to 80% in AIDS related (DLBCL) patient.

Antiretroviral therapy decreases the incidence of NHL—mainly DLBCL, but incidence of Burkitt lymphoma and centroblastic type DLBCL is not affected by HAART (highly active antiretroviral therapy).

Etiology

Main factor is translocation and/or mutation of immunoglobulin gene loci which is responsible for development of lymphoma.

Factors associated with NHL are:
1. *Congenital immunodeficiency:*
   i. Ataxia—telangiectasia
   ii. Wiskott-Aldrich syndrome
   iii. X-linked combined immunodeficiency (? EBV infection)
2. *Acquired immunodeficiency:*
   i. Immunosuppressive drugs
   ii. Transplantation
   iii. HIV infection
3. *Infection:*
   i. HTLV-1
   ii. Epstein-Barr virus (Burkitt lymphoma, Hodgkin lymphoma, immunodeficiency related high grade lymphoma)
   iii. *Helicobacter pylori* gastric mucosa associated (MALT) lymphoma.
4. *Environmental toxin:* Association with exposure to pesticides—herbicides, fertilizers.
5. *Familial risk* ↑ 2–3-fold increase

Classifications

B Cell Lymphoma

I. **Precursor B cell lymphoma:** Precursor B cell lymphoblastic leukemia/lymphoma.
II. **Mature B cell lymphoma:**
   1. B cell CLL/small lymphocytic lymphoma
   2. B cell prolymphocytic leukemia
   3. Lymphoplasmacytic lymphoma (Fig. 5.92)
   4. Splenic marginal zone B cell lymphoma
   5. Hairy cell leukemia (Fig. 5.93)
   6. Plasma cell myeloma/plasmacytoma (Fig. 5.94)
   7. Extranodal marginal zone B cell lymphoma of MALT type

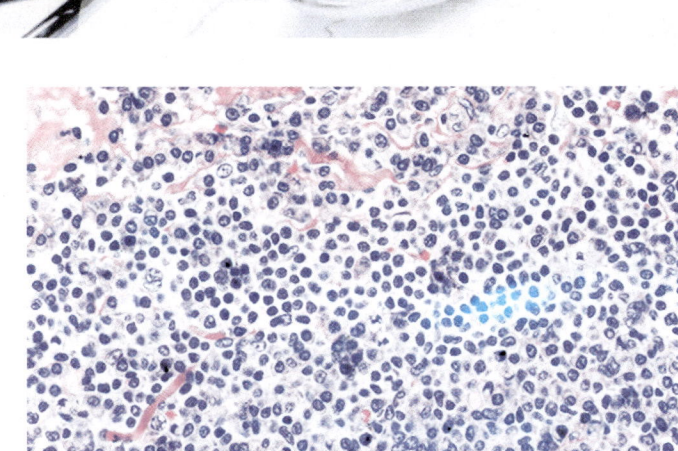

Fig. 5.92: Lymphoplasmacytic lymphoma

8. Nodal marginal zone B cell lymphoma
9. Follicular lymphoma (Fig. 5.95)

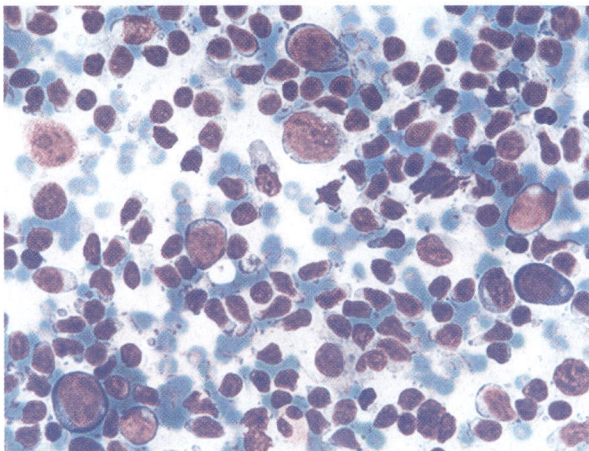

Fig. 5.95: Follicular lymphoma

10. Mantle cell lymphoma (Fig. 5.96)

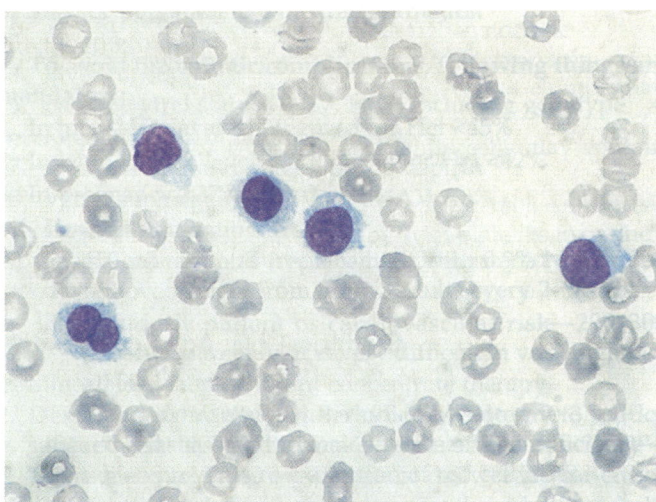

Fig. 5.93: Hairy cell leukemia

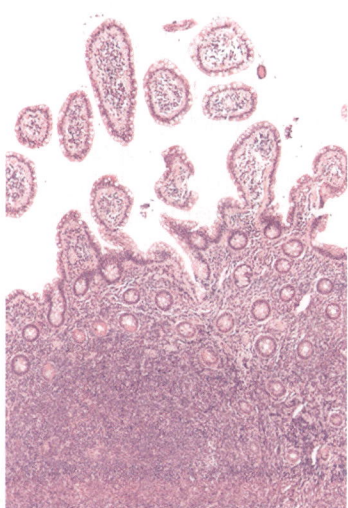

Fig. 5.96: Mantle cell lymphoma

11. Diffuse large B cell lymphoma (Fig. 5.97):
    i. Mediastenal large B cell lymphoma
    ii. 1st degree effusion lymphoma

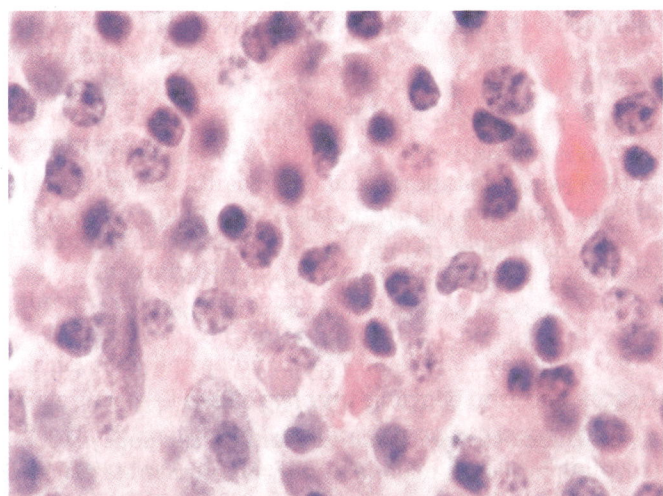

Fig. 5.94: Plasmacytoma

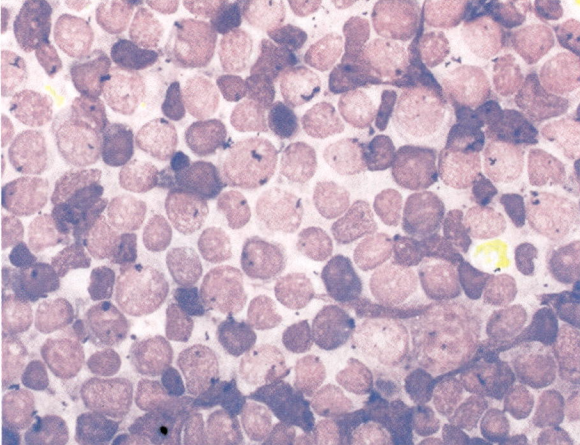

Fig. 5.97: Diffuse large B cell lymphoma

12. Burkitt lymphoma/leukemia (Fig. 5.98)

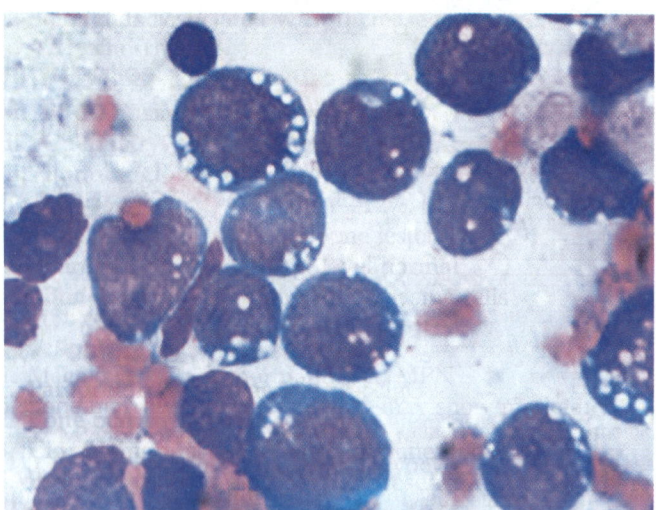

Fig. 5.98: Burkitt lymphoma

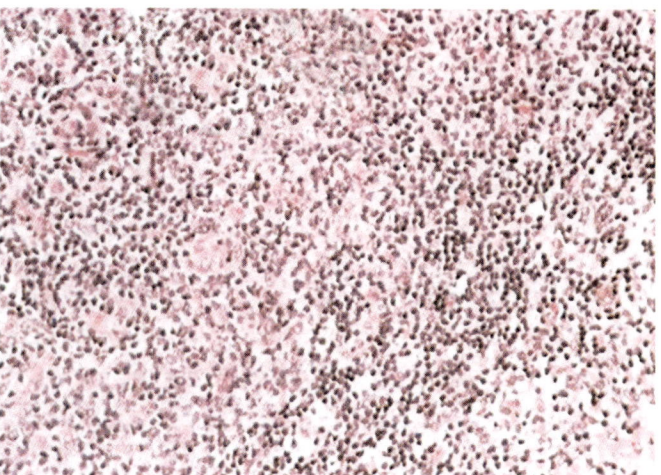

Fig. 5.99: Low-grade lymphoma

T Cell Neoplasm

I. Precursor T cell neoplasm
  i. Precursor T cell lymphoblastic leukemia/lymphoma
  ii. Blastoid NK cell lymphoma

II. Mature T cell and NK cell neoplasm:
   i. T cell prolymphocytic leukemia
   ii. T cell large granular lymphocytic leukemia
   iii. Aggressive NK cell leukemia
   iv. Adult T cell leukemia/lymphoma
   v. Extra nodal T cell/NK cell lymphoma, nasal type
   vi. Hepatosplenic T cell lymphoma
   vii. Subcutaneous panniculitis like T cell lymphoma
   viii. Mycosis fungoides/Sezary syndrome
   ix. Peripheral T cell lymphoma
   x. Anglo immunoblastic T cell lymphoma
   xi. Primary systemic anaplastic T cell lymphoma

Clinical Grade of Lymphomas: REAL Classification

Diagnosis

A. Indolent lymphoma (low risk) (Fig. 5.99):
  1. Follicular lymphoma (grade I and grade II)
  2. Marginal zone B cell, MALT lymphoma
  3. Chronic lymphocytic leukemia/small lymphocytic lymphoma.
  4. Marginal zone, B cell, nodal
  5. Lymphoplasmacytic lymphoma

B. Aggressive lymphoma (intermediate risk):
  1. Diffuse large B cell lymphoma
  2. Mature (peripheral) T cell lymphoma
  3. Mantle cell lymphoma
  4. Mediastinal large B cell lymphoma
  5. Anaplastic large cell lymphoma
  6. Follicular lymphoma (grade III)

C. Very aggressive lymphoma (Fig. 5.100):
  1. Burkitt lymphoma
  2. Precursor T lymphoblastic

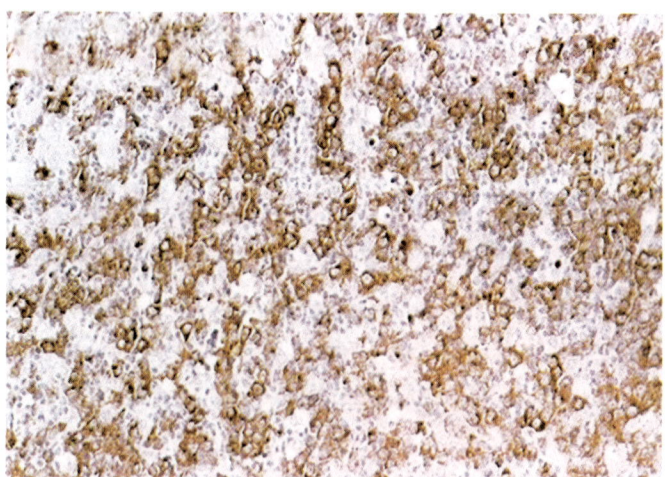

Fig. 5.100: High-grade lymphoma

D. Other lymphomas

Presentation: Patient may present in **wide-spectrum** having low grade lymphoma (wide dissemination non-destructive, indolent course at diagnosis) at one end and very high-grade lymphoma (localized rapidly progressive lymphadenopathy ± constitutional symptom—night sweat, >10% loss of body weight, or fever, destructive growth pattern) at other end.

Patient may present with the following:
1. 75% nodal superficial painless lymphadenopathy
2. 25% extranodal disease:
    i. Oropharyngeal involvement (Waldeyer's ring)
    ii. Gastro intestinal involvement
    iii. Central nervous system involvement
    iv. Skin i8nvolvement (T cell lymphoma)
    v. Autoimmune cytopenia

Diagnostic and Staging Investigations

  I. Diagnostic confirmation from tissue biopsy
    A. Sufficient material is critical for accurate diagnosis.
    B. *Needle biopsy should be avoided*, because amount of material is very small

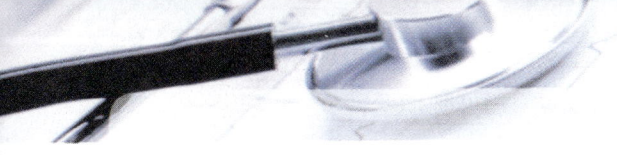

C. *Important studies for diagnosis confirmation:*
1. Assessment of clonality.
2. Immunophenotypic, cytogenetics and molecular studies
3. Marker of histogenesis

Oncogenes rearrangements are diagnostically useful:
a. t (8:14) or MYC—Burkitt lymphoma
b. t (14:18) or bcl-2—follicular lymphoma
c. t (2:5) or ALK—anaplastic large cell lymphoma
d. t (11:14) or bcl-1—mantle cell lymphoma
e. Trisomy 3 or trisomy 18—marginal zone lymphoma

D. Some tumors (e.g. T cell rich B cell lymphoma or lymphomatoid granulomatosis) have excess reactive T cells.

II. History and physical examinations:
- History includes also B symptoms
- Physical examination includes Waldeyer's ring examination.

III. Viral testing: If indicated:
A. HIV serology in all aggressive NAL
B. HTLV-1 serology
C. Hepatitis B and C serology

IV. Clinical and laboratory assessment of organ function:
A. *CD4 cell count,* if HIV positive
B. *Routine blood tests:*
1. Full blood count
2. Plasma viscosity
3. Blood film
4. Lactate dehydrogenase (indirect measure of tumor burden and prognosis).
5. Serum B_2 globulin—may be prognosis factor
6. Serum α fetoprotein or β human chorionic gonadotrophin
7. Serum uric acid
8. Liver function tests
9. Serum protein electrophoresis
10. Leukoerythroblastic blood film—if extensive BM infiltration ± pancytopenia

V. Chest radiograph
VI. CT scan of chest, abdomen neck and pelvis to define nodal and extra nodal disease
VII. PET scan or gallium scans
VIII. MRI of head, spine in patient with CNS symptoms.
IX. Bone marrow trephine biopsy
X. Lumbar puncture with cytology in patient with CNS disease in following patients at risks:
A. Diffuse large B cell lymphoma (DLBCL) with elevated LDH and more than one extranodal sites and/or lymphomatous involvement in the marrow.
B. All Burkitt lymphoma
C. All HIV-related lymphoma
IX. Ann Arbor staging systems

Stage-1 Single node region or single extra-lymphatic organ or site (IE)
Stage-2 Two or more lymph node region on the same side of diaphragm or single extra-lymphatic site with adjacent nodes (IIE)
Stage-3 Nodal regions on both sides of the diaphragm (III) or involving single extranodal site with adjacent nodes (IIIE) or spleen (IIIS) or both (III ES)

Stage-4 Diffuse or disseminated involvement of one or more extra nodal organs, bone marrow, liver, brain involvement.

WHO classification recommends FL (follicular lymphoma) is graded histologically based on the average number of centroblasts or large transformed cells (LTCs) in 10 neoplastic follicles at +40 high power field (HPF) examination:
1. Grade-1 — 0–5 LTCs/HPF
2. Grade-2 — 6–15 LTCs/HPF
3. Grade-3 — >15 LTCs/HPF with many residual small cells
4. Grade-4 — >15 LTCs/HPF in mononuclear sheets.

Prognostic Factors

1. Histological grade
2. Performance status
3. Constitutional symptoms (B)—unfavorable
4. Age >60 years—unfavorable
5. Disseminated disease—stage III–IV unfavorable
6. Extranodal disease—unfavorable ≥2 extranodal sites
7. Bulky disease—unfavorable if >10 cm
8. Raised serum LDH—unfavorable
9. Raised β_2 microglobulin level—unfavorable
10. High proliferation rate by Ki–67 immunochemistry—unfavorable
11. BCL-2 expression poor risk in DLBCL (not with R-CHOP treatment)
12. BCL-6 expression favorable in DLBCL (not with R-CHOP treatment)
13. P-53 mutations—unfavorable
14. T cell phonotype—unfavorable
15. High grade transformation from low grade NHL—unfavorable
16. Genetic expression profile in DLBCL

A. International prognostic index (IPI) for aggressive NHL in all clinical grades of NHL as a predictor of response to therapy, relapse and survival.

One point to be awarded for each at the following characteristics:
1. Age >60 years
2. Stage—III or IV
3. ≥ 2 extranodal sites of disease
4. Performance status ≥2
5. Serum LDH raised

	Score	IPI risk group	% CR
1.	0–1	Low	87%
2.	2	Low/intermediate	67%
3.	3	Intermediate/high	55%
4.	4–5	High	44%

B. Age-related IPI in patient <60 years who may be eligible for more intensive therapy

One point to be awarded for each of the following:
1. Stage III or IV
2. Raised serum LDH
3. Performance status ≥2

Score	IPI risk group (pt ≤ 60)	% CR
0	Low	92%
1	Low/intermediate	78%
2	Intermediate/high	57%
3	High	46%

C. **Revised international prognostic index (R-IPI):** Patients with DLBCL treated with CHOP + rituximab have increased survival rate.

D. **Follicular lymphoma IPI:** One point is awarded for each of the following risk factors:
1. Age >60 years
2. Ann Arbor stage III or IV
3. Hemoglobin <12 gm/dl
4. Raised serum LDH
5. Number of nodal sites ≥5.

Score	Risk group	CR (%)
0 or 1	Low	36%
2	Intermediate	37%
≥3	High	27%

Indolent Lymphomas

A. **Follicular lymphoma:**
1. Middle or old age
2. Very slowly progressive
3. Present with painless lymphadenopathy of fluctuating sizes ≥1 sites
4. 70% has bone marrow infiltration at the time of presentation
5. Constitutional symptoms—15–20%
6. Pressure effects of bulky nodes (ureter, spinal cord, and orbit)
7. High proportion of centroblast (>50%) on histology—is indicator of highly aggressive clinical course.

B. **Marginal zone lymphoma:** Three types:
   a. *MALT lymphoma:*
   1. Locally invasive at the site of origin, e.g. stomach, small bowel, salivary gland, lung
   2. Patient may present with dyspepsia, abdominal pain, GI bleeding
   3. It can be diagnosed by endoscopy with biopsy
   4. 80–90% responds to antibiotic treatment for *H. pylori*
   5. Prognosis → 80% 5 years survival
   b. *Nodal marginal zone lymphoma:*
   1. This disease may be associated with – i. Sjogren's syndrome, ii. Hashimoto thyroiditis
   2. This disease is localized to adnexa, thyroid gland, parotid gland, lung, breast
   c. *Splenic marginal zone lymphoma:*
   1. Marked splenomegaly ± hypersplenism
   2. Bone marrow involvement ± villous lymphocytosis
   3. Absent lymphadenopathy

C. **Small lymphocytic lymphoma:**
1. Age >60 years
2. Disseminated peripheral lymphadenopathy
3. Splenomegaly
4. Lymphocyte <4.5 × 10⁹/L
5. Bone marrow involvement (80% of cases)
6. 20% cases—constitutional 'B' symptoms.
7. Serum paraprotein—IgM in 30% cases.

Treatment of Indolent Lymphoma

A. **Stage I/II follicular lymphoma, small lymphocytic lymphoma:**
1. Involved field radiotherapy (35–40 Gy)
2. Recurrence generally occurs outside the area of radiation field.

B. **Stage III/IV advanced lymphoma (FL/SLL):**
   Indication of treatment:
   1. 'B' symptoms—unexplained weight loss, fever, night sweat
   2. Cytopenia
   3. Bulky disease
   4. Steady progression
   5. Threatened end organ function
   6. Transformation
   7. Patient preference

Treatment Option

CVP:
   i. Cyclophosphamide—400 mg/m² orally daily for 5 days
      Total dose—2000 mg (1–5 day)
   ii. Vincristine—1.4 mgm² IV—day-1,
      Total dose cycle 1.4 mg/m²
   iii. Prednisolone—100 mg/m² orally for 5 days (day 1–5)
      Treatment is repealed every 21 days.

Rituximab—is indicated in:
   i. Treatment of patients with relapse/refractory CD 20 +ve FL
   ii. 1st line of treatment of CD-20 +ve FL in combination with CVP
   iii. Treatment of CD—20+ve low grade NHL in stable disease
      a. Less god response with bulky disease
      b. May be useful for elderly patient

Small lymphocytic lymphoma:
   I. Chlorambucil—0.1–0.2 mg/kg/day × 7–14 day of 28 days cycle
   II. Fludarabine—25 mg/m²/day IV for 5 days (day 1–5)
      Total dose 125mg
      Treatment is repeated every 28 days—achieves more or less complete remission
   III. Fludarabine 25 mg/m²/day (day 2, 3, 4)
      +
      Rituximab (375–500 mg/m²/day—IV day 1) } Cycle 1

      In subsequent cycles, Fludarabine—25 mg/m²/day (day 1–3)
      +
      Cyclophosphamide—250 mg/m² orally with Fludarabine—achieves complete remission in 66% of uses
   III. CVP
   IV. CHOP (cyclophosphamide + doxorubicin + vincristine + prednisolone) + Rituximab—Alemtuzumab (CD-52 antibody)—Kill both B and T cells—making patient more immune compromised.

Malt lymphoma:
a. Eradication of *H. pylori* with treatment—achieves complete remission in 80% of cases. But molecular evidence of persistent disease may be present for 12–18 months.
b. Additional therapy in progressive disease is chlorambucil. If combined with rituximab—highly effective.

Mantle cell lymphoma:
A. *In localized disease*—combination chemotherapy followed by radiotherapy.

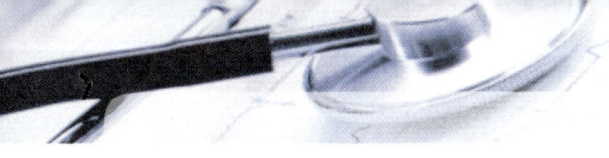

B. *In disseminated disease:*
1. Standard lymphoma therapy is unsatisfactory
2. In younger patient, aggressive combination chemo-therapy followed by autologous or allogenic bone marrow transplantation
3. In elderly asymptomatic patient, observation followed by single agent chemotherapy
4. In younger patient, intensive combination chemo-therapy

   (Cyclophosphamide + Vincristine + Doxorubicin + Dexamethasone + Cytarabine + Methotrexate)

   In combination with rituximab
   ↓
   Better response

5. C-VAD + Rituximab—one regimen
   Rituximab + high dose methotrexate + cytarabine—one regimen.
   Alternate administration of above two regimens may produce complete response in >80% of patient.

Other Treatment Opinions

1. **α-interferon** 9 million units/week for >18 months.
2. **Radioimmunotherapy:** Tositumomab [131]I—radio-labeled murine anti-CD-20 monoclonal antibody—single infusion achieves very good response.
3. Total lymphoid irradiation
4. Autologous stem cell transplantation: 80% complete remission—risk myelodysplasia, 2nd degree malignancy
5. Allogenic SCT; CR >80%, relapse rate is less than autologous SCT: Risk—high treatment related mortality. It should be considered in patient with poor prognosis

   Treatment of relapsed FL/SLL: It is important to rule out DLBCL (↑ LDH, rapidly enlarging lymph node, constitutional symptoms, and extranodal disease).

Treatment Goals

a. Palliative vs potentiality curative
b. Performance status
c. Previous treatments
   1. **In recurrent indolent NHL**—if patient disease has free survival >12 months, with previous therapy—it should be continued.
   2. **Rituximab:** As single agent—50% OR (overall response) in chlorambucil/CHOP treated patient.
      In UK, it is recommended for patient when all options have be exhausted.
   3. **R-CHOP**—offers higher OR (85% vs 72%) over CHOP: Again maintenance rituximab offers further improvement.
   4. Fludarabine ± cyclophosphamide/± mitoxantrone + Dexamethasone achieve good response in relapsed CVP treated patient.
   5. **Radioimmunotherapy**—in case rituximab refractory patient achieves very good response
   6. **Autologous SCT**—offers OS 71–79% vs. 46% in conventional chemotherapy in relapsed FL.

Regimens for advanced stage indolent lymphoma:
FL (follicular lymphoma):
1st line: RCVP, R-CHOP; F±R; FMD ± R; rituximab, chlorambucil

2nd line: F±R; FC±R; radioimmunotherapy
Autologous SCT, rituximab, allogenic SCT

Small lymphocytic lymphoma (SLL):
1st Line: Chlorambucil prednisolone; CVP ± R
CHOP ± R; F±R;' FC ± R.
2nd line: Chlorambucil ± Prednisolone; CVP ± R
F ± R; FC ± R, CHOP ± R, Alemtuzumab

High grade transformation:
i. 50% patients can transform into DLBCL or other indolent NHL
ii. Median time of transformation is 3.5 years
iii. Risk factors:
   a. Grade 3 histology;
   b. High-risk FLIPI score
   c. High B2 microglobulin
   d. Low albumin
   e. Absence of CR with initial therapy

Diffuse large B cell lymphoma: It may present with:
1. Primary as nodal disease
2. Extra nodal involvement
   a. Most common sites are—gastrointestinal tract and bone marrow
   b. Pancreas—left has better prognosis than pancreatic carcinoma
   c. DLBCL in brain—diagnosed with increasing frequency
   d. Pleural effusion lymphoma
   e. Intravascular lymphoma—very poor prognosis.

Investigations followed by staging evaluation show:
1. 50% stage I and stage II disease
2. 50% disseminated disease

Treatment stage I and stage II:
A. *For stage I and stage II non-bulky disease:*
   1. CHOP + R – 3 cycles followed by involved field radiotherapy (30 – 36 Gy) = 99% overall survival
   2. 6 cycles of R – CHOP may be superior to above interest of survival
B. *Patient with stage-II bulky disease:* 6–8 cycles CHOP + involved field radiotherapy
C. *Patient with localized testicular DLBCL:* 6–8 cycles of CHOP + intrathecal therapy followed by scrotal radio-therapy because those in risk of CNS involvement and controlateral testicular relapse.

For stage III and stage IV disease:
1. R-CHOP—6–8 cycles—1st line of therapy in CD 20+ve DLBCL stage III, IV
2. Patient with testicular, bone marrow, epidural, sinus involvement—should receive:
   i. Intrathecal-MTX
      ±
   ii. Cytarabine (4–8 doses)
   iii. Radiotherapy for bulky disease (>10 cm) at diagnosis

Response can be predicted by IPI:
Patients with low IPI score—5 years survival >70% patients with high IPI score 5 years survival ≅ 20%

Prognosis can be further dictated by:
i. Molecular features of the tumor
ii. Level of circulatory cytokines
iii. Soluble receptors and other surrogate markers

In case of relapse or refractory to therapy:
1. Salvage therapy—long-term disease free survival <10%.
2. Autologous bone marrow transplantation superior to salvage chemotherapy—DFS ≅ 40%.

BURKITT'S LYMPHOMA

It is of two types:
1. **Epidemic**—presents in childhood or adolescent, in Africa
2. **Sporadic**—more in children, rare in adult

It is 30% of childhood NHL.

Endemic variety presents with extranodal tumors of jaw, abdominal viscera. 9% associated with EBV infection. It is aggressive (Fig. 5.101).

Sporadic: It presents with:
i. Rapidly growing lymphadenopathy
ii. Intra-abdominal masses arising from Payer's patches or mesenteric lymph node
iii. Bone marrow involvement
iv. CNS involvement
v. Blood involvement.

Diagnosis

i. Morphologically—homogeneous cells in size and shape (Fig. 5.102)
ii. Demonstration of high proliferative fraction—this can differentiate from DLBCL
iii. Presence of t (8:14) or one of its variant t (2, 8) (c-myc and λ light chain gene) or t (8:12) (c-myc and κ light chain gene)—are confirmatory.
iv. **Burkitt's leukemia is recognized by:** Typical monotonous mass of medium-sized cells with round nuclei, multiple nucleoli and basophilic cytoplasm with cytoplasmic vacuoles.

Demonstration of surface expression of immunoglobulin and one of the above noted cytogenic abnormalities is confirmatory.

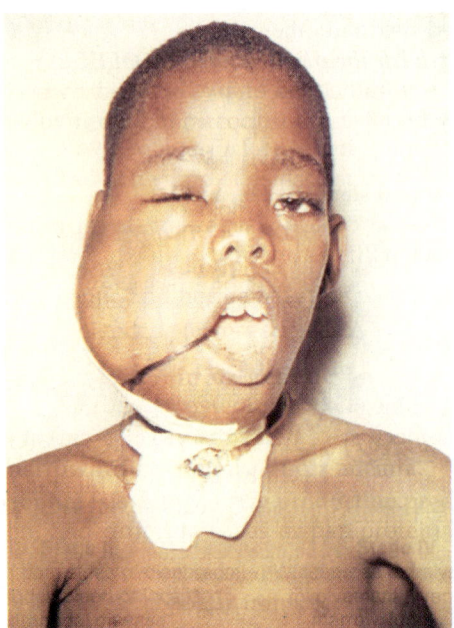

Fig. 5.101: Tumor of jaw

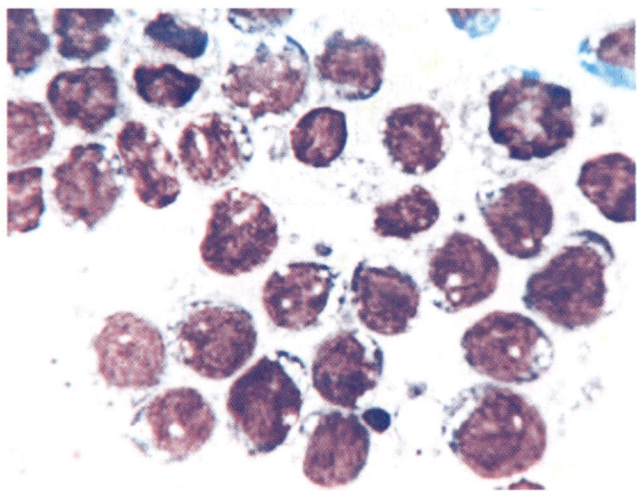

Fig. 5.102: Homogeneous cells in size and shape in Burkitt's lymphoma

Treatment

Treatment should be started within 48 hours of confirmatory diagnosis.

Therapy regimen includes: Intense short duration (3–6 months) with high dose MTX, high dose cytarabine, etoposide, ifostamide and CNS prophylaxis.

Now cure rate is 70–80% in children or adult with effective therapy.

POLYCYTHEMIA VERA

Polycythemia vera (PV) is a neoplastic clonal disorder of bone marrow stem cell causing excessive proliferation of the erythroid, myeloid and megakaryocytic lineage and carries a risk of thrombotic complications.

PV may evolve from: Proliferative phase of increased marrow activity with splenomegaly to **spent phase** characterized by leukoerythroblastic blood smear and extramedullary hematopoiesis producing massive hepatosplenomegaly.

Epidemiology

i. Median age of presentation is 60 years.
ii. It is male predominant disease, occurs in all races.

Causes of Erythrocytosis (Fig. 5.103)

I. **1st degree erythrocytosis:**
   A. *Congenital:* Familial and congenial polycythemia
   B. *Acquired:*
      i. Polycythemia rubra vera
      ii. Proliferative polycythemia
II. **2nd degree erythrocytosis** due to increased endogenous EPO production:
   A. *Congenital:*
      i. High O_2 affinity hemoglobinopathy
      ii. Congenital 2, 3, DPG deficiency
   B. *Acquired:*
      i. Hypoxemia:
         a. Chronic lung disease
         b. Cyanotic congenital heart disease
         c. Living at high attitude

```
Pleuripotent          ┌→ Basophil  →  CBL
stem cell             │
   │    ↘             │  Eosinophil →  CEL
   │    Myeloid ──→ Myeloblast
   │    stem cell     │  PMN       →  CNL
   │    ↙      ↘      │
   │ Erythroblast Megakaryoblast   Monocyte  →  CMML
   ↓      │           │
  CML     ↓           ↓
        RBC        Platelet
         │            │
         ↓            ↓
    Polycythemia  Essential
       vera       thrombocythemia
```

Fig. 5.103: Bone marrow hematopoiesis

ii. Causes of impaired tissue O$_2$ delivery: Smoking, ↑ carboxyhemoglobin

iii. Renal disease:
　　a. Polycystic kidney
　　b. Renal tumor
　　c. Renal artery stenosis

iv. Tumor causing pathological EPO production:
　　a. Hepatoma
　　b. Cerebellar hemangioblastoma
　　c. Bronchial carcinoma
　　d. Adrenal tumor
　　e. Parathyroid carcinoma

v. Liver disease:
　　a. Cirrhosis
　　b. Hepatitis

vi. Drugs:
　　a. Androgens
　　b. EPO

III. Idiopathic erythrocytosis: Persistent increased red cell mass, no evidence of MPN, no cause found

IV Relative erythrocytosis:
A. Decreased plasma volume
B. Dehydration
C. Diuretic therapy
E. Gaisbock's syndrome
F. Alcohol
G. Hypertension
H. Obesity.

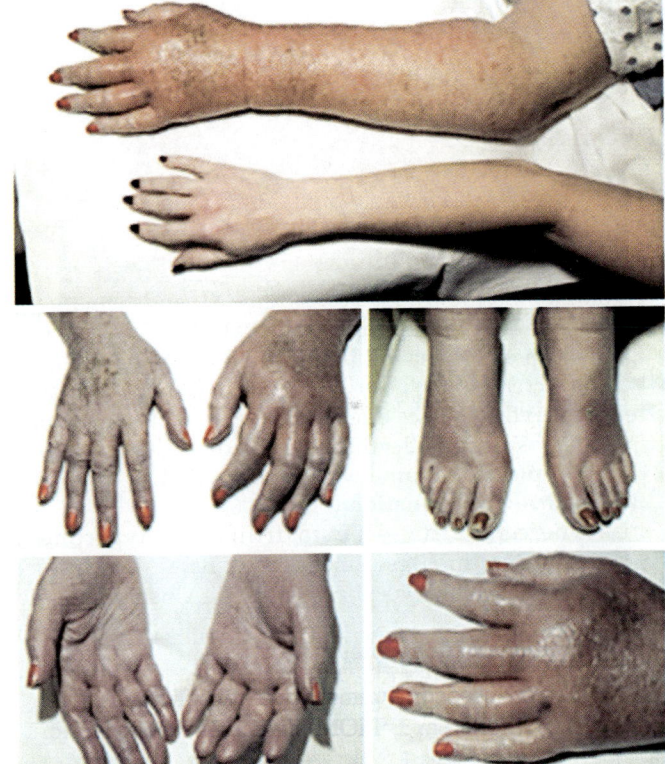

Fig. 5.104: Erythromyalgia

Clinical Features

1. Pruritus—aggravated by bathing—distinctive feature in 50% patients.
2. Erythromyalgia (Fig. 5.104)—a burning sensation in fingers and toes with erythema, pallor and cyanosis—often responds to aspirin therapy.
3. Gout and kidney stones—due to increased cellular turnover, producing joint pain, pain in loin.
4. Evidence of bleeding episodes and hemorrhage in different vital organs is the cause of death in 2 to 10% patients:
5. Thrombosis (coronary, cerebrovascular events, deep vein, pulmonary embolism, mesenteric thrombosis and in many others)—major complication of PV. The risk factors are:

i. Age >65 years
ii. Hct >45%
iii. Leukocytosis ≥15 × 10^9/L
iv. Prior history of thrombosis, atherosclerotic disease
v. Thrombocytosis—these patients should be treated with hydroxyurea to ensure platelet count <600,000/μL.

6. Ruddy cyanosis
7. Tinnitus
8. Vertigo
9. Facial plethora associated with 2nd degree erythrocytosis
11. Hypertension
12. Visual disturbance? Due to retinal vein thrombosis.

13. Headache
14. Epigastric pain.

Arterial thrombosis in 66% of PV and venous thrombosis in 30% .

Investigations

a. Full blood count and peripheral blood film (Fig. 5.105): ↑↑RBC, ↓MCV, neutrophilia and platelets are frequently raised.

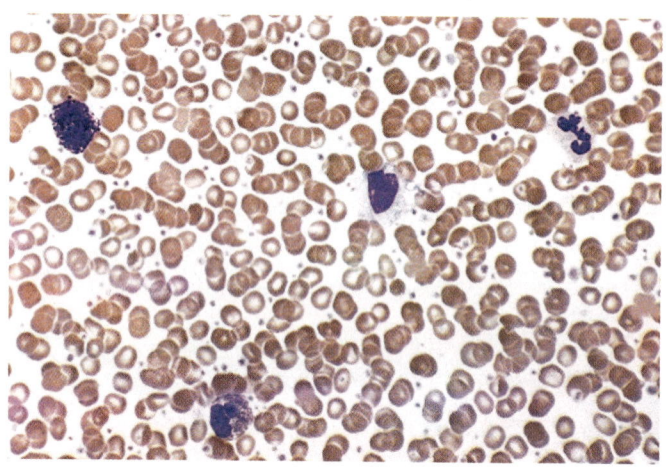

Fig. 5.105: Peripheral blood picture

b. Hemoglobin level must be >20 gm/dl, and hematocrit > 60%, this is in case of true erythrocytosis.
c. **Estimation of plasma volume and red cell volume**—both will be increased in true erythrocytosis (PV) but **in case of relative erythrocytosis** due to reduction in plasma volume (stress or spurious erythrocytosis) or Gaisbock's syndrome)—**plasma volume will be contracted.**
d. **Bone marrow examination** (Fig. 5.106):
    i. Hypercellularity—due to trilineage hyperplasia (mainly erythroid and megakaryocyte)
    ii. Atypical megakaryocytic hyperplasia, clustering round sinusoid
    iii. Decreased ferritin stores
    iv. Increased reticulin fibrosis.

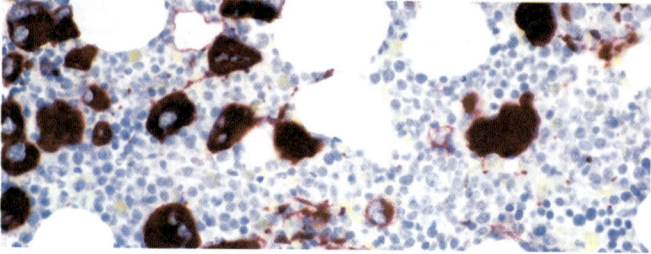

Fig. 5.106: Bone marrow picture

e. **Blood biochemistry:**
    i. Serum ferritin—decreased in overt iron deficiency
    ii. Serum uric acid raised
    iii. Leukocyte alkaline phosphatase raised.
    iv. LDH—raised
    v. Elevated vitamin B_{12} in 40% patients—due to increased transcobalamin release—reflecting associated granulocytosis.

Three situations cause microcytic erythrocytosis: RBC count, MCV, RDW:
1. β-thalassemia trait
2. Hypoxic erythrocytosis
3. PV

RDW—normal in β-thalassemia trait.
RDW—increased in hypoxic erythrocytosis and PV—due to iron deficiency anemia
f. **Diagnostic studies to find etiologies:**
    i. Serum erythropoietin:
        a. Decreased in PV idiopathic erythrocytosis
        b. Increased in secondary erythrocytosis
    ii. Abdominal ultrasound:
        a. Hepatosplenomegaly
        b. Stones in urinary system
    iii. Sleeps studies—as indicated by history of snoring somnolence.
    iv. Pulmonary function test—in case of lung disease–obstructive type
    v. O_2 dissociation curve—to determine patient with erythrocytosis with high affinity for hemoglobin
g. **JAK mutation analysis:** JAK2—V617F mutation found in 95% of patients—differentiates PV from SE and RE but not from PMF and ET (58% +ve)

Diagnostic Criteria—2008 WHO Diagnostic Criteria

Meeting of **both major criteria and one minor criterion**/or **one major criterion and 2 minor criteria**.
A. **Major criteria:**
    1. Hemoglobin >18.5 gm/dl (male), >16.5 gm/dl (female)
       Or
       Hb or Hct >99th percentile of reference range for age, sex or attitude or residence
       Or
       Hb >17 gm/dl (men), >15 gm/dl (women) if associated with a sustained increase of >2 gm/dl from baseline that cannot be attributed to correction of iron deficiency
       Or
       Elevated red cell mass >25% above mean normal predicted value
    2. Presence of JAKV617F or similar mutation
B. **Minor criteria:**
    1. Bone marrow trilineage
    2. Subnormal serum erythropoietin level
    3. EEC (endogenous erythroid colonies) growth in vitro.
Risk stratification in PV to inform treatment decisions:
1. Platelet count: >1500 × 10⁹/L-risk factor for bleeding
2. Leukocyte count >15 × 10⁹/L
3. JAK2—V617F risk factors for thrombosis

Risk category	Age >60 years or H/o thrombosis	Cardiovascular risk factor
1. Low	No	No
2. Intermediate	No	Yes
3. High	Yes	Not applicable

Complications

1. Sudden increase in spleen size can be associated with splenic infarction.
2. Myelofibrosis—it may be
    a. Reactive, reversible process—does not impede hematopoiesis and of no prognostic significance.

b. Accompanied by significant extramedullary hematopoiesis, hepatosplenomegaly and transfusion dependant anemia—manifestations of stem cell failure.
3. Organomegaly produces portal hypertension, cachexia
4. Acute nonlymphocytic leukemia—it is related to:
   i. Extramedullary hematopoiesis
   ii. Organomegaly
   iii. Transfusion dependant anemia
   iv. Exposure to chemotherapy—mainly in hydroxyurea
5. Erythromelalgia: It is associated with thrombocytosis. Involves lower extremities—manifested by erythema, warmth, pain, occasionally digital infarction
6. Ocular migraine
7. Thrombosis of vital organs—heart, brain, lungs.

Treatment

Goals are:

1. Relief of clinical symptoms that result from elevated red cell mass.
2. Decreased thrombotic risk
3. Slow or prevent leukemic transformation

To avoid thrombotic complications, following things are mandatory:

1. In men—Hb level <14.0 gm/dl or Hct <45%
2. In women—Hb level <12.0 gm/dl or Hct <42%
3. In pregnancy <37%.

I. *Venesection:*
   i. 450 ml of blood (replacement with 0.9% NS) can be removed safely from young adults every 2–3 days.
   ii. In elderly patient or cardiovascular risk—200–300 ml—twice weekly. It is very difficult in very high Hct >0.60.
      Maintenance therapy: Periodic phlebotomy to reduce red cell mass and to make a state of iron deficiency—which prevents re-expansion of red cell mass.
II. *Aspirin*—75–10 mg/day—to prevent thrombotic complications
III. *Allopurinol*—In asymptomatic hyperuricemia—it should not be administered. But it can be given in: When chemotherapy is employed to reduce splenomegaly or leukocytosis or to treat pruritus.

Additional Treatment to Patients with High Risk of Thrombosis

1. **Interferon α:** It directly inhibits fibroblast progenitors and antagonizes platelet derived growth factor, tumor growth factor-α—those may be involved in myelofibrosis.
   It can control erythrocytosis, decrease leukocytosis, thrombocytosis and splenomegaly.
   Dose: 3 million units SC daily, when Hct <0.45 is achieved, followed by lowest dose as maintenance.
   Side effects—Flu-like syndrome, myalgia, weakness.
2. **Pegylated interferon**—0.5 µg/kg/week to begin with.
   If no response—double the dose after 12 weeks → followed by maintenance dose.
3. **Hydroxycarbamide**—Ribonucleotide reductase inhibitor

To start with—15–29 mg/kg/day—until Hct <0.45
↓
Adjust the dose to preserve response
↓
Review every 2 weeks initially → when steady state is achieved—full blood count every 3 months

Side effects:
a. GI side effects, skin pigmentation, and leg ulcers—it does not heal until HC is discontinued.
b. In spent phase—HC causes anemia.

Action:
i. Decreased expression of endothelial adhesion molecules
ii. Increased nitric oxide generation

4. **Radioactive phosphorus and busulfan:**

   32P–2.3 mci/m² IV every 12 weeks as necessary, Busulfan 0.5–1 mg/kg orally single dose, if required after 3–6 months.

   ↓

   i. Reduces red cell mass—6–12 weeks after commencement of therapy

   ii. Reduce thrombocytosis
   iii. Reduce myelofibrosis.

   Toxicity—risk of acute myeloid leukemia. Hence, it must be recommended in >75 years age patient.

5. **Anagrelide:**
   i. Anti-cyclic-AMP phosphodiesterase activity, profound effect on megakaryocyte maturation resulting in decreased platelet production.
   ii. It has no effect on PV progression, erythrocytosis or splenomegaly.
   Dose: To start with 500 µg twice daily → weekly increment of 500 µg/day—usual therapeutic dose is 2–3 mg/day.
   Therapeutic effect starts within 14–21 days.

   Side effects: Headache, forceful heart beat; arrhythmia, fluid retention.

Splenectomy: Indications:
i. Massive splenomegaly
ii. Unresponsive to therapy
   Associated with intractable weight loss.

Allogenic bone marrow transplantation: It is curative in young patient.

Under trial: 1> JAK-2 inhibitors:
i. It reduces constitutional symptoms
ii. It rapidly reduces the spleen size without significant effect on blood continents.
   Diagnostic algorithm of polycythemia vera has been shown in Figs 5.107 and 5.108.

Pathogenesis

A mutation in the autoinhibitory, pseudokinase domain of tyrosine kinase JAK 2—that replaces valine with phenylalanine (V617fF) causing constitutive activation of the kinase—it is responsible for central role in the pathogenesis of PV.

JAKV617F is the basis for many of the phenotypic and biochemical characteristics of PV such as elevation of leukocyte alkaline phosphatase score.

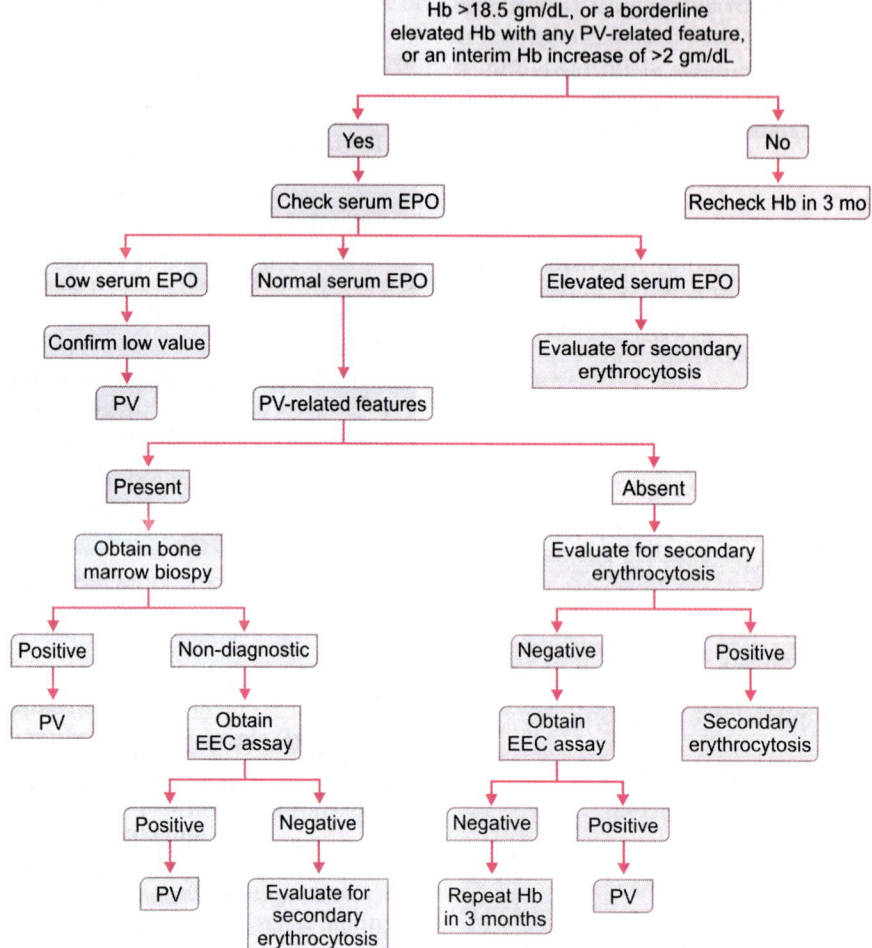

Fig. 5.107: Diagnostic algorithm of polycythemia vera

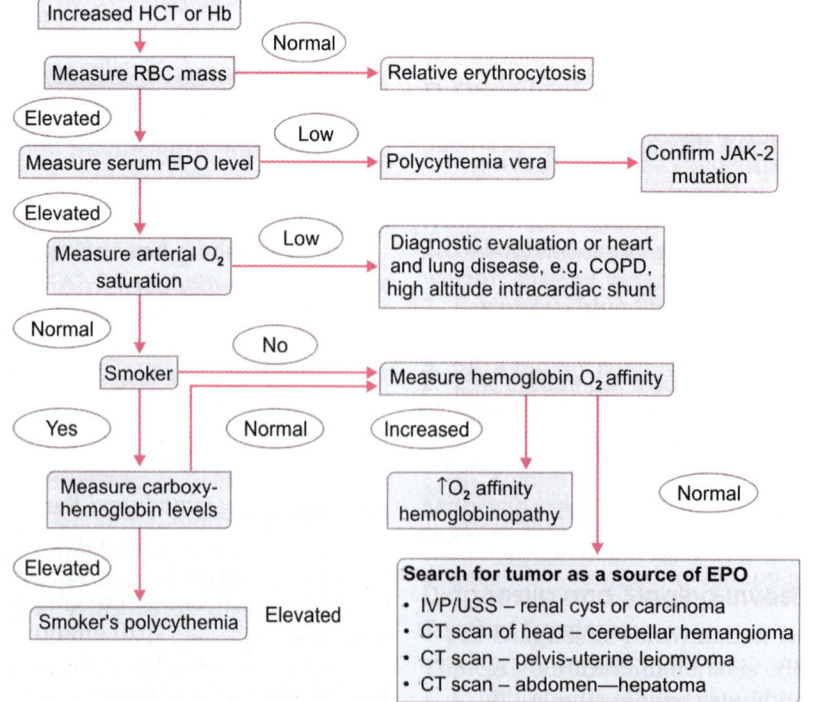

Fig. 5.108: Approach to diagnosing patient with polycythemia vera

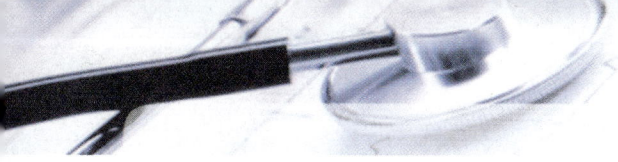

PRIMARY MYELOFIBROSIS

Primary myelofibrosis (idiopathic myelofibrosis, myelofibrosis with myeloid metaplasia, angiogenic myeloid metaplasia) is myeloproliferative neoplasm, **characterized by:**
  i. Marrow fibrosis
 ii. Splenomegaly
iii. Extramedullary hematopoiesis
 iv. Tear drop poikelocytes, and leukoerythroblastosis in peripheral blood picture.

Epidemiology

  i. Median age is 65 years
 ii. Male female ratio—1:1
iii. Median survival 3–5 years
 iv. It is worst of all myeloid neoplasm.

Etiology and Pathogenesis

  i. Marrow fibroblasts are not derived from abnormal clone, rather, increased level of platelet derived growth factor, transforming growth factor β and other cytokines produced by megakaryocytes are responsible for fibrosis.
 ii. Cytogenic abnormalities present in 50% of patients include—13q, 20q, 12p, and trisomy 8, and trisomy 9, high level of CD34 in circulation.
iii. JAK 2 V 615F mutation found in myelofibrosis—associated with PV or ET, or it may present in PMF.

Clinical Features

  i. **20% patient may be asymptomatic**, diagnosed on routine examination (splenomegaly) and full blood count.
 ii. **70–80% patient with symptoms** of progressive anemia, upper abdominal fullness, hypercatabolic features like, fatigue, weight loss, night sweat, low grade fever.
iii. **Abdominal heaviness** in felt upper quadrant or dyspepsia from pressure effects of splenic enlargement.
 iv. **Symptoms of marrow failure**—anemia, bleeding, infection
  v. **Findings:**
   a. Moderate to massive splenomegaly
   b. Variable hepatomegaly
   c. Evidence of portal hypertension
   d. Joint swollen and tenderness
   e. Evidence of plural effusion.

Investigations

1. **Full blood count:**
   i. Hb% ↓ to <10 gm/dl
  ii. Normochromic normocytic anemia
 iii. Leukocytosis or leucopenia
  iv. Thrombocytosis or thrombocytopenia
2. **Blood films:**
   a. *Prefibrotic stage* (Figs 5.109 and 5.110):
      i. Thrombocytosis
     ii. Mild leukocytosis
    iii. Leukoerythroblastic blood picture
     iv. Tear drop cell.
   b. *Fibrotic stage:*
      i. Leukoerythroblastic anemia (nucleated red blood cells, myelocytes)
     ii. Tear drop poikelocytes
    iii. Polychromasia
     iv. Giant platelet
      v. Giant megakaryocyte

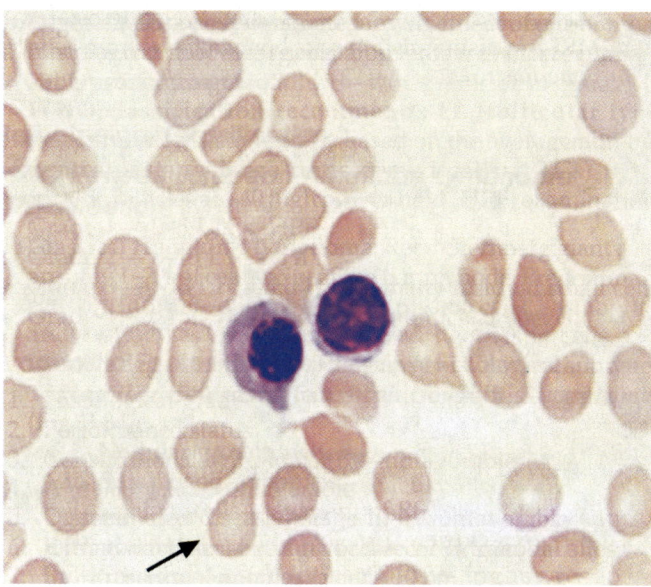

Fig. 5.109: Leukoerythroblastic blood picture

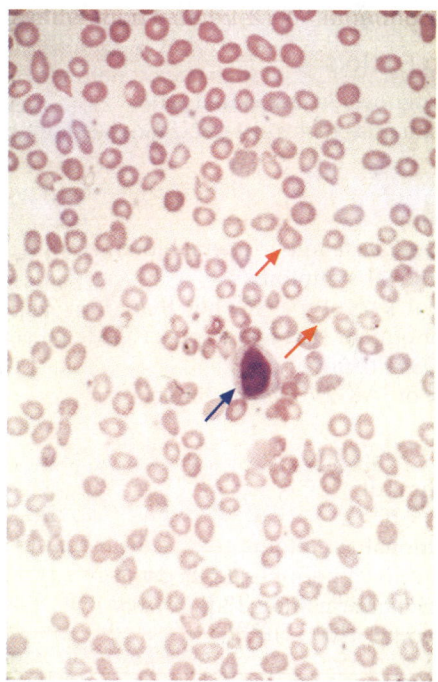

Fig. 5.110: Peripheral blood picture of idiopathic myelofibrosis

   c. *Bone marrow*—aspiration—dry tap
   d. *Bone marrow trephine biopsy* (Fig. 5.111)
      i. Patchy hemopoietic cellularity
     ii. Increased small to large irregular megakaryocytes with aberrant nuclear—cytoplasmic ratio, irregular folded nuclei—cytoplasmic ratio, irregular folded nuclei and dense clustering
    iii. Reticulin fibrosis and/or collagen fibrosis
     iv. Distended marrow sinusoids
   e. JAK2-mutation in 50% cases
   f. Coagulation screen—DIC—15% it may produce problem in surgery.
   g. Cytogenic abnormalities
   h. LDH—due to ineffective erythropoiesis
   i. Serum ferritin—decreased

j. Skeletal radiology—to assess osteomyelosclerosis
k. MRI—to distinguish fibrotic bone marrow from cellular bone marrow.

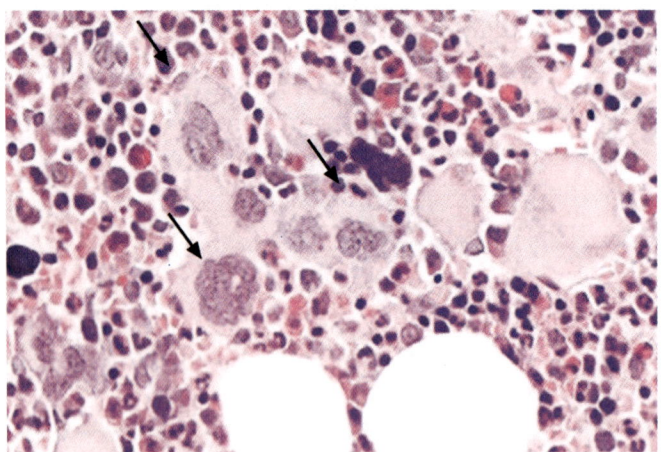

Fig. 5.111: Bone marrow biopsy

Prognostic Factors

Adverse prognosis is associated with:

1. Marked anemia—it is must important factor for patient with PMF
2. Old age
3. WBC count
4. Number of blasts in peripheral blood
5. Constitutional symptoms
6. Abnormal karyotype—(other than 13q, 20q)—stronger predictor of poor survival in post PV-MF or post ET-MF
7. High CD34+ count
8. Presence of JAK-2V617F mutation.

Adverse Factors

1. Hb <10 gm/dl,
2. WBC <4 × 10⁹/L
3. Constitutional symptoms
4. 1% blast cells in peripheral blood
5. Cytogenic abnormalities 13q-, or 20q
6. Platelet count <100 × 10⁹/L

Treatment (Fig. 5.112)

Treatment is mainly palliative.

A. Anemia can be improved with:

  1. *Combination of:*
    i. *Androgen—oxymethalone—*(50 mg four times per day or **fluoxymesterone** 10 mg three times per day)
        +
    ii. *Prednisolone* (30 mg/day)—response is brief.
  2. *EPO*—dose 10,000 units thrice weekly—achieves good response in 40–50% of patients followed by maintenance dose for >12 months.

B. Antiangiogenic agents:

  1. *Thalidomide (50 mg/day)* in combination with *prednisolone (0.5 mg/kg/day)*—improve anemia, thrombocytopenia and reduce spleen size.
  2. *Lenalidomide—(10 mg/day* for 3–4 months)—improves anemia, thrombocytopenia and splenomegaly.

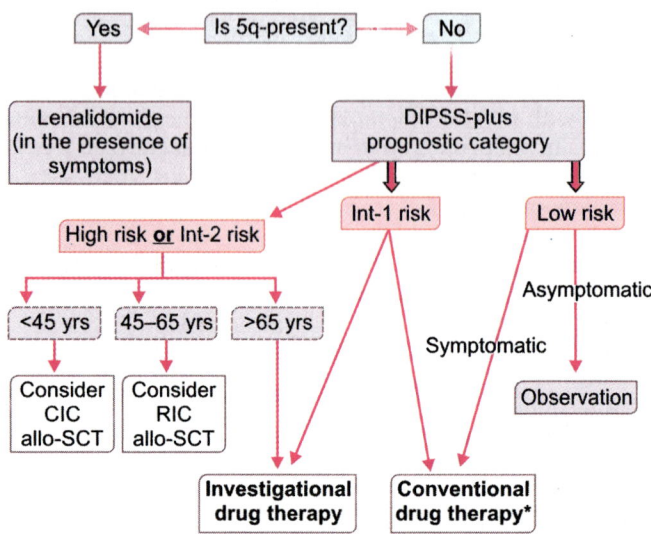

Fig. 5.112: Treatment algorithm of myelofibrosis

C. Cytoprotective therapy:

  1. *Hydroxycarbamide*
  2. *Low dose melphalan*
  3. *Busulfan*
    All reduce leukocytosis, thrombocytosis, splenomegaly and constitutional symptoms.
  4. *Cladribine*—recommended for symptomatic patients refractory to other agents—useful for management of thrombocytosis, leukocytosis, progressive hepatomegaly after splenectomy.
  5. *Interferon α*—it is indicated in younger patients due to least chance of leukemogenesis
  6. *Anagrelide:* It is used to control thrombocytosis in patients intolerant to other cytoprotective therapy.

D. Splenectomy: Indicated in:

  i. Massive splenomegaly
  ii. Excessive transfusion requirement
  iii. Refractory thrombocytopenia
  v. Hypermetabolic symptoms unresponsive to cytoreduction.
    Contraindication—thrombocytosis

E. Radiotherapy:

  1. *Splenic irradiation*—reduce spleen size in patient unfit for splenectomy—risk of severe pancytopenia, increased risk of post-splenectomy bleeding.
  2. *Hepatic irradiation:* Contraindicated
  3. *Involved field irradiation*—in extramedullary hemopoietic sites, paraspinal sites, pericardium, pleural and pericardial cavities (caressing effusion or ascites), whole lung irradiation.

F. Allogenic stem cell transplantation in all patients ≤65 years with high risk features at diagnosis.
Myeloablative SCT is associated with high transplant related mortality (60%)

G. Newer therapies:

  1. JAK-2-V617F inhibitors
  2. Bortezomib—proteosome inhibitor—it hibits NF K
  3. Azacidine and decitabine
  4. Inhibitors of vascular endothelial growth factor.

CHEDIAK-HIGASHI SYNDROME

Etiopathogenesis

LYST gene mutation
↓
Abnormal intracellular protein transport and vacuole formation
↓
Fusion of intracellular granules
↓
Uneven distribution of giant granules in the cytoplasm of neutrophils and many other cells (platelets, melanocytes, renal tubular cells, Schwann cells, thyroid follicular cells and mast cells)
↓
Impaired functions of these cells

Clinical Manifestations

i. Recurrent bacterial infections
ii. Bleeding or easy bruising
iii. Hypopigmentation of skin, eyes, and hair
iv. Peripheral nerve defect (neuropathy, nystagmus)

Diagnosis

Large granules in neutrophils in peripheral smear

Treatment

i. Symptomatic therapy
ii. Antibiotic prophylaxis with trimethoprim—cotrimoxazole
iii. Vitamin C can alter the cellular defect.

Complications

1. Progressive peripheral neuropathy in third decade of life.
2. Lymphoma like syndrome—can be treated by bone marrow transplantation

CLOTTING SYSTEM IN OUR BODY

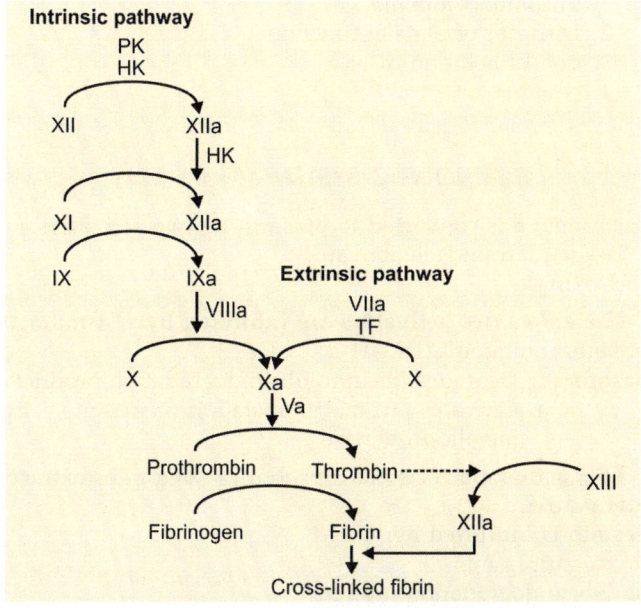

Fig. 5.113: Clotting pathways

COAGULATION SYSTEM

Coagulation factors are synthesized in liver.
1. Factors II, VII, IX, X, XI, XII are proteases—usually inactive immediately after synthesis.

↓ ← Cleaved by other proteins

Acquire enzymatic capability

2. Tissue factor and factors V and VIII are not enzyme but act as co-factor during coagulation reactions.
3. Factors II, VII, IX, X, protein C, protein S–vitamin K modified amino terminal end of each factor to enable vitamin to function.

Coagulation Pathways (Fig. 5.113)

It comprises of:
1. Extrinsic pathway or tissue injury pathway
2. Intrinsic pathway or contact pathway

Extrinsic Pathway

Binding of tissue factor with activated factor VII, (VIIa)
↓
Tissue factor + activated factor VII (TF + VIIa)
↓
Activates factors X to Xa
↓
Xa complexes with Va, phospholipid in presence of Ca^{++} forms prothrombinase complex
Prothrombinase complex is formed—it comprises of Xa + Va (activated factor V) + Phospholipid (PL)
↓
All the above factors in presence of Ca^{++}
↓
Converts prothrombin (factor II) to thrombin (IIa)
↓
Prothrombinase complex cleaves prothrombin (II) to thrombin IIa

Intrinsic Pathway

Activation of contact factors at the site of vascular injury
↓
Converts factor XII to XIIa
↓
Convert factor XI to XIa
↓
Convert factor IX to IXa
↓
Convert factor VIII to VIIIa
↓
Factor IXa complexes with VIIIa in presence of phospholipids and Ca to form Tenase complex
↓
Activates factor X to Xa
↓
Xa complexes with Va, phospholipid in presence of Ca^{++} forms prothrombinase complex
Prothrombinase complex is formed—it comprises of Xa + Va (activated factor V) + Phospholipid (PL)
↓
All the above factors in presence of Ca^{++}
↓

(Contd.)

(Contd.)

Convert prothrombin (factor II) to thrombin (IIa)

↓

Prothrombinase complex cleaves prothrombin (II) to thrombin IIa

Common Pathway

Tissue injury and contact pathway converge to common pathway, where:
1. Factor X will be activated to factor Xa
2. Factor II (prothrombin) will be cleaved to thrombin

Then thrombin cleaves fibrinogen to fibrin

↓

These fibrins will be cross-linked in presence of factor XIII

Common Coagulation Tests

1. **Prothrombin time:** This comprises reactions of coagulation that occurs in—i. tissue pathway, ii. common pathway of coagulation. So **activity of factors II, V, VII, X or fibrinogen deficiency** prolongs the prothrombin time. Normal PT = 11–14 second
2. **Activated partial thromboplastin time (APTT): Normal APTT** = 32–38 seconds depending on the type of contract factor activated used.
3. **Fibrinogen level low in:**
   i. DIC
   ii. Dilutional coagulopathy
   iii. Advanced liver disease
   iv. Following thrombolytic therapy
   v. Congenital hypofibrinogenemia
   vi. Acquired dysfibrinogenemia
4. **Thrombin time—prolonged by:**
   i. Unfractionated heparin
   ii. Hypofibrinogenemia
   iii. FDP

   TT is the time in seconds for a citrated blood sample to clot after addition of thrombin.
5. **Reptilase time (RT):** It is prolonged by low fibrinogen level, but not by heparin.
   So **comparison between thrombin time (TT) and reptilase time (RT)** is useful for determining a **prolonged APTT is due to heparin** (prolonged TT with normal reptilase time in heparin).
6. **Factor assay:** Different factors should be assayed to estimate the level of that factor
7. **Mixing studies:** If PT or APTT is prolonged, **then mixing with normal plasma and repeat the test:**
   i. If it is due to factor deficiency—mixing will correct the abnormality.
   ii. If it is due to heparin or specific factor inhibitor—the mixing will not correct the abnormality.
8. **Bleeding time:** It involves a controlled incision in soft tissue and measuring the time to cessation of bleeding.

   Prolongation of bleeding time:
   i. Abnormalities in platelets
   ii. Abnormalities in vasculature
9. **Anti-Xa assay:** It provides the information about the degree of anticoagulation after addition of heparin into patient's plasma.

Here blood should be drawn 4–6 hours after LMWH administration to plasma.

Specialized Coagulation Tests

1. **Anti-Xa assay**—provides information about the degree of anticoagulation that has occurred in patient's plasma due to the effect of heparin on factor Xa.
2. **Two common test for lupus anticoagulant:**
   i. ***Dilute Russell's viper venom time (DRVVT):***
      Russell's viper venom directly activates factor X in patient's sample—leading to conversion of fibrinogen to fibrin
      Lupus anticoagulant inhibits DRVVT leading to prolongation of clotting time.
   ii. ***Staclot assay:*** It involves performance of APTT with or without hexagonal phase phospholipid (HPE)
      If lupus anticoagulant is present, APTT will be shorter in HPE containing sample because of neutralization of the LA by HPE.
3. ***Bethesda assay:*** For factor VIII assay.

Common Causes of Abnormal Coagulation Studies

I. **Prolonged APTT:**
   1. Lupus anticoagulant,
   2. Heparin in sample (at clinically relevant concentration)
   3. Deficiency of, or inhibitor to factors VII, IX, X, XI
   4. Deficiency of high molecular weight kininogen
   5. Hypofibrinogenemia or dysfibrinogenemia
   6. Traumatic venipuncture
   7. Liver disease
   8. Inhibitors to or deficiency of V, II, X
   9. DIC
II. **Prolonged prothrombin time:**
   1. Lupus anticoagulant
   2. Liver disease
   3. Vitamin K deficiency
   4. Deficiency of II, VII, X
   5. Hypo- or dysfibrinogenemia
   6. Heparin at high concentration only.
III. **Prolonged BT**
   1. Thrombocytopenia
   2. Disorder of platelet function
   3. von Willebrand disease
   4. Anemia

FIBRINOLYTIC SYSTEMS (Fig. 5.114)

Plasminogen is converted to plasmin by two activators:
1. Tissue plasminogen activator
2. Urokinase

The above two activators are inhibited by: Plasminogen activator inhibitor-1 (PAI-1)

Plasmin: i. Degrades fibrin to fibrin degradation product
        ii. Activates pro-matrix metalloproteinase to active metalloproteinase

This active matrix metalloproteinase degrades extracellular matrix.

Plasmin is inhibited by:
i. α_2 antiplasmin
ii. Fibrin degradation product
iii. Tissue inhibitors of metalloproteinase

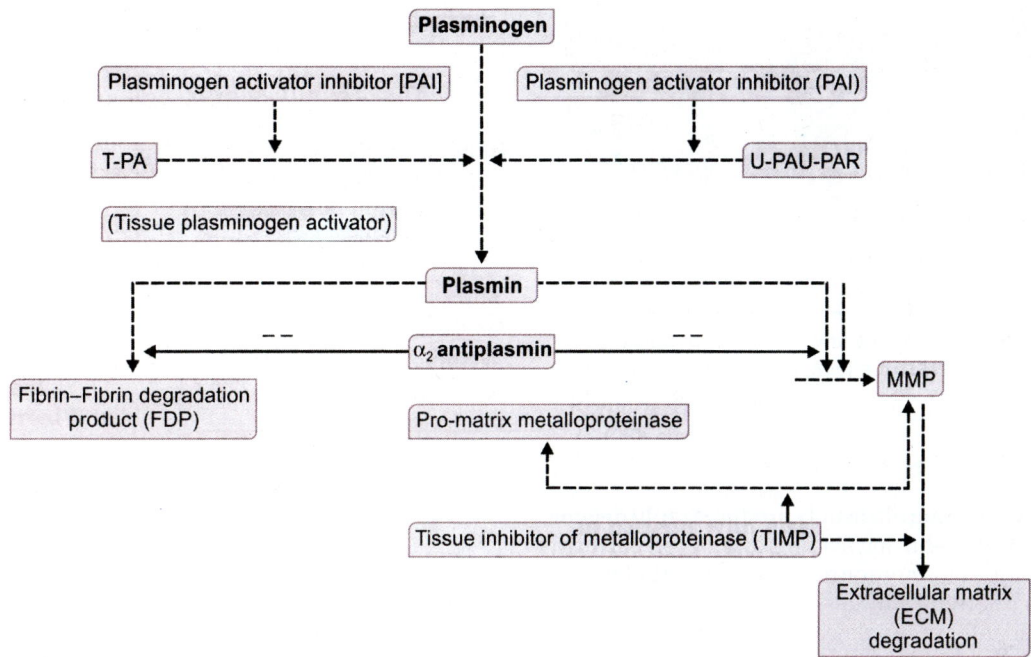

Fig. 5.114: Fibrinolytic system

HYPOFIBRINOGENEMIA

Normal fibrinogen level—2–4 gm/L
Fibrinogen is produced by liver.
It is acute phase protein.

Fibrinogen is raised in:
i. Inflammatory reaction
ii. Pregnancy
iii. Stress

Abnormalities of fibrinogen are mainly acquired than inherited. Inherited defect are usually quantitative. It may be:
i. Heterogeneous hypofibrinogenemia
ii. Homogeneous hypofibrinogenemia

Clinical Presentation
i. Patient may be asymptomatic.
ii. Bleeding following trauma or after surgery, if fibrinogen level <0.5 g/L.
iii. In case of afibrinogenemia (<0.2 gm/L)—patient may present with spontaneous bleeding, umbilical stump bleeding, cerebral or gastrointestinal hemorrhage.
iv. Hemarthrosis is less common.
v. Epistaxis, menorrhagia, and postpartum bleeding are common.

Diagnosis
i. Prolonged PT, APTT, thrombin time
ii. Fibrinogen level—measured by Clause assay

Treatment
Since fibrinogen half-life is 3–5 days, hence prophylactic injection with fibrinogen concentrate, fresh frozen plasma or cryoprecipitate

Aim: Fibrinogen level should be raised to 0.5–1 gm/L to achieve hemostasis.

Factor XIII (Fibrin Stabilizing Factor Deficiency)

Clinical Presentation
i. Delayed postoperative bleeding (6–24 hours later)
ii. Neonatal umbilical stump bleeding more common
iii. High risk of cerebral hemorrhage

Diagnosis
i. PT and APTT one normal
ii. Clot solubility test with thrombin is insensitive
iii. Elisa test to measure factor XIII antigen (a subunit)

Treatment
Since t½ life of factor XIII is very long, one monthly prophylactic replacement of factor XIII concentrate is sufficient.

HEMOPHILIA A AND B

Definition
These are congenital bleeding disorders due to:
i. Low level of factor VIII—producing hemophilia A
ii. Low level of factor IX—producing hemophilia B (Christmas disease)

Clinical Presentation
The symptoms severities depend upon the factor level in blood:
i. Bleeding occurs into muscle
ii. Spontaneous bleeding into arms, legs, iliopsoas muscles
iii. Hematoma in any site—producing nerve compression muscle contracture
iv. Hematuria—1 to 2 episodes per patient per decade.
v. Retroperitoneal bleeding
vi. Bleeding into central nervous system
vii. Bleeding into joints (Figs 5.115 and 5.116):
 a. **Blood in highly irritant**—producing synovial hypertrophy and hyperemia—so there is tendency to rebleed.

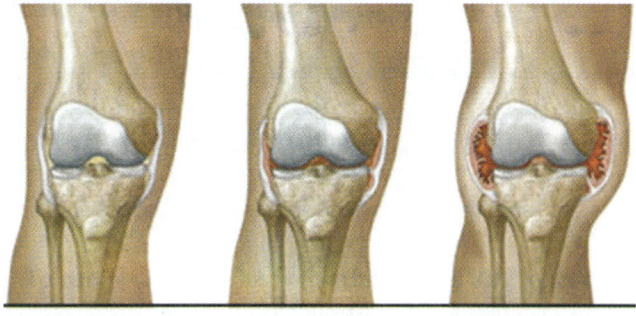

Fig. 5.115: Bleeding into the knee joint

b. **Repeated bleeding ultimately produces rapid degenerative arthritis**—having features of both **osteoarthritis** (mechanical pain, more on movement) and **rheumatoid arthritis** (morning stiffness, worse after rest)

c. Predominantly in hip, knees, and elbows.

viii. **Pseudotumors:** Progressive cystic enlargement of an encapsulated hematoma.

Recurrent subperiosteal bleeding and reactive new bone formation

↓

Destruction of bone (long bone in adults)

Muscles involved is ileopsoas.

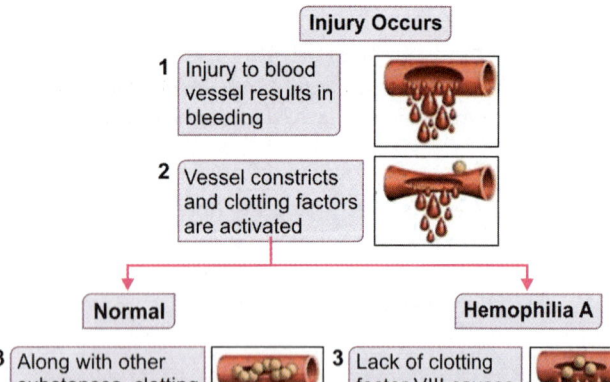

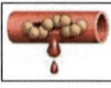
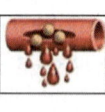
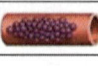
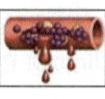

Fig. 5.116: Continuous bleeding into the joint

Pathophysiology

$\left\{ \begin{array}{l} \text{Factor VIIIa} \\ \text{Factor IX activated by tissue factor/factor VIIa complex} \end{array} \right.$

+

Activate factor X

↓

Activate prothrombin to thrombin

↓

Converts fibrinogen to fibrin

In hemophilia A and B disorders:

i. Inability to generate intrinsic pathway associated activated factor Xa.

ii. One-third of hemophilia B patients have dysfunctional factor IX molecules (type II defect).

Genetic Abnormalities (Fig. 5.117)

i. Inversion within intron 22 of factor VIII gene

ii. Point mutation

iii. Deletion

Gross genetic alteration occurs in hemophilia A but infrequent in hemophilia B.

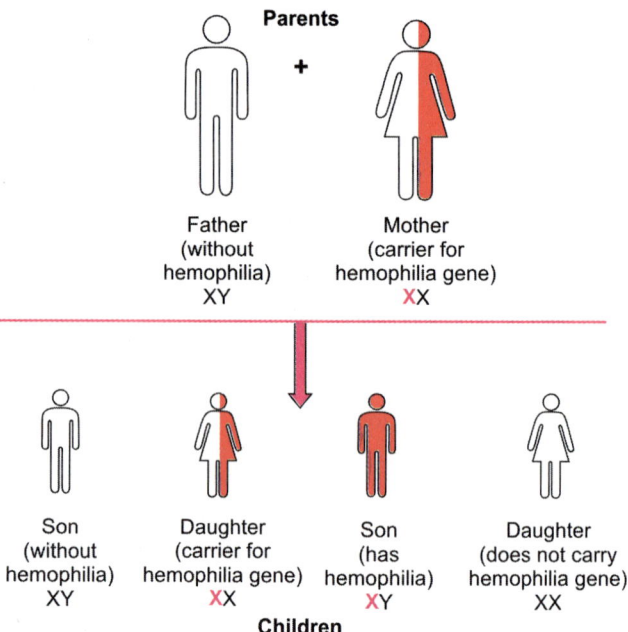

Fig. 5.117: Gene distribution in hemophilia

Epidemiology

i. No obvious family history is present, as it occurs due to genetic mutation. So newborn baby may present with severe umbilical cord bleeding or cephalhematoma

ii. Haemophilia B occurs in 1:50000.

Laboratory Investigations

I. Blood:

1. Prothrombin time—normal

2. APTT—prolonged depending on degree of deficiency

3. Factor VII:

   i. Mild disease—>0.050/ml

   ii. Moderate disease—0.01–0.05 u/ml

   iii. Severe disease—<0.01 u/ml.

II. Radiology:

i. In acute cases—ultrasound and CT scan

ii. In chronic cases—chronic synovitis, arthropathy

Complications

A. Factor VIII inhibitors: These occur after 15–20 episodes of treatment. This antibody acts against:

1. Amino-terminal component of C_2 domain of factor VIII. Or
2. Carboxy-terminal component of C_2 domain of factor VIII

This inhibitor is detected by: Inhibitory screen quantified by Bethesda assay. Patient may present with bleeding.
50% patients have low titre of antibody (<58 u/ml)
50% patients have high titre of antibody (<58 u/ml)

Diagnosis:
  i. Prolonged APTT—which fails to responds with plasma
  ii. Inhibitor—Bethesda assay
  iii. Inhibitor screen: APTT of mix patient's plasma and normal plasma.

Treatment of this complication: Factor VIII by passing agent for treatment of acute bleed and desensitization by immune tolerance with factor VIII for high titre inhibitors.
B. **Transmission of HIV, HCV, HBV**

Treatment of Hemophilia

Investigations

1. Factor level
2. Factor inhibitor screen
3. Blood group
4. Liver function test
5. Baseline viral status—HIV, HCV including genotype
6. Regular check of inhibitor status.
7. Avoidance of antiplatelet drugs, aspirin
8. Vaccination against HBV and HAV
9. Prophylactic antibiotics
10. Factor concentrates need to be administered every 2–3 days.

Hemophilia—Specific Treatment

1. Minor bleed stops without concentrate therapy
2. **Desmopressin** for minor surgery—dose 0.3 μg/kg subcutaneously, or intravenously or nasal spray
3. **Tranexamic acid**—15 mg/kg thrice daily orally for cut or dental procedure
4. **Severe disease**—factor VIII concentrate therapy necessary.

Products: Recombinant products are now treatment of choice—it does not contain any human material in product.

Human donor derived products are subject to multiple virus inactivation step:
  i. Lyophilization (dry heat)
  ii. Pasteurization (wet heat)
  iii. Solvent detergent
  iv. Nanofiltration

Principles of Treatment

To raise the factor VIII level:
  i. 0.15–0.25 U/ml for minor bleed
  ii. 0.25–0.50 U/ml for moderate bleed
  iii. >0.5 U/ml for severe bleed

Formula: 1 U/kg of body weight raise plasma concentration by about 0.02 U/ml
  t½ = 6–12 hours
So for major surgery, replacement therapy may be required up to 10 days.

Specific Treatment for Hemophilia B

Recombinant factor IX is the treatment of choice.
  Formula: 1U/kg—raise plasma concentration by 0.01 U/ml, t½ = 12 hours.

  Antenatal diagnosis: At 10–12 weeks of gestation—chorionic villus sampling—mutation analysis. Nowadays pregnancy termination is usually not done, because of improved treatment and prognosis.

DISSEMINATED INTRAVASCULAR COAGULATION

Definition

This is characterized by uncontrolled local or systemic activation of coagulation because of underlying disorders.
It may be:
  i. Acute or chronic
  ii. Localized or diffuse
  iii. Accompanied by thrombosis or hemorrhage

Causes

Conditions	Examples
1. **Tissue damage**	Trauma, burns
2. **Sepsis**	Gram –ve or +ve bacterial infection Viral infection
3. **Shock**	Cardiogenic shock, septic shock
4. **Pregnancy related**	Placental abnormalities (abortion or previa), amniotic fluid embolism, Retained uterine placenta
5. **Vascular stasis**	Carenernous hemangioma Abdominal aortic aneurysm
6. **Fat embolism**	Fracture of long bones, sickle cell crisis
7. **Malignancy**	Acute promyelocytic leukemia. Adenocarcinoma (Trousseau syndrome)
8. **Injection of toxic procoagulant**	Snake bite

Pathophysiology (Fig. 5.118)

Main pathology of DIC is uncontrolled progression of intravascular coagulation (Fig. 5.120).

Initiating events are: Overwhelming release of tissue factor, by:
  i. Cellular, vascular or hypoxic injury
  ii. Presence of endogenously or exogenously—derived procoagulant molecules (e.g. bacterial lipopolysaccharide, protein produced by neoplastic cells or snake venom.

As the coagulation process continues
↓
Excessive consumption of coagulation factors and platelets
↓
Intravascular bleeding commensurate with the degree of consumption of coagulation factors

If activation of coagulation is chronic and of low grade, clotting factors and platelets may be replenished sufficiently so as to avoid bleeding. So in this case, hypercoagulability predominates—resulting thrombosis.

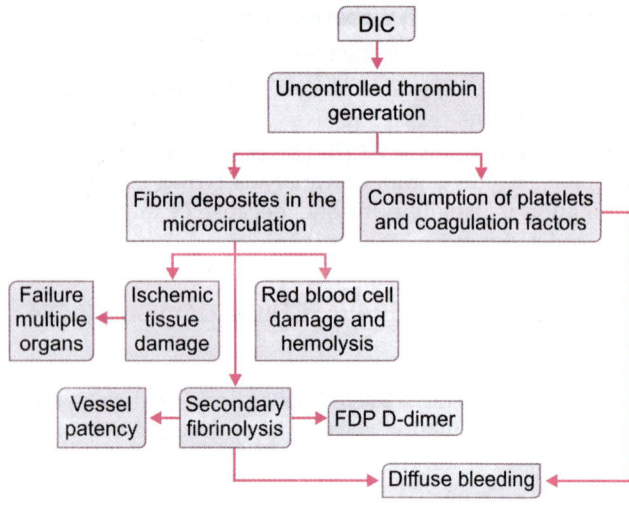

Fig. 5.118: Pathophysiology of DIC

3. Acral cyanosis, petechial, echymotic lesions may occur.
4. Widespread DIC may be associated with—truncal and extremity bruising (**purpura fulminans**) (Fig. 5.119).
5. Patient occasionally asymptomatic—laboratory investigation may clinch the diagnosis.
6. **Severe systemic DIC**—may produce multiorgan dysfunction syndrome—involving hepatic, neurologic, renal or cardiac systems.

Laboratory Parameters (Fig. 5.120)

1. Increased PT, APTT, TT—because of consumption of clothing factors
2. Decreased fibrinogen—because of consumption

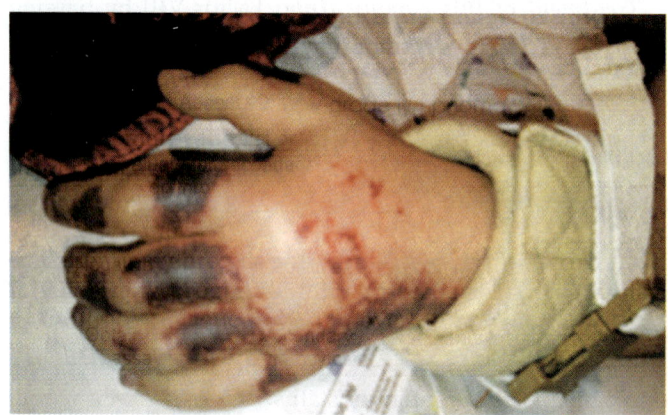

Fig. 5.119: DIC feature

Clinical Presentation (Fig. 120)

1. Appearance of DIC always indicates serious underlying disorders.
2. **Patient may present with**—bleeding from any site and in any system, e.g.
   i. Vascular access catheter
   ii. Urinary catheters
   iii. Pulmonary
   iv. Central nervous system
   v. Cutaneous

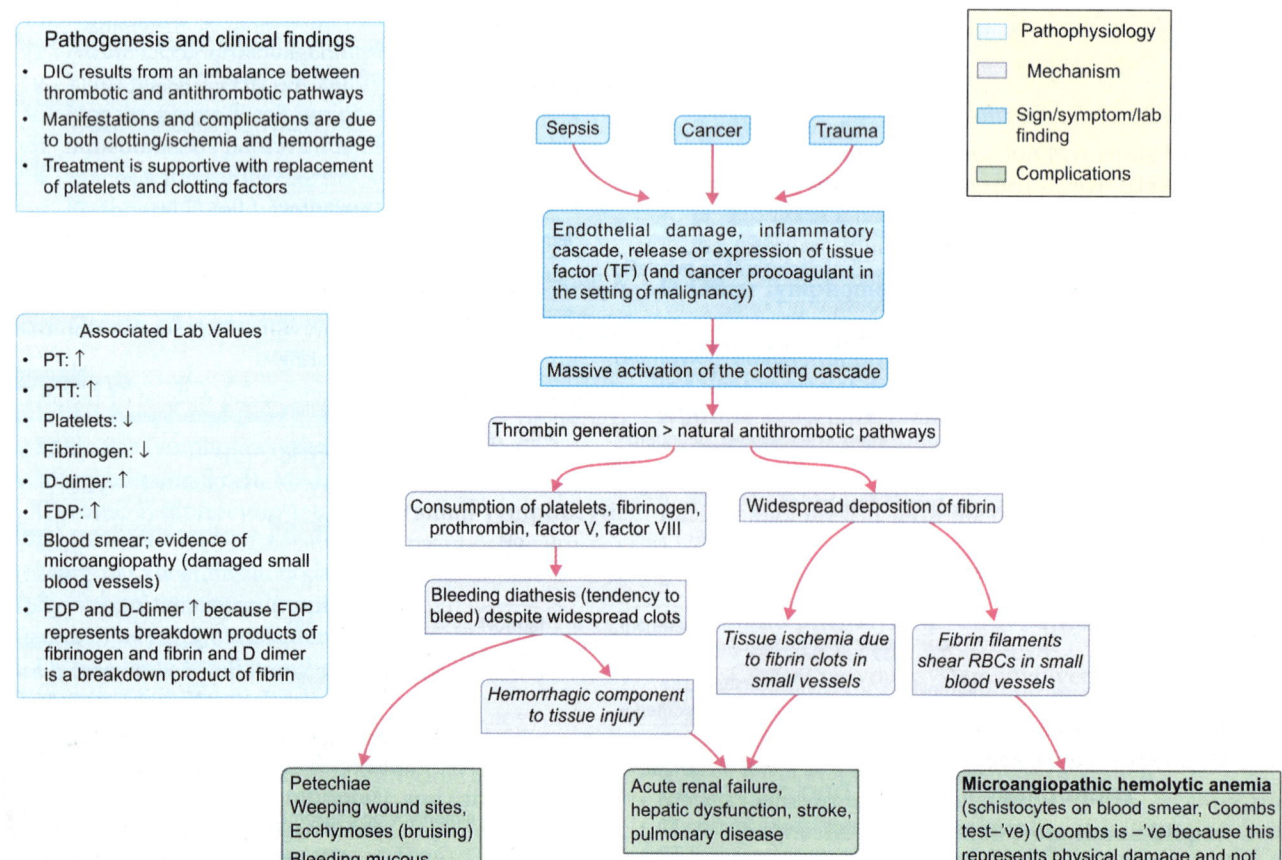

Fig. 5.120: Pathophysiology with clinical manifestation and laboratory parameters

3. Increased fibrinogen degradation product (FDP)—D-dimer assay measures FDP.
4. Decreased platelet count—because of clearance resulting from activation and agglutination at the site of reaction.
5. Fragmented red blood cells (schistocytes) on peripheral blood smear.

Treatment

I. Treatment of cause:
   i. Administration of antibiotic for treatment of sepsis.
   ii. Treatment of malignancy.
   iii. Surgery to repair aneurismal dilatation.
   iv. Removal of conceptus and placenta.
   v. Treatment of multiorgan dysfunction syndrome in intensive care unit.

II. Blood product should not be administered on patient with DIC unless:
   i. Clinically significant bleeding
   ii. Risk of bleeding is very high:
      a. *If bleeding is present:* Platelet transfusion to maintain count, 20000–30000/μl, or >50000/μl (intracranial or life-threatening hemorrhage)
      b. *Cryoprecipitate*—if bleeding is associated with consistently low (80–100 mg/dl).
      c. *Fresh frozen plasma* to be given in patient with prolonged PT or APTT.
      d. *Heparin* should be considered in acute DIC, where bleeding continues in spite of appropriate treatment

   Caution:
      i. No central nervous system bleeding
      ii. No gastrointestinal bleeding
      iii. Platelet count <50000/μl

Dose: Low dose infusion 6–10 mU/kg/hr, no bolus dose is recommended.

Indication of improvement:
   i. Improvement of platelet count
   ii. Improvement on fibrinogen concentration

Contraindication:
   i. Placental abruption
   ii. Other obstatric conditions requiring surgery

Every 6 hours PT, APTT, fibrinogen level, platelet count should be monitored.

HELLP syndrome:
- Hemolysis
- Elevated liver enzyme
- Low platelet—affects women in peripartum period.

Feature:
   i. Severe form of DIC
   ii. Hemolytic anemia
   iii. Hepatocellular injury

It can be differentiated from TTP: Presence of hepatic dysfunction—suggest HELLP.

ESSENTIAL THROMBOCYTOSIS

Essential thrombocytosis—it is also called hemorrhagic thrombocythemia.

Epidemiology

1. According to age—there are two peaks:
   i. One at 30 years—more common in women
   ii. Second peak at 50–60 years—no gender predilection
2. Median survival—10 years.

Pathophysiology

1. **X-chromosome inactivation** study suggests polyclonal disorder.
2. **JAK2-V617F found in 30–50% patient with ET**—this mutation is associated with elevated hemoglobin and neutrophil count, lower EPO levels, venous thrombosis increased progression to polycythemia.
3. **In case of familial case**—disorder is due to mutation of thrombopoietin gene.

Clinical Features (Fig. 5.121)

1. **50% patients are asymptomatic**—they can be diagnosed on routine blood count.
2. **Vasomotor symptoms (in 40% patient):** Headache, light headedness, syncope, atypical chest pain, visual upset, livedo reticularis, erythromyalgia (erythema and burning discomfort in hands and feet due to occlusion in digital microcirculation)
3. **Hemorrhagic symptoms (in 25% of patient):** Easy bruising, mucosal gastrointestinal bleeding, unexplained and prolonged bleeding after trauma or surgery
4. **Thrombosis (in 20% of patients):** Arterial thrombosis is more common than venous thrombosis.
   Organ involved—brain, lung, heart.
5. **Splenomegaly** in <40 marked than other myeloproliferative disorders
6. **Splenic atrophy** due to repeated microvascular infarction.
7. **Recurrent abortion or fetal growth retardation** due to multiple placental infarctions.

Investigation

1. **Full blood count** (Fig. 5.122)
   i. Platelet count > 450×10^9/L. It cannot differentiate ET from RT
   ii. ↓ Hb%, ↓ MCV—due to chronic blood loss
   iii. Mean platelet volume—normal. But platelet distribution width is increased.
2. **Blood film** (Fig. 5.122)
   i. *Platelet thrombocytosis*—platelet anisocytosis, giant platelet, platelet clumps, and megakaryocytes, fragments basophil.
   ii. *Hypochromic, microcytic RBC*—in case of iron deficiency.
   iii. *Howell-Jolly bodies*
3. **Peripheral blood mutation screening for JAK2-V617F mutation** (Fig. 5.123)—excludes reactive thrombocytosis, but absence does not exclude essential thrombocytosis.
4. **Bone marrow:** It is helpful:
   i. Differentiate ET from RT in JAK2—V617F –ve patient
   ii. Differentiate ET from other MPNs (myelodysplastic syndrome, prefibrotic stage of primary myelofibrosis.

Aspiration shows:
   i. Increased platelet dumps
   ii. Large megakaryocytic with hypermature appearance
   iii. Increased nuclear lobulation and large cytoplasm
   iv. Erythroid hyperplasia

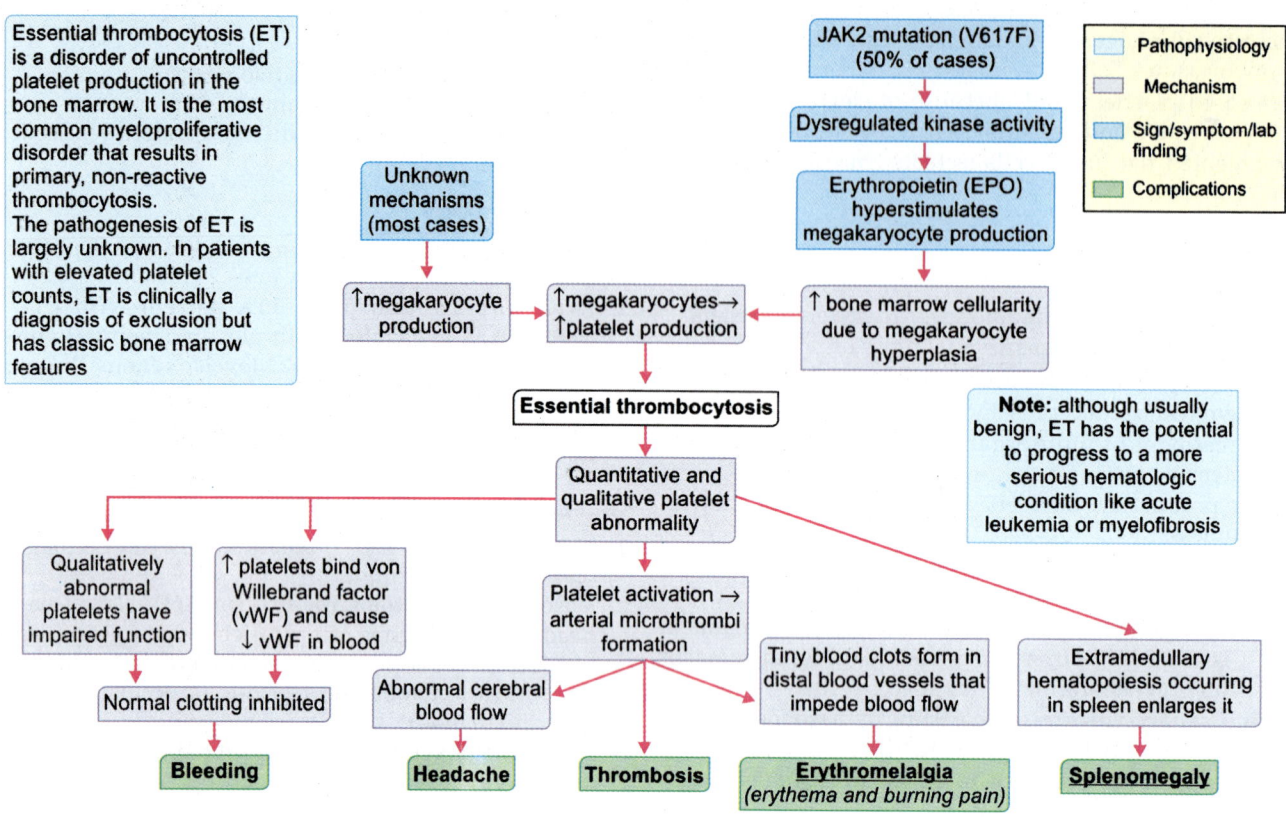

Essential thrombocytosis (ET) is a disorder of uncontrolled platelet production in the bone marrow. It is the most common myeloproliferative disorder that results in primary, non-reactive thrombocytosis.
The pathogenesis of ET is largely unknown. In patients with elevated platelet counts, ET is clinically a diagnosis of exclusion but has classic bone marrow features

JAK2 mutation (V617F) (50% of cases)

Dysregulated kinase activity

Erythropoietin (EPO) hyperstimulates megakaryocyte production

Pathophysiology

Mechanism

Sign/symptom/lab finding

Complications

Unknown mechanisms (most cases)

↑megakaryocyte production

↑megakaryocytes→ ↑platelet production

↑ bone marrow cellularity due to megakaryocyte hyperplasia

Essential thrombocytosis

Quantitative and qualitative platelet abnormality

Note: although usually benign, ET has the potential to progress to a more serious hematologic condition like acute leukemia or myelofibrosis

Qualitatively abnormal platelets have impaired function

↑ platelets bind von Willebrand factor (vWF) and cause ↓ vWF in blood

Platelet activation → arterial microthrombi formation

Tiny blood clots form in distal blood vessels that impede blood flow

Extramedullary hematopoiesis occurring in spleen enlarges it

Normal clotting inhibited

Abnormal cerebral blood flow

Bleeding

Headache

Thrombosis

Erythromelalgia *(erythema and burning pain)*

Splenomegaly

Fig. 5.121: Essential thrombocytosis: Pathogenesis and clinical findings

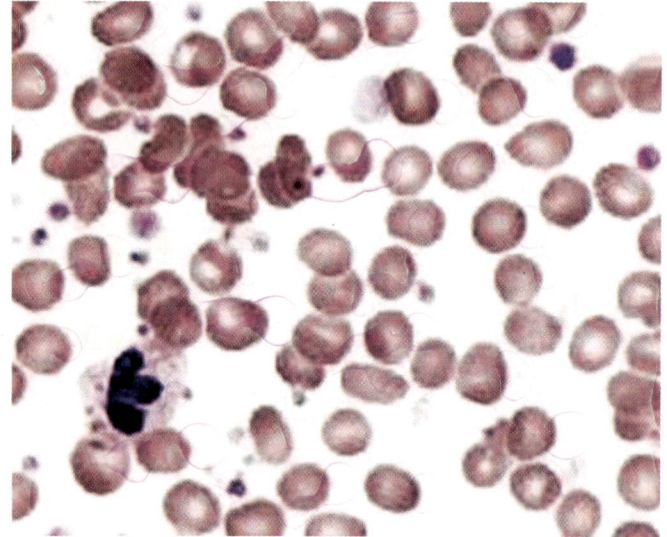

Fig. 5.122: Peripheral blood picture in essential thrombocytosis

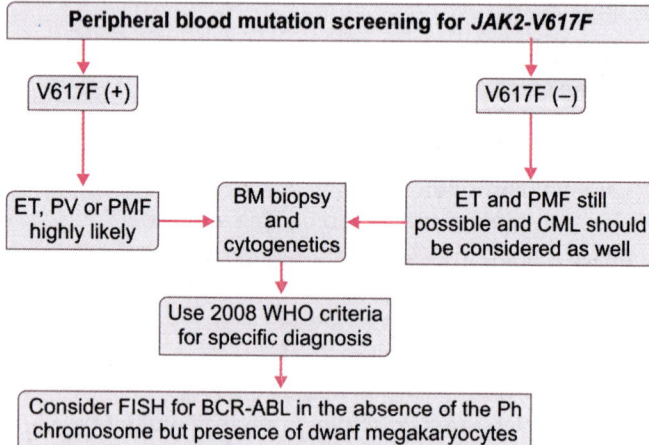

Peripheral blood mutation screening for *JAK2-V617F*

V617F (+)

V617F (−)

ET, PV or PMF highly likely

BM biopsy and cytogenetics

ET and PMF still possible and CML should be considered as well

Use 2008 WHO criteria for specific diagnosis

Consider FISH for BCR-ABL in the absence of the Ph chromosome but presence of dwarf megakaryocytes

Fig. 5.123: Screening for JAK2-V617F

Trephine biopsy shows:
  i. Increased megakaryocytic dispersed throughout marrow.
 ii. Large hypermature with deeply lobulated and hyper-lobulated nuclei
iii. Bizarre atypical forms seen in PMF
 iv. Normal or minimal reticulin, no fibrosis, no dysplastic features

WHO Diagnostic Criteria for ET

Meeting of all major criteria:

1. Persistent elevation of plated count $\geq 450 \times 10^9/L$
2. Megakaryocyte proliferation with large and mature morphology, no or little granulocyte or erythroid proliferation.

3. Not meeting WHO criteria for CML, PV, PMF, MDS or other myeloid neoplasm.
4. Demonstration of JAK2-V617F or other clonal marker or in absence of clonal marker, no evidence of thrombocytosis.

Risk Stratification in ET

A. Low risk:
1. Age <60 years
2. No history of thrombocytosis
3. Platelet count <1500 × 10⁹/L
4. No cardiovascular risk factor (smoking, obesity, hypertension, hyperlipedemia, diabetes mellitus)

B. Intermediate risk: Neither low nor high risk

C. High risk:
1. Age >60 years
2. Previous history of thrombosis.

Management

Aims

1. To alleviate the symptoms of microvascular disturbance
2. To decrease the risk and incidence of thrombotic and hemorrhagic complications.
3. To normalize the platelet count <400 × 10⁹/L

   Non-pharmacological therapy: Lifestyle changes (smoking, obesity and exercise)—to reduce risk of thrombosis and atherosclerosis.

Low-risk patients:
1. Observation with platelet want at regular interval
2. No added risk with pregnancy or surgery
3. Aspirin—75 mg/day—if no contraindication
4. In erythromyalgia—aspirin—loading dose 300–500 mg/day followed by 75 mg/day as maintenance.

Intermediate risk:
1. Aspirin therapy, if there is no contraindication
2. Lifestyle changes
3. Cytoprotective therapy—in patient with marked thrombocytosis
   (>1500 × 10⁹/L) or with risk of hemorrhage
   Interferon α or anagrelide therapy

   Aim is to reduce the platelet count to <400 × 10⁹/L

High-risk patient:
1. *Aspirin* is recommended:
   i. In patient with previous thrombotic event or high risk of thrombosis.
   ii. In patient with erythromyalgia.
      Its use is safest when platelet count <1000 × 10⁹/L
   It is contraindicated in:
   i. Marked thrombocytosis (>1500 × 10⁹/L) with hemorrhagic complications.
   ii. History of peptic ulcerations
      Alternate to aspirin is dipyridamole
2. *Hydroxycarbamide*
   Indication:
   i. Age >60 years, marked thrombocytosis >1500 × 10⁹/L
   ii. Age <60 years, but intolerant to anagrelide or interferon-α
   iii. Some patients require it with interferon-α and anagrelide
   Dose: High initial dose followed by maintenance dose to maintain platelet count <400 × 10⁹/L

Side effect:
i. Myelosuppression
ii. Oral ulceration
iii. Rash
iv. Risk of leukemia increased
Contraindicated:
i. In pregnancy
ii. Breastfeeding

3. **Interferon α:**
   Indication:
   i. Age >60 years, intolerant to HC
   ii. Age <60 years, intolerant to anagrelide
   iii. It is not leukemogenic

   Dose: To start with 3 million units thrice weekly SC followed by maintenance dose 1.5 million units × thrice weekly.
   It decrease platelet count <400 × 10⁹/L
   Reduction in size of splenomegaly
   Peg-interferon is more convenient as it is usually given once weekly.

4. **Anagrelide**
   Indication:
   i. It is preferred in younger patient <60 years.
   ii. It is preferred in patient with child-bearing potential.
   Dose: 500 µg—twice daily with increase in dose weekly 500 µg/day—to reach its therapeutic dose 2–3 mg/day. Therapeutic effects start from 14–21 days.

   Complications:
   i. Headache
   ii. Palpitation
   iii. Fluid retention
   iv. Diarrhea

5. *Busulfan:*
   i. It produces prolonged decrease in platelet count
   ii. Increased risk of AML
   iii. It is used in patient >75 years of age
   Dose: 4–6 mg/day for 2–6 weeks until response can be repeated after 2–3 months, if required.

6. **Radioactive phosphorus**

FLOWCHART IN HEMATOLOGY

Sickle cell anemia

Glutamic acid ⟶ Valine
HbA   [HbS]
↓
Passage through microcirculation in spleen
↓
Low oxygen tension
↓
Reversible sickling occurs → Membrane changes
                            increase adhesiveness
↓   ↓
Cells pass through   Vaso-occlusion in cells
microcirculation   with sluggish flow
with good oxygen
tension
↓   ↓
Desickling   Vaso-occlusion crisis
                            in microcirculation of hand
↓   feet, spleen, head of femur
Various sickling and   renal papillae
desickling
↓   ↓

(Contd.)

(Contd.)

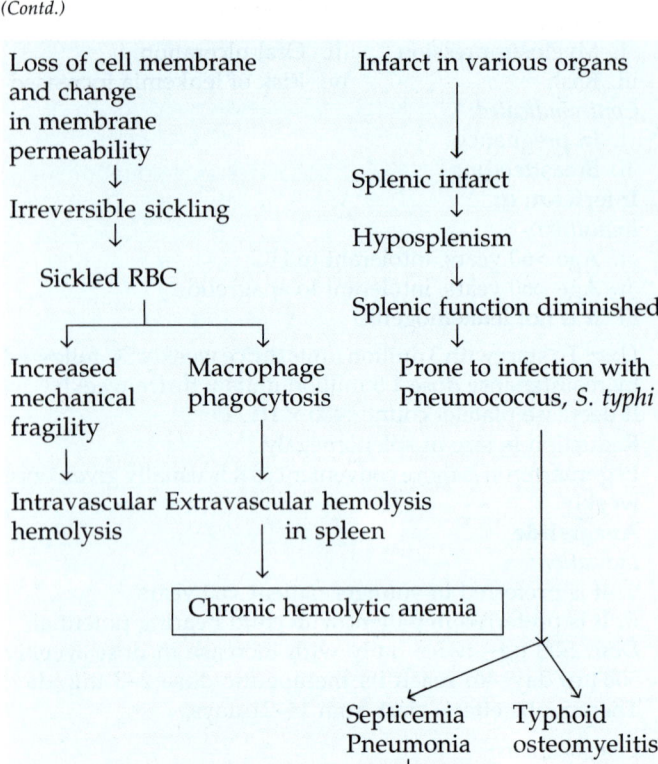

Loss of cell membrane
and change
in membrane
permeability
↓
Irreversible sickling
↓
Sickled RBC
┌────────┴────────┐
Increased   Macrophage
mechanical   phagocytosis
fragility
↓   ↓
Intravascular   Extravascular hemolysis
hemolysis   in spleen

Infarct in various organs
↓
Splenic infarct
↓
Hyposplenism
↓
Splenic function diminished
↓
Prone to infection with
Pneumococcus, *S. typhi*

Chronic hemolytic anemia

Septicemia   Typhoid
Pneumonia   osteomyelitis
↓
Death

Myelofibrosis

Early in the course of disease there is hyperplasia of all
three major cellular elements
↓
Erythroid and granulocytic precursors are normal but
megakaryocytes are large and dysplastic
↓
Abnormal megakaryocytes synthesize platelet desired
growth factor
(PGDF and TGF-β)
↓
Cytopenia ← produce extensive fibrosis of bone marrow
↓
As marrow fibrosis progresses, circulating
hematopoietic stem cells take up residence in secondary
hematopoietic organs such as spleen, liver and lymph
nodes
↓
Blood cell production from extramedullary sites is also
defective.

Following are some algorithm required for diagnosis (Figs 5.124 to 5.127):

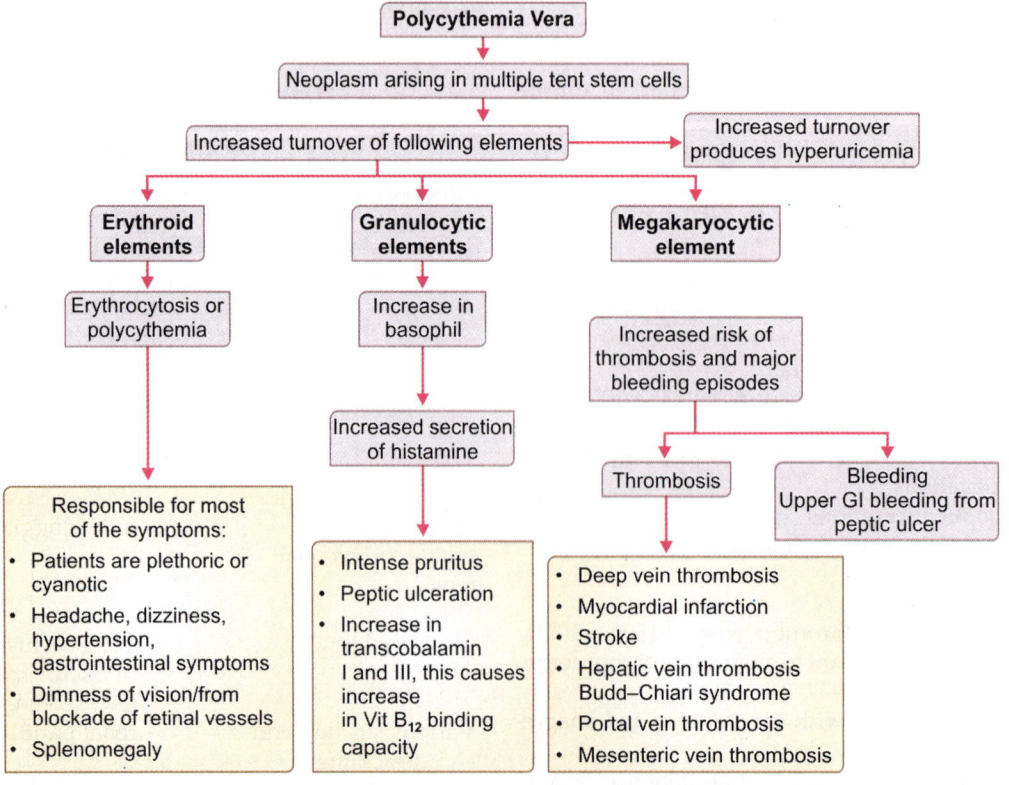

Fig. 5.124: Algorithm of clinical picture of PV

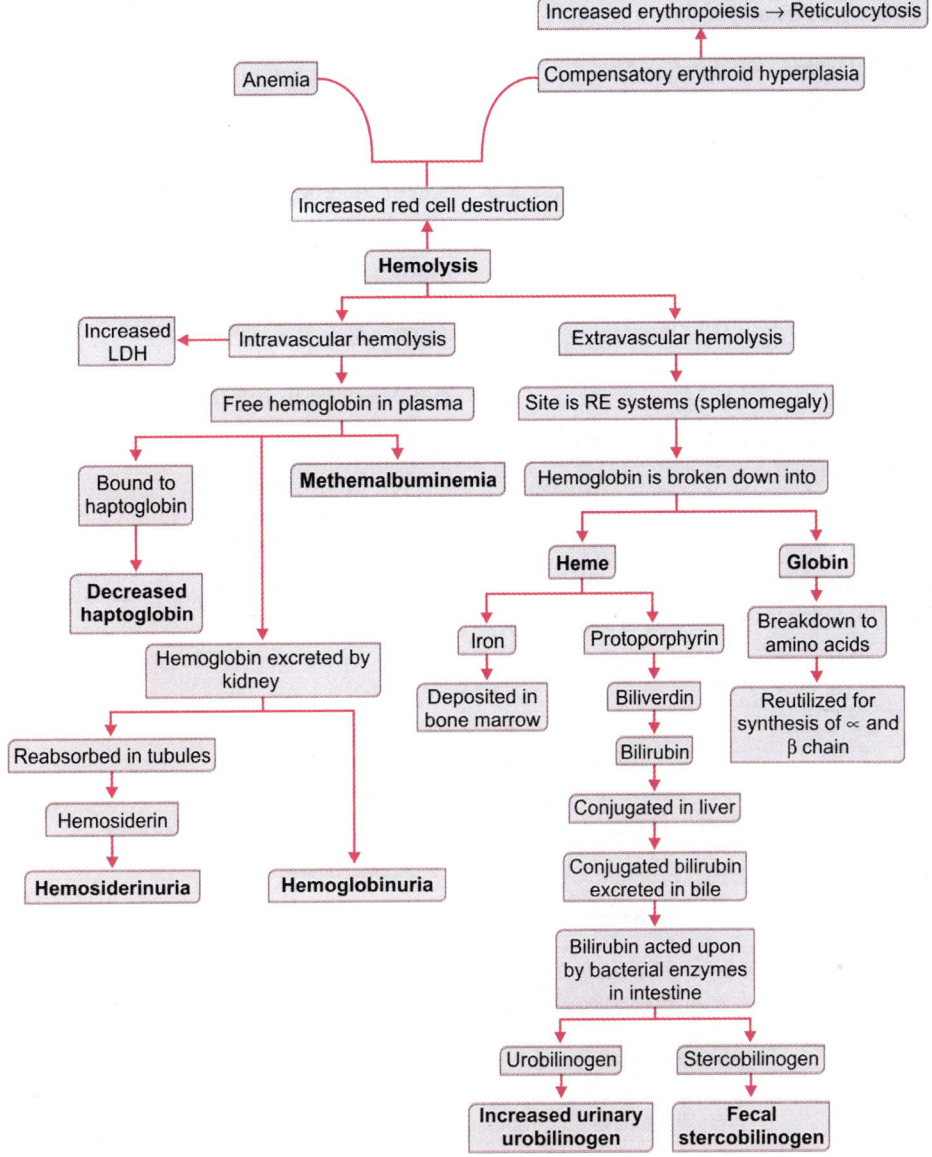

Fig. 5.125: Algorithm of diagnosis of hemolytic anemia

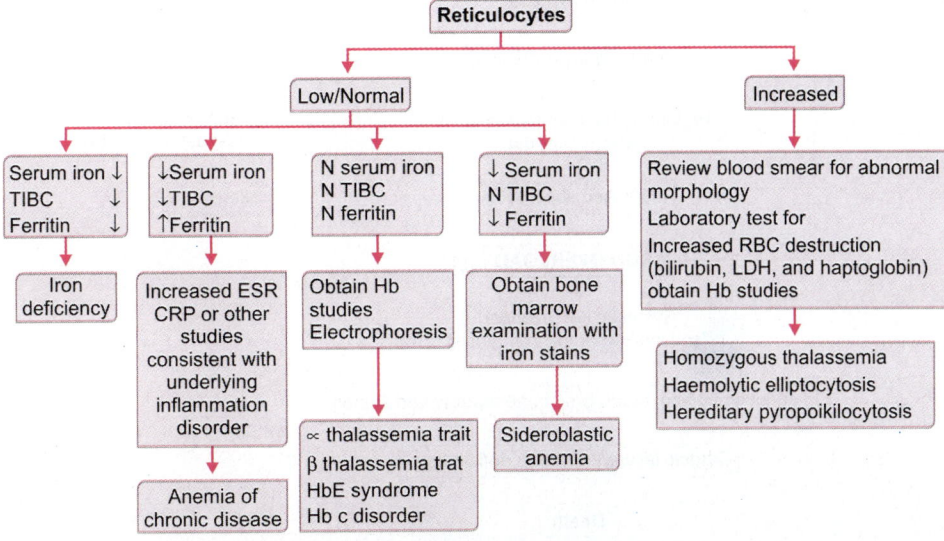

Fig. 5.126: Algorithm of diagnosis on the basis of reticulocytes

Hereditory Spherocytosis (Contd.)

Ankyrin, spectrin deficiency
↓
Reduced membrane stability
↓
Spontaneous loss of red cell membrane
↓
To compensate the loss of surface areas, RBC be come spherical
↓
Cells become microspherocytes
↓
Spherocytosis → Reduced deformability
→ Reduced membrane plasticity
↓
Difficulty in passing through the interendothelial fenestrations of the venous sinusoids of spleen
↓ ↓

Slow passage of spherocytes
↓
Lactic acid accumulates around cells
↓
Inhibition of glycolysis
↓
ATP generation falls
↓
Failure of sodium pump
↓
Accumulation of water in red blood cells
↓
Abnormal red blood cells
↓
Phagocytosed by RE cells lining the sinusoid

Phagocytosis by RE cells → splenomegaly. Lining the sinusoid of the spleen
↓
Extravascular hemolysis → Anemia reticulocytosis

(Contd.)

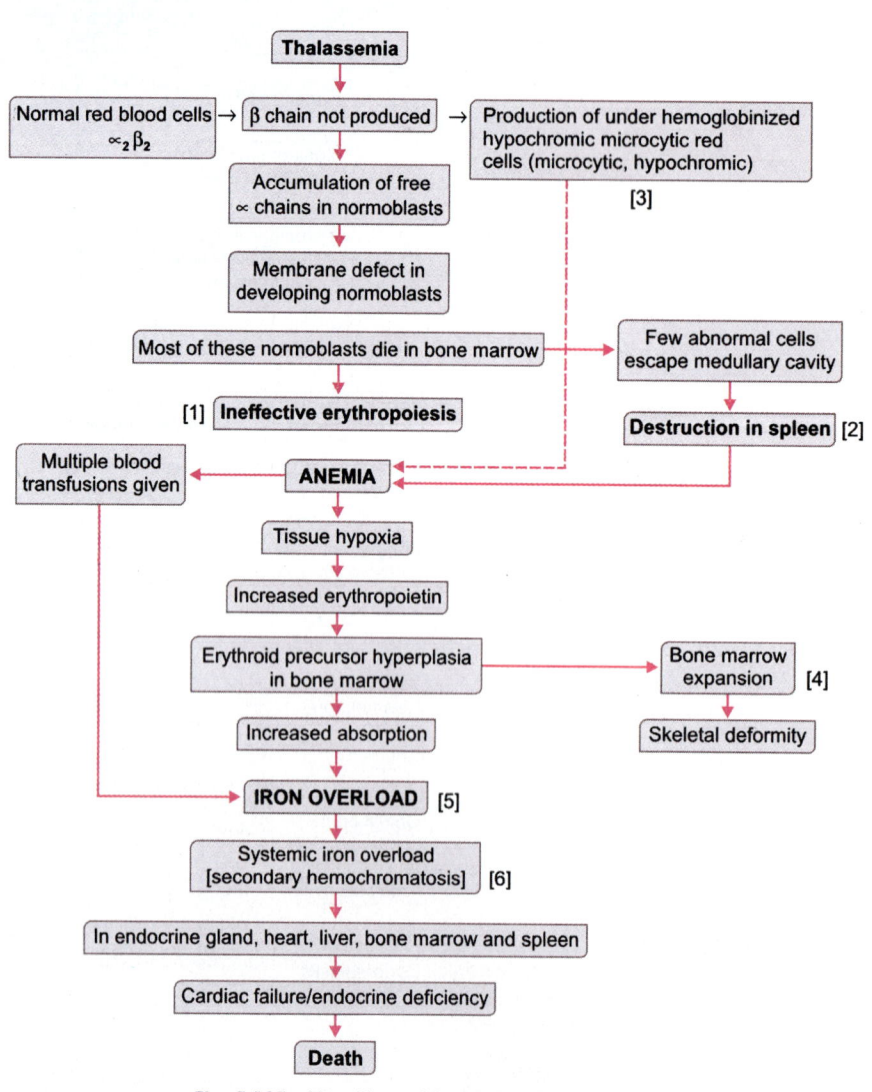

Fig. 5.127: Algorithm of features of thalassemia

PLATELETS

Following laboratory tests should be performed to assess platelet function:

I. Platelet count:
   i. Normal range—150–450 × 10⁹/L
   ii. Adequate function is maintained until platelet count <80 × 10⁹/L
   iii. If platelet count <20 × 10⁹/L—easy bruising, petechial hemorrhage or more serious bleeding.

   Degree of bleeding depends upon causes of thrombocytopenia:
   a. In case of marrow failure syndrome—severe bleeding
   b. In case of peripheral destruction of platelet or immune thrombocytopenia—less bleeding.

II. Platelet size: Larger platelets are biologically more active, high mean platelet volume (MPV>10 fl)—less severe bleeding in patient with severe thrombocytopenia.
The congenital disorders associated with alteration in platelet size:
1. High MPV >10 fl—May-Hegglin anomaly, gray platelet syndrome
2. Low MPV <7 fl—Wiskott-Aldrich syndrome

III. Platelet morphology: Pseudothrombocytopenia—may be due to in vitro platelet dumping—these clumps may be visible in blood film.
Abnormal platelet size and white cells may contain inclusions—in **May-Hegglin anomaly.**

IV. Platelet function at high shear rate (PFA-100): Automated technique that measures the ability of platelets to occlude an aperture at high shear rate.
Test performed on citrated blood sample with 48 hours of sample collection.
This test is abnormal in:
   i. von Willebrand disease
   ii. Platelet function defect

V. Platelet function at low shear rate (platelet aggregation): Platelet rich plasma prepared by slow centrifugation of citrated blood sample.
   i. Agonists used for aggregation studies—ADP, collagen, arachidonic acid, adrenaline.
   ii. Response to restocetin—is an agglutination response, it depends on conformational changes in platelet membrane protein and promoting interaction with VWF.
   iii. Restocetin-induced platelet aggregation—at low restocetin concentration, is abnormal—observed
   In type 2B VWD and with very high VWF level in pregnancy.

Platelet Biology

Megakaryocytic, multinucleated hemopoietic cells in bone marrow
↓
Release platelet into circulation

Thrombopoietin is necessary for platelet function and release. Platelets are removed from circulation by
   i. When activated and utilized at the sites of vascular injury
   ii. When they become senescent.

THROMBOCYTOPENIA

   i. Normal count 150000–3,50,000/μl
   ii. 80000–100000/μL—is adequate for hemostasis
   iii. 20,000–30,000/μL without bleeding—do not require immediate treatment to increase platelet count
   iv. Spontaneous bleeding with count 10000–20000/μl—require platelet transfusion

Causes of Thrombocytopenia

Decreased Production of Platelets

I. Bone marrow failure syndrome
   1. *Congenital:*
      a. Amegakaryocytic thrombocytopenia—isolated
      b. Thrombocytopenia—absent radius thrombocytopenia
      c. Fanconi's anemia—depression of all blood cell lineages
      d. Dyskeratosis congenita.
      e. Shwachman-Diamond syndrome
      f. Wiskott-Aldrich syndrome

      X-linked recessive disorder is characterized by thrombocytopenia, eczema and immunodeficiency. Thrombocytopenia is due to decreased megakaryocytosis and increased destruction of abnormal platelets. Treatment—1. Splenectomy, 2. Allogenic hemopoietic stem cell transplantation.

   2. *Acquired:*
      a. Aplastic anemia
      b. Amegakaryocytic thrombocytopenia.

II. Myelodysplasia
III. Marrow infiltration (neoplastic, infection)
IV. Chemotherapy induced
V. Irradiation induced
VI. Cyclic thrombocytopenia
VII. Folate and vitamin B₁₂ deficiency
VIII. Ethanol

Disorders due to Increased Clearance of Platelets

   i. Immunothrombocytopenic purpura
   ii. Heparin-induced thrombocytopenia
   iii. Thrombotic thrombocytopenia purpura
   iv. Hemolytic uremic syndrome
   v. Disseminated intravascular coagulation
   vi. Post-transfusion purpura
   vii. von Willebrand disease type IIB
   viii. Antiphospholipid antibody syndrome
   ix. Mechanical destruction (aortic valvular dysfunction)

Disorders due to Increased Sequestration of Platelets

   i. Hypersplenism
   ii. Drug induced
   iii. Gestational thrombocytopenia
   iv. HIV associated thrombocytopenia
   v. Sepsis
   vi. Qualitative platelet disorder (Bernard-Soulier disease, Grey platelet syndrome, May-Hegglin anomaly).

Cyclic Thrombocytopenia

1. Cyclic episodes of thrombocytopenia every 3–6 weeks
2. Thrombocytopenia is frequently severe, associated with severe bleeding

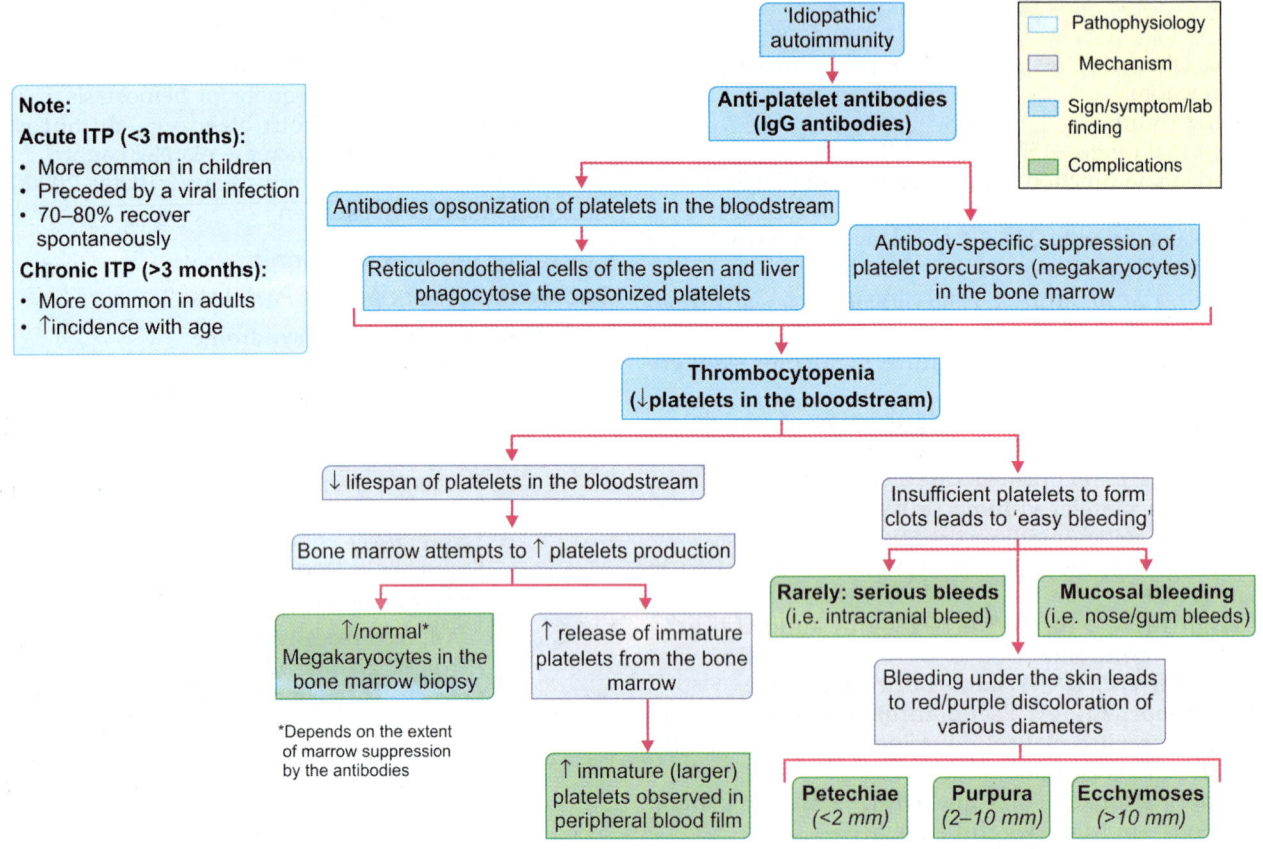

Note:

Acute ITP (<3 months):
- More common in children
- Preceded by a viral infection
- 70–80% recover spontaneously

Chronic ITP (>3 months):
- More common in adults
- ↑incidence with age

Legend:
- Pathophysiology
- Mechanism
- Sign/symptom/lab finding
- Complications

'Idiopathic' autoimmunity

Anti-platelet antibodies (IgG antibodies)

Antibodies opsonization of platelets in the bloodstream

Reticuloendothelial cells of the spleen and liver phagocytose the opsonized platelets

Antibody-specific suppression of platelet precursors (megakaryocytes) in the bone marrow

Thrombocytopenia (↓platelets in the bloodstream)

↓ lifespan of platelets in the bloodstream

Bone marrow attempts to ↑ platelets production

↑/normal* Megakaryocytes in the bone marrow biopsy

*Depends on the extent of marrow suppression by the antibodies

↑ release of immature platelets from the bone marrow

↑ immature (larger) platelets observed in peripheral blood film

Insufficient platelets to form clots leads to 'easy bleeding'

Rarely: serious bleeds (i.e. intracranial bleed)

Mucosal bleeding (i.e. nose/gum bleeds)

Bleeding under the skin leads to red/purple discoloration of various diameters

Petechiae *(<2 mm)*   **Purpura** *(2–10 mm)*   **Ecchymoses** *(>10 mm)*

Fig. 5.128: Clinicopathogenesis in ITP

3. **Treatment:**
   - Oral contraceptives (female patient)
   - Androgens, immunosuppressive agents (azathioprine)
   - Thrombopoietic growth factor—may produce response in some cases.

Immune Thrombocytopenic Purpura

Definition: It is an autoimmune disorder characterized by increased isolated destruction producing thrombocytopenia due to production of antiplatelet antibodies.

Epidemiology: (Fig. 5.128)
   i. Annual incidence—2 cases/100000 population
   ii. Its incidence increases with age.

Pathophysiology:

Antibodies directed against platelet glycoprotein Complexes IIb/IIIa and/or Ib/IX

↓

Antibody-coated platelets are destroyed by reticuloendothelial macrophages in liver and spleen

↓

Reduced lifespan of platelets (2 to 7 days)

ITP in adult is due to:
   i. *Idiopathic*—and becomes chronic
   ii. *Lymphoproliferative disorder* (lymphoma, CLL)
   iii. *Immune dysregulation*—(SLE, HIV)

ITP in children:
Viral infection—resolves spontaneously without specific therapy

Presentation:
1. Petechial bruising (Fig. 5.129)
2. Bleeding from mucous membrane: Conjunctival hemorrhages (Fig. 5.130), gingival bleeding, epistaxis—in severe cases
3. Milder cases (>50000/μl)—patient is asymptomatic.

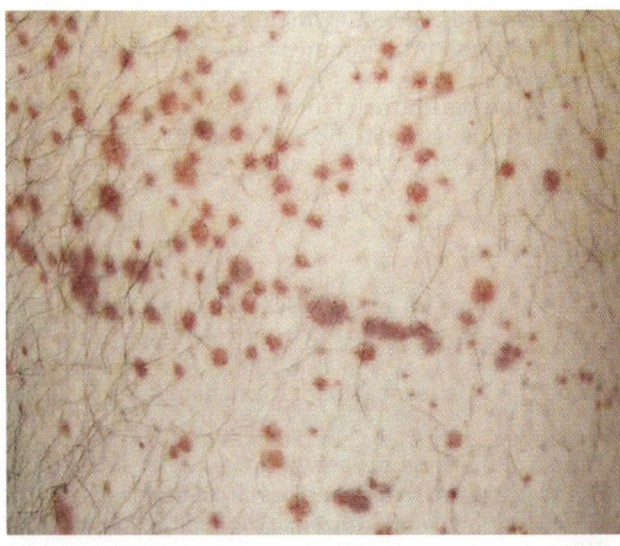

Fig. 5.129: Purpura

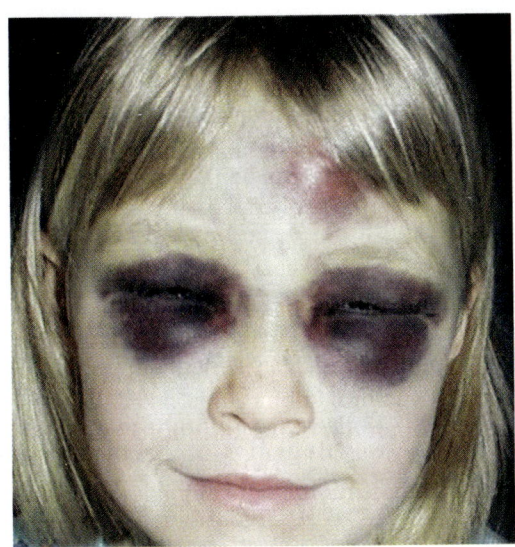

Fig. 5.130: Conjunctival hemorrhage

Diagnosis

1. **New onset isolated thrombocytopenia—without any apparent cause (including drug) in an asymptomatic adult**—should be regarded as patient of ITP until proved otherwise.
2. The presence of other cytopenias: Age >60 years, or failure of primary therapy (corticosteroid trial for one week)—**should prompt for bone marrow examination before commencement of therapy**.
3. Patient should be screened for hepatitis B, C and HIV infection

Treatment (Fig. 5.131)

Prednisolone 1 mg/kg/day × 7–10 days.

+

Pulse methylprednisolone (dexamethasone) 40 mg daily × 4 days

↓

If there is response (increase in platelet count in 3–7 days)

↓

Prednisolone rapidly tapered until dose 20 mg/day

↓

Then the tapering process progresses more slowly (by dose decrement 5 mg per stage at every 2–3 weeks

In patients with severe bleeding and/or severe thrombocytopenia (<5000–1000/µl)

Intravenous immunoglobulin 1 gm/kg/day for 2 days or Anti-D 75 mg/kg/dose in Rh+ve patient

Response is generally seen within 3–5 days of IVIG or anti-D administration.

Chronic Treatment

Despite initial response (60 to 75%)—majority of patients relapse—or patient may become refractory to above agents.

Treatment is appropriate for patients with platelet counts <30000/µL or clinically severe bleeding.

a. **Intravenous immunoglobulin or anti-D (in Rh+ve patient only):** There will be rapid rise in platelet count within a few days, but the effect is transient, so the agents must be re-administered every 2–3 weeks.

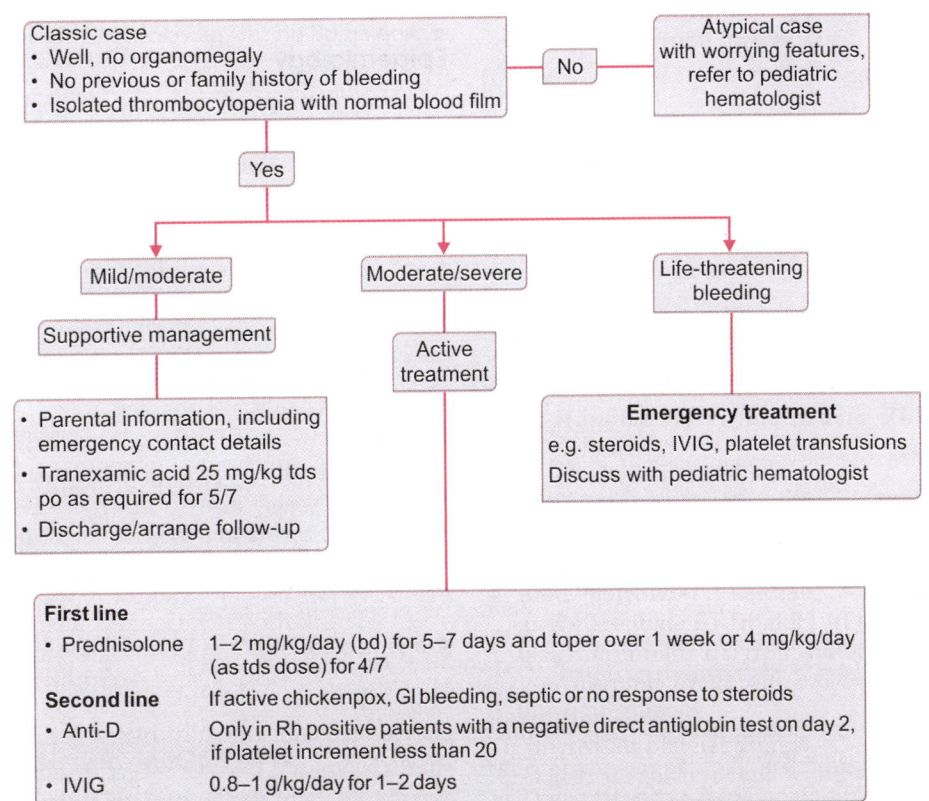

Fig. 5.131: Algorithm of treatment of ITP

Indications:
  i. Intermittent elevation of the platelet count for surgical procedure
  ii. Other periods of increased bleeding risk.
b. **Monoclonal anti-B cell antibody rituximab (anti-CD 20 antibody):** 375 mg/m^2—weekly for 4 weeks in adult with severe chronic ITP.
c. **In case of steroid and/or splenectomy refractory ITP—drugs include:**
  i. High dose pulse dexamethasone
  ii. Single agent vincristine
  iii. Cyclosporine
  iv. Danazol
  v. Mycophenolate mofetil
  vi. Dapsone
  vii. Azathioprine
  viii. Vitamin C
  ix. Plasma exchange
  x. Immunoadsorption over staphylococcal protein A column

  Combination chemotherapy with autologous stem cell transplantation—results in complete remission.
d. **Splenectomy:**

Indications:
- Severe thrombocytopenia
- Failed to respond to 2nd or 3rd line of treatments
- Complicated by severe bleeding

Response rate:
a. 65 to 75% immediate b. 60 to 70% long-term response

  All patients must receive immunization against encapsulated bacterial organisms several weeks prior to splenectomy:
a. *Pneumococcus*   b. *Haemophilus influenzae*
c. *Meningococcus*

Recent Treatment of ITP

TPO-RA: It is thrombopoietin receptor agonist which is responsible for increased platelet production as opposed to the conventional regimen responsible for decreased platelet destruction. It is highly effective in case of refractory ITP with response rate of 95%. They are considered for lifelong treatment of ITP. The drugs are:
a. Eltrombopag—it is orally administered small molecule.
b. Romiplostim—it is subcutaneously administered peptide antibody fusion protein called peptibody.

Risk associated with this drug:
a. Rebound thrombocytopenia—after discontinuation of this drug there may be endogenous depression of the platelet production by already elevated level of platelets. As a result, rebound thrombocytopenia will occur.
b. Abnormalities in liver function test
c. Bone marrow fibrosis, but this condition is reversible because after discontinuation of this drug fibrosis will reverse.
d. Thromboembolic events
e. Cataract
f. Development of anti-TPO antibodies.

  Combination of this drug along with immunosuppressive drugs will address both the pathologic mechanisms and efficacy of the treatment will be enhanced.

  Table 5.5 demonstrated staging and management of ITP.

THROMBOTIC THROMBOCYTOPENIC PURPURA/HUS

Definition

This disorder is characterized by:
  i. Microangiopathic hemolytic anemia, and
  ii. Platelet rich thrombi in the arterial and capillary microvasculature producing thrombocytopenia

Epidemiology

  i. Female preponderance
  ii. HUS occurs in children
  iii. HUS is related to infection with enteropathogenic bacteria

Table 5.5: ITP: Staging and management

Stages	Skin/mucosa	Bleedings	Platelet (× 10⁹/L)	Management
1. Minor/mild, normal lifestyle	Few petechiae and small bruises	• Occasional epistaxis (nose bleeds), stopped by applied pressure • Buccal blood blisters • No other bleeding	>10–150	Consent for observation
2. Moderate, troublesome lifestyle	Numerous new petechiae and large bruises (> 5 cm diameter)	• Intermittent epistaxis longer than 15 min despite applied pressure • Intermittent bleeding from gums, lips, buccal, oropharynx, or gastrointestinal • Hypermenorrhagia, hematemesis, hematuria, melena	>10–20	Punctual intervention to reach stage 1
3. Severe, life-threatering	Extensive petechiae and large bruises	• Continuous bleeding form gums, buccal, oropharynx • Suspected internal hemorrhagia (brain, lung, muscle, joint, others)	<10–20	Intervention

Pathophysiology

Toxins, cytokines, drugs, deficiencies in the function of von Willebrand factor cleaving protease
↓
Directly or indirectly cause platelet aggregation and on endothelial cell damage
↓
Formation of microvascular thrombi
↓
Ischemia of involved organs
Red cells try to negotiate through the thrombotic obstruction and fibrin strands in the microvasculature
↓
Microangiopathic hemolytic anemia due to destruction of RBC.
+
Consumption of platelets—leading to thrombocytopenia and bleeding

Patient with Congenital TTP

von Willebrand factor cleaving protease (metalloproteinase)
↓
Cleave newly synthesized ultra-large vWF multimers (ULvWF)

As a result of congenital deficiency of vWF cleaving protease
ULvWF binds tightly to platelets than smaller vWF molecules
↓
Initiate platelet aggregation

In Sporadic TTP

Acquired deficiency of vWF cleaving protease as a result of production of autoantibody against vWFCP
↓
Accumulation of ULvWF in the circulation
↓
Binds avidly to platelet
↓
Initiate platelet aggregation

In Pregnancy Associated TTP/HUS

In 3rd trimester of pregnancy—decrease level of vWFCP—may be due to **antibody to vWFCP** in some cases.

Drugs: Produces endothelial cell injury and platelet aggregation. The drugs are:
i. Cyclosporine
ii. Quinine
iii. Ticlopidine
iv. Clopidogrel
v. Mitomycin C.

Presentations

a. Microangiopathic hemolytic anemia
b. Fever
c. Purpura
d. Renal manifestations—evidenced by—elevated creatinine, azotemia, proteinuria, hematuria and oliguria
e. Neurological manifestations: Headache, somnolence, confusion, seizures, paresis and coma.

Diagnosis

i. Low hemoglobin
ii. ↑LDH
iii. ↓ Haptoglobin
iv. Red cell fragments
v. Fibrin degradation products
vi. Thrombocytopenia
vii. Raised indirect bilirubin
viii. Increased reticulocyte count
ix. Negative direct antiglobulin test
x. Peripheral blood film shows >3 schistocytes/HPF

Treatment

1. **Plasma exchange:** It should be performed—once daily until LDH and platelet count are normal for 2–3 days. Up to 3 weeks of treatment may be required.

If once daily treatment is unhelpful—twice daily treatment may be given
↓
If LDH and platelet counts indicate proper response
↓
Switch back to once daily treatment
↓
LDH and platelet count comes to normal in 2–3 days
↓
Treatment should be discontinued.

2. Platelet transfusion is **usually not required**. But **it may be given when:**
   i. CT scan proved severed intracranial bleeding.
   ii. Other life-threatening bleeding in any site.

   Usually platelet transfusion **is contraindicated because** it may propagate the formation of platelet rich microthrombi
3. **Packed red cells**—may be transfused commensurate with the:
   i. Pace of microangiopathic hemolytic anemia
   ii. Degree of bleeding
4. **Refractory and relapsing thrombotic microangiopathy**
   a. Addition of steroid or intravenous immunoglobulin with plasma exchange
   b. In selected cases—immunosuppressive agents—cyclophosphamide, vincristine, cyclosporine
   c. Splenectomy
5. **Hemodialysis**

RENDU-OSLER-WEBER DISEASE (HEREDITARY HEMORRHAGIC TELANGIECTASIA)

1. Autosomal dominant disorder
2. Multiple mucocutaneous and skin telangiectasia which bleeds easily (Fig. 5.132).
3. Recurrent epistaxis, menorrhagia, gastrointestinal bleeding producing iron deficiency anemia.
4. Presentation in later life

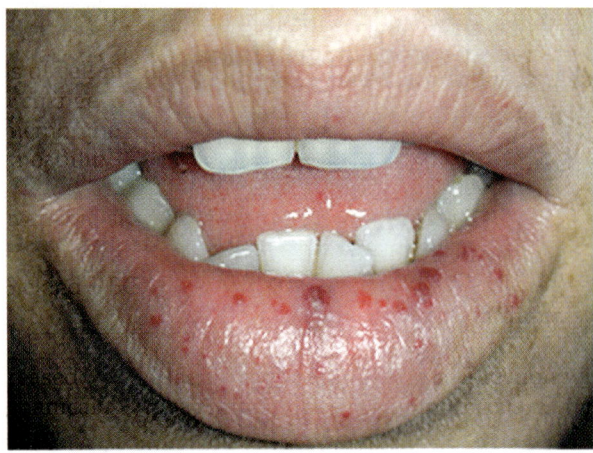

Fig. 5.132: Multiple mucocutaneous telangiectasia

5. There is development of pulmonary and cerebral arterio-venous malformations. Pulmonary AVM enlarges in pregnancy.
6. Positive family history
7. Full blood count—hypochromic microcytic anemia, decreased serum ferritin
8. Angiography of mesenteric circulation—to see ectatic vessels
9. CT scan to identify pulmonary AV malformation
10. **Treatment:**
    i. *Iron supplementation* in case of iron deficiency
    ii. *Tranexamic acid*, if menorrhagia
    iii. *Antibiotics* for dental or surgical procedure because risk of cerebral abscess due to bacteremia and shunting in the lung.
    iv. *Estrogen* may reduce bleeding episodes.

von WILLEBRAND DISEASE

von Willebrand factor is **produced in endothelial cells and megakaryocytes**. Molecular weight 250 kDA.

High molecular weight multimers up to 20×10^6 Da are particularly homeostatically active.

vWF has two functions:
1. Its homeostatic function is to act as ligand for platelet adhesion.
2. It acts as carrier protein for factor VIII protecting it from degradation.

Causes of von Willebrand Disease

1. Genetic mutation at the vWF locus
2. Some may be due to defects in other genes which affect vWF levels (epigenetic factors such as ABO blood group).

von Willebrand disease is classified into 3 main types:
1 *Type-1:* Quantitative deficiency of vWF—majority of which do not have causal mutation of vWF gene, located on chromosome 12.
Patient has mild to moderate bleeding (75% of cases)
2. *Type-2:* Qualitative deficiency of vWF (20% of cases). It has four subtypes:
    i. *Type-2A:* Due to *mutation of vWF gene*—there may be:
        a. Defect in intracellular transport (2A type 1)
        b. Render the molecule more susceptible to proteolysis (2A type-2)

ii. *Type-2B:* Due to mutation, there is an abnormal structure in the binding site for platelet GPIb. Here patient may present with features of thrombocytopenia due to removal of vWF bound platelet aggregates.
iii. *Type-2N:* Due to mutation vWF decreases, its ability to bind and protect factor VIII from its clearance, result in decreased factor VIII level in plasma, producing clinical picture of hemophilia—soft tissue and joint bleeding are very common

The presence of affected female in the family is an important clue to the diagnosis.
iv. *Type-2M:* Due to mutation, vWF decreases its ability to bind with platelets.
3. *Type-3 (rare):* Due to a variety of mutation in vWF molecules, patient may present with severe bleeding since childhood.

Clinical Presentation

Symptoms—mild to moderate intermittent bleeding probably due to fluctuating vWF levels.

So repeated vWF factor assay is necessary to come to a diagnosis of von Willebrand disease.

Bleeding type: Mucocutaneous, easy bruising, nose bleeds (Fig. 5.133), prolonged bleed from cuts, dental extraction, trauma, surgery, **hemarthroses occur in type 3 vWBD, type 2N.**

Patient may present at 2nd or 3rd decade.

Type 2B von Willebrand disease produces thrombocytopenia.

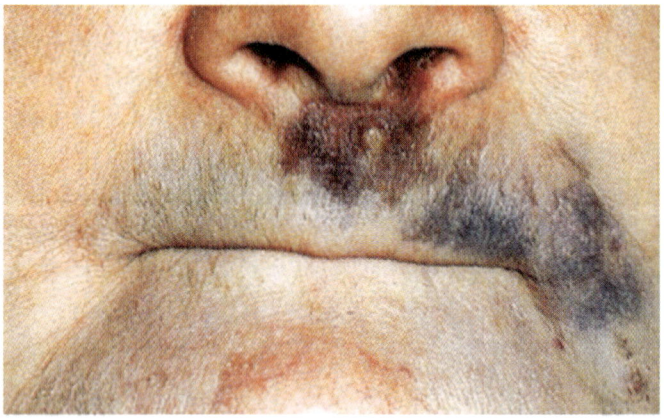

Fig. 5.133: Nose bleed

Laboratory Diagnosis

Laboratory test	Method	Indication
1. vWF antigen	Binding to anti-vWF antibody quantitative measure vWF in plasma	Initial workup
2. vWF activity	**Restocetin promotes binding of patient's plasma vWF to normal platelets** (via GPIb)	Initial workup

(Contd.)

(Contd.)

Laboratory test	Method	Indication
	Decreased platelet aggregation indicates abnormal or reduced vWF in patient's plasma	
3. Factor VIII activity level	Factor VIII levels are reduced in moderate to severe vWFD.	Initial workup
4. Ristocetin-induced platelet aggregation	Type 2B mutation results in increased aggregation of patient's platelet rich plasma with low concentration of ristocetin.	Diagnosis of vWD type 2B
5. vWF multimer assay	Assess distribution of vWF multimers by electrophoresis	Diagnosis type 2A and type 2B
6. Platelet associated vWF activity or antigen	Patient's platelets are lysed to assess amount and activity	

Interpretation in different von Willebrand disease:

Type	VIII	vWF antigen	vWF activity	RIPA low dose	HMW indicator
1	↔/↓	↓	↓	↓/↔	↔
2A	↔/↓	↔/↓	↓	↓/↔	↓
2M	↔/↓	↔/↓	↓	↓/↔	↔
2B	↔/↓	↔/↓	↓	↑	↓
2N	↓	↔	↔	↔	↔
3	↓↓	↓↓	↓↓	↓↓	Usually undectable

1. **Factor VIII level**   normal or low in type 1, 2A and 2B type low
   in 2N type
   Very low in type 3
2. **vWF antigen**   low in type 1; very low in type 3
3. **vWF activity**   low in type 1, type 2A, B and N, very low in type 3
4. **RIPA low dose**   (Ristocetin includes platelet agglutination)—RIPA is increased in type 2B due to high affinity variant vWF—which produces thrombocytopenia and reduced circulations vWF.
5. **High molecular weight multimer**   Decreased in type 2A and 2B
6. **Type 2 is often diagnosed** when:
   i. vWF level is low
   ii. vWF.RCO/vWF antigen ratio <0.7

Treatment of von Willebrand Disease (Table 5.6)

1. **DDAVP:** Dose schedule:
   i. 0.3 mg/kg IV, in 50ml of saline over 20 minutes or
   ii. Nasal spray 150 μg in each nostril—if weight >50 kg or
   iii. 150 mg in one nostril if weight <50 kg
   Duration: Over 8–12 hours
   Doses—minimum 2–3 doses in 48 hours period
   Monitor: Hypoglycemia
2. **Replacement vWF concentrates**
   Indication:
   i. Very severe von Willebrand disease
   ii. Major bleeding from any sites.
      Dose: 20–30 IU/12 hourly for 3–10 days
      Intermediate purity plasma-derived factor VIII concentrates contain VBWF.
      Monitor clinical status and vWF antigen and activity to determine the efficacy.
3. **Antifibrinolytic—Epsilon amino caproic acid** 50 mg/kg 4 times daily for 3 to 5 days.
   This is often used in conjunction with other therapies.
   This is usually effective in case of mucosal bleeding.

Table 5.6: Treatment of von Willebrand disease

Type	Treatment	Comment
1	DDAVP; vWF replacement concentrate	DDAVP effective in most patients
2A	DDAVP, vWF replacement concentrate	DDAVP effective in most patients
2B	Possibly DDAVP, vWF replacement concentrate	DDAVP may worsen thrombo cytopenia
2N	DDAVP, vWF replacement concentrate	Factor VIII half life may be shortened because of lack of binding by abnormal VWF
2M	DDAVP, vWF replacement concentrates	—
3	DDAVP, vWF replacement concentrates, platelet transfusion, if response to vWF replacement inadequate	Increase initial dose of VWF replacement concentrate

Table 5.7 describes classification, mechanism and treatment of von Willebrand disease.

WHITE BLOOD CELLS

Normal Count

1. Total WBC count	4–$11 \times 10^9/L$
2. Neutrophil	2–$7.5 \times 10^9/L$
3. Lymphocytes	1.5–$4.5 \times 10^9/L$
4. Eosinophil	$0.04 \times 0.4 \times 10^9/L$
5. Basophil	0.0–$0.1 \times 10^9/L$
6. Monocytes	$0.2 - 0.8 \times 10^9/L$

Leukocytosis: It can be defined as elevation of WBC >2 standard deviation above the mean.

Leukomoid reaction: Leukocytosis >50 × 10⁹/L—with evidence of neutrophilia with marked left shift (band forms,

Table 5.7: Classification, mechanism, and treatment of von Willebrand disease

Type	Mechanism	vWF activity*	RIPA**	Multimer pattern***	Treatment
Type 1	Partial quantitative deficiency of vWF	Decreased	Decreased	Uniform decreased all present	Desmopressin or factor VIII-vWF concentrate
Type 2	Qualitative defects				
Type 2A	Defective platelet-dependent vWF functions	Decreased	Decreased	Decreased large multimers	Factor VIII-vWF concentrates
Type 2B	Increased platelet-dependent vWF function	Decreased	Decreased	Decreased large multimers	Factor VIII-vWF concentrates
Type 2M	Defective platelet-dependent vWF function	Decreased	Decreased	Uniform large multimers	Factor VIII-vWF concentrates
Type 2N	Defective vWF binding to factor VIII	Normal	Normal	Normal	Factor VIII-vWF concentrates
Type 3	Severe deficiency of vWF and moderate factor VIII deficiency	Markedly decreased or absent	Markedly decreased or absent	Undetectable	Factor VIII-vWF concentrates or recombinant factor VIII

*vWF activity: Ristocetin cofactor activity; it can be performed on plasma as well as platelet vWF; **RIPA: Ristocetin-induced platelet aggregation; ***Multimer pattern; vWF multimer pattern assay on gel electrophores

metamyelocytes, myelocytes, occasionally promyelocytes and myeloblast in blood film). This is found in:
i. Infections
ii. Stressed neonates
iii. Seriously ill patients

Leukoerythroblastic picture: It shows:
i. Metamyelocytes
ii. Other primitive granulocytes
iii. Nucleated red cells
iv. Tear drop red blood cells

It occurs due to:
a. Bone marrow invasion by: i. Tumor, ii. fibrosis, iii. granuloma formation
b. Anorexia
c. Hemolysis

Neutrophilia—causes are:
a. Increased production:
1. Idiopathic
2. Drug-induced—glucocorticoid, granulocyte colony stimulating factor
3. Infections—bacterial, fungal, viral
4. Inflammation—myocardial interaction, pulmonary infarction, collagen vascular disease
5. Myeloproliferative disease—polycythemia vera, myeloid leukemia, myeloid metaplasia
b. Increased marrow release:
1. Glucocorticoid excess
2. Acute infection
3. Inflammation
c. Decreased defective migrations:
1. Drugs—epinephrine, glucocorticoid, NSAID
2. Stress—vigorous exercise, excitement
3. Leukocyte adhesion deficiency type 1, type 2, type 3

d. Miscellaneous:
1. Metabolic disorder
2. Drugs—lithium
3. Metastatic carcinoma

Lymphocytosis

1. Lymphocytosis $>4.5 \times 10^9$/L
2. Normal infants and young children <5 years have higher proportion and concentration of lymphocyte than adult.
3. Rare in acute bacterial infection except in pertussis ($>50 \times 10^9$/L)
4. Acute infections lymphocytosis seen in children, usually associated with transient lymphocytosis.
5. Characteristics of infections lymphocytosis but there lymphocytes are often large and atypical, and diagnosis is confirmed by heterophil agglutination tests
6. Similar atypical cells in CMV and hepatitis A infection
7. Chronic infection with brucellosis, tuberculosis, secondary syphilis and congenital syphilis
8. CLL, ALL, occasionally NHL
9. Post-splenectomy
10. Vigorous exercise
11. β thalassemia intermedia
12. Adrenaline

Bone marrow examination is needed, if:
i. Neoplasia is strongly suspected
ii. Associated with concomitant neutropenia, anemia or thrombocytopenia
iii. Constitutional symptoms—sweat, weight loss

Neutropenia

Defined when neutrophil count $<2 \times 10^9/L$

Clinical significance:

	Neutrophil count	Risk of infection
1.	$1.0–1.5 \times 10^9/L$	No significance, increased risk of infection
2.	$0.5–1.0 \times 10^9/L$	Increased risk of infection, can be treated as out patient
3.	$<0.5 \times 10^9/L$	Major risk, treat with broad-spectrum antibiotics

Types of infections are determined by:

i. Degree of neutropenia
ii. Duration of neutropenia
iii. Ongoing chemotherapy—it increases the risk of fungal and bacterial opportunistic infection
iv. Increased risk of infection with coagulase positive staphylococci and skin commensals

In chronic neutropenia:

a. Recurrent stomatisis
b. Gingivitis
c. Oral ulceration
d. Sinusitis
e. Perioral infections

Bone marrow examination is indication of:

i. Concomitant neutropenia or thrombocytopenia
ii. History of significant infection
iii. Lymphadenopathy or organomegaly on examination
iv. Cytogenetics

Other blood test:

i. Viral serology
ii. Collagen diseases
iii. Antineutrophil antibodies
iv. Immunoglobulin

Causes are:

1. Isolated neutropenia—may be presenting features of:
   a. Myelodysplastic syndrome
   b. Aplastic anemia
   c. Fanconi anemia
   d. Acute leukemia
2. Post-infections—usually post-viral?—Last for several weeks may be followed by prolonged immune neutropenia
3. Severe sepsis
4. Drugs:
   i. Cytotoxic agent
   ii. Phenothiazine
   iii. Antibiotics
   iv. NSAIDs
   v. Antithyroid agents
   vi. Psychotropic drugs
5. **Autoimmune neutropenia**—due to presence of antineutrophil antibodies associated with hemolytic anemia.
6. **Felly syndrome**—is accompanied by rheumatoid arthritis and splenomegaly.
7. **Chronic benign neutropenia**—in infancy and childhood associated with fever and infection, resolves by the age of 4 years.
8. **Benign familial and racial neutropenia.** In certain racial groups (Negroes), mild neutropenia, propensity to infection.
9. **Chronic idiopathic neutropenia** is a diagnosis by exclusion.
10. **Cyclic neutropenia** usually in childhood onset and dominant inheritance characterized by:
    i. Severe neutropenia
    ii. Fever
    iii. Stomatitis
    iv. Other infections at 4 weeks interval
11. **Hereditary causes:**
    i. Kostmann syndrome
    ii. Shwachman-Diamond-Oski syndrome
    iii. Chediak-Higashi syndrome
    iv. Reticular dysgenesis
    v. Dyskeratosis congenital

Lymphopenia

When count $<1.5 \times 10^9/L$

Causes

i. Acute infections
ii. Cardiac failure
iii. Pancreatitis
iv. Tuberculosis
v. Uremia
vi. Lymphoma
vii. Carcinoma
viii. LE and other collagen diseases after corticosteroid therapy
ix. Radiation, chemotherapy
x. Anti-lymphocyte globulin therapy
xi. Anorexia nervosa
xii. Cushing's disease
xiii. Sarcoidosis

Most common cause of chronic severe lymphopenia in recent years:

i. HIV infection   ii. HIV infection and AIDS

The infective agents in chronic severe lymphopenia $<0.5 \times 10^9/L$

i. *Candida* species
ii. *Pneumocystis jirovecii*
iii. CMV
iv. Herpes zoster
v. *Mycobacterium sp*
vi. *Cryptosporidium*
vii. Toxoplasmosis

Neoplasias are:

i. NHL
ii. Kaposi's sarcoma
iii. Skin carcinoma
ix. Gastric carcinoma

Thrombocytosis

$> 50 \times 10^9/L$

Causes

I. **Associated with myeloproliferative neoplasm:**
   1. 1st degree thrombocythemia
   2. Polycythemia

3. Chronic granulocytic leukemia
4. Idiopathic myelofibrosis

II. Disorders associated with increased platelet:
1. Hemorrhage
2. Trauma
3. Surgery
4. Iron deficiency anemia
5. Malignancy—carcinoma lung, breast, Hodgkin's disease
6. Acute and chronic infections
7. Inflammatory disease
8. Post-splenectomy

Investigation

Bone marrow examination—shows:
i. Megakaryocytic abnormalities in MPN
ii. Bone marrow trephine biopsy—may show marked:
   a. Myeloid hyperplasia
   b. Clusters of abnormal megakaryocytes
   c. Increased reticulin or fibrosis in MPN

Eosinophilia

I. **Common cause:**
   A. *Drugs:*
      i. Gold
      ii. Penicillamine
   B. *Drug reactions:* Erythema multiforme (Stevens-Johnson syndrome)
   C. *Parasitic infestation:* Hookworm, ascariasis, tapeworm, filariasis, amebiasis
II. **Least common causes:**
   a. Pemphigus
   b. Dermatitis herpetiformis
   c. Polyarteritis nodosa
   d. Sarcoidosis
   e. Irradiation
III. **Rare**
   a. Hypereosinophilic syndrome
   b. Eosinophilic leukemia
   c. AML with eosinophilia

PAN: Renal failure neuropathy, angiography, and ANCA positivity.

Sarcoid: Multisystem features with non-caseating granulomas in biopsy in affected tissue on bone marrow biopsy, high serum ACE.

Hypereosinophilic syndrome:
i. History of allergy
ii. Cough
iii. Fever
iv. Pulmonary infiltrates on chest X-ray
v. May be cardiac involvement
vi. Eosinophil on peripheral blood film—normal morphology and granulation

Eosinophilic leukemia
i. Eosinophil on blood film—abnormal morphology, hyperlobular, and hypergranular form
ii. Bone marrow heavily infiltrated with same abnormal cells

Basophil

i. Lifespans of basophil—1–2 days
ii. Degranulation produces hypersensitivity reaction

Basophilia *(Blood Basophil >0.1 × 10⁹/L)*

Causes:
1. Myeloproliferative disorders
2. AML
3. Hypothyroidism
4. IgE mediated hypersensitivity reaction
5. Inflammatory disorders (rheumatoid disease ulcerative colitis)
6. Drugs—estrogen
7. Infections
8. Irradiations
9. Hyperlipedemia

Basopenia *(Blood basophil <0.1 × 10⁹/L):*

1. As a part of generalized leukocytosis
2. Thyrotoxicosis
3. Hemorrhage
4. Cushing syndrome
5. Allergic reactions
6. Drugs—progesterone

Monocytosis *(peripheral blood monocytes > 0.8 × 10⁹/L)*

A. **Common:**
   1. Malaria, trypanosomiasis, typhoid
   2. Post-chemotherapy
   3. Stem cell transplantation
   4. Tuberculosis
   5. Myelodysplasia
B. **Less common:**
   1. Infective endocarditis
   2. Brucellosis
   3. Hodgkin's lymphoma
   4. AML
   • *Malaria*—peripheral blood film, thick and thin slides
   • *Trypanosomiasis*—Parasites in blood film, lymph node biopsy, blood culture
   • *Typhoid*—blood culture, urine culture, stool culture
   • *Infective endocarditis*—cardiac sign, blood culture
   • *Tuberculosis*—AFB seen and culture in sputum; early morning urine, blood or bone marrow, tuberculosis positivity, caseating granulomas in biopsy of affected tissue or bone marrows
   • *Brucellosis*—blood culture and serology
   • *Hodgkin's disease*—hepatosplenomegaly, lymph adenopathy, eosinophilia

Biopsy of Node and Bone Marrow

Monocytopenia (peripheral blood monocytes <0.2 × 10⁹/L)
1. Autoimmune disorders, e.g. SLE
2. Hairy cell leukemia
3. Drugs, e.g. glucocorticoids, chemotherapy